P9-AOP-581

Sports Medicine
A Comprehensive Approach

Second Edition

Giles R. Scuderi, MD
Assistant Clinical Professor, Orthopedic Surgery
Albert Einstein College of Medicine
Bronx, New York
Chief, Adult Knee Reconstruction
Department of Orthopedics
Beth Israel Medical Center
Director
Insall Scott Kelly Institute for Orthopedics and Sports Medicine
New York, New York

Peter D. McCann, MD
Assistant Clinical Professor, Orthopedic Surgery
Albert Einstein College of Medicine
Bronx, New York
Associate Chair, Department of Orthopedic Surgery
Beth Israel Medical Center
Director, Fellowship Program
Insall Scott Kelly Institute for Orthopedics and Sports Medicine
New York, New York

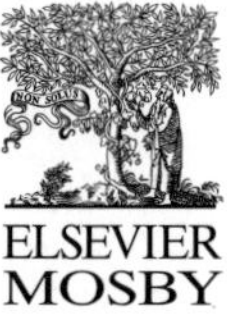

ELSEVIER
MOSBY

ELSEVIER
MOSBY

An Affiliate of Elsevier

The Curtis Center
170 S Independence Mall W 300E
Philadelphia, Pennsylvania 19106

SPORTS MEDICINE: A COMPREHENSIVE APPROACH ISBN: 0-323-02345-2
Second Edition

NOTICE

Sports Medicine is an ever-changing field. Standard safety precautions must be followed, but as new research and clinical experience broaden our knowledge, changes in treatment and drug therapy may become necessary or appropriate. Readers are advised to check the most current product information provided by the manufacturer of each drug to be administered to verify the recommended dose, the method and duration of administration, and contraindications. It is the responsibility of the licensed prescriber, relying on experience and knowledge of the patient, to determine dosages and the best treatment for each individual patient. Neither the publisher nor the authors assume any liability for any injury and/or damage to persons or property arising from this publication.

The Publisher

Previous edition copyrighted 1997.

Library of Congress Cataloging-in-Publication Data

Sports medicine : a comprehensive approach / [edited by] Giles R. Scuderi, Peter D.
McCann. – 2nd ed.
p. ; cm.
Includes bibliographical references and index.
ISBN 0-323-02345-2
1. Sports medicine. I. Scuderi, Giles R. II. McCann, Peter D.
[DNLM: 1. Athletic Injuries–therapy. 2. Sports Medicine–methods. QT 261 S7655 2005]
RC1210.S76 2005
617.1′027–dc22 2004040332

Acquisitions Editor: Daniel Pepper
Publishing Services Manager: Joan Sinclair
Project Manager: Cecelia Bayruns

Printed in the United States of America

Last digit is the print number: 9 8 7 6 5 4 3 2 1

Dedication

To our families, who continue to support us through all our endeavors.

GRS
PDM

Contents

Section I

General Principles of Sports Medicine

Section II

The Systems

Section III

Common Injuries

Contributors

David Abramson, MD, FACS
Clinical Professor of Ophthamology, Weill Medical College of Cornell University; Chief Opthalmic Oncology Service, Memorial Sloan Kettering Cancer Center; Attending Staff, New York Eye and Ear Infirmary; New York, New York
Eye Injuries

Christopher S. Ahmad, BS, MD
Assistant Professor of Orthopedic Surgery, Columbia University; Attending Orthopedic Surgeon, New York Presbyterian Hospital; New York, New York
The Shoulder

Jens O. Andreasen, DDS
Department of Maxillofacial Surgery, University Hospital, Copenhagen, Denmark
Dental Injuries

Steven Arsht, MD
Attending Orthopedic Surgeon, Beth Israel Medical Center, New York, New York
Basketball Injuries, Baseball Injuries, Soccer Injuries, Swimming Injuries

Anne R. Bass, MD
Assistant Professor of Clinical Medicine, Weill Medical College of Cornell University; Assistant Attending Physician, Hospital for Special Surgery; Assistant Attending Physician, New York Presbyterian Hospital; New York, New York
Medical Considerations for Sports and Exercise Participation in the Older Athlete

Adam J. Berman, BA, MD
Urology Resident, Beth Israel Medical Center, New York, New York
Genitourinary Injuries

Jacqueline R. Berning, PhD, RD
Assistant Professor, Department of Biology, University of Colorado, Colorado Springs, Colorado
Nutrition

Louis Bigliani, AB, MD
Frank E. Stinchfield Professor, Columbia University; Chairman of Orthopedic Surgery, New York Presbyterian Hospital; New York, New York
The Shoulder

Edward C. Brown, MD, LCDR, MC, USNR
Staff Surgeon, Department of Orthopedics, Sports Medicine and Adult Reconstruction Services, National Naval Medical Center, Bethesda, Maryland
The Leg, Credentials and Responsibilities for Team Physicians

Peter Bruno, MD
Clinical Instructor in Medicine, New York University School of Medicine; Assistant Attending Physician, Beth Israel Medical Center—North Division; Attending Physician, Lenox Hill Hospital; New York, New York
Cardiopulmonary Conditions

Joe H. Camp, DDS, MSD
Adjunct Associate Professor, University of North Carolina School of Dentistry, Chapel Hill, North Carolina; Private Practice in Endodontics, Charlotte, North Carolina
Dental Injuries

Jerome D. Chao, MD
Attending Physician, Albany Medical Center, Albany, New York
The Wrist

Gail S. Chorney, MD
Assistant Professor, Department of Orthopedic Surgery, New York University School of Medicine, Hospital for Joint Diseases; New York, New York
The Spine

Seth A. Cohen, MD
Attending Physician, Beth Israel Medical Center, New York, New York
Gastrointestinal System

Kathleen Cook
Department of Bioengineering, Duke University, Durham, North Carolina
Upper Extremity Injuries in the Female Athlete

Frances Cuomo, MD
Assistant Professor of Orthopedic Surgery, Albert Einstein College of Medicine, Bronx, New York; Chief, Shoulder and Elbow Service, Insall Scott Kelly Institute for Orthopedics and Sports Medicine, Beth Israel Medical Center, New York, New York
Upper Extremity Injuries in the Female Athlete

Fred D. Cushner, MD
Assistant Clinical Professor, Albert Einstein College of Medicine, Bronx, New York; Director, Insall Scott Kelly Institute for Orthopedics and Sports Medicine, New York, New York
Preparticipation Physical Evaluation, Fluid Balance

Gilbert B. Cushner, MD
Assistant Clinical Professor, George Washington University, Washington, DC; Holy Cross Hospital, Wheaton, Maryland
Preparticipation Physical Evaluation, Fluid Balance

Jeffrey E. Deckey, BS, MD
Attending Spine Surgeon, St. Joseph's Hospital; Attending Spine Surgeon, Children's Hospital of Orange County; Orange, California
The Thoracic and Lumbar Spine

David Diduch, MD, MS
Associate Professor of Orthopedic Surgery; Fellowship Director, Sports Medicine; Orthopedic Team Physician; Co-Director, Sports Medicine; University of Virginia, Charlottesville, Virginia
Knee Injuries

Michael S. Ferrara, PhD, ATC
Professor and Program Director of Athletic Training, Department of Exercise Science, University of Georgia, Athens, Georgia
Sport for the Athlete with a Physical Disability

Matthew E. Fink, MD
Professor, Departments of Neurology and Internal Medicine, Albert Einstein College of Medicine, Bronx, New York; Director of Neurosciences Continuum Health Partners; Co-Director, Institute for Neurology and Neurosurgery; Beth Israel Medical Center; New York, New York
Head Trauma

Laura Forese, MD, MPH
Clinical Associate Professor of Orthopedic Surgery, Columbia University College of Physicians and Surgeons; Vice President of Medical Affairs, New York Presbyterian Hospital; New York, New York
The Upper Extremity

Peter G. Gerbino II, MD, MS
Instructor, Harvard Medical School; Assistant in Orthopedic Surgery, Children's Hospital Boston; Boston, Massachusetts
The Lower Extremity

Dennis J. Gleason, BS
Credentialed Prevention Professional, New York State Office of Alcoholism and Substance Abuse Services
Substance Abuse

David A. Gold, MD
Orthopedic Surgeon, Chilton Memorial Hospital, Wayne, New Jersey
Rehabilitation Techniques and Therapeutic Modalities

Robert T. Goldman, MD
Attending Orthopedic Surgeon, Morristown Memorial Hospital, Morristown, NJ
The Elbow and Forearm

Robert S. Gotlin, DO
Assistant Professor, Rehabilitation Medicine, Albert Einstein College of Medicine, Bronx, New York; Director, Orthopedic and Sports Rehabilitation, Beth Israel Medical Center, New York, New York
The Lower Extremity, The Upper Extremity, The Spine

Alex M. Greenberg, DDS
Assistant Clinical Professor, Division of Oral and Maxillofacial Surgery, Columbia University School of Dental and Oral Surgery; Clinical Instructor, Division of Oral and Maxillofacial Surgery, The Mt. Sinai School of Medicine; Associate Attending Physician, Division of Oral and Maxillofacial Surgery, St. Luke's/Roosevelt Hospital; Assistant Attending Physician, Division of Oral and Maxillofacial Surgery, Beth Israel Medical Center; Assistant Attending Physician, Division of Oral and Maxillofacial Surgery, Columbia University Medical Center; Assistant Attending Physician, Division of Oral and Maxillofacial Surgery, The Mt. Sinai Hospital; New York, New York
Craniofacial Injuries

Letha Y. Griffin, MD, PhD
Team Physician and Adjunct Professor, Department of Kinesiology and Health, Georgia State University; Member, Peachtree Orthopedic Clinic; Atlanta, Georgia
Lower Extremity Injuries in the Female Athlete

Robyn J. Hakanson, MD
Orthopedic Surgeon, Tri-County Orthopedic and Sports Medicine, P.A., Mt. Airy, North Carolina
Metabolic Conditions in the Female Athlete

Steven F. Harwin, MD, FACS
Associate Clinical Professor of Orthopedic Surgery, Albert Einstein College of Medicine, Bronx, New York; Chief of Adult Reconstructive Surgery and Surgical Director, New York Medical Center for Bloodless Medicine and Surgery, Beth Israel Medical Center, New York, New York
Pelvis, Hip, and Thigh

Richard H. Haug, DDS
Professor of Oral and Maxillofacial Surgery and Executive Associate Dean, University of Kentucky Medical Center, Lexington, Kentucky
Craniofacial Injuries

David C. Helfgott, MD
Clinical Assistant Professor, Department of Medicine, Weill Cornell Medical College; Assistant Attending Physician, New York-Presbyterian Hospital; New York, New York
Infectious Diseases

David L. Herbert, BBA, JD
Senior Partner, Herbert, Benson and Scott, Canton, Ohio
Legal Issues in Sports Medicine

Christopher E. Hubbard, MD
Attending Foot and Ankle Service, Department of Orthopedic Surgery, Insall Scott Kelly Institute for Sports Medicine and Orthopedic Surgery, Beth Israel Medical Center, New York, New York
The Foot and Ankle

Gordon Huie, PA
Senior Physician Assistant, Insall Scott Kelly Institute for Sports Medicine; Supervising Physician Assistant, Beth Israel Medical Center—North Division; New York, New York
Rehabilitation Techniques and Therapeutic Modalities

Joshua Hyman, MD
Clinical Assistant Professor of Orthopedic Surgery, Columbia University, College of Physicians and Surgeons; Attending Orthopedic Surgeon, New York Presbyterian Hospital, Children's Hospital of New York; New York, New York
The Upper Extremity

Paul M. Juris, EdD
Adjunct Assistant Professor, Teachers College, Columbia University; Research Coordinator, Beth Israel Medical Center; New York, New York
Muscle and Exercise Physiology

Barbara A. Kahn, BS, RN, ONC
Orthopedic Nurse Clinician, The Hospital for Special Surgery, New York, New York
Why Sports Medicine?

Stuart B. Kahn, MD
Assistant Clinical Professor of Rehabilitation Medicine, Albert Einstein College of Medicine, Bronx, New York; Director of Spine Pain and Rehabilitation, Spine Institute, Department of Orthopedics, Beth Israel Medical Center, New York, New York
Sports Medicine and Sports Injuries in the Older Population

Daniel J. Kane, MD
Attending Physician, Chester County Hospital, West Chester, Pennsylvania; Attending Physician, Brandywine Hospital, Coatesville, Pennsylvania; Attending Physician, Montgomery County Medical Center, Department of Physical Medicine and Rehabilitation, Norristown, Pennsylvania
Sports Medicine and Sports Injuries in the Older Population, The Upper Extremity

Susan M. Kaschalk, MS, PA-C
Physician Assistant, St. Joseph Mercy—Oakland Hospital; Physical Assistant, Pontiac Osteopathic Hospital; Pontiac, Michigan
Sport for the Athlete with a Physical Disability

Michael A. Kelly, MD
Director, Insall Scott Kelly Institute for Orthopedics and Sports Medicine; Chief, Sports Medicine Services, Beth Israel Hospital, New York, New York
The Leg

Nancy Kim, MD
Attending Physician, Christiana Hospital, Newark, Delaware
Sports Medicine and Sports Injuries in the Older Population, The Upper Extremity

Gwen S. Korovin, MD
Clinical Assistant Professor of Otolaryngology, New York University School of Medicine; Attending Physician, Lenox Hill Hospital; Attending Physician, Manhattan Eye, Ear and Throat Hospital; Attending Physician, New York University Hospital; New York, New York
Otorhinolaryngology

Michael D. Kurtz, DDS
Former Lecturer in Sports Dentistry, Columbia University, School of Dental and Oral Surgery, New York, New York
Dental Injuries

Ulla Kristiina Laakso, MD
Assistant Clinical Professor of Psychiatry, Albert Einstein College of Medicine, Bronx, New York; Attending Psychiatrist, Beth Israel Medical Center; Attending Psychiatrist, Lenox Hill Hospital; New York, New York
Sports Psychology

Richard A. Marder, MD
Professor of Orthopedic Surgery, Chief Sports Medicine Service, University of California, Davis, Davis, California; Team Physician, Sacramento Kings (NBA), Sacramento, California
On-Field Emergencies

Nino Marino, MD
Physician-in-Charge, Echocardiography Laboratory, Lenox Hospital; Consultant in Cardiology, New York Knicks; New York, New York
Cardiopulmonary Conditions

Peter D. McCann, MD
Assistant Clinical Professor of Orthopedic Surgery, Albert Einstein College of Medicine, Bronx, New York; Associate Chair, Department of Orthopedic Surgery, Beth Israel Medical Center; Director, Fellowship Program, Insall Scott Kelly Institute for Orthopedics and Sports Medicine; New York, New York
Why Sports Medicine?, The Elbow and Forearm, Basketball Injuries, Baseball Injuries, Swimming Injuries, Football Injuries, Running Injuries, Racquet Sports Injuries, Injuries in Alpine Skiing, Soccer Injuries

Michelle McTimoney, BSc, MD, FRCPC
Lecturer, Department of Pediatrics, Dalhousie University; Pediatrician, Emergency Department, Izaak Walton Killam Health Centre; Sports Physician, Orthopedic and Sport Medicine Clinic of Nova Scotia; Halifax, Nova Scotia, Canada
Spinal Injuries in the Female Athlete

Pietro A. Memmo, MD
Assistant Clinical Professor, Department of Orthopedics, University of Connecticut School of Medicine; Attending Physician, Hartford Hospital; Attending Physician, University of Connecticut Medical Center; Attending Physician, Orthopedic Associates of Hartford; Hartford, Connecticut
The Spine

Mary Mendelsohn, MD
Attending Staff, The Valley Hospital, Ridgewood, New Jersey; Attending Staff, Pascack Valley Hospital, Westwood, New Jersey
Eye Injuries

Lyle J. Micheli, AB, MD
Associate Clinical Professor of Orthopedic Surgery, Harvard Medical School; Director, Division of Sports Medicine, Boston Children's Hospital; Boston, Massachusetts
Spinal Injuries in the Female Athlete, The Lower Extremity

Harris M. Nagler, MD, FACS
Professor of Urology, Albert Einstein College of Medicine, Bronx, New York; Chairman, Department of Urology and Chief, Graduate Medical Education, Beth Israel Medical Center, New York, New York
Genitourinary Injuries

Michael A. Palmer, MD, MA
PreMed Preceptor, Princeton University; Physiatrist, University Medical Center of Princeton, Princeton Orthopedics and Rehabilitation Associates; Princeton, New Jersey
The Spine

Andrew H. Patterson, MD
Professor Emeritus of Orthopedic Surgery, Columbia University; Emeritus Attending Orthopedic Surgery, St. Luke's Roosevelt Hospital Center; New York, New York
Medicolegal Issues

Stuart H. Popowitz, BA, MD
Practicing Urologist, Boca Raton, Florida
Genitourinary Injuries

Martin A. Posner, MD
Clinical Professor of Orthopedic Surgery, New York University School of Medicine;
Chief of Hand Service and Director of Fellowship, Department of Orthopedic Surgery, New York University Hospital for Joint Diseases; New York, New York
The Hand

Kenneth J. Richter, DO
Clinical Associate Professor, Michigan State University, E. Lansing, Michigan; Clinical Associate Professor, Wayne State University, Detroit, Michigan; Medical Director, Rehabilitation Programming and Services, St. Joseph Mercy-Oakland; Medical Director, Inpatient Rehab Unit, Pontiac Osteopathic Hospital; Pontiac, Michigan
Sport for the Athlete with a Physical Disability

Andrew L. Rosen, MD
Attending Orthopedic Surgeon, Beth Israel Medical Center, New York, New York
Football Injuries, Running Injuries, Injuries in Alpine Skiing, Racquet Sports Injuries

Melvin Rosenwasser, MD
Carroll Professor of Orthopedic Surgery, Columbia University Medical Center; Attending Orthopedic Surgeon and Director, Hand and Trauma Service, New York Presbyterian Hospital, Columbia Campus; New York, New York
The Wrist

Michael Saunders, RPT, ATC
Trainer for New York Knicks; Faculty, Insall Scott Kelly Institute for Sports Medicine, Beth Israel Hospital—North Division; New York, New York
Rehabilitation Techniques and Therapeutic Modalities

Robert S. Scheinberg, MD
Clinical Professor, Department of Medicine, University of California, San Diego, School of Medicine, San Diego, California
Dermatologic Conditions

Susan Craig Scott, MD
Attending Physician, Plastic Surgery, Beth Israel Medical Center and Lenox Hill Hospital, New York, New York
Wound Healing

W. Norman Scott, MD
Clinical Professor of Orthopedic Surgery, Albert Einstein College of Medicine, Bronx, New York; Chairman, Department of Orthopedics, Beth Israel Medical Center; Director, Insall Scott Kelly Institute for Orthopedics and Sports Medicine; New York, New York
Wound Healing, Knee Injuries, Credentials and Responsibilities for Team Physicians

Giles R. Scuderi, MD
Assistant Clinical Professor of Orthopedic Surgery, Albert Einstein College of Medicine, Bronx, New York; Chief, Adult Knee Reconstruction, Department of Orthopedics, Beth Israel Medical Center; Director, Insall Scott Kelly Institute for Orthopedics and Sports Medicine; New York, New York
Why Sports Medicine?, Knee Injuries, Basketball Injuries, Baseball Injuries, Football Injuries, Running Injuries, Soccer Injuries, Injuries in Alpine Skiing, Swimming Injuries, Racquet Sports Injuries, Credentials and Responsibilities for Team Physicians

V. Franklin Sechriest II, MD
Fellow, Insall Scott Kelly Institute, New York, New York
Return to Play After Musculoskeletal Injury

Jerome H. Siegel, MD
Clinical Professor of Medicine, Albert Einstein College of Medicine, Bronx, New York; Chief, Endoscopy, Beth Israel Medical Center—Singer Division, New York, New York
Gastrointestinal System

Andrew G. Sikora, MD, PhD
Teaching Assistant, New York University School of Medicine, New York, New York
Otorhinolaryngology

Stephen G. Silver, MD
Beth Israel Medical Center, New York, New York
Return to Play After Musculoskeletal Injury

Stefano M. Sinicropi, BS, MD
Medical Doctor, Post-Graduate Residency Training Program, New York Presbyterian Hospital, New York, New York
The Thoracic and Lumbar Spine

Joseph S. Torg, MD
Professor of Orthopedic Surgery, Temple University School of Medicine, Philadelphia, Pennsylvania
The Cervical Spine, Spinal Cord, and Brachial Plexus

Mark Weidenbaum, MD
Associate Professor of Clinical Orthopedic Surgery, Columbia University College of Physicians and Surgeons; Associate Attending Surgeon and Director, Orthopedic Spine Surgery, Milstein, New York Presbyterian Hospital; New York, New York
The Thoracic and Lumbar Spine

Robert H. Wilson, MD
Assistant Professor, Howard University College of Medicine; Attending Physician, Howard University Hospital; Washington DC
The Wrist

Sara M. Wiskow, MS, ATC
Assistant Athletic Trainer, United States Military Academy, West Point, New York
Metabolic Conditions in the Female Athlete

Ira Wolfe, BA
Consultant to Center for Shoulder, Elbow and Sports Medicine, New York, New York
The Shoulder

Ken Yamaguchi, MD, MA, BS
Associate Professor of Orthopedic Surgery and Chief of Elbow Service, Washington University School of Medicine; Chief of Shoulder and Elbow Service, Barnes Jewish Hospital, Washington University School of Medicine; Staff Physician, Shoulder and Elbow Surgery, John Cochran Veterans Administration Hospital, St. Louis, Missouri
The Shoulder

Preface

The factors that led us to develop the first edition of this book remain relevant today. The general public's interest and participation in organized recreational sports continue to expand. New prevention and treatment options continue to develop. Managed care continues to be a major vehicle for the delivery of medical services.

The first edition's main focus was to offer the primary care provider a comprehensive reference to aid in the diagnosis and initial management of sports injuries. In this second edition, we hope to continue to meet the needs of the primary care provider but also expand our initial focus to include orthopedic surgeons in training and in general practice. To that end, we have updated the content of each chapter to include advances in treatment developed in the past five years and have added new chapters of increasing interest, such as specific sports injuries in the female athlete, osteoporosis in the older female athlete, and sports and exercise in the geriatric population.

Once again, we gratefully acknowledge the tremendous efforts of the authors who contributed to this second edition as well as the continued guidance of our editors. We hope that this second edition will be a helpful guide for both the primary care provider and the general orthopedic surgeon in the management of patients with sports-related injuries.

Giles R. Scuderi, MD
Peter D. McCann, MD

I

General Principles of Sports Medicine

1 Why Sports Medicine?

Barbara A. Kahn, Giles R. Scuderi, and Peter D. McCann

The increased understanding of the relationship between physical fitness and health among the current growing population has led to a reevaluation of the importance of sports and physical activity in our daily lives. Although this has led to a decrease in certain medical conditions such as heart disease, it has also increased sports related injuries. Consequently, this has created the need for improved and specialized medical care. Advances in the field of sports medicine have provided the techniques necessary to prevent, cure, and recover from injuries which detract and often terminate participation in physical activity and athletics.

HISTORY

Throughout history, human beings' ability to survive and take care of their families have depended on their physical capabilities. Speed, strength, and skill were essential survival tools during early civilization. Progress led to the transformation of these physical attributes to organized contests where highly trained members began competing in a team-like fashion.

Therapeutic exercise has been in existence as far back as 1000 BC. Milo, an Olympic wrestler in ancient Greece, used to lift a calf every day until it reached adulthood. This marked the beginning of strength training using progressive resistance exercises. Herodicus became known as the first sports physician to treat injuries with therapeutic diet and exercise. Although his methods were criticized at first, other physicians came to observe and utilize his techniques, leading to the specialization of sports medicine. In the second century AD, Galen became the first appointed team physician. His purpose was to cure injured gladiators so that they could return to battle. Galen was followed by Oribasius of Pergamum, who claimed that the body's organs had greater function while being physically stressed. Aurilianus in the fifth century was the first physician to institute postoperative exercise programs to promote healing.

Physical education in the United States started at Amherst College in Massachusetts with the appointment of Edward Hitchcock Jr. as professor of physical education and hygiene in 1854. He developed a program incorporating the Swedish and German methods of gymnastics and running with the American games of football, basketball, and track. Dr. Hitchcock also served as the school physician for Amherst College, enabling him to record the prevalence of injury and disease among the student population. He published several books on athletics which earned him the titles of America's first team physician and founder of physical education in the United States.

In 1885 the American Alliance of Health, Physical Education, and Recreation (AAHPER) was founded. Dance was added in 1977 and the organization became known as AAHPERD, which it remains to this day. Its purpose was to promote research in exercise and maintain high standards for physical education. After President John F. Kennedy was inaugurated, he took an interest in promoting physical education and formed the President's Council on Physical Fitness. This ensured the standardization of the school system to promote and educate youngsters about the advantages of regular physical exercise.

The evolution of athletic training and sports medicine occurred from the expansion of intercollegiate athletics. The National Collegiate Athletic Association (NCAA), founded in 1906, standardized team sports among colleges and universities. Its purpose, then and now, has been to promote intercollegiate athletics, govern national championships, and enforce rules for sport safety and competitiveness.

As the number of participating athletes grew during the 1950s, the demand for clinicians to care for medical needs and athletic injuries increased. Physicians were called on to provide immediate treatment to otherwise young, healthy individuals. Aggressive treatment with a rapid return to competition created the need for a highly specialized and challenging field of medical care.

WOMEN IN SPORTS

The acceptance of female athletes, both professionally and recreationally, added a new dimension to both sports medicine and sports in general. During the 1800s women were forbidden to engage in any type of physical activity. Frailty and pallor were symbols of a woman's status in society, for only poor, working-class females showed any signs of physical well-being or strength. Doctors in the late 1800s felt that females were an inherently ill species due to their reproductive cycles and felt that most diseases, regardless of origin, were diseases of the womb.[14]

The Women's Suffrage Movement of the 1870s introduced women into the collegiate system, which was a cause for major concern for many physicians. It was believed that the stress brought about by studying would cause infertility and uterine atrophy because the brain was in direct competition with the uterus.[14] To prevent this from happening, women were encouraged to engage in noncontact activities such as walking, swimming, tennis, and golf. In 1896 the bicycle was invented. Women abandoned all sense of morals and sexual taboos that had been bestowed on them to participate in bicycle riding.

World Wars I and II forced women to enter the workforce to support the war effort. They worked long hours, mostly in factories. To compensate for poor working conditions, recreational and team sports were organized by factory owners to alleviate stress. In the 1940s Philip Wrigley, owner of the Chicago Cubs, formed a professional female baseball league to fill the void left by the absence of men's professional baseball. It was tremendously popular, but no further advancement in women's athletics came about once the men returned after the war ended.

In 1972 Title IX was enacted, which prohibited discrimination on the basis of sex in any educational institution receiving federal funding. Under Title IX, women were to receive a percentage of funding high enough to give them equivalent uniforms, playing fields, coaches, and budgets to that of their male counterparts. Title IX opened the door for women to enter competitive sports at the high school and college levels. This had a major effect on the field of sports medicine for young women.

DISABLED ATHLETES IN SPORTS

Women were not the only group experiencing exclusion from recreational and competitive sports. Until the late 1950s persons with either physical or mental disabilities were unable to become involved in physical activity at all. At present, it is estimated that 2 to 3 million people with disabilities participate in sports each year in the United States.[8] Part of the reason for this is the advancement in special equipment needed for the disabled to participate in a wide variety of activities. Disabled athletes now compete in basketball, skiing, swimming, and many other sports. The advent of sport-specific wheelchairs became the catalyst for competitive sports for the disabled about 35 years ago. In the late 1970s special committees were formed to represent disabled athletic participants. This included organizations on the national and international level to include the deaf, blind, wheelchair bound, dwarfed, and cerebral palsied, among many others. Health care personnel realize the benefits of physical activity for individuals with disabilities and are developing ways to treat and prevent injuries incurred by these athletes. Burnham et al.[3] in 1991 found that injuries sustained during the 1988 Canadian Paralympics occurred most often in the musculoskeletal, general medical, and disability-related groups. Richter and his colleagues studied injury patterns of athletes with cerebral palsy at the same paralympic games and found that 60% of the athletes with cerebral palsy reported an injury or illness, as compared with 75% of participants from the 1988 Olympic Games.[16] The study also found that of these reported injuries the most commonly traumatized region was the shoulder and respiratory tract in the disabled athlete.

Sports medicine physicians have needed to adapt their practice to treat disabled athletes differently from other groups because they are prone to specific injuries. For example, athletes who are blind tend to injure their lower extremities most often. Those athletes with cerebral palsy and spinal cord injuries have a tendency toward urinary retention, infections, and dehydration. Because prolonged immobilization leads to bone loss, wheelchair athletes are at an extreme risk for sustaining fractures. In addition, these athletes are prone to developing pressure sores or ulcers due to increased friction and loss of sensation.[16] It is apparent, then, how the field of sports medicine has needed to advance and become more specialized over the past 40 years.

SPORTS AND THE ELDERLY POPULATION

In 1989 there were 25 million Americans over the age of 65. It is expected that this number will rise to 65 million in the year 2030, which will equal approximately 20% of the population.[7] In 1900 the average life expectancy was only 48.2 years for males and 51.1 years for females. By 1987 these numbers had increased to 72.2 years and 78.9 years, respectively, with individuals older than 85 years of age becoming the largest growing portion of the American population.[18]

Researchers have found that moderate-intensity physical activity such as walking, stair-climbing, cycling, and gardening convey health benefits. Epidemiologic studies have shown a decrease in cardiovascular morbidity/mortality and increased longevity in people who participate in moderate activity on a regular basis. It is estimated that at least 6 million Americans have coronary artery disease and that 500,000 patients will undergo coronary artery bypass grafting or angioplasty each year.[9] Even with these findings, there has been a 30% decrease in coronary artery disease in the United States since 1960.[9] This decrease can be attributed to a change in the lifestyles of middle-aged and elderly people. The United States Masters Swimming Association (USMS) serves as the national governing body for aquatic athletes competing in organized events over the age of 20. In 1989, there were 28,600 athletes registered in the USMS. Of these, 34% were between the ages of 30 and 39, and 23% were between 40 and 49.[17] Other moderate-intensity cardiovascular activities done by middle-aged and elderly athletes include cycling, jogging, golfing, rock climbing, and tennis. Bicycling is an excellent sport for athletes of any age. It offers cardiovascular benefits comparable with those of jogging yet relies on smooth motion, which does not overstress the muscles and joints. Eighty-six million Americans will ride a bicycle this year, with 30% of these being older than 30 years of age.[15]

In 1975 the United States Tennis Association (USTA) established a seniors division to include athletes desiring to play tennis competitively up through age 85.[13] This was in response to the growing number of senior athletes wanting to play competitive tennis. It has been shown that senior athletes who play tennis regularly suffer fewer injuries than the intermittent recreational athlete of the same age. The same is true for the jogger, rock climber, bicycler, and so on. All mature athletes need to be involved in a proper conditioning program to include stretching, warm-up, endurance, and strength training to avoid injury. Since this is not always possible or done properly, it is important for the sports medicine physician to be able to recognize and treat mature athletes. Physiologic changes such as osteoporosis, decreased elasticity of articular cartilage, and spinal disc degeneration need to be addressed when treating an older person but should not be considered factors that necessarily end an individual's athletic career.

EFFECTS OF EXERCISE ON PSYCHOLOGIC WELL-BEING

In today's society, sports and physical fitness play an important role in physical well-being. Great emphasis has been placed on living longer, disease prevention, and holistic treatment through diet and exercise. Over the past several years, more and more studies have been conducted in the area of exercise and physical health. As we will discuss later in this chapter, many serious health problems can be controlled or obliterated through moderate, consistent physical activity.

There is a growing amount of evidence to support the fact that exercising regularly can heighten intellectual acuity and self-concept while decreasing anxiety and levels of depression. Exercise promotes release of serotonins and endorphins, which are natural pain killers and antidepressants produced by the brain. Release of these substances into the blood produces a euphoric sense intrinsically. Hilyer and Mitchell[10] studied three groups of college students in regard to self-concept and found that the most positively affected group had both exercise and mental counseling as opposed to counseling alone. To support these results, a study was conducted by Eickhoff et al.,[6] which proved that young women with low self-concept who became involved in a 10-week aerobic dance program showed greater improvement in self-concept and self-esteem than any other group involved. Additional studies have been conducted in the area of mental acuity. Bowers et al. showed that reaction time in a mental task involving memory could be significantly reduced following a 10-week aerobic exercise program in middle-aged adults.[2] Similarly, it has been demonstrated that cognition was improved either during or immediately after physical activity in both the younger adult and the geriatric patient.

In terms of anxiety, there is a direct correlation between stress levels and high blood pressure, heart attack, and stroke. Reducing the stress level of a "type A personality" would greatly decrease the risk of severe health ailments. Many studies have been conducted on this subject. Of those that included physical activity as a parameter, anxiety levels have been shown to decrease significantly in the groups engaging in exercise programs.

For many years it has been noted that chronic psychologic and emotional disturbances are associated with deterioration of one's health status. Therefore, it appears that the converse must also be true; improving one's physical health can improve psychologic wellness. Depression affects thousands of people in the United States alone and accounts for the majority of cases seen by psychotherapists daily. It has been proven that exercise of any type helps alleviate depression, with the longest programs having the greatest effect. When comparing exercise programs with relaxation techniques and psychotherapy, exercise was proven to be more effective at decreasing depression than relaxation techniques and equally as effective as psychotherapy.[2] We can therefore conclude that moderate, consistent physical activity can promote physiologic and psychologic health.

CONDITIONING

DeLorme[4] in 1940 introduced a way to increase muscular strength using cables and pulleys systematically while gradually increasing resistance. This method of conditioning became known as progressive resistance exercise. In 1978 the American College of Sports Medicine (ACSM) updated their recommendations for exercise in adults to include muscular strengthening and endurance exercises.[5] They defined physical fitness as being composed of cardiorespiratory fitness, body composition, muscular strength, endurance, and flexibility.

Flexibility can be defined as the range of motion of a joint or a series of joints that are influenced by muscles, tendons, ligaments, bones, and bony structures.[1] Flexibility varies in accordance with several intrinsic and extrinsic factors. Aging causes a decrease in flexibility, with the only increase being seen from birth to adolescence. Males are, in general, less flexible than females. The level and type of activity performed, rest intervals between activities, temperature, and specific joint involvement all have strong influences on flexibility. Adequate flexibility helps to prevent soft tissue injuries. As tendons and ligaments are stretched repeatedly, lengthening occurs, giving way to free movement with less stiffness. Because sprains, strains, and tears of both muscle and connective tissue are common sports-related injuries, it is important to present proper stretching and conditioning techniques to the recreational and professional athlete. These injuries generally respond well to a therapeutic program of rest with stretching and nonsteroidal anti-inflammatory medications. When patient compliance to this regime is poor or when athletes ignore symptoms of overuse injuries, more serious injuries can occur.

Conditioning for sports is no longer restricted to those athletes playing team sports. Participants at all levels in every sport should be engaged in a conditioning program to help reduce the risk of injury during sporting activity. Maximum performance in athletic activity can best be obtained by conditioning the body with a sport-specific series of exercises designed to maximize the body's ability to withstand the demands inherent within a sport.[11,12] The role of conditioning to modify sports injuries and risk of injury is still being researched. Injuries of the skeletal muscle and musculoskeletal junction are common causes of pain and disability. Improved understanding of normal physiologic mechanisms and pathologies will lead to new strategies for injury prevention and treatment. For example, resistive training strengthens the structures surrounding a joint. This is a positive influence because it spares the joint which is most susceptible to injury, prevents osteoporosis, improves posture, assists in weight control, and rehabilitates and prevents injury.

ADVANCES IN SPORTS MEDICINE

The field of sports medicine grew rapidly during the 1970s, with increased numbers of participants in both recreational and competitive athletics. Family practitioners and internists contributed to the welfare of the athlete by conducting physicals and treating medical conditions in conjunction with the orthopedist. Additionally, orthopedic surgeons were required to attend many organized sporting events to treat injuries on the field or sidelines. The foundation of the American Orthopaedic Society for Sports Medicine (AOSSM) in 1972 confirmed the existence of sports medicine as its own medical specialty. The American Medical Society for Sports Medicine (AMSSM) arose as more nonorthopedic physicians who were interested in sports medicine saw the benefits of the AOSSM. These primary care physicians found that the ACSM was too heterogeneous and research oriented to satisfy their needs. Members of the AMSSM are board certified physicians in primary care who have completed a fellowship in sports medicine or meet certain practice requirements and have passed a standardized exam that leads to a Certification of Qualifications. The interaction between the AOSSM and the AMSSM is instrumental in maintaining the excellence of sports medicine care.

Current research is also going beyond evaluation of specific injuries and various treatment measures. Epidemiologic studies are now directed at surveying the injury patterns of the athlete, the sporting activity, and the environment in which the event occurs. These studies shift some investigations from treatment modalities to possible preventive measures. In fact, this type of investigation can be undertaken as a multicenter study with a single epidemiologic team, which establishes a single protocol and uniform definitions. With this common interest, multicenter studies can acquire larger amounts of more diverse information. As more information is gathered, changes or modifications in a specific sports venue may reduce the injury rate.

CURRENT ISSUES

Over the last decade the concept of team physician has evolved from the original model of an orthopedic surgeon taking complete responsibility for the medical needs of a sports team. Many nonorthopedic physicians, including family practitioners, internists, and pediatricians, are now actively involved in many sports medicine programs. The ideal team physician is a combination of a primary care physician and an orthopedic surgeon. This permits complete care of the athlete, dealing with all the aspects of medical care and traumatic injuries. Since many sports injuries do not necessarily require surgery, primary care physicians are at the forefront of prevention and treatment. The AMSSM, in recognizing this fact, has qualified sports medicine primary care physicians. Working closely with consulting orthopedic surgeons, these physicians ensure that the athlete will receive the optimal care.

One of the most challenging problems in the current state of health care is the role of the team physician in the managed care environment. Many find it difficult to care for players because a player's coverage is not a plan with which the physician participates. Prompt diagnosis and treatment remain the most cost-effective means of returning the athlete to competition. It is for this reason that as health care changes, health care providers and legislators realize that the best treatment for sports related injuries is provided by team physicians with an expertise in sports medicine. This will maintain the continuity of care with these athletes, enable the team physician to make decisions regarding return to competition, and is probably the most cost-effective means of delivering health care to these athletes.

In this time of health care reform, it appears that the primary care physician will have the initial responsibility of administering treatment to the injured athlete. Following recommended treatment plans or algorithms, these physicians should be able to manage many of the injuries. However, it behooves them to refer the athlete to a specialist as soon as it becomes apparent that the injury is not improving or is beyond the scope of their expertise.

REFERENCES

1. Anderson B, Burke ER: Scientific, medical and practical aspects of stretching. Clin Sports Med 10(1): 63–86, 1991.
2. Anthony J: Psychologic aspects of exercise. Clin Sports Med 10(1):171–180, 1991.
3. Burnham R, Newell E, Steadward R: Spartle medicine for the physically disabled: The Canadian team experience at the 1988 Seoul Paralympics games. Clin J Sports Med 1(3):193–196, 1991.
4. DeLorme T, Watkins A: Techniques of progressive resistance exercise. Arch Phys Med 29:263, 1948.
5. DiNubile NA: Strength training. Clin Sports Med 10(1):33–62, 1991.
6. Eickoff J, Thorland W, Ansorge C: Selected physiological and psychological effects of aerobic dancing among young adult women. Sports Med Phys Fitness 23:278, 1983.
7. Elia, EA: Exercise in the elderly. Clin Sports Med 10(1):141–155, 1991.
8. Ferrara MS et al: The injury experience of the competitive athlete with a disability: Prevention implications. Med Sci Sport Ex 24(2):184–188, 1994.
9. Gordon NF, Scott CB: The role of exercise in the primary and secondary prevention of coronary artery disease. Clin Sports Med 10(1):87–103, 1991.
10. Hilyer J, Mitchell W: Effect of systematic physical fitness training combined with counseling on the self-concept of college students. Counsel Psychol 26:427–436, 1979.
11. Kibler WB: Clinical implications of exercise: Injury and performance. In Schafer M (ed): American Academy of Orthopaedic Surgeons 43:17–24, 1994.
12. Kibler WB, Chandler TJ, Reuter BH: Advances in conditioning. In Griffen LY (ed): Orthopaedic Knowledge Update Sports Medicine. American Academy of Orthopaedic Surgeons 1:65–72, 1994.
13. Leach RE, Abramowitz A: The senior tennis player. Clin Sports Med 10(2):283–290, 1991.
14. Lutter MJ: History of women in sports. Clin Sports Med 13(2):263–279, 1994.
15. McLennan JG, McLennan JC: Cycling and the older athlete. Clin Sports Med 10(2):291–299, 1991.
16. Peck DM, McKeag DB: Athletes with disabilities. Phys Sports Med 22(4):59–62, 1994.
17. Richardson AB, Miller JW: Swimming and the older athlete. Clin Sports Med 10(2):301–318, 1991.
18. Seto JL, Brewster CE: Musculoskeletal conditioning of the older athlete. Clin Sports Med10(2):401–429, 1991.

2 Muscle and Exercise Physiology

Paul M. Juris

Tradition, or perhaps convention, has it that a discourse on exercise physiology would focus on the subject of muscle ultrastructure and the various energy producing systems that allow for muscle contraction. The importance of such a discussion cannot be overstated, yet a slightly different perspective might be more appropriate when addressing the issues of sports medicine and rehabilitation.

From a more global approach, one might consider that the essential role of muscle is to either move or fixate the skeleton so that purposeful behavior can occur. This broad concept has led to numerous discussions of the musculoskeletal system and the interaction between muscle and bone. Absent from this model, however, is the nervous system, which is primarily responsible for the coordination of muscular activity.

Conventionally, neural and muscular behavior have been treated separately as either muscle physiology or neurophysiology. This scientific dichotomy is problematic in that one system does not function appropriately without the other. Although muscles act directly on the skeleton, they cannot do so unless there is neural input instructing them on how to function. On the other hand, although the nervous system provides the primary impetus for muscles to contract, its activity would be immaterial without intact musculature. Thus, the discussion of physiology from this perspective will explore the intact neuromuscular system, focusing on the essential functional element of this system, the motor unit.

THE MOTOR UNIT

The principle component of the neuromuscular system, as seen in Figure 2-1, is the motor unit. The motor unit is defined as the cell body and dendrites of a motor neuron, its axon and branches, and all of the muscle fibers that it innervates. Motor units can generally be classified as either fast-twitch or slow-twitch, referring to their twitch characteristics. Likewise, they can be characterized according to their resistance to fatigue, in which case they are referred to as fast-fatigable (FF), fast-fatigue resistant (FR), or slow-fatigue resistant (S). In all cases, the linkage between the motor neuron and the muscle cell is closely related to the character of the motor unit.

Cell diameter, for example, relates directly to the type of motor unit and is consistent with both neural and muscular components. In general, FF type units have larger axon diameters than do S units, and the muscle cells also tend to be larger.[6] Motor axon diameter bears a direct relationship to nerve conduction velocity. This is simply because the larger the area of the axonal cylinder, the less resistance there is to the flow of electrons. Thus, fast-twitch motor neurons tend to have higher conduction velocities than slow-twitch nerve cells. These findings have been reported in studies of cat hindlimb alpha motoneurons wherein the conduction velocities of FF nerve cells were more than 15 msec faster than those of S neurons.[7,8]

Another contributor to conduction velocity is the nature of conduction along the nerve cell. Motor neurons are covered in an insulating sheath called myelin (Fig. 2-2). The myelin is interrupted periodically along the axon by nodes, which cause the depolarized signal to jump from one node to the next in wavelike fashion. This form of signal conduction is referred to as saltatory conduction after the Latin *saltare*, meaning "to leap." The wider the nodal spacing, the more rapidly the signal jumps from node to node, and consequently, the faster the rate of transmission. Fast-twitch motor units have greater internodal distances than slow-twitch units, contributing to their faster conduction velocity.[23]

In addition to their signal transmission characteristics, motor units can be separated into groups with different excitatory potentials. In other words, the strength of the input required to evoke an action potential along the nerve cell varies between fast and slow-twitch motor units. Although slow-twitch neurons are more readily excited (have a lower firing threshold), fast-twitch neurons require more input to overcome a higher excitatory threshold.

Muscle fiber characteristics in motor units closely parallel their associated nerve cells. Muscle fibers can be categorized histochemically according to the level of myosin-ATPase associated with the cell. Myosin-ATPase is bound to the myosin heads and is related to twitch speed. Fast-twitch muscle fibers have higher levels of myosin-ATPase and consequently, stain darkly in slide preparations. Slow-twitch fibers, on the other hand, have low levels of myosin-ATPase and thus appear very light under stain (Fig. 2-3).

Muscle twitch responses are also clearly distinguishable between FF, FR, and S motor unit types. Enoka[13] describes three such motor units from the medial

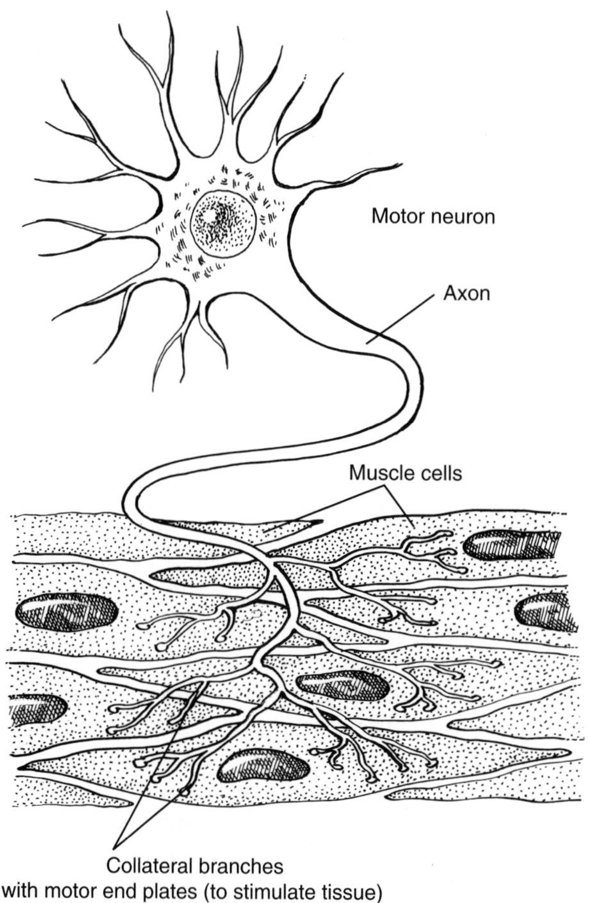

FIGURE 2-1. Motor unit.

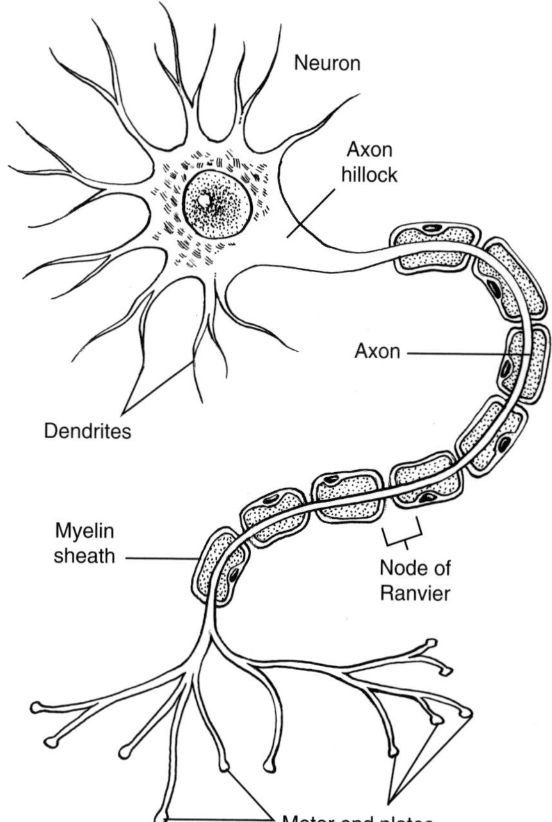

FIGURE 2-2. Myelination/nodes of Ranvier.

gastrocnemius of the cat. Muscle fibers from the FF motor unit produce nearly 50 grams of force with a twitch time of less than 100 ms. Twitch tension from FR fibers was recorded at less than 20 gm, with a twitch duration of greater than 100 ms. Fibers from the S motor unit achieved a tension of less than 10 gm over a period of more than 200 ms. Thus, the diversity of motor unit types provides the neuromuscular system with a fairly precise means of controlling contractile activity, thus influencing the nature of motor coordination.

MOTOR-UNIT RECRUITMENT

The gradation of muscle contraction is necessary for purposeful movement to occur. The force required to hold a 12-pound bowling ball, for example, is greater than that needed to hold a crystal goblet. The higher force may serve both conditions, but in the latter case is unnecessary and may result in damage or injury. Through a diverse motor-unit pool, the neuromuscular system has a means of controlling not only the amplitude of muscle activity, but also the rate of change in tension. These are accomplished through motor-unit recruitment strategies.

It is first necessary to understand that motor-unit activity adheres to the "all-or-none" principle. That is, once the firing threshold of a motor-unit is reached, depolarization of the nerve cell proceeds, resulting in the stimulation of all of the associated muscle fibers. Those fibers will respond by contracting fully, meaning that they will produce the maximal amount of force that they are capable of producing. Thus, a motor-unit can be viewed as either quiescent or fully contracting; there are no other possibilities.

The gradation of muscle contraction, therefore, must account for this phenomenon, and accordingly, there are two essential means by which force modulation is accomplished. These are sometimes referred to as recruitment or frequency strategies. Under a recruitment strategy, the nervous system recruits a progressive number of motor-units until the appropriate level of force output is achieved. Frequency strategies involve the repeated stimulation of a fixed number of motor-units, contributing to tension development with each successive twitch response.

Either an isolated or combined application of these strategies will result in graded muscle tension. It is generally reported, however, that recruitment is the predominant strategy for a stepwise or gross increase in

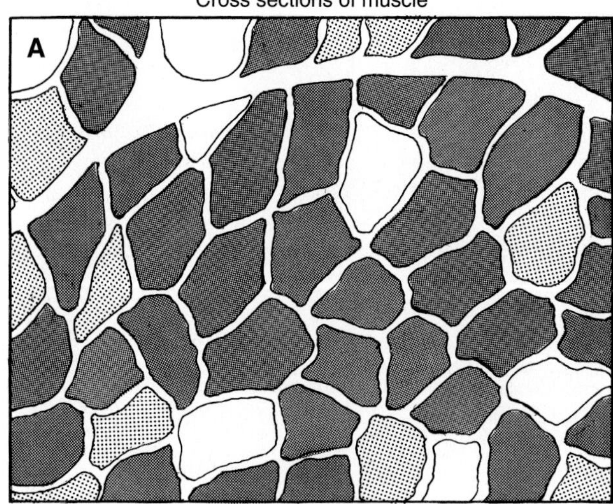

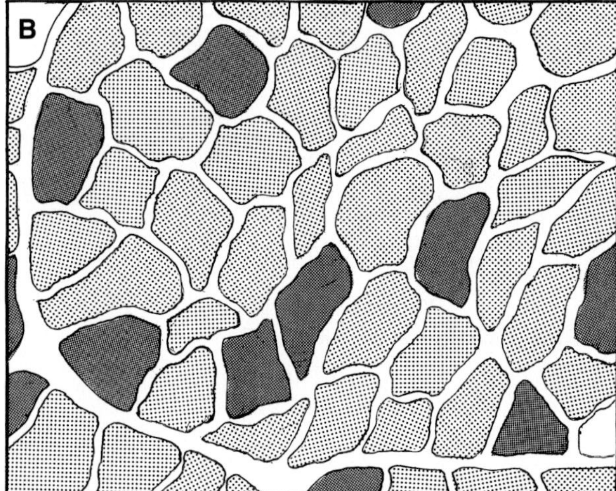

FIGURE 2-3. **A,** Myosin-ATPase stains dark in the predominantly type II muscle. **B,** Type I muscle shows little staining.

muscle force, and smooth changes or minor fluctuations in twitch tension emanate from frequency control schemes.[10,26,35] Milner-Brown and Stein[29] suggest that recruitment occurs under low-level muscular contractions, but the manipulation of firing rate becomes more critical at higher force levels. Regardless of their specific manner of activation, the presence of these two strategies and the associated variety of muscle torque profiles that can be generated suggest that a high degree of variability exists in the recruitment of motor-units. Yet, evidence exists suggesting that the recruitment of motor-units follows a quite orderly pattern.

Henneman's Size Principle

Through decades of research in the area of motor control, many hypotheses have emerged to explain the nature of motor activity and the systematic activation of motor-units. One theory presented over 35 years ago, however, remains relatively unchallenged in its explanation of the governing of muscle force output. Henneman's size principle[15] states that the activation of motor units at the spinal cord level follows an orderly progression from the low threshold, slow-twitch nerve cells, to the higher threshold, fast-twitch motor neurons.

Low force contractions, therefore, will involve only slow-twitch motor units, but high force muscle activity will result from the sequential activation of first slow then fast-twitch nerve cells. More specifically, Komi and Viitasalo[26] suggest that the contribution of fast-twitch motor units begins when force output reaches 60% of an individual's maximal volitional contraction (MVC). Thus, for contractions below this level, recruitment strategies may be employed exclusively to the low-threshold motor units. Tension requirements above 60% MVC, on the other hand, will be met by applying combined recruitment and frequency schemes to the entire available motor unit pool (this scheme is presented graphically in Figure 2-4).

This model of motor unit activation offers a logical interpretation of the dynamic control of muscle force output. It is not, however, the solitary explanation, and may only partially explain the diverse mechanisms controlling motor outflow. For example, 20 years ago Milner-Brown, Stein, and Lee[30] introduced the notion of motor-unit synchronization, wherein individuals demonstrated a propensity to group discharges from different motor units. Most of the subjects falling into this category

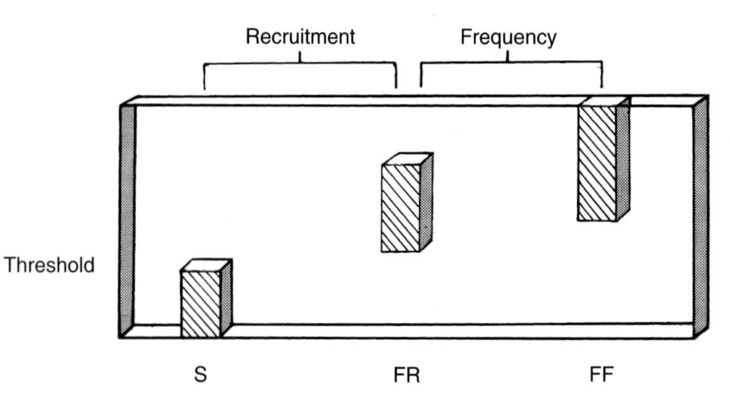

FIGURE 2-4. Illustration of recruitment strategies.

were either weight lifters or were involved in manual jobs requiring the exertion of large, briefly applied forces. Ostensibly, synchronization is an efficient strategy by which one can develop high forces through the combined output of various motor-unit pools.

Although motor-unit synchronization offers an alternative explanation to the control of motor outflow, it does not necessarily conflict with Henneman's premise. It is quite possible that the clustering of motor units follows a similar progression along the threshold hierarchy, wherein low-threshold units are grouped first and high-threshold units enter the cluster in response to greater force demands. In this sense, synchronization is not an alternative strategy, but rather a different method of employing the size principle. Instead of recruiting individual motor units in a specified sequence, the nervous system can engage groups of motor units simultaneously to achieve high force levels more efficiently. This concept is supported by De Luca,[10] whose notion of a "common drive" suggests that individual motor units are not individually controlled but that motoneuron pools are controlled as a whole.

In essence, the synchronized output of a set of clustered slow-twitch motor units may equal the force generated by single fast-twitch motor units. It follows, then, that the combined force output of synchronized motor-unit pools may exceed the sum force generated by sequentially activated individual motor units. The result is not only an extension of the potential range of muscle force output, but a more finite degree of control over the development and disposition of muscle force.

It is worth repeating that Henneman's size principle has been largely unchallenged during the past four decades. There is evidence, however, suggesting that additional recruitment schemes exist, not necessarily as replacements for the size principle but perhaps as coexisting strategies for the control of motor neurons. Person,[34] for example, examined the activity of motoneuron pools during submaximal isometric contractions when individuals were either in a "fixed body" position or in a "free posture." The author reports that while subjects were "fixed" the recruitment of motor units followed an orderly sequence, as described by Henneman. Under "free posture" conditions, on the other hand, subjects demonstrated significant variability in the recruitment and deactivation of motor units.

This variability in the pattern of muscle activation is apparently related to the nature of the neuromuscular activity. Person argues that under normal movement conditions, the recruitment of motor units and their differential control are coordinated by the combination of afferent and supraspinal structures. In other words, the process of neuromuscular coordination is generated from higher levels in the central nervous system (CNS) from which a choice of inputs to independent motoneurons or motoneuron pools can be made. Consequently, the CNS may be capable of selective recruitment resulting in movement-specific motor-unit firing patterns.

The method by which selective recruitment occurs has been partially explained by Burke et al.,[7] who postulated that during voluntary contractions a neural switching mechanism can redirect the excitation of motor units toward high-threshold neurons, while simultaneously depressing slow-twitch units. Basmajian[1] also discusses the selective inhibition of superfluous motor pathways, resulting in the excitation of only those motor-unit pools that will yield the appropriate muscle activity for specific tasks. Both of these authors support Person's notion of high-level control mechanisms. Belanger and McComas,[3] however, in addressing Burke's hypothesis, failed to detect evidence of selective control of motor units under conditions of isometric ankle plantar and dorsiflexion. So the evidence associated with selective recruitment is not altogether certain.

The lack of consistency in the various findings may relate to the nature of the experimental task rather than the absolute presence or absence of recruitment selectivity. Much of the work focusing on motor-unit recruitment involves simple tasks performed under highly regulated conditions. It is quite possible that under these circumstances the innervation of motor units follows a tightly regulated linear pattern, as described by Henneman. Person's investigation, on the other hand, compared a simplistic condition in which coordinated muscle activity for postural control was not required, to one that involved the dual task of having to perform muscular contractions while simultaneously maintaining posture and equilibrium. In this case, the difference in task complexity might explain the varied findings. The implication, although somewhat speculative, is that the CNS has the ability to vary the strategy by which motor units are recruited, adhering to a regulatory pattern under more simple movement conditions and switching to a more adaptable combination of linear recruitment, synchronization, and selective recruitment as movement complexity increases (Fig. 2-5).

The Extent of Motor-Unit Activation

The nature of the movement may also influence the extent to which motor units can be recruited. To pose this as a question, one may ask under what conditions can motor units be maximally recruited? It is often suggested, for instance, that moderate-level prolonged contractions will involve the complete recruitment of available motor units. This assumption, however, is flawed in its logic and is not supported scientifically.

In essence, the activation of motor units is influenced by three principle factors. The first involves the force levels inherent in the muscular contractions. Second is the contraction rate, or velocity of shortening. Third is the type of contraction itself, that is, whether the muscle

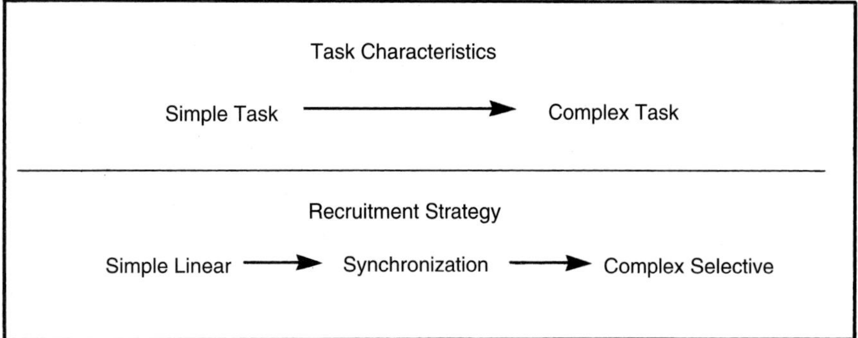

FIGURE 2-5. Change in recruitment strategy with task complexity.

is developing tension isometrically, concentrically, or eccentrically.

As discussed previously in relating Henneman's size principle, the contribution or innervation of high-threshold, fast-twitch motor units is associated with increased force levels. Prolonged contractions that involve moderate loads may not possess the characteristic force requirements that would elicit a response from fast-twitch motor units, and there is little scientific evidence to suggest that such muscular activity would involve the activation of high-threshold units. To the contrary, there is ample evidence to indicate a direct relationship between the type of motor-unit activity witnessed during a contraction and the velocity, force, and shortening characteristic of that contraction.

Moritani and Muro,[33] for example, have demonstrated a linear relationship between EMG amplitudes, mean power frequencies, and the level of muscular contraction. This suggests that higher-threshold motor units are activated only when enhanced levels of force production are attempted.

Motor-unit recruitment associated with various force levels has also been investigated by Hannerz.[21] Motor units recruited at 15% MVC fired at a rate of 10 per sec. At 60% MVC, the rate increased to 20 per sec, and at 90% MVC, firing rate reached 35 per sec. These findings represent the gradual change from slow-twitch to fast-twitch motor units as the level of contraction rises. Hannerz also discovered an interesting alteration in firing behavior when comparing isometric and isotonic contractions. During a 20% static contraction, low-frequency motor units fired continuously. When the level of muscular work was increased to 25%, new motor units were recruited. During a low-level twitch contraction involving a higher velocity of shortening, only the new motor units were activated, indicating a direct relationship between the speed of the muscle contraction and the recruitment of high-threshold motor units.

Further comparisons between the two contraction types were performed by Grimby and Hannerz[17] in 1977. Using wire electrodes, the authors distinguished between two types of motor units. The first was labeled *continuously firing long interval motor units* (CLMUs) and could discharge at long intervals. During maximum sustained efforts, CLMUs fired at 30 to 50 ms intervals. With twitch contractions, the intervals decreased, reducing to 10 msec during maximum twitches. Alternating movements were characterized by intervals of 15 to 20 msec.

The second motor unit type isolated by Grimby and Hannerz was an *intermittently firing short interval motor unit* (ISMUs). These units were inactive during weak or moderately sustained efforts and fired only occasionally during maximal isometric contractions. During rapid alternating movements, however, these motor units fired in high-frequency bursts with intervals between 20 and 40 ms. Both CLMUs and ISMUs were then recorded simultaneously. Prolonged sustained contractions involved only CLMUs, but during rapid accelerations both fired. These results indicate that there is a clear difference in the way that motor units are recruited when one develops tension either isometrically, isotonically, or at different rates of shortening. It is only in the rapid moving condition that both types of motor units fired.

Finally, Enoka and Fuglevand[14] have demonstrated that isometric contractions will not involve maximal motor-unit recruitment. Their subjects were instructed to produce a maximal volitional contraction on top of which was introduced an electrical stimulus. The authors discovered that muscle force output increased with added stimulation. Arguably, the MVC could not have involved maximal motor-unit recruitment because under those conditions no additional stimulus would have increased force output. The inability of the system to recruit high-threshold motor units during isometric contractions has been explained by Tax and colleagues,[39] who demonstrated that recruitment thresholds were lower during isotonic contractions than they were under isometric conditions.

From the combined scientific evidence then, it can be argued that the maximal recruitment of motor units cannot be achieved under conditions of sustained maximal isometric or prolonged moderate-level isotonic contractions. Rather, it is only when rapid, forceful movements are attempted that motor-unit populations are fully recruited.

Strength Development

It is noteworthy that exercise physiology chapters exploring strength development focus primarily on changes at the muscular level. In context with this discussion, however, adaptations in strength will be examined from the neuromuscular level. A change in strength implies that not only has the muscle improved its contractile capability, but that the motor drive has evolved as well. This notion is supported by studies utilizing an electromyograph (EMG) as an instrument by which nervous system activity can be explored. Häkkinen and Komi,[18] for example, show that EMG amplitude rises linearly with muscle tension. By itself, this only shows an immediate change in neural drive to increase muscle output. But there is evidence depicting a more lasting change in the integrated EMG (IEMG) over the course of training programs.[18,25,32,41] These studies demonstrate training induced changes not only in maximal tension development, but in maximal IEMG as well. These results do depict learning at the nervous system level. The role of the neuromuscular system in learning becomes more evident in examining the time course of strength development.

Several authors have demonstrated strength improvement within a relatively short period of time. Ishida, Moritani, and Itoh,[22] for example, documented a 31% increase in maximal volitional contraction in their training subjects. All but 1% of this change occurred within the first 4 weeks of training. Moritani and deVries[32] demonstrated an average strength gain of 17% within 7 weeks, and others showed maximal strength increases within 4 weeks.[18,25] These results are significant not by virtue of the fact that subjects experienced a gain in strength but because their strength improvement came in the absence of muscular hypertrophy. Thus, the enhanced muscle tension experienced by their subjects could not be related to increased contractility. Rather, a change in the pattern of muscle activation was most likely the impetus for improved strength.

The phenomenon of "neural learning" has also been demonstrated in studies in which the effects of training on one limb are seen in the contralateral untrained limb. Such bilateral transfer was noticed, for example, by Komi et al.,[27] whose subjects experienced a 20% increase in isometric knee extension strength in their trained limbs and an 11% increase in MVC in their nontrained limbs. Moritani and deVries[32] found similar results in comparisons of elbow flexor strength, but remarkably, increases in MVC on the untrained side were greater than those of the trained side (21% versus 17%). Once again, these results can hardly be attributed to muscle hypertrophy. It is more likely that subjects experienced a reorganization of the efferent systems that are responsible for the muscle activity under investigation.

Besides increased strength as an end product of weight training, changes in the actual patterns of neuromotor behavior have been documented. In the previously discussed study by Milner-Brown, Stein, and Lee,[30] for example, 2 out of 10 subjects who exercised their first dorsal interosseous muscle showed a tendency for the synchronization of discharges. It is quite possible that the firing of motor units had become synchronized as a function of resistance training. Synchronization, therefore, may be one means by which the nervous system can effect a permanent increase in muscle tension without a concomitant change in muscle mass.

This is not to suggest that muscle hypertrophy bears no significance to strength development. Strength training studies have clearly demonstrated muscle mass changes as a consequence of the strengthening paradigms. The role of the central nervous system, however, cannot be overlooked and may in fact be the most critical determinant of the nature of hypertrophic gains at the muscle level.

Morphologic Adaptation and Neural Drive

Traditional theory suggests that the types of loads employed during training dictate the nature of the muscular response. For instance, light loads and high repetitions create muscle tone, and heavy loads lifted with few repetitions induce increases in muscle mass. This very simplistic view overlooks key factors, such as the recruitment of motor units that would contribute to specific morphologic adaptation. In addition, it fails to consider the difference in training responses among slow-twitch and fast-twitch muscle fibers. On a more scientific level, one might suggest that any exercise that invokes motor-unit recruitment throughout the threshold scale would result in hypertrophy of all of the muscle fibers recruited. In other words, if all of the motor units are recruited in the manner described by Henneman, then both slow-twitch and fast-twitch muscle cells should experience equal levels of hypertrophy. Although this concept might address the issue of total muscular development, it does not distinguish between different characteristics of adaptation, such as tone or mass. Furthermore, it has not been supported scientifically, as evidenced in the findings of studies involving strength or power training.

One should begin with an operational definition of strength and power. *Power* is defined as force applied over a given distance for a specific period of time. More simply stated, power is force times velocity. It follows that exercises involving high, rapidly achieved force levels would constitute power-training exercises. An example of such an exercise is weighted jumping.

Strength, on the other hand, is not so easily defined and, in fact, is somewhat nebulous because of the variety of measures used for its assessment. For instance, strength is often measured as one's maximal volitional isometric contraction (MVC) or as a one-repetition maximum (1 RM). Strength can also be characterized as isokinetic peak torque. All of these make the exact meaning of strength unclear because they yield different results. An interesting interpretation of strength was issued by Bohannon,[5] who claimed that strength was simply "one's ability to bring force to bear on the environment." This is an attractive definition because it places strength into a task-specific context. In theory then, any exercise that improves one's ability to apply force in a task-specific context can be considered a strength-developing exercise (this includes, of course, power-training exercises). To distinguish between strength and power exercises, strength-training exercises will be limited to loaded movements that do not involve high velocities, such as a leg press done at a relatively slow, consistent pace.

Two strength-training studies warrant mention, not so much for their demonstration of strength gains, but for the absence of morphologic adaptation despite the demonstrated strength gains. Dons and colleagues[11] in 1979 examined strength changes in subjects performing controlled squat exercises over a 7-week interval. In addition, they monitored the number and size of slow and fast-twitch fibers before and after training. Subjects exercising at 80% of their 1 RM experienced a 42% increase in strength after 7 weeks. Interestingly, there was no change in the relative number of fast or slow-twitch fibers, nor did the area of those fibers or the ratio between fast-twitch and slow-twitch fibers change.

The results of this study mirrored those of Moritani and deVries[32] and serve to reinforce the notion that early strength gains are most likely the end product of adaptation within the central nervous system. It is possible that with training beyond 7 weeks the subjects of both studies would have experienced changes in the area and ratio of fast-twitch and slow-twitch fibers. Häkkinen et al.[20] addressed this issue by investigating strength and muscle changes in various groups engaged in "high intensity" strength-training programs over a 12-month period. Curiously, none of the subjects demonstrated a change in fast-twitch or slow-twitch fiber area. Perhaps it is not the duration of exercise but the nature of the exercise that contributes most significantly to changes at the muscle level. Several studies, in fact, support this contention.

Thorstensson et al.,[41] for instance, investigated the effects of 8 weeks of squat and jump training. Their subjects demonstrated an increase in FT/ST area ratio from 1.20 to 1.37 over the training period. Although the training interval of 8 weeks was similar to those of the previously mentioned strength studies, clearly the nature of the activity was different. Likewise, Häkkinen et al.[19] examined the effects of 24 weeks of "explosive" jumping and noticed an increase in the area of fast-twitch muscle fibers and a decrease in the area of slow-twitch cells. The result was an increase in FT/ST area ratio. Again, the principle difference between this study and their 1987 work was the nature of the training involved.

Similar results have been reported in isokinetic training studies. Costill et al.[9] witnessed a decrease in the percent of ST area and an increase in the percent of FT area after 7 weeks of isokinetic training at 180°/sec. More recently, Bell and colleagues[4] detected a 5% increase in FT cross-sectional area and a 10% increase in myosin-ATPase activity after a course of "high velocity" isokinetic training.

The findings of these studies clearly suggest that the type of training in which one engages has a marked influence on the muscular response. Specifically, it has been demonstrated that power training results in an increase in FT/ST area ratio or a selectively greater increase in the area of fast-twitch muscle fibers. Strength training, on the other hand, does not seem to affect this ratio. This is a curious phenomenon. If Henneman's size principle holds true, then clearly there ought to be equal development of both ST and FT fiber populations, because the recruitment of these fibers progresses systematically along the motor unit scale. Assuming, for instance, that power training involves more fast-twitch muscle fibers than strength training, one might expect more hypertrophy among the fast-twitch muscle cells in power trained subjects. Slow-twitch fibers, however, should also experience some growth, because they are presumably recruited first. Yet, these do not seem to change.

Two theories may explain this behavior. First, the neuromuscular system might actually experience a form of selective recruitment during power-training exercises. This concept was presented by Schmidtbleicher and Haralambie[38] in a study in which the push-off time of the upper extremity was studied in low- and high-intensity training groups. The high-intensity group experienced a significant reduction in push-off time, but the low-intensity group did not improve, prompting the authors to suggest that high-intensity training involved only fast-twitch motor units, and low-intensity training employed both ST and FT units. In this case, the selective activation of type II motor units would lead to the hypertrophy of only fast-twitch muscle fibers.

Although this theory does provide an explanation for selective hypertrophy, it is somewhat problematic. The assumption that only FT motor units, and hence fibers, would be recruited during an ongoing exercise is not, in itself, without fault. In light of the fact that fast-twitch muscle cells are easily fatigued, it is arguable that the selective recruitment of these cells would be impossible, because they would fatigue rapidly and leave the neuromuscular system with no force generating mechanism. If they were selectively recruited and subsequently fatigued, then the system would, out of necessity, be forced to employ slow-twitch units to maintain some level of motor activity. In that case, ST muscle cells should experience some growth.

The second explanation behind selective hypertrophy is not only interesting but is also quite possibly the driving mechanism behind muscle growth. Studies comparing strength training to power training, or isotonic training to isometric training, have yielded a fascinating result. Referring to the study by Häkkinen and others,[19] the authors noted a 24% increase in the rate at which tension was developed in the power-trained group. This increase correlated positively with the detected increase in FT fiber area in that population of subjects. Peak isometric torque, on the other hand, experienced only a 10% improvement, which was deemed not significant by the authors.

A study conducted by Duchateau and Hainaut[12] reported similar findings. Subjects who trained isometrically experienced an increase in peak torque, while those undergoing isotonic training increased their rate of tension development. Rate of tension development may actually be the single most significant factor in the production of strength and power. It may also be the most significant contributor to the selective hypertrophy of muscle fibers. Komi[25] suggests that "the degree of hypertrophy may follow the effects of the motor input," citing rate of tension development as the primary factor. The mechanism behind the rate of tension development is clearly elucidated.

The time course of tension development is depicted in Figure 2-6. On the left is a slowly developing muscle tension curve with its associated IEMG activity. It can be seen that peak EMG activity precedes peak muscle tension. This occurs naturally, as the muscle responds to the neural drive with a slight delay. To the right is a tension curve that is increasing at a faster rate. Notice that the IEMG activity has shifted in time, and like the tension curve, has a markedly increased slope. This phenomenon was presented in Komi's work in 1986, depicting the change in the rate of tension development and the shift in IEMG activity that accompanies power training.

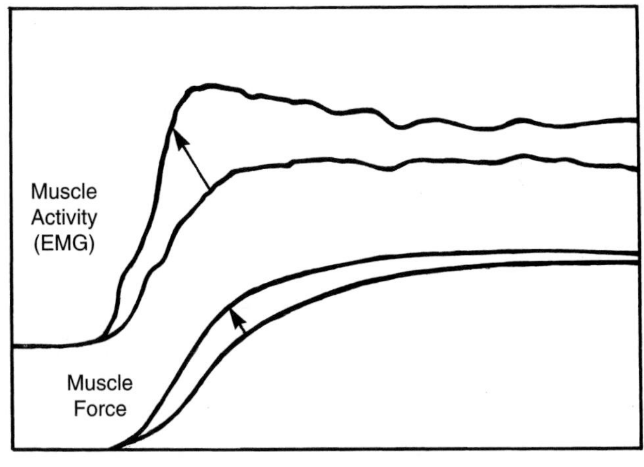

FIGURE 2-6. Increase in slope of neural drive, as seen in EMG profile, is reflected by an increase in rate of tension development, producing strength increases.

It has been suggested that the characteristic shape of the EMG profile, and hence the nature of the neural drive to the muscle, is actually responsible for creating the hypertrophic muscular response. More simply stated, if the pattern of neural drive to the muscle follows a gradual rise to peak, then training in this fashion might produce a general hypertrophy of ST and FT fibers, regardless of the level of tension developed. If, however, neural input rises rapidly, as depicted in an EMG trace with a high slope, then the musculature might experience a selective recruitment of FT muscle cells following training.

Speed Specificity

A quarter century ago, Moffroid and Whipple[31] presented a study examining the effects of exercise speed on increases in isokinetic torque. The authors noted that torque increases were specific at and below the speed of exercise, which touched off a flurry of research activity leading to one of the more controversial issues involving strength development. How specifically are strength gains related to the speed at which exercises are performed? The answer to this question has been elusive at best, given the contradictory scientific literature.

Moffroid and Whipple's study provides evidence that strength gains do not occur at speeds above those employed during training and thus are speed specific. One should note, however, that their training speeds of 6 and 18 revolutions per minute are comparable to 36° and 108°/sec, neither of which could truly be considered a high velocity. Thus, it is difficult to determine from this study whether similar training responses would exist if exercises were performed at higher speeds. This issue was addressed in a study by Ewing and colleagues,[16] who trained their subjects at 60° and 240°/sec. When tested at the slow speed, only the slowly trained group exhibited torque increases. At the fast speed, on the other hand, torque improvements were noted only in the fast-trained group, indicating a speed-specific response.

These results, however, are hardly consistent throughout the literature. Bell at al.,[4] for example, trained their subjects at 180°/sec but found strength improvements at test speeds ranging from 90°/sec to 240°/sec. Contrary to Moffroid and Whipple, this study does indicate that strength gains can transcend training speeds, particularly when training is slow and testing is fast. Other studies have presented similar findings after evaluating a variety of movement speeds. For example, subjects who trained at either 60°/sec or 180°/sec demonstrated strength gains at all testing speeds from 60°/sec to 300°/sec, but those whose training was performed at 300°/sec experienced gains only at higher angular velocities.[24,36] Evidently, speed specificity is related only to high training velocities, at least as indicated by these works. Still, the issue of specificity of velocity is somewhat obscured.

Perhaps the most significant work to emerge during the last decade is the 1993 study presented by Behm and Sale.[2] In this investigation subjects trained one limb by attempting rapid contractions at resistances that prevented motion entirely (isometric), and the other limb at resistances that allowed movement to occur at a high rate of speed (300°/sec). At the conclusion of the 16-week training period, both limbs experienced the same high-velocity-specific training response. The authors concluded that the stimulus for a high-velocity training response was the repeated attempt to produce a high-speed movement, rather than the actual movement speed. The results of this study have far-reaching implications.

Because of the difficulty involved in the control of limb pacing, the majority of the studies examining speed specificity have employed isokinetic devices. Such devices allow the experimenter to apply an external regulatory constraint on movement speed by the selection of a preset velocity that can not be exceeded by the performer. It is here that Behm and Sale's findings have their greatest impact. During isokinetic exercise or testing, one is instructed to exert as much force as possible against the machine, which in turn will constrain the movement to its preset speed of 60°/sec, for example. One can well imagine, however, that in the absence of such constraints, an attempt to move a limb with maximal force would produce a motion far in excess of 60°/sec. In essence, the intention on an isokinetic device is to move as rapidly as possible, but the actual motion occurs at a slower rate.

This would explain the common finding among isokinetic studies that training at a slow speed can lead to increased strength at fast testing velocities. Because the intention at all training speeds is to move as rapidly as possible, a carryover in strength from one rate of motion to another is clearly feasible. Unfortunately, the most important implication to emerge from Behm and Sale's work is lost in isokinetic testing. Strength gains are specific to the speeds at which training occurs. If one desires to move quickly with maximum force production, then one should adopt a training regime that requires such motion.

RECOMMENDATIONS FOR STRENGTH TRAINING

In 1957, Rasch and Morehouse[37] conducted a study that would eventually become a landmark in strength-training literature. In this investigation 49, subjects trained their biceps for a period of 6 weeks. At the end of the training period the subjects were evaluated for strength under familiar and unfamiliar positions. The subjects demonstrated strength gains in the familiar positions, but not when the position was unfamiliar. These results indicate that isolated muscle training does not necessarily lead to strength gains, but that strength really involves the acquisition of skill in a movement specific manner.

The mechanism underlying this phenomenon of task-specific strength changes appears to be related to the recruitment of motor units. It has been demonstrated, for example, that in multifunctional muscles the order of recruitment can be varied continuously by changing the task and consequently the direction of movement and the mechanical properties acting on the joints and limbs.[40] This results in a "directional programming" of muscle forces that, when done repeatedly, results in strength gains specific to that movement and body position.

This theory has been advanced by Loeb,[28] who not only addresses the recruitment of motor units, but suggests that the physical composition of the neuromuscular system is influenced by movement dependency. Referring once again to the discussion of motor-unit activation, one can infer that the recruitment of motor units is influenced by the desired speed of movement and the force requirements of the task. Loeb, on the other hand, in following ter har Romeny and colleagues,[40] suggests that motor units are recruited in a manner that befits the task at hand. In fact, he goes further to suggest that motor units are organized into "task groups" that may comprise a combination of slow-twitch, fast-twitch, and intermediate units. These motor-unit groupings are developed as one's movement repertoire grows.

Indeed, Loeb argues that not only are motor units grouped according to task, but that the physical orientation of muscle fibers is also task related, rather than simply organized according to motor-unit type. For instance, it is generally accepted that muscle fibers are bundled into homogeneous groupings so that motor units of similar type will occupy a common region within the muscle. Loeb, on the other hand, suggests that the grouping of motor units is task related, and that fibers from motor units may actually traverse several areas within a single muscle. It is also possible, Loeb argues, that fibers from motor-unit task groups may actually span different muscles as well. The development of strength, therefore, may well require the activation of various motor-unit task groups involving several muscles, with specifically applied movement patterns.

Strength development, therefore, requires considerably more than the simple repeated contractions of isolated muscle groups. If we return to the original premise of this chapter, that the functions of muscle are to stabilize or move the skeleton, then strength development should involve one or both of these functions. Stabilization and movement, however, are also task dependent. Thus the activation of motor units or task groups will also depend on the nature of the movements. In essence, strength enhancement can be achieved through the application of various natural resisted movements that incorporate different speeds and loading conditions. In this way the subject will most likely activate all of the appropriate motor units for those given tasks, not only developing isolated muscle strength but coordination and skill as well. A concern for skill, rather than muscle tone or mass, will lead to more effective functional strength gains that translate from the gym or rehabilitation center to the real world.

REFERENCES

1. Basmajian JV: Motor learning and control: A working hypothesis. Arch Phys Med Rehabil 58:38–41, 1977.
2. Behm DG, Sale DG: Intended rather than actual movement velocity determines the velocity-specific training response. J App Physiol 74(1):359–368, 1993.
3. Belanger AY, McComas AJ: Extent of motor unit activation during effort. J App Physiol 51(5): 1131–1135, 1981.
4. Bell GH, et al: Effect of high velocity resistance training on peak torque, cross sectional area and myofibrillar ATPase activity. J Sports Med Phys Fit 32:10–18, 1992.
5. Bohannon RW: The clinical measurement of strength. Clin Rehab 1:5–17, 1987.
6. Burke RE: On the central nervous system control of fast and slow twitch motor units. In Desmedt JE (ed): New Developments in Electromyography and Clinical Neurophysiology, 3:69–94, Basel, Karger, 1973.
7. Burke RE, et al: Physiological types and histochemical profiles in motor units of the cat gastrocnemius. J Physiol 234:723–748, 1973.
8. Burke RE, Rymer WZ, Walsh JV: Relative strength of synaptic input from short-latency pathways to motor units of defined type in cat medial gastrocnemius. J Neurophysiol 39: 447–458, 1976.
9. Costill DL, et al: Adaptations in skeletal muscle following strength training. J App Physiol 46(1): 96–99, 1979.
10. De Luca CJ: Control properties of motor units. J Exp Biol 115:125–136, 1985.
11. Dons B, et al: The effect of weight-lifting exercise related to muscle fiber composition and muscle cross-sectional area in humans. Eur J App Physiol 40(2):95–106, 1979.
12. Duchateau J, Hainaut K: Isometric or dynamic training: Differential effects on mechanical properties of a human muscle. J App Physiol 56(2): 296–301, 1984.
13. Enoka RM: Neuromechanical Basis of Kinesiology. Champaign, IL, Human Kinetics Books, 1988.
14. Enoka RM, Fuglevand AJ: Neuromuscular basis of the maximum voluntary force capacity of muscle. In Grabiner MD (ed): Current Perspectives in Biomechanics. Champaign, IL, Human Kinetics Publishers, 1991.
15. Enoka RM, Stuart DG: Henneman's size principle: Current issues. Trends Neurosci 7:226–228, 1984.
16. Ewing JL, et al: Effects of velocity of isokinetic training on strength, power, and quadriceps muscle fiber characteristics. Eur J App Physiol 61:159–162, 1990.
17. Grimby L, Hannerz J: Firing rate and recruitment order of toe extensor motor units in different modes of voluntary contraction. J Physiol 264:865–879, 1977.
18. Häkkinen K, Komi PV: Electromyographic changes during strength training and detraining. Med Sci Sports Exerc 15(6):455–460, 1983.
19. Häkkinen K, Komi PV, Alén M: Effect of explosive type strength training on isometric force and relaxation time, electromyographic and muscle fibre characteristics of leg extensor muscles. Acta Physiol Scand 125:587–600, 1985.
20. Häkkinen K, et al: EMG, muscle fibre and force production characteristics during a 1-year training period in elite weight-lifters. Eur J App Physiol 56:419–427, 1987.
21. Hannerz J: Discharge properties of motor units in relation to recruitment order in voluntary contraction. Acta Physiol Scand 91:374–384, 1974.
22. Ishida K, Moritani T, Itoh K: Changes in voluntary and electrically induced contractions during strength training and detraining. Eur J App Physiol 60: 244–248, 1990.
23. Kandel ER, Schwartz JH: Principles of Neural Science, 2nd ed. New York, Elsevier, 1985.
24. Kanehisa H, Miyashita M: Specificity of velocity in strength training. Eur J App Physiol 52:104–106, 1983.
25. Komi PV: Training of muscle strength and power: Interaction of neuromotoric, hypertrophic, and mechanical factors. Int J Sports Med 7(Suppl):10–15, 1986.
26. Komi PV, Viitasalo HT: Signal characteristics of EMG at different levels of muscle tension. Acta Physiol Scand 96: 267–276, 1976.
27. Komi PV, et al: Effect of isometric strength training on mechanical, electrical, and metabolic aspects of muscle function. Eur J App Physiol 40:45–55, 1978.
28. Loeb GE: Hard lessons in motor control from the mammalian spinal cord. Trends Neurosci 10(3): 108–113, 1987.
29. Milner-Brown HS, Stein RB: The relation between the surface electromyogram and muscular force. J Physiol 246: 549–569, 1975.
30. Milner-Brown HS, Stein RB, Lee RG: Synchronization of human motor units: Possible roles of exercise and supraspinal reflexes. Electro Clin Neurophysiol 38:245–254, 1975.

31. Moffroid MT, Whipple RH: Specificity of speed of exercise. Physical Therapy 50(12):1692–1700, 1970.
32. Moritani T, deVries HA: Neural factors versus hypertrophy in the time course of muscle strength gain. Am J Phys Med 58(3):115–129, 1979.
33. Moritani T, Muro M: Motor unit activity and surface electromyogram power spectrum during increasing force of contraction. Eur J App Physiol 56:260–265, 1987.
34. Person RS: Rhythmic activity of a group of human motoneurons during voluntary contraction of a muscle. Electro Clin Neurophysiol 36:585–595, 1974.
35. Person RS, Kudina LP: Discharge frequency and discharge pattern of human motor units during voluntary contraction of muscle. Electro Clin Neurophysiol 32:471–483, 1972.
36. Petersen SR, et al: The influence of velocity-specific resistance training on the in vivo torque-velocity relationship and the cross-sectional area of quadriceps femoris. J Ortho Sports Phys Ther May: 456–462, 1989.
37. Rasch PJ, Morehouse LE: Effect of static and dynamic exercises on muscular strength and hypertrophy. J App Physiol 11(1):29–34, 1957.
38. Schmidtbleicher D, Haralambie G: Changes in contractile properties of muscle after strength training in man. Eur J App Physiol 46:221–228, 1981.
39. Tax AAM, et al: Differences in the activation of M. biceps brachii in the control of slow isotonic movements and isometric contractions. Exp Brain Res 76:55–63, 1989.
40. ter har Romeny BM, Denier van der Gon JJ, Gielen CCAM: Changes in recruitment order of motor units in the human biceps muscle. Exp Neurol 78:360–368, 1982.
41. Thorstensson A et al: Effect of strength training on EMG of human skeletal muscle. Acta Physiol Scand 98:232–236, 1976.

3 Preparticipation Physical Examination

Gilbert B. Cushner and
Fred D. Cushner

The preparticipation physical examination (PPE) is a fluid situation depending on the age of the athlete, the sport involved, and setting of the examination. Just as a preoperative examination should not be considered a comprehensive annual physical exam, the PPE should only identify the athlete at risk for injury, illness, or death consequent to his or her participation in this specific sport. Overzealous disqualification is to be avoided.

Secondary objectives that have been proposed include general health examination, bringing the participant to the optimal level of performance, size and maturity evaluation, and furthering the doctor–patient relationship.[7] It is our feeling that although on occasion these will be touched upon during the PPE, they are not mandatory or universally accepted. In our society, legislative, legal, and insurance requirements also have to be considered.

LEGISLATIVE REQUIREMENTS

With the exception of Rhode Island, all states and the District of Columbia require some screening of athletes engaged in formal high school athletics. However, 8 of the 51 do not have an approved universal form. It is of some concern that 21 out of 51 jurisdictions permit nurses or physician assistants to do the PPE and in 11 in 51 chiropractors can do the evaluation.[9,21]

LEGAL ISSUES

Legal action has addressed the issues of unjust disqualification as well as failure to disqualify. Metzl describes a patient who unsuccessfully sued for being disqualified because of structural heart disease.[21] Also discussed is the Hank Gathers case in which a physician was sued for clearing the athlete who later died of cardiac arrest while playing basketball.

VALIDITY AND OUTCOMES

Smith and Laskowski[29] reviewed 10 studies involving 26,247 student athletes (Table 3-1): 9.5% were cleared for sport participation with follow-up recommendations but only 0.99% were not cleared. An estimated 200,000 student athletes would have to be examined to find the 1,000 at risk, and of these only one that would experience sudden death.[6] Is screening financially feasible? Risser[26] found the cost-benefit ratio to be $4,537 per athlete. He considered this to be clearly "unfavorable."

Although not proven to alter significantly mortality or morbidity, the PPE does identify health issues that need further evaluation in 10% of those examined. This, the occasional achieved secondary objective, and legal and legislative issues justify our continued use of the PPE.

SITE

Most examinations are either single physician office-based or station type. The assembly line examination, although the least expensive and most rapid, has largely been discontinued. Problems with this type of examination include lack of individual attention, insufficient history taking, and lack of continuity of care.[29] In addition, the quality of this examination is questionable and unproven.[1]

Table 3-2 compares the pros and cons of office versus station examination. The office exam will work only if the examining physician has specific knowledge of sports medicine, and if the exam is not a rushed last minute evaluation because of a deadline to have forms submitted. Many forms are completed based on a physician–patient encounter within 6 months, but not necessarily with a sports medicine focus.

In the best of all worlds, the exam would be performed by a kindly "Marcus Welby" type physician with the expertise of a sports medicine specialist. Unfortunately, this usually isn't the case. The advantages of having the exam performed by a nonspecialist can include better physician–athlete interaction, family and past history awareness, and guaranteed continuity of care. This is, of course, balanced by incomplete knowledge, lack of consistency, and the incomplete nature of the exam.

STATION EXAM

The set-up for the station exam as done at Mayo Clinic[29] is shown in Table 3-3. Advantages of this system are the ability to use specialized personnel, time and cost effectiveness, the large number of participants that can be evaluated, and adaptability. Disadvantages are a noisy environment, no preexisting physician–patient relationships, and no guarantee of continual care (Fig. 3-1). One study comparing the two approaches has been reported by DuRant.[5] He found that the station approach yielded significantly higher abnormalities, particularly in the musculoskeletal area.

TABLE 3-1 Summary of Published Studies on Sports Preparticipation Physical Examination in Students*

Reference	Method	Duration of Study (yr)	Athletes Examined (no.)	CEU Group No.	CEU Group %	NC Group No.	NC Group %	Comment
Goldberg et al,[10] 1980	Station	1	701	95	13.6	9	1.3	MSK #1 abnormality
Linder et al,[14] 1981	Station	2	1,268	64	5.0	2	0.2	Male students only MSK #1 abnormality
Tennant et al,[30] 1981	Assembly line	4	2,719	217	8.0	32	1.2	Male students only MSK #4 abnormality
Thompson et al,[31] 1982	Station	1	2,670	256	9.6	31	1.2	MSK #1 abnormality
Risser et al,[27] 1985	Station	2	2,114	75	3.1†	6	0.3†	MSK #1 abnormality
DuRant et al,[16] 1985	Single physician	1 (?)‡	170	4	2.4	0	0.0	MSK #1 abnormality
	Station	1 (?)‡	752	48	6.4	3	0.4	MSK #1 abnormality
Magnes et al,[24] 1992	Station	4	10,540	1,070	10.2	47	0.4	HTN #1 abnormality MSK #6 abnormality in NC group MSK #3 abnormality in CFU group
Rifat et al,[22] 1995	Single physician	7	2,574	325	12.6	66	2.6	MSK #1 abnormality§
Current study	Station	3	2,739	327	11.9	53	1.9	MSK #1 abnormality in NC group MSK #2 abnormality in CFU group
Total			26,247	2,481	9.5	249	0.9	

*CFU = cleared for participation in sports but follow-up recommended; HTN = hypertension; MSK = musculoskeletal; NC = not cleared for participation in sports.

†This study did not distinguish between CFU and NC groups initially; numbers are from available data.

‡Duration of study not specified in methods.

§MSK #1 when abnormal historical and examination findings were combined.

TIMING

The exam should be approximately 6 weeks prior to the start of the particular sport season, allowing time for further evaluation and possible correction of defects.[11]

FREQUENCY

A yearly examination is required in some jurisdictions, and some even require exams before each sport (pity the triple letter man!). A more reasonable approach is to have comprehensive exams at middle school, high school, and college entrance, with an interval exam yearly focusing on injuries, new illnesses, and so forth.

HISTORY

To paraphrase Sir William Osler, "Listen to the patient, they're telling you what is wrong with them." The history is without question the most important part of the PPE. Up to 75% of all orthopedic and medical problems are detected on history review.[15]

Both parents and athletes should review the history form (Fig. 3-2). Carek et al.[3] have found significant discrepancies when the forms are completed separately, particularly in the cardiovascular and musculoskeletal areas. A focused history as proposed by Fields and Delaney[7] seems to be a logical approach to obtaining an appropriate history. This approach covers the basic areas that need exploration, including cardiovascular risks, musculoskeletal injuries, and neurological history. Also included are the recently emphasized areas of exercise-induced asthma, heat injury, and general medical review.

Cardiovascular Risks

1. Has anyone in the athlete's family died of heart disease or sudden death before age 50?

TABLE 3-2

Potential Advantages and Disadvantages of Office-Based and Station Screening PPEs

Office-Based PPE	Station Screening PPE
Advantages	**Advantages**
Established physician-patient relationship	Low cost
Privacy (HIPAA)	Specialized personnel
	Availability of coaches/ athletic staff
	Efficiency
	Standardization
Disadvantages	**Disadvantages**
Busy offices	Privacy concerns (HIPAA)
No primary care physician	Continuity of care
Cost	Follow-up can be difficult
Lack of health insurance	
No established relationship with coaches	

From American Academy of Family Physicians, American Academy of Pediatrics, American Medical Society for Sports Medicine, American Orthopaedic Society for Sports Medicine, American Osteopathic Academy for Sports Medicine: Preparticipation Physical Evaluation Monograph, 1992.

2. Has the athlete ever experienced chest pain, shortness of breath, dizziness, syncothe, or palpitations with exercise?
3. Is there a history of heart murmur, hypertension, or high cholesterol?

TABLE 3-3

Stations for Administering the Sports Preparticipation Physical Examination

Station	Function	Suggested No. of Staff
1	Check-in, height, weight	2
2	Vision assessment	1
3	Blood pressure	1
4	Cardiopulmonary, HEENT, skin, genitalia, hernia (male)	2†
5	Neuromusculoskeletal	1 or 2†
6	Review, disposition assignment, dietary and psychology follow-up	2†

*HEENT = head, eyes, ears, nose, and throat.
†Physicians.

Question #1 probes for a family history that might suggest hypertrophic cardiomyopathy, an autosomal dominant disorder that has been consistently the leading cause of cardiovascular sudden death in athletes accounting for up to one third of cases.[18] Question #2 screens not only for hypertrophic cardiomyopathy but possible coronary artery malformation, arrhythmias, and cardiovascular risk factors.

Exercise-Induced Asthma

4. Does the patient have wheezing or coughing spells after exercise?

Exercise asthma is not uncommon, with 11% of Olympic hopefuls at the Colorado Springs Training Center found to suffer from this in 1984.[25] Because this is a readily treatable disease, early diagnosis is warranted.

Musculoskeletal Injury

5. Has the athlete ever broken a bone, injured a joint, or worn a cast?

This is the most common cause of disqualification, and obviously must be explored. The most common involved joint is the knee, followed by the ankle.[10,24,26] Joint injury tends to repeat itself. Robey[28] noted a 71% injury rate in football players injured in the previous season compared with a 43% injury rate in players without a previous injury. A positive response to this question will enable the examiner to more carefully evaluate this area and pursue further rehabilitation if necessary.

Neurological Injury

6. Has the athlete ever had a concussion (been knocked out)?

The athlete with recurrent concussions falls into a specified category with clearance requiring a thorough evaluation and referral.

Heat-Related Illness

7. Has the athlete ever suffered a heat-related illness?

Athletes who have suffered a bout of heat-related illnesses are at increased risk for recurrence.[23] Although not necessarily grounds for disqualification, it would be prudent to observe these athletes more carefully when their sport is performed in a hot, humid environment.

General Health Survey

8. Does the athlete have any chronic illnesses requiring regular medical follow-up?
9. Does the athlete take any medications?
10. Is there a history of allergy to medicine or bee stings?

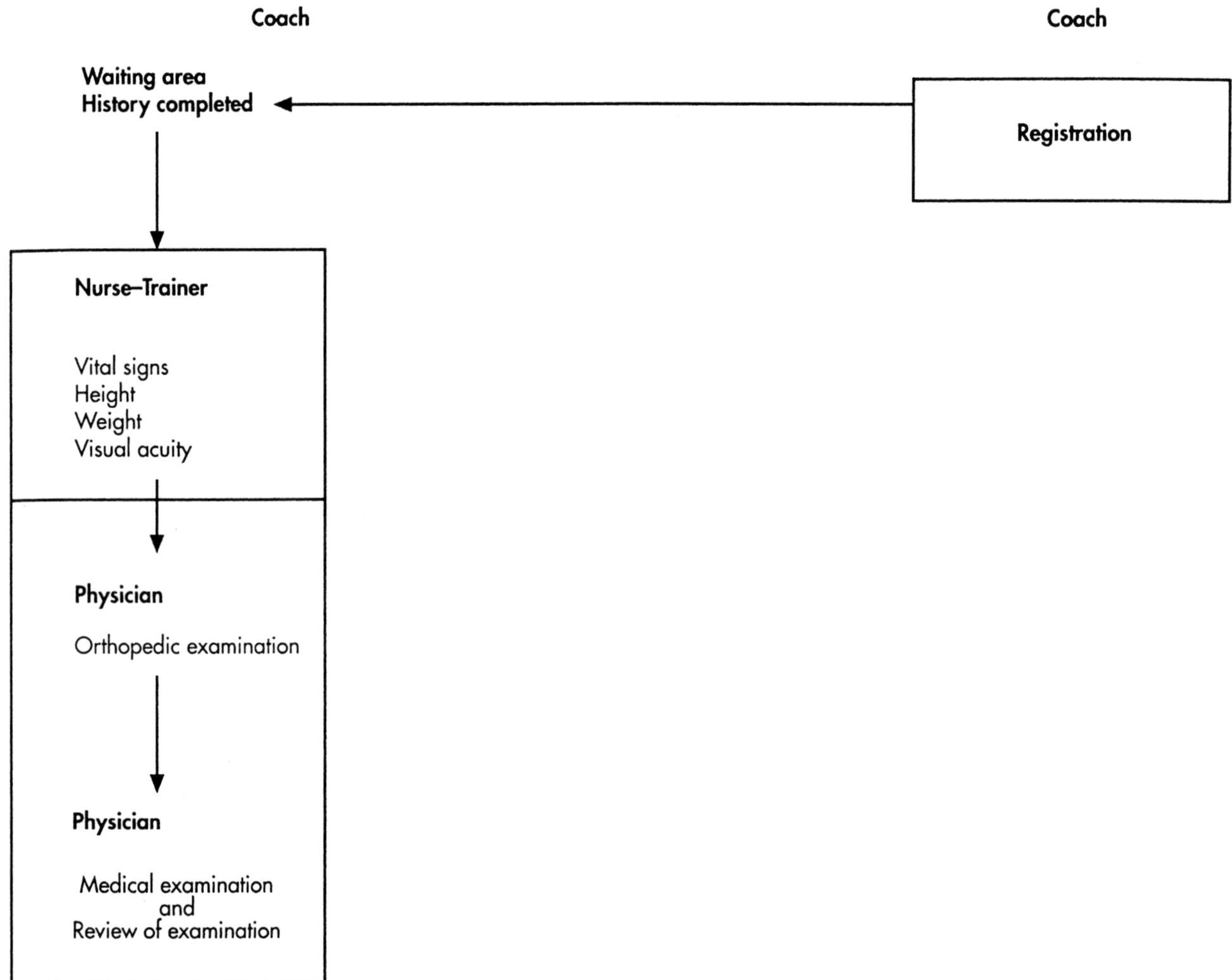

FIGURE 3-1. Typical station layout for screening examinations.

11. Does the athlete have only one of any paired organs? (eyes, ears, kidney, testicles, ovaries)
12. When was the last tetanus shot?
13. (Females) When was the athlete's last menstrual period?

Positive responses obviously require the examiner to further evaluate these areas, obtaining further studies and examinations to fully define the problem.

PHYSICAL EXAMINATION

The areas of the physical examination of greatest diagnostic utility are musculoskeletal, cardiovascular, and blood pressure.

Musculoskeletal Concerns

A history of injury should elicit a detailed evaluation of the joint involved (the knee and ankle are most common). An example of a screening musculoskeletal exam is shown in Table 3-4. This examination would evaluate range of motion and joint strength.

Blood Pressure

Unrecognized hypertension has been found in most studies of adolescent athletes; 1.5% to 6% of athletes have had significant elevations.[12] Upper limits of normal are 125/75 for athletes younger than 10 years and 135/85 for athletes older than 10 years.[12] Moderate or severe hypertension will limit safe athletic participation, but those with mild elevation can safely play.[7] There is no documented increased evidence of sudden death in hypertensive athletes.

Cardiovascular Concerns

Although occasionally a significant arrhythmia may be detected on cardiac examination, the main purpose of the exam is to detect significant murmurs, particularly those suggestive of hypertrophic cardiomyopathy, the leading cause of cardiac sudden death.[18] This cardiac disease is characterized by an asymmetrically hypertrophied but not dilated left ventricle occurring with an incidence of 1 in 500 persons in the general population.[17]

Date of Exam_____ /_____ /_____
School Official ______________
Exam Doctor ______________

Cleveland Clinic Foundation

PREPARTICIPATION SPORTS EXAM

A B C

Contact: Coach ☐
School Nurse ☐
Family Doctor ☐
Family Dentist ☐

THIS IS NOT A SUBSTITUTE FOR A REGULAR PHYSICAL EXAM PERFORMED BY YOUR FAMILY DOCTOR

Name______________ Grade ______ Age ______ Birthdate _____ /_____ /_____
School ______________ Sport ______________ Sex ______
Parents ______________ Address ______________ Phone ______
Family Doctor ______________ Address ______________ Phone ______

HISTORY: Answer **No** or **Yes** with details and dates. Use reverse side if necessary.

I. Have you ever sustained **an injury** which prevented you from playing sports for **more than one day and** have you had any injuries **such as** (circle): skull fracture - **brain surgery concussion** - knocked out, **neck pain**/injury - arm/finger **numbness**, **back pain**/injury - leg/toe numbness, heatstroke/fainting - exhaustion, broken bone - **fracture**, joint **dislocation** - out of place, **deep bruise** - muscle pull, ligament **sprains**, tender kneecap/shin, **trick knee** - catching/locking,
____
____

II. Do you have a history of **and/or** take medicine (specify) for any medical problems **such as** (circle): **asthma** - allergy - wheezing - short of breath, heart **murmur**/palpitation - rheumatic fever - **high blood high blood pressure**, diabetes - high/low **sugar**, fainting - **seizure**, yellow jaundice - **hepatitis**, severe influenza/cold - **mononucleosis** - weakness, **anemia** - bruise easily - bleeding - sickle cell, loss of eyesight, hearing, testicle, kidney, etc., **hernia** - rupture - bulging, skin disease - boils - **rash**, or other?
____
____

III. Are you allergic to any medicine such as (circle) penicillin, iodine, novocaine or other?
____

IV. Any family history of medically unexplained or cardiac caused sudden death under age 50?
____

V. L.M.P. ______________

BP___/___ P_____ Ht_____ Wt_____ Gross Vision: R_____ L_____, Pupils R_____ L_____ LAB: UA_____

EXAM:

1. Upper Extr: AC jts ______
   Symm ______
   ROM ______
2. Spine: Neck ______
   Fwd Bend ______
   Curve ______
3. Lower Extr: Gait ______
   1-Hop ______
   Duck ______
   Symm ______
   ROM ______
4. Heart: ______
5. Lungs: ______
6. Skin: ______
7. Abdo: Spleen ______
   Liver ______
8. GU: Hernia ______
   Testicles ______
9. Dental ______
10. Other ______
   ______
   ______

IMPRESSION:

☐ Satisfactory Exam
☐ Recommend further evaluation/rehabilitation regarding: ______________

Contact your: School Nurse — Coach — Family Doctor — Family Dentist

CLEARANCE:

A — Cleared for: Collision — Contact — Noncontact sports
B — Cleared for: Collision — Contact — Noncontact sports after completing eval/rehab
C — NOT cleared for: Collision — Contact — Noncontact sports due to: ______________
____

2285570 Rev. 9/90

FIGURE 3-2.

TABLE 3-4

Example of a Screening Musculoskeletal Examination

Athletic Activity (Instructions)	Observations
1. Stand facing examiner	AC joints; general habitus
2. Look at celling, floor, over both shoulders, touch ears to shoulder	Cervical spine motion
3. Shrug shoulders (examiner resists)	Trapezius strength
4. Abduct shoulders 90° (examiner resists at 90°)	Deltoid strength
5. Full external rotation of arms	Shoulder motion
6. Flex and extend elbows	Elbow motion
7. Arms at sides, elbows at 90° flexed; pronate and supinate wrists	Elbow and wrist motion
8. Spread fingers; make fist	Hand and finger motion and deformities
9. Tighten (contract) quadriceps; relax quadriceps	Symmetry and knee effusion, ankle effusion
10. "Duck walk" four steps (away from examiner)	Hip, knee, and ankle motion
11. Back to examiner	Shoulder symmetry; scoliosis
12. Knees straight, touch toes	Scoliosis, hip motion, hamstring tightness
13. Raise up on toes, heels	Calf symmetry, leg strength

From McKeag DB: Preparticipation screening of the potential athlete. Clin Sport Med 8(3): 373, 1989.

The murmur of hypertrophic cardiomyopathy is a systolic ejection murmur heard best at the left sternal border and that is accentuated by maneuvers that reduce blood flow to the left side of the heart, such as changing from a lying to a standing position.[4] Causes of sudden cardiac death compiled by Maron[18] are listed in Table 3-5. Most sudden deaths in the United States occur while athletes are playing football or basketball. The male-female ratio of 9:1 reflects the sex distribution of athletes playing those sports.

When a murmur is not present, there are usually no tell-tale physical findings to identify the athletes with these other abnormal states. Exceptions might be the physical characteristics of Marfan syndrome (tall, high, arched palate, pectis excavartum, long fingers and toes), which is associated with aortic abnormalities that account for 3% of sudden deaths.

MISCELLANEOUS EXAMINATIONS

Certain sports require more specific examinations. Ear, nose, and throat examination is necessary in swimmers and divers to rule out chronic ear problems. Skin screenings may be meaningful in wrestlers, who often have chronic skin infections. Pulmonary examination to rule out wheezing and an abdominal exam to rule out splinomeglia can quickly be accomplished. Needless to say, areas of abnormality found on the history should be explored.

LABORATORY TESTS

Routine laboratory testing plays no role in the PPE. Hemoglobin and urine screenings have not been found to identify those athletes who need to be disqualified.[7] Laboratory testing is necessary when the history suggests certain illnesses such as anemia or diabetes.

An important question to be answered is whether the use of electrocardiograms and/or echocardiograms as screening tools would decrease the incidence of cardiac sudden death. In a retrospective study, only 3% of trained athletes who died suddenly of heart disease were suspected of having cardiovascular abnormalities in their PPE history, and physical exam and none were disqualified.[20]

The Italian government has mandated 12-lead electrocardiograms as part of the PPE. Although this program has permitted the identification of many athletes with previously undiagnosed hpertrophic cardiomyopathy,[17] similar studies in smaller population have had less productive results.[8,13,19] Portable echocardiograms have been used to screen high school athletes in the field.[22]

As stated by Maron,[18] in a large population the value of preparticipation screening with noninvasive testing is limited by the large numbers of false positive and false negative results (the echocardiogram will not show the classic findings of hypertrophic cardiomyopathy in patients younger than 14).[17]

CLEARANCE

At the conclusion of the PPE, the examiner must decide on one of four courses of action:

1. The athlete is cleared for the sport requested.
2. The athlete is cleared for the sport requested but abnormalities were found that need further evaluation.
3. The athlete is not cleared, pending evaluation of a medical problem needing further study.
4. The athlete is not cleared.

The athlete, family, and coach should be notified of the decision. Tables 3-6 and 3-7 are useful tools in decision making. The latter classifies sports as to degree of contact and exertion. The former shows useful tests and examinations for evaluation of the athlete.

When cardiac disease is diagnosed, further input can be obtained from the recommendations of the Twenty-sixth

TABLE 3-5

Causes of Sudden Death in 387 Young Athletes*

Cause	No. of Athletes	Percent
Hypertrophic cardiomyopathy	102	26.4
Commotio cordis	77	19.9
Coronary-artery anomalies	53	13.7
Left ventricular hypertrophy of indeterminate causation†	29	7.5
Myocarditis	20	5.2
Ruptured aortic aneurysm (Marfan syndrome)	12	3.1
Arrhythmogenic right ventricular cardiomyopathy	11	2.8
Tunneled (bridged) coronary artery‡	11	2.8
Aortic-valve stenosis	10	2.6
Atherosclerotic coronary artery disease	10	2.6
Dilated cardiomyopathy	9	2.3
Myxomatous mitral-valve degeneration	9	2.3
Asthma (or other pulmonary condition)	8	2.1
Heat stroke	6	1.6
Drug abuse	4	1.0
Other cardiovascular cause	4	1.0
Long-QT syndrome§	3	0.8
Cardiac sarcoidosis	3	0.8
Trauma involving structural cardiac injury	3	0.8
Ruptured cerebral artery	3	0.8

*Data are from the registry of the Minneapolis Heart Institute Foundation.
†Findings at autopsy were suggestive of hypertrophic cardiomyopathy but were insufficient to be diagnostic.
‡Tunneled coronary artery was deemed the cause in the absence of any other cardiac abnormality.
§The long-QT syndrome was documented on clinical evaluation.

TABLE 3-6

Components of the Orthopedic Screening Portion of the Sports Preparticipation Physical Examination*

Test Maneuver	Focus of Observation
Spread fingers, make a fist	Hand and finger motion or deformity
Tighten quadriceps	Symmetry, effusion, patellar tracking
Duck walk 4 steps	Hip, knee, and ankle ROM
Stand with back to examiner	Shoulder asymmetry, scoliosis
Touch toes and keep knees straight	Scoliosis, hip ROM, tight hamstrings
Raise toes and heels	Calf asymmetry, leg strength
Stand and look forward	Shoulder asymmetry, general habitus
Look at ceiling, floor, other sites	Cervical ROM
Shrug shoulders against resistance	Trapezius strength
Abduct shoulders against resistance	Deltoid strength
Perform full-shoulder external rotation	Shoulder ROM
Flex and extend elbows	Elbow ROM
Flex and extend wrists	Wrist ROM

*ROM = range of motion.

TABLE 3-7 Classification of Competitive Sports by Degree of Contact and Exertion

Contact/Collision	Limited Contact/Impact	Noncontact: Strenuous	Noncontact: Moderately Strenuous	Noncontact: Nonstrenuous
Boxing	Baseball	Aerobic dancing	Badminton	Archery
Field hockey	Basketball	Crew	Curling	Golf
Football	Bicycling	Fencing	Table tennis	Riflery
Ice hockey	Diving	Field		
Lacrosse	Field	Discus		
Martial arts	High jump	Javelin		
Rodeo	Pole vault	Shot put		
Soccer	Gymnastics	Running		
Wrestling	Horseback riding	Swimming		
	Skating	Tennis		
	Ice	Track		
	Roller	Weight lifting		
	Skiing			
	Cross-country			
	Downhill			
	Water			
	Softball			
	Squash, handball			
	Volleyball			

Bethesda Conference. Their guidelines for athletic eligibility or disqualification are predicated on the premise that strenuous training and competition with the risk of sudden death should be discouraged in susceptible athletes.[18]

CONCLUSIONS

In spite of probably no cost-effectiveness and a low degree of disqualification, the PPE will continue to exist with ethical, legal, and insurance justification. Goals for the future include improving techniques for the identification of those most at risk for significant injury and sudden death.

REFERENCES

1. Altemeier WA 3rd, Robinson DP: Preparticipation screening by assembly line. Pediatric Ann 29(3): 139–140, 2000.
2. American Academy of Pediatrics Policy Statement: Recommendation for participation in competitive sports. Pediatrics 81(5):739, 1998.
3. Carek PJ, Futrell M, Hevston WJ: The preparticipation physical examination history: Who has the correct answers? Clin J Sports Med 9(3):124–128, 1999.
4. DeGowin EL, DeGowin RL: Bedside Diagnostic Examination. London, Macmilian, 1969, p 365.
5. DuRant RH, Seymore C, Linder CW, Jay S: The preparticipation examination of athletes: Comparison of single and multiple examiners. Am J Dis Child 139:657, 661, 1985.
6. Epstein SE, Maron BJ: Sudden death and the competitive athlete: Perspectives on preparticipation screening studies. J Am Coll Cardiol 7:230, 1986.
7. Fields KB, Delaney M: Focusing the preparticipation sports examination. J Fam Prac 30(3):304–312, 1990.
8. Fuller CM, McNulty CM, Spring DA, et al: Prospective screeing of 5,615 high school students for risk of sudden cardiac death. Med Scr Sports Exec 29:1131–1138, 1997.
9. Glover DW, Marow BJ: Profile of preparticipation cardiovascular screening for high school athletes. JAMA 279:1817–1819, 1998.

10. Goldberg B, Saranti A, Witman P, et al: Preparticipation sports assessment: An objective evaluation. Pediatrics 66(5):736–745, 1980.
11. Johnson MD: Preseason sports examination for women, In Agostini R: Medical and Orthopedic Issues of Active and Athletic Women. Philadelphia, Hanley & Befus, 1994, p 38.
12. American Academy of Family Physicians, American Academy of Pediatrics, American Medical Society for Sports Medicine, American Orthopaedic Society for Sports Medicine, American Osteopathic Academy of Sports Medicine: Preparticipation Physical Evaluation, 1992.
13. Lewis JF, Maron BJ, Diggs JA, et al: Preparticipation echocardiology screening for cardiovascular disease in a large predominated black population of collegiate athletes. Am J Cardiol 6:1024–1033, 1989.
14. Linder CW, Du Rent RH, Sakiecki RM, Strong WB: Preparticipation health screening of young athletes: Results of 1268 examinations. Am J Sports Med 9:187–193, 1981.
15. Lombardo JA, Grogan JW: Preparticipation screening and performance assessment. In Giana WA, Kalenak A (eds): Clinical Sports Medicine. Philadelphia, WB Saunders, 1991, pp 79-99.
16. Magnes BA, Henderson JM, Hunter SC: What conditions limit sports participation? Experience with 10,540 athletes. Phys Sports Med 20:143–158, 1992.
17. Maron BJ: Hypertrophic cardiomyopathy: A systematic review. JAMA 287:1308–1330, 2002.
18. Maron BJ: Sudden death in young athletes. N Eng Med 349(11):1064–1075, 2003.
19. Maron BJ, Bodison SA, Wesley XE, et al: Results of screening a large group of inter collegiate athletes for cardiovascular disease. J Am Coll Cardiol 10:1214–1221, 1987.
20. Maron BJ, Shirani K, Poliack LC, et al: Sudden death in young competitive athletes: Clinical, demographic and pathological profiles. JAMA 276:199–204, 1996.
21. Metzl JD: The adolescent preparticipation physical examination: Is it helpful? Clin Sports Med 19(4):577–592, 2000.
22. Morahed MR, Ahmodi-Kashani M, Sabnes M, et al: Left ventricular hypertrophy correlates with body surface area and body mass index in healthy teenage athletes. Circulation 106: Supp II-II–352, 2002.
23. Position Stands. AMD Opinion Statements (1975–1984). Indianapolis, American College of Sports Medicine, 1983.
24. Rifat SF, Roffin MT, Govenflo DW: Disqualifying criteria in preparticipation sports evaluation. J Fam Prac 41:42–50, 1995.
25. Risser WL: Exercise for children. Pediatr Rev 10(5):131–139, 1988.
26. Risser WL, Hoffman HM, Bellah GG Jr: Frequency of preparticipation sports examination in secondary school athletes: Are the University Interscholastic League guidelines appropriate? Texas Med 81:35–39, 1985.
27. Risser WL, Hoffman HM, Bellah GG Jr, et al: A cost-benefit anaylsis of preparticipation sports examination of adolescent athletes. J School Health 55:270–273, 1985.
28. Robey JM, Blythe CS, Mueller F: Athletic injuries: Application of epidemiologic methods. JAMA 27:184–188, 1971.
29. Smith J, Laskowski ER: The preparticipation physical examination: Mayo Clinic experience with 2,739 examinations. Mayo Clinic Proc 73(5):419–429, 1998.
30. Tennant MB Jr, Berenson KE, Day CM: Benefits of preparticipation sports examinations. J Fam Pract 13:287–288, 1981.
31. Thompson TR, Andrish JT, Bergfeld JA: A prospective study of preparticipation sports examinations of 2570 young athletes: Method end results. Cleve Clin Q 49:225–233, 1982.

4 On-Field Emergencies

Richard A. Marder

The recent tragic deaths of several high-profile athletes from heatstroke, coupled with alleged concomitant use of ephedrine, provide only too vivid a reminder of the paramount importance of having a medical team poised to deliver effective emergency treatment. Of added significance is that the initial treatment may positively or negatively affect the final outcome. Although serious accidents are most likely in contact sports such as football, every team physician must be prepared to deal with a catastrophic occurrence.[24,32]

"Sudden death" head and neck injuries with and without cardiopulmonary arrest, heatstroke, blunt chest and abdominal trauma, open fractures, and limb-threatening dislocations are among the serious injuries the medical staff must be able to handle. Up-to-date knowledge of emergency treatment, proper and functioning resuscitative equipment, and ancillary emergency services are vital components of medical preparedness. In addition, the successful management of on-field emergencies requires a well-organized preinjury plan developed and executed by the medical staff.

PRINCIPLES

Prior to the start of the season, the team physicians and trainers identify potential emergencies for their sport and establish or review treatment protocols. New equipment and treatments are discussed. For example, a new helmet recently introduced by Riddell (Riddell Corporation, Elyria, Ohio) was designed with increased side and facial protection and greater shell offset to decrease the incidence of cerebral trauma. In addition, the cost of automatic external defibrillators (AEDs) has dropped under $2,000, making them more affordable. Preseason is the time to determine whether or not such additions to the medical armamentarium are to be made.

Athletes on the team with a particular injury or illness risk are identified ahead of time, and responses to specific on-field emergencies are coordinated with the selected emergency medical personnel. Potential hospital services also are arranged at this time.

The medical team must be capable of providing emergent care to the athlete in cardiopulmonary arrest. The ability to provide basic life support (BLS) procedures is an absolute necessity, and two or more members of the medical staff must be trained to do so; ideally, at least one member of the medical team will be certified in advanced cardiac life support (ACLS) techniques.

Basic Life Support

The foremost goal of basic life support is to provide oxygen to the brain and heart until definitive medical treatment can restore normal cardiac and pulmonary functions. Cardiopulmonary resuscitation (CPR) consists of three components—airway, breathing, and circulation (the "ABC")—and can be performed without any equipment.[10]

Advanced Life Support

Advanced life support improves on the organ perfusion accomplished during basic life support by securing adequate ventilation and maintaining cardiac output and blood pressure through correction of cardiac arrhythmias.[11] Essential components of therapy include early defibrillation of those athletes with ventricular tachycardia or fibrillation, tracheal intubation and ventilation with oxygen, intravenous fluid replacement, and appropriate resuscitative medications as indicated. The ability to defibrillate the heart in ventricular tachycardia or fibrillation within minutes of cardiac arrest greatly improves the odds of survival.[6,7] In advance of an emergency, the medical staff should divide and assume the component responsibilities of ACLS: leader of the resuscitation effort; airway, ventilation, and intubation; cardiac compression; cardiac monitoring/defibrillation; and intravenous access and administration.

EMERGENCY PERSONNEL, EQUIPMENT, AND TRANSPORTATION

Before the season begins, the medical staff will decide what emergency equipment to maintain during games and practices and will need to contract with an ambulance or emergency medical service to provide on-field coverage and transport of the seriously injured athlete to a hospital or medical center. If the selected hospital facility is not a Level I center, the medical team should make arrangements to have appropriate specialists readily available by call.[1] At each away game, the visiting team physicians and trainers should meet with their counterparts from the home team to review standard emergency procedures, including the level of training of emergency medical personnel, location and method of obtaining the assistance of such personnel during the game, and evacuation of the seriously injured player requiring hospital services.

Providers of emergency medical services differ markedly in their levels of training.[12,39] An Emergency Medical Technician-Ambulance (EMT-A) is trained in basic life support only and has skills in routine splinting, use of oxygen, and transport. More highly trained EMTs have experience in defibrillator use, tracheal airways, and central lines. Whenever possible, especially in high-risk sports, emergency personnel trained in ACLS, such as an EMT-P (Paramedic), should be utilized. The medical staff, through a prearranged signal, must be able to immediately call the emergency medical services personnel onto the field or court. Familiarity of the medical staff with the abilities and equipment of the emergency services personnel, in conjunction with a preemergency plan for resuscitation and transport, can optimize treatment of the injured athlete.

Equipment for dealing with on-field injuries varies by sport and medical staff preferences. Although no standards exist, by reviewing the potential injuries to each organ system, each medical staff can develop a checklist of useful equipment (see box, Emergency Medical Equipment and Medications). This is in addition to the usual medications and equipment available for nonemergencies.[26] Experience and advances in therapy will result in season-to-season modifications. Depending on individual circumstances, the medical staff may decide to maintain their own equipment for advanced life support (cardiac defibrillator, oropharyngeal and endotracheal airway tubes, intravenous set-ups, cardiac medications, etc.) or have these items provisioned by the emergency medical service. Certain equipment should be carried "on-person" by one of the medical staff, including a pocketknife, scissors, a penlight, and a padded tongue blade. All other equipment must be immediately available on the sidelines.

CHECKLIST

Emergency Medical Equipment and Medications

For resuscitation:

Airway: oropharyngeal and nasopharyngeal airways, endotracheal tubes, laryngoscope, 14-gauge catheter for cricothyrotomy

Other: bolt cutters in sports with obstructing face mask

Breathing: supplemental oxygen, mask with oxygen inlet, bag-valve mask, epinephrine kit, albuterol inhalers, aminophylline

Circulation: cardiac monitor/defibrillator, intravenous catheters, tubing, and solutions (crystalloid), cardiac drugs (epinephrine, atropine, lidocaine, etc.)

Other: PASG if hospital transit time excessive

For transport:

Spine board, rigid cervical collar, sandbags, ambulance bed or stretcher, blankets

Diagnostic equipment: stethoscope, sphygmomanometer, penlight, combination oto-opthalmascope, thermometer, reflex hammer

For fracture care:

Splints (air, plaster, prefabricated), Thomas (per Dorland's) or Hare femoral traction splints, knee immobilizers, cast padding, finger splints, ace and bias bandages, slings, clavicle loops, shoulder immobilizers, crutches, and cervical collars (rigid and soft)

Other:

Minor surgical and suture sets, scalpels, eye patches, fluroscein, irrigation sets, alcohol, betadine, lidocaine, ethyl chloride spray, tongue blades, adhesive tape, sterile gloves, needles, syringes, sponge pads, drapes, bandages, etc.

INJURY PATTERNS

As observed from the sidelines, injuries that occur during sporting events can be categorized according to one of the following presentations: 1) athletes down from contact and not moving, 2) athletes down from contact and moving, 3) athletes down without contact, and 4) athletes injured but moving to the sidelines under their own power (Fig. 4-1). Examination begins with an assessment of the level of consciousness, the airway, breathing, and circulatory status. Subsequently, a secondary survey is performed to evaluate potential neurologic, chest, abdominal, and extremity injuries.

ATHLETE DOWN FROM CONTACT AND NOT MOVING

A sense of urgency is quickly detected as fellow players frantically motion to the sidelines for help. The previously designated medical staff who will provide the initial assessment runs to the player without delay. This may be the team trainer(s) alone or with the team physician, depending on preference. A number of possibilities must be considered: concussion and other cerebral trauma, fracture or dislocation of the spine, blunt chest trauma, and cardiopulmonary arrest. The medical team must be prepared to initiate resuscitation on the field. On reaching the player, the injury plan goes into action.

Assessment

Without moving the player, the designated medical staff member kneels, lightly touches the player with a hand, and asks, "Are you okay?" or "Where are you hurt." Even in a prone position, it is usually possible to determine if there is spontaneous breathing by either observing chest expansion or feeling air movement during exhalation. Three possible scenarios exist: the player is a) unconscious

Down without contact
Sudden death
Seizure
Heatstroke
Drug or alcohol reaction
Anaphylaxis

Down from contact, not moving
Cardiopulmonary arrest
Cerebral trauma
Fracture-dislocation, cervical spine

Down from contact, moving
Musculoskeletal injury
Chest trauma
Abdominal injury

Injured, moving off field
Musculoskeletal injury

FIGURE 4-1. Basic injury patterns.

and not breathing, b) unconscious but breathing, or c) conscious and breathing.

Player Unconscious and Not Breathing

Upon determining that a player is unconscious and is not breathing, the on-field examiner raises his or her hand in a prearranged signal to the other sidelines medical staff, who will start onto the field with the emergency medical equipment. If one of the medical staff is not ACLS trained, the emergency medical crew should be signaled to come onto the field. Using the universal algorithm for adult emergency cardiac care, CPR is started (Fig. 4-2). At this point, the predetermined leader for CPR assumes control. The player must be positioned supine using techniques to protect the cervical spine, which must be presumed injured. While a physician or trainer applies gentle longitudinal traction to the head to maintain the head and neck in line with the body, at least three other staff members, positioned at the shoulders, hips, and legs, logroll the athlete into the supine position onto a rigid, long spine board.[36] If there is no spontaneous breathing, CPR must be initiated. If not already present, the emergency medical services personnel should be notified by signal to assist on the field.

Airway and Breathing. The faceguard blocks access to the airway. Without removing the helmet, a window in the face mask can be cut using a bolt cutter, or when present, the helmet anchoring plastic loops can be detached by a knife. Newer helmets have a special t-nut anchoring the faceguard to the helmet which allows for quick release in an emergency. In general, it is preferred to leave the helmet on because it facilitates better control of the head and neck. If it is deemed necessary to remove the helmet, the neck and head should be stabilized by a rescuer inserting his or her hands under the helmet from below. If the helmet is removed, placement of a rigid cervical collar with adjunctive immobilization using towel rolls, sandbags, and/or forehead taping to the spine board is performed at this time. A rigid collar, by itself, is unable to control motion of the occipital–cervical junction or the upper two cervical segments.

The most common cause of airway obstruction in the unconscious patient is the tongue. Opening the airway using the jaw-thrust maneuver protects the cervical spine. This method (Fig. 4-3) relies on forward displacement of the mandibular angles by the resuscitator with minimal backward tilt of the head.[27] Using the chin-lift, head-tilt method, however, may improve the effectiveness of opening the airway and should be used if needed to ensure adequate ventilation (Fig. 4-4).[9] If present, remove the mouthguard and clear vomitus or foreign material from the airway using the index finger to sweep in a hooking motion along the base of the tongue. An oral (oropharyngeal) airway can be inserted.

Ventilation is started with two initial breaths, followed by a rate of 10 to 12 breaths/min, using either mouth to mouth, mouth to sealed mask, or a bag-valve to mask device.[10,11] Evidence indicates that the risk of HIV or HBV cross-infection is minimal with mouth to mouth breathing.[28] In vitro studies have shown that mouth to mask ventilation may deliver greater tidal volumes than do bag-valve to mask devices.[19] Nevertheless, bag-valve devices are commonly employed.

Inability to ventilate may be due to an aspirated tooth, blood, or chewing gum, as well as laryngeal edema or fracture. Laryngeal fracture is suggested by subcutaneous emphysema of the anterior neck. If laryngeal fracture is suspected and the player is not breathing, careful orotracheal intubation or emergency tracheostomy is necessary.[17,33] To relieve intraluminal obstruction, perform up to five manual upper abdominal thrusts (Heimlich maneuver).[18] If this is unsuccessful, laryngoscopy can be used to remove the object or cricothyrotomy done to perform bypass ventilation.[21]

Circulation. After the airway is opened and two initial breaths have been given, determine whether or not cardiac arrest has occurred by noting the presence or absence of the carotid pulse. If the athlete is pulseless, cardiac compression is started using sternal compression at a rate of 80 to 100 compressions/min with a compression-to-ventilation ratio of 5:1.[10,11]

Cardiac monitoring is the next priority. Attachment of the cardiac monitor/defibrillator unit allows rhythm monitoring through "quick-look" paddles. Rhythm recognition is an essential component of ACLS training. Inability of the rescuer to analyze cardiac rhythms

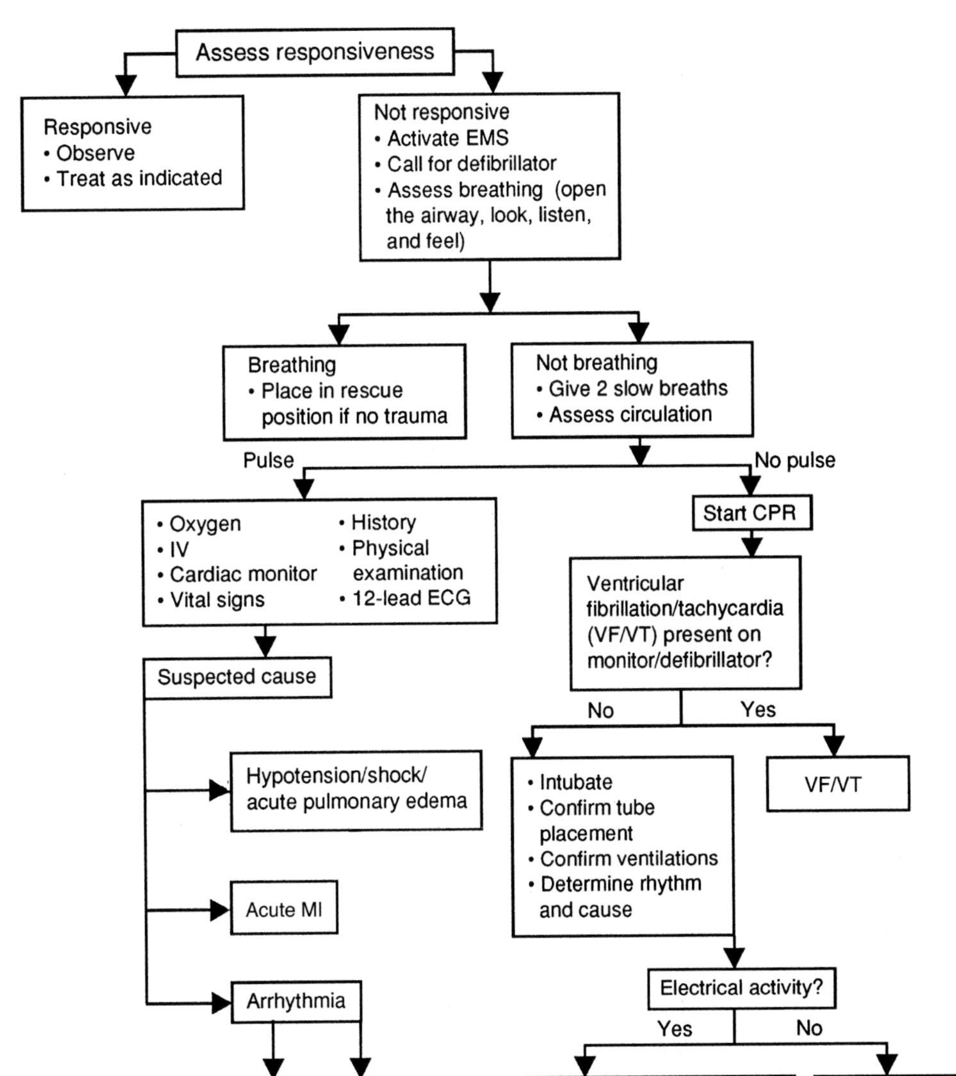

FIGURE 4-2. Universal algorithm for adult emergency cardiac care (ECC). (From Emergency Cardiac Care Committee and Subcommittees, American Heart Association: Guidelines for cardiopulmonary resuscitation and emergency cardiac care, III: Adult advanced cardiac life support, JAMA 268:2199–2241, 1992; with permission.)

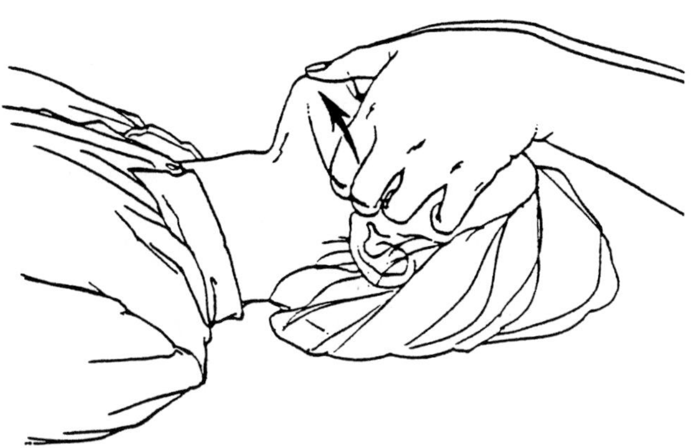

FIGURE 4-3. Jaw-thrust maneuver for opening airway in player with suspected cervical spine injury. (From American Heart Association: Basic Life Support for Healthcare Providers, Dallas, American Heart Association, 1994; with permission.)

does not, however, preclude defibrillation. Automatic external defibrillators (AEDs) detect ventricular tachycardia and fibrillation, discharging automatically (Fig. 4-5). The success of AEDs compares favorably with trained personnel using manual defibrillators.[5]

Prior to defibrillation, manual cervical stabilization must be replaced (if not already done) by a hard cervical collar supplemented by additional immobilization. Once ventricular tachycardia or fibrillation has been detected, defibrillation is carried out using up to three sequentially stacked shocks of increasing energy (Fig. 4-6). Early defibrillation takes precedence over endotracheal intubation and intravenous therapy due to the responsiveness of ventricular tachycardia and fibrillation to early shocking.[11]

The presence of electrical activity without a pulse (electromechanical disassociation) is most often due to hypovolemia. Other causes include tension pneumothorax and cardiac tamponade. Relieving hypoxemia and

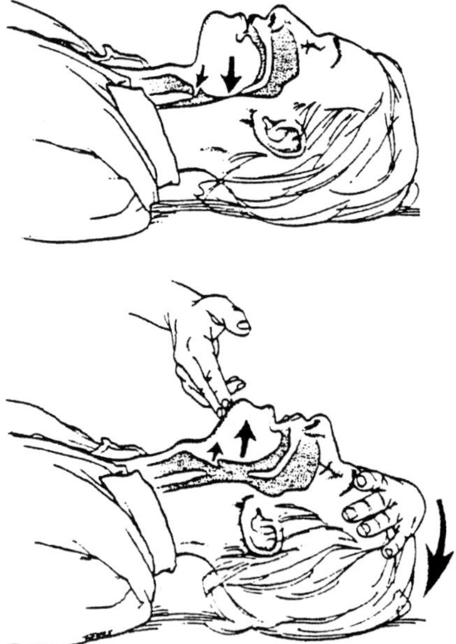

FIGURE 4-4. Head-tilt, chin-lift method of opening airway. (From American Heart Association: Basic Life Support for Healthcare Providers. Dallas, American Heart Association, 1994; with permission.)

hypovolemia may reverse this condition. Therefore, endotracheal intubation and rapid intravenous fluid replacement are indicated. If spontaneous circulation does not return following these measures, epinephrine 1 mg is administered intravenously and repeated every 3 to 5 minutes.[11] Atropine is used for bradycardia.

If ventricular tachycardia or fibrillation persists or recurs after initial attempts at defibrillation, endotracheal intubation and intravenous access are necessary.[11] Epinephrine is administered and defibrillation repeated with an energy of 360 J. Intravenous bolus followed by drip infusion of an antiarrhythmic drug (lidocaine and/or bretylium) is indicated for persistent ventricular tachycardia or fibrillation in conjunction with repeated defibrillation attempts following drug administration (see Fig. 4-6).

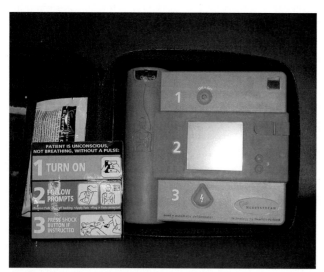

FIGURE 4-5. Automatic external defibrillator.

Following cardioversion, the athlete may be responsive and breathing spontaneously. The athlete is transported to the hospital, receiving supplemental oxygen and intravenous fluids. A lidocaine or bretylium infusion is continued or started when the cause of cardiac arrest is ventricular tachycardia or fibrillation.

Player Unconscious But Breathing

Assume the player has sustained a severe head and/or neck injury. If in the prone position, the player is logrolled to the supine position for further evaluation, while medical personnel manually maintain the head and neck in line to the body using gentle, longitudinal traction.

Airway and Breathing. Secure an open airway with the neck in a neutral position; if present, remove the mouthguard. The jaw-thrust maneuver can be used for improved airway patency. Be alert to the potential for respiratory arrest, depression, or aspiration.

Circulation. The adequacy of circulation (systolic blood pressure) is first estimated by the ability to palpate the radial (80 mm Hg or >), femoral (70 mm Hg or >), and carotid (60 mm Hg or >) pulses. Note the pulse rate and quality. An absent or thready radial pulse, extremity coolness, or delayed capillary refill (>2 seconds) suggests hypovolemic shock. Measure the blood pressure using a sphygmomanometer. The combination of elevated blood pressure and bradycardia suggests increasing intracranial pressure, whereas spinal shock accompanying cervical fracture or dislocation is more likely to produce a decrease in both pulse and blood pressure due to the loss of sympathetic tone.[8]

Neurologic. The neurologic exam is directed at determining the level of consciousness and the presence of any focal neurologic deficits. Continue to monitor breathing and circulation. Do not reduce the head or neck to align with the long axis of the body, but manually maintain their position relative to the body. Rotary dislocation of C1-C2 and unilateral facet dislocations may produce asymmetric positioning of the neck. Note any unusual flexion (decorticate) or extension (decerebrate) posturing of the extremities. Determine the best eye, verbal, and motor responses according to the Glasgow Coma Scale (Table 4-1).[29] Coma is defined as the absence of any eye opening, motor, and sensory responses (Glasgow score of 3). Measure pupillary diameters and response to light. Differences in diameter greater than 1 mm and asymmetry of reactivity to light are abnormal.[38] Lateralized extremity motor weakness is difficult to

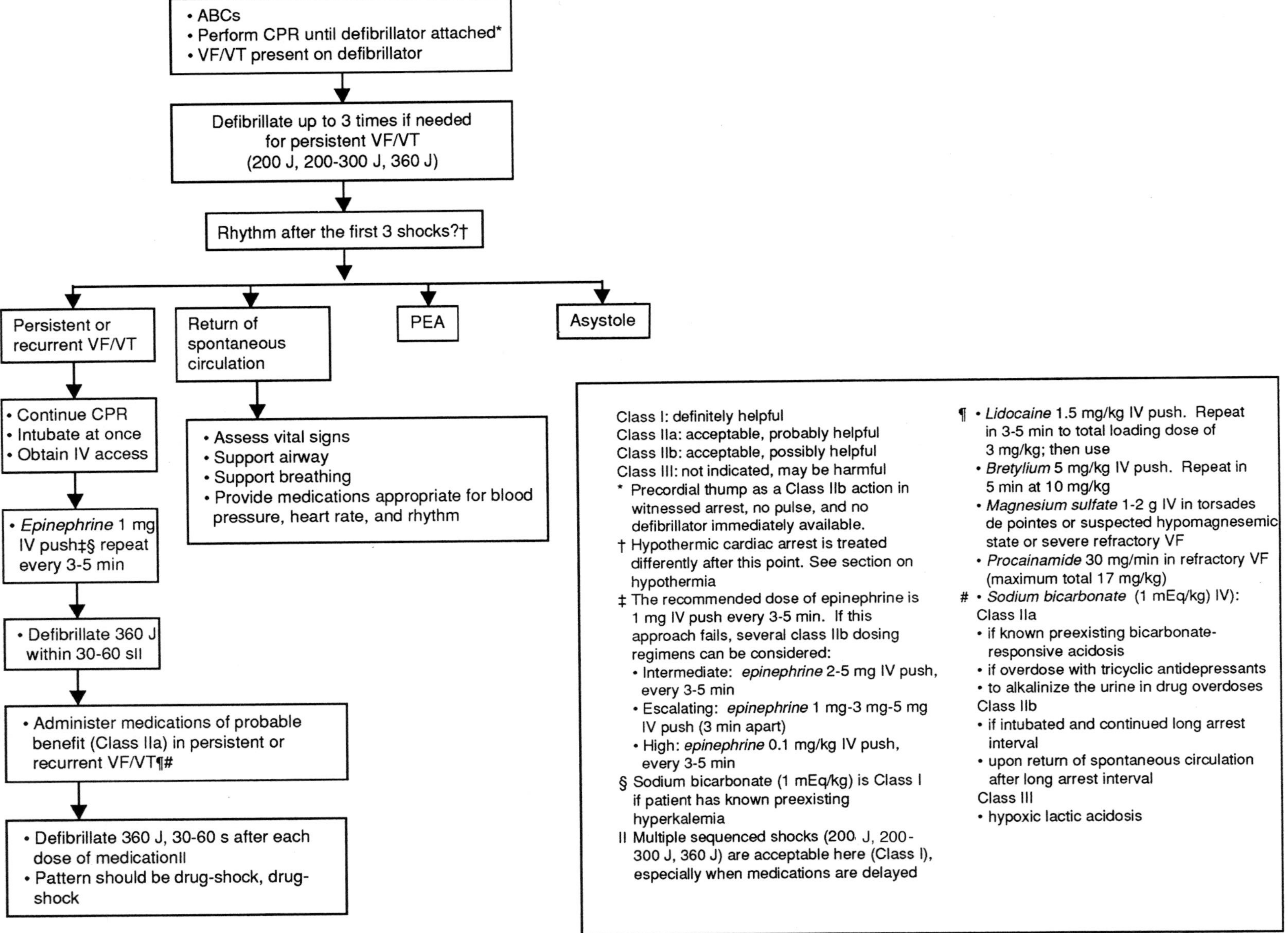

FIGURE 4-6. Algorithm for ventricular fibrillation and pulseless ventricular tachycardia (VF/VT). (From Emergency Cardiac Care Committee and Subcommittees, American Heart Association: Guidelines for cardiopulmonary resuscitation and emergency cardiac care, III: Adult advanced cardiac life support. JAMA 268:2199–2241, 1992; with permission.)

TABLE 4-1 **Glasgow Coma Scale**

Eye Opening	
Spontaneous	4
To voice	3
To pain	2
None	1
Motor Response	
Obeys commands	6
Purposeful movement	5
Withdraws to pain	4
Flexion posturing	3
Extension posturing	2
None	1
Verbal Response	
Oriented	5
Confused	4
Inappropriate words	3
Incomprehensible sounds	2
None	1
Possible Score	3–15

detect in the unresponsive patient. Subtle differences in extremity response to stimuli may be the only finding. A palpable depressed skull fracture or signs of a basilar skull fracture (orbital ecchymosis, mastoid ecchymosis, or cerebrospinal fluid leaking from the ear or nose) may be evident.

The presence of abnormal posturing, lateralized weakness, pupillary asymmetry, vomiting, prolonged unconsciousness, bradycardia, and elevated blood pressure are symptoms and signs of increasing intracranial pressure and portend imminent cerebral herniation. If any of these are noted or subsequently develop, immediately transport the athlete, with the head and neck securely immobilized, to an alerted neurosurgical team for evaluation and treatment. Adjunct measures to combat rising intracranial pressure may be performed en route so as not to delay transport. These include endotracheal intubation for hyperventilation to reduce pCO_2 to between 25 to 30 mm and intravenous Mannitol (50 to 100 g).[20] If the player regains consciousness while being attended, proceed with the screening neurologic examination. Inquire about the presence of neck pain or headache as well as numbness, tingling, or weakness of the extremities. Perform a mental status check to determine orientation and if there is amnesia, either post-traumatic or retrograde. Test extraocular movement. Palpate the cervical spine for any tenderness or hematoma and step-off of the lower cervical and upper thoracic spinous processes. Prolonged unconsciousness (>3 to 5 min), retrograde amnesia, focal neurologic deficit, abnormal cervical finding, complaints of neck pain, numbness, tingling, and/or extremity weakness are indications for immediate hospital transfer, while maintaining spinal immobilization.

If the cervical and screening neurologic exams are negative, the player is allowed to perform active range of motion of the neck. If no pain or limitation of cervical motion is noted, the player, with assistance, can walk off the field. After suffering a concussion, the player may experience headache, confusion, blurred vision, amnesia, and unsteadiness. The player who has sustained only a mild concussion may usually return to the same game after resolution of all symptoms and signs.[20,36,37] However, cognizant of the significant number of sports fatalities from cerebral trauma and the difficulty of performing close and frequent observation along the sidelines, the team physician may prefer to have a player hospitalized for evaluation and further observation.

Player Conscious and Breathing But Not Moving

Injury may range from having the "wind knocked out" of a player from a blow to the upper abdomen causing temporary paralysis of the diaphragm, to a fracture or dislocation of the cervical spine with quadriplegia and potential respiratory arrest. The trainer and/or physician, as they arrive, should kneel by the player, touching the player to provide reassurance. Even if the player complains of abdominal pain, for example, proceed with the standard protocol (the ABCs) for evaluating the injured player. Manually immobilize the head and neck whether the player is supine or prone while the assessment is started. Determine the player's level of consciousness and then assess the airway and breathing status.

Airway and Breathing. Without moving the player, the trainer and/or team physician observe respiratory rate and pattern. If dyspnea, stridor, wheezing, or a respiratory rate above 30 breaths/min are noted, ventilatory support is needed. Before proceeding, the player needs to be logrolled to the supine position onto the spine board, protecting the cervical spine as described earlier. If the player is helmeted, the face mask will need to be cut away to provide airway access. Remove the mouthguard. If respirations are abnormal, check the chest for asymmetrical chest wall motion, palpate for crepitus and tenderness over the sternum and ribs, and auscultate the chest, listening for diminished breath sounds. Stridor, hoarseness, and/or subcutaneous emphysema of the anterior neck should alert the examiner to the possibility of laryngeal fracture.

If a flail chest (paradoxical wall motion due to multiple rib fractures) is noted, initial management consists of direct pressure manually or with a sandbag over the flail segment, which can improve the efficiency of ventilation. Intubation and mechanical ventilation may be necessary. If a tension pneumothorax develops (progressive respiratory distress, tracheal shift, and shock with distended neck veins), immediate decompression of the affected lung by inserting a 14-gauge needle in the second intercostal space in line with the midclavicle is necessary. Simple pneumothorax although causing tachypnea and pain usually does not require on-field decompression.

Control of the airway is a dilemma in the player with suspected laryngeal fracture. Although milder injury may be manageable without the need for airway intervention, there is a risk of complete airway loss. Careful orotracheal intubation has been used to ventilate successfully in some cases, but emergency tracheostomy is recommended for severe laryngotracheal separation.[17,33]

Circulation. Palpate the radial pulse, noting its quality and rate. Use a sphygmomanometer to follow blood pressure. If shock is present, start treatment as described previously while continuing with the neurologic examination. Compression may be needed to control external hemorrhage.

Neurologic. Ask if the player has any head, neck, or back pain. Determine whether the player has active movement of each extremity and note if sensation is present or absent. If neck or back pain is present or the player has abnormal or lost sensation, weakness or loss of active extremity motion, great caution must be exercised by the medical team to prevent further injury to the injured spine. While maintaining manual control of the head and neck, palpate for any cervical tenderness, soft tissue swelling, or deformity.

Once there is symptomatic or physical evidence of a cervical injury, immobilization in preparation for transport should be performed before proceeding with additional examination of the player. Securing the player to the spine board together with continued manual traction to maintain the neck in a neutral position may prevent additional cervical trauma. Although respiratory failure occurs quickly in cervical lesions above C4 due to paralysis of the diaphragm, even in lower-level injury airway and breathing need to be monitored due to the potential for respiratory insufficiency. Without unduly delaying transport, an adequate peripheral neurologic examination is done to establish a baseline. The player who is less than fully responsive must be checked with a comprehensive cranial examination as discussed previously.

A stretcher or ambulance bed should be used for transport. A neurosurgical and orthopedic spine team should be on alert at the receiving hospital. One of the team physicians should accompany the injured player.

In the fully responsive player with a negative screening examination, active cervical spine motion can be assessed. Again, any limitation of motion or pain requires continued protected immobilization and transport for further evaluation. In this case, if no limitation of motion or pain is experienced during active motion, the player can walk off the field without immobilization and undergo more detailed examination on the sidelines.

Secondary Survey. If present, the abdominal or extremity injury is now addressed by the examiners.

ATHLETE DOWN FROM CONTACT AND MOVING

The player writhing on the field or court after a collision is likely to have sustained a musculoskeletal, chest, or abdominal injury. The athlete may be clutching the injured area or deformity of an extremity may be readily apparent.

Assessment

The trainer kneels and establishes verbal contact with the player. The level of responsiveness is quickly established.

Airway, Breathing, and Circulation

Remove the mouthguard, if present. Observe the player's breathing rate and pattern; check the adequacy of circulation by palpating the peripheral pulse. If respiratory or circulatory distress is present, initiate CPR as described previously. If vital signs are stable, proceed to the neurologic and secondary survey.

Neurologic

Start by reviewing the level of responsiveness of the athlete. Inquire as to head or neck pain, presence of any numbness, tingling, or weakness of the extremities. Palpate the neck. If no neurologic abnormalities are present, proceed to the area of complaint.

ATHLETE DOWN ON THE FIELD WITHOUT CONTACT

A number of potentially life threatening conditions present in this manner, including "sudden death," anaphylaxis from an insect bite or drug reaction, seizure, heatstroke, and nonemergent, noncontact musculoskeletal injuries of the lower extremity (e.g., ACL tear, ankle sprain).

Assessment

As in the preceding examples, the trainer approaches the player, kneels, and, without moving the player, determines responsiveness to the question, "Are you okay?" or "Where are you hurt?" If the player is not breathing, the trainer signals to the sidelines for help from the other medical staff. In this situation, where the athlete has been seen to collapse without contact, the likelihood of cervical injury is minimal. Therefore, the player can quickly be turned supine to secure a patent airway and prepare for resuscitation.

Airway and Breathing

The patient experiencing "sudden death," may be semiconscious, and agonal respirations may be noted. Using the chin-lift, head-tilt method, open the airway. Remove the mouthguard and any foreign matter. Give two initial breaths and begin ventilation.

Circulation

Without a palpable carotid pulse, sternal compressions are initiated as described previously. The rapidity with which the cardiac monitor/defibrillator is attached in the player presenting in this manner cannot be overemphasized. As Maron et al. have reported, hypertrophic cardiac myopathy is the most common condition associated with "sudden death" in the athlete.[22] A potential sequence of arrhythmia occurrence is ventricular tachycardia, progressing to ventricular fibrillation, and finally to asystole if untreated.[16] Defibrillation is performed as described previously.

ATHLETE INJURED BUT MOVING OFF THE FIELD UNDER HIS OR HER OWN POWER

Most of these injuries are nonemergent, consisting of a variety of musculoskeletal conditions such as shoulder and finger dislocations, ankle and knee injuries, and acute muscle strains. However, a number of potentially serious injuries, including transient quadriparesis,[31] acute brachial plexus traction injuries,[3] pneumothorax, or aspiration of a foreign body may also present in this fashion.

OTHER SPECIFIC EMERGENCIES

Anaphylaxis

Antibody (IgE) mediated systemic reactions can result from exposure of a sensitized individual to pollens, insect stings, or drugs. Shock due to decreased peripheral resistance, and pulmonary distress due to bronchospasm and/or laryngeal edema, may develop quickly. Local erythema and edema from a bite or sting and generalized urticaria and pruritis may be present. There may be no known history or previous episodes.

Management. The first line of treatment is epinephrine, oxygen, and fluid replacement.[34] Epinephrine in a dose of 3 to 5 cc (1:1000 dilution) is administered subcutaneously and repeated as necessary. Prefilled syringe kits (e.g., Ana-Kit, EpiPen) facilitate emergent use. If shock is severe and the player markedly dyspneic, epinephrine can be used intravenously (3 to 5 ml of a 1:10,000 dilution) or delivered through an endotracheal tube.[8,34]

The airway must be ensured. Laryngeal stridor dictates immediate need for ventilation by intubation or cricothyrotomy. Wheezing and dyspnea from bronchospasm not responsive to initial epinephrine and supplemental oxygen is managed with a beta-agonist inhaler (albuterol), followed by intravenous aminophylline (250 to 500 mg over 20 to 40 minutes) if necessary.[8,34]

Rapid fluid resuscitation using crystalloid is started and the patient is transported to the hospital for observation and further treatment as necessary.

Heat Illness

A number of heat-related disorders can affect the athlete, the most serious of which is heatstroke.[25] Heatstroke results from a derangement of the normal sweating response which maintains the core body temperature. If fluid lost from sweating is not replaced, the hypovolemia that develops may result in cerebral mediated cessation of sweating to preserve circulatory volume. This in turn causes a rapid rise in internal body temperature.

Clinically, heatstroke can present with lightheadedness, nausea, confusion, uncoordination, or most dramatically, loss of consciousness with collapse. Characteristic are the findings of hot and dry skin, indicating shutdown of the normal sweating response associated with tachycardia. Body temperature is markedly elevated and, due to unreliability of oral temperature readings, is best followed with rectal temperatures.

Management. If the player is not breathing, CPR is started. Further treatment is directed at immediate lowering of body temperature to prevent permanent damage to the brain, kidneys, and liver. Rapid cooling with ice packs, immersion in cold water, and rapid intravenous fluid replacement should be started immediately, with transport to the hospital for further treatment.

Abdominal Injury

Intraabdominal injuries may occur in contact sports. A direct blow to the abdomen or flank can cause injury to the abdominal wall itself (e.g., rectus abdominis contusion) or to an underlying organ, usually the spleen, liver, and kidney. Abdominal wall injuries are associated with localized pain and tenderness, especially with active muscle contraction, but may be difficult to differentiate from intraabdominal injury in certain cases. Characteristically, intraabdominal injuries exhibit diffuse abdominal pain and tenderness, signs of peritoneal irritation, and shock from bleeding.

If the abdominal injury consists of solid organ bleeding, and especially with retroperitoneal (kidney) injury, early clinical findings may be minimal, and diagnosis may depend on a high index of suspicion.[14] When assessed on the field immediately after injury, pain and abdominal tenderness may be the only significant clinical findings in the patient with a serious abdominal injury. Bleeding, either intracapsular of the organ involved or even intraperitoneal, may not initially result in signs of peritoneal (pain with body motion, referred and rebound tenderness, guarding, loss of bowel sounds) or diaphragmatic (referred shoulder pain) irritation. Additionally, blood loss of 15% or less total volume may produce only slight tachycardia (Class I shock),[4] which may be difficult to determine in the acutely injured athlete. Renal injury may go undetected until gross hematuria is subsequently noted by the player after the game.

Management. Obviously, nothing should be given orally to the player with a suspected intraabdominal injury. If shock is developing (tachycardia and hypotension) or if there are abdominal symptoms and signs such as nausea, vomiting, referred shoulder pain, guarding, rebound tenderness, or diminished bowel sounds, then start resuscitation and prepare for immediate transport to the hospital. If there are no neck complaints, turn the head and neck to the side in case of vomiting to prevent aspiration. Keep the airway clear as necessary. Record the pulse rate and quality and determine the blood pressure with a sphygmomanometer. Without delaying transport, insert a 16-gauge catheter and start intravenous therapy with a crystalloid fluid challenge, maintaining the systolic blood pressure above 90 mm Hg. Cover the player with warm blankets, elevate the lower extremities, and transport. For shock not responding to rapid infusion of 2 to 3 L of intravenous crystalloid solution, a pressurized antishock garment (PASG) may be used to stabilize the player en route to the hospital, although its use remains controversial.[23]

If the player has localized abdominal pain in the absence of other symptoms and signs, the medical staff must decide whether to monitor the player on the sidelines or in the hospital setting. The importance of serial examinations and immediate transport because of a change in status cannot be overstated.

Knee Dislocation

Dislocation of the tibiofemoral joint is infrequent but is associated with a high incidence of vascular injury that can lead to amputation above the knee if circulation cannot be restored.[15] Disruption of the popliteal artery is most likely with posterior dislocations (tibia displaced posteriorly), whereas intimal injury with in situ thrombosis is noted more often with anterior dislocation due to stretching of the artery (Fig. 4-7). It is important to remember that vascular injury can occur in the dislocated knee with spontaneous reduction, potentially lulling the examiner into a false sense of security. Whereas an unreduced dislocation will be readily apparent (Fig. 4-8), a probable dislocation (dislocation with spontaneous reduction) requires careful examination. Probable dislocation should be suspected when one of the following is noted: greater than 30° of genu recurvatum (knee hyperextension), more than 1 cm of anterior–posterior tibial excursion on knee laxity exam (indicating probable anterior and posterior cruciate ligament rupture), and rapid hemarthrosis or soft tissue swelling.[35]

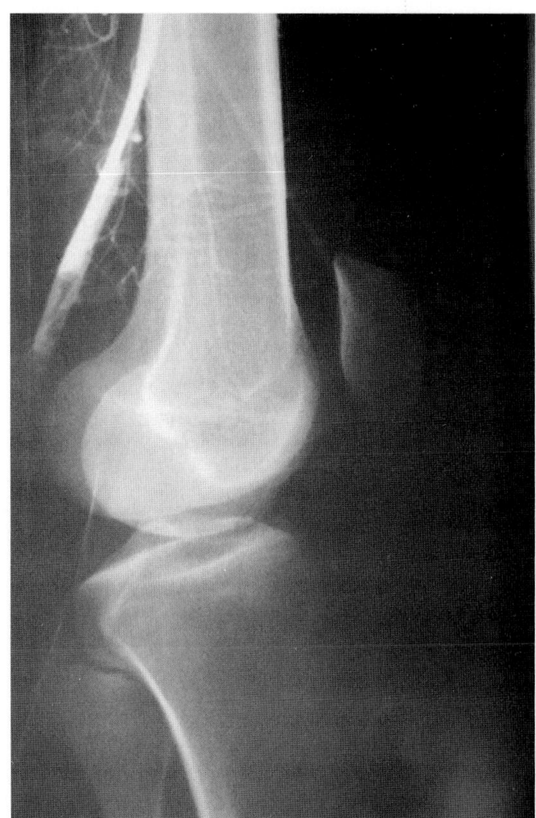

FIGURE 4-7. Arteriogram demonstrating in situ thrombosis of popliteal artery following knee dislocation.

Management. Attention is first directed at determining adequacy of distal circulation and noting any impairment of distal motor and sensory function due to associated peroneal nerve injury. Check the dorsum of the first webspace to detect subtle peroneal nerve injury. If gross deformity is present and pedal pulses are absent, reduction should be attempted on the field. Longitudinal traction is usually sufficient to effect reduction of both anterior and posterior dislocations. For anterior dislocations, longitudinal traction may be combined with gentle lifting of the femur anteriorly. Hyperextension of the knee should be avoided to prevent further injury to the popliteal structures. Infrequently, a posterior dislocation may be irreducible.

After reduction, the knee may be stable in 5° to 10° of flexion with an immobilizer or posterior splint. If not, maintain longitudinal traction during transport. Repeat the distal neurovascular examination. The return of pedal pulses does not eliminate the need for immediate transport of the player to the hospital for vascular study with arteriography. Limited ligamentous surgery can be performed at the time of vascular repair, if needed, or delayed safely until 7 to 10 days after the injury, at which time delayed primary ligamentous repairs and/or reconstructions can be performed with the expectation of improved extremity perfusion and diminished soft tissue swelling.[13]

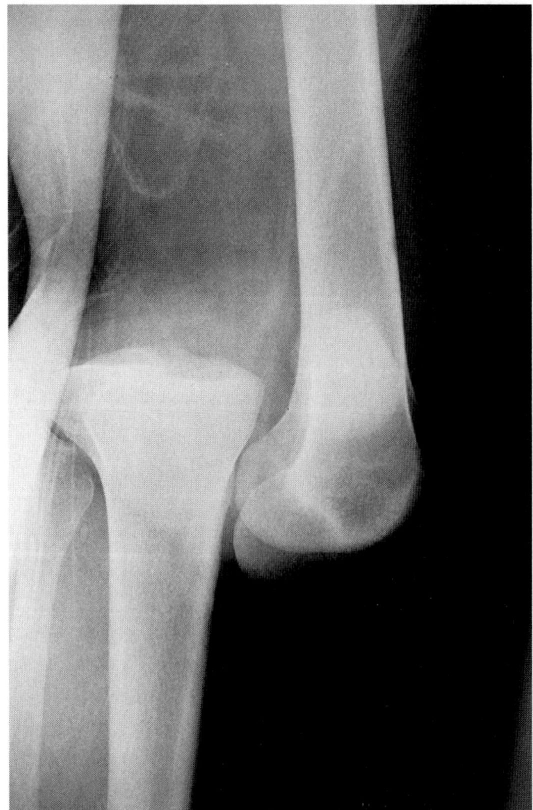

FIGURE 4-8. Lateral radiograph of an unreduced posterior knee dislocation.

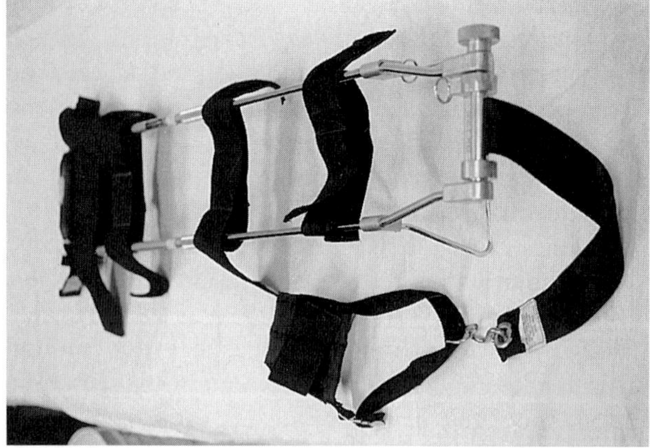

A

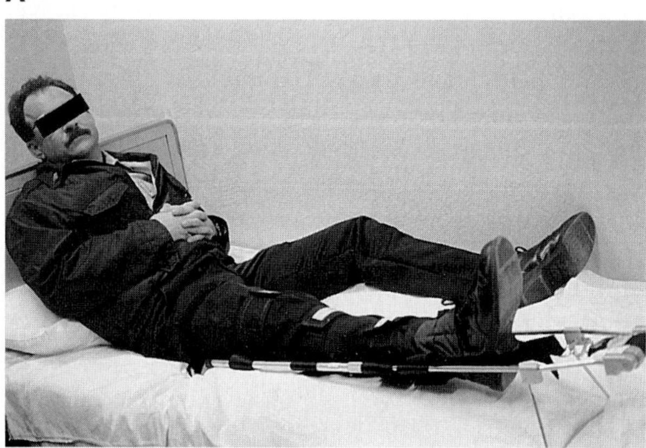

B

FIGURE 4-9. Commercial traction splint (**A**) for immobilization of femur fractures showing traction applied to the foot through the ankle hitch counterbalanced by padded ring at the ischial tuberosity of the pelvis (**B**).

Extremity Fractures

After routine assessment of the overall physical condition of the athlete (ABCs), the first priority is to determine the status of distal pulses and peripheral neurologic function. Adjacent joint injury may be present, especially in fractures of the tibia and femur.[30] Bleeding from long bone fractures can be significant, leading to shock, especially in the already dehydrated athlete. Pelvic and femoral shaft fractures can result in blood loss of 2 L or more. Bleeding from fractures of the elbow, forearm, thigh, and leg rarely can lead to acute compartment syndromes.

Management. If pulses are absent and marked deformity exists, longitudinal traction is applied to improve alignment of the distal extremity without necessarily attempting to reduce the fracture. Otherwise, the fractured extremity is not manipulated but is splinted in its position. A diligent examination of the skin about the fracture site is necessary to recognize the potential open fracture. In open fractures, no attempt is made to replace exposed bone within the soft tissue envelope. Open fracture-dislocations and open dislocations of the ankle, subtalar, knee, and elbow joints, however, are best treated by early reduction.[2] The open wound is covered using sterile gauze soaked with povidone-iodine solution secured with a gently compressive, sterile gauze bandage roll. The fracture should be splinted, with the joints immediately above and below also immobilized. Most fractures can be splinted with an inflatable air splint or plaster, if preferred. Femoral shaft fractures are best immobilized with a commercial traction splint (Fig. 4-9) to maximize stability en route to the hospital. Observe the player for any signs of shock. Use blankets to warm the player and, if indicated, insert a peripheral, large bore intravenous catheter for crystalloid infusion during transport.

REFERENCES

1. American College of Surgeons: Resources for the Optimal Care of the Injured Patient. Chicago, American College of Surgeons, 1990.
2. Chapman MW: Open fractures. In Chapman MW (ed): Operative Orthopaedics, 3rd ed. Philadelphia, Lippincott, Williams and Wilkins, 2001, p 383.
3. Clancy WG, Brand RL, Bergfeld JA: Upper trunk brachial plexus injuries in contact sports. Am J Sports Med 5:209–216, 1977.

4. Committee on Trauma, American College of Surgeons: Advanced Trauma Life Support Course. Chicago, American College of Surgeons, 1985.
5. Cummins RO, et al: Automatic external defibrillators used by emergency medical technicians: A controlled clinical trial. JAMA 257:1605–1610, 1987.
6. Cummins RO, et al: Improving survival from sudden cardiac arrest: The "chain of survival" concept. A statement for health professionals from the Advanced Cardiac Life Support Subcommittee and the Emergency Cardiac Care Committee, American Heart Association. Circulation 83: 1833–1847, 1991.
7. Cummins RO: From concept to standard-of-care? Review of the clinical experience with automated external defibrillators. Ann Emerg Med 18: 1269–1275, 1989.
8. Eisenberg PR, Schuller D: Shock. In Stine RJ, Chudnofsky CR (eds): A Practical Approach to Emergency Medicine, 2nd ed. Boston, Little, Brown, 1994.
9. Elam JO, et al: Head-tilt method of oral resuscitation. JAMA 172:812–815, 1960.
10. Emergency Cardiac Care Committee and Subcommittees, American Heart Association: Guidelines for cardio-pulmonary resuscitation and emergency cardiac care, II: Adult basic life support. JAMA 268:2184–2198, 1992.
11. Emergency Cardiac Care Committee and Subcommittees, American Heart Association: Guidelines for cardiopulmonary resuscitation and emergency cardiac care, III: Adult advanced cardiac life support. JAMA 268:2199–2241, 1992.
12. Emergency Medical Services System Act of 1973. Laws of the 93rd Congress. Public Law 93-154, Washington, DC, 1973.
13. Ertl JP, Marder RA: Traumatic knee dislocations. In Chapman MW (ed): Operative Orthopaedics, 2nd ed. Philadelphia, JB Lippincott, 1993.
14. Freeman MB, Anderson CB: Abdominal emergencies. In Stine RJ, Chudnofsky CR (eds): A Practical Approach to Emergency Medicine, 2nd ed. Boston, Little, Brown, 1994.
15. Green NE, Allen BL: Vascular injuries associated with dislocation of the knee. J Bone Joint Surg 59A: 236–239, 1977.
16. Greene HL: Sudden arrhythmic cardiac death: Mechanisms, resuscitation, and classification. Am J Cardiol 65:4B–12B, 1990.
17. Gussack GS, Jurkovich GJ: Treatment dilemmas in laryngotracheal trauma. J Trauma 28:1439–1444, 1988.
18. Heimlich HJ: The Heimlich maneuver to prevent food choking. JAMA 234:398–401, 1975.
19. Hess D, Baran C: Ventilatory volumes using mouth-to-mouth, mouth-to-mask, and bag-valve-mask devices. Am J Emerg Med 3:292–296, 1985.
20. Lehman LB, Ravich SJ: Closed head injuries in athletes. Clin Sports Med 9:247–261, 1990.
21. Mace SE: Cricothyrotomy. J Emerg Med 6:309–319, 1988.
22. Maron BJ, Epstein SE, Roberts WC: Causes of sudden death in competitive athletes. J Am Coll Cardiol 7:204–214, 1986.
23. Mattox KL, et al: Prospective MAST study in 911 patients. J Trauma 29:1104–1112, 1989.
24. Mueller FO, Blyth CS: Fatalities from head and cervical spine injuries in tackle football. Clin Sports Med 6:185–196, 1987.
25. Murphy RJ: Heat illness in the athlete. Am J Sports Med 12:258–261, 1984.
26. Ray RL, Feld FX: The team physician's medical bag. Clin Sports Med 8:139–146, 1989.
27. Safar P: Cardiopulmonary Cerebral Resuscitation. Philadelphia, WB Saunders, 1981.
28. Sande MA: Transmission of AIDS: The case against casual contagion. N Engl J Med 314: 380–382, 1986.
29. Teasdale G, Jennett B: Assessment of coma and impaired consciousness: A practical scale. Lancet 2:81–83, 1974.
30. Templeman DC, Marder RA: Injuries of the knee associated with fractures of the tibial shaft. Detection by examination under anesthesia: A prospective study. J Bone Joint Surg 71A:1392–1395, 1989.
31. Torg JS, et al: Neuropraxia of the cervical spinal cord with transient quadriplegia. J Bone Joint Surg 68A:1354–1370, 1986.
32. Torg JS, et al: The National Football Head and Neck Injury Registry: 14-year report on cervical quadriplegia, 1971 through 1984. JAMA 254: 3439–3443, 1985.
33. Trone TH, Schaefer SD, Carder HM: Blunt and penetrating laryngeal trauma: A 13 year review. Otolaryngol Head Neck Surg 88:257–261, 1980.
34. Valentine MD: Anaphylaxis and stinging insect hyper-sensitivity. JAMA 268:2830–2833, 1992.
35. Varnell RN, et al: Arterial injury complicating knee disruption. Am Surg 55:699, 1989.
36. Vesgo JJ, Lehman RC: Field evaluation and management of head and neck injuries. Clin Sports Med 6:1–15, 1987.
37. Wilberger JE, Maroon JC: Head injuries in athletes. Clin Sports Med 8:1–9, 1989.
38. Wilberger JE: Emergency care and initial evaluation. In Cooper PR (ed): Head Injury. Baltimore, Williams & Wilkins, 1993.
39. Williams KA: Emergency medical services system. In Stine RJ, Chudnofsky CR, eds: A Practical Approach to Emergency Medicine, 2nd ed. Boston, Little, Brown, 1994.

5 Return to Play After Musculoskeletal Injury

V. Franklin Sechriest II and Stephen G. Silver

INTRODUCTION

One of the goals of sports medicine is to get the injured athlete back into the game as soon as possible without putting that individual at risk. After a musculoskeletal injury, the time for an athlete's recovery and return to play cannot be easily defined as these endpoints are affected by many factors including the athlete's pre-injury condition,[21,23,30,38,52] the type of tissue injured, the response to treatment, the need for surgical intervention, the demands of the sporting activity, and the psychological impact of the injury.[1] Additionally, the individual athlete's motivation and/or any external pressures for performance must be considered. Overuse syndromes,[44,51,54] reinjury,[16,39] and even long-term disability[18,43] may occur when athletes return to play before adequate recovery. Although established guidelines are not available for most of the dilemmas that arise when caring for the injured athlete, successful return to play can be achieved by combining the principles of musculoskeletal care with an organized and multidisciplinary process of evaluation, treatment, rehabilitation, functional testing, and training in sport-specific skills. Such a return-to-play process may greatly assist the team physician in the complex decision making process of returning an athlete to play after musculoskeletal injury.

GENERAL PRINCIPLES

After a musculoskeletal injury, an athlete may think he or she is ready to return to play as soon as the limp or the swelling subsides. However, a full recovery is not assured unless joint range of motion (ROM), flexibility, strength, coordination, general fitness, endurance, and sports-specific skills are optimized. Musculoskeletal tissue healing has defined limits that cannot be shortened without risking the consequence of reinjury or tissue failure. The phases of tissue healing and recovery are well established[9,32,36,41,64] and include acute response to tissue damage with localized hemorrhage, inflammation, and edema; resolution of inflammation and proliferation of immature repair tissue; remodeling with tissue regeneration and maturation; and restoration of tissue function. The greater the severity of the injury, the greater the time required for each of these phases. A treatment regimen that incorporates the general principles of musculoskeletal care and that follows the rational progression of these phases not only lessens the chance of reinjury but also supports that an athlete will be able to perform at his or her best after return to play.

During the acute phase after any musculoskeletal injury, use of the RICE formula (rest, ice, compression, and elevation) to control swelling and pain is most effective.[7] Additionally, judicious use of oral anti-inflammatory medications for pain management may be considered as an adjunctive therapy.[6,26] The rationale for use of anti-inflammatory medications is that by controlling inflammation, the amount of damage to the injured tissue will be limited. It should be recognized, however, that inflammation is the precursor to tissue repair. Without some initial inflammation, healing cannot progress, and overuse of anti-inflammatory medicines may be detrimental.[2,65] Use of steroids in the treatment of acute sports injuries remains extremely controversial.[8,14,22,24,59] Although corticosteroids are potent inhibitors of inflammation, they also have a catabolic effect that can impair tissue healing.[63]

With the resolution of inflammation, early ROM should be initiated. Concurrent use of isometric exercises to promote strengthening may also be beneficial. Prolonged immobilization and/or non–weight bearing must be avoided because this may delay recovery and adversely affect normal tissues.[5,42,49,57,62] As the recovery process continues with tissue healing, remodeling, and maturation, the athlete should progress with rehabilitation consisting of weight-bearing and dynamic strengthening exercises (both isotonic and isokinetic) within the limits of pain.

Basic scientific and clinical investigations have shown that musculoskeletal tissues respond to repetitive use and load by increasing matrix synthesis and in many instances by changing the composition, organization, and mechanical properties of their matrices.[10] The effects of motion and loading on healing tissues have been studied less extensively, but the available evidence indicates that repair and remodeling tissues respond favorably and may be more sensitive to cyclic loading and motion than mature healthy tissues.[11,12] Of course, early motion and loading of injured tissues is not without risk. Excessive or premature loading and motion of repair tissue can inhibit or stop healing. Although the optimal methods for facilitating healing by early and controlled motion and loading have not been defined, experimental studies and newer clinical investigations document significant benefits in the treatment of musculoskeletal injuries.[13,27]

Throughout the recovery and rehabilitation period, it is critical to look beyond the injury, toward keeping the rest of the body as fit as possible. It is important to recognize the systemic effects of deconditioning that may otherwise result from time out of sports participation.[4] Early and continued emphasis must be placed on maintenance of aerobic status, muscle mass, and bone density. Designing a treatment program in which the athlete can stay physically fit while recovering can improve his or her outlook, both physiologically and psychologically.[15] Whether through alternative sports, cross-training, or water exercise, the patient can preserve the integrity of the injured extremity, keep the noninjured muscles active, and maintain cardiovascular fitness.

The endpoint for tissue healing may or may not imply sports readiness. Return to play requires not only healing the injury, but also a functional recovery and, ultimately, recovery of sports-specific skills. Adequate healing implies the relief of pain, the absence of swelling/effusion, weight bearing without difficulty, and, when dealing with skeletal injury, evidence of radiographic union. Adequate functional recovery implies a return of stability, full flexibility, full range of motion, and muscle strength that is ideally to within 80% to 100% of the contralateral extremity.[40] A functional assessment using objective measurement tools such as the goniometer and dynamometer will validate the athlete's subjective sense of recovery.[20] Finally, adequate recovery of quickness, agility, coordination, and mechanics must be assured before return to play is considered. For most athletes, this will include general abilities such as running, cutting, and/or jumping. In this final phase of recovery, athletes perform higher-level functional tests and drills that incorporate sport-specific movement patterns on the field or court such as blocking, throwing, rebounding, and backpedaling. This is a transition time from the sideline back to the field of play. Athletes should demonstrate relatively pain-free and normal skill performance in their sport with minimal post-activity swelling. The athlete must be monitored closely with special attention given to pre-activity warm-up and post-practice condition (i.e., presence of pain, swelling). The athlete should rehearse his or her skill level in multiple practice sessions before returning to competition. Use of protective taping or bracing to prevent reinjury may offer some benefit and may be a logical consideration based on the individual case.[25,31,53,61]

ESTABLISHING A RETURN-TO-PLAY PROCESS

Before an injury ever occurs, it is prudent to have an existing strategy for returning the athlete to play that is understood and accepted by the athletes and the organization of which they are a part. The team physician should take responsibility for developing and coordinating this basic process of player evaluation, medical and/or surgical care coordination, functional and sport-specific rehabilitation, and information documentation and communication. Above all else, the process must protect the athlete's health and safety and should be in compliance with existing local, school, and/or governing body safety regulations.[3,47] When a musculoskeletal injury does occur, the fundamentals of this process for return to play may be promptly communicated to the player, family, allied health professionals, coaches, athletic trainers, and other individuals relevant to the athlete's care. The basic process can then be customized according to the individual's injury and circumstances.

Because the injured athlete's care may be provided by a number of different medical specialists, surgeons, therapists, athletic trainers, and others, three concepts are crucial to a successful and smooth return-to-play process. First, a clear chain of command regarding the decision making process for the injured athlete must be in place. The team physician is at the top of this chain of command and is ultimately responsible for decisions regarding treatment, rehabilitation, and return to play. Second, channels of communication among the physician, athlete, trainers, therapists, and coaches should be established to enhance care through a common understanding of the athlete's condition, treatment regimen, activity restrictions, and rehab expectations. If necessary, a system for release of privileged information regarding an athlete's medical condition and return to play should be in place. Confidentiality of the patient/athlete must always be protected, and release of any information by the physician requires the athlete's expressed consent in accordance with the Health Insurance Portability and Accountability Act.[19] Third, a uniform system of documentation of diagnosis, treatment, and the athlete's response to treatment must be maintained. Adequate record keeping is essential to the success of any management program and plays a significant role in the present medical and legal environment.

EVALUATING THE INJURED ATHLETE

The successful return of an athlete to play after musculoskeletal injury depends largely on the early, accurate, and ongoing evaluation of his or her injury. The evaluation process is used in all phases of athletic injury management. Evaluation of the injured athlete may occur on the field, in the training room, in the office, or in the rehab setting. Another common setting for evaluation of the injured athlete is during the preseason examination (PSE), when the dilemma regarding an athlete's return may arise before play even begins. Because prevention of sports-related injury is the ideal, it is important to have a comprehensive system of injury surveillance, part of which is the PSE. The goal of the PSE is not to disqualify athletes but to ensure that their participation in sports does not unnecessarily increase their risk of injury.[45] The examination should be conducted many weeks prior to the beginning of the season and at the beginning of each new level of competition. A well-designed PSE may prevent some of the musculoskeletal injuries associated with sports participation by identifying the presence of preexisting conditions that have not yet been fully rehabilitated.[28,37]

During the athletic season, strategies for prevention of injury include regular inspection of the athlete's protective equipment, emphasis on pre-activity stretching and warm-up,[55] attention to potentially hazardous field/surface playing conditions, and a constant surveillance for any performance dysfunction on the field such as a limp, poor technique, or loss of condition. Recognizing that the majority of athletic injuries occur during practice sessions, making an effort to observe practice workouts will enhance the physician's ability to make timely and appropriate medical decisions and safety interventions.

When an injury is suspected, prompt medical evaluation is appropriate. A thorough evaluation includes identifying and grading the injury as well as assessing its potential impact on the athlete's overall health status. In addition to making an evaluation of the injured extremity, it is important for the physician to evaluate the potential for a prolonged period out of practice or competition that might put the athlete at risk for physical deconditioning. Psychological impact should also be assessed. Significant adverse psychological responses to injury and time out of competition may have adverse effects on the athlete's recovery as well as reinjury patterns.[34,35,56,60] Thus, a comprehensive approach to the evaluation process may involve not only physicians and physiotherapists, but also consultation with sports psychologists.

Based on the results of the evaluation process, the team physician may develop a plan and organize a network to carry out the treatment and rehabilitation of the injured athlete. Early evaluation of the injury and ongoing evaluation of the efficacy of treatment promote the safe and timely return to play.

TREATING AND REHABILITATING THE INJURED ATHLETE

Treatment should be initiated as early as possible. An explanation of the injury and care plan must be communicated to the athlete to obtain his or her consent to receive treatment. At the outset of treatment, a general timetable should be established. Short-term and long-term goals should be set for the athlete. During treatment and rehabilitation, if the short-term goals are not met, the athlete may need to undergo reevaluation and/or the treatment plan may need to be revised.

As stated previously, the key principles of treating any musculoskeletal injury are early control of inflammation, minimizing the period of immobilization, and early active motion utilizing flexibility, strengthening, and endurance exercise programs. Passive physical treatments such as heat, ice, and manual therapy, as well as anti-inflammatory medications and psychological interventions, are used as adjunctive therapies.[29,46] Coexisting and/or underlying medical conditions (i.e., managing a stress fracture in an athlete with an eating disorder, amenorrhea, and osteoporosis) should be addressed and treated at the same time as the acute injury.

Comprehensive treatment must include an appropriate rehabilitation regimen. For the injured athlete, a rehabilitation network consisting of a team of experts in sports medicine, physical therapy, and athletic training is invaluable. This network should develop an individualized plan designed to restore function of an injured extremity, restore overall musculoskeletal health and general fitness, and provide sport-specific assessment and training.[33] Additionally, the rehabilitation plan should include reinjury prevention training.[58]

The athlete's compliance with the rehabilitation plan must be monitored and encouraged. A key component to promoting compliance is providing a realistic estimate of the length of disability with milestones for recovery. Achievement is especially good for increasing an athlete's self-confidence and motivation to continue with rehabilitation. During rehabilitation, outlining a number of goals (i.e., full ROM, walking without assistance) helps to keep the athlete focused on progress. These intermediate goals provide direction for the day-to-day efforts of the injured athlete. Therapists can also help to provide short-term goals in the form of daily exercises that should be performed by the athlete. These markers are the stepping stones that pave the way to achieving the ultimate goal of return to play. This approach can help combat any feelings of self-doubt that can arise when an athlete focuses purely on the long process of rehabilitation and return to play.[17] Continued monitoring of an athlete's rehabilitation is necessary to ensure efficacy of treatment, monitor progress, allow for ongoing tailoring of the regimen, and keep the injured athlete on the proper path to recovery.

RETURNING THE INJURED ATHLETE TO PLAY

Safely returning the injured athlete to sporting activity after injury is the desired result of the return-to-play process of evaluation, treatment, and rehabilitation. Although decisions regarding the athlete's return to play will always depend on the individual and the specific circumstances, definite criteria must be met. Tissue healing and restoration of functional capacity of the extremity must be confirmed. The ability to play safely with restoration of sport-specific skills must be assured.

The presence of or risk for chronic injury must be determined, documented, and discussed with the athlete in terms of the risk for ongoing and/or permanent disability. The psychological state of the athlete and his or her state of mental preparedness must be understood and optimized. Finally, any decision to return an athlete to play must be in compliance with all applicable local, state, and/or governing body regulations.[48,50]

CONCLUSION

After a musculoskeletal injury, a successful return-to-play process depends largely on the early, accurate, organized, and ongoing evaluation of an athlete's injury and response to treatment and rehabilitation. The decision on whether or when an athlete should return to play is best determined by the team physician in active consultation with the medical, surgical, and rehabilitation specialists involved in the return-to-play process. Unfortunately, scientific recommendations and published guidelines are not available for most of the return-to-play dilemmas. Individual decisions regarding when to return an injured athlete will depend on the specific facts and circumstances presented to the team physician and the network of consultants.

The return-to-play decision may be thought of as risk management. A physician making a decision for an injured athlete must therefore use the best available information and communicate the inherent limitations of this decision making process to the athlete and all parties involved. Ultimately, the team physician must guide the athlete to understand and accept the risks of reinjury, additional injury, or even permanent impairment. Ideally, these risks are minimized by following a comprehensive return-to-play process designed to fully rehabilitate the athlete and to optimize his or her physical and mental condition.

REFERENCES

1. Ahern DK, Lohr BA: Psychosocial factors in sports injury rehabilitation. Clin Sports Med 16(4): 755–768, 1997.
2. Almekinders LC, Gilbert JA: Healing of experimental muscle strains and the effects of nonsteroidal anti-inflammatory medication. Am J Sports Med 14(4):303–308, 1986.
3. American Academy of Family Physicians, American Academy of Orthopaedic Surgeons, American College of Sports Medicine, American Medical Society for Sports Medicine, American Orthopaedic Society for Sports Medicine, and the American Osteopathic Academy of Sports Medicine: The team physician and return-to-play issues: A consensus statement. Med Sci Sports Exerc 34(7):1212–1214, 2002.
4. Arnaud SB: Effects of inactivity on bone. In: Sandler H, Vernikos J (eds): Inactivity: Physiological Effects. Orlando, FL, Academic Press, 1986, pp 49–76.
5. Baker JH, Matsumoto DE: Adaptation of skeletal muscle to immobilization in a shortened position. Muscle Nerve 11:231–244, 1988.
6. Baldwin LA: Use of nonsteroidal anti-inflammatory drugs following exercise-induced muscle injury. Sports Med 33(3):177–185, 2003.
7. Baumert PW Jr: Acute inflammation after injury. Quick control speeds rehabilitation. Postgrad Med 97(2):35–36, 1995.
8. Bentley S: The treatment of sports injuries by local injection. Br J Sports Med 15(1):71–74, 1981.
9. Best TM, Hunter KD: Muscle injury and repair. Phys Med Rehabil Clin N Am 11(2):251–266, 2000.
10. Buckwalter JA, Grodzinsky AJ: Loading of healing bone, fibrous tissue, and muscle: implications for orthopaedic practice. J Am Acad Orthop Surg 7(5): 291–299, 1999.
11. Buckwalter JA: Effects of early motion on healing of musculoskeletal tissues. Hand Clin 12(1):13–24, 1996.
12. Buckwalter JA: Activity vs. rest in the treatment of bone, soft tissue and joint injuries. Iowa Orthopaed J 15:29–42, 1995.
13. Carter DR, Beaupre GS, Giori NJ, Helms JA: Mechanobiology of skeletal regeneration. Clin Orthop 355(Suppl):S41–S55, 1998.
14. Cox JS: Current concepts in the role of steroids in the treatment of sprains and strains. Med Sci Sports Exerc 16(3):216–218, 1984.
15. Croce P, Gregg JR: Keeping fit when injured. Clin Sports Med 10(1):181–195, 1991.
16. Croisier JL, Forthomme B, Namurois MH, et al: Hamstring muscle strain recurrence and strength performance disorders. Am J Sports Med 30(2): 199–203, 2002.
17. Crossman J: Psychological rehabilitation from sports injuries. Sports Med 23(5):333–339, 1997.
18. Dekker R, van der Sluis CK, Groothoff JW, et al: Long-term outcome of sports injuries: Results after inpatient treatment. Clin Rehabil 17(5):480–487, 2003.
19. Dinkins CR, Gilbreath AF: HIPAA in Daily Practice. Memphis, TN, Kerlak Publishing, 2003.
20. Edwards RH, Hyde S: Methods of measuring muscle strength and fatigue. Physiother 63(2):51–55, 1977.
21. Ekstrand J, Gilquist J: The avoidability of soccer injuries. Int J Sports Med 4:124–128, 1983.
22. Fadale PD, Wiggins ME: Corticosteroid injections: Their use and abuse. J Am Acad Orthop Surg 2(3): 133–140, 1994.
23. Feiring DC, Derscheid GL: The role of preseason conditioning in preventing athletic injuries. Clin Sports Med 8(3):361–372,1989.

24. Fredberg U: Local corticosteroid injection in sport: Review of literature and guidelines for treatment. Scand J Med Sci Sports 7(3):131–139, 1997.
25. Gerrard DF: External knee support in rugby union. Effectiveness of bracing and taping. Sports Med 25(5):313–317, 1998.
26. Glick JM: Therapeutic agents in musculoskeletal injuries. J Sports Med 3(3):136–138, 1975.
27. Hayashi K: Biomechanical studies of the remodeling of knee joint tendons and ligaments. J Biomech 29(6):707–716, 1996.
28. Hershman E: The profile for prevention of musculoskeletal injury. Clin Sports Med 3(1):65–84, 1984.
29. Hillman SK, Delforge G: The use of physical agents in rehabilitation of athletic injuries. Clin Sports Med 4(3):431–438, 1985.
30. Hunt A: Musculoskeletal fitness: The keystone in overall well-being and injury prevention. Clin Orthop Rel Res 409:96–105, 2003.
31. Hunter LY: Braces and taping. Clin Sports Med 4(3):439–454, 1985.
32. Hyman J, Rodeo SA: Injury and repair of tendons and ligaments. Phys Med Rehab Clin N Am 11(2): 267–288, 2000.
33. Irrgang JJ, Delitto A, Hagen B, et al: Rehabilitation of the injured athlete. Orthop Clin N Am 26(3): 561–577, 1995.
34. Junge A: The influence of psychological factors on sports injuries. Review of the literature. Am J Sports Med 28(5 Suppl):S10–S15, 2000.
35. Kaforey GR, Stricker PR: The psychological effects of athletic injury. Clin J Sport Med 9(4):191–192, 1999.
36. Kellett J: Acute soft tissue injuries—A review of the literature. Med Sci Sports Exerc 18(5):489–500, 1986.
37. Kibler WB, Chandler TJ, Uhl T, Maddux RE: A musculoskeletal approach to the preparticipation physical examination. Preventing injury and improving performance. Am J Sports Med 17(4): 525–531, 1989.
38. Knapic JJ, Bauman CL, Jones BH, et al: Preseason strength and flexibility imbalances associated with athletic injuries in female collegiate athletes. Am J Sports Med 19:76–81, 1991.
39. Kralinger FS, Golser K, Wischatta R, et al: Predicting recurrence after primary anterior shoulder dislocation. Am J Sports Med 30(1):116–120, 2002.
40. Lephart SM, Henry TJ: Functional rehabilitation for the upper and lower extremity. Orthop Clin North Am 26(3):579–592, 1995.
41. Loitz BJ, Frank CB: Biology and mechanics of ligament and ligament healing. Exer Sport Sci Rev 21: 33–64, 1993.
42. MacDougall JD, Elder GCB, Sale DG, Moroz JR, Sutton JR: Effects of strength training and immobilization on human muscle fibers. Eur J Appl Physiol 43:25–34, 1980.
43. Marchi AG, Di Bello D, Messi G, Gazzola G: Permanent sequelae in sports injuries: A population based study. Arch Dis Child 81(4):324–328, 1999.
44. McKeag DB: The concept of overuse. The primary care aspects of overuse syndromes in sports. Primary Care; Clin Office Pract 11(1):43–59, 1984.
45. McKeag DB: Preseason physical examination for the prevention of sports injuries. Sports Med 2(6): 413–431, 1985.
46. Meeusen R, Lievens P: The use of cryotherapy in sports injuries. Sports Med 3(6):398–414, 1986.
47. Mitten MJ: Legal issues affecting medical clearance to resume play after mild brain injury. Clin J Sport Med 11(3):199–202, 2001.
48. Mitten MJ, Maron BJ: Legal considerations that affect medical eligibility for competitive athletes with cardiovascular abnormalities and acceptance of Bethesda Conference recommendations. Med Sci Sports Exerc 26(10 Suppl):S238–S241, 1994.
49. Montgomery RD: Healing of muscle, ligaments, and tendons. Sem Vet Med Surg 4(4):304–311, 1989.
50. National Collegiate Athletic Association: Sports Medicine Handbook. Mission, KS, 1998.
51. O'Neill DB, Micheli LJ: Overuse injuries in the young athlete. Clin Sports Med 7(3):591–610, 1988.
52. Orchard J, Marsden J, Lord S, et al: Preseason hamstring muscle weakness associated with hamstring muscle injury in Australian footballers. Am J Sports Med 25:81–85, 1997.
53. Osternig LR, Robertson RN: Effects of prophylactic knee bracing on lower extremity joint position and muscle activation during running. Am J Sports Med 21:733–737, 1993.
54. Renstrom P, Johnson RJ: Overuse injuries in sports: A review. Sports Med 2:316–333, 1985.
55. Safran MR, Seaber AV, Garrett WE Jr: Warm-up and muscular injury prevention. An update. Sports Med 8(4):239–249, 1989.
56. Sanderson FH: The psychology of the injury-prone athlete. Brit J Sports Med 11(1):56–57, 1977.
57. Sargeant AJ, Davies CTM, Edwards RHT, et al: Functional and structural changes after disuse of human muscle. Clin Sci Mol Med 52:337–342, 1977.
58. Scott SG: Current concepts in the rehabilitation of the injured athlete. Mayo Clin Proc 59(2):83–90, 1984.
59. Scott WA: Injection techniques and use in the treatment of sports injuries. Sports Med 22(6):406–416, 1996.
60. Smith AM: Psychological impact of injuries in athletes. Sports Med 22(6):391–405, 1996.
61. Teitz CC, Hermanson BK, Kronmal RA, et al: Evaluation of the use of braces to prevent injury to the knee in collegiate football players. J Bone Joint Surg 69A:2–9, 1987.

62. Thornton GM, Shrive NG, Frank CB: Healing ligaments have decreased cyclic modulus compared to normal ligaments and immobilization further compromises healing ligament response to cyclic loading. J Orthopaed Res 21(4):716–722, 2003.
63. Wiggins ME, Fadale PD, Barrach H, Ehrlich MG, Walsh WR: Healing characteristics of a type I collagenous structure treated with corticosteroids. Am J Sports Med 22(2):279–288, 1994.
64. Woo SL, Vogrin TM, Abramowitch SD: Healing and repair of ligament injuries in the knee. J Am Acad Orthop Surg 8(6):364–372, 2000.
65. Youlten LJ: Effects of drugs on prostaglandin synthesis. Rheumatol Rehab Suppl:47–52, 1978.

The Systems

6 Cardiopulmonary Conditions

Nino Marino and Peter Bruno

THE HEART AND ITS FUNCTION

As the central organ of the cardiovascular system, the heart acts as a continuously self-regulating pump. This pump's function is crucial to the supply of blood to every organ of the body. The vessels of the arterial system deliver oxygenated blood with other nutrients throughout the body. Clearing of blood depleted of its oxygen is mediated via the vessels of the venous system.

Of vital importance, especially in sports-related activity, is the heat transport or cooling function of the blood via the blood vessels to maintain a core body temperature within a precise and critical range. It is not far-fetched to consider the skin surface and mucosa of the body as "radiators." Without the blood's cooling function, the athlete's body would likely fail during exercise as enzyme systems and other proteins were denatured or "cooked" by undissipated heat.

Finally, the cardiovascular system performs a vital messenger function as it carries important hormones in the blood that act as distant mediators of metabolic processes.

We traditionally have measured the parameters of the heart's pump function by, among others, terms such as *stroke volume*, *ejection fraction*, *cardiac output*, and *cardiac index*. The following is a short glossary of terminology.

- *Stroke volume* is a measure of the quantity of blood, in cubic centimeters, that is ejected from the ventricles of the heart with each contraction.
- *Ejection fraction* is a measure of that quantity of diastolic blood volume that is pumped from the ventricles during systole or contraction. This measure is expressed as a percentage.
- *Cardiac output* is a measure, usually in liters per minute, of the volume of blood circulated by the heart.
- *Cardiac index* is a measure of the cardiac output divided by the subject's body surface area in square meters.
- *Myocardial oxygen consumption* (MVO_2) is the amount of oxygen consumed by the heart per contraction.

The foregoing are perhaps the most important and widely used measures of cardiac function.

THE HEART IN EXERCISE

The cardiovascular systems adapt to increasing loads of activity by first displaying an anticipatory response, which will be initiated by the central nervous system. Higher cortical brain centers will stimulate a catecholamine surge before the actual activity begins. This surge of neural hormones (epinephrine and norepinephrine) acts on the heart. By causing the sinoatrial node to depolarize more rapidly, the impulse for heart muscle contraction will become more frequent. In the highly trained athlete, heart rate may go from a low of 30 to 35 beats per minute to more than 200 beats per minute via catecholamine mediation. This increase in heart rate (and contractile force of the heart) is mediated by the sympathetic nervous system, which signals for the pumping of catecholamines.[20]

Whereas sympathetic discharge is increased, there is an inhibition of parasympathetic discharge. The heart begins to free itself of parasympathetic restraints and prepares itself for higher performance.

PERIPHERAL VASCULAR RESPONSES

To understand the heart in exercise, we must view it as the central organ of an exquisitely adaptable vascular system. With the anticipation of exercise, higher cortical stimulation is accompanied by stimulus from other brain centers, such as the diencephalon and vasomotor areas of the medulla. The result of this stimulation is a constriction of resistance and capacitance (arteries and veins) vessels. This mechanism allows blood to flow "downhill" to the right atrium. As a result, the more active heart will be adequately supplied by sufficient venous return.

Although the previously mentioned mechanisms may predominate just before exercise begins, other factors come into play during exercise. Contraction of muscles and intensifying neural discharge will increase cardiac output. Muscle contractions serve to "milk" veins to increase venous return to the right heart, further priming the heart.

Local vascular changes enhance delivery of oxygen and metabolic substrates to muscles. There are local vasodilator responses mediated by hypoxemia and, in some vessels, enabled by substances such as nitric oxide generated by the vascular endothelium.

The increasing sympathetic discharge that continues into the active phase of exercise serves to redistribute blood throughout the body. Vasoconstriction in the splanchnic organs (liver, spleen) and skin surface shunts blood volume to exercising muscles. It is in this manner that blood pressure increases and cardiac output can be made to match muscular demands. Local muscle vascular dilations facilitate increased blood delivery to the muscles involved in any particular athletic endeavor.

Whether or not there is a true anticipatory phase in a particular situation, as the exercise phase is undertaken a steady state in cardiac output soon develops. There may be small variations and adjustments in preload, afterload, and mean arterial pressure. For a relatively fixed exercise task, a very efficient interplay of peripheral variables appears to adjust delivery of blood to the left ventricle. Stroke volume is not fixed but will vary to accommodate for changes in heart rate. With a slight increase in heart rate or stroke volume, metabolic needs of mild exercise can be met. As the exercise advances beyond moderate, increase in heart rate added to stroke volume increase will supply the fivefold or greater increase in cardiac output required.

Larger stroke volumes are observed in subjects performing supine exercise. In erect exercise, stroke volume increases that measure more than double the resting volumes can be observed.

Several neurogenic adjustment mechanisms that may alter cardiac output originate not only from central neurologic impulses but also from sympathetic afferents from working muscle. These impulses will result in increases in heart rate, contractility, and peripheral vascular tone (Table 6-1).

Volume Status in Exercise

In the early phase of exercise, there is an alteration in intravascular volume that allows for flow of plasma from capillaries into the interstices of muscles involved. Lymphatic drainage generally returns plasma back to the intravascular space, and intravascular fluid loss remains at 10% to 45% early on.

It is almost intuitive that as the period of vigorous athletic activity increases, the steady state becomes less "steady." Heart rate tends to increase to compensate for any further drop in intravascular volume and central venous pressure. Stroke volume and arterial pressure continue to fall gradually. The body continues, with heart-rate increase, to try to maintain a constant cardiac output.

Temperature Regulation

As mentioned previously, vasoconstriction in vessels of the skin during exercise serves to shunt blood to working muscles. With prolonged intense activity and generation of heat, the body begins to be less able to dispose of this heat. Thermoregulatory centers in the brain respond by

TABLE 6-1 Summary of Integrated Chemical, Neural, and Hormonal Adjustments Before and During Exercise

Condition	Activator	Response
Preexercise "anticipatory" response	Activation of motor cortex and higher areas of brain causes increase in sympathetic outflow and reciprocal inhibition of parasympathetic activity.	Acceleration of heart rate; increased myocardial contractility; vasodilation in skeletal and heart muscle (cholinergic fibers); vasoconstriction in other areas, especially skin, gut, spleen, liver, and kidneys (adrenergic fibers); increase in arterial blood pressure
Exercise	Continued sympathetic cholinergic outflow; alterations in local metabolic conditions resulting from hypoxia, ↓ pH, ↑ PCO_2, ↑ ADP, ↑ Mg^2, ↑ Ca^3, and ↑ temperature.	Further dilation of muscle vasculature.
	Continued sympathetic adrenergic outflow in conjunction with epinephrine and norepinephrine from the adrenal medullae.	Concomitant constriction of vasculature in inactive tissues to maintain adequate perfusion pressure throughout arterial system.
		Venous vessels stiffen to reduce their capacity. This venoconstriction facilitates venous return and maintains the central blood volume.

From McArdle WD, Katch FI, Katch VL: Exercise Physiology: Energy, Nutrition, and Human Performance. Philadelphia, Lea and Febiger, 1981. Reprinted by permission of the publisher.

dilating the skin vessels. The "radiator" function of the skin performs well but at a certain cost. Blood volume shunted to skin vessels diminishes mean circulatory pressure and central venous pressure.[19] The heart's stroke volume diminishes, and heart rate increases. An unchanging cardiac output under these circumstances supplies skin vessels at the expense of blood flow to working muscles. It is this mechanism that helps to explain the time course of the drift phase and eventual fatigue.

TRAINING AND THE HEART

Endurance training seems to make the cardiovascular system more efficient. After prolonged (several months) endurance activity, the athlete's heart becomes slow at rest and during exercise. This bradycardia may become diagnostic and include benign forms of heart block. Athletes who endurance train the leg muscles enjoy a greater bradycardic response than those who do upper body training. There may be a change in autonomic balance emanating from conditioned musculature. After long-term endurance training, intravascular blood volume is higher.

With an increase in oxygen extraction at the muscle level, cardiac output may not need to be so high to maintain a certain level of performance. The acclimatization response also will see that metabolic heat is dissipated efficiently (Table 6-2).

TABLE 6-2 Physiologic Adjustments During Heat Acclimatization

Acclimatization Response	Effect
Improved cutaneous blood	Transports metabolic heat flow from deep tissues to the body's shell
Effective distribution of cardiac output	Appropriate circulation to skin and muscles to meet demands of metabolism and thermoregulation; greater stability in blood pressure during exercise
Lowered threshold for start of sweating	Evaporative cooling begins early in exercise
More effective distribution of sweat over skin surface	Optimum use of effective surface for evaporative cooling
Increased sweat output	Maximizes evaporative cooling
Lowered salt concentration of sweat	Dilute sweat preserves electrolytes in extracellular fluid

With the improvement of oxygen extraction at the cellular level of muscle fibers, exercise of up to 50% of maximal oxygen consumption (VO_2 max) does not induce a rise in heart rate. It is speculated that increased vagal tone resulting from training explains these observations. If exercise becomes more intense in the aerobically conditioned athlete, sympathetic discharge is relatively reduced.

In the trained athlete, stroke volume is increased. This increase probably occurs as a secondary function of bradycardia (longer filling time). It does not seem that there are primary myocardial charges that increase stroke volume. Stroke volume is a secondary or dependent variable. Whereas ejection fraction may remain constant, maximal cardiac output in the trained athlete will reflect an increase in end-diastolic volume. It is likely that the Frank-Starling mechanism may be operative in maximal exercise. This mechanism is operative as preload (venous return) increases with high-intensity activity.

Diastolic properties of left ventricular function become more important in athletes as they age. We are becoming more aware of concepts such as active and passive filling characteristics of the ventricles. Abnormal diastolic properties of the left ventricle can cause the heart to fail during increasing activity. In the aging heart, it is often the diastolic filling properties that will be altered. An understanding of these alterations is helping us better understand the inexorable decline in cardiac performance observed in aging athletes.

CARDIOVASCULAR SCREENING OF THE ATHLETE

Perhaps because the athlete is considered to be the one who carries the standard of which we all would like to become, his or her sudden unexpected death is a heavy blow to us. Although less dramatic, his or her long-term health and the effect that participation in certain sports could have on the athlete should also be our concern. At the outset, it is imperative that the highest level of importance be rendered to the good of the athlete. As a principal decision maker regarding participation screening, it is vital that pressures that might be brought by team organizations, scholastic or otherwise, be resisted if they place the athlete at risk.[12] A sample cardiac screening questionnaire including questions proposed by the American Heart Association is shown in Figure 6-1.

Although preexercise cardiovascular screening for sedentary men aged 40 or older has been a general rule, the presentation of acute myocardial infarction, especially in men aged 35 or younger, prompts us to advise taking a detailed cardiovascular history to include suggestive risk factors such as family and smoking history. In this age group, a careful cardiac examination to search for abnormal murmurs and heart sounds should be followed by an electrocardiogram (ECG) and screening stress test.

Have you ever become dizzy or passed out during or after exercise?
Have you ever had chest pain during or after exercise?
Do you get tired more quickly than your friends do during or after exercise?
Have you ever had racing of your heart or skipped beats?
Have you had high blood pressure or high cholesterol?
Have you ever been told you have a heart murmur?
Has any family member or relative died of heart problems or sudden death before the age of 50?
Have you had a severe viral infection such as mononucleosis within the last month?
Has a physician ever denied or restricted your participation in sports for any heart problems?
Have any of your relatives ever had any of the following conditions?
- Hypertrophic cardiomyopathy
- Dilated cardiomyopathy
- Marfan's syndrome
- Long QT syndrome
- Significant heart arrhythmia

FIGURE 6-1. Cardiac preparticipation questionnaire. (Adapted from Seto CK: Clin Sports Med 22:23–35, 2003. With permission.)

Should the results of cardiovascular examination, ECG, or stress test prove to be equivocal or abnormal, one should refer the patient to a cardiologist for additional evaluation or exercise prescription. The task for the cardiologist is not totally clear. In some series, most highly trained young athletes have audible murmurs. Furthermore, many of our testing modalities may be too sensitive.

In the young athlete, the cardiovascular abnormalities that threaten health are overwhelmingly congenital; however, many times more middle-aged athletes die each year while exercising because of acquired coronary heart disease. Nevertheless, although in numbers exercise-related death in the young is rare, we are compelled to do all that we can to identify those at great risk. The task is difficult because we are not certain of the prevalence of certain congenital cardiac abnormalities in the general population. We do not have reliable statistics regarding mortality rates for participating athletes who carry congenital cardiovascular abnormalities.

The revised eligibility recommendations for competitive athletes with cardiovascular abnormalities set forth at the 26th Bethesda Conference held January 6, 1994, are an indispensable guide to screening the competitive athlete. We frequently consider its recommendation when evaluating athletes who may have cardiac abnormalities.

Congenital Cardiac Abnormalities

In screening for the presence of significant cardiac abnormalities, care must be taken to establish whether the subject has ever experienced cardiac symptoms. Although not yet carrying a cardiac diagnosis, he or she may have experienced syncope or chest pain that could represent the first warning of grave events to follow. Careful questioning about sudden death and cardiac disease in the subject's kin is vital.

The following sections provide a brief review of the most important cardiac abnormalities to consider in a preexercise screening.

Hypertrophic Cardiomyopathy. With the growth of echocardiography, we have become increasingly aware of this congenital heart muscle disease that Maron confirmed to be a major cause of sudden cardiac death in the young athlete.[15] With echocardiography, we are able to identify those subjects with this disordered heart muscle morphology, although the obstructive nature of this disease had been described during cardiac catherizations before the widespread use of echocardiography.

The primary screening of hypertrophic cardiomyopathy (HCM) can be difficult because the subject may have never complained of suggestive symptoms. Such symptoms could include unexplained chest pain, dizziness, palpitations, frank syncope, or, more frequently, exertional dyspnea. It is probable that he or she never has undergone more than a cursory heart examination. If such an examination had been conducted, the subject might either not have had an audible murmur or had a murmur dismissed as "functional." It is common for HCM to produce a murmur of varying intensity from examination to examination. During screening, a changing murmur should raise the suspicion of HCM.

The gradient developing within the left ventricle in HCM is dynamic and has to do with acceleration of blood through an ever-narrowing left ventricular outflow tract. Certain maneuvers can change the outflow gradient and alter its resultant murmur. By having the subject perform a Valsalva maneuver (straining against a closed glottis or blowing against the thumb placed in the mouth), the systolic outflow murmur's intensity will increase. The increase in systolic murmur loudness results from the reduction of preload on the left ventricle, making its internal diameter smaller, which accelerates the blood being ejected, drawing the mitral valve leaflets into the path of the blood by a Venturi effect (Fig. 6-2).

Extensive study of HCM also has elucidated its important diastolic abnormalities. In many subjects, these diastolic abnormalities appear to predominate in symptom generation. Inadequate and slowed diastolic filling is the most important abnormal mechanism to obtain, especially when the subject has tachycardia (Fig. 6-3). These diastolic abnormalities may result from the characteristic disordered morphology of myofibrils found on myocardial biopsy specimen. Called *myofibrillar disarray*, it is considered histologically characteristic of HCM. Of note, although evidence for a left ventricular outflow gradient may be absent in as many as half of subjects with HCM, diastolic abnormalities are common to all sufferers of HCM. It has been postulated that these diastolic abnormalities may further result from a disorder of

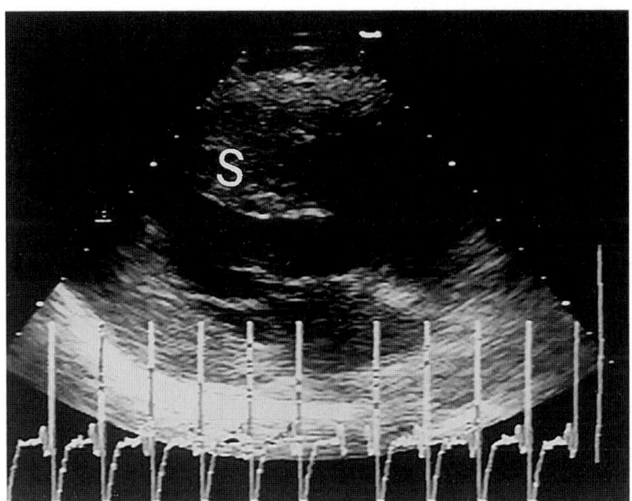

FIGURE 6-2. Long axis view of a heart with hypertrophic obstructive cardiomyopathy. Note the markedly thickened interventricular septum (S).

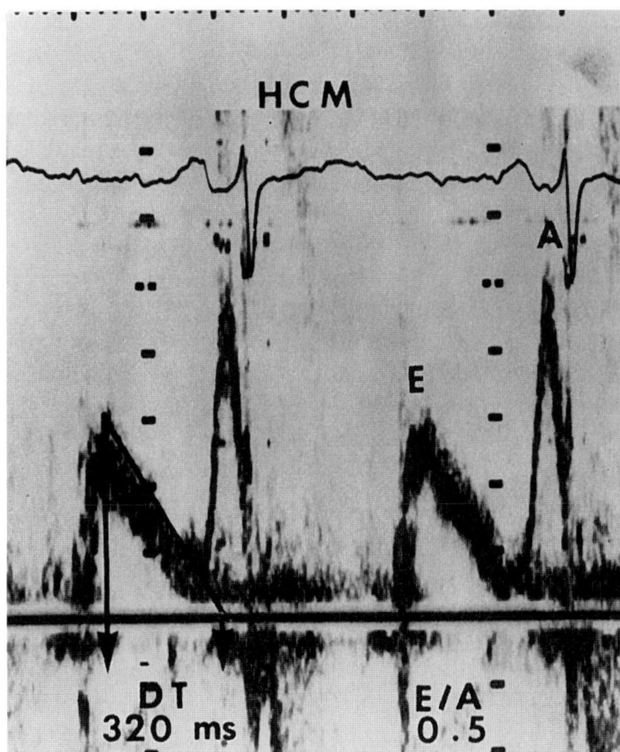

FIGURE 6-3. Doppler tracing hypertrophic obstructive cardiomyopathy below mitral valve in diastole reveals abnormal relaxation in a patient with hypertrophic obstructive cardiomyopathy. Note the prolonged deceleration time (DT). HCM, hypertrophic obstructive cardiomyopathy; E, passive left ventricular filling phase; A, filling wave during left atrial contraction. (From Oh JK, Seward JB, Tajik JA: The Echo Manual. Boston, Little Brown, 1994. Reproduced with permission.)

calcium metabolism in the myocardial cells of the left ventricle and sometimes the right ventricle. Small coronary vessel and conduction abnormalities may contribute to symptom generation in HCM.

DNA testing is increasingly being used with some success in screening of subjects suspected of having HCM. Unfortunately, we are learning that HCMs are a whole spectrum of diseases with multiple genetic determinants. There are those who believe that certain other types of testing, such as electrophysiologic testing, may be able to stratify those with HCM according to risk. We someday may be able to screen and prescribe with greater confidence. The more widely followed approach prohibits participation in most competitive sports for those who carry the diagnosis of HCM.

Coronary Artery Disease. A second relatively important cause of sudden cardiac death in young athletes is coronary artery disease. In one study by Corrado et al.[6] 23% of deaths in young athletes appeared to result from coronary artery disease. Most appeared to have lesions of the proximal left anterior descending coronary artery. We should be suspicious of coronary artery disease in subjects aged 10 to 29 years. In younger patients, Kawasaki disease, an acquired childhood febrile disorder, may leave coronary lesions in as many as 25% of subjects.

Congenital anomalies of the coronary arteries can cause sudden death in young subjects. Diagnosis of an aberrant coronary artery should be suspected in the subject who complains of anginal pain on exertion or exercise-induced syncope. Patients who present with such symptoms should undergo echocardiographic evaluation of their coronary ostia, thallium or echo stress testing, and coronary angiography, if necessary.

Complaints of chest pain related to position, respiration, or palpation are common in the young athlete and rarely suggest coronary artery disease. They often can be managed with explanation and reassurance. Conversely, exertion-related chest pain, sometimes accompanied by near-syncope or syncope, must be given careful scrutiny.

Complex Congenital Disorders. When considering sudden death from the time of birth, congenital valvular cardiac abnormalities play a large role. The young athlete arriving for screening will have been diagnosed with many of the severe complex malformations that would limit his or her activity. Also because of the subject's symptoms, the diagnosis is less likely to be missed.

When chest pain or syncope are the subject's complaints, there often will be no gross and obvious congenital cardiac abnormality detected, and the possibility of abnormal coronary arteries must be entertained. About 50% of young sufferers of sudden cardiac death will have reported previous prodromal symptoms.

Marfan Syndrome. Marfan syndrome, a congenital disease with the aorta as its most important target organ, has been implicated in the sudden cardiac death of some star athletes. Recently, there has been more awareness of this disorder, especially because it appears to present in tall, slender athletes. There have been high-profile sudden deaths of volleyball players and basketball players who seemed apparently well until their deaths.

Marfan syndrome is believed to be a fibrillin disorder that weakens the walls of the major vessels and may lead to aortic rupture. Some affected subjects may have very long, spidery fingers and lax joints. There apparently are many grades of the clinical expression of this disease. Some subjects might have aortas so dilated that on reaching a certain diameter, prophylactic replacement of the aortic root must be undertaken. This course might be recommended after close regular follow-up evaluation, even if the young subject is asymptomatic (Fig. 6-4).

Competitive sports for those with Marfan syndrome are believed to increase the shear stress on the ascending aorta resulting from the augmented hemodynamic shear force that results from increased cardiac contractility during exercise.

Myocarditis. Myocarditis, or inflammatory disease of the heart muscle, is a potential cause of sudden death in young athletes and in older athletes. Whereas myocarditis might be implicated in infant deaths, severe pump impairment and arrhythmia generation sometimes strike adult athletes with this disorder. The patient may or may not be aware of a recent bout of gastroenteritis or "flu" symptoms. The disease may present with recent dyspnea on exertion. The athlete might complain only of unexplained palpitation or lightheadedness. These latter symptoms might represent potentially dangerous ventricular or atrial arrhythmia. On examination, the findings could be minimal, but a pericardial rub suggesting coexistent pericarditis or a displaced apex heartbeat should prompt the prohibition of exertion. An echocardiogram would reveal reduced ejection fraction and perhaps a pericardial effusion. The most important viral agent responsible for myocarditis is *Coxsackie B* virus.

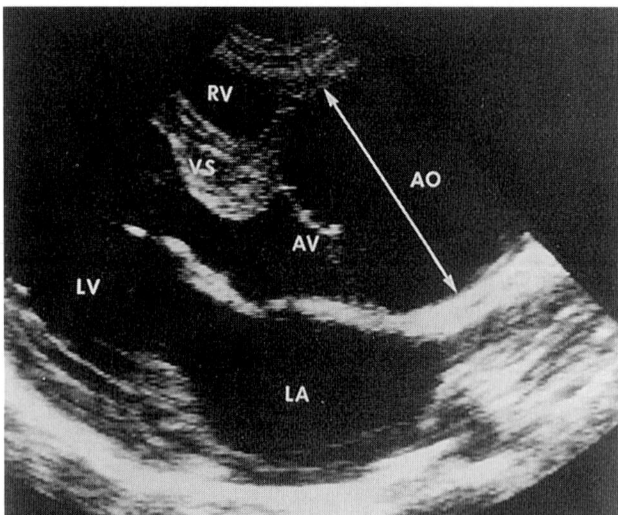

FIGURE 6-4. Two dimensional long axis view of a typically dilated aortic root (AO) in a patient with Marfan syndrome. RV, right ventricle; LV, left ventricle; AV, aortic valve. (From Oh JK, Seward JB, Tajik JA: The Echo Manual. Boston, Little Brown, 1994. Reproduced with permission.)

Dilated Cardiomyopathy. Dilated cardiomyopathy may be the final result of myocarditis, although there are some cardiomyopathies that may be familial. The diagnosis is relatively straightforward with echocardiography and careful history, although the etiology may be unclear. Systolic left ventricular function may be severely impaired. With exertion, this patient might experience an arrhythmia death.

Right Ventricular Dysplasia. In some sudden death series, particularly in one representing sudden death in northern Italy, right ventricular dysplasia, a congenital cardiomyopathy, predominates as an etiology.[6] On echocardiography, this patient, who may have a only right bundle branch block pattern on ECG, will have a thinned right ventricular wall. The patient may have syncope and death on exertion. This subject would require extensive electrophysiologic testing, perhaps combined with repeated stress testing to stratify his or her sudden death risk. Increasingly, magnetic resonance imaging (MRI) has become the preferred diagnostic modality for arrhythmogenic right ventricular dysplasia (ARVD), although this imaging method is relatively expensive and not always widely available.

Commotio Cordis. Commotio cordis is the event after which a young athlete will fall to the ground unconscious after a blow to the precordium. Maron,[14] in a recent study, described the disturbing scenario. A young athlete, perhaps playing sandlot baseball, will sustain a blow to the precordium and collapse immediately or briefly thereafter. Most notable is how little force will appear to have been delivered, but the subject will collapse and die. The subject appears remarkably resistant to resuscitation attempts. It does not appear that the integrity of the chest wall or mediastinal structures are compromised. Instead, it is postulated that a force is transmitted to the heart during its electrically vulnerable period, which apparently triggers a lethal ventricular arrhythmia.[14] Work is ongoing in attempting to protect young athletes from these tragedies by redesigning chest padding and the missiles that the athlete might encounter during sporting events.

Mitral Valve Prolapse. Mitral valve prolapse is a rare cause of sudden death in young athletes. Nevertheless, there are some series in sudden death in young adults that implicate this etiology. This malformation of the mitral valve forces the leaflet farther into the left atrium in systole and is more often present in women. It may be symptomatic.[4,12] It may generate atrial or, more importantly, ventricular arrhythmias that could lead to sudden death.[5] Careful history taking may reveal a family history of this disease. Physical examination may reveal a midsystolic click or a late systolic blowing murmur. Sometimes mild or severe mitral regurgitation will be present. Echocardiography is perhaps the most sensitive test for the establishment of the diagnosis (Fig. 6-5). In the subject who wishes to exercise vigorously, stress testing and Holter monitoring is in order. Abstention from stimulants, such as caffeine and tobacco, is recommended. Some patients will become more symptomatic, requiring the use of beta-blocker medications. Good hydration of these patients is an important rule to follow. Perhaps lengthening of the mitral apparatus relative to the left ventricular dimension may worsen mitral valve prolapse. Hydration, increasing intravascular volume and preload, may tighten up on this apparatus and reduce ventricular irritability and any mitral regurgitation.

Other Cardiac Anomalies. Careful history taking and physical examination will screen many of the remaining major anomalies. As with mitral prolapse, congenital aortic valvular disease has not been incriminated as among the important causes of sudden death in the athlete. Congenital aortic valvular disease in the relatively asymptomatic patient will most often be detected by careful auscultation. Although congenital (or acquired) aortic stenosis may be mimicked by coarctation of the aorta, an aortic abnormality will be the rule-out. The subject should be scheduled for an echocardiogram to clarify the issue. Significant aortic regurgitation also may produce a loud systolic murmur and a diastolic "blow." The important issue is that the athlete be screened and scheduled for additional testing to more clearly identify the problem.

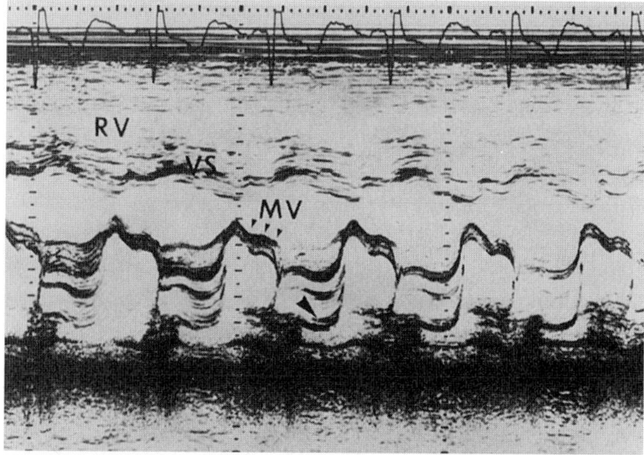

FIGURE 6-5. Note the thickened appearing mitral valve (MV) prolapsing posterior mitral leaflet (*large arrow*) in this subject with mitral valve prolapse. RV, right ventricle; VS, ventricular septum. (From Oh JK, Seward JB, Tajik JA: The Echo Manual. Boston, Little Brown, 1994. Reproduced with permission.)

The same is true for most other congenital or acquired cardiac abnormalities. Although the examiner may have difficulty deciding whether the systolic murmur heard is aortic stenosis or pulmonic stenosis, he or she will know that the issue deserves additional investigation. An echocardiogram, ECG, and cardiology consultation will be needed before clearing the subject for competitive athletic activity. In congenital aortic stenosis, peak instantaneous Doppler gradients are of value, whereas in acquired aortic stenosis mean gradients are measured.[10]

After a careful history is taken and a careful cardiac examination is performed (at rest and after exercise), the need for noninvasive testing may arise if the diagnosis is in doubt. The basic tests should include an ECG, an echocardiogram, and a stress test. Additionally, ambulatory rhythm monitoring (Holter monitoring), chest radiograph, and, in rare cases, coronary angiography or arrhythmia testing in an electrophysiology laboratory may be required.

Although the absolute number of sudden cardiac deaths in young athletes is few, one can only imagine the effect general screening with echocardiography would have on this number. Most epidemiologists and public health authorities agree that general echocardiographic screening of athletes would be a huge expenditure. The hope is that the cost of these studies will come down, and a more general application of cardiac sonography in the screening of athletes could be the positive result.

DIAGNOSTIC TESTING MODALITIES

The Electrocardiogram

The resting ECG, although not part of the standard screening examination for the athlete, can be a vital tool. In those athletes who were victims of sudden death, review of any ECGs in their history would have pointed to the need for additional examinations.[15] Most patients with hyperthropic cardiomyopathy could be readily screened by a standard 12-lead ECG. As mass ECG testing would not be cost-effective, reserving these traces for any subject with dizziness, syncope, or chest pain on exertion could reduce sudden athletic death by as much as 50%.

Typically, the ECG of the patient with hypertrophic cardiomyopathy would show high voltage resulting from characteristic wall thickening. Often, there also are abnormal q waves and t waves. The abnormal q waves and t waves are sometimes referred to as *pseudo infarct* patterns. Not uncommonly, the ECG might vary considerably.

Other important abnormalities, including those of rhythm disorders, might be detected by the 12-lead ECG. In the athlete complaining of rapid heart action, irregular heartbeat, dizziness, or shortness of breath, an ECG could be diagnostic. Ventricular premature beats can signal more serious sustained ventricular arrhythmias.

A short PR interval could warn of Wolff-Parkinson-White syndrome, which sometimes can cause life threatening atrial arrhythmias.

Atrioventricular block, from generally benign first-degree atrioventricular block and Type 1 second-degree (Wenkeback) atrioventricular block to more important second-degree and complete heart block and congenital long QT interval, can be revealed by ECG techniques.

To further investigate ventricular and atrial arrhythmias and their daily frequencies, 24-hour ambulatory ECG monitoring is useful. The newest models of these devices are very light and can be worn during vigorous athletic activity. We are now able to monitor the athlete with arrhythmias while he or she is performing most sports at high intensity. In the event that the athlete suffers from arrhythmias that require medical therapy, ambulatory monitoring will enable us to monitor the effectiveness of the antiarrhythmic therapy as he or she performs exercise at various intensities to measure effectiveness of arrhythmia suppression.

Cardiac Stress Testing

Cardiac stress testing is used frequently to screen patients in populations in which there is a high incidence of coronary disease, particularly in men aged more than 35 years. Its reliability is greatest in this group when stress ECG is used. Greater sensitivity is afforded by the use of echocardiography and nuclear isotope techniques that attempt to add information about left ventricular wall motion to each test. The subject's tendency to develop arrhythmias with increasing workloads is addressed by an ECG-graded stress test.

The standard ECG stress test can be performed by using any one of several well-known protocols (Bruce, Naughton) or custom protocols that address the particular needs of a testing population. Tests could be modified to most closely reproduce the loads the athlete would encounter when engaging in his or her sport. Information about the subject's fitness or aerobic capacity can be obtained by calculating the subject's double product. This value can be obtained by multiplying the peak systolic blood pressure times peak heart rate.

In preparation for the test, the subject is asked to fast. Before testing, ECG electrodes are attached to the chest. The subject is requested to exercise to exhaustion. Blood pressure and ECG are monitored periodically throughout the test. Currently, some exciting work is being performed with an echocardiographic technique called tissue Doppler imaging. This ultrasound method beams Doppler signal at the heart muscle to measure its relaxation properties. This technique promises to help us discriminate between the appropriately hypertrophied heart of certain athletes and the pathologically thickened ventricular walls of hypertensives and subjects with cardiomyopathies.

The stress test is stopped only if the subject requests to stop or shows dangerous arrhythmias or ECG changes. An inappropriate drop in blood pressure, heart rate, pallor, or diaphoresis may also prompt cessation of the test. When echocardiography or radionuclide studies are part of the test, the images are reviewed to render more information about myocardial perfusion and dynamics.

There are treadmill-based tests and bicycle-ergometer tests. Both techniques have their proponents. Treadmill testing has the advantage of more easily achieving higher peak heart rates, although echocardiographic image acquisition is delayed momentarily. We have not found this to be a problem. Bicycle stress testing has the advantage of image acquisition without delay, but the subject must be coached (and familiar with cycling) to best use this technique and achieve the desired end point.

The use of Doppler wave techniques during echo–stress testing can add useful information and is an interesting investigational tool that helps better elucidate mechanics during exercise.

Echocardiography

The use of ultra-high-frequency sound waves to render an ultrasound picture of cardiac structures has become an indispensable tool in the evaluation and screening of the athlete's heart. Without echocardiography, we would still have to rely on invasive or nuclear techniques to screen and measure the heart and major vessels. Echocardiography enjoys the combined unique advantages of sensitivity, technique, safety, repeatability, and portability. A major and ever-growing part of what we know about cardiac morphology and function in the healthy and at-risk athlete is because of echocardiography and Doppler echocardiography.

In the diagnosis of hypertrophic cardiomyopathy, Marfan syndrome, right ventricular dysplasia, mitral valve prolapse, congenital abnormalities of the heart valves and great vessels, myocarditis, and pericarditis, echocardiography is an essential diagnostic tool. We also are able to evaluate wall thickness, systolic thickening, diastolic properties, and changes in these parameters over time and how these vary with type and intensity of sport in the training athlete.

Hemodynamics are evaluated by Doppler techniques that project a beam of ultra-high-frequency sound waves into flowing blood. Erythrocytes act as Doppler beam reflectors that inform us of the direction and speed of the blood flow being interrogated. With these methods, we can readily determine whether there is a dynamic intraventricular or left ventricular outflow tract obstruction in the subject being screened. Doppler echocardiography also is useful in noninvasively determining cardiac output in varying loading conditions during exercise. With this testing modality we can detect and evaluate intracardiac shunts and stenosis and regurgitation of any of the cardiac valves.

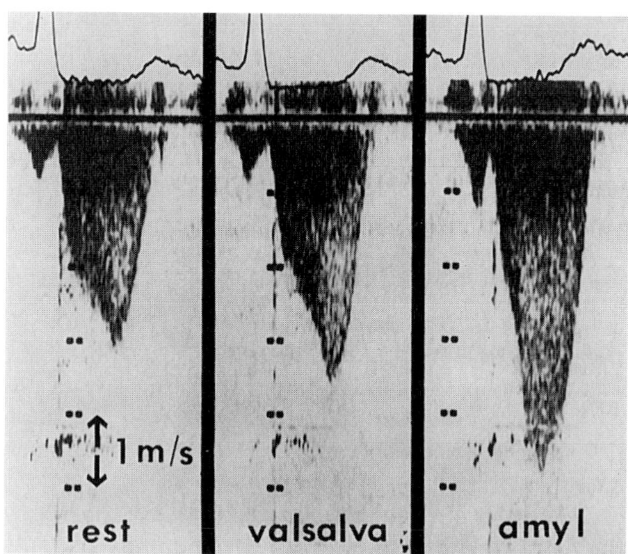

FIGURE 6-6. Dynamic left ventricular outflow tract (LVOT) gradients recorded from the cardiac apex with continuous wave Doppler. During the Valsalva maneuver and after inhalation of amyl nitrate, outflow velocities increase, suggesting dynamic increase in obstruction under different loading conditions. (From Oh JK, Seward JB, Tajik JA: The Echo Manual. Boston, Little Brown, 1994. Reproduced with permission.)

Figure 6-6 represents a Doppler study revealing a typical dynamic obstructive left ventricular outflow tract obstruction that worsens with provocation by Valsalva maneuver and by the inhalation of amyl nitrate, which dramatically decreases afterload.

Despite the powerful noninvasive techniques we now can use readily, sometimes more invasive techniques are the tests of last resort to be used in evaluating cardiac abnormalities in the athlete, from the "semiinvasive" modality called transesophageal echocardiography (TEE) to the clearly invasive cardiac catherization and electrophysiologic studies. With TEE, complex congenital abnormalities, aberrant coronary arteries, and cardiac and aortic trauma are evaluated. In catherization tests, coronary arteries and assessing conduction velocities in the heart clarify causes of supraventricular arrhythmias and heart block. Ventricular stimulation techniques attempt to induce potentially lethal sustained ventricular arrhythmias in a controlled setting. These tests appear to be useful in stratifying athletes with ventricular arrhythmias as high or low risk for life threatening cardiac events.

GENERAL EXERCISE CLASSIFICATION

We generally have categorized exercise into the large general groups of static and dynamic. As Mitchell has described,[16] static exercise includes athletic activity that involves a large mass of muscle with little movement through space of bones and joints. Dynamic exercise produces movement of joints and changing muscle lengths, often performed rhythmically.

Many studies have elucidated the hemodynamic changes that occur during each type of exercise. Dynamic exercise increases cardiac output and oxygen consumption without greatly increasing systolic and mean arterial blood pressure. Total peripheral resistance is reduced. Static exercise increases systolic, diastolic, and mean arterial pressure while heart rate and cardiac output remain unchanged. Oxygen consumption is increased only mildly. Clinically, jogging would be considered dynamic, whereas isometric weight exercises would be considered static because static exercise places a pressure load on the heart; the walls of the heart thicken, whereas the chamber dimension does not significantly increase. Echocardiography assessments of these hearts are characteristic.

As dynamic exercise generates a volume load on the heart, the ventricular chamber will enlarge without dramatic wall thickening or hypertrophy. Nature's correlates of these circumstances yield a concentrically hypertrophied left ventricular wall in pressure-load lesions. An obvious example would be the left ventricular hypertrophy of severe aortic stenosis. Where the volume to be ejected by the heart increases (as in mitral regurgitation), the left ventricular chamber becomes enlarged with proportionately little wall thickening. As opposed to the pressure-loaded heart that has concentric hypertrophy, the volume-loaded heart with eccentric hypertrophy is associated with a high maximal oxygen uptake during exercise. If we consider the determinants of myocardial oxygen consumption, we can understand how exercise can increase it. Heart rate, myocardial wall tension, and contractility are these determinants. The product of these three determinants yields maximal oxygen consumption in exercise.

Certain cardiac abnormalities cannot safely sustain the load that certain sport-related activities can place on the heart. Certain sports such as cycling share a high dynamic and static character. Other sports may involve a mostly static sports load on the heart. All the high-static sports should be contraindicated for the subject with heart abnormalities intolerant of static loads.

In subjects with some degree of aortic stenosis, for example, dynamic exercise would be contraindicated. Such exercise depends on an increase in heart rate to maintain cardiac output. An increase in heart rate increases the gradient across the stenotic valve, thus unacceptably increasing myocardial oxygen demand and decreasing perfusion of the brain and other vital organs.

In subjects with hypertrophic cardiomyopathy, competitive high-intensity athletics generally are to be prohibited. As there is a very large gray zone in the disease, especially where the left ventricular thicknesses may not be dramatically increased, a very exhaustive history (including family history), physical examination, and noninvasive (and perhaps even invasive) work-up is required. Presently, we do not have a fool-proof method of stratification of risk in these patients.

Athletes with Marfan syndrome often present the dual problems of aortic regurgitation, which requires prescription of exercise according to severity, and dilated aorta. The potential for aortic dissection is real. Static exercise and any exercise that would increase myocardial contractility may pose increased risk to the athlete.

Because the primary care physician may be called on to generally screen athletes before sport participation, an understanding of the principles governing cardiac clearance is essential. Final patient-by-patient recommendations should be undertaken only after an in-depth history, physical examination, and noninvasive evaluation in consultation with a cardiologist.

CARDIAC BENEFITS OF EXERCISE

We are well aware that regular exercise benefits all levels of fitness; there also is evidence to suggest regular exercise may help reduce coronary death. Regular aerobic exercise has been labeled cardioprotective. Bassler once postulated that marathon runners who completed a full marathon were granted a certain immunity to coronary death,[1] but this claim has been disputed. Nevertheless, regular vigorous exercise appears to raise the favorable component of serum cholesterol, called HDL-C.[11] Perhaps, through increased insulin sensitivity in tissues, lipase activity and HDL-C levels increase.

More recently, direct rheologic effects of accelerated blood flow in coronary arteries have been studied. There is an enhanced efficiency of the natural arterial dilating system mediated by nitric oxide that results from vigorous exercise. Finally, the development of rich collateral arterial coronary networks seems to be the result of graded regular exercise when performed by patients with known symptomatic coronary artery disease.

Exercise in the athlete, whether amateur, scholastic, or professional, is beneficial to the cardiovascular system. It increases fitness and quality of life and perhaps promotes cardioprotective mechanisms.[17]

THE LUNGS AND THEIR FUNCTION

As the heart is the pump of the vascular system, the respiratory system is responsible for the delivery of oxygen contained in the air to the blood and the removal of waste products such as carbon dioxide back to the air. Any medical condition that alters this delivery will either increase or decrease the ability of exercising muscles and the athlete to perform. Changes in the oxygen and carbon dioxide content of the air and changes in the intraerythrocytic concentration of 2,3-biphosphoglyceric acid (2,3-BPG) will cause shifts in the oxygen dissociation curve.

The respiratory system includes the lungs, the central nervous system, the chest wall, and pulmonary circulation. When needed, this system can increase ventilation by more than 12 times its baseline. Therefore, exercise is usually not limited by pulmonary factors in normal healthy athletes.

RESPIRATORY SYMPTOMS

Dyspnea

Dyspnea is defined as an abnormally uncomfortable awareness of breathing. Normally, our pattern of breathing is controlled by mechanisms that can vary ventilation to meet the demands of physical exertion. In addition, emotional states such as anxiety and fear can cause a change in normal ventilatory patterns. When evaluating the degree of dyspnea in a patient, one must take into consideration factors such as the overall level of fitness of the subject and the individual's perception of how bad the shortness of breath is.

Dyspnea may be related directly to the amount of physical exertion or may be sudden and related to specific underlying conditions, such as pulmonary embolism, spontaneous pneumothorax, or anxiety. In any athlete with dyspnea, it is important to look thoroughly for the cause.

Types of Dyspnea. *Orthopnea* is defined as dyspnea on assuming the supine posture. *Paroxysmal nocturnal dyspnea* is defined as attacks of dyspnea that usually occur at night and awaken the patient from sleep. It also is known as *cardiac asthma*. *Tripopnea* describes dyspnea only in the left or right lateral decubitus position, which usually occurs in patients with congestive heart failure. *Platypnea* describes dyspnea that only occurs in the upright position, specifically in situations where the abdominal viscera has no diaphragmatic support because of herniation when the individual stands. Platypnea would be managed with an abdominal binder or surgical repair.

The actual mechanism of dyspnea is unknown, and the differential diagnosis of dyspnea is included in the box, Causes of Dyspnea.

Hypoxia

Arterial hypoxia is a fall in the oxygen content in the arterial blood, noted as a fall in the partial pressure of oxygen or the $PaCO_2$.

Cyanosis

Cyanosis is a dark bluish or purplish coloration of the skin and mucous membrane resulting from deficient oxygenation of the blood in the lungs or from an abnormally great reduction of the blood in its passage through the capillaries. It appears when the reduced hemoglobin in

CAUSES of Dyspnea

Obstructive disease of airways
- Extrathoracic airway obstruction
  - Aspiration of food or a foreign body (gum, dental prosthesis)
  - Angioedema of the glottis or acute allergic reaction
  - Fibrotic stenosis of trachea
  - Acute respiratory infections (intermittent)
- Obstruction of intrathoracic airways
  - Asthma
  - Chronic bronchitis
  - Bronchiectasis
  - Chronic obstructive pulmonary disease

Diffuse parenchymal lung diseases
- Pneumonia
- Sarcoidosis
- Pneumoconiosis
- Carcinoma

Pulmonary vascular occlusive diseases
- Pulmonary embolism

Diseases of the chest wall
- Kyphoscoliosis
- Pectus excavatum
- Spondylitis

Heart disease
- Congestive heart failure
- Mitral stenosis
- Cardiogenic pulmonary edema

Anxiety neurosis

Noncardiogenic pulmonary edema
- Liver disease
- Nephrotic syndrome
- Protein-losing enteropathy
- Narcotic overdose
- Exposure to high altitude
- Neurogenic

Anemia

Obesity

the minute blood vessels is 5 mg or more per 100 mL. A false cyanosis can be caused by the presence of an abnormal pigment such as methemoglobin (carbon monoxide poisoning). It usually is most marked in the lips, nail beds, ears, and malar eminences.

When hypoxia occurs as a result of a respiratory problem, the $PaCO_2$ level usually rises and displaces the oxygen dissociation curve to the right, which allows the percentage saturation of the hemoglobin in the arterial blood at a given level of alveolar oxygen tension (PaO_2) to decline. Thus, arterial hypoxia and cyanosis are likely to be more marked in proportion to the degree of depression of PaO_2 when such depression results from pulmonary disease.

Clubbing

Clubbing is the broadening and thickening of the ends of the fingers. Although in some patients, the cause may be unknown, it may be inherited or seen with a variety of diseases. The mechanism of clubbing is unclear, but it appears to be secondary to humoral substance, which caused dilatation of the vessels of the fingertip. As part of the physical examination, the presence of clubbing should elicit a differential diagnosis. See the box, Causes of Clubbing.

Clubbing in patients with primary and metastatic lung cancer, mesothelioma, bronchiectasis, and hepatic cirrhosis may be associated with hypertrophic osteoarthropathy. Hypertrophic osteoarthropathy is the subperiosteal formation of new bone in the distal diaphyses of the long bones of the extremities, which causes pain and symmetric arthritis-like changes in the shoulders, knees, ankles, wrists, and elbows. It may be confirmed by radiography.

Cough

Coughing is a form of violent exhalation by which irritant particles in the airways can be expelled. Stimulation of the cough reflexes results in the glottis being kept closed until a high expiratory pressure has built up, which suddenly is released. The causes are listed in the box, Causes of Cough.

Chest Pain

Chest pain or tightness is a common sign of many diseases and is important in the diagnosis of pulmonary-related disorders. See the box, Common Causes of Chest Pain.

Ventilatory Function

Ventilation is the process of exchange of air in the lungs with atmospheric air, which has higher oxygen and lower carbon dioxide contents. Measurement of ventilatory function includes total lung capacity (TLC), which is the volume of gas contained within the lungs after a maximal expiration, and residual volume (RV), which is the volume of gas remaining within the lungs at the end of a maximal expiration. Vital capacity (VC) is the volume

CAUSES of Clubbing

Primary lung carcinoma
Metastatic lung carcinoma
Bronchiectasis
Lung abscess
Cystic fibrosis
Mesothelioma
Regional enteritis
Ulcerative colitis
Cirrhosis

CAUSES of Cough

Acute
- Upper respiratory infections
- Aspiration
- Asthma
- Bronchitis
- Bronchogenic carcinoma
- Foreign body inhalation
- Gastro esophageal reflux (GERD)
- Left ventricular failure/angina

Chronic
- Post-nasal drip/sinusitis
- Asthma/exercise-induced asthma
- Chronic bronchitis
- Cocaine usage
- Gastro esophageal reflux (GERD)
- Post-infective cough/bronchospasm
- Psychogenic
- Carcinoma
- Interstitial lung disease
- Benign tumors of the lung
- Drugs (e.g., ACE inhibitors)

of gas that is exhaled from the lungs when going from the TLC to the RV (Fig. 6-7). Minute ventilation is the tidal volume × frequency of respiration. A typical example might be a tidal volume of 500 with a respiratory rate of 12, which would equal 6000 ml air/minute.

Healthy patients are able to augment their minute ventilation (VE) to exercise loads in large part as a response to increased carbon dioxide production (VCO_2). In patients with chronic obstructive pulmonary disease, the PCO_2 has been up chronically, so it is no longer the driving force behind increased ventilation. O_2 becomes this motivation. Therefore, if we place these individuals on higher concentrations of O_2 (greater than about 2 liters per minute via nasal cannula), they will lose their drive to ventilate and slow down respirations until they go into respiratory failure.

COMMON CAUSES of Chest Pain

Asthma
Exercise-induced asthma
Infection
Chest wall injuries
Referred pain from the thoracic spine
Cardiac ischemia
Carcinoma
Interstitial lung disease
Herpes zoster (shingles)

Circulatory Function

Circulatory function depends on cardiac output and pulmonary vascular resistance. The peripheral vascular resistance (PVR) typically is obtained in an intensive care unit using a flow-directed pulmonary arterial catheter (Swan-Ganz). The normal value for PVR is approximately 50 to 150 dyn.s/cm^5.

A healthy individual at rest inspires 12 to 16 times per minute, each breath having a TV of approximately 500 ml. A portion of each breath (about 30%) never reaches the alveoli; this portion is known as the *dead space*.

The most commonly used measures of gas exchange are the partial pressures of O_2 and CO_2 in the arterial blood (PaO_2 and $PaCO_2$). The alveolar–arterial O_2 difference (PAO_2–PaO_2), or the A–a gradient, is a useful calculation. The alveolar and, hence, arterial PO_2 can be expected to change depending on the level of alveolar ventilation, reflected by the arterial PCO_2.

Pulse oximetry is a recent practical development in respiratory care which allows continuous monitoring of the patient's state of oxygenation. It is more practical than arterial puncture, which is required to measure the $PaCO_2$. Using a probe clipped to a patient's finger, it measures the absorption of wavelengths of light by hemoglobin in arterial blood. Because of differential absorption of the two wavelengths of light by oxygenated and nonoxygenated hemoglobin, the percentage of

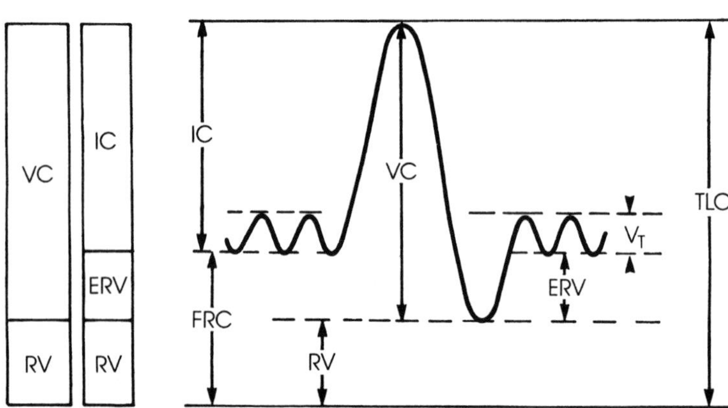

FIGURE 6-7. Lung volumes, shown by block diagrams (*left*) and by a spirographic tracing (*right*). TLC, total lung capacity; VC, vital capacity; RV, residual volume; IC, inspiratory capacity; ERV, expiratory reserve volume; FRC, functional residual capacity; V_t, tidal volume. (From Weinberger SE: Principles of Pulmonary Medicine, 2nd ed. Philadelphia, WB Saunders, 1992.)

hemoglobin that is saturated with oxygen can be displayed instantaneously.

Radiologic testing and other diagnostic procedures have become more state-of-the-art and include many modalities. See the box, Radiologic and Diagnostic Procedures Available. In all patients, a simple history and physical examination is important to make a diagnosis. A simple posteroanterior chest radiograph may suffice as an inexpensive diagnostic procedure. The examiner should always review the films him- or herself because the examiner has the best knowledge of the clinical state of his or her patient. Portable films are a necessary evil in some situations but never as reliable in quality.

Computed tomography (CT) has added amazing clarity to studies, and magnetic resonance imaging (MRI) is superior to differentiating pulmonary vessels versus lymph nodes. However, the added cost of these procedures must be considered. Lung scans are important in the diagnosis of pulmonary embolisms.

CLINICAL DISEASE STATES

There are three groups of individuals who experience asthma-like symptoms after exercise.

1. Athletes with chronic asthma, 90% of whom will experience symptoms after exercise.
2. Athletes with allergic rhinitis or atopic dermatitis who have a positive exercise challenge.
3. Athletes who do not have underlying allergies or asthma and only experience symptoms of asthma after exercise.

Asthma

Asthma is an obstructive disease of airways that is characterized by increased responsiveness of the tracheobronchial tree resulting from a variety of stimuli. The airways narrow by contraction of their smooth muscle, by a swelling of the mucous membrane, and by edema of the bronchial wall and an increase in the production of mucus. Recurrent attacks of difficult breathing, particularly on exhalation caused by an increased resistance to airflow through the respiratory bronchioles, are typical of the disease. Status asthmaticus is the persistence of severe airway obstruction for days or weeks.

Asthma may be induced by exercise. Sports vary in their tendency to induce asthma, with running having the highest tendency, cycling a moderate tendency, and gymnastics and swimming a low tendency. Paradoxically, many sufferers gain relief from their bronchospasm by regular exercise, and exercise is not seen as negative in the management of asthma. Many drugs help to control asthma, but team physicians must be aware that some are on the International Olympic Committee list of banned substances.

The National Institute of Allergy and Infectious Disease estimates that 41 million Americans have asthma and allergies. Asthma is said to be found in 4% to 5% of the general population in the United States. Half of the cases occur in patients before age 10 years, and another one third in those before age 40 years. In children, there is a 2:1 male preponderance, which equalizes by age 30 years.

Allergy is a state of altered reactivity in the host that results from interaction between antigen and antibody. An antigen is an agent that stimulates the production of an antibody. An allergen is defined as an antigen that has been shown to initiate an allergic response. The antibody classically associated with allergy is the IgE immunoglobulin. After inhalation of an allergen, it penetrates the respiratory epithelium and combines with pairs of IgE molecules attached to underlying mast cells, thus signaling release of mediators that initiate an inflammatory response. Individuals who readily make IgE antibody are prone to allergic reactions of the respiratory tract.

Allergic asthma often is associated with a family history of allergic diseases, such as rhinitis, urticaria, and eczema. These individuals will have positive skin reactions to intradermal injections of allergens and a positive response to the inhalation of the antigen. As many as 40% of patients with allergic rhinitis will have asthma.

Idiosyncratic asthma refers to those individuals without a history of allergy, negative skin testing results, and normal levels of IgE.

Environmental and occupational factors may be potent bronchial irritants, such as ozone and the oxides of sulfur and nitrogen. Metal salts, wood and vegetable dusts, pharmaceutical chemicals and plastics, biologic enzymes, and animal and insect dusts can cause problems. The house dust mite (*Dermatophagoides pteronyssinus*) or fungal spores (e.g., *Aspergillus fumigatus*) can cause bronchial hyperactivity. Fumes from paint and household cleaners may precipitate an acute attack of asthma, as may some perfumes. A drop in temperature at night can trigger asthma and may be prevented by heating the bedroom at night.

CHECKLIST

Radiologic and Diagnostic Procedures Available

Pulmonary imaging
- ☐ Chest radiographs
- ☐ Portable chest radiographs
- ☐ Computed tomography
- ☐ Magnetic resonance imaging
- ☐ Ultrasound
- ☐ Ventilation/perfusion (V/Q) lung scan
- ☐ Interventional (computed tomography–guided biopsy)

Diagnostic procedures
- ☐ Skin tests (ppd, candida, RAST, etc.)
- ☐ Bronchoscopy/biopsy

Obesity is on the rise in the United States. The rise in obesity has been most in middle-aged women, in whom the prevalence has increased by 65%. Most notably, the prevalence of asthma among middle-aged women has increased by 80% of the past 2 decades. This data suggests a potential link between obesity and asthma.[9,13]

The most common stimulus for an asthmatic attack is a respiratory infection. Exercise and emotional stress also can be stimuli.

The symptoms of dyspnea, cough, and wheezing are the hallmarks of asthma. One must be careful to differentiate asthma (see boxes on cough and dyspnea).

Every new patient with asthma should be examined. See the box, Asthma Medical History. The diagnosis is made by demonstrating reversible airway obstruction, which is defined as a 15% or more increase in FEV1 after two puffs of a beta-adrenergic agonist. Once the diagnosis is confirmed, the course of the illness and the effectiveness of therapy can be followed by measuring the peak expiratory flow rates (PEFR) or the FEV1.

Therapy should be aimed at elimination of the cause of the attack.

CHECKLIST

Asthma Medical History

Evaluate the following areas with every new patient with asthma.

1. Current symptoms
- ☐ Cough, wheeze, dyspnea, chest tightness, sputum production, exercise-related symptoms

2. Patterns of symptoms
- ☐ Perennial, seasonal, or perennial with seasonal exacerbation
- ☐ Continuous or episodic
- ☐ Onset, duration, and frequency of symptoms
- ☐ Diurnal variation (with special reference to nocturnal symptoms)
- ☐ Relation to exercise

3. Precipitating or aggravating factors (trigger factors)
- ☐ Viral respiratory infections
- ☐ Exposure to known allergens, e.g., dust mite, pollens, animal dander, molds
- ☐ Exposure to chemicals or other occupational sensitizers
- ☐ Exposure to irritants, e.g., cigarette smoke, perfume
- ☐ Drugs, e.g., aspirin and beta-blockers
- ☐ Foods
- ☐ Food additives—colorings, metabisulphite, monosodium glutamate
- ☐ Changes in weather, exposure to cool air
- ☐ Exercise

Continued

CHECKLIST

Asthma Medical History—cont'd

4. Development of disease
- ☐ Age of onset, age at diagnosis
- ☐ Progress of disease with time (better or worse)
- ☐ Previous treatments and response
- ☐ Frequency of symptoms
- ☐ Frequency of exacerbations
- ☐ History of accident and emergency room visits and admissions
- ☐ History of life threatening attacks and intensive care unit admissions
- ☐ Limitation of physical activity

5. Present management
- ☐ Current medication
- ☐ Response
- ☐ Current action plan

6. Profile of a typical exacerbation
- ☐ Trigger
- ☐ Usual time course, especially the amount of time between the first signs or symptoms and sudden deterioration
- ☐ Usual management
- ☐ Usual outcome

7. Home environment
- ☐ Smoking
- ☐ Other factors including clinically relevant allergens—dust mite, pollens, animal danders, molds, birds

8. Impact of the disease
- ☐ Time off school or work
- ☐ History of life threatening asthma
- ☐ Emergency room visits and admissions
- ☐ Limitation of physical activity
- ☐ Effect on work, schooling, or physical activity
- ☐ Effect on growth and development of children
- ☐ Impact on the family when either a child or an adult family member is affected

9. Assessment of the patient's knowledge and self-assessment ability

10. Related atopic disorders
- ☐ Family history of asthma, eczema, allergic rhinitis
- ☐ Personal history of eczema or allergic rhinitis

11. General health, other medical conditions, and other prescribed medications. Inquire specifically about
- ☐ Medications known to aggravate asthma, e.g., beta-blockers for hypertension or glaucoma, aspirin, and nonsteroidal anti-inflammatory drugs
- ☐ Sinusitis, nasal polyps

Drug Treatment. There are five basic drug categories.

1. Beta-adrenergic agonists/adrenergic stimulants
2. Methylxanthines
3. Glucocorticoids
4. Mast cell stabilizing agents
5. Anticholinergics

Adrenergic stimulants include epinephrine and isoproterenol, which are not beta-2 selective and have considerable side effects (palpitations and tremulousness). They are effective only as an inhalation or parentally. The usual dose is 0.3 cc of a 1:1000 solution administered subcutaneously.

The most commonly used inhalers are metaproterenol (Alupent, Boehringer Ingelheim Pharmaceuticals, Ridgefield, CT), albuterol (Proventil, Schering Corporation, Kenilworth, NJ), salbutamol (Ventolin, Allen & Hanburys, Research Triangle Park, NC), and salmeterol (Serevent, Allen & Hanburys, Research Triangle Park, NC). With the exception of metaproternol, these inhalers are highly selective for the respiratory tract and virtually devoid of significant cardiac effects except in high doses. The major side effect is jitteriness because of the stimulation of the beta receptors on skeletal muscles. They also may cause headaches and insomnia.

Inhalation is the preferred route because fewer side effects occur. The dose is up to two puffs every 4 hours while awake. Oral forms also are available; however, the International Olympic Committee has approved only *inhaled* albuterol, terbutaline, metaproterenol, and bitolterol. There is some debate whether these drugs improve performance in athletes without bronchospasm.

Methylxanthines (theophyllines) are medium-potency bronchodilators and are best used in maintenance therapy. Their dose has to be reduced in elderly patients. The most common side effects are nervousness, nausea, vomiting, anorexia, and headache. Because of a need for blood level monitoring, they have been less popular recently.

Glucocorticoids are not bronchodilators and have most benefit in patients with acute illness with severe airway obstruction that is not resolving. The usual dose is 6 mg/kg/day of hydrocortisone, and higher doses do not improve patients' symptoms.

Inhaled glucocorticoids are sometimes combined with beta-adrenergic agonist inhalers. The most popular of these is Advair, a combination of Serevent (salmeterol) and Flovent (fluticasone). This product is best used in those athletes who have chronic lung disease and use the medication on a chronic, not emergent or episodic, basis. Although albuterol will work immediately, Serevent (salmeterol) will take 20 minutes to take effect and therefore is not for use in emergent asthmatic attacks, rather for long-term treatment. This inhaler can be left at home as it is only used twice a day. The Alupent is what should be carried along for episodic asthmatic attacks. Combivent is a combination of atrovent (ipratropium bromide) and albuterol sulfate inhalation aerosol (Boehringer Ingelheim).

Mast cell stabilizing agents, cromolyn sodium (Intal) and nedocromil sodium (Tilade), are not bronchodilators. They inhibit degranulation of mast cells, preventing the release of the chemical mediators of anaphylaxis. They are most useful in atopic patients. A therapeutic trial of two puffs daily for 4 to 6 weeks frequently is necessary. Nedocromil may cause an unpleasant bitter taste about 10 to 15 minutes after inhalation.

Anticholinergics such as atropine sulfate can cause bronchodilation, but their side effects limit their usefulness. Inhaled anticholinergics such as ipratropium bromide (Atrovent) are somewhat useful but not as useful as they are in the management of chronic obstructive pulmonary disease.

Any athlete who is prescribed a new medication should be asked to report any deterioration in his or her asthma. Beta-adrenergic blocking agents, either oral or in eye drop form, aspirin, and other nonsteroidal anti-inflammatory drugs may cause or worsen asthma and should be avoided or used cautiously. Nonproprietary preparations, such as Royal Jelly, are contraindicated in athletes with asthma.

There is evidence that microaspiration of stomach acid, or reflux of stomach acid over an inflamed lower esophagus, can lead to bronchospasm in patients with asthma. Asthma control may be better in these athletes if the reflux is managed.[7] Nearly half of patients with asthma experience GERD symptoms regularly.[8] The best way to manage this is with diet (reduced acidity in the diet) and proton pump inhibitors (PPIs). These include Prevacid, Nexium, Aciphex, and Protonix.[7]

Athletes with asthma should not smoke, and friends and relatives should be asked to avoid smoking around them.

The need for influenza vaccine in adults should be assessed. Influenza vaccine is not indicated routinely for children with asthma.

Emergent Therapy. Aerosolized beta-2 agonists can be given every 20 minutes by a hand-held nebulizer for three doses in an emergency situation. This then can be followed by use of up to every 2 hours until the attack has stabilized. Aminophylline can be added to the regimen after the first hour to speed resolution. Salmeterol (Serevent) takes 30 minutes to work, and it should not be used in emergencies. In general, there is a correlation with the severity of the episode and the speed of resolution.

The mortality of asthma is small, less than 5000 deaths per year, but it is rising, especially in inner cities. The number of children having asthma 7 to 10 years after diagnosis is 26% to 78%. Arterial blood gases are essential in severe asthma. An increase in respiratory rate results in a decrease in PCO_2. An increase of the PCO_2

above 40 mm/Hg may constitute a medical emergency, and intubation may be necessary. Important indications for hospital admission of patients with asthma include cyanosis, exhaustion, difficulty speaking, and pulsus paradoxus more than 20 mm/Hg. Pulsus paradoxus is an exaggeration of the normal variation in the pulse volume with respiration, becoming weaker with inspiration and stronger with expiration. Pulmonary function testing is an important part of diagnosis, but it should be performed when the patient is not in the midst of an acute attack.

Chest radiography usually will show hyperaeration, but it should be done to rule out concurrent infection or pneumothorax. Skin prick tests and radioallergosorbent tests (RAST) may be helpful in confirming the patient's atopic status and in establishing certain allergies. They have no usefulness in testing for food allergies.

Drugs may be implicated in the production of asthma, especially beta-blocking agents and prostaglandin inhibitors such as aspirin.

Exercise-Induced Bronchospasm

Exercise-induced bronchospasm (EIB) is a condition in which vigorous physical activity triggers acute airway narrowing in people with heightened airway reactivity. The pathogenesis of EIB is associated closely with fluxes in heat and water that develop within the tracheobronchial tree during the conditioning (warming and humidification) of large volumes of air. It is more likely to occur in cold, dry environments and in the presence of environmental pollution. Twelve percent to 15% of the general population are affected by EIB. Seventy percent to 80% of patients with asthma have it. It occurs at any age, although 40% of children will have it at some time. It is distributed equally between male patients and female patients.

Vigorous exercise induces an initial bronchospasm, reaching a maximum in 5 to 10 minutes. Pulmonary function returns to normal in 20 to 60 minutes, which usually is followed by a refractory period lasting several hours (30 minutes to 120 minutes). Bronchospasm will not recur during this period, and an athlete may take advantage of this in timing his or her play. Warm-up exercises (either 20 minutes of submaximal exercise or 7 30-second sprints 30 minutes before exercise) are effective in diminishing EIB.

During the acute attack, the athlete may present with dyspnea, chest tightness, cough, and fatigue more than expected for the type of exercise performed. Recovery may be slow. If the testing is equivocal, an exercise challenge test using methacholine may be done. Methacholine is an inhaled bronchoconstrictor.

Criteria for Diagnosis. A history should be taken for the types and levels of exercise that produce the problem, the timing, and the nature of the symptoms. Laboratory criteria for diagnosis and for severity are found in Table 6-3. The severity of the disease is influenced by the same factors that affect asthma: the type, intensity, and duration of the exercise; the environmental conditions; the level of fitness of the athlete; the intercurrent infections; and time since the athlete's last bronchospastic episode.

Exercise Testing for Exercise-Induced Bronchospasm. Assessment by exercise testing is an integral part of pulmonary testing in the athlete. When performing the calculations, it is important to use a reputable laboratory to ensure that the results may be reproducible and easily comparable. When establishing a baseline, a 10% change in some results is enough to make a diagnosis, so that reproducibility is paramount.

The athlete should be told to sustain vigorous exercise for at least 5 minutes continuously, and the heart rate should exceed 70% of his or her maximum rate. Treadmills and cycle ergometers have had standard exercise programs developed for testing. It is important to note that for EIB, treadmill running is more asthmagenic than cycling.

Inexpensively, peak flow meters can be used to assess pulmonary function. Standardized readings should be taken immediately before and after exercise and at 1-, 3-, 5-, 10-, and 15-minute intervals after exercise. Spirometry is more sensitive but more expensive (Fig. 6-8). In more sophisticated laboratories, histamine or methacholine challenge can be performed. Also, drugs used for therapy can be assessed running these tests with or without the various bronchodilators.

Therapy. Patients with EIB will benefit from good conditioning, which will, however, reduce the severity of EIB but not prevent it.

Exercising with submaximal exercise will induce EIB. After waiting 30 minutes, one can restart exercising during the refractory period. About 50% of people who get EIB will have no more attacks for 1 to 2 hours after the first attack. These warm-up times are important for the athlete with EIB, as is the cool down afterward. Patients should avoid hyperventilation, try to use slow nasal breathing when possible, and wear a scarf or mask

TABLE 6-3 Severity of Exercise-Induced Bronchospasm

Category	Criterion
Mild	15–20% fall in FEV1
Moderate	20–30% fall in FEV1
Severe	> 30% fall in FEV1

From McArdle WD, Katch FI, Katch VL: Exercise Physiology: Energy, Nutrition, and Human Performance. Philadelphia, Lea and Febiger, 1981. Reprinted by permission of the publisher.

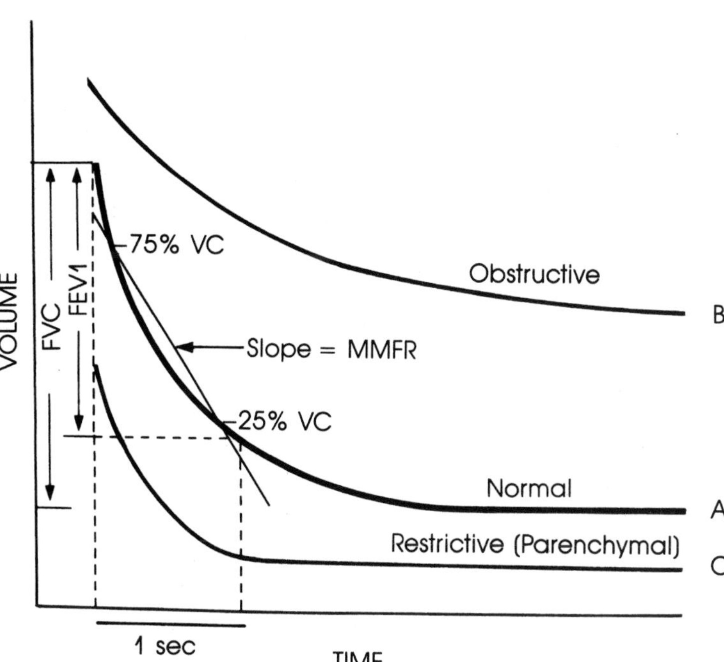

FIGURE 6-8. Spirographic tracings of forced expiration, comparing a normal tracing (A) and tracings in obstructive (B) and parenchymal restrictive (C) disease. Calculations of FVC, FEV1, and FEF25–75% are shown only for the normal tracing. Because there is no absolute starting volume with spirometry, the curves are positioned artificially to show the relative starting lung volumes in the different positions. (From Weinberger SE, Drazen JM: Disturbances of respiratory function. In Isselbacher KJ, et al [eds]: Harrison's Principles of Internal Medicine, 13th ed. New York, McGraw-Hill, 1994, p 1152.)

in the winter to warm the air and keep in the humidity. The cold, dry air is a precipitant of EIB. Exercising in a warm, more humidified environment will help minimize symptoms. Also trying to avoid exercise during times of high pollen counts is helpful. If one has the luxury of picking a sport, swimming and water sports are among the least asthmagenic. Baseball and volleyball are relatively easy for patients with EIB. Running is one of the hardest for these individuals, but long-distance running is better than sprinting.

Drug therapy remains the mainstay of management. Most physicians would prescribe an aerosolized selective beta-2 agonist, such as salbutamol or albuterol, one to two puffs, 5 to 20 minutes before exercise. This usually provides effective prophylaxis against the development of EIB for 2 to 3 hours. Alternatives include an inhaled cromoglycate (Intal) or nedocromil sodium (Tilade), two to four inhalations a few minutes before exercise. These drugs are used in athletes who do not tolerate the side effects of the inhaled beta-2 agonists, in those who appear to experience late-phase responses to exercise, and in those whose EIB is not prevented by beta-2 agonist therapy. Some athletes will need two to four inhalations of bronchodilators plus the same dose of cromoglycate (Intal) or nedocromil sodium (Tilade). Ipratropium bromide (Atrovent), an anticholinergic agent, may be beneficial, but for most athletes, it is less effective than the other classes of inhalers.

As in patients with asthma, beta-blockers and sedatives are contraindicated, and their use can be fatal. Long-acting bronchodilators such as Serevent should be taken 30 minutes before exercise, preferably 2 hours before. Athletes should be told to keep their bronchodilators handy while exercising. If they have an attack, they should take two to four inhalations. If the attack is severe, the dose should be repeated 5 to 10 minutes later. Medical help should be sought if the attack does not go away.

Inhaled steroids do not prevent EIB if taken before exercise. If an inhaled steroid is taken regularly, the EIB will be less severe. Also, less bronchodilator medication or mast cell stabilizing agents will be needed before exercising. Oral forms of bronchodilators used to manage asthma may not prevent EIB.

If these management strategies are not successful, consider the following possibilities.

- Poor drug delivery—check technique
- Combining beta-2 agonist with four inhalations of cromoglycate sodium (Intal) or nedocromil sodium (Tilade)
- Poor cardiopulmonary fitness—some patients will need a graduated exercise program to develop fitness
- Poor asthma control—check peak expiratory flow rates at home over a 2-week period
- Check for another cause of breathlessness on exertion

If symptoms still are occurring during or after exercise, the athlete should cease activity, rest, and use a short-acting beta-2 agonist. Inhaled steroids do not prevent EIB if taken immediately before exercise.

Sinus-Related Symptoms

Sinusitis is a common disorder in athletes. In its acute state, it is easily recognized. Allergic rhinitis occurs in about 15% to 20% of the general population. Viral infections are common, but about 50% of these infections result from *Hemophilus influenzae* and *Streptococcus pneumoniae.* Other bacteria such as *Branhamella catarrhalis* and mixed oral anaerobes can cause this problem.

Chronic sinusitis may be a more subtle cause of respiratory difficulty in the athlete. Symptoms may present as facial pain, headache, toothache, post-nasal drip, cough, rhinorrhea, nasal obstruction, fever, and epistaxis.

Diagnosis is made on history and physical examination and supplemented by radiographs of the sinuses, looking for opacification or fluid levels. CT scan of the sinus also is a good, albeit more expensive, way to make the diagnosis. Cultures of the nasal sinus often will just show normal flora and are not that helpful in diagnosis or management.

Management is aimed at hydration of the athlete, adequate humidification of the air, and appropriate antibiotic therapy. Decongestants are of some value. The use of intranasal steroids such as fluticasone propionate (Flonase, Glaxo Pharmaceuticals, Research Triangle Park, NC), budesonide (Rhinocort, Astra Pharmaceutical Products, Westboro, MA), and flunisolide (Nasarel, Roche Laboratories, Nutley, NJ) is widely advocated in the acute situation, but there is a latent period of about 24 hours before these are effective.

The presence of polyps or anatomic deformity may be a reason for medical failure, and surgery may be required in these patients.

Exercise-Induced Anaphylaxis

Exercise-induced anaphylaxis is characterized by a sensation of warmth, pruritis, cutaneous erythema, angio-edema, urticaria (giant, more than 1 cm), upper respiratory obstruction, and occasionally vascular collapse. Risk factors include previous atopic history, family atopic history, food ingestion (shellfish, celery, nuts, alcohol), weather conditions (heat, high humidity), and drug ingestion (aspirin, nonsteroidal anti-inflammatory drugs).

Management includes decreasing the intensity of exercise, avoiding exercising on warm, humid days, and stopping exercise at the earliest sign of itching. Also, avoiding meals 4 hours before exercise will help. Drug therapy includes antihistamines, cromglycate and epinephrine. Pretreatment does not prevent the onset of exercised-induced anaphylaxis.

Cholinergic Urticaria

Cholinergic urticaria is an exaggerated cholinergic response to body warming. The athlete will develop urticarial papules after exposure to heat and humidity and exercise. Generally, the papules appear first on the wrist or upper thorax and spread to the limbs. Antihistamines are used in management.

Exercise-Induced Angioedema

Exercise-induced angioedema is a nonitchy swelling occurring in the deep dermis and subcutaneous tissue. It tends to involve the face and oral region. Attacks may be life threatening if the airway is involved. Prevention may be achieved with modification of exercise programs or with the use of antihistamines (diphenhydramine). In addition, selective H2-receptor blockers, such as cimetidine (Tagamet, SmithKline Beecham, Philadelphia, PA), ranitidine (Zantac, Glaxo Pharmaceuticals), famotidine (Pepcid, Merck & Co., West Point, PA), lansoprazole (Prevacid, TAP Pharmaceuticals, Deerfield, IL), omeprazole (Prilosec, Astra Merck, Wayne, PA), and nizatidine (Axid, Eli Lilly and Company, Indianapolis, IN), have been used in the management of this condition.

Chronic Obstructive Pulmonary Disease (COPD)

COPD is defined as progressive airflow limitation that is not fully reversible. It is characterized by airway inflammation and mucus hypersecretion.

It has been shown repeatedly that exercise programs, although not accompanied by measurable improvement in lung function, result in increased exercise tolerance and an improved sense of well-being. Arm exercises are poorly tolerated. If there is any evidence of malnutrition, improvement will yield dividends. The use of bronchodilators will be helpful for those who have some evidence of reversible bronchospasm on PFTs. Cardiopulmonary testing is the best way to correlate the symptoms of COPD with objective evidence of limitations. Usually, to increase exercise endurance, exercise must be at least at 60% of VO_2 max, three times a week.

Allergic Rhinitis

Allergic rhinitis is a common chronic condition, which can cause significant discomfort in affected patients, but will also affect performance times in elite athletes. In addition, sleep disturbances and fatigue can impair performance. Treatment as outlined earlier in this chapter is important to keep the nasal passages clear and allow maximum oxygen transport to the lungs and to decrease susceptibility to upper respiratory infections. This is especially true of athletes who often are exposed to many other individuals who may harbor viruses, which will more easily cause disease when they can enter through the disturbed mucous membranes of the nasal cavities.

Pulmonary Embolism

Pulmonary embolism is a leading cause of morbidity and mortality. Any athlete with dyspnea or chest pain and with a history of recent trauma or surgery to the lower extremities or history of deep vein thrombophlebitis should be suspect. Female athletes receiving estrogen therapy or birth control pills have a higher incidence of phlebitis.

Sleep Apnea

Sleep apnea is intermittent obstruction of airflow during sleep. It is no more common in athletes than in the general population, but its diagnosis should be entertained when an overweight recreational athlete who snores is having trouble with alertness during the day. There are easy to use sleep study kits, which patients can take home to get an easy assessment of their sleep habits.

Severe Acute Respiratory Syndrome (SARS)

SARS is a viral infection caused by a coronavirus called SARS-associated coronavirus (SARS-CoV), which was first reported in Asia in February 2003. It was reported by the World Health Organization to have been seen in 30 countries worldwide. The first outbreak centered in China and Hong Kong, although large outbreaks occurred in Toronto, Canada, and Singapore. In general, SARS begins with a high fever and other symptoms may include headache, an overall feeling of discomfort, and body aches. Some people also have mild respiratory symptoms at the outset. About 10% to 20% of patients have diarrhea. After 2 to 7 days, SARS patients may develop a dry cough. Most patients develop pneumonia.[3]

SARS seems to spread by close person-to-person contact. It is thought to be transmitted most readily by respiratory droplets. A recent study showed that SARS might be deadlier to patients born with a gene found in 10% to 15% of people of southern-Chinese ancestry. BMC Medical Genetics, an online biomedical-research journal, first published this. The gene is known as HLA B-46. Although initial research appeared to indicate a high fatality rate for this disease, it appears to be in line with influenza epidemics. Physicians should be suspect of sudden onset of dyspnea and high fevers in athletes flying to or from endemic areas. Treatment is symptomatic.

Hot Tub Lung

The use of hot tubs is growing in popularity in the United States. Humidifier lung has been previously described (hypersensitivity pneumonitis associated with a humidifier caused by various fungi).[2]

Hot tub lung is an incompletely characterized disease associated with Mycobacterium avium complex (MAC) growing in hot tub water.[18] Patients present with progressively worsening respiratory symptoms and pulmonary function along with diffuse x-ray changes consisting primarily of ground-glass opacities (noncaseous granulomas). Treatment with discontinuation of hot tub use, without antimycobacterial therapy, seems to lead to prompt improvement in symptoms, pulmonary function, and radiographic abnormalities. Hypersensitivity to MAC, rather than an infection, is the likely underlying mechanism of hot tub lung.

BIBLIOGRAPHY

The Bantam Medical Dictionary. New York, Bantam Books, 1990.

Barnes PJ: Drug therapy: Inhaled glucocorticoids for asthma. N Engl J Med 332(13):868–875, 1995.

Bennett JC, Plum F (eds): Cecil Textbook of Medicine, 20th ed. Philadelphia, WB Saunders, 1996.

Brukner P, Khan K: Clinical Sports Medicine. Sydney, McGraw-Hill, 1993.

Cantu RC, Micheli LJ (eds): ACSM's Guidelines for the Team Physician. Philadelphia, Lea and Febiger, 1991.

Cishek MB, Moser KM, Amsterdam EA: Chest pain: Working up nonemergent conditions. J Respir Dis 17(7):560–575, 1996.

Harries M, Williams C, et al (eds): Oxford Textbook of Sports Medicine. New York, Oxford University Press, 1994.

Harrison's Principles of Internal Medicine, 13th ed. New York, McGraw-Hill, 1994.

Leff AR (ed): Cardiopulmonary Exercise Testing. Orlando, FL, Grune and Stratton, 1986.

Mahler DA, Horowitz MB: Perception of breathlessness during exercise in patients with respiratory disease. MSSE 26(9):1078–1081, 1994.

McFadden ER: Exercise-induced airway obstruction. Clin Chest Med 16(4):671–682, 1995.

McFadden ER, Gilbert IA: Current concepts: Exercise-induced asthma. N Engl J Med 330(19):1362–1367, 1994.

Rupp N: Diagnosis and management of exercise-induced asthma. Phys Sports Med 24(1):77–87, 1996.

Spector SL: Update on exercise-induced asthma. Ann Aller 71(6):571–577, 1993.

Sports Medicine for the Primary Care Physician. Boca Raton, FL, CRC Press, 1994.

Stedman's Medical Dictionary, 21st ed. Baltimore, Williams & Wilkins, 1966.

REFERENCES

1. Bassler TJ: Better life expectancy and marathon running. Am J Cardiol 45:1292–1297, 1980.
2. Baur X, Behr J, Dewair M, et al: Humidifier lung and humidifier fever. Lung 166:113–124, 1988.
3. CDC Basic Information about SARS Fact Sheet. September 29, 2003.
4. Cheitlin MD: Mitral valve prolapse: Key references. Circulation 59:610–612, 1979.

5. Chester E, King RA, Edwards E: The myxomatous mitral valve and sudden death. Circulation 67: 632–639, 1983.
6. Corrado D, Thiene G, Nava A, et al: Sudden death in young competitive athletes: Clinicopathologic correlations in 22 cases. Am J Med 89:588–596, 1990.
7. Field SK, Sutherland LR: Does medical antireflux therapy improve asthma in asthmatics with gastro esophageal reflux? A critical review of the literature. Chest 114:275–283, 1998.
8. Field SK, Underwood M, Brant R, Cowie RL: Prevalence of gastro esophageal reflux symptoms in asthma. Chest 109:316–322, 1996.
9. Flegal KM, Carroll MD, Ogden Cl, Johnson CL. Prevalence and trends in obesity among US adults, 1999–2000. JAMA 288:1723–1727, 2002.
10. Graham TP Jr, Bricker TJ, James FW, Strong WB: 26th Bethesda conference: Recommendations for determining eligibility in athletes with cardiovascular abnormalities. J Am Coll Cardiol 24:867–873, 1994.
11. Hartung GH, Squires WG, Gotto AM: Effects of exercise training on plasma high density lipoprotein cholesterol coronary disease patients. Am Heart J 101(2):181–184, 1981.
12. Hutter AM Jr: Cardiovascular abnormalities in the athlete: Role of the physician. Keynote address 26th Bethesda Conference: Recommendations for determining eligibility in athletes with cardiovascular abnormalities. J Am Coll Cardiol 24:851–852, 1994.
13. Mannino DM, Homa DM, Pertowski CA, et al: Surveillance for asthma—United States, 1960–1995. MMWR 47:1–27, 1998.
14. Maron BJ, Poliac LC, Kaplan JA, Mueller FO: Blunt impact to the chest leading to sudden cardiac arrest during sports activities. N Engl J Med 333(6): 337, 1995.
15. Maron BJ, Roberts WC: Sudden death in young athletes. Circulation 62(2):218–229, 1980.
16. Mitchell JH, Blomqvist CG, Haskill WL, et al: Classification of sports. 16th Bethesda Conference. Cardiovascular abnormalities in the athlete: Recommendations regarding eligibility for competition. J Am Coll Cardiol 6:1198–1199, 1985.
17. Paffenberger RS, Laughlin ME, Gina AS, et al: Work activity of long-shoreman as related to death from coronary heart disease and stroke. N Engl J Med 282:1109–1114, 1970.
18. Rickman OB, Ryu JH, Fidler ME, et al: Hypersensitivity pneumonitis associated with Mycobacterium avium complex and hot tub use. Mayo Clin Proc 77:1233–1237, 2002.
19. Rowell LB: Human cardiovascular adjustments to exercise and thermal stress. Physiol Rev 54:75–159, 1974.
20. Rushmer RF, Smith O, Franklin D: Mechanisms of cardiac control in exercise. Circ Res 7:602–627, 1962.

7 Head Trauma

Matthew E. Fink

EPIDEMIOLOGY OF SPORTS-RELATED HEAD INJURIES

Sports-related head injuries, except those incurred during boxing or combat sports, are accidental, and great efforts are being made to reduce their frequency. Unlike the more common musculoskeletal injuries associated with athletic activities, head injuries may first appear trivial; but there may be a progression of disability or the start of a lifelong process of neurologic impairment, which, if not recognized early with the appropriate interventions, can result in serious disability in later life.

The magnitude of the problem can be appreciated best from statistics compiled by the National Football Head and Neck Injury Registry.[19] It is estimated that there are 250,000 concussions in this country each year in football alone.[7] In the years between 1971 and 1984, there was a documented yearly average of eight deaths due to head injuries. At the high school level, about 20% of football players sustain a concussion during a single season, and some suffer two or more. In football, the risk of sustaining a concussion is four times greater for the player who has a history of concussion than for a player who has never sustained a previous concussion.[8] In Great Britain, a recent survey of 544 rugby players found that 56% had suffered at least one head injury associated with post-traumatic amnesia; this lasted more than an hour in 58 players, of whom only 38 had been admitted to the hospital for evaluation and treatment.[15] Repeated concussions, best documented in professional boxers, can cause long-term impairments in cognitive functions (dementia pugilistica) and have been associated with pathological changes in the brain on imaging studies.[9,11,20] Recent epidemiologic studies have also suggested that head injury with concussion is an independent and additive risk factor for the development of Alzheimer's disease in later life.[14] For all of these reasons, it is crucial that a standardized program be instituted for the prevention and treatment of all head injuries during sports activities to prevent the long-term consequences.

In the United States, the sports associated with the highest incidence of head injury are football, horseback riding, and bicycling, especially in children. In Glasgow, Scotland, a survey revealed that golf (club injuries), horseback riding, and rugby were the most common causes of head injury, reflecting the relative frequency of different sports in different countries.[13] The use of hard-shell helmets significantly reduces the risk of head injury during sports activities, and major efforts are underway to encourage their universal use by both children and adults.[3,10,16]

CLASSIFICATION AND PATHOLOGY OF HEAD INJURIES

Primary Brain Damage

Concussion, the most common brain injury during sports, refers to a syndrome of brief loss of consciousness (LOC) with a variable period of post-traumatic amnesia (PTA) and confusion. Some injuries do not have a documented period of unconsciousness, but there is a clear period of PTA; these episodes should also be defined as concussion because it is likely that the period of LOC was too brief to be recognized. Although there has been controversy regarding the underlying neuropathology of concussion, animal studies and recent neuroimaging studies in humans confirm that there are pathological lesions associated with concussion, specifically axonal swelling in subcortical white matter.[12,17]

The hallmarks of concussion are a period of post-traumatic confusion and amnesia for recent events. The severity of the concussion has been graded according to the duration of LOC and PTA, according to the scheme of Cantu.[7]

Grade 1 (mild): No LOC, PTA less than 30 min
Grade 2 (moderate): LOC less than 5 min or PTA more than 30 min
Grade 3 (severe): LOC for 5 min or PTA for 24 hours or more

This classification is important in determining when athletes may return to play after acute injury.

Cerebral contusions, or bruising of the surface of the brain, can occur as a result of a direct blow to the skull. Contusions may be focal underneath a skull fracture after direct impact to the head, or multifocal due to slamming of the whole brain against the interior of the skull and rigid dural membranes. Multifocal contusions generally occur during a rapid deceleration injury, such as occurs when the athlete falls to the ground and strikes the head against a hard surface. The most common locations are the anterior tips of the frontal and temporal lobes and the occipital poles. Although these lesions may not result immediately in loss of consciousness or focal neurologic signs, they can cause significant impairments in cognitive functions and personality and create a risk for post-traumatic epilepsy. Brain contusions in eloquent areas may cause focal deficits or aphasia. Brain imaging studies will reveal the extent of these lesions immediately.[4]

Diffuse axonal injury is caused by a combination of deceleration and rotational forces that cause shearing of large areas of white matter from the overlying cerebral cortex. This results in immediate coma and has a poor prognosis for recovery. This serious injury may occur in the absence of any external injuries or skull fractures, and initial brain imaging studies may appear normal.[4]

Secondary Brain Damage

Contusions and diffuse axonal injuries may secondarily cause brain edema; increased intracranial pressure; and subarachnoid, intracerebral, or subdural hematomas. A skull fracture across the path of meningeal arteries may cause an acute epidural hematoma. About half of all patients who develop coma from epidural and subdural hematomas are initially brought to the hospital awake and talking but deteriorate 6 to 24 hours later. Close observation, neuroimaging studies, and emergency neurosurgical consultation is required for any athlete who shows a decline in alertness after a lucid period.

Post-traumatic epilepsy may occur in patients with cerebral contusions with or without an underlying skull fracture. Overall, the incidence is about 5% in patients with these lesions. If a seizure occurs within the first week following injury, there is a high risk of recurrent seizures, and antiepileptic medication is usually required on a long-term basis.

The "second impact syndrome" is the development of malignant brain edema after a second concussion occurs before the injured athlete has fully recovered from the first.[18] This syndrome is most common in young children but also occurs in teenagers and young adults.[5] The mechanism is thought to be persistence of vasomotor paralysis in the brain from the first concussion, resulting in severe vasogenic edema after the second insult. This potentially fatal disorder is a major reason for enforcing a period of rest and abstinence from play until the athlete has fully recovered from the effects of a concussion.

The "postconcussive syndrome" refers to a constellation of symptoms that may persist for weeks or months after a concussion—loss of intellectual capacity, poor recent memory, personality changes, headaches, dizziness, lack of concentration, and fatigue. In the past, many of these symptoms were thought to be psychologically based. However, it is now accepted that these symptoms represent the subacute and chronic effects of brain injury and reflect the underlying neuropathology of concussion.

EVALUATION AND TREATMENT ON THE FIELD

Following head injury, there may be a scalp wound with extensive bleeding. Hemorrhage should be controlled with pressure and players immediately removed from the field because of the risk of HIV transmission. Using sterile gloves, the wound should be explored to determine if there is a fracture. A depressed skull fracture may cause underlying brain contusion without loss of consciousness, but could result in a delayed epidural or subdural hematoma. An athlete with a scalp laceration, even without LOC, should be immediately moved to a hospital for neuroimaging studies and observation.

If the athlete is unconscious on the field, the cervical spine should be immobilized, and before any movement, the athlete should be examined for chest and abdominal injuries and limb fractures. The injured player should be placed in a semiprone position to protect the airway, and neurologic assessment on the field should be based on the Glasgow Coma scale (Table 7-1); pupil size and responses to light; examination of the ears and nose for blood, cerebrospinal fluid, and hemotympanum; and tests for perception of pain, tendon reflexes, and plantar responses. Search for an associated spinal injury should be paramount in the mind of the examiner. After examination, the injured athlete should be rapidly transported to the nearest trauma hospital.

TABLE 7-1 Glasgow Coma Scale

Glasgow Coma Scale	Score 3–15
Eye Opening	
Spontaneous	4
To voice	3
To pain	2
None	1
Best Verbal Response	
Oriented	5
Confused	4
Inappropriate	3
Incomprehensible	2
None	1
Best Motor Response	
Obeys command	6
Localizes pain	5
Withdraws from pain	4
Flexes to pain	3
Extends to pain	2
None	1

Fortunately, most players have a brief LOC and are awake by the time a physician arrives on the field. The mental status examination should consist of tests for orientation (time, place, person, situation), concentration (digits forward and backward, the months of year in reverse), and memory (names of teams in prior games, the president, the governor, or the mayor; recent newsworthy events; 3 words at 0 and 5 minutes; details of current contest). Neurologic tests should include symmetry and light reactivity of pupils, coordination tests with finger-nose-finger and heel-shin tests, heel to toe standing with eyes open and closed, and standing on one foot. Challenge tests may include a 40-yard sprint, 5 push-ups, 5 sit-ups, and 5 deep knee bends. If the above activities cause headaches, dizziness, nausea, unsteadiness, photophobia, blurred or double vision, emotional lability, or mental status changes, the athlete should be transferred immediately to a hospital for brain imaging studies and observation. If there are no other abnormalities on the examination other than post-traumatic amnesia, the player should undergo brain imaging studies to look for a fracture or contusion. If these studies are normal, the athlete may return home for observation by family members for any change in neurologic condition, as instructed by the medical staff. It is useful to provide instructions on a Head Injury Card similar to the one described in the box.

CHECKLIST

Head Injury Card

This patient has received an injury to the head. A careful examination has been made, and no sign of any serious complication has been found.

It is expected that recovery will be rapid, but in such cases it is not possible to be quite certain.

If you notice any change of behavior, vomiting, dizziness, headache, double vision, or excessive drowsiness, please telephone the hospital at once.

No alcohol. No analgesics. No driving.

From McLatchie G: ABC of sports medicine. Head injury in sport. Brit Med J 308:1620–1624, 1994.

RECOMMENDATIONS FOR RETURN TO ATHLETIC ACTIVITIES

The decision to allow an athlete to return to play is based on empiric guidelines rather than scientifically based knowledge. The guidelines are designed to ensure that the athlete has fully recovered from the head injury before allowing return to play, recognizing that there is a cumulative effect from recurrent brain injuries. According to the criteria developed by Cantu, guidelines are as follows[1,6,7]:

1. Grade 1 Concussion (Mild)
   - First Concussion: May return to play if asymptomatic for 1 week
   - Second Concussion: Return to play in 2 weeks if asymptomatic at that time for 1 full week
   - Third Concussion: Terminate season; may return to play next season if asymptomatic
2. Grade 2 Concussion (Moderate)
   - First Concussion: Return to play if asymptomatic for 1 week
   - Second Concussion: Minimum of 1 month of no play; may then return if asymptomatic for 1 week; consider terminating season
   - Third Concussion: Terminate season; may return next season if asymptomatic
3. Grade 3 Concussion (Severe)
   - First Concussion: Minimum of 1 month of no play; may then return if asymptomatic for 1 week
   - Second Concussion: Terminate season; may return next season if asymptomatic
   - Third Concussion: Terminate season; consider permanent retirement from contact sports

PREVENTION OF HEAD INJURIES

In 1904 President Theodore Roosevelt urged the formation of the National Collegiate Athletic Association after 19 athletes were killed or paralyzed from football injuries.[2] Since then, prevention of head injuries in sports has been a high priority, although this may be impossible in boxing and other combat sports. Contact sports such as football, rugby, and basketball have a significant risk that can be reduced with the use of headgear, and this has already been well established in motorcycle and autoracing accidents.

In children younger than 16, accidental injuries are the leading cause of death, and head injuries from skateboarding, bicycling, horseback riding, rollerblading, and rock-climbing are a major cause of death and disability. Most states in the United States now require children to wear helmets while riding bicycles; similar helmets should be worn for other activities where there is a risk for head injury.[3,10,16] Golf club injuries among children younger than age 16 are common and point to the need for stronger rules of play on golf courses to ensure that spectators stand clear of players.

Boxing represents a special situation, since the goal of professional boxing is to cause a concussion (i.e., a knockout). Professional boxers enter the ring voluntarily. knowing the risks. But we certainly have an obligation to protect amateur athletes, and we should ensure that headgear is always used in amateur competition to prevent head injuries. In addition, professional boxers should have their total number of fights limited if they have sustained repeated knock-outs or dazed states. In other combat sports, the use of padded and spring flooring may protect against serious injuries during falls.

REFERENCES

1. Akau CK, Press JM, Gooch JL: Sports medicine. 4. Spine and head injuries. Arch Phys Med Rehabil 74:S443–446, 1993.
2. Albright JP, McCauley E, Martin RK, et al: Head and neck injuries in college football: An eight-year analysis. Amer J Sports Medicine 13:147–152, 1985.
3. Ashbaugh SJ, Macknin ML, Medendorp SV: The Ohio Bicycle Injury Study. Clin Pediatrics 34:256–260, 1995.
4. Becker DP, Gudeman SK: Textbook of Head Injury. Philadelphia, WB Saunders, 1989.
5. Bruce DA, et al: Diffuse cerebral swelling following head injuries in children: The syndrome of "malignant brain edema." J Neurosurg 54:170–178, 1981.
6. Cantu RC: Guidelines for return to contact sports after cerebral concussion. Physician and Sports Medicine 14:75–83, 1986.
7. Cantu RC: When to return to contact sports after a cerebral concussion. Sports Med Digest 10:1–2, 1988.
8. Gerberich SG, et al: Concussion incidences and severity in secondary school varsity players. Amer J Public Health 73:1370–1375, 1983.
9. Gronwall D, Wrighttson P: Cumulative effects of concussions. Lancet 2:995–997, 1975.
10. Hamilton MG, Tranmer BI: Nervous system injuries in horseback-riding injuries. J Trauma 34:227–232, 1993.
11. Jordan BD, Zimmerman RD: Computed tomography and magnetic resonance imaging comparisons in boxers. J Amer Med Assoc 263:1670–1674, 1990.
12. Levin HS, et al: Magnetic resonance imaging and computerized tomography in relation to the neurobehavioral sequelae of mild and moderate head injuries. J Neurosurg 66:707–713, 1987.
13. Lindsay KW, McLatchie GR, Jennett B: Serious head injury in sport. Brit Med J 281:789–791, 1980.
14. Mayeux R, et al: Genetic susceptibility and head injury as risk factors for Alzheimer's disease among community-dwelling elderly persons and their first-degree relatives. Ann Neurol 33:494–501, 1993.
15. McLatchie G, Jennett B: ABC of sports medicine. Head injury in sport. Brit Med J 308:1620–1624, 1994.
16. Nelson DE, Bixby-Hammett D: Equestrian injuries in children and young adults. Amer J Dis Child 146:611–614, 1992.
17. Ommaya AK, Gennarelli TA: Cerebral concussion and traumatic unconsciousness. Correlation of experimental and clinical observations on blunt head injuries. Brain 97:633–654, 1974.
18. Saunders RL, Harbaugh RE: The second impact in catastrophic contact sports head trauma. J Amer Med Assoc 252:538–539, 1984.
19. Torg JS, et al: The national football head and neck injury registry. 14-year report on cervical quadriplegia, 1971 through 1984. J Amer Med Assoc 254:3439–3443, 1985.
20. Unterharnscheidt F: About boxing: Review of historical and medical aspects. Texas Reports Biol Med 28:421–495, 1970.

8 Gastrointestinal System

Seth A. Cohen and Jerome H. Siegel

Gastrointestinal problems are common among athletes, especially in those who participate in endurance events such as long-distance running. Although much is not yet understood about the effects of exercise on the gastrointestinal tract, a large amount of new information has come to light in the past 15 years. The most common gastrointestinal complaints reported by athletes include diarrhea, fecal urgency, abdominal pain, bloating, nausea, vomiting, heartburn, chest pain, and occult or overt gastrointestinal hemorrhage. In this chapter we will review the pathophysiology, clinical presentation, and treatment for the various problems affecting the gastrointestinal tracts of athletes.

GENERAL OVERVIEW

Gastrointestinal symptoms are common among athletes, but the problems vary widely according to the specific sport, level of exertion, degree of anxiety, and possibly gender of the athlete. Most studies reporting these problems are in general agreement in terms of the spectrum of gastrointestinal symptomatology. Studies have concentrated on endurance athletes—long-distance runners and triathletes—but specific recreation or competitive team sports such as football and tennis have not been studied. All studies report that the incidence of gastrointestinal symptoms is proportional to the level of exertion, and some studies have found more than 80% of endurance athletes experience frequent or occasional gastrointestinal symptoms. This high incidence of gastrointestinal symptomatology is remarkable even though it reflects some selection bias. Lower GI symptoms—watery bowel movements, fecal urgency or incontinence, cramps, or GI bleeding—are more commonly reported than upper GI symptoms—nausea, vomiting, belching, heartburn—which are perceived as more intermittent and milder.

Most studies of endurance athletes have focused on men; less information is available concerning women. Women, however, appear to experience more frequent GI problems (40% to 70%) than men, and this is exacerbated during menses. More information on female athletes is needed. Younger runners (age less than 35) and less experienced runners experience a high incidence of GI symptoms compared to those reported by older and more experienced runners. Anxiety concerning performance is a well-recognized factor in provoking or exacerbating GI symptoms among athletes.

Most athletes note a "training effect" on gastrointestinal symptoms; that is, the symptoms occur more commonly during the initial training period and diminish as the athletes "get into shape." However, exercise exceeding an athlete's usual threshold provokes GI symptoms again. Paradoxically, there are reports that preexisting functional GI complaints (such as the irritable bowel syndrome) improve in athletes after they have been in training.

TRAUMA

Contact sports can lead to traumatic injury of the abdominal organs. The most serious injuries include laceration or rupture of the spleen, laceration of the liver, and contusion or disruption of the pancreas. Typically, affected individuals will develop signs and symptoms of an acute abdomen, possibly with vascular collapse. Persons with these injuries require immediate referral for resuscitation and surgical evaluation. Further discussion will not be included here.

GASTROESOPHAGEAL REFLUX

Belching, regurgitation, heartburn, chest pain, or acid reflux are common, occurring intermittently in about 10% of the general population. Symptoms of reflux are provoked by vigorous exercise. Of long-distance runners, 20% to 25% experience symptoms. Belching and regurgitation are more common than heartburn. Although the mechanism for belching and regurgitation is not known, it is probably related to aerophagia, large volumes of liquids or food contained in the stomach, gastric agitation, and, possibly, increased intragastric pressures generated during exertion. Esophageal spasm is another possible cause for chest pain and is often misinterpreted as heartburn. Abnormal relaxation of the lower esophageal sphincter does not occur with exercise, so does not explain reflux symptoms. Athletes are more likely to develop reflux symptoms if they eat just before exertion. Some athletes, however, experience heartburn if they eat after exercise, especially if they imbibe foods that either relax the lower esophageal sphincter or are acidic (e.g., alcohol, citrus drinks). Heartburn is also reported among anxious competitive players of team sports either before or during games.

Treatment of reflux symptoms is empiric and is based on clinical judgment. Young people who complain of only intermittent symptoms can be treated empirically without undergoing investigation. If, on closer questioning, patients report frequent or persistent symptoms or other abnormalities such as weight loss or dysphagia, they should be evaluated with endoscopy. Older patients with new or persistent symptoms should be referred for evaluation to exclude significant esophagitis or neoplasia. In middle-aged men and women who are at risk for coronary artery disease, the complaint of exertional chest pain should always prompt a consideration of angina. Acid perfusion of the esophagus can lead to chest pain and myocardial ischemia. Most patients, and physicians, cannot accurately distinguish between esophageal pain and angina. Exclusion of coronary disease should take priority in patients at risk.

Patients should be counseled not to eat for several hours prior to exercise. They should also be cautioned not to "gulp" down fluids when drinking, as this action increases aerophagia. Simple symptoms of heartburn are readily treated with antacids. An alginate-based antacid, such as Gaviscon (SmithKline Beecham), is preferred by many authorities. Care must be taken with magnesium-containing antacids, as they can precipitate or exacerbate diarrhea. On the other hand, while calcium-based antacids are a good source of this essential element, they may lead to constipation. Patients with more severe symptoms can take an antisecretory agent such as a histamine type 2 receptor antagonist (H-2 blocker) before exercising, but this approach should not be necessary for most athletes. The optimal treatment for peptic esophagitis and refractory symptoms of reflux is a proton pump inhibitor, a new class of gastric antisecretory medication (Table 8-1).

TABLE 8-1 Medicines Available for Peptic Ulcer Disease (PUD) and Gastroesophageal Reflux Disease (GERD)

H-2 Blockers
Cimetidine (Tagamet) 400 mg BID or 800 mg qhs
Famotidine (Pepcid) 20 mg BID or 40 mg qhs
Nazitidine (Axid) 150 mg BID or 300 mg qhs
Raniditine (Zantac) 150 mg BID or 300 mg qhs
Antacids
Calcium carbonate
Magnesium hydroxide
Aluminum carbonate
Aluminum hydroxide and alginic acid
Proton Pump Inhibitors
Esomeprazole (Nexium) 40 mg qd
Lansoprazole (Prevacid) 30 mg qd
Omeprazole (Prilosec) 20 mg qd
Pantoprazole (Protonix) 40 mg qd
Rabeprazole (Aciphex) 20 mg qd
Cytoprotective Agents
Misoprostol (Cytotec) 100 or 200 mcg QID
Sucralfate (Carafate) 1 gm QID

NAUSEA, CRAMPING, VOMITING

Symptoms of nausea, cramping, and vomiting commonly occur in athletes who are not in shape, exceed their exertional capacity, or have eaten too soon before exertion. Of endurance runners, 5% to 10% vomit and retch after finishing a hard run. Gastric emptying is retarded during severe exertion, but, clinically, this phenomenon is not relevant to most athletes. Symptoms are inversely related to aerobic training capacity and may be exacerbated by dehydration as the result of prolonged exercise in hot weather. Treatment consists of rest and oral rehydration. Rarely, patients with severe dehydration will require parenteral hydration.

ABDOMINAL PAIN

A "stitch" in the side is frequent among athletes. It is characterized as a sharp, subcostal pain which may occur on either side and is exacerbated by breathing and relieved by rest. The frequency and severity of a stitch diminishes with aerobic training endurance. Although the cause of a stitch is unknown, speculative causes include ischemia, a trapped gas bubble in the intestine, or spasms of the diaphragm. Clinical diagnosis is evident and no treatment is required. Other types of abdominal pain that do not meet the criteria for a stitch should be evaluated systematically as they would be in a nonathlete. There are rare reports of cecal volvulus, ischemic bowel, incarcerated or strangulated hernia, colon cancer, or Crohn's disease presenting as abdominal pain during exercise. Evaluation of abdominal pain in the athlete is the same as in other patients: What is the nature of the pain? What are the associated symptoms? Over what period of time does the pain present?

IRRITABLE BOWEL SYNDROME

The irritable bowel syndrome (IBS) is common among the general population. It is characterized by altered bowel habits with abdominal pain or bloating in the absence of organic disease. IBS generally affects younger people and women more than men. The pathophysiology remains unknown, but possible explanations include disordered intestinal and colonic motility, increased sensitivity to colonic distension, exaggerated gastrocolic reflexes, carbohydrate intolerance, psychoneurotic disorders, and stress. The physiologic abnormalities and symptoms of IBS are believed to be common, but only a minority of people seek medical evaluation. Those patients who do seek medical help have significantly more psychoneurotic disorders. There appears to be an association between functional abdominal pain and a history of physical and sexual abuse, but this remains debatable. Some studies have noted a higher frequency of IBS among athletes, but exercise ameliorates the symptoms. IBS is a clinical diagnosis of exclusion. Treatment options include dietary restrictions (e.g., excluding lactose products and including high residue foods), fiber supplementation, antispasmodic agents, and medical and psychological counseling.

PSYCHOGENIC ABDOMINAL PAIN

Psychogenic abdominal pain is seen among young, anxious athletes. Although it is a diagnosis of exclusion, it does have certain characteristics. It can be a sharp, epigastric pain without radiation or it can be associated with symptoms of nausea, vomiting, fever, or altered bowel habits. It has no relationship to food intake or other physiologic stimuli but may be associated with stress and anger. On examination, the abdomen is flat and soft, with normal bowel sounds and no guarding or peritoneal irritation. Generally, the history is chronic and repetitive. Acute presentation of epigastric pain in a young person could represent, among other causes, gastroenteritis, esophagitis, appendicitis, peptic ulcer disease, pancreatitis, or bowel obstruction, but these are unusual. The patient's history, associated symptoms, physical examination, and laboratory results along with observation will identify those people with organic disease. The most important aspect of treatment is recognition of the nonorganic cause of the pain to avoid unnecessary and costly testing.

DIARRHEA

Watery bowel movements, cramps, fecal urgency, and incontinence are the most common and troubling gastrointestinal symptoms among athletes who exercise strenuously. As many as 50% to 60% of marathon runners experience one or more of these symptoms. The urge to defecate is the most common reason for endurance runners to interrupt a race. Interestingly, in a survey of triathalon athletes, lower gastrointestinal symptoms were significantly reduced during the swimming and cycling portions of the event compared to during running. This observation highlights the fact that running specifically triggers colonic symptoms.

Although there is no proof that running increases intestinal transit, it is widely believed that running increases the frequency of bowel movements. The jarring of repetitive footfalls during running may stimulate mass movements in the colon or alter the absorption of fluids and electrolytes. Alternative hypotheses include the release of various prokinetic gastrointestinal hormones or inflammatory mediators such as prostaglandins. Runners note that the frequency and intensity of lower gastrointestinal symptoms are proportional to the level of exertion, their aerobic training capacity, and their level of anxiety. Symptoms are significantly more common in women than in men and among younger runners than in older runners.

Athletes who experience diarrhea and/or fecal urgency associated with running, and not at other times, do not require a work-up. Most runners have adopted their own approach to handling exercise-induced diarrhea. The majority of runners abstain from eating 3 to 6 hours before running. Many consciously evacuate their bowels before running. Others always know where they can find a toilet on their usual running route. Individual runners may take fiber supplements to "bulk up" the stool to prevent a watery bowel movement, and others take an antimotility agent such as Loperamide or a nonsteroidal anti-inflammatory agent. The goal of treatment for exercise-induced diarrhea is to control symptoms to avoid interrupting the person's performance.

A patient with an alteration of bowel habits independent of exercise should be evaluated as any other patient would be: What is the pattern of bowel movements—a colitis pattern (urgency, tenesmus, bloody) or a small bowel pattern (less frequent, large volume, watery)? Is the onset of the problem acute or chronic? Are blood or fecal leukocytes present in the stool? Are there any risk factors for infectious causes of diarrhea? After obtaining a complete history and physical examination, the work-up of diarrhea includes a stool sample for fecal leukocytes and occult blood, a complete blood count, and an erythrocyte sedimentation rate (ESR). If fecal leukocytes are present, this finding suggests colitis, which can be infectious or idiopathic. Stool cultures will diagnose bacterial etiologies. Pseudomembranous colitis should always be considered in any patient who has taken antibiotics in the past several months; a stool specimen for *Clostridium difficile* toxin is the best test to establish the diagnosis. *Giardia lamblia*, the only parasitic infestation commonly seen in practice, produces large-volume liquid stools and weight loss, and can be diagnosed on examination for ova and parasites. An elevated ESR will help identify patients who have inflammatory bowel disease. A flexible sigmoidoscopy is important in diagnosing colitis, and, often, the combination of the endoscopic findings and the mucosal biopsies can be diagnostic of Crohn's disease, ulcerative colitis, or pseudomembranous colitis. Treatment consists of supportive care and specific treatment for the illness (Table 8-2).

TRAVELER'S DIARRHEA

Athletes who travel to foreign countries to compete are always at risk for contracting traveler's diarrhea. This syndrome occurs predominantly as a result of exposure to

TABLE 8-2

Etiologies and Treatment of Diarrhea

Etiology	Diagnosis	Treatment
Toxigenic *E. coli*	Clinical dx, exclusion	Bismuth subsalicylate, loperamide, fluids
*Salmonella, Shigella, Yersinia,** *Campylobacter*	Stool culture	Ciprofloxacin 500 mg BID or erythromycin 500 mg BID × 5 days
Pseudomembranous colitis, *Clostridium difficile*	Stool for toxin Sigmoidoscopy	Metronidazole 250 mg QID or vancomycin, 125 mg QID × 10 days
Irritable bowel syndrome	Clinical dx, exclusion	Fiber supplements, antispasmodics, antidiarrheals
Runner's diarrhea	Clinical dx	See text
Inflammatory bowel disease	Sigmoidoscopy Barium radiography	Sulfasalazine, Mesalamine, glucocorticoids

Clinical dx = clinical diagnosis, exclusion = diagnosis of exclusion.
**Yersinia* is not sensitive to erythromycin.

the different strains of toxigenic *Escherichia coli* present in foreign areas. The best measures are preventative: encouraging travelers to avoid tap water, ice cubes, and fresh vegetables. It is best to drink bottled water or carbonated beverages and eat only thoroughly cooked or peeled foods. Bismuth subsalicylate (Pepto-Bismol, Proctor & Gamble) taken four times a day has been shown to be effective in preventing traveler's diarrhea, but such a regimen is impractical. The administration of prophylactic antibiotics to protect against diarrhea (e.g., ciprofloxacin or trimethoprim-sulphamethoxazole) is effective, but the benefit does not justify the incidence of side effects, and it is not cost effective. A better strategy is to counsel the travelers in preventive measures and have them carry an antidiarrheal agent and antibiotics in case symptoms arise. At the onset of the first liquid bowel movement, the patient should be instructed to take loperamide 4 mg once and ciprofloxacin 500 mg by mouth twice a day for several days. Loperamide 2 mg can be taken as needed several times a day. If the patient has persistent fever or blood is present in the stool, the patient should seek medical consultation.

LACTOSE INTOLERANCE

Lactose (milk sugar) is a disaccharide that requires enzymatic hydrolysis by lactase before it can be absorbed in the small intestine. Inherited lactose intolerance results when lactase is deficient, leading to carbohydrate malabsorption and osmotic diarrhea. Lactase deficiency occurs in 50% to 80% of adult African Americans and Asians and 5% to 15% of Caucasians. Typically, affected persons develop bloating, abdominal pain, and foul-smelling watery diarrhea shortly after ingesting milk products. Similar symptoms can be provoked in all people by the ingestion of nonabsorbable disaccharides such as sorbitol or mannitol, which may be found in medicinal elixirs and sugar-free products. Lactase deficient individuals should either abstain from lactose or use lactase supplements to enzymatically split the lactose into absorbable components.

GASTROINTESTINAL BLEEDING

Gastrointestinal bleeding is uncommon among athletes, with the exception of long-distance runners. Up to 20% of marathon runners have occult blood in their stools after competition when tested by the guaiac reagent. More sensitive assays for hemoglobin have shown that almost all long-distance runners experience occult GI blood loss. A much smaller percentage of patients will experience overt gastrointestinal bleeding either as hematochezia (bright red blood per rectum) or melena (black, tarry stool). It is not clear why runners experience gastrointestinal bleeding and other athletes do not. Two major theories are proposed. The first is related to intestinal ischemia. During marked exercise, splanchnic blood flow decreases 60% to 80%, and this may provoke a low-flow ischemia to vulnerable areas of the bowel, especially if patients become dehydrated and hypovolemic. The second theory suggests that bleeding is related to the trauma of repetitive footfalls and consequent jarring during running. This explanation is similar to that of runners' hematuria, which probably results from trauma to the bladder. Most episodes of bleeding are self-limited. There are, however, well-reported cases of ischemic colitis associated with running involving significant bleeding and, at times, colonic infarction requiring surgical resection. There is one case report of fatal hemorrhagic gastritis of unknown etiology that occurred in a marathon runner.

Evaluation and Treatment

All gastrointestinal bleeding should be interpreted in the complete clinical setting. Clinical decision making always begins with a good history and physical examination. Any athlete may suffer from organic gastrointestinal disease such as peptic ulcer, inflammatory bowel disease, or colonic neoplasm. As with any patient with gastrointestinal symptoms, if orthostatic hypotension, signs of peritoneal irritation, melena, or significant or persistent bleeding are present, the patient should be urgently referred for evaluation. The amount of blood loss, hemodynamic parameters, physical examination, and laboratory assessment dictate whether the patient should be admitted to the hospital or treated as an out-patient. Young, fit patients without any remarkable history who experience minimal blood loss related to strenuous exercise, particularly endurance events, probably can be observed without evaluation. Young patients with gross hematochezia are best evaluated by performing a flexible sigmoidoscopy. Almost all cases of hematochezia are benign and self-limited. Ischemic colitis is unusual and is usually self-limited. Occult blood loss needs to be interpreted on the basis of the person's age and risk factors for colon cancer. Patients younger than 40 with no family history of colon cancer probably do not require colonic evaluation. Older people and those with a family history of colon cancer should be evaluated with colonoscopy. Guidelines now recommend that if an average risk patient has had a normal colonoscopy without any colon polyps, another examination is not necessary for at least 5 years.

Athletes with iron-deficiency anemia should have serial fecal occult blood testing after light exercise and independent of exercise; if occult blood loss is present, evaluation is indicated. Bloody diarrhea with urgency, tenesmus, fever, and lower abdominal pain suggests colitis that is either infectious, idiopathic, or ischemic. These patients should be referred for evaluation and treatment.

Bleeding from the stomach or duodenum leads to melena, the by-product of bacterial degradation of hemoglobin as it passes through the intestine. Melena indicates a significant amount of upper GI bleeding, and the affected person should be referred urgently for resuscitation and evaluation (i.e., endoscopy).

EATING DISORDERS

Anorexia nervosa and bulimia are prevalent and serious problems among adolescent women. It is estimated that 5% to 20% of female college students suffer from eating disorders, and it has been suggested that participation in competitive athletics may contribute to the development of eating disorders. Anorexia nervosa is characterized by a severely distorted body image with pathologic fear of food and weight gain. Psychologic disturbances that often accompany anorexia include feelings of inadequacy and lack of control, perfectionism, interpersonal distrust, and maturity fears. Bulimia is characterized by episodes of uncontrolled binge eating, followed by vomiting. Affected women often have a pathologic fear of not being able to voluntarily control their eating or control their weight, have low self-esteem, and experience episodes of depression. Both disorders can seriously impair a person's health, resulting in malnutrition, growth retardation, electrolyte abnormalities, and even death.

Anorexia and bulimia are most prevalent among well-educated young women who are achievement oriented. Thus, it is found frequently among high school and college female athletes. One study analyzed the tendency toward eating disorders in three groups of college women: 1) nonathletes, 2) athletes in sports that do not emphasize thinness (swimming, track and field, and volleyball), and 3) athletes in sports that do emphasize thinness (ballet, cheerleading, gymnastics). The study found an exceptional preoccupation with weight or a tendency toward eating disorders in 6% of nonathletes, 10% of all athletes, and 20% of athletes in sports that emphasize thinness. Anorexia athletica is characterized by symptoms of early anorexia nervosa prevalent among young female athletes. The relationship between competitive athletics and eating disorders may not be causal, however, because specific sports may attract women who already have eating disorders.

Many athletes occasionally use vomiting as a form of weight reduction, such as a wrestler who has to "make weight." This is not classified as bulimia because these people do not have a morbid fear of becoming obese, nor do they experience uncontrolled binging. Persistent vomiting, however, even when not part of bulimia, can be harmful, leading to electrolyte abnormalities, myopathies, muscular weakness and esophageal laceration, bleeding (Mallory-Weiss syndrome), or perforation. Laxatives and enemas also are abused by some individuals as a form of weight control. Such activity is also associated with electrolyte imbalance such as hypokalemia and contraction alkalosis, which can lead to weakness, postural hypotension, and syncope.

It is imperative that coaches and physicians who care for young athletes, particularly women, be aware of the prevalence and severity of eating disorders. These disorders are easiest to treat when detected early, before they become serious. Furthermore, coaches can supply the ultimate motivation for these young people by not making inclusion on the team dependent on specific behavior or minimum weight. Conversely, misguided coaches who place competitive performance above the health and well-being of their athletes place additional stresses on these women, exacerbating the eating disorders and leading to serious consequences.

NSAID-RELATED GASTROINTESTINAL PROBLEMS

Nonsteroidal antiinflammatory drug (NSAID) use is common in the United States, mostly among people with arthritis, but also among athletes. This class of medication provides moderate analgesia and good antiinflammatory action appropriate for treating bruises, strains, and sprains. NSAIDs inhibit the production of prostaglandins that are mediators of inflammation and pain. There are more than 20 varieties of nonaspirin containing NSAIDs, several of which are now available over the counter. Acutely, aspirin and NSAIDs induce superficial gastric erosions (NSAID gastropathy or erosive gastritis) in most people, which are typically located in the antrum of the stomach. These erosions are not clinically significant and cause neither symptoms nor gastrointestinal bleeding. The gastric mucosa adapt, and the lesions heal spontaneously. When people take NSAIDs on a continuous basis for more than 4 to 5 days, up to 50% of users begin to experience symptoms of abdominal pain, dyspepsia, heartburn, and nausea. The presence of symptoms does not correlate well with significant mucosal abnormalities such as ulcers, and, conversely, patients with ulcers can be asymptomatic. Although short-term NSAID use can lead to superficial gastric erosions, chronic NSAID users (longer than 4 weeks) are at risk for developing significant peptic ulcers and their complications. Young, healthy patients who take NSAIDs intermittently have only a slightly increased risk of ulcer disease.

Concern about the gastrointestinal toxicity of traditional NSAIDs has led to the development of more selective medications. Standard NSAIDs inhibit both cyclooxygenase-1 (COX-1) and cyclooxygenase-2 (COX-2), isoenzymes involved in the production of prostaglandins. COX-1 is constitutively expressed and generates prostaglandins involved in the maintenance of the integrity of the gastrointestinal mucosa and platelet aggregration, whereas in areas of inflammation COX-2 is induced and leads to production of prostanoids which mediate inflammation and pain. Traditional nonselective NSAIDs are believed to act by disabling COX-2 activity, and the gastrointestinal toxicity results from inactivation of COX-1. A new class of NSAIDs that selectively inactivate only COX-2 enzymes theoretically should treat the pain and inflammation while reducing the incidence of serious GI toxicity of complicated ulcer disease. Two large randomized controlled trials have shown that the use of celecoxib and rofecoxib results in significantly fewer serious GI events than does the use of nonselective NSAIDs. It should be noted, however, that the mild symptoms of gastrointestinal intolerance were similar and patients at risk for cardiovascular disease lose the protective effect of the antiplatelet activity of traditional NSAIDs.

Evaluation and treatment of NSAID-associated symptoms includes identifying the indication for NSAID use and the other risk factors for peptic ulcer disease. Established risk factors for ulcer disease and their complications include prior history of ulcers, age greater than 60, concomitant use of corticosteroids or anticoagulants, higher dose NSAID use, coexisting serious systemic disorder, and probably *Helicobacter pylori* gastritis. For patients with self-limited inflammatory conditions, discontinuing the NSAID is the most effective treatment for relieving symptoms and healing mucosal disease. In patients taking NSAIDs simply for analgesia, acetaminophen or mild narcotics can be substituted. For people who have a chronic need for NSAIDs (e.g., osteoarthritis), treatment options include changing to an alternative agent (because symptoms can be idiosyncratic to a specific agent), reducing the agent to the lowest effective dose, administering NSAIDs with meals, or treating the person with antiulcer medication (see Table 8-1). Misoprostol and proton pump inhibitors are the most promising for the treatment of NSAID-associated ulcers when ongoing NSAID use is obligatory. A minimal amount of data is available concerning the treatment of symptomatic NSAID gastropathy, but antacid use as needed is the most cost-effective method. High-risk patients who require ongoing treatment with NSAIDs should be prescribed a COX-2 inhibitor or anti-ulcer prophylaxis with a proton pump inhibitor or misoprostol in addition to the anti-inflammatory agent. Symptomatic older patients and those at high risk for ulcers or with persistent symptoms require endoscopic evaluation.

Rarely, chronic NSAID use can lead to small bowel ulceration, chronic GI blood loss, and stricture formation. There are also reports of colonic ulceration and colitis induced by NSAIDs, but, again, these entities are uncommon.

ELEVATED LIVER CHEMISTRIES

Mild elevations of liver chemistries are commonly detected incidentally during routine examination with the use of multichannel analyzers and automated chemistry profiles. The most common pattern is the isolated elevations of alanine aminotransferase (ALT or SGPT) and aspartate aminotransferase (AST or SGOT) in an asymptomatic person. The history should focus on any prior liver disease, episodes of hepatitis, prior abnormal blood tests, rejection as a blood donor, hemolytic disorders, blood transfusion, intravenous substance use, alcohol intake, and medication use, including NSAIDs, anabolic steroids, and acetaminophen. Physical examination should look for icterus, stigmata of chronic liver disease, and hepatosplenomegaly. The most common etiologies for mild elevations of the AST and ALT are obesity, alcohol use, and NSAID use. Suspected medications should be discontinued and blood chemistries should be repeated in 3 to 4 weeks. Abnormal liver chemistries due to fatty liver require no treatment. Serologies to exclude hepatitis C and, less commonly, hepatitis A and B, may be appropriate in people with an unremarkable history and physical examination. Chronic hepatitis C tends to be an indolent disease, but it is increasingly being diagnosed. The mode of acquisition of hepatitis C is unknown in 80% to 90% of patients, but a number of affected patients will progress to chronic liver disease, so patients should be referred for evaluation.

Anabolic steroids, which are used by some athletes for muscle growth and strength, can cause a reversible cholestasis similar to that caused by estrogens. Chronic anabolic steroid use is associated with peliosis hepatis (blood lakes in the liver), hepatic adenoma, and malignant neoplasms. The use of these agents is to be discouraged, and they are banned in many competitive sports.

HELICOBACTER PYLORI

Helicobacter pylori infection of the stomach was first described in 1983 in association with chronic active antral gastritis. *H. pylori* is now recognized as the most important treatable risk factor for peptic ulcer disease, present in 90% and 60% of duodenal and gastric ulcers, respectively. Infection with *H. pylori* is common and increases with age to about a 50% prevalence in the United States among people 60 years old or older. The vast majority of these patients, however, are asymptomatic and do not have ulcers. For patients with ulcer disease and *H. pylori*, treatment to eradicate this infection is recommended to reduce ulcer recurrence (Table 8-3). Treatment of *H. pylori* has no proven benefit in patients with nonulcer dyspepsia and, at this time, is not recommended.

TABLE 8-3 Treatment Regimes for *Helicobacter Pylori*

Regimen	Duration
Tetracycline (500 mg QID)… Metronidazole (250 mg QID)… Bismuth subsalicylate (2 tabs QID)… A proton pump inhibitor also may be added…	10–14 days
Amoxicillin (1 gm BID) or Metronidazole (500 mg BID) and Clarithromycin (500 mg BID) and Omeprazole (20 mg BID) or Lansoprazole (30 mg BID for 10–14 days)	

BIBLIOGRAPHY

Borgen JS, Corbin CB: Eating disorders among female athletes. Physician Sports Med, 15:89–95, 1987.

Kam LW, Pease WE, Thompson PD: Exercise-related mesenteric infarction. Am J Gastroenterol 89: 1899–1900, 1994.

McCabe ME, Peura DA, Kadakia SC, et al: Gastrointestinal blood loss associated with running a marathon. Dig Dis Sci 31:1229–1232, 1986.

Mellow MH, Simpson AG, Watt L, et al: Esophageal acid perfusion in coronary artery disease: Induction of myocardial ischemia. Gastroenterology 85: 306–312, 1983.

Moses FM: The effect of exercise on the gastrointestinal tract. Sports Med 9:159–172, 1990.

Moses FM, Berer TG, Peura DA: Running-associated proximal hemorrhagic colitis. Ann Int Med 108: 385–386, 1988.

Peters HP, Bos M, Seebregts L, et al: Gastrointestinal symptoms in long-distance runners, cyclists, and triathletes: Prevalence, medication, and etiology. Am J Gastroenterol 94:1570–1581, 1999.

Peters HPF, De Vries WR, Vanberge-Henegouwen GP, Akkermans LMA: Potential benefits and hazards of physical activity and exercise on the gastrointestinal tract. Gut 48:435–439, 2001.

Riddoch C, Trinick T: Gastrointestinal disturbances in marathon runners. BJ Sports Med 22:71–74, 1988.

Silverstein FE, Faich G, Goldstein JL, et al: Gastrointestinal toxicity with celecoxib vs nonsteroidal anti-inflammatory drugs for osteoarthitis and rheumatoid arthritis: The CLASS study: a randomized controlled trial: Celecoxib Long-term Arthritis Safety Study. JAMA 284:1247–1255, 2000.

Smith NJ: Excessive weight loss and food aversion in athletes simulating anorexia nervosa. Pediatrics 66:139–142, 1980.

Wolfe MM, Lichtenstein DR, Singh G: Gastrointestinal toxicity of nonsteroidal anti-inflammatory drugs. N Engl J Med 340:1888–1899, 1999.

Worobetz LJ, Gerrard DF: Gastrointestinal symptoms during exercise in Enduro athletes: Prevalence and speculations on the aetiology. NZ Med J 98: 644–646, 1985.

9 Genitourinary Injuries

Adam J. Berman, Stuart H. Popowitz, and Harris M. Nagler

Participation in team sports and individual exercise for health and recreation has assumed increasing importance in our society. Aerobics, running, swimming, bicycling, racquet sports, and "pick-up" ball games can all produce significant physiologic stresses on the body by forcing the body to go from rest to intense physical exercise. In addition to these physiologic stresses and their effects, exercise may result in pathologic stress from falls, collisions with individuals or objects, and sudden changes in stress applied to joints, tendons, and muscles. The genitourinary tract is one of the many organ systems susceptible to the effect of these extremes. This chapter will review the potential effect of these physiologic and pathologic processes on the kidneys, bladder, and reproductive organs.

SPORTS-RELATED HEMATURIA

Incidence

The most visible sign of injury to the genitourinary tract of athletes is hematuria, either gross or microscopic. Gross hematuria in runners, the first reported exercise-induced urinary abnormality, was noted in 1793 by Italian physician Bernaedini Ramazziani.[23] Later, Collier in 1907 and Barach in 1910 reported similar findings in athletes following both rowing and long-distance running.[8,31] Hematuria subsequently has been reported as a consequence of a variety of sporting activities.

Hematuria in athletes has been well documented in contact and noncontact sports. Alyea and Parish[4] published an in-depth review of urinary findings in a wide variety of sporting activities. They found that 60% to 80% of all athletes had red blood cells, albumin, and casts in their urine after exercise. Surprisingly, there was no significant difference in the incidence of hematuria in athletes involved in contact as compared to noncontact sports; however, gross hematuria was more likely to occur as a consequence of contact sports. Thus, it appears gross hematuria is caused by direct trauma. The significance of direct trauma in inducing gross hematuria was supported by Boone et al. in a study of urine samples from football players. The incidence of hematuria paralleled the players' participation in games and was more prevalent immediately following game day. Of the 37 players who participated in this study, 60% had hematuria, 16% of which was gross.[15] All hematuria resolved with bed rest. A similar study by Fletcher reported the results of urine samples obtained from 15 hockey players immediately after a game, and 24, 48, and 72 hours thereafter. All players had some degree of hematuria that resolved within 72 hours.[32] Amelar and Solomon studied 103 boxers who gave urine samples before and after their fights. Microhematuria was noted in 73% of the boxers after their bouts. The only significant factor associated with hematuria was the length of the fight. Surprisingly, the location and number of blows to the flank had no predictive value. In fights that lasted less than six rounds, 65% of the fighters had hematuria compared to 89% of the fighters in bouts lasting beyond six rounds. Gross hematuria was found only in boxers whose fights lasted longer than six rounds.[5]

Hematuria can also result from noncontact sports. Again, the the presence of hematuria is directly correlated with the duration and intensity of the activity. Kachadorian, who exercised male subjects on a treadmill, originally documented this relationship. As the treadmill speed increased, so did the number of episodes of microscopic hematuria.[45] There have also been numerous reports on the effect of long-distance running on both microscopic and gross hematuria.[6,14] Fassett et al. reported that 69% of athletes completing runs of 9 and 14 km had hematuria.[31] Siegel studied 50 physicians with no preexisting medical or renal disease who ran the Boston Marathon. Of these doctors, 18% developed hematuria immediately after the race.[68]

Pathophysiology

There are several potential mechanisms by which sports-related hematuria may occur.The most obvious mechanism is direct trauma to the kidneys, bladder, or urethra. However, exercise also results in complex pathophysiologic effects on renal function that cause sports hematuria (Fig. 9-1). The kidney at rest receives approximately 20% of the cardiac output or close to 1200 ml/min. Renal plasma flow is approximately 700 ml/min. Thus, the blood flow to the kidney exceeds by three- to fivefold that to other metabolically active organs such as the brain, liver, and heart. When the body is stressed, the skeletal muscles, heart, and lungs require increased blood flow. As a result, there is a concomitant decrease in kidney and splanchnic blood flow. The renal

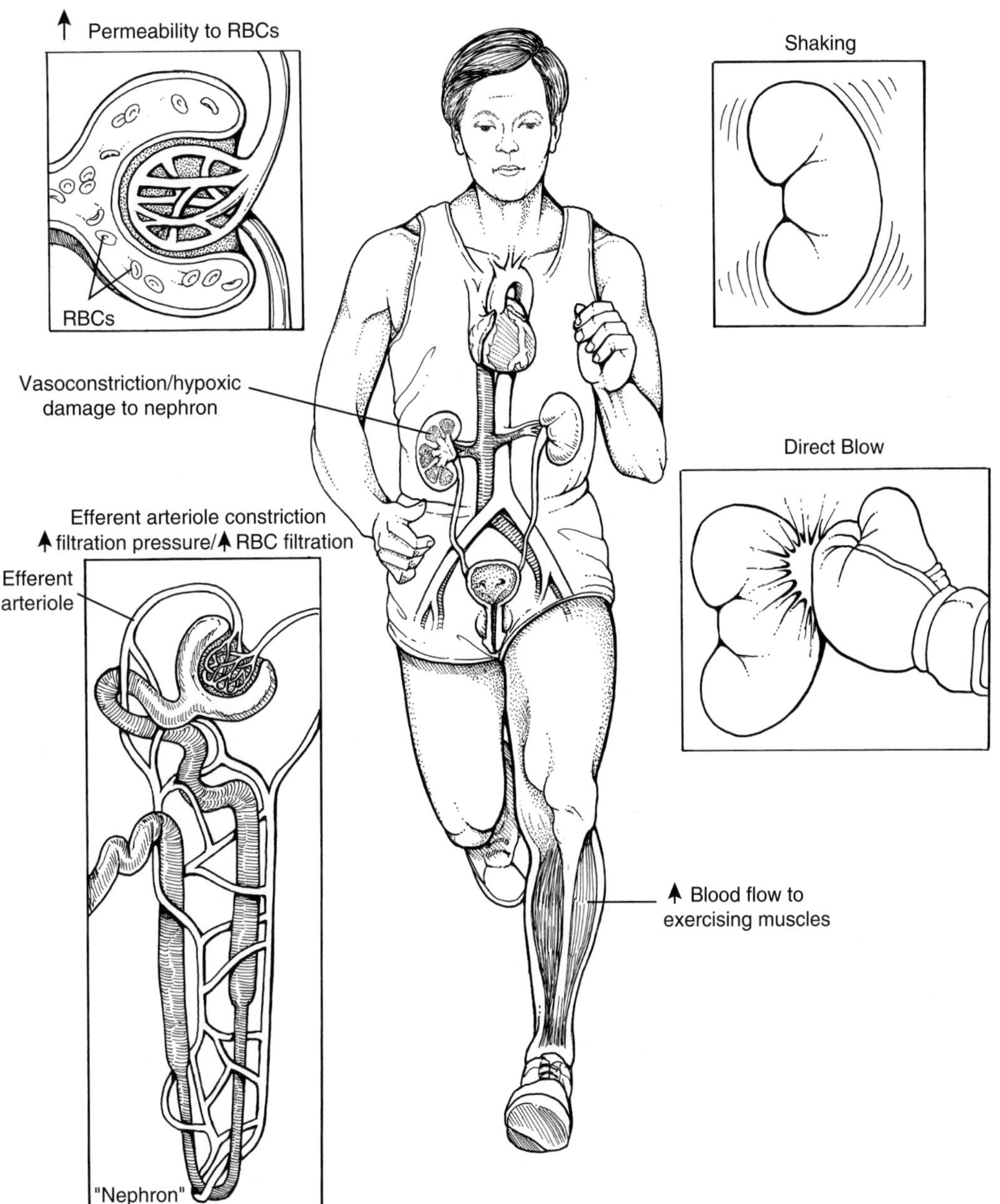

FIGURE 9-1. Mechanisms of sports hematuria in the kidney. (Modified from Abarbanel J, et al: Sports hematuria. J Urol 143:887, 1990.)

plasma flow decreases to approximately 200 ml/min.[46] The decrease observed is proportional to the intensity of the exercise. Poortman demonstrated that moderate exercise resulted in a 30% reduction in plasma flow, whereas heavy exercise resulted in a 75% reduction.[64] The decreased flow that accompanies vigorous exercise causes hypoxic damage to the nephrons, resulting in an increased permeability of the glomerulus, thereby allowing blood cells to pass through into the urine.[46]

Vasoconstriction also results from exercise and is a second pathophysiologic mechanism by which exercise may result in hematuria. Vasoconstriction resulting from exercise is more prominent in the efferent arteriole vasculature. This results in an increased filtration pressure, thereby producing stasis within the glomerular capillaries and allowing red blood cells to escape into the urine.[22] These physiologic hypotheses help to explain why 80% of swimmers, noncontact athletes, had hematuria compared to 55% of the football players in Alyea and Parish's study. Despite football's traumatic nature, the amount of exercise and physiologic stress involved in swimming is more profound.

Hemoglobinuria and Myoglobinuria

Not all exercise-associated hematuria, however, is an innocuous pathophysiologic response. The differential diagnosis of exercise-associated hematuria is identical to that of nonexercise-associated hematuria (see box, Causes of Hematuria). The physician must also be aware of two entities that present with red-colored urine yet fail to demonstrate red blood cells on urinalysis. The first is *march hemoglobinuria*. This entity occurs 1 to 3 hours after exercise in an upright position. Marching or running on hard surfaces results in mechanical trauma to the red blood cells in the feet. Hemolysis results, releasing hemoglobin which then binds to haptoglobin. The excess unbound hemoglobin is cleared into the urine, giving the urine a reddish appearance.[17,63]

Exercise myoglobinuria is the second entity causing red-colored urine without the presence of red blood cells. Exercise myoglobinuria appears 24 to 48 hours after the event and is the result of muscle fiber breakdown that releases myoglobin into the plasma. Myoglobin is readily cleared into the urine, resulting in the red discoloration.[27]

CAUSES of Hematuria

Kidney
- Acute renal failure
- Cystic disease
- Glomerulonephritis
- Hemorrhagic disorders: Hemophilia
- Hydronephrosis
- Infectious diseases: Tuberculosis
- Ischemia
- Neoplasm
- Pyelonephritis
- Renal calculus
- Renal infarct
- Trauma
- Vascular diseases

Ureter
- Neoplasm
- Strictures
- Trauma
- Ureteral calculus

Bladder
- Bladder calculus
- Cystitis
- Neoplasm
- Trauma

Prostate
- Benign prostatic hypertrophy
- Neoplasm
- Prostatitis

Urethra
- Foreign body
- Neoplasm
- Stricture
- Trauma
- Urethral calculus
- Urethritis: Sexually transmitted disease

The important complications of sports hematuria that demand medical attention include anemia and renal failure. Anemia has been noted in athletes who are involved in daily exercise.[18] Renal dysfunction may result from prolonged strenuous exercise in the heat. The resultant dehydration will further decrease the renal blood flow, which is already diminished in response to the exercise. This lowers the perfusion pressure below the critical threshold of the kidney, producing renal ischemia. Additionally, exercise results in muscle injury causing rhabdomyolysis and myoglobinuria, either of which can cause renal dysfunction by obstructing the renal tubules. Hemoglobinuria from intravascular hemolysis (march hemoglobinuria) may also contribute to renal dysfunction by causing tubular necrosis.[38] Adequate fluid replacement to maintain urine output is critical to prevent acute renal failure.

There are also concerns about hematuria as a result of exercise-enhancing supplements. The use of diet supplements to aid in athletic performance has gained a great deal of attention recently.[25] One such substance with great potential to effect the genitourinary system is creatine phosphate. During the initial stages of exercise, phosphocreatine is broken down in skeletal muscle to form creatine and ATP. This source of ATP provides energy during the first 10–20 seconds of maximal anaerobic exertion. This initial expenditure of phosphocreatine is quickly replenished once aerobic activity is activated. At this point a great deal of ATP and phosphocreatine can be generated. Athletes generally take 20 grams of creatine per day for one week, followed by 2 grams per day, with maximal benefit seen in high-energy repetitive workouts.[43]

Creatine phosphate supplementation has been reported to be associated with renal dysfunction. Urinary and serum creatinine levels do increase by up to 20% in some studies.[44] Concerns about hematuria secondary to nephritis are generally unfounded. Small studies have shown that this rise in urinary and serum creatinine does not impair renal function.[65] Only one case report exists in which a healthy athlete had an adverse renal effect from creatine supplementation. This individual had biopsy-proven interstitial nephritis after consuming 20 grams per day of oral creatine for 4 weeks, followed by complete resolution after discontinuation of the substance.[48] The current ACSM guidelines are that athletes with renal disease should avoid creatine, and healthy individuals must stay well hydrated while taking the supplements.[6]

Management

Management of "physiologic" sports hematuria begins with recognition of this condition. A careful history is of paramount importance in rendering the appropriate diagnosis. Any history of contact injury requires further diagnostic intervention in the setting of gross hematuria (see the following paragraph). In the absence of the potential for contact injury, the anxious athlete should be reassured of the benign nature of this process. In the acute setting, dehydration should be corrected. The initial consultation should consist of a proper history and physical, a urinalysis, and a urine culture. The urinalysis should be repeated 48 to 72 hours after the insult. A normal urinalysis will essentially exclude significant renal and urologic disease. If the hematuria fails to resolve, further investigation is warranted. Sports hematuria should never be assumed to be the cause of hematuria in an athlete, rather it is a diagnosis of exclusion. Radiologic evaluation and cystoscopy are reserved for persistent hematuria. Additional investigation for intrinsic renal causes is indicated if the patient continues to exhibit hematuria or a change in renal function.

No clear guidelines exist for the resumption of activity after an episode of gross hematuria. Some authors advocate bedrest until the hematuria has completely resolved. Most authors recommend that the athlete should not exercise until the gross hematuria has resolved; activity may resume if only microscopic hematuria persists. If all athletes adhered to the dictum that bedrest was required until hematuria resolved completely, numerous athletes, including possibly the entire starting lineup of your local football, lacrosse, or swim team, would be sidelined. It appears that as long as gross hematuria becomes microscopic hematuria within 24 to 72 hours, activity may be resumed without adverse sequelae.[1]

RENAL INJURIES

The growing participation in sports has resulted in the increased frequency and diagnosis of sports-related injuries. Abdominal and genitourologic trauma literature report that 5% to 10% of all trauma is related to sporting activities.[10,11,19,30,49,53,61,66] Sports-related injuries to the genitourinary system may be the result of blunt or penetrating forces to the chest, abdomen, pelvis, perineum, or external genitalia. Genitourinary injury should be suspected when gross anatomical pathology is apparent. The severity of the hematuria, however, has not proven to be indicative of the severity of the injury. In the absence of visible signs or symptoms, the recognition and subsequent treatment requires a fundamental knowledge of the mechanism of injury, the anatomy and pathophysiology of the organs involved, and the appropriate diagnostic tests and treatment.

The kidney and its vasculature are well protected in the retroperitoneum surrounded by the abdominal wall, abdominal viscera, ribs, and back musculature (Fig. 9-2). A significant blow to the abdomen or flank is normally necessary to cause visible injury. Organs adjacent to the kidney may also be injured when trauma is sufficient to injure the kidney. The left kidney, proximal ureter, and adrenal gland are surrounded by Gerota's fascia. Adjacent structures include the spleen, diaphragm, tail of the pancreas, posterolateral chest wall, lower three ribs, and descending colon. The right kidney, proximal ureter, and adrenal gland within Gerota's fascia are displaced approximately 1 to 2 cm below the left kidney by the liver and are in close proximity to the duodenum.

The kidney is the most common urologic organ injured from both blunt and penetrating trauma, and in certain sports such as skiing may be the most commonly injured thoracoabdominal organ.[66] The exact incidence of renal trauma due to sports injuries has not been well defined. The trauma literature for children and adults report an incidence of renal injuries due to sports of between 10% and 33%. A review of all urologic trauma in the Pacific Northwest by Krieger et al. found 184 urologic injuries, of which 154 injuries included the kidney. Of these renal injuries, 20% were directly sports related.[49] Similarly, researchers at the University of San Diego found that of 14,763 patients enrolled in the trauma registry, 3% had a diagnosis of renal or testis injury and 92% of these were renal in origin. In this study, only 4% of injuries sustained during team sports were renal injuries.[56] Bergqvist reported on all abdominal trauma over a 30-year period in Sweden and found that 29% of the injuries involved the kidney.[11] Renal trauma in children is related to sports activities in 10% to 25% of the cases.[19,40,53,61] Virtually every sporting activity has been associated with renal trauma and its consequences.[10,11,15,19,30,35,42,47,53,66,71]

Renal injuries are classified as minor (Grade I and II) or major (Grade III–V) based on the severity of damage to the parenchyma, collecting system, and vasculature. Minor injuries include contusions and perirenal hematomas (Grade I), and parenchymal lacerations confined to the cortex (Grade II) (Fig. 9-3). The kidneys are quite mobile within Gerota's fascia, and a direct blow to the flank or abdomen can cause parenchymal lacerations or contusions by compression of the kidney against the surrounding musculature or vertebral bodies.[24] The result of these contusions or lacerations is local extravasation of blood beneath the renal capsule. These injuries are not usually serious and complete recovery is expected. Infection of the hematoma is a rare late complication.

Major injuries, which are rarely seen in sporting events, include deep parenchymal disruption (Grade III) with extension into the collecting system (Grade IV), a vascular injury, or a shattered kidney (Grade V) (Fig. 9-4). These injuries are usually caused by associated fractures of the lower ribs or transverse processes. A severe laceration may extend into the collecting system or cause the renal capsule to rupture with subsequent development of a perirenal hematoma. The most violent injuries cause either avulsion or thrombosis of the renal artery and/or vein. Because the kidney is quite mobile, deceleration injuries result in the stretching of the renal vessels, producing a tear in the renal vein or intimal tears in the

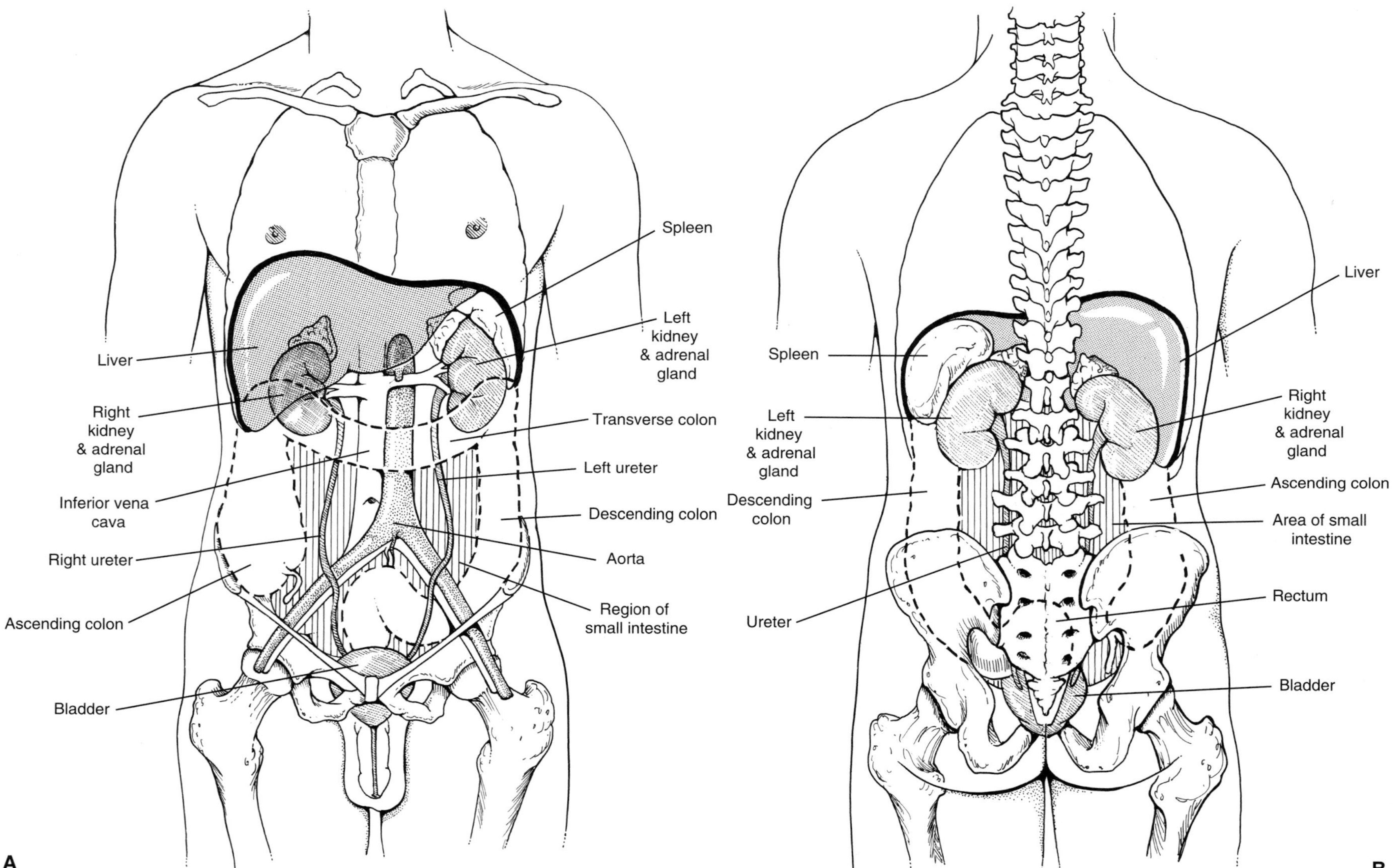

FIGURE 9-2. Anatomic relationships of the kidneys and ureters. **A,** Anterior anatomic positions of frequently injured organs. **B,** Posterior anatomic positions of frequently injured organs.

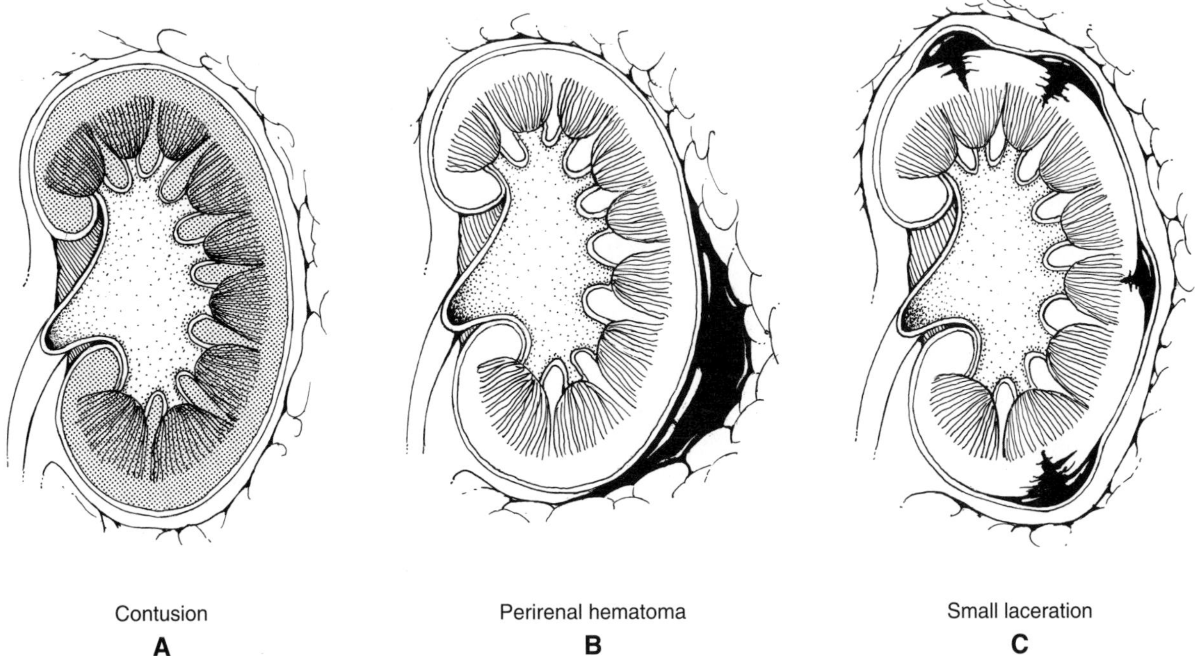

FIGURE 9-3. Classification of minor renal injuries. **A,** Contusion; **B,** Perirenal hematoma; **C,** Small parenchymal laceration less than 1 cm in length that does not extend into the collecting system.

artery with subsequent spasm and thrombosis.[28] Injuries of this magnitude usually require exploration and an attempt to salvage the kidney, depending on the status of the patient and the associated injuries. Unfortunately, these injuries may be overlooked because they may not be associated with hematuria.

It is important to realize that abnormal organs are more susceptible to injury. Thus renal cancer, ureteropelvic junction obstructions, renal cysts, horseshoe kidneys, and duplex or ectopic kidneys will usually require less trauma to cause significant injury.[55] The incidence of renal abnormalities in children is reported to range between 1% and 23%,[54] making children more likely to experience renal injury after apparently minor trauma. Furthermore, as discussed by Kuzmarov, children have less perirenal fat, weaker abdominal musculature, and proportionately larger kidneys relative to abdominal size when compared to an adult. Therefore, children deserve special attention, as they are more prone to renal injury after blunt trauma than adults. The child may also still have fetal lobulations that are more susceptible to parenchymal laceration.[51] This point was highlighted by Sparnon and Ford's article on bicycle handlebar injuries. In this report no child showed signs or symptoms immediately following the trauma. Subsequently, five children presented with severe renal lacerations requiring three nephrectomies.[71]

Evaluation begins with a history, detailed physical exam, and appropriate laboratory studies. Because the kidneys are so well protected by the ribs and surrounding musculature, the magnitude of force required to injure the kidney may also result in injuries to other organs. Associated injuries are observed in 60% to 80% of patients with blunt renal injuries and 90% of penetrating injuries.[28] Fractures of the extremities, injuries to the head, and lacerations of the liver and spleen are the most common concurrent injuries.

The most common presenting sign in renal injury is gross or microscopic hematuria. A minor renal injury may present without hematuria if the collecting system is not involved. However, it cannot be emphasized enough that the absence of hematuria does not exclude the possibility of a severe renal injury. A major injury such as an avulsed ureter or a lacerated or thrombosed renal vessel may also present without gross or microscopic hematuria. Dixon and McAninch reported that 19% to 36% of renal pedicle injuries have normal urinalyses.[28] The diagnosis of renal injury thus requires a high index of suspicion. Even without significant signs or symptoms, any injury to the lower chest, abdomen, or flank warrants attention to the genitourinary tract.

The signs or symptoms that may be associated with renal injury include a palpable mass, muscle tenderness or spasm, rib fractures, flank pain, or colic. Severe injuries may have similar findings; however, these patients are often in clinical shock and become surgical emergencies.

The initial diagnostic study in a stable patient should be a CT scan or excretory urography with tomograms. An abdominal film may show loss of renal contour or psoas shadow, a fractured rib or transverse process, bowel displacement, or elevation of the hemidiaphragm. Intravenous pyelography (IVP) will detect most major renal injuries, including diminution or nonvisualization

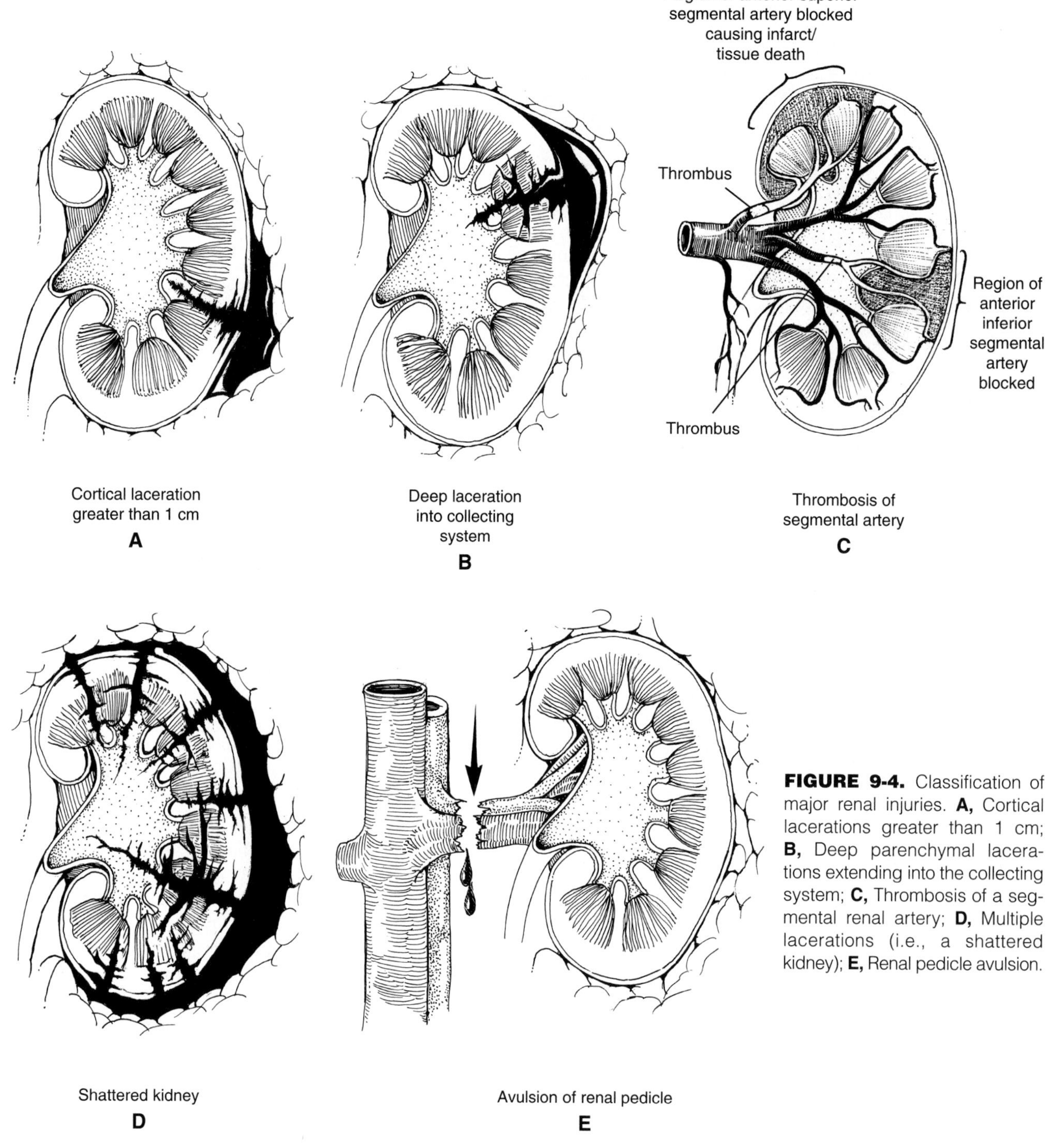

FIGURE 9-4. Classification of major renal injuries. **A,** Cortical lacerations greater than 1 cm; **B,** Deep parenchymal lacerations extending into the collecting system; **C,** Thrombosis of a segmental renal artery; **D,** Multiple lacerations (i.e., a shattered kidney); **E,** Renal pedicle avulsion.

of a portion of or the entire renal unit, pelvicalyceal displacement, cortical mass defects, or extravasation of contrast, but may not provide adequate staging information when expectant treatment is planned for high-risk patients. In fact, as many as 33% to 60% of IVPs may not be adequate to exclude a major renal injury.[28] In these cases, a CT scan of the abdomen and pelvis is warranted. Additionally, because patients with urologic trauma frequently have associated injuries, a CT scan is usually the first test of choice. The CT scan is more accurate in differentiating between minor and major renal injury (Figs. 9-5 and 9-6). Renal nuclear scans are of limited value, but may be used in patients with contrast allergies when there is concern about renal perfusion. Angiography is utilized only when there is evidence of a vascular injury severe enough to require surgical intervention in an otherwise stable patient.

The majority of sports-related trauma to the kidneys results in minor injuries such as contusions and small lacerations, which can be treated conservatively with

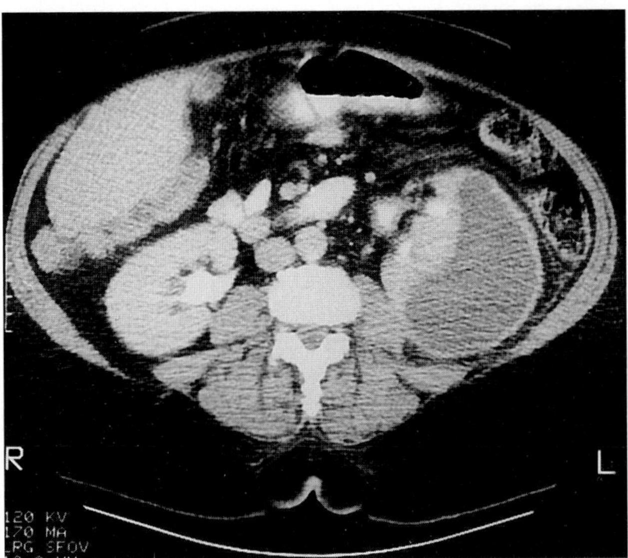

FIGURE 9-5. A CT scan demonstrating a large subcapsular hematoma.

bedrest and supportive therapy. The athlete with a parenchymal laceration should abstain from contact sports for 6 weeks with a repeat IVP at 3 months. Of patients with blunt trauma and minor injuries, 97% can be managed in this manner.[28] Surgical intervention is rarely required for sports-related trauma and is reserved for a major laceration, fracture, vasculature, or pedicle injury (Fig. 9-7). All patients with severe renal trauma should be followed at 3-month intervals with a urinalysis and an IVP for at least 1 year. Athletes with severe renal trauma should not return to contact sports for 6 to12 months, if at all.[23]

URETERAL INJURIES

Ureteral injuries secondary to external trauma are exceedingly rare, accounting for less than 1% of all urologic trauma.[26] The right ureter lies behind the duodenum proximally and the mesentery, terminal ileum, and appendix distally. The right colic, ileocolic, and gonadal vessels cross the ureter anteriorly. The left ureter lies behind the sigmoid colon, and the gonadal, left colic, and sigmoid colon vessels. The ureter, with its narrow caliber and retroperitoneal location, is surrounded by fat and muscle and is well protected from injury (see Fig. 9-2).

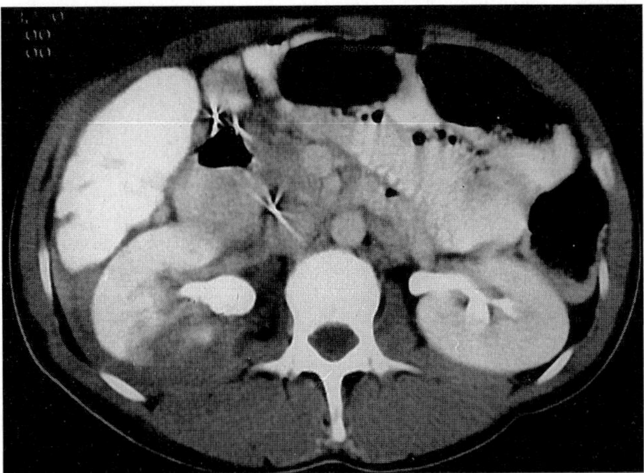

FIGURE 9-6. A 20-year-old male with right flank pain while playing football. The CT scan demonstrates a fracture of the posterior medial parenchyma of the kidney.

Ureteral trauma is most often the result of penetrating injury, rarely occurring from blunt trauma. Due to associated abdominal injuries and mechanism of the injury, diagnosing a ureteral injury is usually not an immediate concern. Signs and symptoms of ureteral injury are not specific but instead are common to abdominal, renal, and bladder injuries. An IVP is the study of choice for documenting ureteral injuries, followed by retrograde pyelography if the IVP is indeterminate. Abdominal exploration is often required due to the associated injuries. When ureteral injuries are diagnosed, they may be treated with urinary diversion via percutaneous nephrostomy or with endoscopic placement of a nephroureteral stent. Alternatively, if the ureteral damage is noted during exploration for other injuries, the ureter can be reconstructed over a ureteral stent. Nephrectomy is rarely necessary (Fig. 9-7).

BLADDER INJURIES

The incidence of bladder injury is also extremely uncommon in sports. The bladder is a pelvic organ behind the pubic symphysis. In children, the bladder assumes an abdominal position and, thus, is more susceptible to injury. The bladder is protected anteriorly and laterally by the pubic arch, supported inferiorly by the pelvic diaphragm and superiorly by the peritoneum and intraperitoneal structures. The superior surface of the bladder is in close contact with the uterus and ileum in the female and with the ileum and portions of the colon in the male. The base of the bladder is separated from the rectum by the uterus and vagina in the female and by the seminal vesicles, vas deferens, and ureter in the male (Figs. 9-8*A* and *B*).

There is approximately a 5% to 10% incidence of bladder injury in the trauma literature.[10,11,19,42,49,74] Bladder rupture is rarely an isolated injury, and associated injuries are found in 94% to 97% of the cases.[74] Blunt trauma accounts for up to 80% of all bladder injuries, with the remainder due to penetrating injuries. Although up to 80% of patients with blunt injuries to the bladder will have an associated pelvic fracture, only 10% to 16% of patients with pelvic fractures will have an associated bladder injury.[29,74]

Bladder injuries are classified as contusions, extraperitoneal ruptures, intraperitoneal ruptures, or a combination of both extra- and intraperitoneal ruptures.

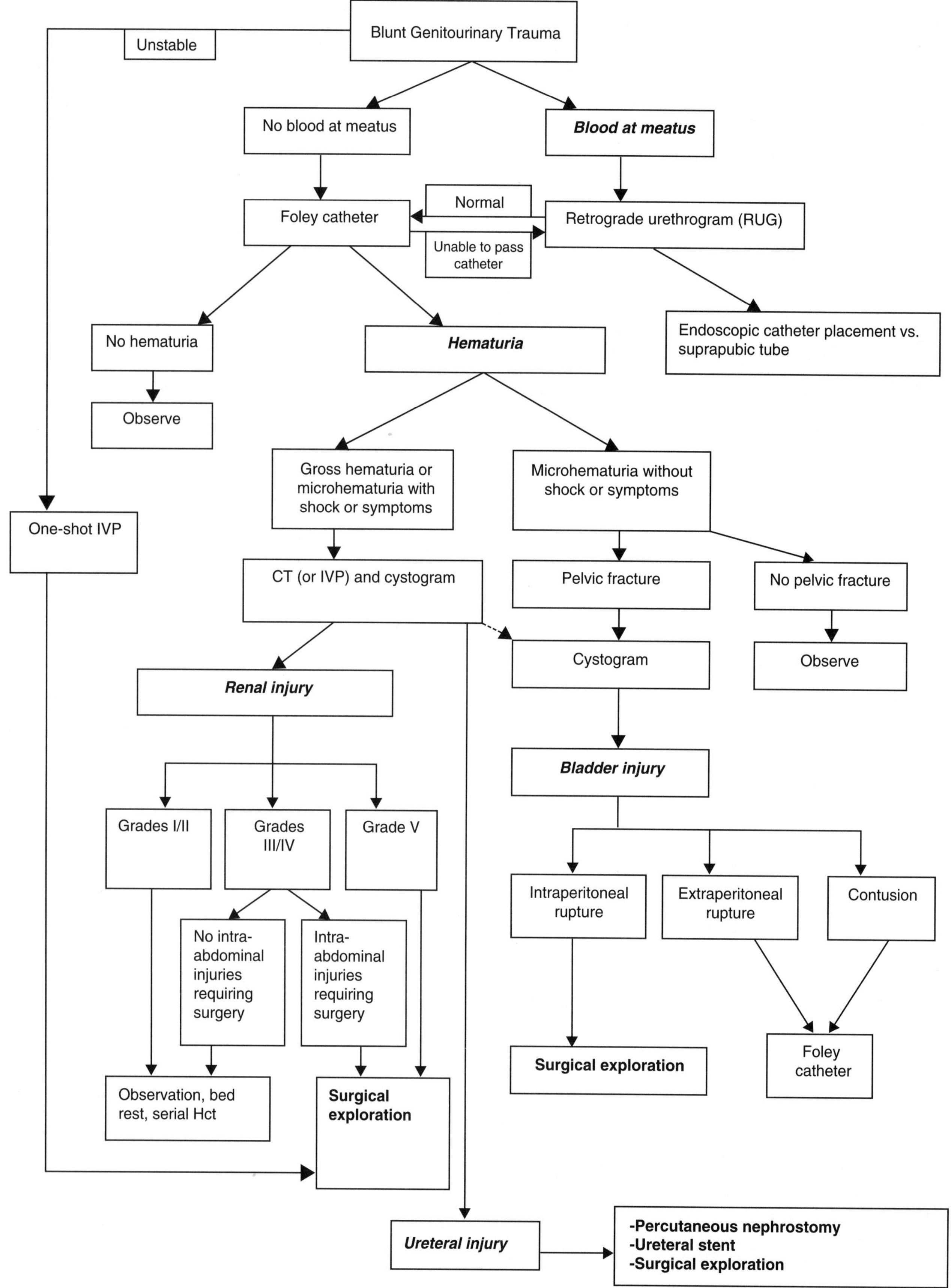

FIGURE 9-7. Renal trauma algorithm for sports-related injuries. (Adapted from McAninch J: Smith's General Urology, 14th ed. Appleton and Lange, 1995, p 315.)

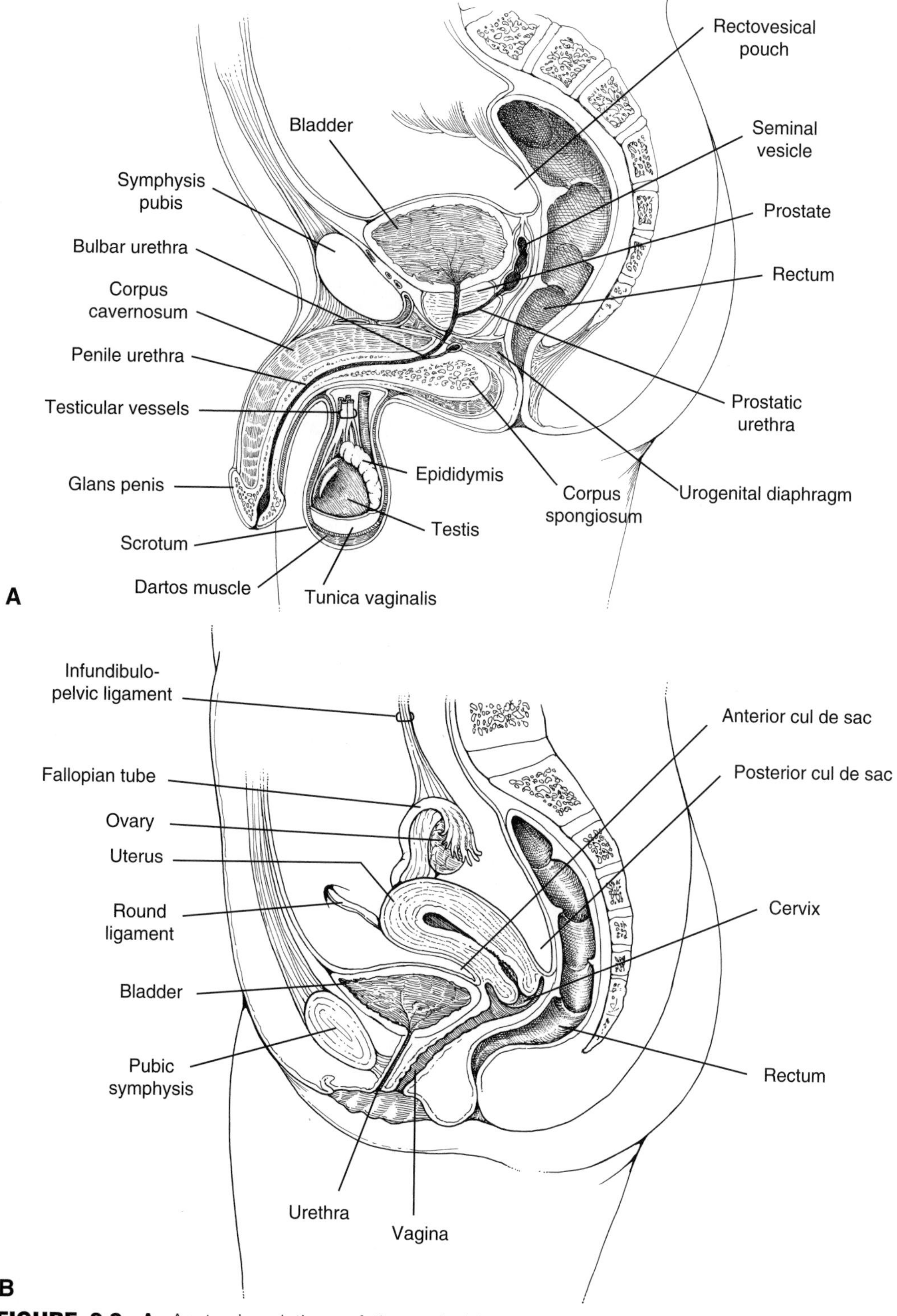

FIGURE 9-8. A, Anatomic relations of the male bladder, prostate, penis, urethra, and scrotum. **B,** Anatomic relations of the female bladder, urethra, uterus, ovaries, and vagina.

Extraperitoneal rupture is twice as common as intraperitoneal rupture, with both occurring in 12% of bladder injuries. Contusions of the bladder are diagnosed after the exclusion of more severe injuries in patients with hematuria and account for 45% of bladder injuries.[16]

The mechanism of bladder injury differs between adults and children. In the child, the bladder is an abdominal organ; in the adult, the bladder is a pelvic organ. Therefore, bladder injuries in children are usually intraperitoneal. Abdominal pain in a child after trauma may indicate a bladder injury.

Bladder rupture from blunt trauma occurs by three mechanisms. Intraperitoneal rupture may occur secondary to the hydraulic forces resulting from compression of a full bladder. The bladder thus ruptures at its weakest point—the dome. A direct blow to a full bladder may cause a bladder wall contusion and result in urinary extravasation into the extraperitoneal perivesical space or intraperitoneally. Pelvic fractures may result in the formation of bony spicules that lacerate the bladder and lead to extraperitoneal urinary extravasation. Additionally, shear forces may cause the ligaments attached to the bladder to forcefully disengage and lacerate the bladder.[74]

The diagnosis of bladder injuries may be delayed due to the associated major trauma. An inability to void is frequently observed. The first indication of a bladder rupture may be a nonpalpable bladder with absence of urine output after placement of a Foley catheter. Intraperitoneal urine will irritate the peritoneum, causing tenderness, muscle guarding, and abdominal rigidity. There may be ecchymosis of the lower abdomen, pubic region, or perineum. Gross or microscopic hematuria is present in 82% to 97% of the cases. Of patients with gross hematuria, 50% have significant bladder injuries compared with 2% with microscopic hematuria.[74]

A cystogram with a postdrainage film is the diagnostic test of choice in patients suspected of having bladder injuries. If a pelvic fracture is diagnosed on the basis of clinical findings or x-ray findings, a retrograde urethrogram should be performed to rule out urethral pathology prior to the insertion of a urethral catheter. After placement of the Foley catheter, the initial plain abdominal x-ray may show free air. A properly performed cystogram with instillation of up to 400 cc of contrast by gravity filling can achieve close to 100% diagnostic accuracy. The bladder should be completely filled, thus stretching the bladder and dislodging blood clots that may have sealed off a bladder tear. A postdrainage film is essential, and by itself will result in the diagnosis of small extraperitoneal ruptures in 13% of the cases (Fig. 9-9). Extraperitoneal ruptures are seen as "flamelike" or "starburst" areas of contrast extravasation. Another common finding is the "tear drop" or "spindle shape" bladder due to the compression of the bladder by a large pelvic hematoma (Fig. 9-10).[74] Intraperitoneal rupture will be demonstrated by contrast around loops of bowel within the peritoneal cavity. Contrast may also be visualized streaming along the "gutters" of the posterior peritoneum along the psoas muscles (Fig. 9-11). A CT scan, usually performed to aid in the diagnosis of the associated injuries, may demonstrate both intraperitoneal and extraperitoneal extravasation. Cystography is rarely warranted in patients with blunt trauma without gross hematuria, because the incidence of a significant bladder injury is less than 2% with microscopic hematuria.

The most common sports-related bladder injury is the bladder contusion. Cystography is usually normal or may demonstrate clots in the bladder. Generally, no treatment is required, although a urethral catheter may be placed if the patient experiences difficulty in voiding. Bladder contusions were first described by Blacklock, who noted characteristic cystoscopic findings in long-distance runners with hematuria, in whom no upper tract pathology was noted. Within 48 hours of the injury, bladder contusions appeared on specific areas of the dome and base of the bladder and the bladder neck. These observations suggest that the contusions are the result of the posterior bladder wall striking the base of the empty bladder. Running with even a small amount of urine to absorb the trauma can prevent this type of benign hematuria.[13]

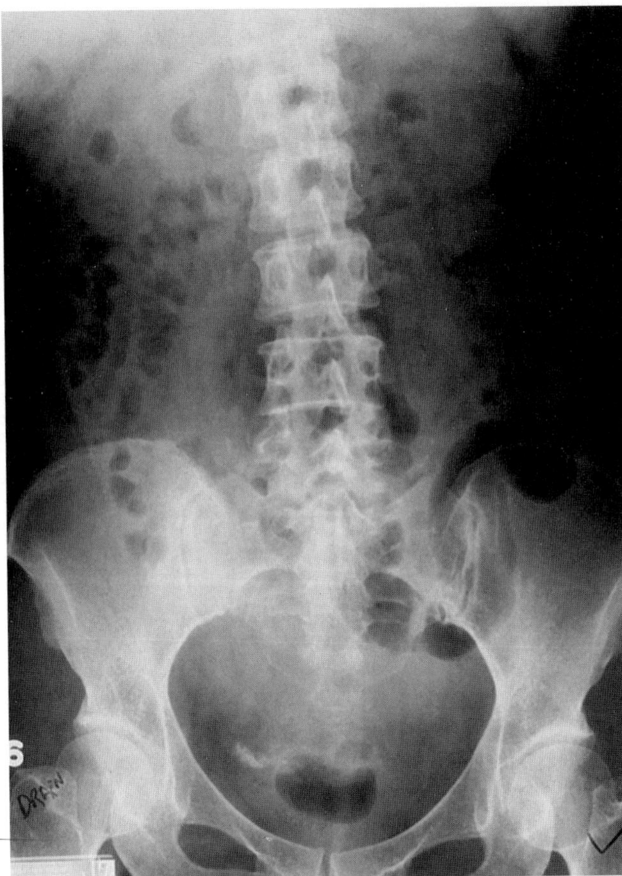

FIGURE 9-9. A posturinary drainage film documenting a small extraperitoneal bladder rupture.

Extraperitoneal bladder ruptures should be treated with drainage by a urethral catheter for 10 to 14 days. Intraperitoneal rupture, however, requires surgical exploration, repair of the laceration, and catheter drainage (see Fig. 9-7). If the patient is to undergo surgical exploration for associated injuries, an extraperitoneal laceration may then be concurrently repaired.[74] Bladder contusions require no treatment.

URETHRAL INJURIES

Urethral injuries are more common in sports than one would expect. These injuries are the result of straddle injuries to the perineum and are commonly seen in gymnastics, bicycling,[34,52,83] horseback riding,[33] and winter

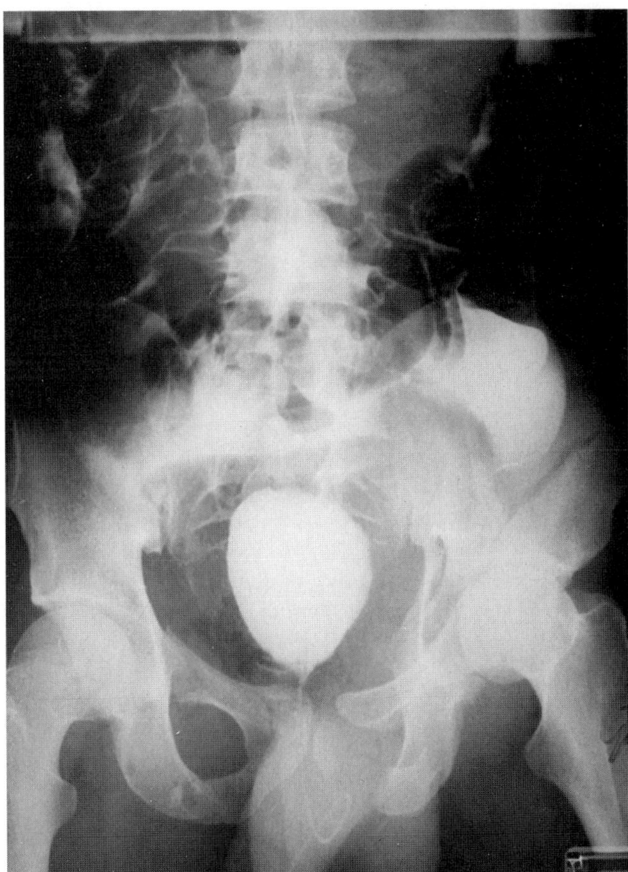

FIGURE 9-10. A tear-drop-shaped bladder resulting from the compression of a large extraperitoneal hematoma.

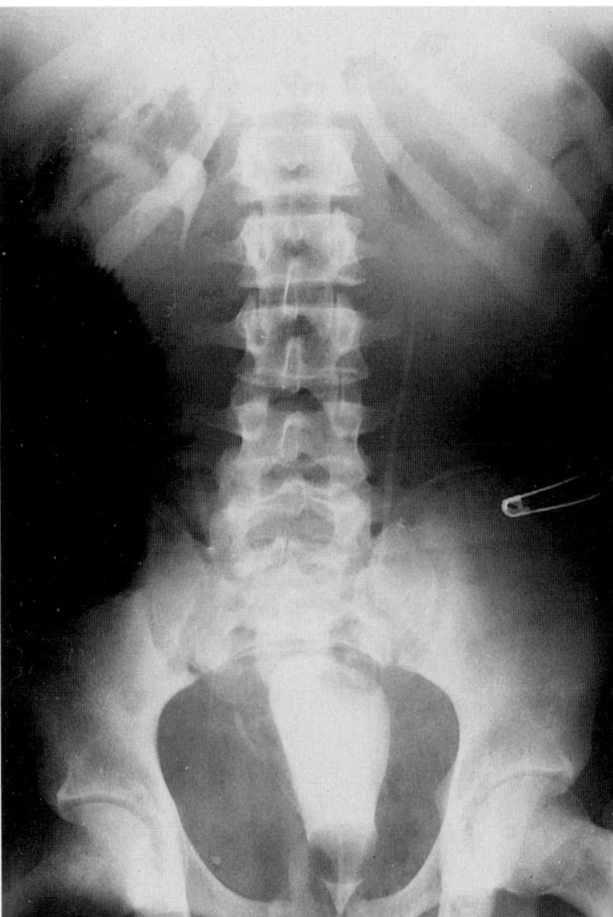

FIGURE 9-11. Intraperitoneal bladder rupture with contrast extravasating throughout the peritoneum. Of note is the pubic rami fracture.

sports accidents.[41,42,75] A urethral injury may present with blood at the urethral meatus or hematuria (see Fig. 9-7).

Males are far more likely than females to sustain a urethral injury. The male urethra is divided into anterior and posterior portions (see Fig. 9-8*A*). The anterior urethra is distal to the urogenital diaphragm, which surrounds the external sphincter. The anterior urethra includes the bulbar and pendulous or penile urethra. In spite of its mobility, the anterior urethra, which is contained within the corpus spongiosum, is most commonly injured by blunt trauma. In straddle-type injuries, the bulbar urethra is crushed against the undersurface of the pubic rami. Reports of even minor trauma to the urethra such as occurs from hard, banana-type bicycle seats can cause urethral pathology.[34,52,60] Hematuria is the common presenting sign to these injuries. Anterior urethral injuries can usually be avoided with proper use of genital supporters and protectors.

The posterior portion of the urethra is above the urogenital diaphragm and includes the membranous and prostatic urethra. The membranous urethra is muscular and comprises both smooth muscle and skeletal muscle that form the external sphincter. The proximal prostatic urethra enters the bladder neck that constitutes the internal sphincter. Rupture of the posterior urethra is usually associated with pelvic fractures. Significant shearing forces are required to tear the prostate and prostatic urethra from the fixed membranous urethra. These will not only avulse the urethra but may damage the erectile neurovascular bundles alongside the prostate, causing hemorrhage and potential impotence. Whenever a pelvic fracture is present, a urethral injury should thus be suspected. An inability to void, blood at the meatus, a distended bladder out of the pelvis, and a high-riding prostate gland on rectal exam are all indications of a posterior urethral injury.

The fascial planes of the perineum, penis, and scrotum help limit and delineate the boundaries of blood and urine extravasation that are associated with lower genitourinary tract injuries (Fig. 9-12*A*). The corporal bodies of the penis are surrounded by Buck's fascia. Colles' fascia is attached to the triangular ligament and fascia lata of the thigh and is continuous with Scarpa's fascia of the abdominal wall. Buck's fascia will limit urinary and blood extravasation associated with an injury to the anterior urethra to the penile shaft. The result is a

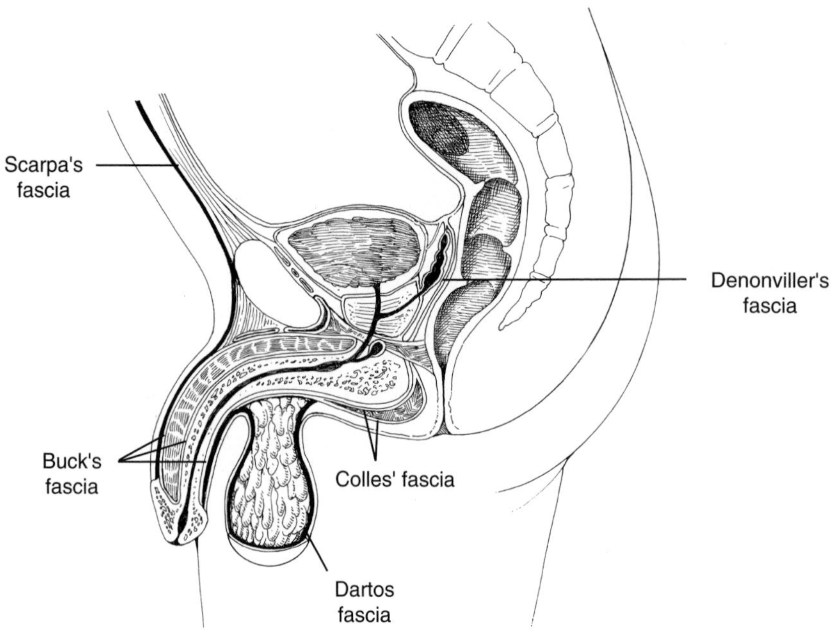

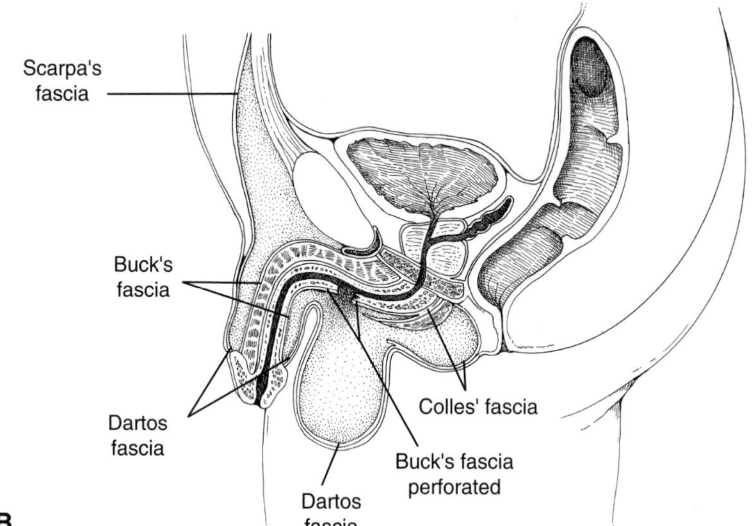

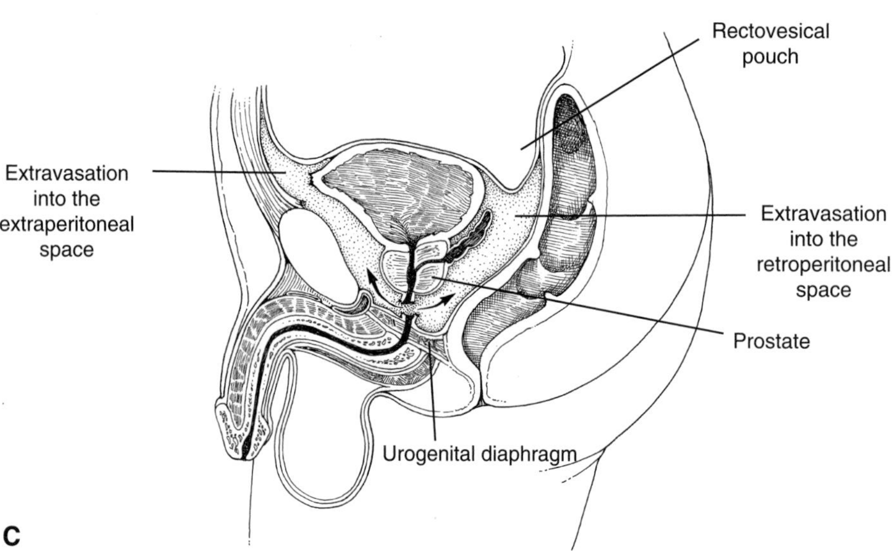

FIGURE 9-12. A, The fascial planes of the male perineum, penis, and scrotum. **B,** An anterior urethral injury through Buck's fascia will allow extravasation of blood and urine into the perineum, scrotum, and anterior abdominal wall being limited by Colles' fascia. **C,** A posterior urethral injury will be contained within the extraperitoneal and retroperitoneal space as long as there are intact fascial planes. The scrotum may be swollen if the extravasation extends along the spermatic cord into the scrotum.

swollen, ecchymotic, distorted phallus. Because of the strong fascial planes of the urogenital membrane, an injury limited by Buck's fascia is not usually associated with extravasation of blood and urine into the scrotum or perineum. If an injury to the urethra is severe enough to violate Buck's fascia, blood and urine may reach the perineum, scrotum, and abdominal wall, being limited only by Colles' fascia (Fig. 9-12*B*).

In a posterior urethral injury, blood and urine will be contained within the extraperitoneal or retroperitoneal space due to the strong fascial planes. With posterior urethral injuries, there should be no perineal ecchymosis unless there is disruption of the fascial planes. However, extravasation above the level of the membranous urethra may track along the spermatic cord into the scrotum, causing a swollen, ecchymotic scrotum without disruption of normal fascial planes (Fig. 9-12*C*).

A retrograde urethrogram is the most important diagnostic study to establish the presence of a partial or complete disruption of the urethra. Partial tears in the anterior urethra can be adequately managed with urethral catheter drainage; however, complete urethral disruptions will require placement of a suprapubic catheter and a formal repair at a later date. The widespread availability of flexible cystoscopy has enhanced the ability of urologists to traverse partial disruptions in an atraumatic fashion. Most authors favor delayed repair of posterior urethral injuries to allow for the resorption of the associated pelvic hematoma. With resorption, the distance between the two portions of the urethra is shortened.[21] Recently, there has been a renewed enthusiasm for primary repair of posterior urethral injuries. This is particularly favorable in patients with associated bladder neck or rectal injuries.[57] The long-term complications of the injury and the repair include impotence, urethral stricture, incontinence, diverticula, and fistulas.[54]

In the female, most injuries to the urethra involve lacerations from prolonged labor, instrumentation, or pelvic trauma. These injuries often go unrecognized, with the only presenting signs and symptoms being an inability to void or labial or vulvar edema. A successful urethral catheter placement does not rule out pathology. A cystoscopy is necessary for definitive diagnosis because a retrograde urethrogram may not be diagnostic. There have also been reports of urethral injuries in women with genital injuries during water sporting activities.[40,50,58,62] Urethral catheter drainage is usually sufficient treatment.[36]

GENITAL INJURIES

Male Genital Injuries

Injuries to the male genitalia are the most common genitourinary injuries in sports trauma, with an incidence of 10% to 15%.[3,20,42] With the increasing participation of females in sports, there will certainly be more case reports of female genital injuries. Genital injuries are the most anxiety provoking of all genitourologic trauma for many reasons. Because most injuries occur in children, teenagers, and young adults in whom sexual identity is evolving, it is most important that the physician must be prepared to deal with not only the injury but the emotional concerns of the individual.

The testicle lies within the scrotal sac consisting of skin, dartos muscle, and external and internal spermatic fascia, and is suspended by the spermatic cord that contains the testicular vessels (see Fig. 9-8*A*). The tunica albuginea is a tough, resilient capsule that encompasses the entire testicle. The tunica vaginalis, which was once continuous with the peritoneal cavity, surrounds the testicle, except posteriorly, where the epididymis attaches to the testicle.

Due to their mobility, the testes are not generally injured unless they are trapped against a fixed structure, as may occur in a straddle injury. In this circumstance the testicle is caught between a forceful object and the pubic bone or ischial rami. This is less common in the infant and young child due to the small size of the testicles. The right testicle is more often injured than the left, perhaps due to the higher position of the right testicle within the scrotum.[54]

Scrotal and testicular trauma have been widely reported in active team sports such as football, rugby, soccer, and baseball. Individual sports have also resulted in severe genital injuries. Children have sustained severe scrotal injuries on the handlebars of BMX bicycles while jumping over obstacles. Severe scrotal skin avulsion are more common in industrial or agriculture accidents, but may become more common with the expansion of motorized sports. These injuries are challenging. The exposed testicle may be repaired with split-thickness skin grafts.[72]

Testicular rupture may occur after forceful blunt trauma or penetrating trauma. The severe scrotal pain and swelling may make a physical examination very difficult to perform. Ecchymosis in the overlying scrotal skin or a hematocele or hematoma within the tunica vaginalis may be associated with testicular rupture or trauma. This renders palpation of the testicle very difficult.[67] Severe scrotal trauma may produce hematoceles, traumatic hydroceles, dislocation, contusion, and/or testicular rupture. Testicular torsion has also been attributed to testicular trauma, with approximately a 10% incidence.[54] One must also be aware that testicular tumors may present with scrotal pain after minor trauma. Therefore, patients with severe scrotal injuries should be evaluated carefully with ultrasonography and followed until the swelling and hematoma have subsided to be certain that there are no underlying testicular abnormalities.

Ultrasound examination, a relatively quick, noninvasive test, is extremely helpful in differentiating between contusion, hematoma, and testicular rupture.

If testicular torsion is suspected, a duplex ultrasound or radionuclide scan will provide a definitive answer in up to 95% of the cases.

Not all scrotal and testicular trauma is quite so dramatic. Adno reported on marathon runners who presented with perineal pain due to "jogger's testicles."[2] Vuong et al. observed perineal nodular indurations in cyclists that were referred to as "accessory" or third testicles. These developed from chronic microtrauma to the perineum and histologically consisted of pseudocysts with central areas of necrosis.[76] Mandell et al. discussed the "highball syndrome" seen in lacrosse players and other athletes. The resulting testicular trauma occurred because of perineal trauma causing a forceful cremasteric contraction that drew the testicle into the inguinal region. The athlete subsequently complained of inguinal pain that resulted from the testicle pushing against the external ring. The treatment was orchiopexy.[55]

Treatment of testicular injuries is individualized according to the history, physical, and diagnostic tests. Testicular dislocation that results from a severe blow to the scrotum displaces the testicle to the inguinal, perineal, penile, pubic, or crural regions. This can usually be treated by manual reduction and rarely requires exploration and orchiopexy.[55] A contusion of the testicle will tamponade within the hydrocele sac and can be followed, with return to physical activity as the signs and symptoms abate.

In all cases of hematoceles and ecchymosis of the scrotum after trauma, a ruptured testicle should be suspected. The diagnosis of testicular rupture can often be confirmed by ultrasound. Scrotal exploration is warranted in cases of testicular rupture.[67] A hematocele or contusion of the testicle presents minimal risk to the patient. Blood clots and necrotic or nonviable tissue should be removed and the remaining tunica albuginea closed over the defect. Ruptured testicles can be salvaged by exploration when accomplished within 3 days of injury. Morbidity and duration of bedrest are decreased with early exploration.[37] These athletes should not return to athletic participation until completely recuperated from surgery. Any injury to the testicle should be taken seriously because it has recently been reported that there is an unexpected increased incidence of infertility in men who sustained testicular trauma in adolescence.[59]

The penile shaft is composed of two cavernosa corpus and a corporus spongiosum that surrounds the urethra. The three corporal bodies are surrounded by Buck's fascia, a dense, fibrous layer of tissue. Each corpora cavernosum is separately attached to the pubic arch. This attachment along with the suspensory and fundiform ligaments provide fixation and stability to the erect penis. The corporus spongiosum surrounds the urethra and expands at its distal end to form the glans penis.

Most penile injuries are not sport related. The most common injuries are zipper injuries and fractures of the erect penis during a sexual act. There have, however, been various individual reports of sports-related penile trauma. Penile insensitivity and impotence have both been reported as a result of bicycling on a standard, narrow, hard leather seat. Both vascular and neural compression have been implicated in these cases.[39,70] Perineal trauma associated with impotence was reported in a young basketball player, who while descending after dunking a basketball, slammed his perineum into an opponent's knee. Work-up revealed a total occlusion of his deep and dorsal penile arteries from either an intimal tear or disruption of the vessels.[73] Weakening of the corporal bodies secondary to the trauma of horseback riding has also been implicated as a cause of impotence.[12] Finally, two soccer players in one report presented to the physician with partial skin thickness burns of the penis, scrotum, and inner thigh as a result of the soda lime used to mark the lines on the playing field.[9]

Trauma to the penis may affect one or all of the corporal bodies. The physical examination may show a subcutaneous hematoma. Penile deviation and swelling may be prominent and occasionally result in voiding difficulties. Urethral injuries coexist in approximately 20% of patients with penile trauma.[36] The physical findings are determined by the fascial compartments. With an intact Buck's fascia, ecchymosis will be limited to the penis, while violation of the fascial plane may allow extravasation of the hematoma into the perineum or abdomen, as seen with urethral injuries (see Figs. 9-12*A* and *B*). Cavernosography usually identifies the site of extravasation and the fracture. A retrograde urethrogram is performed if a urethral injury is suspected. The treatment is individualized. A skin injury can be primarily repaired. If the corpora and urethra have been injured, then a primary surgical repair is warranted.

Female Genital Injuries

Female external or internal genital injuries are rare occurrences in conjunction with athletics, and are associated with straddle-type injuries seen in horseback riding, bicycling, and gymnastics. These injuries include labial contusions or lacerations, clitoral tears, vaginal and cervical lacerations, and urethral injuries. A variety of genital tract injuries have also been reported in association with water sports, particularly waterskiing and jetskiing. These include injury to the cervix, vaginal lacerations, perineal lacerations, salpingitis, tubo-ovarian abscess, and incomplete abortion.[50,58,62] In one case report, Haefner et al. describe a vaginal laceration requiring pudendal artery ligation when a jet skier fell behind the jet ski and the full force of the jet nozzle was directed into the vagina.[40]

Because these patients are usually quite anxious and in a state of shock due to the tremendous bleeding associated with this injury, a sufficient initial assessment is usually very difficult. The patient may present with urinary retention requiring placement of a suprapubic catheter. Contusions or minor lacerations to the external genitalia can usually be controlled by manual compression. Deeper lacerations involving the vagina or cervix will require exploration and repair under general anesthesia. On exploration, the surgeon must be aware of the possibility of both rectal and urethral injuries. Urethral injuries can usually be treated with catheter drainage. Long-term complications include vesicovaginal fistulas and urethral strictures.

THE ATHLETE WITH A SOLITARY PAIRED ORGAN

Having reviewed the genitourinary system with regard to sports trauma, one is left with the question of whether the athlete with a solitary testicle or kidney should be allowed to participate in contact sports. All too often physicians are approached by athletes, their parents, and coaches asking for recommendations and advice on this subject. Whether the absence of the testicle or kidney is the result of a congenital malformation or due to a previous injury, there is always the possibility of injury to the remaining organ.

Historically, physicians have recommended that the individual with the absence of one of the paired organs avoid participation in contact sports. However, current epidemiologic studies of sports injuries, clinical experience, and changing attitudes toward sports have prompted most physicians to avoid this attitude and instead to provide informed counseling to prospective athletes and their parents regarding risks, equipment for protection, and sports alternatives.[69]

However, even today, a consensus at all levels of athletic participation is still lacking. To gain some insight into the attitudes of college team physicians and athletic directors, Mandell et al. conducted a survey of 40 major universities across the country. This study found varied philosophical and individualized opinions. First, there was a broad interpretation of what was a contact or collision sport. Only five universities had unrestricted athletic participation, and seven opposed any participation. Some schools required waivers to be signed by the athlete and the parents. Almost 80% of the respondents stated that they would advise directing the athlete with a single paired organ into an alternative noncontact sport. The authors concluded from the study that the single organ athlete can compete, even at the college level, as long as the athlete and parents are correctly counseled as to the dangers of possible loss of the organ in question and the appropriate protective measures.[55]

A more recent survey of close to 200 pedatric urologists showed that 68% of physicians would advise against contact sports for the athlete with a solitary kidney. When these results were further stratified, 27% strongly advised against participation, 30% advised against, with rare exceptions, 14% had no recommendation either way, 25% would allow participation, and 4% would make no restrictions. In this study, 88% of the respondents felt that the risk of renal injury in this circumstance is less than 1% and 8% felt that the risk of medical renal disease in this population is less than 2%.

When a child with a solitary organ wishes to compete in athletics today, several considerations must be addressed. The child and parents should first be counseled in the pros and cons of contact sports and if possible should attempt to direct the child into a noncontact sport. If the child still wishes to participate in contact sports, proper counseling regarding the use of protective equipment and close supervision are warranted.

As discussed in the preceding section, abnormal kidneys are more likely to suffer injury from otherwise innocuous trauma. Therefore, it is imperative that the normalcy of the solitary paired organ be assessed prior to participation in a contact sport. Although the possibility of loss of the organ in question is low, this complication and its consequences should be discussed with the parents, child, and coach. Those athletes with a solitary kidney or testicle and an anatomical variant, such as ureteropelvic junction abnormality, ectopic location, or a functional abnormality should not be allowed to participate in contact sports due to the increased susceptibility to injury.[55]

The overall incidence of genitourologic trauma in sporting events is low. In general terms, the prevention of serious urologic injuries, as with any injuries, includes proper athletic physical conditioning, use of protective equipment, and reliable supervision. Successful management requires prompt assessment, diagnosis, and treatment.

CONCLUSIONS

There are a myriad of mechanisms by which the genitourinary tract can be injured by athletic endeavors. Most injuries can be successfully managed when the diagnosis is entertained and appropriate diagnostic and management strategies are invoked in a timely fashion.

REFERENCES

1. Abarbanel J, et al: Sports hematuria. J Urol 143: 887–890, 1990.
2. Adno J: "Jogger's testicles" in marathon runners. S Afr Med J 65:1036, 1984.
3. Altarac S, et al: Testicular trauma sustained during football. Acta Med Croatica 47:141–143, 1993.
4. Alyea EP, Parish HH Jr: Renal response to exercise: urinary findings. JAMA 167:807, 1958.
5. Amelar RD, Solomon C: Acute renal trauma in boxers. J Urol 72:145–148, 1954.

6. American College of Sports Medicine: The physiologic and health effects of oral creatine supplementation. Med Sci Sports Exerc 32: 706–717, 2000.
7. Anonymous: The hematuria of a long distance runner. Br Med J 2:159, 1979.
8. Barach J: Physiological and pathological effects of severe exertion (marathon race) on circulatory and renal systems. Arch Intern Med 5:382, 1910.
9. Benmeir P, et al: Chemical burn due to contact with soda lime on the playground: A potential hazard for football players. Burns 19:358–359, 1993.
10. Bergqvist D, et al: Abdominal injuries in children: An analysis of 348 cases. Injury 16:217–220, 1985.
11. Bergqvist D, et al: Abdominal trauma during thirty years: Analysis of a large case series. Injury 13:93–99, 1981.
12. Bissada NK: Penile joint, (letter) South Med J 85: 1266–1267, 1992.
13. Blacklock NJ: Bladder trauma in the long-distance runner: "10,000 metres hematuria." Br J Urol 49: 129–132, 1977.
14. Boileau M, et al: Stress hematuria: Athletic pseudonephritis in marathoners. Urology 15: 471–474, 1980.
15. Boone AW, Haltiwanger E, Chambers RL: Football hematuria. JAMA 158:1516, 1955.
16. Brosman SA, Fay R: Diagnosis and management of bladder trauma. J Trauma 13:687–694, 1973.
17. Buckle RM: Exertional (march) haemoglobinuria. Reduction of haemolytic episodes by use of sorbo-rubber insoles in shoes. Lancet 1:1136, 1965.
18. Carlson DL, Mawdsley RH: Sports anemia: A review of the literature. Am J Sports Med 14:109–112, 1986.
19. Cass AS: Blunt renal trauma in children. J Trauma 23:123–127, 1983.
20. Cass AS: Testicular trauma. J Urol 129:299–300, 1983.
21. Cass AS: Urethral injury in the multiple-injured patient. J Trauma 24:901–906, 1984.
22. Castenfors J: Renal function during prolonged exercise. Ann N Y Acad Sci 301:151–159, 1977.
23. Cianflocco AJ: Renal complications of exercise. Clin Sports Med 11:437–451, 1992.
24. Coady C, Stanish WD: Emergencies in sports: The young athlete. Clin Sports Med 7:625–640, 1988.
25. Congeni J, Miller S: Supplements and drugs used to enhance athletic performance. Ped Clin N Amer 49:435–461, 2002.
26. Corriere JN Jr: Ureteral injuries. In Gillenwater JY (ed): Adult and Pediatric Urology. St Louis, Mosby Year Book, 491–497, 1991.
27. Demos MA, Gitin EL, Kagen LJ: Exercise myoglobinemia and acute exertional rhabdomyolysis. Arch Intern Med 134:669–673, 1974.
28. Dixon AM, McAninch JW: Traumatic renal injuries, Part 1: Patient assessment and management. AUA Update Series 11:274–279, 1991.
29. Dretler SP, Schiff SF: Urologic emergencies. In Earle Wilkins Jr (ed): Emergency Yearbook, 674–700, 1989.
30. Emanuel B, Weiss H, Gollin P: Renal trauma in children. J Trauma 17:275–278, 1977.
31. Fassett RG, et al: Urinary red-cell morphology during exercise. Br Med J 285:1455–1457, 1982.
32. Fletcher DJ: Athletic pseudonephritis. Lertter to the editor. Lancet 1:910–911, 1977.
33. Flynn M: Disruption of symphysis pubis while horse riding: A report of two cases. Injury 4:357–359, 1973.
34. Frey JJ: Banana-seat hematuria (letter). N Engl J Med 287:938, 1972.
35. Fujita S, et al: Perirenal hematoma following judo training. NY State J Med 88:33–34, 1988.
36. Gill IS, McRoberts JW: New directions in the management of GU trauma. Mediguide to Urology 5:1–8, 1992.
37. Goldman MS: Repair of shattered solitary testicle. Urology 24:229–231, 1984.
38. Goldzer RC, Siegel AJ: Renal abnormalities during exercise. In Straus R (ed): Sports Medicine. Philadelphia, WB Saunders, 1984.
39. Goodson JD: Pudendal neuritis from biking (letter). New Engl J Med 304:365, 1981.
40. Haefner HK, Anderson F, Johnson MP: Vaginal laceration following a jet ski incident. Obstet Gynecol 78:986–988, 1991.
41. Hildreth TA, Cass AS, Khan AU: Winter sports-related urologic trauma. J Urol 121:62–67, 1979.
42. Jakse G, Madersbacher H: Winter sports injuries in the urogenital tract. Urologe A 16:315–319, 1977.
43. Juhn MS, Tarnopolsky M: Oral creatine supplementation and athletic performance: A critical review. Clin J Sport Med 8: 286–297, 1998.
44. Juhn MS, Tarnopolsky M: Potential side effects of oral creatine supplementation. Clin J Sport Med 8: 298–304, 1998.
45. Kachadorian WA, Johnson RE: Athletic pseudonephritis in relation to rate of exercise. Lancet 1:472, 1970.
46. Kachadorian WA, Johnson RE: Renal response to various rates of exercise. J Appl Physiol 28:748–752, 1970.
47. Kleinman AH: Hematuria in boxers. JAMA 168: 1633–1640, 1958.
48. Koshy KM, Griswold E, Schneeberger EE: Interstitial nephritis in a patient taking creatine. N Engl J Med, 340: 814–815, 1999.
49. Krieger JN, et al: Urological trauma in the Pacific Northwest: Etiology, distribution, management and outcome. J Urol 132:70–73, 1984.
50. Kuntz WD: Water-ski spill and partial avulsion of the uterine cervix. N Engl J Med 309:990, 1983.
51. Kuzmarov IW, Morehouse DD, Gobson S: Blunt renal trauma in the pediatric population: A retrospective study. J Urol 126:648–649, 1981.

52. LeRoy JB: Banana-seat hematuria (letter). New Engl J Med 287:311, 1972.
53. Linke CA, et al: Renal trauma in children. NY State J Med 72:2414–2420, 1972.
54. Livine PM, Gonzales ET: Genitourinary trauma in children. Urol Clin North Am 12:53–65, 1985.
55. Mandell J, et al: Sports related genitourinary injuries in children. Clin Sports Med 1:483–493, 1982.
56. McAleer IM, Kaplan GW, LoSasso BE: Renal and testis injury in team sports. J Urol 168: 1805–1807, 2002.
57. Morey AF, Hernandez J, McAninch JW: Reconstructive surgery for trauma of the lower urinary tract. Urol Clin North Am 26:49–60, 1999.
58. Morton DC: Gynaecological complications of water-skiing. Med J Aust 1:1256–1257, 1970.
59. Nolten WE, et al: Association of elevated estradiol with remote testicular trauma in young infertile men. Fertil Steril 62:143–149, 1994.
60. O'Brien KP: Sports urology: The vicious cycle (letter). N Engl J Med 304:1367–1368, 1981.
61. Persky L, Forsythe WE: Renal trauma in childhood. JAMA 132:709, 1962.
62. Pfanner D: Salpingitis and water-skiing. Med J Aust 1:320, 1964.
63. Pollard TD, Weiss IW: Acute tubular necrosis in a patient with march hemoglobinuria. N Engl J Med 283:803–804, 1970.
64. Poortmans JR: Exercise and renal function. Sports Med 1:125–153, 1984.
65. Poortmans JR, Francaux M: Long-term oral creatine supplementation does not impair renal function in healthy athletes. Med Sci Sports Exer 31: 1108–1110, 1999.
66. Scharplatz D, Thurleman K, Enderlin F: Thoracoabdominal trauma in ski accidents. Injury 10:86–91, 1978.
67. Schuster G: Traumatic rupture of the testicle and a review of the literature. J Urol 127:1194–1196, 1982.
68. Siegel AJ, et al: Exercise related hematuria. Findings in a group of marathon runners. JAMA 241:391–392, 1979.
69. Smith NJ: Participation of athletes with one testicle (letter). Am J Dis Child 140:89–90, 1986.
70. Solomon S, Cappa KG: Impotence and bicycling: A seldom reported connection. Postgrad Med 81:99–102, 1987.
71. Sparnon AL, Ford WDA: Bicycle handlebar injuries in children. J Pediatr Surg 21:118–119, 1986.
72. Sparnon T, Moretti K, Sach RP: BMX handlebar: A threat to manhood? Med J Aust 2:587–588, 1982.
73. St Louis EL, et al: Basketball-related impotence (letter). N Engl J Med 308:595–596, 1983.
74. Thomas CL, McAninch JW: Bladder trauma. AUA Update Series 8:242–246, 1989.
75. Towers RJ: Complete transection of urethra: A urogenital ski injury. Rocky Mount Med J 74: 81–82, 1977.
76. Vuong PN, Camuzard P, Schoonaert M: Perineal nodular indurations ("Accessory testicles") in cyclists. Acta Cytol 32:86–90, 1988.

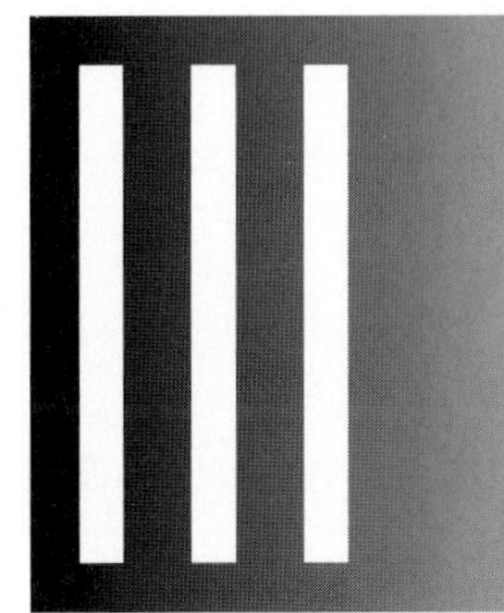

III Common Injuries

10 Wound Healing

Susan Craig Scott

GENERAL CONSIDERATIONS

Primary wound healing is the goal of management in all wounds; scar tissue composed of collagen is the material that the body uses to repair wounds. In optimal circumstances, the body is able to heal a wound in the predictable orderly sequence of events commonly known as wound healing. Certain local and systemic factors can influence wound healing. To the extent that physicians are able to control these factors, a durable healed wound will result.

Initial wound assessment begins with an accurate history and a careful physical examination. If the patient is able to respond adequately, he or she must be questioned carefully regarding the time and the mechanism of injury. The physician makes every effort to elicit factors that might influence the decision regarding how and whether to proceed with wound closure, such as severe contamination from a human bite or crush from a garbage compactor. With this accomplished, the physician taking the patient's history addresses questions of systemic factors—clotting abnormalities, diabetes, and immune compromise—that will influence how the wound and the patient will be treated.

Attention is then turned to the wound itself, which is examined for bleeding, contamination, and foreign bodies. Control of bleeding by local pressure is indicated. Local contamination must be eliminated before a wound can be closed. A careful inspection for shards of glass or pieces of dirt or gravel is done, and any other obvious contaminants are removed; this inspection is followed by vigorous irrigation.

Bleeding vessels ordinarily stop bleeding spontaneously as vasospasm and the formation of a platelet plug herald the beginning of the clotting cascade. Under certain circumstances, bleeding can be difficult to control. If a vessel is only partially transected and cannot contract adequately to allow the cessation of bleeding, or if a vessel is rigid with atherosclerotic plaque and is unable to contract sufficiently, persistent bleeding may be a problem. In both instances, although control is of the essence, clamps must never be blindly stabbed into a wound in an attempt to halt bleeding. This will injure tissue unnecessarily and add to the burden of debris that must be cleared for healing to progress. Pressure should be maintained until adequate help—sufficient personnel, adequate anesthesia, and proper equipment—is available. When these conditions are met, the vessel responsible for bleeding can be precisely clamped and irrigated or repaired as necessary. After bleeding is controlled, the wound is examined. Wound margins are inspected, and any crushed components are evaluated for viability; crushed tissue beveled edges and missing tissue present specific problems (Fig. 10-1). As the physician gains experience in wound management, he or she does not hesitate to debride severely crushed tissue, which will invariably be a source of contamination and a nidus for infection. The beveled wound requires attention to detail to coapt accurately (Fig. 10-2). Missing tissue requires a decision to allow for healing by secondary intention or to proceed with coverage (Fig. 10-3). The coverage decision is best made in conjunction with a plastic surgeon.

WOUND HEALING PHASES

Our current knowledge of how an acute wound heals has been broadened in the last decade by advances in molecular biology. The body's messenger systems, which direct the healing sequence, are now more fully understood. Although the five phases of wound healing overlap with one another significantly, understanding the process illustrates how the clinician can maximize the final outcome.

The five phases of wound healing are: 1) hemostasis, 2) inflammation, 3) cellular migration and proliferation, 4) protein synthesis and wound contracture, and 5) remodeling.[10] Skin penetration and the disruption of blood vessels is the initial event that signals, via vasoactive amines and epinephrine, the local vessels to constrict. Exposed endothelium in the vessel wall causes platelets to adhere, and these fuse and release elements that further the process of hemostasis and initiate the intrinsic and extrinsic cascade which results in clot formation. These messengers at the same time usher in the second phase, inflammation.

Within minutes of the initiation of hemostasis, vascular permeability, the hallmark of the inflammatory phase, is under way as gaps develop in the cells lining the blood vessels. Plasma begins to leak into the surrounding soft tissue, rapidly followed by polymorphonuclear leukocytes and monocytes to begin their work of clean-up of local debris and contaminants, including bacteria, in preparation for wound repair.

This process is overseen and regulated by those all-important mediators and wound generals produced by the accumulating platelets and transformed monocytes

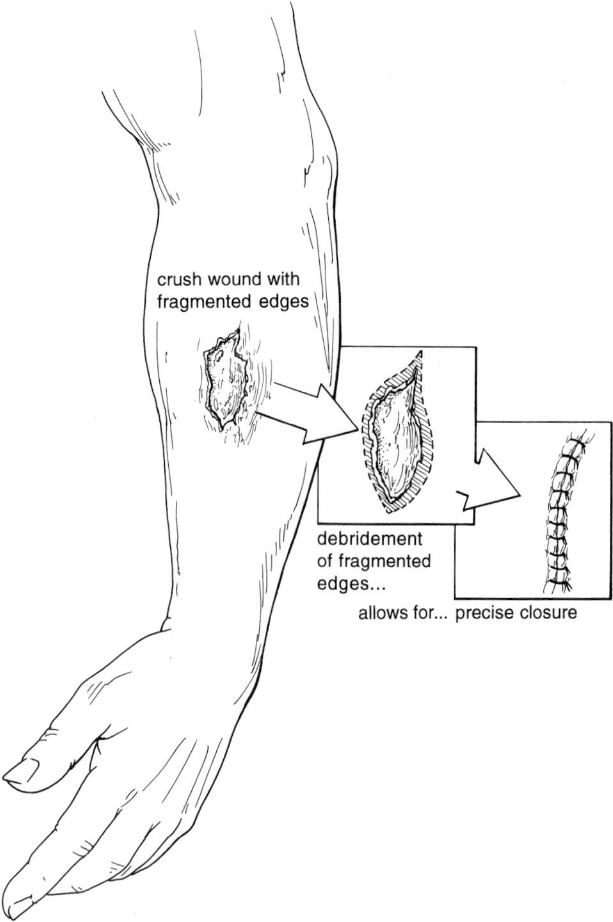

FIGURE 10-1. Crushed or damaged wound edges may be judiciously debrided to provide clear edges for suturing.

known as macrophages, cytokines. Cytokines are involved in virtually every phase of wound healing; these fascinating compounds coordinate the activities of different cell types, and can influence a single cell's activity in one direction or another simply by the concentration of cytokine in the reparative milieu.

As the inflammatory phase progresses, cells that are important for wound repair, such as fibroblasts and endothelial cells, begin to accumulate in the wound, initiating the phase of cellular migration and proliferation. Fibroblasts are stimulated to migrate by the activation of certain compounds on the walls of local cell membranes known as integrins, which must be switched on and active so that compounds that encourage cell migration such as platelet-derived growth factor (PDGF) and transforming growth factor-β (TGF-β) can become active.[11] In addition, the revascularization of the wound known as angiogenesis and the advancement of epithelial cells from the wound margin are both regulated by cytokines to effect wound closure. It is in this phase that local tissue oxygenation is crucially important, for proliferating cells consume oxygen 3 to 5 times faster than cells that are in a resting phase.

It is in this phase that T-lymphocytes play a crucial role as well; summoned by cytokines from the injured tissues, T-lymphocytes are required for their ability to destroy cells containing viruses and other foreign elements, and are the primary directors of cell-mediated immunity.

These first three phases of wound healing occur rapidly within the first five days after wounding. Toward the end of the first week, the predominant activity in the acute wound is protein synthesis, which is responsible for the strength of wound repair. It is in this phase of wound healing that surgeons are best able to see the clinical effects of a variety of illnesses, and is the phase that the clinician is best able to influence. The effects of impairment in patients' nutrition, technical details of wound closure, patient age, systemic illness, and medications are most evident in this fourth phase in which the building blocks of a healthy wound are formed and strengthened.

Wound contracture is affected by wound location; pretibial skin contracts much more slowly than the more lax skin of the abdomen. Although the clinician relies on wound contracture to minimize the areas of healing, and most times this process is beneficial, there are situations in which contracture is undesirable, such as wounds that cross mobile joints. In this situation, splinting during this phase of contracture, or skin grafting if necessary, can minimize the unfavorable effect of contracture.

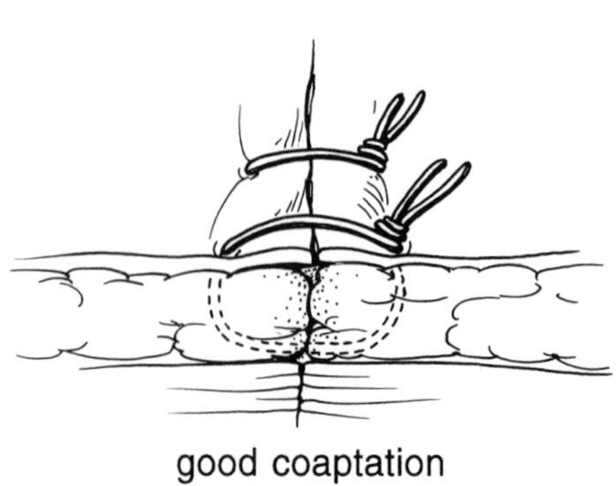

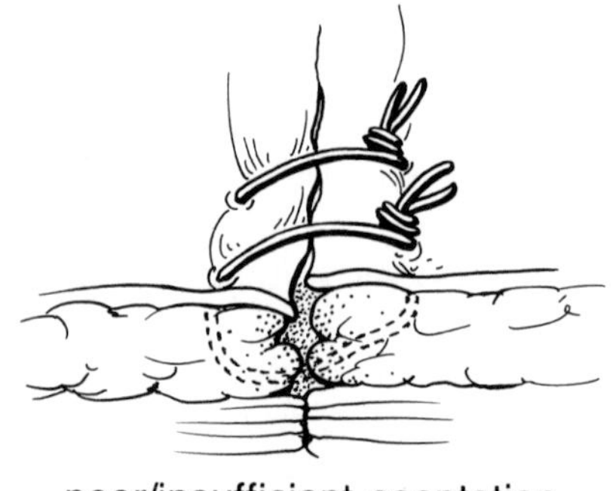

FIGURE 10-2. Perfect edge-to-edge suturing is necessary for most satisfactory wound healing.

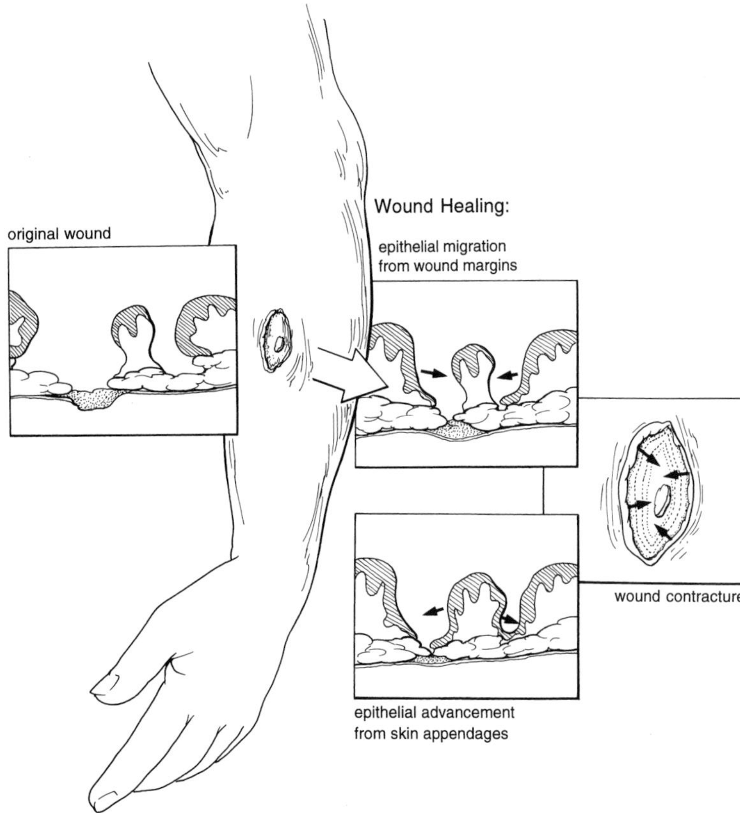

FIGURE 10-3. Healing by secondary intention proceeds inward from the periphery and outward from the center.

The final phase of wound healing, the phase of remodeling and scar formation is fully active by about three weeks after wounding as collagen synthesis and breakdown begin to reach a steady state. Embryonic collagen, type III, is gradually replaced by type I collagen and the multiple cross-links of this more stable and mature collagen forge a wound that can withstand mechanical stresses comparable with the strength of intact skin.[1,8] Although strength gains are greatest in these early weeks, the wound continues to gain strength for many months after injury as it responds to mechanical stresses placed upon it.

FACTORS THAT AFFECT WOUND HEALING

Although most wounds heal normally and uneventfully, a reason must be sought when healing does not proceed as expected. A brief review of the factors that influence wound healing is in order.

Wound-Related Factors

Local tissue oxygenation (pO_2, tissue partial pressure of oxygen) is the single most important factor in wound healing. It is poor local pO_2 that ultimately accounts for healing problems in irradiated tissue or in a patient with diabetes mellitus, peripheral vascular disease, chronic infection, and pressure sores.[7]

Interestingly, the fibroblast, which lays down the collagen for wound healing, is oxygen sensitive. Collagen synthesis requires a pO_2 in the range of 90 to 95 mm Hg; in patients on a normal diet with adequate vitamin C, the availability of O_2 to the fibroblast is the rate-limiting cofactor for collagen production.

Adequate local pO_2 depends on several factors. There must be adequate inspired O_2, and hemoglobin must be adequate in level and normal in structure to allow the transfer of O_2 on demand by local tissue. From this, it is easy to infer the types of systemic illness that may predictably interfere with O_2 delivery to healing tissue and, by extrapolation, interfere with wound healing.

Infection. Local accumulations of bacteria can overwhelm the body's ability to fight infection. Certain virulent organisms, such as beta hemolytic streptococcus, can cause greater damage in smaller numbers than less-virulent organisms. A bacterial inoculation of 10^5 mg per gram of tissue is necessary for infection with most organisms.[13]

Patient-Related Factors

Diabetes mellitus predisposes to poor healing of soft tissue because of impaired microcirculation, associated neuropathy, and predisposition to infection. Excellent control of blood glucose is especially helpful in delaying and decreasing these known complications of the disease and is essential when wound healing is critical in the postsurgical period.[12]

Nutritional Status. Nutritional status must be severely impaired, with a serum protein below 2 gm %, before any effect on wound healing is seen. Isolated nutritional deficiencies, such as the vitamin C deficiency that causes scurvy or severe elemental zinc deficiency, are well-known and commonly accepted causes of deficient healing. Interestingly, vitamin E, commonly touted as an aid to healing, has no known beneficial healing properties, and given systemically in large doses, it can lower the collagen accumulation and decrease the tensile strength of a healing wound.

Smoking. Smoking has been blamed as a culprit in wounds that fail to heal; its mechanism seems to be via the sympathetic nervous system, causing severe vasoconstriction that impairs the oxygenation of healing tissues. In addition, carbon monoxide present in inhaled smoke has predictable effects on the oxygen–hemoglobin dissociation curve, shifting the curve to the left and at the same time forming carboxyhemoglobin. The effect can impair local pO_2 levels enough to cause skin necrosis.[3]

Anemia. There is no evidence that hematocrit levels that fall to even 50% of normal levels significantly decrease the tensile strength of the healing wound. The crucial importance of local tissue oxygenation for adequate healing would argue that a low hematocrit level will at least delay wound strength gain, but the evidence for this is controversial.[4]

Medication-Related Factors

Steroid Administration. Steroid administration orally or by injection results in the arrest of the inflammatory phase of wound healing; wound macrophages, fibrogenesis, angiogenesis, and wound contraction are halted by the administration of steroids. Anabolic steroids and vitamin A can reverse this effect of steroids; although the exact dose of vitamin A is unknown, 25,000 IU per day orally or 200,000 IU of ointment applied topically is usually effective.[5,6] Vitamin A is an essential ingredient for normal wound healing; its absence impairs the macrophages' role in wound repair.

Chemotherapeutic Agents. Chemotherapeutic agents decrease the proliferation of fibroblasts in the healing wound; certain agents, such as Actinomycin D and Bleomycin, are more detrimental than others to the gains of tensile strength in a healing wound. The question of wound healing arises when chemotherapy is planned in the postoperative period. Timing is important: in general, when chemotherapy treatment is begun 10 to 14 days after surgery, there is very little long-term effect on wound healing.[2]

Growth Factors. Growth factors such as fibroblast growth factors and platelet growth factors are proteins that appear to play an enormous role in cell synthesis and division; they also play a role in wound healing and are responsible for attracting collagen-synthesizing fibroblasts into the healing wound and stimulating their proliferative and division. Growth factors are being used experimentally and with great success to heal open wounds, burns, and skin graft donor sites.[9]

SUMMARY

Circumstances that support satisfactory wound healing are known; the physician's role is to minimize those conditions that negatively affect the healing process. Careful attention to detail in wound care, careful history taking, and an accurate, current understanding of factors that might benefit the healing wound work to support this normal series of events.

REFERENCES

1. Chapman JA, Kellgren JH, Steven FS: Assembly of collagen fibrils. Fed Proc 25:1811, 1966.
2. Falcone RE, Nappi JF: Chemotherapy and wound healing. Surg Clin North Am 64:779, 1984.
3. Forrest CR, Pang CY, Lindsay WK: Dose and time effects of nicotine treatment on the capillary blood flow and viability of random pattern skin flaps in the rat. Br J Plast Surg 40:295, 1987.
4. Heughan C, Grislis G, Hunt TK: The effect of anemia on wound healing. Ann Surg 179:163, 1974.
5. Hunt TK: Vitamin A and wound healing. J Am Acad Dermatol 15(42):817, 1986.
6. Hunt TK, et al: Effect of vitamin A on reversing the inhibitory effect of cortisone on healing of open wounds in animals and man. Ann Surg 170:633, 1969.
7. Johnson K, et al: Tissue oxygenation, anemia, and perfusion in relation to wound healing in surgical patient. Ann Surg 214:605, 1991.
8. Madden JW, Peacock EF: Studies on the biology of collagen during wound healing. III. Dynamic metabolism of scar collagen and remodeling of dermal wounds. Ann Surg 174:511, 1974.
9. McGrath MH: Peptide growth factors and wound healing. Clin Plast Surg 17(3):421, 1990.
10. Monaco JL, Lawrence WT: Acute wound healing. Clin Plast Surg 30:1, 2003.
11. Monaco JL, Lawrence WT: Acute wound healing. Clin Plast Surg 30:6, 2003.
12. Morain WD, Colen LB: Wound healing in diabetes mellitus. Clin Plast Surg 17(3):493, 1990.
13. Robson MC, Stenberg BD, Heggers JP: Wound Healing alterations caused by infection. Clin Plast Surg 17(3):485, 1990.

11 Dermatologic Conditions

Robert S. Scheinberg

The athlete may get any of the dermatologic conditions seen in the sedentary individual. However, trauma, perspiration, and prolonged exposure to sunlight, cold, water, and protective equipment make the athletic patient particularly vulnerable to a number of dermatoses and neoplasms.

SKIN PROBLEMS CAUSED BY TRAUMA

Blisters, Erosions, and Scrapes

Repeated shearing force against a relatively small area of skin will cause epidermal separation and fluid accumulation. If such a blister breaks, a sensitive eroded area is uncovered, which may become a portal to secondary infection. A sudden shearing force will result in a scrape.

The best management is prevention of blisters with properly fitted equipment and shoes. The use of absorbent cellulose powder such as Zeasorb and absorbent acrylic rather than cotton socks decreases friction, as does petroleum jelly applied to the feet or areas of rubbing such as the thighs and nipples of runners. Incipient blisters can be covered with moleskin. Alternatively, tincture of benzoin or tannic acid soaks (use strong tea) can "toughen" the skin to prevent blister formation. If a blister forms and is intact, it should be drained with a sterile lancet or needle in several places and then dressed with antibiotic ointment and gauze several times a day. If the blister roof has been sheared off, peroxide or antiseptic scrub followed by antibiotic ointment and gauze will speed healing. Alternatively, several of the newer occlusive or semipermeable dressings (i.e., Duoderm, ConvaTec, Princeton, NJ; OP Site; Vigilon; Second Skin, etc.) can be used right over lanced blisters and erosions and, most impressive, over painful scrapes (such as the infamous "strawberry" on the thighs and buttocks of base stealers and on Astroturf burns) with almost immediate pain relief and accelerated reepithelialization.

Subungual Hematoma, Cauliflower Ear, and Talon Noir

Subungual hematoma, cauliflower ear, and talon noir all result from bleeding into or under the skin. The painful subungual hematoma is best managed by draining the blood through a small hole made in the nail by repeatedly twisting a 11 blade until it breaks through the nail or by heating a paper clip until it is red hot and then melting a hole in the nail. Pain relief is instantaneous, and the squirting blood prevents burning of the nail bed with the hot paper clip.

A cauliflower ear (Fig. 11-1) results from bleeding into the thin, subcutaneous space between the skin and the ear cartilage. The resulting hematoma organizes into fibrous tissue, which may calcify. Incision and drainage of the hematoma and pressure dressings should prevent the disfiguring sequelae. Recently, swimmer's noseclips applied over collodion-soaked cotton has been advocated as a simple way to provide constant compression on the pinna postaspiration of the hematoma.

Talon noir (black heel) occurs from repeated rapid movement of the calcaneal area against an athletic shoe. It needs no treatment but can be irregular and black, perfectly mimicking a malignant melanoma. Management consists of making an accurate diagnosis by paring away the surface of the skin and finding the pigment removed (chronic subungual hematoma can also mimic a subungual melanoma). If diagnosis is in doubt, drill through the nail and hematest the black material. Melanin will be negative, whereas dried blood will be strongly positive. Tache noir is a similar black hemorrhagic lesion on the palms of weight lifters, gymnasts, golfers, baseball and tennis players, and mountain and rock climbers.

Corns and Callouses

Corns and callouses consist of thickened stratum corneum. Callouses are nontender and show the dermatoglyphic skin markings on the surface. They result as an adaptation to repeated shearing forces on the skin surface not strong enough to cause blisters, erosions, or scrapes. They need not be treated except for cosmetic reasons, and there is no reason to change shoes because large callouses have formed. Corns, also known as clavi, are tender compactions of stratum corneum resulting from compression of skin or callous between two unyielding surfaces. Paring a tender area of thickened skin (most typically under a prominent metatarsal head) reveals a translucent yellowish "kernel," which can be further

---

Text and illustrations adapted with permission from Scheinberg RS: Exercise-related skin infection: Managing bacterial disease. Phys Sports Med 22(6): 47–58, 1994; and Scheinberg RS: Stopping skin assailants: Fungi, yeast and viruses. Phys Sports Med 22(7):33–39, 1994.

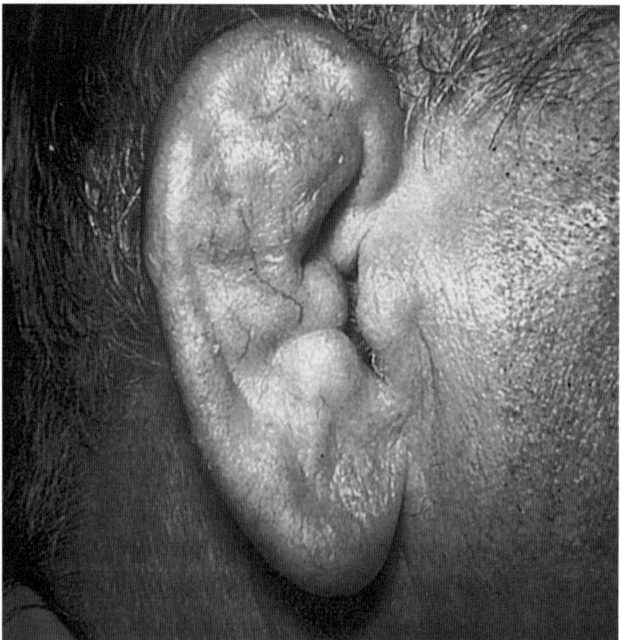

FIGURE 11-1. Cauliflower ear.

pared away to give pain relief. Repeated parings or the use of corn plasters (40% salicylic acid; Trans-vers-sal, Tsumura Medical, Shakopee, MN; or Trans-Plantar, Tsumura Medical) or keratolytics such as 20–40% urea cream can make the area asymptomatic, but frequently new shoes or orthotics are needed to change the biomechanics of the area so the corns will not reform. Very painful and unresponsive corns may require surgery to realign foot bones. Collagen also can be injected as a cushion around a prominent metatarsal head, but the resulting pain relief usually lasts for only 4 to 12 months until the collagen is metabolized.

Fibrous Nodules

Fibrous nodules are firm bumps that feel like part of the skin but are elevated and are frequently a red or brown color. They result from repeated blunt trauma which causes dermal fibroblasts to produce more collagen. They are seen most frequently on the shins (usually termed *dermatofibromas*) and on the knuckles, dorsal feet, and sacral areas. Depending on the sport, they have been called surfer's nodules, knuckle pads, foot bumps, and rower's bumps. No treatment is necessary, but the nodules sometimes persist long after the activity is stopped, making knowledge of a patient's past athletic activities helpful in arriving at the proper diagnosis.

Piezogenic Papules

Piezogenic papules are smooth, dome-shaped 2–10 mm skin-colored papules extending outward from the lateral and medial skin of the heel, which may be asymptomatic or painful. They consist of herniations of subcutaneous fat through the fibrous band of connective tissue surrounding the heel that stretch the overlying skin. Painful piezogenic papules can be treated with heel cups and taping to push the fat back through the herniations. Unfortunately, this treatment is not always successful and surgical procedures have not been developed to correct the problem. The athlete who cannot run because of the pain may have to take up cycling or swimming.

Frostbite

As a response to cold, cutaneous blood vessels constrict and shunt blood away from the skin in an attempt to keep up the core body temperature. Ice crystals form in the extracellular space, dehydrating the cells and resulting in irreversible injury. Wind accelerates heat loss from the skin, as does direct contact with metal (such as a ski pole). If clothing is saturated with perspiration, it loses most of its insulating properties, so covered areas can experience severe cold injury.

The clinical signs of mild frostbite (also called frostnip) include a grayish white color to the skin and loss of sensation. Frostnip occurs most commonly on the nose, cheeks, hands, and feet. Once the diagnosis is made, the affected skin should be rewarmed rapidly as long as it is certain that the area will not be exposed again to the cold. The rewarming can be done with tepid soaks or warm body parts applied to the frostnipped skin. The area will become warm and swollen and frequently severely painful, requiring analgesia. Blisters may form in 12 to 24 hours, and throbbing and burning may persist for days to weeks. Ultimately, healing is almost always complete with minimal scarring or functional impairment; however, deep frostbite is analogous to a third-degree burn with full-thickness loss of skin and possible damage to underlying muscle and bone, sometimes requiring amputation. Initial management is the same as for frostnip, but the area frequently remains anesthetic, indicating irreversible nerve damage, and the patient should be transported to the hospital immediately.

SKIN PROBLEMS CAUSED BY INFECTIOUS AGENTS

Heat and humidity are increased on the skin surface of athletes because exertion causes increased blood temperature, dilated cutaneous blood vessels, and copious sweating. The occlusion caused by uniforms, pads, and footwear worn for prolonged periods of time; direct contact with competitors; and cuts and abrasions on the skin surface create an almost ideal environment for bacterial proliferation and invasion of the skin. The most common cutaneous bacterial infections are those caused by *Staphylococcus aureus*, beta hemolytic *streptococcus*, and gram negative rods. These infections vary in clinical appearance and symptoms, depending on the part of the skin infected, the extent of the infection, and whether the athlete irritates the area by continued sports participation.

The best management is preventive measures such as loose-fitting clothing of breathable fabric changed frequently when saturated, dusting powder or antiinfective creams applied prophylactically before exercise, and blow-drying moist skin surfaces after exercise.

If an infection is suspected, it is best to make a precise diagnosis by means of wet mount, fungal and yeast, or bacterial culture. However, intertrigo, which is macerated and very malodorous, frequently consists of a mixed infection, and the best treatment is to dry the area with cool compresses such as acetic acid (one part vinegar to ten parts water) or Burow's solution, followed by blow-drying the area until it is no longer sticky, and applying antiseptic solutions such as povidine.

Dermatophytic and other fungal conditions such as athlete's foot, jock itch, and related infections cause much discomfort, but they usually respond well to treatment and prevention. However, skin lesions caused by viruses such as herpes simplex, herpes zoster, warts, and molluscum contagiosum can be tougher to manage because they often require long-term therapy and activity restrictions.

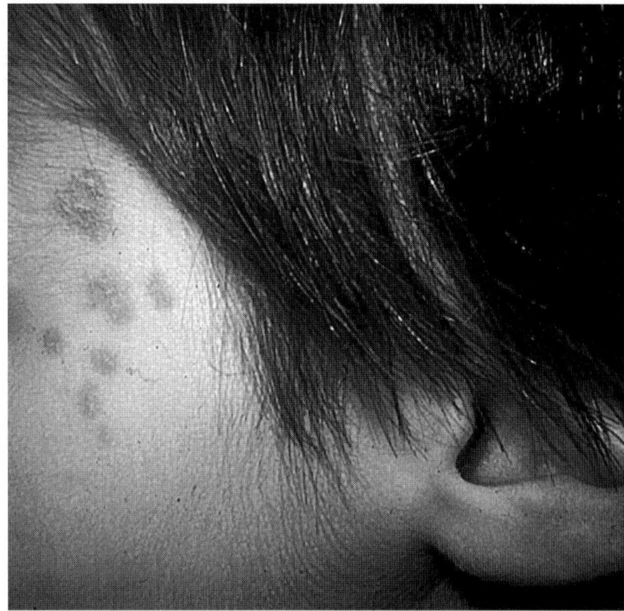

FIGURE 11-2. This variation of impetigo appears as vesicles and bullae on this patient's cheek. (From Scheinberg R: Exercise-related skin infection: Managing bacterial diseases. Phys Sports Med 1994.)

Bacterial Infections

Impetigo and Ecthyma. Impetigo consists of honey-colored crusts with little surrounding redness. Symptoms may include itching or burning, and removal of crusts leaves a raw base with a tendency to weep. It may be caused by coagulase positive *S. aureus* alone or as a mixed infection including beta hemolytic *streptococcus*. One variant of impetigo (Fig. 11-2), produced by *S. aureus* phage type II, produces vesicles and bullae that may be centimeters in diameter and can be mistaken for poison oak or ivy, blistering insect bite reactions, herpes simplex or zoster, bullous drug eruptions, or blistering diseases such as pemphigus or pemphigoid.

Impetigo tends to favor body folds (Fig. 11-3) and areas subject to friction and occlusion such as thighs and axillae. It also may complicate abrasions or areas of dermatitis such as atopic dermatitis (the patient will have a history of asthma, hay fever, or eczema, and the crusts frequently will be on the face, popliteal, or antecubital fossae), contact dermatitis (especially from shoe materials and rubberized pads), and irritant dermatitis (such as hands chapped from frequent immersion or handling irritating substances as occurs when cleaning fish). Secondary impetiginization may complicate other infections such as herpes simplex. Fifteen percent to 20% of people carry coagulase positive *S. aureus* in their nares. Some will have a tiny fissure at the most anterior aspect of the nares, representing very localized impetigo. In impetigo, bacterial toxins cause a split near the cutaneous surface where the living epidermal cells are connected to the acellular stratum corneum.

Ecthyma is caused by the same organisms as impetigo, but it differs from impetigo in that the bacteria cause destruction of the entire epidermis and part of the superficial dermis, resulting in erosions or shallow ulcers surrounded by erythema (Fig. 11-4).

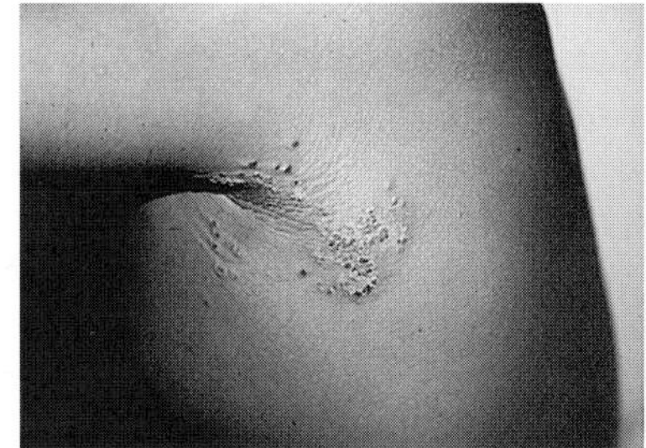

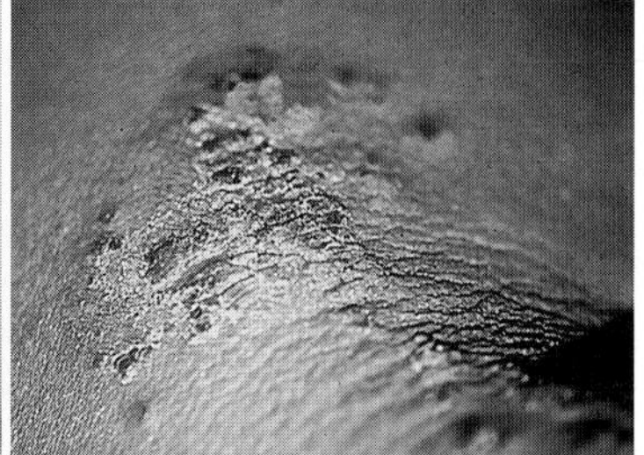

FIGURE 11-3. Most commonly, impetigo consists of honey-colored crusts with little surrounding redness. (From Scheinberg R: Exercise-related skin infection: Managing bacterial diseases. Phys Sports Med 1994.)

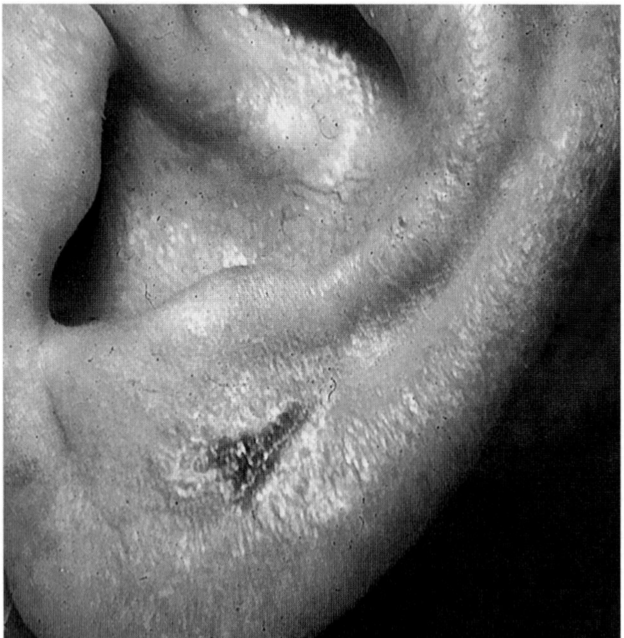

FIGURE 11-4. The same organism that causes impetigo, *Staphylococcus aureus,* causes ecthyma, which appears as erosions or shallow ulcers on this patient's ear. (From Scheinberg R: Exercise-related skin infection: Managing bacterial diseases. Phys Sports Med 1994.)

Diagnosis of impetigo and ecthyma is made by the clinical appearance, supplemented by a culture showing the causative organism, and its sensitivities whenever possible. Management with systemic antibiotics, such as dicloxacillin, cephalothin, and erythromycin, is preferable to topical therapy because the medication will be transported by the bloodstream to the whole cutaneous surface, making uninvolved skin resist the spread of infection. The organisms are highly contagious, and athletic competition quickly can make a mild infection widespread or transfer the bacteria to other competitors. Skin-to-skin contact must be avoided while crusts are present. Gentle cleansing with soap and water is valuable in removing the crusts. Uniforms and towels from infected individuals must be laundered in hot water to prevent inoculation back to the patient or to other individuals. Very localized impetigo or ecthyma may be managed with mupirocin (Bactroban, SmithKline Beecham, Philadelphia, PA) cream or ointment applied to the skin three times daily if the athlete is finished with competition or is participating in a noncontact sport. Recurrent impetigo may mean that a family member, competitor, or the patient is a carrier. Mupirocin in the nostrils three times daily for 1 week each month and regular use of antibacterial soap (Lever 2000, Dial, Safeguard, Irish Spring) may prevent future recurrences.

Cellulitis. The term *cellulitis* refers to an infection in the deep dermis and subcutaneous tissues. It is very painful and tender and is primarily caused by beta hemolytic *streptococcus* and *S. aureus,* which are almost impossible to culture from the surface of the skin. Cellulitis is recognized as a somewhat ill-defined plaque of tender erythema of the trunk or extremities, usually appearing around a break in the skin from antecedent trauma or from bacteria entering a fissure caused by athlete's foot. The patient may have malaise and fever with intense pain and may have streaks along pathways of lymphatic drainage (blood poisoning or lympangitis). The athlete must be kept from competition to avoid systemic dissemination, because additional trauma to an area of cellulitis can cause bacteremia. Hospitalization for intravenous antibiotics administration may be necessary, as was the case with Michael Jordan, who missed several games during the 1992–1993 season because of cellulitis around a foot corn. Milder cases of cellulitis can be managed with oral antibiotics such as dicloxacillin or erythromycin, warm tapwater compresses for 15 minutes three times daily, elevation, and bedrest.

If the erythema is sharply defined and if the skin surface has a peau d'orange appearance, a *streptococcus* infection of the upper dermis termed *erysipelas* is present. Management is the same as for cellulitis, but if erysipelas is in the periorbital area, ophthalmologic consultation should be obtained on an emergency basis because blindness can result from intense pressure on the globe or spread of the infection to the eye itself.

Folliculitis, Acneiform Lesions, and Miliaria. The same forces of friction, heat, and humidity that can cause impetigo, ecthyma, and cellulitis will frequently cause occlusion of the skin's adnexal structures, and bacteria will proliferate behind the obstruction to cause folliculitis (hair follicle infection), acneiform lesions (pilosebaceous gland inflammation and infection frequently termed *acne mechanica* if rubbing and other mechanical factors are aggravating the condition), and miliaria (sweat gland and duct inflammation and infection).

Follicular papules and pustules are found most commonly on the scalp, chest, back, buttocks, and thighs (Fig. 11-5). If a pustule is surrounded by a small erythematous halo, it is most likely caused by coagulase-positive *S. aureus.* Dome-shaped follicular papules and pustules can be caused by *staphylococcus, streptococcus,* or gram negative organisms. Very extensive folliculitis may occur from women shaving their legs and after total body shaving by men and women competitive swimmers, which is presumably because an infective focus is seeded to other follicles by the razor. Furuncles (boils) are deep-seated inflammatory nodules resulting from rupture into the tissues of preexisting folliculitis.

Carbuncles occur when several furuncles merge in the subcutaneous tissue. Furuncles and carbuncles occur most commonly on the buttocks, neck, face, and axillae as complications of folliculitis subject to friction and

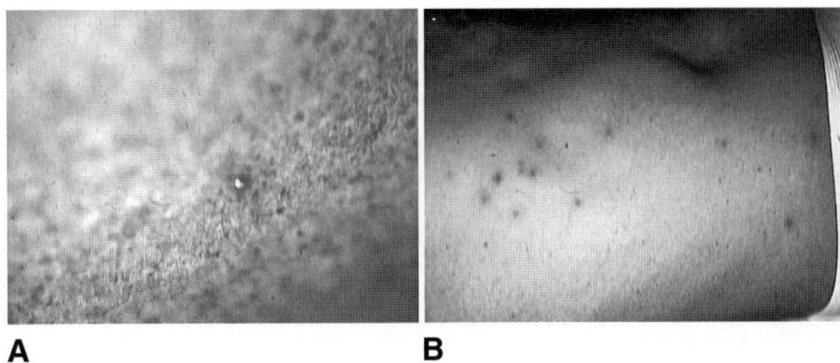

FIGURE 11-5. Folliculitis and pustular forms of acne and miliaria often are impossible to differentiate from one another. A pustule surrounded by a halo of erythema **(A)** that appears on this patient's trunk **(B)** is typical of staphylococcal folliculitis. (From Scheinberg R: Exercise-related skin infection: Managing bacterial diseases. Phys Sports Med 1994.)

repeated blunt trauma of athletic competition. Several weeks of systemic antibiotic therapy should be instituted and, in patients with severe cases, immobilization, incision and drainage, and hospitalization may be necessary.

Pseudomonas organisms can produce a widespread folliculitis if there is a heavy innoculum of the organism while the patient is bathing in a hot tub that has inadequate chlorination; "hot tub dermatitis" (Fig. 11-6). Other gram negative organisms can cause folliculitis, especially if the patient has been receiving antibiotics with a primarily gram positive spectrum as treatment for acne. The pustular forms of acne and miliaria can be impossible to distinguish from folliculitis. If the patient with widespread presumed folliculitis has no systemic signs such as malaise or fever, he or she should be treated empirically with a systemic antibiotic such as erythromycin, tetracycline, or minocycline to cover for gram positive folliculitis and acne and miliaria pustulosa. In addition, the patient should be advised to begin measures to avoid maceration of the skin, such as the use of absorbent powders (Zeasorb, which contains cellulose to prevent caking like pure talcum powder and does not act as a nutrient medium, such as cornstarch, is preferred), changing clothing frequently, and decreasing sweating with aluminum chloride (Xerac AC, Person & Covey, Inc., Glendale, CA). Regular use of antiseptic soaps may also prevent recurrences (in addition to the soaps used to prevent impetigo, bar or liquid soap with benzoyl peroxide, which can penetrate follicles and sweat ducts, is recommended). Very localized folliculitis can be managed with the topical antibiotics developed for acne, such as erythromycin (Erycettes, Ortho Pharmaceutical Corporation, Raritan, NJ; Emgel, Glaxo Dermatology, Research Triangle Park, NC; TStat) and clindamycin (Cleocin T, Upjohn Company, Kalamazoo, MI). Folliculitis is stubborn, and cultures and even skin biopsies are needed to establish the diagnosis and causative organism for appropriate antibiotic coverage. However, if the culture grows *Pseudomonas* organisms, topical therapy with acetic acid (1:10 vinegar solution) and meticulous drying, along with avoiding underchlorinated hot tubs, should clear the infection without having to resort to systemic antibiotics.

Some patients with folliculitis, acne mechanica, and miliaria pustulosa will not see their symptoms resolve until the competitive season ends and until the local factors that predispose the patient to the adnexal occlusive disease are finished.

Other Bacterial Infections. Corynebacteria, in addition to being the main pathologic organism implicated in acne, can cause two other common infections. Well-defined, slightly scaling plaques in the inguinal folds and between the toes may result from *Corynebacterium minutissimae*, the causative organism of erythrasma. Diagnosis is confirmed by putting the patient under a Woods black light, which will cause the area to glow with a coral red fluorescence. The organism responds to topical erythromycin or clindamycin or systemic erythromycin. Well-demarcated 1- to 15-mm pits on the soles of patients with very sweaty, macerated, and malodorous feet are diagnostic of pitting keratolysis (Fig. 11-7) in which a corynebacterium or micrococcus species lyses the very thick stratum corneum of the soles, giving a dramatic appearance. Treatment consists of 20% aluminum

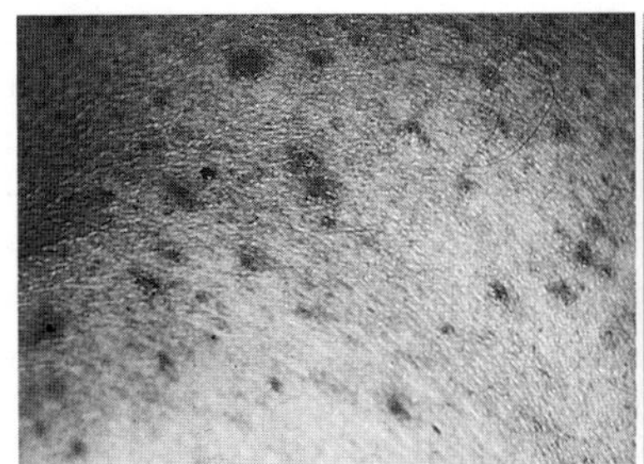

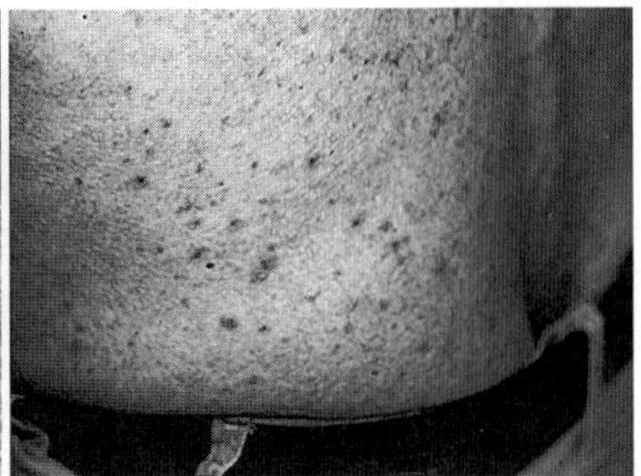

FIGURE 11-6. Widespread folliculitis, as on this patient, can result from *Pseudomonas,* which thrive in underchlorinated hot tubs. (From Scheinberg R: Exercise-related skin infection: Managing bacterial diseases. Phys Sports Med 1994.)

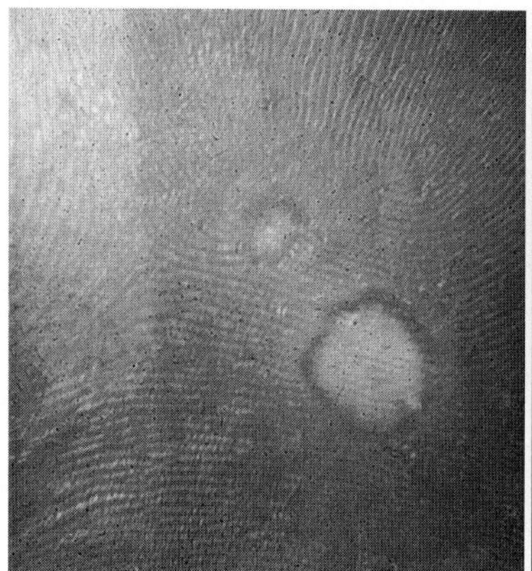
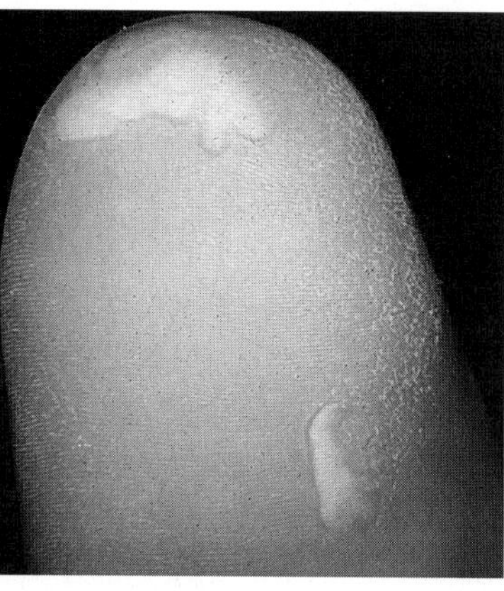

FIGURE 11-7. Pitting keratolysis appears on this patient's heel and sole. (From Scheinberg R: Modern Med 1993.)

chloride tincture (Drysol) or topical antibiotics such as clindamycin and erythromycin as prescribed for acne or erythrasma. In addition, the patient should be instructed to soak in a 1:10 vinegar solution for 5 minutes twice daily, followed by blow-drying the skin, dusting the feet with absorbent cellulose powder (Zeasorb), and wearing absorbent acrylic socks to make the environment less hospitable to the bacteria. Footgear should be changed frequently when wet or sweaty.

Erysipeloid looks like cellulitis but is somewhat more purple and typically occurs on the hands of people who fish and have been exposed to *Erysipelothrix rhusipathiae*, a gram positive rod commonly found on fish. It responds to penicillin and erythromycin. A more serious fish-borne infection is caused by *Vibrio vulnificus*, which can cause hemorrhagic bullae progressing to gangrenous-type lesions and sepsis if it enters the skin through a cut or abrasion. The organism is most prevalent in the Gulf coast and also may produce a severe gastroenteritis and severe skin infections after ingestion of raw fish and shellfish. Most susceptible are persons with poor liver function resulting from cirrhosis, in whom bacteria is not cleared from the bloodstream. Mortality in these individuals approaches 50%.

Rickettsial Disease

The major rickettsial disease to which athletic patients have increased risk is Lyme borreliosis. In endemic areas, hikers, golfers, hunters, and ballplayers who retrieve balls in areas of heavy grass may be exposed to infected ticks. If the tick is not removed within 24 hours, the rickettsia can get into the patient's bloodstream, causing Lyme disease. The majority of patients (but certainly not all) get a rash consisting of a ring of erythema, which may be mildly itchy, in the area of the tick bite. This ring may appear 3 to 12 days after the bite and may be associated with fever and malaise. Months to years later, peripheral and central neuropathies, arthritis, and cardiomyopathy may occur. Preferred management is a 21-day course of amoxicillin or doxycycline, although erythromycin and tetracycline also may be used. Most practitioners will treat persons bitten by ticks in endemic areas, but this treatment is controversial. All patients with the characteristic rash (erythema chronicum migrans) should be treated with antibiotics because the blood tests for Lyme disease are presently unreliable, and the causative organism has been cultured from cutaneous lesions repeatedly after negative results on blood tests.

Fungal and Yeast Infections

Dermatophytes and yeasts thrive in the same warm, moist environment that makes active patients susceptible to bacterial skin infections. Although fungus is the most common etiology of athlete's foot and jock itch, it is essential to recognize that infections in intertrigenous areas may be caused by different organisms. Conversely, active, sweaty persons are particularly susceptible to extensive fungal infections in nonintertrigenous areas. Athlete's foot, when presenting as dry and scaly and involving the toe webs and sole, is most commonly caused by dermatophyte fungus *(tinea pedis)* (Fig. 11-8). This diagnosis can be confirmed by collecting a scale with a scalpel blade and performing a potassium hydroxide microscopic examination or by culturing the scale in DTM (dermatophyte test medium), which turns red in the presence of dermatophytes. Blisters on the instep also may be caused by dermatophytes, which may be distinguished from contact dermatitis by potassium hydroxide and culture. The macerated toe web infection, also called athlete's foot, usually is a mixed infection caused by *Candida* or gram negative rods in addition to or replacing the original dermatophyte. Likewise, jock itch, when forming pruritic, scaly rings involving the inguinal folds and sparing the scrotum and penis, is invariably dermatophytic, whereas a tender and itchy bright red plaque with pustules peripheral to it (satellites) that does involve the penis and scrotum most commonly is caused by *Candida albicans* (Fig. 11-9). Gram negative and gram positive bacteria also may cause a macerated inguinal intertrigo. As mentioned previously, erythrasma can form a dry, finely scaling infection in this area.

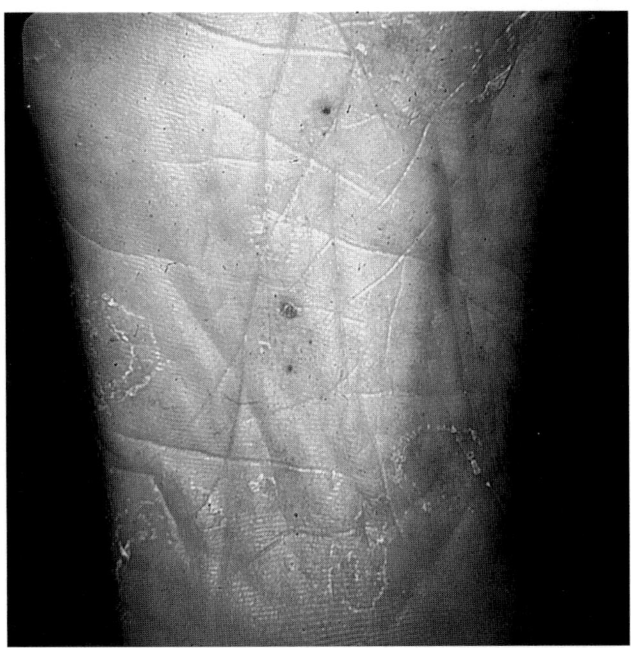

FIGURE 11-8. Athlete's foot appears as scaling on the sole and blistering on the instep of a patient's foot. (From Scheinberg R: Fungal, yeast, and viral infections. Phys Sports Med 1994.)

Management of athlete's foot and jock itch depends on recognizing the probable etiologic organisms and modifying the environment that is conducive to their growth. The dry dermatophyte infections can be cured with topical antifungal medication. Imidazoles such as clotrimazole (Lotrimin, Schering Corporation, Kenilworth, NJ; Mycelex, Miles Inc., Elkhart, IN), miconazole (Micatin), econazole (Spectazole, Ortho Pharmaceutical Corporation), ketoconazole (Nizoral, Janssen Pharmaceutica, Inc., Titusville, NJ), sulconazole (Exelderm, Westwood-Squibb Pharmaceuticals, Inc., Buffalo, NY), and Oxistat (Glaxo Dermatology), which have a spectrum including yeast and some bacteria, are recommended. For recalcitrant scaling of the sole caused by fungus (sandal *t. pedis*), the allylamines naftifine (Naftin, Allergan Herbert, Irvine, CA) and terbinafine (Lamisil), and the benzylamine butenafine (Mentax, LotriminUltra) are especially effective and may induce longer fungus-free periods than the imidazoles. Allylamines and benzyamines, however, are less effective against yeast, therefore, they are best not used if a fungal etiology has not been positively established. Florid inguinal *Candida* and bacterial intertrigo of groin and toe webs can be quickly cooled down with a regimen consisting of cool 1:10 vinegar soaks for 15 minutes three times daily followed each time by blow-drying or fanning the area until it is thoroughly dry and the skin can be touched with a finger that will not stick to the surface when lifted. This can be followed by a moderate-strength corticosteroid (two to three sample tubes of triamcinolone or flucinolone are recommended) and an imidazole cream or lotion. Within 2 to 3 days, the compresses and blow-drying usually can be stopped, and the imidazole can be used alone twice a day.

Active patients may require prolonged topical treatment because the area is continually subjected to the same forces that produced the infection initially. Topical management should be continued until the infection is clinically gone and then for an additional 2 weeks. Drying powders such as Zeasorb, and measures to diminish sweating such as Drysol (Person & Covey), XeracAc, and tannic acid soaks (made by adding two tea bags to a cup of boiling water, letting it steep, and then pouring it into a basin and adding enough water to cool the solution to a tolerable temperature) can prevent future infections. Frequent changes of synthetic socks and changing athletic shoes, bathing suits, and uniforms as soon as possible after athletic activity should be encouraged. If the patient has recurrent infections, daily imidazole cream on the feet and groin may prevent recurrences.

Patients with widespread fungus infections (*tinea corporis*) (Fig. 11-10) or symptomatic onychomycosis (fungus infection of the toenails) should be treated with griseofulvin (Gris-PEG, Albergan Herbert; Fulvicin,

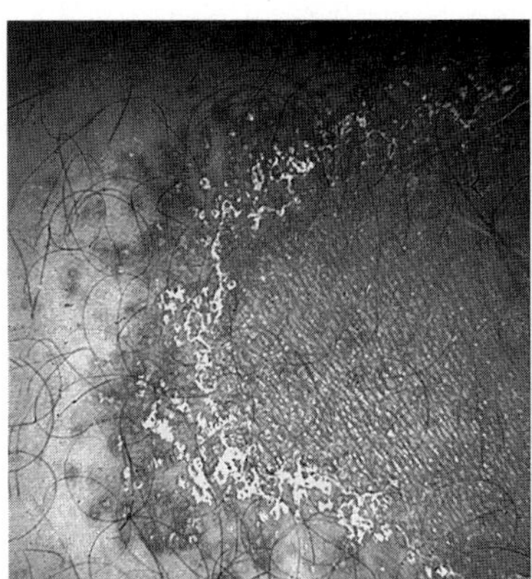

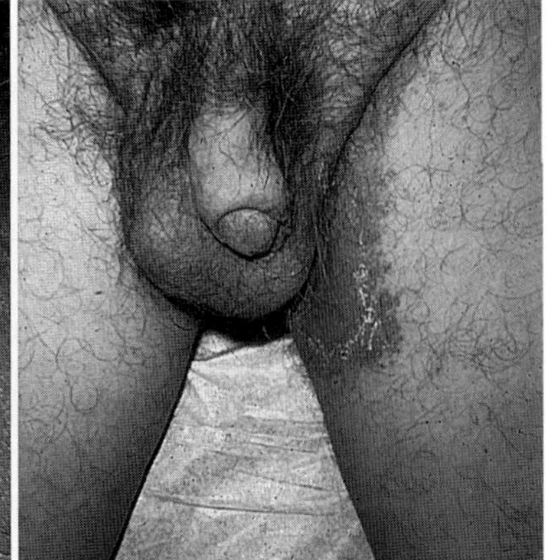

FIGURE 11-9. Jock itch caused by *Candida albicans* appears as a bright red plaque with peripheral pustules. (From Scheinberg R: Fungal, yeast, and viral infections. Phys Sports Med 1994.)

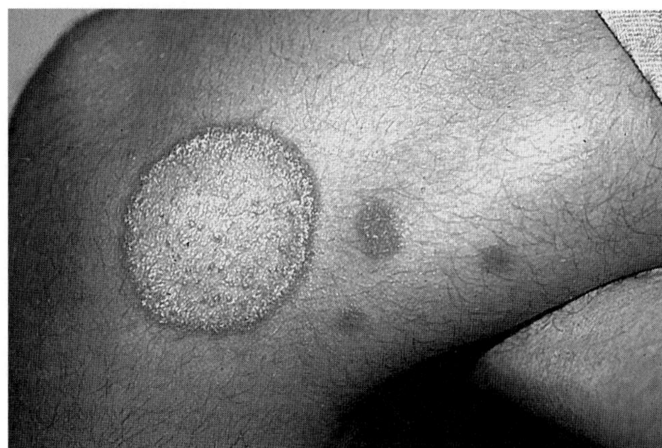

FIGURE 11-10. *Tinea corporis* on a patient's leg demonstrates the typical ringworm pattern of this fungal infection. (From Scheinberg R: Fungal, yeast, and viral infections. Phys Sports Med 1994.)

Schering Corporation) in the newly recommended higher dosing schedules (500 mg twice daily for a large man). Resistant cases may indicate fungal resistance or the patient's immunologic tolerance of the organism (this is especially true of atopics). Systemic ketoconazole (Nizoral, Janssen Pharmaceutica, Inc.), fluconazole (Difulcan, Roering, New York, NY), and itraconazole (Sporonox) have shown excellent results in many of these patients, but they may cause liver toxicity (especially ketoconazole). Before prescribing any of the systemic antifungals, check to see if the athlete is taking any of the many medications that can interact through the cytochrome P450 metabolic pathways. Systemic terbinafine at 200 mg once daily for 2 weeks will cure most *t. corporis* with minimal interaction with other medications and little chance of liver toxicity. Twelve-week courses of both oral itraconazole and terbinafine have higher cure rates for fungal infections of the toenails (onychomycosis) than a year of oral griseofulvin. Since athletes frequently have thickened, cracked, discolored nails due to trauma, and anyone can have dystrophic nails due to skin disease such as psoriasis, systemic antifungal therapy for dystrophic nails should never be given unless there is laboratory confirmation of fungus infection by potassium hydroxide (KOH) examination, fungal culture, or microscopic demonstration of the fungus in a nail plate sent to a pathologist and stained for fungus.

Tinea versicolor commonly affects active individuals because the causative yeast (pityrosporum) is lipophilic and a normal inhabitant of hair follicles and sebaceous glands, which colonize the skin when host factors of heat and moisture are increased. On unexposed skin, the colonies will be rust-colored and asymptomatic or mildly pruritic. They are more dramatic during the summer months when the areas colonized do not tan or sunburn so they appear as well-defined white patches, especially on the chest or back. Woods black-light examination shows yellow fluorescence, and potassium hydroxide examination has a characteristic appearance as spores and hyphae resemble spaghetti and meatballs, whether the patches are white or rust-colored. Extensive cases of *t. versicolor* may involve the entire trunk and extremities. This same pityrosporum organism occasionally is responsible for patients with antibiotic-resistant folliculitis.

Management of pityrosporum can be topical or systemic. Selenium sulfide, 2.5% (prescription strength Selsun, Exel), applied to affected areas for 10 minutes each day for 1 week frequently will be curative (because the areas will remain white until the skin is tanned, a Woods black-light examination showing no yellow fluorescence or a negative potassium hydroxide examination may be needed to assure the physician and the patient that treatment was effective). Topical imidazoles also are effective in this infection, but treatment requires several weeks and is very expensive if large areas of skin are involved. Many clinicians favor systemic ketoconazole for extensive *t. versicolor*, and it frequently will be the only effective treatment for pityrosporum folliculitis. *T. versicolor* can be cured with a single dose of two tablets (400 mg) of ketoconazole taken with a carbonated beverage or cranberry juice to increase absorption. The drug is excreted in the sweat, so patients are advised to work out for 1 hour or more after taking the two pills and to delay showering by an additional hour. This treatment can be repeated in 1 week if Woods black-light or potassium hydroxide examination is still positive. If the patient has no history of liver disease, this minidose has not been associated with liver toxicity. Management of folliculitis may take several weeks of daily medication, and monitoring of liver function tests should be done. Alternatively, itraconazole at 100 mg two times a day for 2 weeks can be prescribed for resistant *t. versicolor* or pityrosporum folliculitis.

Viral Infections

Herpes simplex, herpes zoster, warts, and HIV may be transmitted during or precipitated by athletic participation. Fortunately, however, the risk of transmitting HIV and hepatitis is low if published guidelines are followed. Routine hygienic measures, such as cleansing the skin after athletic competition and removing participants with open cuts on exposed skin from participation involving contact, may reduce or eliminate transmission of these pathogens. The full scope of HIV and athletics is beyond the scope of this chapter and will not be discussed further.

Herpes Simplex and Zoster. Because up to 80% of adolescents already have antibodies directed against herpes simplex, the main role of activity is reactivating the latent virus that resides in dorsal root nerve ganglia

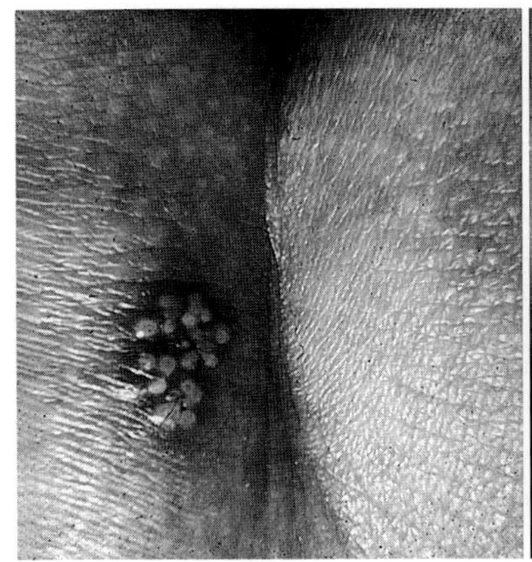
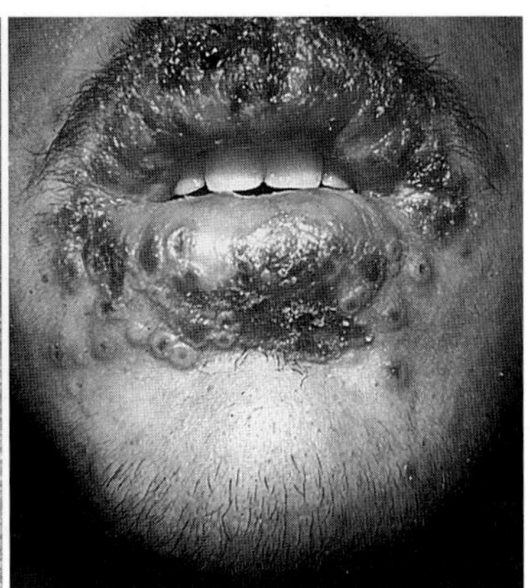

FIGURE 11-11. Herpes simplex.

between attacks. The term *fever blister* has been used to indicate that increased body temperature can trigger an attack of herpes labialis. During many sports activities, body temperature may rise to 102° F or more. This thermal stress, combined with the stress of athletic competition and exposure to ultraviolet light, may precipitate frequent attacks of herpes in susceptible individuals (in labial and genital areas).

Management of recurrent herpes simplex is directed at reducing trigger factors whenever possible by cooling down the skin and taking nonsteroidal anti-inflammatory drugs after competition and wearing sunscreens on a daily basis if attacks are precipitated by ultraviolet light. Acyclovir (Zovirax, Burroughs Wellcome Co., Research Triangle Park, NC) tablets, 200 mg, taken five times a day for 5 days can shorten an episode if taken within 48 hours of the attack. Alternatives are famciclovir (Fanovir, SmithKline Beecham) 125 mg two times a day for 5 days and valacyclovir (Valtrex, Burroughs Wellcome Co.) 500 mg two times a day for 5 days. Ideally, antiviral therapy should be started at the first sign of tingling that presages such an attack. A prophylactic regimen of acyclovir, 400 mg, taken twice daily will prevent most herpes simplex and should be started the day before the active individual expects to be at risk. Topical acyclovir is of no use in these circumstances. Valcyclovir has been found to shorten episodes at a dose of 2 grams two times a day for a single day at the first sign of an outbreak. It can also be used at 500–1000 mg per day as prophylaxis. Other antiherpes drugs may also be effective in a one-day megadose regimen but clinical data is lacking.

Those persons participating in contact sports must be kept away from other participants while they have an active herpetic lesion. The term *herpes Gladiatorum* was coined to describe epidemics of inoculation herpes occurring in wrestlers. Recent outbreaks have occurred in wrestling camps and on football and basketball teams.

Herpes zoster results from reactivation of the varicella (chickenpox) virus, and occasionally can be precipitated by local trauma in contact sports. Infected individuals should be kept from competition and treated with acyclovir, 800 mg, taken five times a day for 7 days, famciclovir, 800 mg every 8 hours for 7 days, or valacyclovir, 1000 mg three times daily for 7 days. Because HIV also can precipitate herpes zoster in a young person, a test for HIV antibodies also is appropriate.

Herpes viruses typically produce clusters of painful blisters. Herpes simplex blisters are 1 to 3 mm in diameter and appear as localized clusters (Fig. 11-11). Herpes zoster blisters may be centimeters in diameter and follow a dermatome. If blisters are broken, shallow erosions may be present.

Warts. Verrucae are caused by dozens of varieties of the human papilloma virus (HPV). They are recognized as papillomatous, flesh-colored, well-defined papules and nodules that occur predominantly on exposed skin parts (Fig. 11-12). Incubation is from several weeks to 5 years after exposure. Plantar warts will be round or

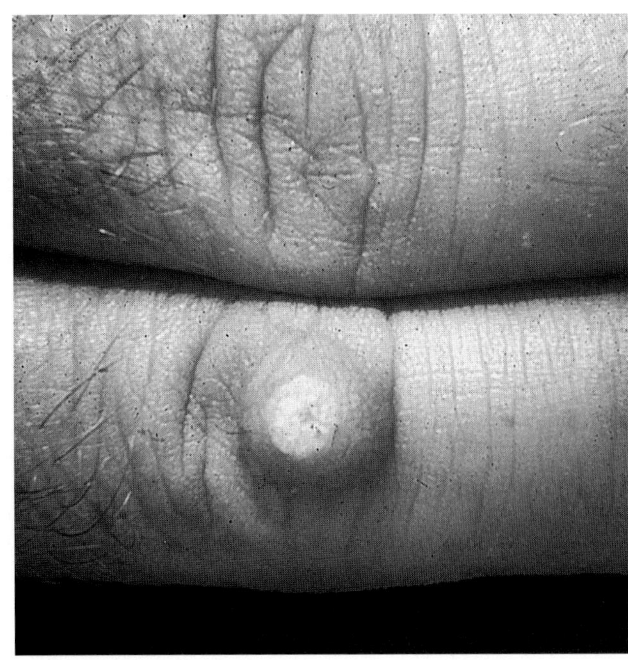

FIGURE 11-12. Wart on right-hand index finger.

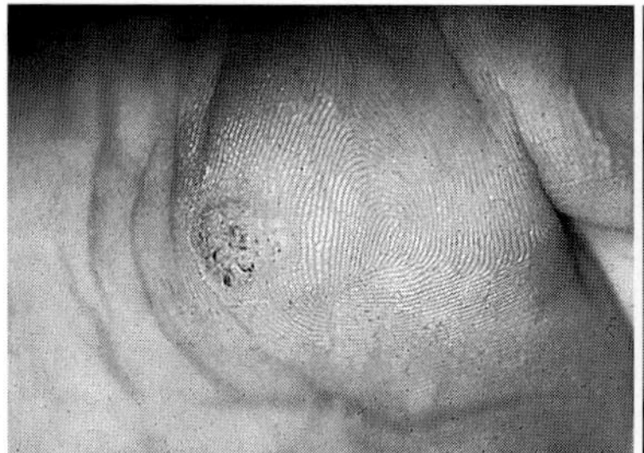
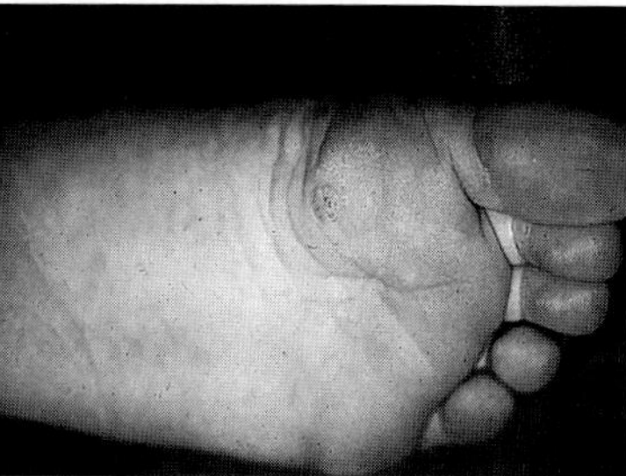

FIGURE 11-13. Plantar wart.

oval, and on close inspection can be seen to interrupt the dermatoglyphic skin lines on the sole (Fig. 11-13). When the thick stratum corneum is pared, tiny bleeding puncta or black dots of dried blood are revealed, representing blood vessels projecting vertically toward the skin surface. In most young individuals, the body will mount an immunologic reaction against the virus within 6 months, so any treatment—including no treatment—may be effective. However, a minority of persons will not mount an effective response to the virus, and almost any treatment will be ineffective. The people frequently are atopic, analogous to the susceptible and hard-to-cure patients with impetigo and fungal and yeast infections.

The goal of therapy in an active individual is to minimize "down time" while maximizing the chance of cure. Treating a patient with one or two warts with liquid nitrogen cryocautery is recommended. A spray is directed at the wart for approximately 10 seconds or a cotton swab is applied to the wart with minimal pressure for the same time. Thicker warts might require a second spray or application during the same visit after they are allowed to thaw. Alternatively, the warts can be curetted or hyfrecated under local anesthesia. Care must be taken not to go too deeply in a misguided attempt to prevent recurrences because excessive morbidity and scarring can result. Most recurrences occur from subclinical infection by the HPV in the surrounding normal-appearing skin. For many competitive athletes who run a high risk of wound infection during their season, topical therapy with keratolytic liquids or pads (Compound W, Whitehall Laboratories, Inc., New York, NY; DuoFilm, 40% salicylic acid plasters, Trans-ver-sal, and Trans Plantar) is prescribed. These medications are all over-the-counter and are especially helpful in keeping painful plantar warts soft so they do not feel like a pebble in the shoe. Liquid nitrogen and surgical treatment of plantar warts should be avoided until the competitive season is over because postoperative pain can be disabling. CO^2 laser excision has the least chance of scarring and minimizes morbidity, but it can occasionally result in significant postoperative pain, and the excision site is an easy portal of entry for secondary bacterial infection if the patient is engaged in competitive sports before the 1- to 3-week healing period is finished. The author has been unimpressed with Bicloroacetic acid applications to plantar warts, but some practitioners use this therapy with success. Intralesional bleomycin by injection and scarification also is used by many dermatologists, but there is severe associated pain and risk of permanent nerve damage. Imiquimod (Aldara 3M Pharmaceuticals) is FDA approved for treatment of genital warts and, when used in conjunction with paring and plasters to enhance skin penetration, may cause warts on nongenital skin to involute by stimulating the immune system locally to produce interferons and antiviral cytokines.

Molluscum Contagiosum. The molluscum virus belongs in the pox family and produces flesh-colored to yellow papules with a tiny punctum on the surface best visualized if the lesion is lightly frozen with liquid nitrogen. It represents a viral folliculitis and is easily spread by children at play, sexual activity, and athletic competition. It is primarily of cosmetic concern, although occasionally a molluscum will rupture from blunt trauma, resulting in a foreign body reaction that can mimic cellulitis and be disabling (Fig. 11-14).

Management is the same as with almost any destructive modality. They are easier to cure than warts because there is no subclinical extension of virus. Curettage, light

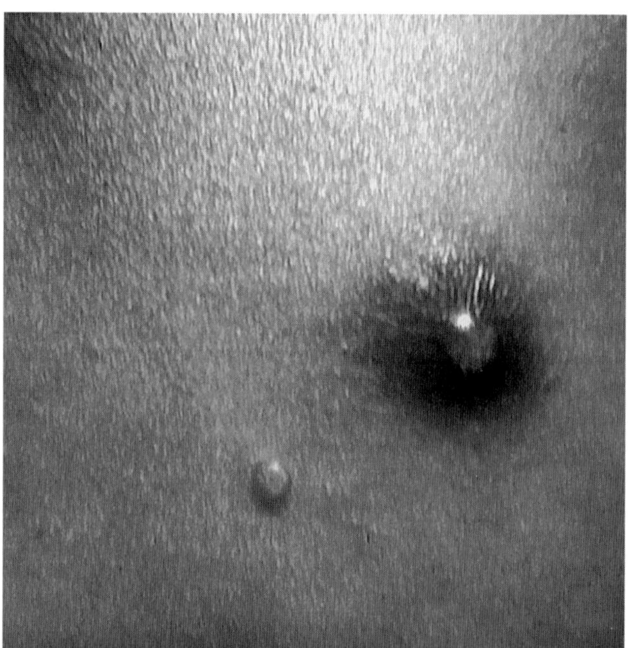

FIGURE 11-14. Molluscum contagiosum papules appear on this patient's cheek. Cellulitis from trauma to the papule on the right induced a foreign-body reaction. (From Scheinberg R: Modern Med 1993.)

hyfrecation, or topical 50% trichloroacetic acid applied only to the surface of the lesions is favored. Topical wart preparations sometimes can be effective, as can tretinoin (Retin-A, Ortho Pharmaceutical Corporation), which is useful especially in uncooperative children. Athletes do not need to be kept from competition because they have warts or molluscum, but the hygienic measures noted earlier should be emphasized, and affected areas should be covered whenever person-to-person contact is to be expected. Imiquimod (Aldara) is used off label to treat molluscum as well as warts.

Summary

A skin condition that is out of control can make participation uncomfortable or even unsafe. Physicians who know when to tell the patient to avoid participation are making sports safer not only for the patient, but also for other competitors.

ALLERGIC AND IRRITANT CONTACT DERMATITIS

Contact dermatitis occurs when the eruption fits an area of exposure to a garment, liquid, medicament, or bandage. Most common causes are sweat (which can cause sweaty sock syndrome); rubber products in shoes, stretch garments, and dressings; fragrances in medications and toiletries; topical antibiotics, herb, and vitamin preparations; sunscreens; and plants such as poison oak. Management consists of making the proper diagnosis and substituting less irritating substances wherever possible, and the use of cool compresses with topical and systemic corticosteroids for relief.

A unique reaction to an environmental agent is green discoloration of the hair of athletes with blond or gray hair who swim in chlorinated pools. This results from copper leached from pipes supplying the pool or from various pool-care products. If the pH of the pool is kept between 7.4 and 7.6, the copper will not attach to the hair. Hair already affected can be treated by application of hydrogen peroxide, 3%, for several hours or copper-chelating shampoos such as UltraSwim and Metalex for 30 minutes.

Abrasions, small lacerations, and callosities on the dorsum of the hand overlying metacarpophalangeal and interphalangeal joints may be a physical sign of bulimia, caused by contact of the incisors with those areas of skin during self-induced vomiting (Russell's sign). This is an extreme form of irritant contact dermatitis.

PHOTODERMATITIS

A common rash in the athlete is the *phototoxic reaction*. The prototype is acute sunburn, which can be prevented with sunscreens that are protective (i.e., Sun Protective Factor of 10 to 50) and substantive (i.e., resist wash-off by sweat and water). Some of the best are Sundown 15, 20, and 24; PreSun 15, 29, and 30 (this last one is nongreasy and waterproof); Eclipse 15; Solbar 15 and 50; Sea and Ski 15; Coppertone Supershade; and Bullfrog. PABA-sensitive patients can use Tiscreen, PABAFree, and PreSun 29. Patients who claim to be sensitive to all sunscreens can be protected by the so-called chemical-free sunscreens, which contain the physical blocker titanium dioxide. Examples are chemical-free Neutragena and Tiscreen. Phototoxic reactions can be precipitated by medications such as thiazide diuretics, sulfonamides (including TMP/SXT), griseofulvin, tetracycline, and Accutane (E.C. Robbins Company, Inc., Richmond, VA). Doxycycline, commonly used to prevent traveler's diarrhea, is a notorious photosensitizer, and patients using this on a trip to sunny Mexico or the Caribbean should be forewarned of this side effect. Phototoxic reactions are caused by the longer UVA ultraviolet light and are best protected against by the chemical-free physical blockers and sunscreens containing parsol, such as UVA-guard.

Management of phototoxic reactions consists of cooling the skin, preferably in a tub of cool water. Ice compresses can be used on blistered areas, and nonsteroidal anti-inflammatory drugs are useful for pain relief. Although they have been used for years, systemic corticosteroids have been found to be no better than placebo in reducing pain and inflammation of sunburn. Topical anesthetics may result in sensitization, so the popular OTC benzocaine-containing products are not recommended. Nonsensitizing pramoxine (Pramasone) is the preferred topical anesthetic.

The athlete who, while exercising, develops intensely itchy 1- to 2-mm papules surrounded by erythematous halos probably has cholinergic urticaria. This condition frequently begins during young adult life and interferes with exercise and any activities that raise body temperature. The etiology of this apparent hyperreactivity to acetylcholine in peripheral nerve endings is unknown, but it frequently responds to antihistamines, especially hydroxyzine. The nonsedating antihistamines loratidine (Clariten), desloratidine (Clarinex), and fexofenadine (Allegra), and the mildly sedating cetirizine (Zyrtec) may be helpful in managing cholinergic urticaria and seasonal rhinitis and urticaria in the athletic patient bothered by drowsiness from the more commonly used antihistamines. Exercise-induced anaphylaxis may result from food allergies and be made more intense by the increased blood flow during exercise or from insect bites occurring during exercise. Dietary elimination of chocolate, nuts, dairy products, and preservatives before exercise may prevent this problem in some patients, although others may require constant availability of an epinephrine-containing anaphylaxis kit during exercise.

NEOPLASMS

Because chronic sun exposure frequently is a part of the life of an athlete, active patients should be warned

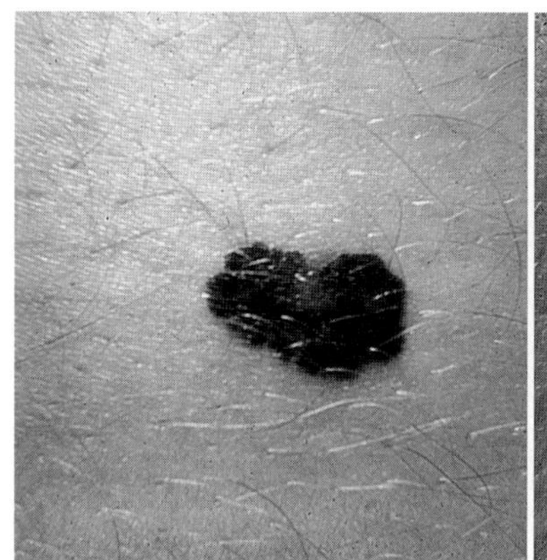
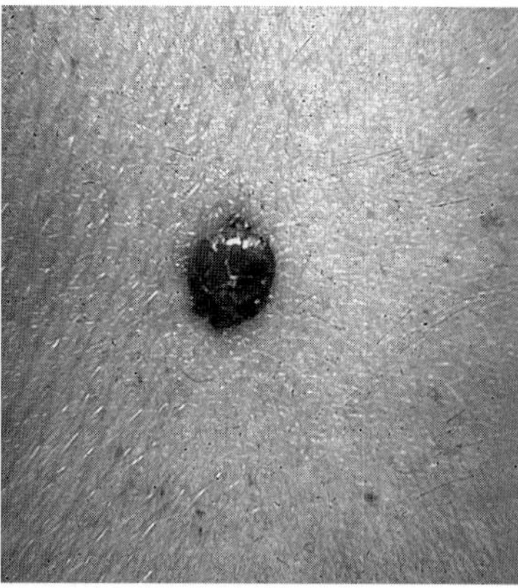

FIGURE 11-15. Malignant melanoma.

about the risks of sun exposure and closely watched for skin cancers (15% of women professional golfers have skin cancers before they are 30 years old). The usual skin cancers are represented, such as basal and squamous cell carcinomas; however, there has been an alarming increase in malignant melanomas (Fig. 11-15), and the skin of outdoor-loving patients should be examined once a year (especially fair-skinned patients) to catch melanomas in their earliest stage (before they have descended into the dermis) when they are virtually 100% curable by simple excision. The use of sunscreens (SPF 10 to 50) should be encouraged to prevent skin cancers and to prevent the aging of the skin caused by the sun. Patients with several large (greater than 7 mm) flat or slightly elevated acquired nevi may have dysplastic nevus syndrome. This syndrome is relatively common but only recently recognized, and patients with this syndrome have a 20% to 100% chance of developing a melanoma during their lifetime (other Caucasians have a 1.25% risk according to the latest figures). These patients should be examined every 3 months for their entire lives and should drastically reduce sun exposure to minimize this otherwise considerable risk.

If the increased risk of skin cancer does not impress athletic patients, the irony of having wrinkled, leathery, old-looking skin from the solar ultraviolet irradiation they were exposed to while keeping their cardiovascular and musculoskeletal systems in a youthful state should be stressed.

BIBLIOGRAPHY

Adams BB: Dermatologic disorders of the athlete. Sports Med 32(5):309–321, 2002.

Adams BB: Tinea corporuis gladiatorum: A cross-sectional study. J Am Acad Dermatol 43(6): 1039–1041, 2000.

Basler RS: Skin lesions related to sports activity. Prim Care 10(3):479–494, 1983.

Basler RS, Basler GC, Palmer AH, Garcia MA: Special skin symptoms seen in swimmers. J Am Acad Dermatol 43(2):299–305, 2000.

Belongia EA, Goodman JL, Holland EJ, et al: An outbreak of herpes gladiatorum at a high school wrestling camp. N Engl J Med 325(13):906–910, 1991.

Bender TW: Cutaneous manifestations of disease in athletes. Skinmed 2(1):34–40, 2003.

Conklin RJ: Common cutaneous disorders in athletes. Sports Med 9(2):100–119, 1990.

Dorman JM: Contagious diseases in competitive sport: What are the risks? J Am Coll Health 49(3):105–109, 2000.

Dover JS: Sports-related dermatoses. Curr Challenges Dermatol Spring:1–9, 1992.

Daluiski A, Rahbar B, Meals RA: Russell's sign: Subtle hand changes in patients with bulimia nervosa. Clin Orthop 343:107–109, 1997.

Fitzpatrick TB, Eisen AZ, Wolff K, et al (eds): Dermatology in General Medicine, 4th ed. New York, McGraw-Hill, 1993.

Levine N: Dermatologic aspects of sports medicine. J Am Acad Dermatol 3(4):415–424, 1980.

Magid DM, Schwartz B, Craft J, et al: Prevention of Lyme disease after tick bites: A cost effectiveness analysis. N Engl J Med 327(8):534–541, 1992.

Pharis DB, Teller C, Wolf JE Jr: Cutaneous manifestations of sports participation, J Am Acad Dermatol 36:448–459, 1997.

Pro basketball power poll. Sporting News 215(11):39, 1993.

Scheinberg RS: Exercise-related skin infection: Managing bacterial disease. Phys Sports Med 22(6): 47–58, 1994.

Scheinberg RS: Summer skin clinic: Recognizing and treating common derm problems in active adults. Modern Med 61(6):48–62, 1993.

Spruance SL, Hamill ML, Hoge WS, et al: Acyclovir prevents reactivation of herpes simplex labialis in skiers. JAMA 260(11):1597–1599, 1988.

12 Eye Injuries

Mary Mendelsohn and
David Abramson

An eye injury can carry significant consequences for vision, disability, and future lifestyle. It is essential that health care professionals, trainers, and others involved in the care of athletes understand how to handle eye injuries. This chapter is organized in four sections. First, we review the anatomy of the eye. Second, we suggest a systematic method for examining the eye after injury. Third, we discuss how to diagnose and manage common ophthalmic injuries encountered in sports activities. Finally, we list useful contents of an emergency eye care kit.

ANATOMY REVIEW

Figures 12-1 and 12-2 show the basic anatomy of the eye. The labeled structures will be referred to throughout the chapter. The *cornea* is the clear covering in the front of the eye. The *sclera* is the visible white layer of the eye. The *limbus* is the junction of the cornea and the sclera. The sclera is covered by the *conjunctiva*, a thin, transparent membrane with fine red blood vessels in it that can become thickened, reddened, and opaque from acute injury. The *iris* is the circular pigmented structure that gives the eye its color (blue, brown, hazel, etc.). The space between the iris and the cornea is called the *anterior chamber*. The anterior chamber is filled with a clear fluid called *aqueous humor*. The black *pupil* is simply a hole bounded by the iris. Behind the pupil and iris sits the *lens*, which is supported by fibers called *zonules*. The zonules run radially from the lens to a structure called the *ciliary body*, which is attached to the inner eye wall. The ciliary body makes the aqueous humor and supports and focuses the lens. The ciliary body is continuous with the iris anteriorly and fuses with the retina and choroid posteriorly. Behind the lens is the large cavity of the eyeball that is filled with a clear gel called *vitreous humor*. The inner lining of the eye is the *retina*, a transparent neurosensory membrane with blood vessels running in it. The retina transforms light to neural impulses and sends that information to the brain via the *optic nerve*. The optic nerve transmits the visual information to the brain. The *macula* is the area of the retina where the sharpest vision occurs. The optic nerve and the macula are posterior structures within the eye that can be identified with the direct ophthalmoscope (Fig. 12-3). Between the retina and the sclera is a middle layer of the eye wall called the *choroid*. The choroid is a blood vessel layer of the eye. Another common anatomic term is the *uvea*; it is a collective name for the three vascular structures of the eye: the iris, ciliary body, and choroid.

EXAMINATION OF THE EYE AFTER TRAUMA

Before attempting to examine an injured eye, protect it from further injury. While at the playing area, place a shield over the eye that rests on the brow and cheek; tape the shield in place. Do not use a patch or device that touches the eye or eyelids because this can worsen conditions such as ruptured globe or foreign body penetration. Do not put pressure on the eye; instruct the player not to rub the eye. If a specific eye shield is not available, taping a paper cup over the eye is an acceptable alternative. Remove the player to the examining area. If a foreign object is penetrating the eye or orbit, do not attempt to remove it; instead, stabilize the object and eye and transfer to the hospital for evaluation. Objects lodged in the orbit might extend into the brain, and further damage might be done if the object is removed in an uncontrolled manner.[5]

Once the eye is protected, take a history. The history will direct the examiner to the kind of injury sustained. Record the time, location, and mechanism of the injury. Was it a scraping, lacerating, chemical, or concussive injury? If concussive (sudden blunt trauma), was the object that hit the eye larger than the size of the orbit (basketball, baseball bat) or smaller than the orbit (elbow, squash ball)? Objects larger than the diameter of the orbital entrance have their forces absorbed by the bones of the orbit and are more likely to cause fracture of these bones. Objects smaller than the orbital entrance are more likely to cause injury to the globe itself. What symptoms does the player have (decreased vision, double vision, photophobia, pain, tearing)? Symptoms can help direct the examiner to the part of the eye that was injured; symptoms are discussed more fully under each diagnosis in the next section. A complete history including allergies, medical illnesses, and other medication used is required before giving any antibiotic, eyedrop, or other medication.

Next, check the vision. Cover each eye and have the patient read an eyechart at 20 feet or a near card to the lowest line he or she can read. It is important to check vision before manipulating the eye in any way. If vision is

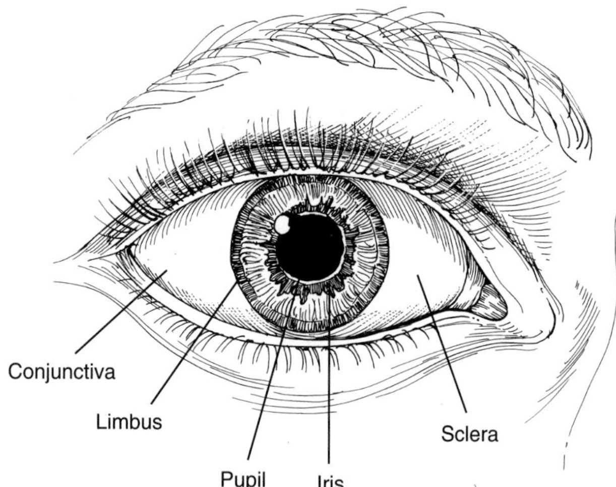

FIGURE 12-1. Eye anatomy, front view.

being checked with a near card and the patient ordinarily uses reading glasses, a substitute pair of over-the-counter reading glasses of +2.50 diopters can be used to assist near vision. If a patient's contact lenses or glasses were damaged or lost, the vision can be better approximated in each eye by having the patient read the chart while looking through a pinhole. (A small hole made in an index card will do if the diameter of the hole is approximately 1.2 mm.[1] This is about the size of a hole made with the end of a paper clip.)

Observe the lids and periorbita (area around the eye). If the lids are swollen shut, a lid speculum can be used to open them without putting pressure on the eye itself, but if this is necessary, it is better to refer to an ophthalmologist for further care. Note any lacerations, facial bone deformities, or irregular positioning of the eye. Test the extraocular movements: have the patient look in all directions of gaze (right, left, up, down, up and right, down and right, up and left, down and left). Note any limitations of movement; can they be explained by local swelling? Have the patient report any double vision seen in any direction. Palpate gently around the orbital rims, feeling for any discontinuity or excessive mobility of the facial bones. Brush a cotton swab on each cheek, testing for diminished sensation. Any findings such as limitation of eye movement, orbital rim discontinuity, or decreased sensation of the cheek can signal orbital fracture.

Check the pupil reactivity, an important indicator of damage to the iris or the optic nerve. Dim the room lights. Have the patient look into the distance (the patient should not look at the examiner or the light), and shine a bright light in one pupil while observing its reaction. It should constrict briskly. Remove the light from the eyes. Next, shine the light on the second pupil. It should also constrict briskly to the same final size as the first pupil. A normal pupillary phenomenon called *hippus* may cause the pupil to slightly "bounce" (constrict and dilate) when light is held on it for an extended time, but its first reaction when a light is brought to it should be constriction.

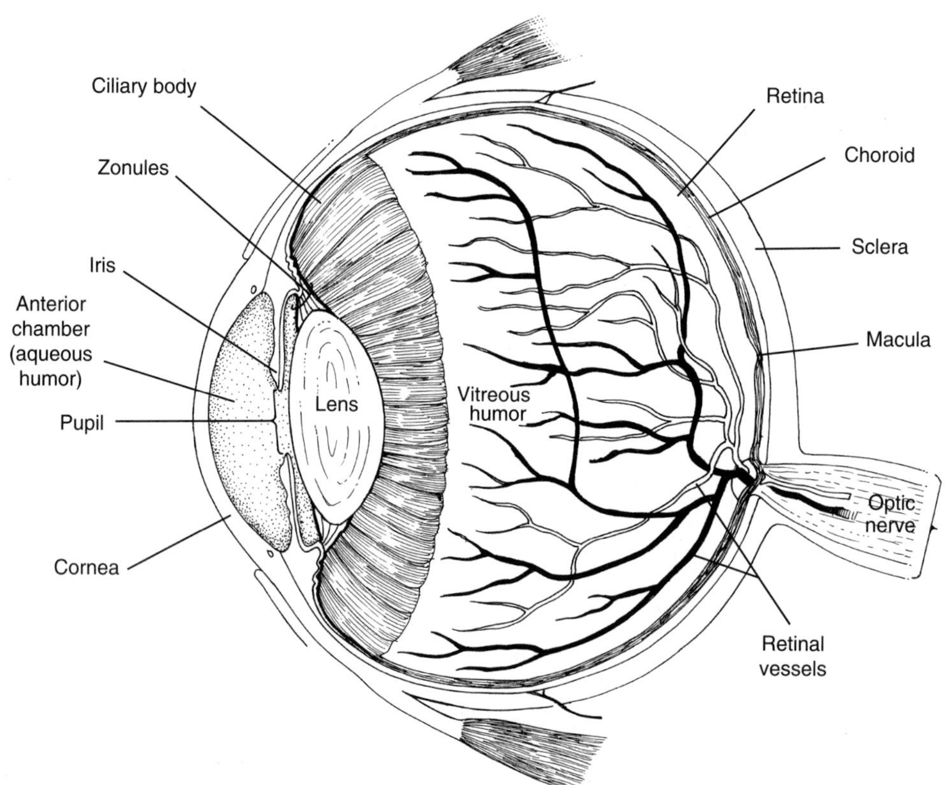

FIGURE 12-2. Eye anatomy, side view.

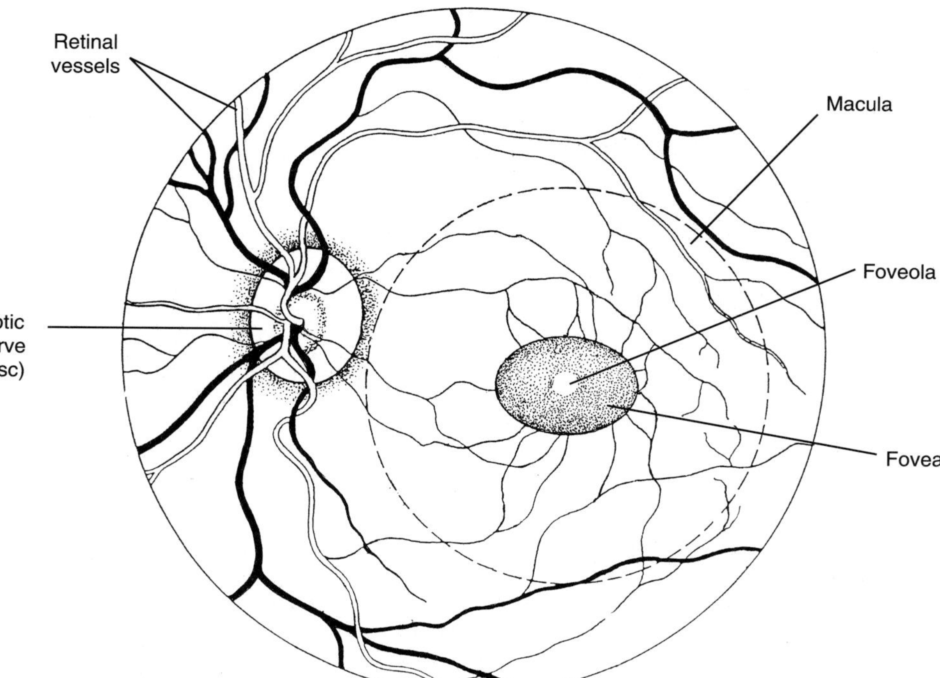

FIGURE 12-3. Posterior structures of the eye: the macula, optic nerve, and retinal blood vessels.

If one pupil is not responding, iris damage or optic nerve damage is likely. Subdural hematoma with herniation of the brain can also cause an ipsilateral, nonreactive, mid-dilated pupil.[12]

Next, do the "swinging flashlight" test, a good method of detecting optic nerve damage. Optic nerve damage diagnosed in this manner is called an *afferent pupillary defect.* The patient should look into the distance. Hold a bright light on the first eye, and watch as the pupil constricts. When it is fully constricted, quickly move the light to the other pupil—it should already be fully constricted and should not change much in size. Quickly return the light to the first pupil—it also should remain fully constricted. With normal eyes, light in one pupil will fully constrict both pupils simultaneously. (You may hold the light on a pupil for as long as you like, but the time spent crossing from one eye to the other should be minimal. You may swing the light to each eye several times to confirm your observations.) If one pupil dilates when the light is quickly returned to it, the eye has optic nerve damage. For example, if the right pupil constricts when the light is swung onto it but the left pupil dilates when the light is swung onto it, the left (dilating) eye has optic nerve damage. Swing the light back to the right pupil, and it will constrict. Swing the light to the left pupil, and it will dilate. This dilation is an abnormal reaction, signaling optic nerve damage of the left eye. However, the constriction of the right eye when the light is swung to it is also abnormal, and it also signals optic nerve damage of the left eye. If the eyes were healthy each pupil would already be constricted when the light was swung to it from the other eye. Suppose the injured eye has blood obscuring the pupil or the pupil is nonreactive because of iris damage. Shine the light on the injured eye; the damaged eye's pupil is obscured or does not move. Quickly swing the light to the fellow eye; if the uninjured eye's pupil constricts when the light is swung to it, the injured eye has suffered optic nerve damage. Any patient with an afferent pupillary defect after trauma must be seen by an ophthalmologist immediately to identify the cause of the optic nerve damage.

Peripheral vision can be quickly checked by the *confrontation* technique to rule out a retinal detachment. Any patient who notes loss of peripheral vision or describes visual loss "like a curtain coming down" into his or her visual field should have a confrontation visual field test performed (Fig. 12-4). The examiner sits directly across from the patient. The patient covers his or her left eye while the right is tested. The examiner aligns his or her own left eye directly across from the patient's right eye about 3 feet away and closes his or her right eye. Each person stares into the other's eye throughout the entire test. The examiner holds his or her hand in a fist halfway between the two eyes but slightly off to the side, briefly raises a number of fingers, and then closes the fist again. The patient must respond by saying how many fingers were shown, which the examiner and patient see with their peripheral vision. The examiner should repeat the test showing different number of fingers while moving his or her hand around all clock hours and at different distances from the center of gaze to test the patient's peripheral vision against the examiner's own. To test the patient's reliability, the examiner should flash some fingers that are so far outside the examiner's

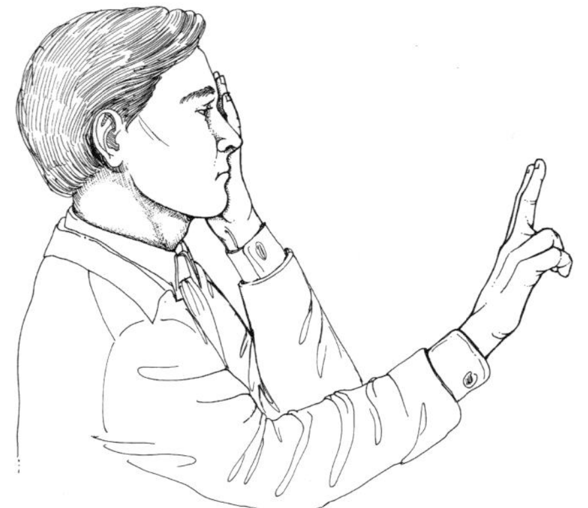
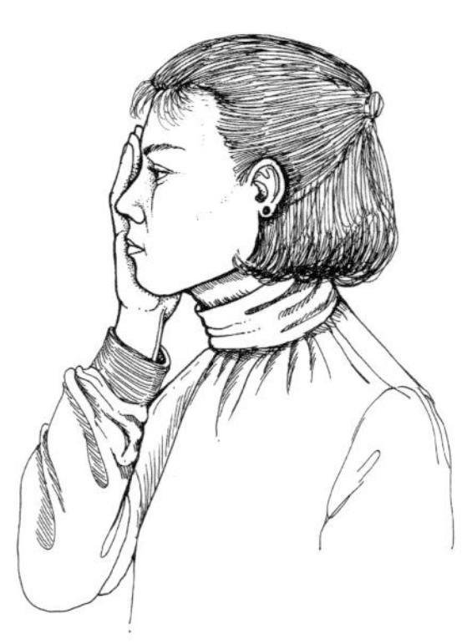

FIGURE 12-4. A confrontational visual field test is done to detect losses of peripheral vision.

peripheral vision that he or she knows they cannot be seen. Test the uninjured eye for comparison.

The conjunctiva and sclera should be examined for hemorrhage, laceration, redness, and swelling. The cornea should be clear—any opacity may indicate ulcer or perforation. A drop of topical anesthetic such as proparacaine 0.5% can be used to facilitate the examination if a ruptured globe has been ruled out. (A ruptured globe is an eye that has a perforating [full-thickness] tear through either the cornea or sclera into the uvea or humors of the inner eye. See the diagnosis section on how to diagnose and manage a ruptured globe. No drops should be used if a ruptured globe is present.) If a slit lamp is available, it can be used for a more magnified and detailed view; however, the procedure is the same whether a slit lamp or penlight examination is done. A fluorescein strip can be used to check for conjunctival abrasions, lacerations, corneal abrasions, or perforation. The fluorescein strip is moistened with water or anesthetic drop and touched briefly to the inside of the patient's lower lid to transfer some orange dye to the lid. The patient blinks to spread the dye evenly across the surface of the eye in a smooth green wash. (The orange dye turns yellow-green in water.) If any geographic patches of dye stain brightly on the cornea because of pick-up of extra dye, the area is a corneal abrasion. Mucous threads and tear debris can also stain brightly, so the examiner should have the patient blink a few times. The items in the tear film will float about, but a corneal or conjunctival abrasion will remain stationary. The fluorescein should remain an even green wash over the cornea. A blue-filtered light or Woods lamp can be used to better visualize fluorescein stain because it causes the dye to fluoresce; any staining areas appear bright green. (Blue filters are available with many penlights, slit lamps, direct ophthalmoscopes, and muscle light attachments.) If there is a question of corneal perforation, the examiner should do the Seidel test. A dry fluorescein strip should be held up to the cornea just below the site in question. If there is a perforation, aqueous humor flowing from the perforation site will cause fluorescein to stream off the strip (Fig. 12-5). If a perforation is present, it must be surgically explored and repaired.

Make sure the iris and pupil are fully visible. If red or black blood is obscuring the view of any part of the iris, the patient has a hyphema, defined as blood in the anterior chamber. If the pupil is irregular or the sclera is obscured by pigmented material, a ruptured globe may be present. Iris tears or iridodialysis (iris disinsertion from its base at the ciliary body) can occur after blunt trauma and can cause irregular pupils.

The pressure in the eye should be checked, usually by Schiotz tonometer or applanation tonometry, if experienced personnel are present. (Any eye with a suspected rupture or possible perforation should not have the pressure checked until examined by an ophthalmologist because pressure on the globe can worsen such situations.) Finger pressure can provide a rough guide to intraocular pressure if no other method is available. This is done by gently pressing on both sides of the globe at once through the patient's closed lids with the index fingers to get an idea of the pressure within the globe. The examiner can compare the firmness of the globe to the patient's uninjured eye and to his or her own to get an idea of normal pressure. An eye that is abnormally soft may indicate a ruptured globe—further examination should be deferred until seen by an ophthalmologist. An eye that is abnormally firm may have glaucoma or retrobulbar hemorrhage, blood collecting behind the eye—a potential ophthalmic emergency. Resistance to retropulsion can also be assessed to evaluate for retrobulbar hemorrhage: the eye should be pushed gently backward into the orbit by pressure on the globe through the closed lids. Healthy eyes can be retropulsed with a mild force; if the eye meets undue resistance, a retrobulbar bleed should be considered. This is especially significant if periocular tissue swelling is not sufficient to explain the degree of resistance.

If a direct ophthalmoscope is available, it can be used by experienced personnel to visualize the optic nerve, macula, and vitreous and to look for optic nerve edema. Optic nerve edema can indicate increased intracranial

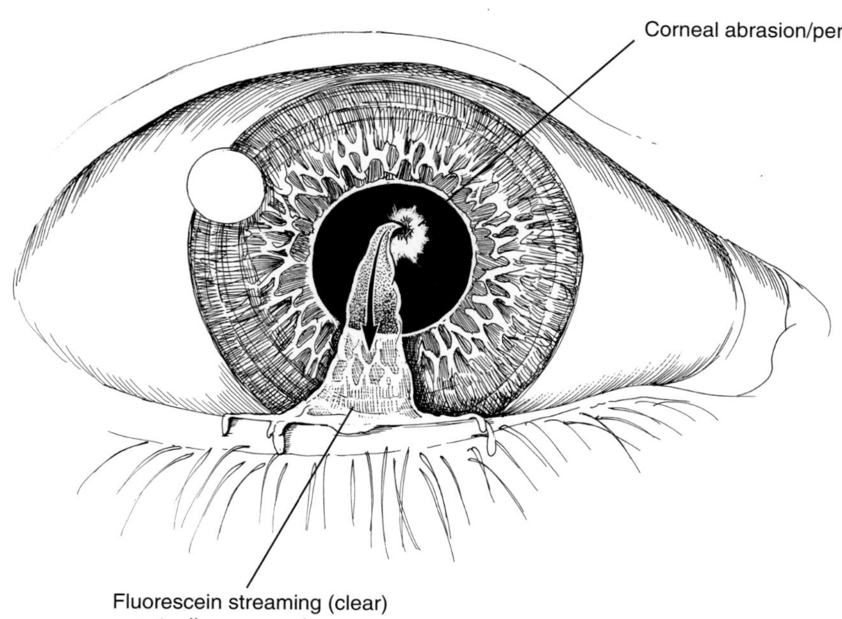

FIGURE 12-5. Seidel test: a corneal perforation detected by fluorescein streaming resulting from aqueous humor outflow.

pressure (from subdural hematoma, usually bilateral) or severe hypotony (from ruptured globe). Retinal or vitreous hemorrhage, posterior retinal tears, or retinal detachment can also be seen. The direct ophthalmoscope can be used easily by following these simple steps. The examiner should set the displayed number to 0 (diopters) and stand facing the patient on the same side as the eye to be examined. The examiner should wear his or her glasses if applicable; the patient should remove his or her glasses. The examiner should ask the patient to look up slightly and to the side away from the examiner. For example, if the patient's right eye is being examined, the patient should look up slightly and to the left. (This brings the optic nerve directly in line with the examiner's view through the pupil.) The ophthalmoscope is held close to the examiner's eye and brought close to the patient's pupil. The patient should be instructed to keep his or her eyes open and still while maintaining gaze up and away, although his or her view will be largely blocked by the examiner's head. The examiner will see the red reflex of the pupil and should come closer, moving his or her head and the scope as one unit and keeping a direct view through the scope, until a linear, red retinal blood vessel is visible. That vessel leads to the optic nerve by following any branching vessel back to its trunk. Vessels branch in a "Y" pattern; the optic nerve is at the base, or bottom, of all the Y's (see Fig. 12-3). The scope can be focused if necessary by slowly turning different plus (black or green) or minus (red) diopter values into the scope while looking at the vessels to get the clearest view. A nearsighted (myopic) patient will have the retina in clearest focus with minus diopters added to the scope; a farsighted patient may require plus diopters in the scope for a clear view. Before the examiner attempts to focus, he or she should be close to the patient and have a retinal vessel or optic nerve in view. Usually no more than 4 diopters need be dialed to achieve focus. The optic nerve, once it is in focus, is generally a little larger than the examiner's field of view with the direct ophthalmoscope, and the examiner will have to move his or her head slightly to assess all of its borders. The margins should be clear and sharp. To see the macula, the examiner turns the scope temporally toward the patient's ear and looks for the area where the blood vessels curve toward a darker area of retina and then stop, not reaching the center. This is the macula—the area of sharpest vision. The examiner should evaluate for blood or pallor and may have the macula brought directly to his or her view by telling the patient to look directly into the light of the scope. A limited examination of the posterior retina can be done by moving slowly around the periphery, looking for tears or blood. To fully evaluate the retina for tears or detachment, a dilated examination by an ophthalmologist is necessary. Naturally, if the symptoms cannot be explained after the initial examination or if any significant finding is encountered, an ophthalmologist should be consulted.

Additional references that offer general descriptions of an eye examination after trauma are noted here.[8,9,11]

COMMON INJURIES: DIAGNOSIS AND TREATMENT

All medications have side effects and contraindications to usage in certain situations; eye medications are no exception. Anyone administering any of the medications recommended in this chapter must be familiar with their restrictions and must ascertain their safety for each patient on a case-by-case basis.

Conjunctiva, Cornea, and Sclera

The most common injuries to this region of the eye are abrasions and lacerations, subconjunctival hemorrhage, entrapped foreign bodies, and chemical injury.

Lacerations and Abrasions. Lacerations and abrasions of the conjunctiva and cornea can be caused by any kind of scraping or wiping across the ocular surface. Lacerations and abrasions often cause symptoms of pain, tearing, a gritty sensation, or photophobia (sensitivity to light). If the central cornea is abraded, vision will be decreased. Signs include conjunctival hyperemia (redness) and conjunctival chemosis (swelling). If of long duration, lid swelling and a reactive ptosis (upper lid droop) may occur. Diagnosis is made by inspection, noting a defect in the conjunctival or corneal surface, and aided by a slit lamp if available. Fluorescein dye should be applied after initial inspection to better visualize any abrasions; they will stain brightly and be seen well with blue light (the technique was described in the previous section).

Simple linear conjunctival lacerations usually heal well. The only treatment required is an antibiotic drop 3 to 4 times a day for 4 days to prevent infection. A broad-spectrum antibiotic ophthalmic drop such as tobramycin 0.3% or sulfacetamide 10% can be used. If a geographic patch of conjunctiva has been removed, an antibiotic ophthalmic ointment (tobramycin or erythromycin) and pressure patch can be applied (patching technique is discussed in the following paragraph). A patch worn for 24 hours is advised; then the area can be reexamined. Conjunctiva usually heals within 24 hours. If the abrasion has healed or become smaller, the patient can use antibiotic drops as discussed previously for several more days. If the conjunctiva is in many shreds, surgical examination and debridement are warranted. The sclera below any conjunctival laceration must be carefully examined to rule out scleral laceration or penetrating injury. Any sign of laceration that involves the sclera requires a fully dilated examination to rule out ruptured globe or underlying retinal injury. If the laceration worsens or becomes purulent, prompt referral to an ophthalmologist is necessary.

Corneal abrasions are superficial lacerations to the cornea that remove the epithelial layer of the cornea. On penlight examination the cornea may look normal, but with fluorescein staining the abraded area will stain bright green (also seen best with a blue light). Corneal abrasions can be managed with an antibiotic ointment (tobramycin, erythromycin) and a pressure patch worn for 24 hours. If the wound is dirty, however, a patch may increase the risk of infection, and some patients cannot tolerate a patch. Corneal abrasions can also be managed with frequent (i.e., every two hours) applications of ophthalmic antibiotic ointment. (Ointments containing neomycin should be avoided, as this can be irritating to the cornea with frequent application.) These abrasions are usually painful because of the ciliary muscle spasm that often accompanies them. If the patient is very uncomfortable, a drop of cycloplegic can be given to relax the ciliary muscle. Such drops, like homatropine 5% (preferred for children; 2% for infants) or cyclopentolate 1%, or 2% for adults, will dilate the pupil and blur the patient's vision of close objects for 24 hours or so. The patient should be warned of this side effect. Atropine drops should not be used because their effects can last 1 to 2 weeks. Nonsteroidal anti-inflammatory drops (such as ketorolac) may be used every 4 hours to decrease pain, although the efficacy varies.[22] The patient may even need prescription pain medication orally for a day or two. If using a pressure patch, the examiner should apply the cycloplegic drop, the ointment directly over the cornea, and then the pressure patch as follows: fold an oval eye pad in half and place over the closed eyelid. Put an unfolded eye pad over this, and place tape on the patient's forehead, across the pads, and onto his or her cheek. The patch should be taped tightly to prevent the eyelid from opening, but should not be uncomfortable for the patient. The next day, the patient should be examined by an ophthalmologist to ensure complete healing or for repatching if necessary. Abrasions can become corneal ulcers if unhealed and will require much more intensive treatment. Any area of white or grey opacity in the normally clear cornea is a possible corneal ulcer and should be examined by an ophthalmologist. Corneal ulcers require intensive antibiotic management, possible scraping and culture, and may worsen if a patch is applied. They do not form in the acute injury period; it takes 1 to 2 days for an ulcer to form after injury.

The sclera is a tougher tissue that does not abrade. It can be lacerated, however, which is usually associated with an overlying conjunctival laceration and subconjunctival hemorrhage. A scleral laceration will appear as a discontinuity in the sclera. If the laceration penetrates the sclera, the underlying reddish-brown uvea may bulge through the wound. (The uvea is the vascular layer of the eye between the retina and sclera, comprising the choroid, ciliary body, and iris.) This bulge is a sign of a ruptured globe. A shield should be placed over the eye and further examination should be done by an ophthalmologist because surgical repair may be required. If there is a possibility of perforating scleral injury but the sclera cannot be adequately visualized because of overlying subconjunctival hemorrhage, the eye needs to be explored surgically.

Subconjunctival Hemorrhage. A subconjunctival hemorrhage can occur with any laceration or blunt injury, but also may result from Valsalva maneuvers during straining, weightlifting, constipation, or vomiting. It can also occur with aspirin use or spontaneously, unassociated with an injury. A subconjunctival hemorrhage is a collection of bright red blood under the conjunctiva but overlying the sclera, obscuring the white of the sclera (Fig. 12-6). The blood stops at the cornea and does not

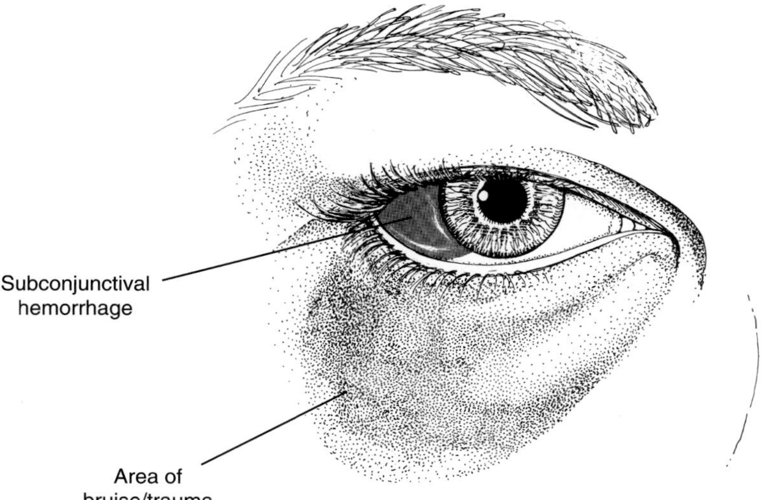

FIGURE 12-6. Subconjunctival hemorrhage: blood does not cross the limbus or obscure the iris.

obscure the cornea, iris, or pupil. This bleeding is often startling, but is painless and not associated with other symptoms. Isolated hemorrhages do not require treatment and will resolve after a few weeks, changing color and clearing in the same manner as a bruise of the skin. The sclera below the hemorrhage should be carefully inspected to rule out laceration or perforation. If associated with other signs or symptoms such as decreased vision, pain, irregular pupils, or scleral irregularity, a dilated examination is needed to discover the cause.

Foreign Bodies. Foreign bodies are usually felt entering the eye. Before any topical anesthetic drop is applied, the patient should be asked to localize where he or she feels the foreign body to direct the examiner's search. Pain is the usual symptom of conjunctival or corneal foreign bodies. Conjunctival foreign bodies often show a localized hyperemia. The longer the time from injury, the more diffuse conjunctival irritation will be seen. A marked papillary reaction can be seen around many conjunctival foreign bodies (the conjunctiva shows many small, elevated bumps, seen with a slit lamp for magnification). Corneal foreign bodies show a perilimbal (encircling the base of the cornea) or diffuse irritation. If lodged in the central cornea, a foreign body may be associated with decreased vision.

If a visible foreign body is located superficially in the conjunctiva, it can be removed with a fine forceps under direct visualization. A slit lamp or surgical loupes can be used to aid magnification. A drop of proparacaine and an antibiotic drop (such as tobramycin 0.3% or sulfacetamide 10%) should be given before and after removal, and an antibiotic drop should be used four times daily for approximately 4 days while the conjunctiva heals. A small amount of conjunctival bleeding is expected and should stop momentarily or at most require local pressure with a cotton swab soaked in proparacaine (or phenylephrine, 2.5%, for hemostasis) for a few minutes.

Any foreign body in the cornea should be removed at a slit lamp by trained personnel. The beveled edge of a 27-gauge needle on a tuberculin syringe makes a useful removal tool (care must be used to avoid perforating the cornea). An antibiotic drop and anesthetic drop should be given before and after removal. A corneal burr can be used to smooth the residual abrasion if necessary. If there are many scattered particles that are difficult to see, such as glass shards, the superficial pieces can be removed, but any that might be penetrating the eye should be left for an ophthalmologist to examine. If there is a possibility of foreign bodies penetrating into the eye, orbit, or lids where they cannot be seen, radiographs or computed tomography (CT) scans can help localize them if they are of radioopaque material.

If there is a possibility of a ruptured globe, a shield should be placed over the eye and orbital rim. No drops, manipulation, or further examination should be done until seen by an ophthalmologist. Ruptured globes require surgical exploration and repair and will be discussed more fully.

The upper lid should be everted to remove any foreign particles that may have become trapped beneath it. (This should not be done if there is a risk of the eye having a perforating laceration because the maneuver puts increased pressure on the eye and may worsen a laceration.) The examiner should apply a drop of proparacaine and ask the patient to look down. The examiner should grasp the upper eyelashes, pull the upper lid toward him- or herself and away from the patient's eye, and then push with a cotton swab or coin edge downward on the skin of the upper lid near the upper lid crease, while folding the lashes upward over the swab, and back toward the brow (Fig. 12-7). The examiner then checks the inner (tarsal) surface of the eyelid exposed in this way and removes or flushes away any particles; sweeping underneath the tarsus can be done with a cotton swab

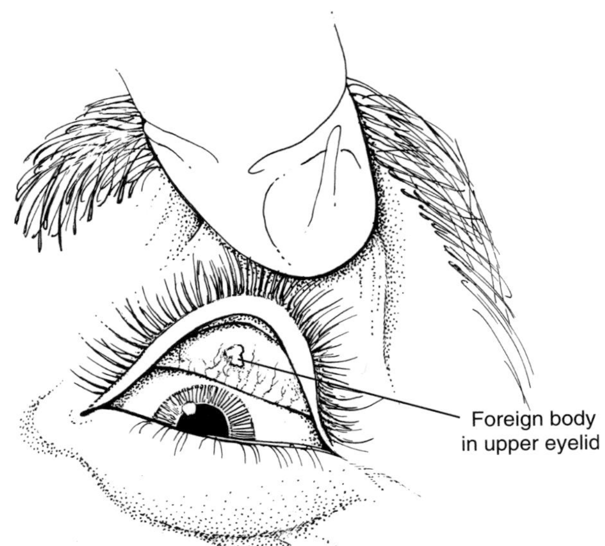

FIGURE 12-7. Everted upper lid.

moistened with an anesthetic drop to ensure that no particles are trapped there. Care should be taken to not rub against the surface of the cornea during this procedure because the patient's natural reaction is to pull away from the swab and to roll his or her eyes upward. The patient should be instructed to look down during this maneuver.

After foreign body removal from the cornea, abrasions inevitably remain. If very small, they can be managed with antibiotic ointment (tobramycin or erythromycin) for 1 night—they should be examined the next day to ensure complete healing. The patient can then use an antibiotic drop (such as tobramycin or sulfacetamide) four times daily for 4 days. If the abrasion is larger, it should be pressure-patched as described previously.

Foreign bodies lodged in the sclera are penetrating injuries; these are most safely explored and removed by an ophthalmologist because of the possibility of ruptured globe.

Chemical Injuries. Chemical injuries occur when a toxic material such as grass lime enters the eye. The history is usually sufficient to diagnose the problem. The injury to most eyes will be painful and will involve varying degrees of photophobia and visual loss. The conjunctiva is usually red and may be chemotic. Even when the eye is white, the risk of damage from acidic or basic substances is high. In severe base burns, the eye is deceptively white because of extensive ischemic damage to the conjunctival and episcleral vessels. The cornea may be abraded, cloudy, or opaque. The eye should be flushed immediately with several liters of fluid. Rinses designed for the eye, sterile normal saline, or Ringer's lactate are preferred, but plain water should be used if it is the only fluid available. A drop of proparacaine in the eye as a topical anesthetic will allow the patient to open his or her eye during flushing, making it easier to get water past the lids, but flushing should begin immediately whether or not the drop is available. The eye should be flushed for 15 minutes with several liters of fluid. This is most easily done using a squeeze bottle, emergency eyewash sinks, or intravenous tubing connected to a bag of solution. The stream of water should not be sprayed directly onto the cornea if possible (to avoid abrasion), but rather rinsed on the sclera and allowed to flow over the cornea. The upper lid should be everted (technique as previously described), and the area beneath the lids should be flushed as well. Any foreign material should be removed. The pH of the tears (normally 7.0 to 7.7) can be tested several minutes after rinsing to ensure that no residual acidic or basic substances remain. Mild chemical injury that has only reddened the conjunctiva can be managed with an antibiotic drop. A small corneal abrasion can be pressure-patched with antibiotic ointment and a cycloplegic drop as described previously. However, if symptoms, signs, or visual disturbances persist for more than a few hours, the patient should be referred to an ophthalmologist. Perilimbal blanching, large abrasions, or elevated intraocular pressure are ominous signs and require referral. Steroid drops are sometimes useful but should be used by an ophthalmologist because they can aggravate some situations, such as infections.[3,13]

Swimmers experience frequent mild injuries to the cornea and conjunctiva from the hypotonicity, pH, chlorine, and chloramines of pool water. They develop conjunctivitis, corneal superficial punctate keratitis, microabrasions, and corneal edema, symptoms of which include eye irritation and halos seen around lights. No treatment is required if symptoms disappear several hours after cessation of swimming. Goggles greatly decrease the incidence of eye irritation.[15] If symptoms or signs persist, the patient should be examined for corneal abrasions and treated as outlined previously. If corneal opacities are noted, the patient should be referred to an ophthalmologist for possible corneal ulcer.

Anterior Segment (Anterior Chamber, Iris, Pupil, Lens)

Iritis (inflammation of the iris) is very common after concussive (blunt) trauma. The most prominent symptom is photophobia, with mildly decreased or normal vision, mild-to-moderate pain, and tearing. The eye is usually red, often more prominently around the limbus. Iritis is diagnosed at the slit lamp by observing cells and flare in the aqueous humor. The injured eye may have a lower intraocular pressure and poorly dilating pupil. It can be managed by steroid drops (prednisolone acetate 1% four times daily for 4 days can resolve a moderately traumatic iritis). Dosage is adjusted depending on severity. A cycloplegic drop (cyclopentolate 1% or homatropine 5%) may be added for comfort and to prevent iris adhesions to the cornea or lens during the period of acute inflammation.

Follow-up evaluation should ensure that the iritis is gone before the drops are no longer administered. Traumatic iritis should resolve within 1 week with drops; if additional treatment is required, the patient should be referred to an ophthalmologist.

Certain kinds of damage to iris structures and the ciliary body can be asymptomatic, with normal vision and general appearance. Examples are iridodialysis (a tear of the iris base from its attachment to the ciliary body) and angle recession (a tear through the muscle layers of the ciliary body). These injuries may not cause symptoms until months after the injury, when a late-onset glaucoma causes permanent visual loss. Patients with severe iridodialysis may appear to have an irregular pupil and have symptoms of iritis (Fig. 12-8). Even patients without symptoms are at risk for late-onset glaucoma. Any patient who had a concussive injury should have an eye examination done to evaluate these structures 1 to 2 weeks after injury.[19]

A hyphema is a serious injury often associated with blunt trauma to the globe. A hyphema is blood in the anterior chamber of the eye collecting behind the cornea and in front of the iris (Fig. 12-9). The blood partially obscures the view of the iris, sometimes the pupil, and layers by gravity. When the patient is sitting up, only the inferior part of the iris may be obscured. The patient may have no symptoms or may experience only the expected pain and photophobia from an associated iritis. A complete, or "eight ball," hyphema fills the entire anterior chamber with blood so that behind the cornea the eye looks like a dark mass, with no iris or pupil seen. Vision is obviously decreased in such cases. Hyphemas are associated with a 10% incidence of rebleeding and risk of severe glaucoma. The patient must be referred immediately to an ophthalmologist and followed daily, usually with bedrest, until the blood clears. He or she may require hospitalization or surgery to clear the blood and control the intraocular pressure. While awaiting referral, the patient should be placed at bedrest with the head of the bed elevated 30° to allow the blood to settle into the inferior part of the eye; the patient should not be given aspirin, which can worsen bleeding. Vomiting can worsen bleeding; an antiemetic should be given if needed. If a ruptured globe can be ruled out, atropine 1% drops can be given every 6 hours. Elevated intraocular pressure can be controlled by topical beta-blocker drops, oral carbonic anhydrase inhibitors (acetazolamide, methazolamide), and intravenous mannitol as needed.

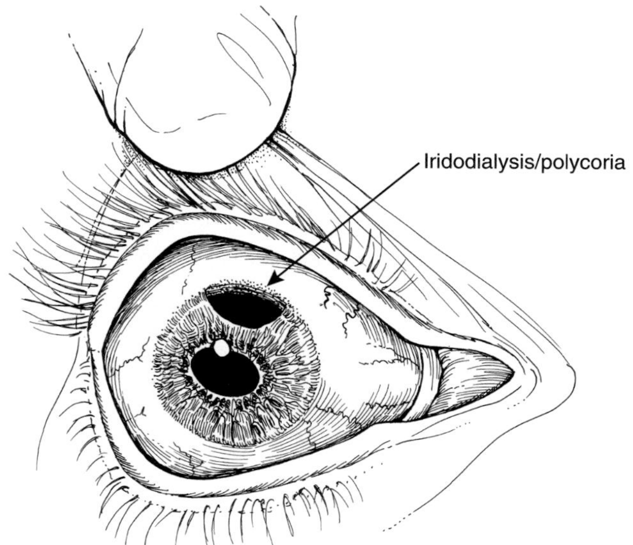

FIGURE 12-8. Iridodialysis causing irregular pupil and polycoria (the appearance of multiple pupils).

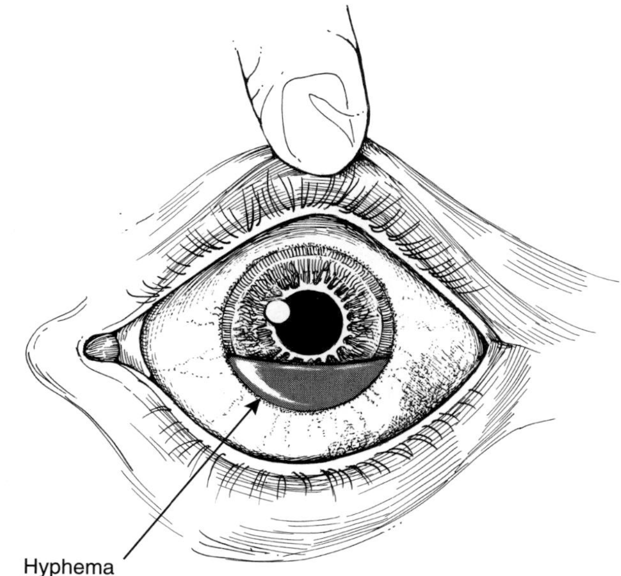

FIGURE 12-9. Hyphema: blood layers in anterior chamber and obscures iris.

Microhyphemas have erythrocytes floating in the anterior chamber but no layering of blood. This diagnosis can only be made with the slit lamp. Care must be taken to distinguish erythrocytes from the pigmented iris cells of iritis. When a microhyphema is present, the patient must also be put at bedrest and observed closely for rebleeding. A complete dilated examination is needed to evaluate for other trauma.

Topical steroid drops are generally indicated (such as prednisolone acetate 1%) to treat the associated iritis. The risk of vision loss increases if a spontaneous rebleed occurs after a patient has suffered a hyphema. To decrease the likelihood of rebleed, the use of topical steroid drops, oral steroids, and oral or topical aminocaproic acid may be considered.[6]

Blunt trauma can sublux (partially dislocate) or completely dislocate the lens of the eye. A symptom is decreased vision. Diagnosis is made by visualizing the lens edge or eccentric center of the lens with a dilated

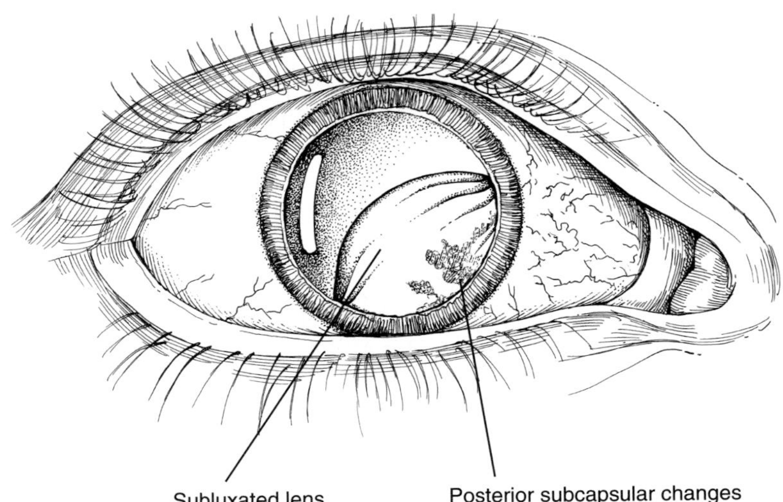

FIGURE 12-10. Subluxed, or partially dislocated, lens. The lens edge can be seen in the pupil.

examination or by observing the lens in the anterior chamber or in the vitreous (Fig. 12-10). Any patient with this problem should see an ophthalmologist. Lenses dislocated into the anterior chamber cause glaucoma and corneal decompensation and need to be removed. Lenses in the vitreous are often well tolerated, and surgery may not be necessary. Cataracts can form from trauma, especially after penetrating injuries when a foreign body enters the lens. Blunt trauma can also cause cataracts. If the lens capsule is intact, these findings can be observed. Rupture of the capsule may require removal to avoid the development of phacoanaphylactic inflammatory response to the lens proteins released inside the eye. Such reactions, which develop days to weeks after the injury, can be severe and can destroy the eye.

Posterior Segment (Optic Nerve, Retina, Vitreous)

Any patient with signs or symptoms of posterior segment trauma (as will be described) requires an immediate dilated examination to adequately evaluate the optic nerve, retina, vitreous, and choroid. In addition, any patient who has suffered concussive trauma but is asymptomatic should have a dilated examination in the next week to rule out asymptomatic injury.

Concussive trauma to the eye can cause retinal swelling called *commotio*, which is often asymptomatic. If the commotio involves the macula, the patient will have decreased vision. When commotio is present, the retina is whitened on examination. This condition is difficult to appreciate with the direct ophthalmoscope I but is more obvious with the indirect ophthalmoscope. Commotio usually resolves completely without treatment, but it can leave areas of retinal pigment changes with some visual loss. A dilated examination should be done for all patients who have commotio because of the possibility of retinal tears.

Retinal tears are important to diagnose because they may lead to detachment. Symptoms of new floating spots in front of the eyes or spontaneous flashing lights require examination by an ophthalmologist. Retinal tears appear as distinct retinal defects with the orange choroidal color showing through (Fig. 12-11). There may be pigment or retinal fragments floating in the vitreous above the tear. Retinal detachments and retinal tears are usually located more peripherally than can be seen with the direct ophthalmoscope; a dilated examination with indirect ophthalmoscopy is necessary. Tears can also occur without signs or symptoms, so after concussive injury a dilated eye examination by an ophthalmologist should be done in the next week to rule out asymptomatic injury.

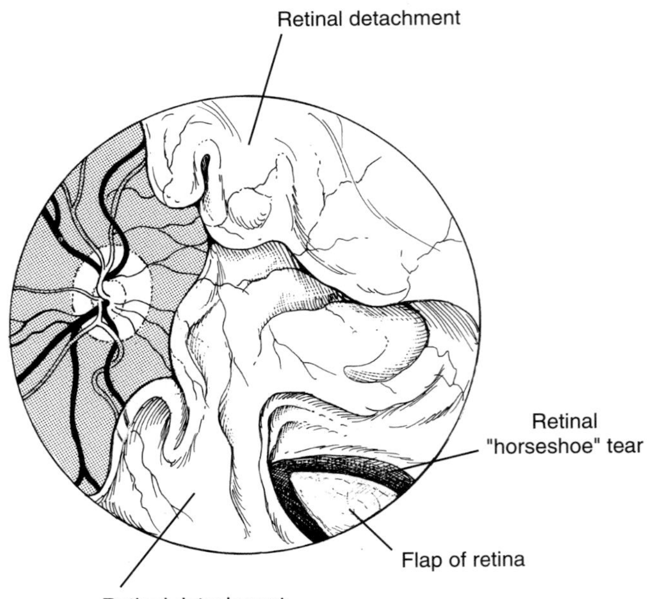

FIGURE 12-11. Retinal detachment.

Laser treatment, cryotherapy, or surgery may be required if tears are present.

Retinal detachment (see Fig. 12-11) can occur without loss of central vision. The patient may notice, when covering one eye, that the other eye has lost part of its peripheral vision. This vision loss is often described as a "curtain coming down" into the patient's field of view. Such symptoms require an immediate dilated eye examination. A confrontation visual field test (as described previously) should be performed after concussive trauma, even for asymptomatic patients. If loss of vision is noticed, a dilated examination is required. Other signs of retinal detachment are pigment in the vitreous, and the transparent membrane of the retina with the retinal blood vessels floating off the surface of the choroid. Retinal detachments require prompt surgical repair. They can progress if untreated and result in permanent visual loss.

Blood in the vitreous will obscure vision or give symptoms of floating spots or lines in front of the vision. Local clumps of heme or a diffuse red haze in the vitreous are seen, often obscuring the view of the optic nerve or macula. Although the blood will often clear without treatment, a dilated examination is needed to identify the source of the bleeding. Retinal tears or choroidal rupture (a tear in the choroid) are common causes of vitreous hemorrhage after trauma.

Optic nerve injury can occur from severe concussive trauma (more commonly seen after automobile collisions than after sports injuries). The vision will be decreased, and the patient will have an afferent pupillary defect. If results of the examination are otherwise normal, the afferent pupillary defect may be caused by compression of the optic nerve at the level of the optic canal. A new afferent pupillary defect should be considered an ophthalmic emergency; imaging studies (CT or magnetic resonance imaging [MRI] scan concentrating on the optic nerve from globe to chiasm and the brain) and an ophthalmologic examination should be obtained. Management may include consideration of high-dose steroid administration to decrease inflammation or surgery to relieve compression.[18]

Optic nerve edema, noted with a direct ophthalmoscope, may occur without symptoms or vision changes. Symptoms, when they occur, include central scotomas, headache, and brief periods (seconds) of visual loss. The margins of the optic nerve appear blurred, either diffusely or focally, with partial obscuration of the blood vessels as they cross the optic nerve margin (Fig. 12-12). An ophthalmologic examination and imaging studies are required because optic nerve edema after trauma can signal increased intracranial pressure such as from subdural or epidural hematoma (usually affecting both optic nerves). Unilateral optic nerve edema may imply severe hypotony from a ruptured globe—this is usually obvious from other signs.

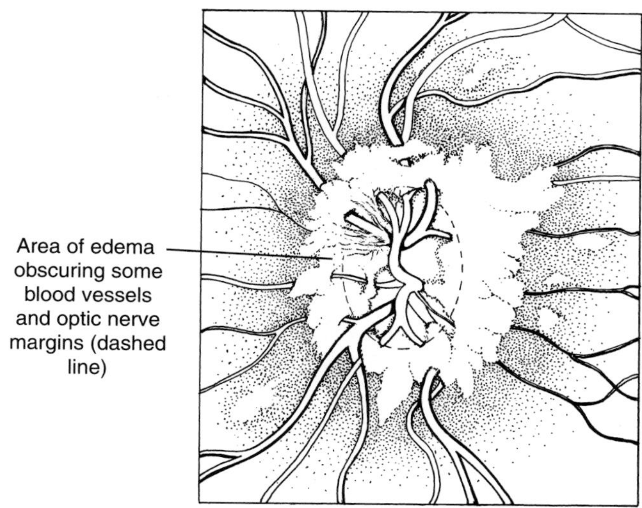

FIGURE 12-12. Edema of the optic nerve. The optic nerve margins are blurred, and the blood vessels may be indistinct as they cross the optic nerve.

Ruptured Globe

A ruptured globe is a perforation of the sclera or cornea. A direct blow with an object smaller than the size of the orbit (a squash ball or an elbow) is the most likely type of injury to cause ragged rupture of the globe. Other common causes of ruptured globe are lacerating injuries (darts, glass shards). The patient usually has poor vision but may not have much pain. The most obvious signs of a ruptured globe are disorganization of anterior structures. Without touching the eye, the sclera should be examined for signs of uvea (dark pigmented tissue) protruding through the sclera (Fig. 12-13).

The weakest points of the sclera are near the insertion of the recti muscles, so ruptures most often occur at these sites (approximately 6 to 7 mm posterior, radially outward, from the limbus, at 12, 3, 6, and 9 o'clock). There is often extensive subconjunctival hemorrhage. The pupil, instead of being round, may be misshapen or elongated as the iris is pulled toward the rupture site. There may be a hyphema that obscures the iris entirely or partially. An afferent defect is sometimes present.

If there is a possibility of ruptured globe, the eye should not be manipulated in any way. Drops should not be used. An eye shield should be placed over the eye and the patient sent immediately to an ophthalmologist. Any pressure put on the eye from patches or examination may cause the rupture to enlarge and the contents of the eye to extrude. The patient should be kept at bedrest and receive no food or drink. Antiemetics should be administered if needed to avoid vomiting, which can worsen a rupture. Tetanus toxoid should be given if needed. Intravenous antibiotics can be administered: for adults, cefazolin 1 g intravenously every 8 hours plus

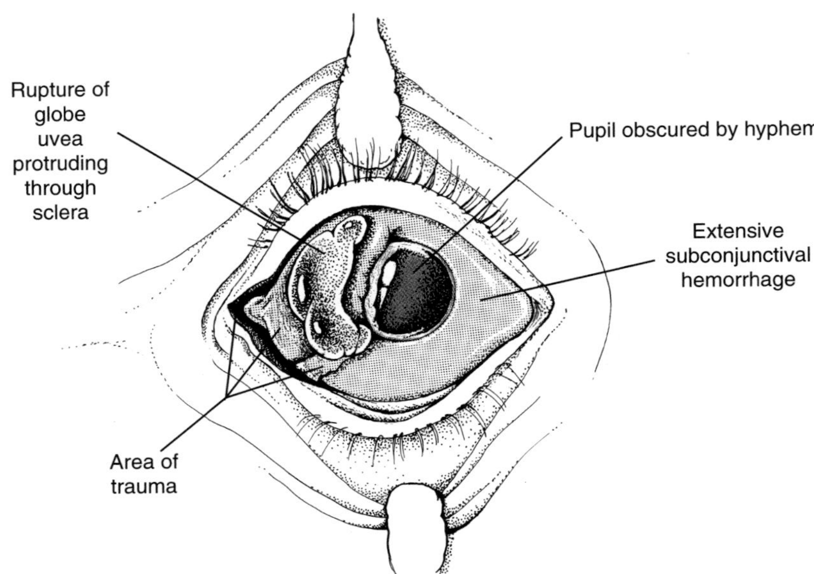

FIGURE 12-13. Ruptured globe. Uvea is seen protruding through sclera from 7 to 9 o'clock just outside limbus. Also present are extensive subconjunctival hemorrhage and the pupil obscured by hyphema.

gentamicin 2.0 mg/kg intravenous load, then cefazolin plus gentamicin, 1 mg/kg intravenously every 8 hours. For children, the dose is cefazolin 50 mg/kg/24 h intravenously in divided doses given every 6 or 8 hours, plus gentamicin, 2 mg/kg intravenously every 8 hours.[7] CT scan may be needed to rule out intraocular foreign body or to localize a rupture site.

A small, localized corneal perforation can be temporarily sealed with cyanoacrylate glue or fibrin glue to maintain eye integrity before an ophthalmologist is available, but a thorough slit lamp examination is necessary to ensure that the injury is localized and amenable to such treatment.[17,21]

Ruptured globes can occur posteriorly and be difficult to see. Findings associated with occult scleral rupture include severe vision loss (less than 20/400), hypotony (low intraocular pressure), extensive subconjunctival hemorrhage, hyphema, vitreous hemorrhage, afferent pupillary defect, abnormally deep or shallow anterior chamber, or unexplained loss of extraocular movement. If the eye looks intact but these findings suggest occult rupture, the patient should be referred to an ophthalmologist rather than risking a missed diagnosis. Imaging studies can sometimes be helpful in such cases. Ruptured globes require surgical repair.[10]

Orbital Bone Fractures

In a blunt injury with an object larger than the orbital opening (basketball or baseball bat), most of the force of the injury is absorbed by the bones of the orbit, often sparing the globe. All the injuries mentioned in the previous section can be seen, but more commonly fractures of the orbital bones occur. Orbital floor fractures and medial wall fractures are the most common because the bones are thinnest at these locations. A greater force is needed to cause inferior orbital rim or lateral rim fractures. High impact forces are required for superior orbital rim fractures and tripod fractures (fractures of the zygoma at its three articulations: the arch, the lateral orbital rim, and the inferior orbital rim).[14]

Symptoms of orbital fracture include local tenderness and binocular double vision (usually worse on upgaze for orbital floor fractures). It should be noted that binocular double vision (with both eyes open) in any field of gaze can be a sign of injury to an extraocular muscle or nerve or a result of soft-tissue swelling displacing the eye. Difficulty chewing or inability to open the mouth widely can indicate a tripod fracture because the coronoid process impinges on the mandible. Key physical findings that suggest a fracture include an irregularity or discontinuity in palpation along the orbital rims (there are normal notches along the inferior and superior rims—compare with the other orbit to detect asymmetry). Swelling and ecchymosis of the overlying eyelid are often present. Decreased sensation to the upper cheek below the injured eye often accompanies an orbital floor fracture, signaling injury to the inferior orbital nerve. Crepitus from emphysema of the lids or periorbital tissues occurs with floor or medial wall fractures, when the orbital wall fractures into a sinus and air from the sinus enters the periorbital tissues. (The patient may notice his or her lids swell after nose blowing. If so, the patient should avoid nose blowing.) An eye that appears enophthalmic (sunken in compared with the other eye) also suggests a floor or medial wall fracture. Limited vertical movement of the involved eye (an inability to look up or down) can mean that a floor fracture has trapped orbital tissue or extraocular muscle within it (Fig. 12-14). Forced ductions can be performed to test eye mobility. A topical

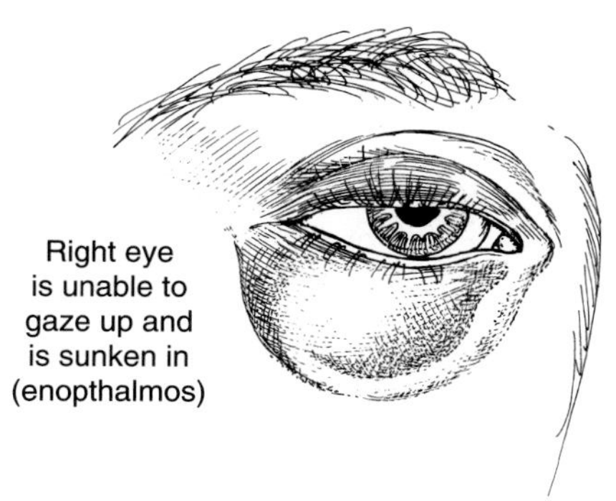
Right eye
is unable to
gaze up and
is sunken in
(enopthalmos)

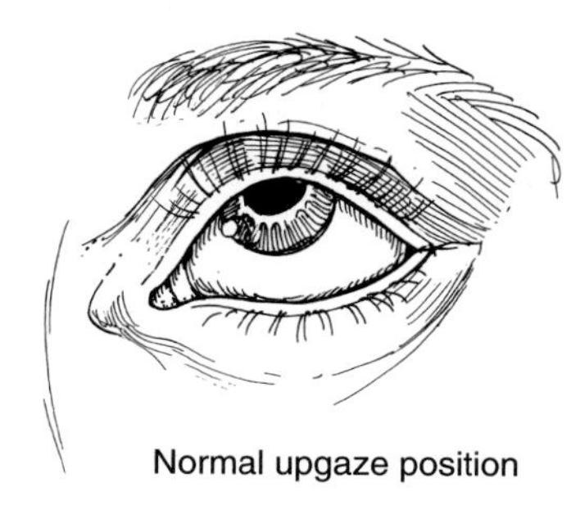
Normal upgaze position

FIGURE 12-14. Right orbital floor fracture. Patient is attempting to look up: note restricted upgaze and enophthalmos of right eye.

anesthetic drop, such as proparacaine, should be given. The conjunctiva should be grasped near the cornea and the eye rotated in any direction. A normal eye is freely movable. If the eye is unable to be elevated with forceps and there is resistance against the pull of the forceps, there may be an orbital fracture. To diagnose any fracture with certainty requires radiographs and, occasionally, CT scans. Large fractures require surgical repair, but small fractures frequently do not. An ophthalmologist should be consulted to determine if surgery is necessary.

Other traumatic causes of binocular diplopia, such as damage to an extraocular muscle or nerve, are rare in sports injuries unless associated with obvious lacerations that require surgical exploration and repair. A binocular vertical diplopia can develop because of concussive trauma resulting from IVth nerve palsy. In this case the double vision is worse (images appear farther apart) in gaze down and toward the nose of the effected side. The patient should be followed; if no resolution occurs when the soft-tissue swelling resolves, he or she should see an ophthalmologist.

Periorbital Injury

Bruising and swelling of the eyelids and tissues around the eye are common after blunt trauma. Localized pain is the usual symptom. Management consists of applying ice packs to the area as frequently as possible during the first 24 hours; after that, bruising will resolve with time. Swollen or lacerated lids should not prevent a thorough examination of the globe itself. The same blunt trauma may have caused a hyphema or other asymptomatic but potentially serious conditions. Obviously, no ice packs should be applied until a ruptured globe has been ruled out; the pressure from the pack can worsen a rupture.

Laceration of the skin around the eye is usually repaired with sutures after cleaning the wound with betadine, as with other wounds. There are several areas of special concern to the eye. The lacrimal drainage system is one such area. If the laceration is between the corner of the eye and the nose, it may have cut the lacrimal apparatus (tear drainage system). Any incision in this area should be cleaned, covered with sterile gauze moistened with saline, and the patient referred for an immediate ophthalmic examination. If the laceration is through the eyelid margin, the repair must be done with a layered technique, first closing the tarsus of the lid, then the skin, to prevent lid notching when healed. The patient should be referred if the field surgeon is not familiar with lid-suturing techniques. Any patient with a laceration associated with poor eye movement (possibly involving an eye muscle), lid droop (damage to eyelid retractor muscles), or unusual anatomic position should be referred to an ophthalmologist. Tetanus prophylaxis should be given if needed for any laceration.

A retrobulbar hemorrhage is a collection of blood behind the eye and within the orbit. It is an ophthalmic emergency that can occur from any deep laceration around the eyelids. If the injury penetrates the orbital septum (the tissue barrier between the eyelids and the deep orbit), blood can collect behind the globe within the orbit, where it cannot be seen. As the bleeding continues, the blood will push the globe forward and the intraocular pressure will be severely elevated. This condition can cause permanent blindness within hours if not detected. The patient may not be aware of the condition, and any pain may be attributed to the laceration. The main symptoms are increasing pain and decreased vision, often rapidly worsening over several hours. Characteristic signs and symptoms of retrobulbar hemorrhage are pain, proptosis (forward protrusion of the eye), eyelid and subconjunctival hemorrhage, resistance to retropulsion, development of an afferent defect, and increased intraocular pressure.

Any patient who has had a laceration around the eyelids should be instructed, after repair, to check the vision in each eye periodically and compare the appearance of the eyes during the first 24 hours; he or she should be sure nothing has worsened. The patient should report any increasing pain. Any surgical repair of a lid laceration should be taped with sterile adhesive strips and not covered by a patch that obscures the eye, so appearance and vision can be monitored. If a retrobulbar hemorrhage occurs, it is an emergency. A lateral canthotomy with inferior cantholysis should be done immediately by an ophthalmologist or trained emergency personnel.[20] The canthotomy is done to allow the accumulated retrobulbar blood to exit and relieve the pressure on the eye. When performed promptly, permanent visual loss can be avoided. While waiting for the canthotomy, the intraocular pressure can be lowered by using topical beta-blocker drops, carbonic anhydrase inhibitors, or intravenous mannitol as needed.

PREVENTION

The best method for managing eye injuries is to prevent their occurrence. Adequate eye protection is essential for any sport in which injury is$_2$ a risk; face and head protection are often needed as well. The standards set by the American Society for Testing and Materials (ASTM) are based on performance testing by committees (composed of physicians, manufacturers, and athletes) and are useful guidelines for minimum recommended protection. Any protective eyewear should have lenses made of polycarbonate, which is more impact resistant than other plastic or glass lenses. Such lenses are recommended for all racquet sports; none of the lensless eye protectors are adequate because balls traveling at high speeds can deform and mold into the opening sufficiently to strike the eye.[2,4,16]

CONTENTS OF AN EYE EXAMINATION KIT

Several useful items should be available to facilitate eye examination and management whether at fieldside or in the emergency room. The following list includes the contents of a basic eye examination kit, with more extensive equipment listed in brackets.

- Emergency phone numbers (emergency room, ophthalmologist)
- Near card for vision testing (usually read at 14 inches) [eye chart for vision testing, preferably read at a 20-foot distance]
- Pinhole occluder for vision testing
- Pair of +2.50-diopter, over-the-counter reading glasses
- Penlight, with bright light [or halogen "muscle light" attachment of direct ophthalmoscope]
- Blue filter for tip of penlight for reviewing fluorescein stain
- Sterile cotton swabs
- Topical anesthetic drop (i.e., proparacaine 0.5%)
- Antibiotic ophthalmic drop (i.e., tobramycin, gentamicin, sulfacetamide)
- Antibiotic ophthalmic ointment (i.e., tobramycin, erythromycin, bacitracin)
- Fluorescein strips
- Sterile, large eye pads
- Paper tape
- Eye shields
- Eye fluid rinse bottle
- Sterile strips for closing lid skin wounds
- Direct ophthalmoscope, which may come with blue filter and bright light for fluorescein viewing, and slit lamp, useful for any examining area or emergency room.

REFERENCES

1. American Academy of Ophthalmology: Basic and clinical science course, section 3—optics, refraction and contact lenses. San Francisco, American Academy of Ophthalmology, 1993.
2. Anderson J: Prescription safety eyewear: Today vs. yesterday. Occ Health Saf 71(10):68–72, 2002.
3. Brodovsky SC, McCarty CA, Snibson G: Management of alkali burns: An 11-year retrospective review. Ophthalmol 107(10):1829–1835, 2000.
4. Chambers A: Safety goggles at a glance. Occ Health Saf 71(10):58–66, 2002.
5. Chang YS, Kao PL, Lee SC, et. al.: Severe stab injury of the eyelid can mimic eyeball perforation. Arch Ophthal 120(10):1410–1411, 2002.
6. Crouch ER Jr, Williams PB, Gray MK, et al: Topical aminocaproic acid in the treatment of traumatic hyphema. Arch Ophthal 115(9):1106–1112, 1997.
7. Cullen RD, Chang B (eds): Wills Eye Hospital: Office and emergency room diagnosis and treatment of eye disease, 3rd ed. Philadelphia, Lippincott, 1998.
8. DeLee JC: DeLee and Drez's Orthopaedic Sports Medicine, 2nd ed. Philadelphia, WB Saunders, 2003.
9. Harlan JB Jr, Pieramici DJ: Evaluation of patients with ocular trauma. Ophthal Clin N Am 15(2):153–161, 2002.
10. Hatton MP, Thakker MM, Ray S: Orbital and adnexal trauma associated with open-globe injuries. Ophthal Plas Recon Surg 18(6):458–461, 2002.
11. Juang PS, Rosen P: Ocular examination techniques for the emergency department. J Emer Med 15(6):793–810, 1997.
12. Koc RK, Akdemir H, Oktem IS, et al: Acute subdural hematoma: outcome and outcome prediction. Neurosurg Rev 20(4):239–244, 1997.
13. Kuckelkorn R, Schrage N, Keller G et al.: Emergency treatment of chemical and thermal eye burns. Acta Ophthalmol Scan 80(1):4–10, 2002.
14. Long J, Tann T: Orbital trauma. Ophthal Clin N Am 15(2):249–253, viii, 2002.
15. Pizzarello L, Haik B (eds): Sports ophthalmology, chapter 6. Springfield, Charles C. Thomas, 1987.
16. Protective eyewear for young athletes: A joint statement of the American Academy of Pediatrics and the

American Academy of Ophthalmology. Ophthal 103:1325–1328, 1996.
17. Sharma A, Kaut R, Kumar S, et al: Fibrin glue versus N-butyl-2-cyanoacrylate in corneal perforations. Ophthal 110(2):291–298, 2003.
18. Steinsapir KD, Seiff SR, Goldberg RA: Traumatic optic neuropathy: Where do we stand? Ophthal Plas Recon Surg 18(3):232–234, 2002.
19. Tumbocon JA, Latina MA: Angle recession glaucoma. Int Ophthal Clin 42(3):69–78, 2002.
20. Vassallo S, Hartstein M, Howard D et al: Traumatic retrobulbar hemorrhage: emergent decompression by lateral canthotomy and cantholysis. J Emerg Med 22(3):251-256, 2002.
21. Vote BJ, Elder MJ: Cyanoacrylate glue for corneal perforations: A description of a surgical technique and a review of the literature. Clin Exper Ophthal 28(6):437–442, 2000.
22. Weaver CS, Terrell KM: Evidence-based emergency medicine. Update: Do ophthalmic nonsteroidal anti-inflammatory drugs reduce the pain associated with simple corneal abrasion without delaying healing? Ann Emerg Med 41(1):134, 2003.

13 Craniofacial Injuries

Alex M. Greenberg and Richard H. Haug

The craniomaxillofacial region is injured frequently by athletes engaged in various forms of sports-related activities. The role of the primary care provider involved in the treatment of athletes, whether as a generalist or specialist, should be to have a well-informed appreciation of the anatomy, pathophysiology, etiology, distribution, and classification of the craniomaxillofacial injuries that may be encountered. This way, preventive and management-oriented approaches to these many problems can be applied to the treatment of these patients. Because contemporary sports activities range from those with minimal interpersonal contact to those with high-energy contact, including high-velocity vehicular and high-altitude–dependent activities,[3,10,31,36,41,54,55,71,43,18,53] possibilities exist for variations in the form of trauma. It is important to begin with a definition of the craniomaxillofacial region and the types of classical injuries that can be sustained. The region is divided into hard- and soft-tissue structures that, because of anatomic position, predilection to traumatic forces, and the presence or absence of protective garb, will have specific types of injuries.

It is important to maintain a hierarchy of prioritization when evaluating these patients because certain head and neck organ systems will be of greater immediate concern than others. Of paramount importance is the central nervous system (CNS), which in the head and neck region consists of the brain and cervical spine column. Injuries to the brain and spinal cord can range from mild concussion to severe paralysis and death. Certain sports activities have higher degrees of risk to the CNS than others, such as boxing, automobile racing, boat racing, and other contact sports.[4,68] The primary sports care provider should be able to perform a basic neurologic examination to determine the integrity of the CNS, associated cranial nerves, and cervical spine structures. This also requires the ability to provide acute care services on the playing field to permit stabilization of the patient before hospitalization. Upon implementation of basic Advanced Trauma Life Support (ATLS) guidelines,[3] when neurologic integrity is determined, a more thorough history and physical examination of the patient may be performed.[3,41]

The most frequently injured organ system for athletes is the integumentary system.[10,31,36,55,71] External soft-tissue structures of the craniomaxillofacial region consist of the scalp, posterior neck, ears, face, and anterior neck. Internal soft tissues include the oral and oropharyngeal mucous membranes, ophthalmologic structures, nasal septum, and auditory canal. These sites are at risk for contusion, abrasion, hematoma formation, laceration, and avulsion. Numerous studies have attempted to categorize and classify the incidence of soft-tissue injuries encountered in sports activities.[36,50,68,71] In the craniomaxillofacial region, certain soft-tissue injuries may have functional and cosmetic implications because of the exposure of this anatomic site. Because many minor soft-tissue injuries are managed on an outpatient basis through on-site repair or in private offices, it is difficult to obtain statistics for other than the more major types of injuries.[10,31,36,55,71] When injuries are classified according to certain parameters, it becomes possible to gain certain information regarding these injuries and whether they may result in any significant disability of a temporary or permanent nature.[4,23,63] The goal of this chapter is to provide information regarding the more commonly encountered American sports as opposed to the least frequent higher-risk types of sports (i.e., bungee jumping, hang gliding, and sky diving). This way, common sport activities related to athletic competition that have a higher rate of injury because of interpersonal contact will be emphasized rather than injuries associated with high-risk individual sports that are machine-dependent activities.

Soft-tissue injuries occur more frequently in some sports activities than others. For example, sports such as hockey and football have a minimal incidence of scalp injuries because of the use of protective helmets.[6,57] Other sports such as soccer and basketball, which have a high degree of physical contact without the use of head and face protective equipment, have higher numbers of scalp lacerations.[7,10,31,55] Facial and ear lacerations occur more frequently in contact sports such as boxing, wrestling, and basketball.[10] Lacerations may be classified as simple, complex, or avulsive, and particular attention must be paid to the specific anatomic site. For example, a depressed skull fracture could be present with a scalp laceration. Ocular soft-tissue injuries may require further ophthalmologic evaluation before treatment. Soft-tissue injuries may mask underlying hard-tissue injuries.

Where indicated or suspected, radiography should supplement the physical examination to determine the presence of underlying skeletal injuries.[24] Plain radiography is useful for the facial skeleton, cervical spine, and dental structures.[24] Computed tomography (CT) and magnetic resonance imaging (MRI) scanning may be indicated in the presence of neurologic symptoms or where neurologic injuries are suspected, especially in the brain and spinal cord.[24]

Injuries of the facial skeleton are generally studied as hospital populations.[10,31,36,55,71] The types of injuries are generally more severe and have a poor prognosis. Therefore, information concerning the distribution and etiology of facial injuries is generally within the context of the hospital emergency room or operating room. Sports injuries, on the other hand, are usually of a minor nature or may be managed at the athletic facility or in private offices. These injuries may include more significant facial lacerations or minor nasal, dentoalveolar, and mandibular fractures.[31] There have been few studies that have been directed toward the etiologies, distribution, and classification of maxillofacial sports injuries.[36,50,54,71] Perhaps the difficulty of engaging in such a study has to do with the large variety of sports activities that are available today at the amateur and professional levels. Sports activities and athletic competitions have become part of daily activities from the school-aged to the elderly. Most studies have examined injuries severe enough to require treatment or cause disability, but the variations seen between amateur and professional athletes make these studies even more difficult. For example, Watson,[71] in studying four types of sports (endurance, contact, noncontact, and explosive) in Irish athletes, found that 6% of all injuries included head (5%) and dental (1%) injuries.[5,6] Therefore, it is more important for the primary care provider to be able to diagnose the various types of injuries that can occur in the craniomaxillofacial region and be able to either treat on a primary basis or be knowledgeable enough to make the appropriate referral to qualified specialists. Unlike orthopedics and sports medicine, there is no singular head and neck discipline that can claim specialty status in sports injuries. Rather, there are interested individuals who attend sporting events as team dentists, oral and maxillofacial surgeons, plastic surgeons, or otolaryngologists.

Many studies document the frequency of certain types of injuries in specific sports. In baseball, basketball, hockey, and football, because of the high level of contact and the relative energies of impact, dental and craniomaxillofacial injuries are predictable.[6,10,50,57,68,72,58,35] Fortunately, these sports have evolved so that protective devices and regulations concerning their use have become more widespread and many of the injuries seen in the past occur less frequently today.[6,57] For example, Torg et al.[68] in the National Football Head and Neck Injury Registry reported a significant reduction in the incidence of quadriplegia between 1975 and 1984. This reduction reflected the change in the "spearing" rule of tackling in 1976, resulting in an immediate reduction in cervical spine injuries.

Of special interest are the pediatric populations between ages 5 and 14 years, in whom facial injuries in sports are frequent because of the learning stages of sports ability, the need for proving fearlessness to peers, and the ignorance of the consequences of taking greater risks.[54] Several recent studies have shown that 15% of pediatric facial fractures were sports related, with 56% having associated soft-tissue injuries.[55] Polytrauma must always be considered as a cofactor, with head injuries comprising 42%.[55] Others have demonstrated that of those having facial fractures, children aged less than 12 years comprise less than 5% of all injuries, and children aged less than 6 years account for less than 1%.[60] Other authors claim a range of 1.5% to 8% of facial fractures in children aged less than 12 years, whereas children aged less than 1 year account for less than 1%.[31] Another study by the U.S. Consumer Product Safety Commission in 1981 indicated a facial injury rate of 11% to 40% in children aged 5 to 14 years, depending on the type of sport.[50] Because of differences between the pediatric and adult facial morphology, there are differences in the fracture patterns. In infants and children, the cranium is large relative to the face. The cranial-to-facial ratio is 8:1 in infants and 2.5:1 in adults.[55] The accessory sinuses are poorly developed in children, and therefore high-energy injuries are less likely to be absorbed by the face than by the frontal bones. McGraw and Cole[46] observed age-related variations in a pediatric population, with a decrease in cranial fractures from 88% (in children aged less than 5 years) to 34% (in children aged 12 to 16 years). Such studies may be skewed, based on the different hospital services that may treat these patients. For example, neurosurgeons may see more of the cranial injuries relative to craniomaxillofacial surgeons.[55]

With development, the paranasal sinuses become aerated and enlarged, and the mandible gains a more prominent position, allowing this structure to be more readily injured.[31,55,61] Maxillary and mandibular fractures increase in occurrence with age. In the younger pediatric population, less-developed sinuses, more-flexible suture lines, and thicker adipose tissues result in fewer midfacial injuries.[31]

Because of soft-tissue edema, presence of lacerations, greater incidence of CNS involvement, poorly pneumatized sinuses, and presence of tooth buds (which can obscure fracture lines), CT axial and coronal scanning is the imaging method of choice in pediatric trauma patients.[31,55] The panoramic radiograph is still a highly cost-effective and accurate method for the determination of the presence of mandibular fractures, especially of the condylar region. Mandibular fractures are the most commonly reported fractures in the pediatric hospital population.[31,55,60]

EXAMINATION AND TREATMENT

It is important for the primary care provider involved in the management of acute sports-related craniomaxillofacial injuries to be able to diagnose, treat, or refer the patient to other specialists. To be able to perform these tasks, it is necessary to be cognizant of the types, distribution, and classification of these injuries and to be able to perform accurate history taking and physical examination, which may include other diagnostic procedures and tests.

Soft-Tissue Injuries

Soft-tissue injuries may be described as clean or contaminated, and classified as contusions, abrasions, punctures, lacerations, and burns. Patients may present with combinations of the previously mentioned classifications and may have associated damage to vital structures and varying degrees of underlying skeletal involvement.

In sports injuries of the face, most soft-tissue injuries can be considered to be contaminated because of the usual conditions under which they occur. If any athlete has a penetrating injury of the skin, tetanus immunization status must be determined, and appropriate tetanus coverage provided. Superficial burns, abrasions, and contusions should be gently washed and examined under good light. If particulate matter is embedded in the soft tissues, it should be meticulously debrided to avoid tattooing. Clean wounds may be dressed with antibiotic ointment preparations such as Neosporin (Burroughs Wellcome, Research Triangle Park, NC), and light dressings may be applied where tissue protection is desired. Superficial lacerations should be cleansed with antimicrobial agents and then repaired primarily, when possible, with sutures or sterile strip dressings or a combination of the two. Deep lacerations may cause greater concern and often require more extensive diagnostic imaging or surgical intervention.

Because traumatic forces can be so variable in sports, ranging from a boxing glove to a flying hockey puck, deep structures such as the CNS, eyes, tongue, ear, and base of skull should be carefully evaluated for damage. Penetrating wounds, especially of the scalp, ocular region, and neck region, have particular anatomic concerns. Depressed skull fractures are easily masked by large scalp lacerations, and their radiographic examination should be carefully considered, rather than performed by blind digital or instrument techniques to avoid iatrogenic injuries. Radiologic examination, involving CT or MRI, may be necessary. Ocular injuries are seen frequently in sports-related trauma and must be carefully evaluated to determine the need for acute intervention.[51,69] Problems such as hyphema, retinal tears, lens dislocation, penetrating globe injuries, optic nerve compression, orbital apex syndrome, superior orbital fissure syndrome, retrobulbar hematoma, and orbital floor and roof blowout fractures with adnexiae entrapment should all be carefully considered. Neck soft-tissue considerations include concern for the major vessels (carotid and jugular) and the laryngeal structures.

Laryngeal injuries, although infrequent, can be devastating catastrophic problems if airway patency is compromised. There can be many indications for intubation, cricothyrotomy, and tracheostomy, depending on the circumstances, environment, and status of the patient. The unconscious athlete may require emergency airway treatment that is separate and distinct from laryngeal trauma. Basic life support considerations must always be considered in the initial assessment of these patients. Salivary gland injuries, although rare, should be considered when a laceration occurs in the midface where the parotid duct can be transected.

The external ear is also of great concern, especially in athletes who engage in high-impact contact sports, such as boxing, wrestling, basketball, and football. Protective headgear should be worn by these athletes, but in certain situations it can be dislodged or not used (i.e., professional boxing). Hematoma and contusion of the external ear should be managed aggressively to avoid "cauliflower ear," and lacerations are best treated immediately.[10]

Skeletal Injuries

Various sports committees have adopted specific guidelines for the prevention of dental and craniomaxillofacial injuries. Sports such as hockey and football have adopted full facial and cranial protective headgear.[6,57] Evolution of these protective devices has significantly reduced many types of head and neck injuries in these sports.[6,57,68]

Dentoalveolar Injuries

The craniomaxillofacial region (Fig. 13-1) can be divided into the cranium, facial bones, and dentition (primary and permanent). Injuries to these sites may be categorized according to the particular anatomy and various classification schemes. Dental injuries range from minor enamel fragments, to complete coronal fractures, to complete tooth avulsion.[4] For further discussion of dental injuries, see Chapter 14.

When the dental fracture involves the alveolar bone, whether in the maxilla or the mandible, these injuries are classified as *dentoalveolar* fractures and may include dental fractures and fractures of the supporting bone. Alveolar region fractures include more highly fragmented jaw fractures. These types of injuries are common in sports and are highly preventable with the use of mouthguards. The diagnosis of an alveolar fracture is made by physical and radiographic examination. Examination requires bimanual palpation and periapical dental or occlusal radiographs. More severe dentoalveolar fractures may involve laceration of the overlying mucosa, and displacement can occur with preservation of a lingual or buccal pedicle. Dentoalveolar fractures also can be completely avulsed. Today, with open reduction and stabilization using techniques of microplate fixation, these fractures

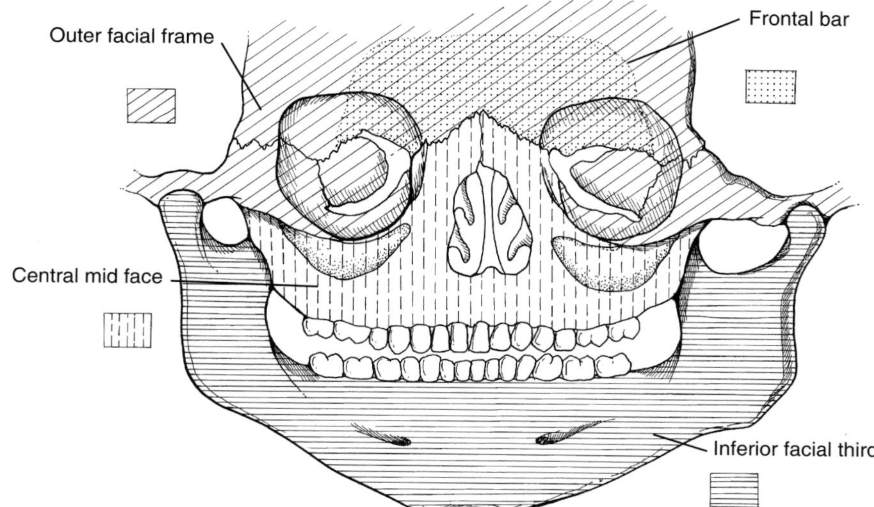

FIGURE 13-1. Pancraniomaxillofacial skeletal regional landmarks. (From Greenberg AM [ed]: Craniomaxillofacial Fractures: Principles of Internal Fixation Using the AO/ASIF Technique. New York, Springer-Verlag, 1993.)

can be managed with retention of even completely avulsed segments.

Facial Skeletal Fractures

Moving beyond dental and dentoalveolar fractures, the various facial bones of the craniomaxillofacial complex may be considered for their etiology, distribution, and classification of fractures. The craniomaxillofacial region may be defined anatomically as the cranium, which consists of the parietal, occipital, temporal, frontal, and sphenoid bones. The frontal, temporal, and sphenoid bones are most commonly associated with facial bone injuries. The facial skeleton is defined by the mandible, maxillae, palatine, zygomatic, nasal, ethmoid, and lacrimal bones.

Mandibular Fractures. The mandible is the most extensively studied facial bone, and there is a well-defined pattern of classically encountered fractures (Table 13-1).[1,2,5,14,23,26,27,30,33,48,59] The particular fracture patterns seen are related to the particular biomechanics of the mandible and the insertions of the muscles of mastication (Fig. 13-2).[17] The frequency of occurrence at various mandibular fracture sites appears to be predominated by the body, followed by the angle, condyle, symphysis, ramus, and coronoid process (in that order).

TABLE 13-1 Mandible Fracture Locations

Study	Location (%)							Number of patients in study
	Symphysis	Body	Angle	Ramus	Coronoid	Condyle	Alveolus	
Rix et al. (1991)[59]	24	24	34	3	0	15	NI	80
Haug et al. (1990)[24]	20	30	27	2	0	21	NI	307
Abiose (1986)[1]	20	59	9	0	0	10	2	87
Bochlogyros (1985)[5]	7	42	24	3	0	23	1	853
Ellis et al. (1985)[13]	8	33	23	3	2	29	1	2137
Hill et al. (1984)[27]	4	14	12	0	0	15	25	214
Olson et al. (1982)[48]	22	16	25	2	1	29	3	580
James et al. (1981)[30]	14	27	31	6	3	19	NI	253
Khalil and Shaladi (1981)[33]	10	20	14	2	0	14	7	187
Adekeye (1980)[2]	26	48	15	1	0	11	NI	1106

From Greenberg AM (ed): Craniomaxillofacial Fractures: Principles of Internal Fixation Using the AO/ASIF Technique. New York, Springer-Verlag, 1993.

NI—not investigated.

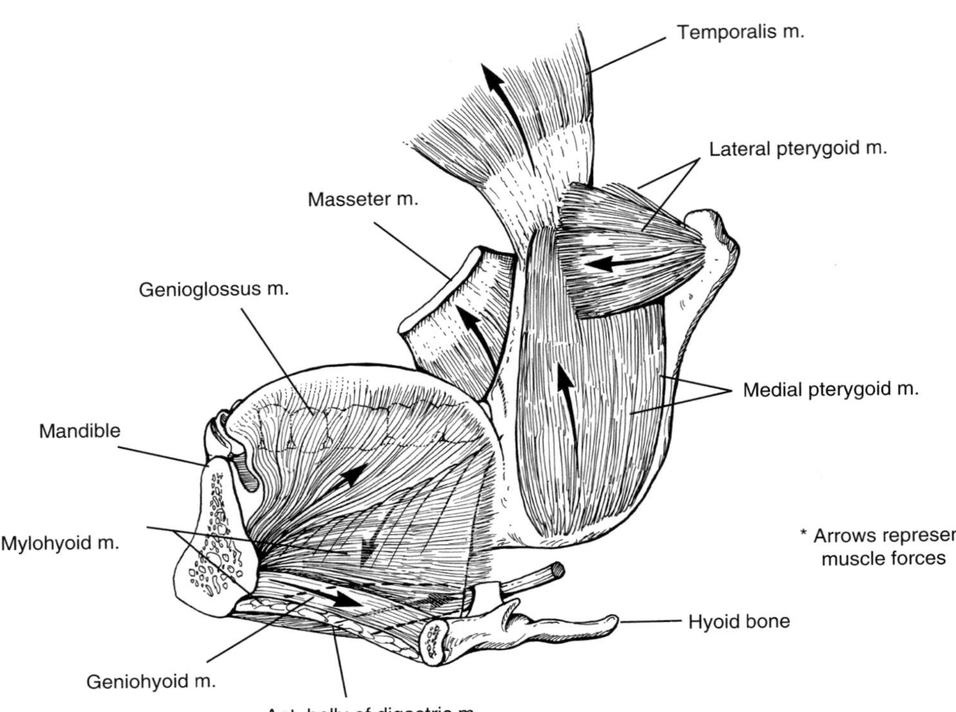

FIGURE 13-2. Diagram indicating muscles of mastication and their vectors of force during contraction. (From Greenberg AM [ed]: Craniomaxillofacial Fractures: Principles of Internal Fixation Using the AO/ASIF Technique. New York, Springer-Verlag, 1993.)

Mandibular fractures may be classified as single, multiple, fragmented, or avulsive according to the Spiessl classification as modified by Haug and Greenberg (Fig. 13-3).[23,63] Localization of fractures is defined by the anatomic site (Fig. 13-4).[63] There are a variety of causes for mandibular fractures (Table 13-2)[5,14,23,26,48,59] predominated by assaults and motor vehicle collisions, with sports as a smaller etiology (2% to 6%).[5,14,23,26,48,59]

Maxillary Fractures. Maxillary fractures were typically referred to in the context of LeFort's early anatomic studies.[38–40] This particular classification was useful in the era when management was by closed reduction (jaw wiring). Current therapy is oriented toward aggressive anatomic open reduction with rigid internal fixation via miniplates and microplates.[22,56,66] Such surgical approaches have revealed to clinicians fracture patterns that differ from the classical LeFort classification system. The forces of function or impact are transmitted through the midfacial skeleton across the facial buttress system, which was well described by Manson and Gruss (Fig. 13-5).[19,20,44] The orientation and level of energy of impact influence the type of fracture pattern that develops. The LeFort system classifies LeFort I fractures at the level of the zygomaticomaxillary buttresses and inferior piriform rim with separation at the pterygoid plates.[38–40]

A LeFort II fracture is defined as fracture lines crossing through the zygomaticomaxillary buttress superiorly through the infraorbital rim and medially to the nasal bridge (naso-orbital-ethmoid complex).[38–40,61] A LeFort III fracture no longer simply involves the maxillary bones, but also the naso-orbital-ethmoid complex and zygomatic bones.[38–40,61] Such a fracture will involve the bilateral frontozygomatic processes, nasofrontal suture, naso-orbital-ethmoid, sphenozygomatic, and zygomaticotemporal processes. LeFort I, II, and III fracture patterns are considered to be general terms to describe collections of bone fractures in close proximity, which at higher levels and as the result of higher energy have greater degrees of complexity and a higher predilection for complications from the injury and management methodologies. Previous studies have noted the distribution and frequency of such injuries (Table 13-3).[1,2,9,23,26,27,32,62,65]

There are four varieties of localized maxillary fractures, which range from high alveolar to the classical LeFort I and II types (Fig. 13-6).[23] We have separated our classification from the typical LeFort to include an individual bone-based system because it facilitates diagnosis and subsequent management-oriented therapies and research methods.[23] Midfacial fractures are rarely equal bilaterally, with variations from one side to the other; for example, a higher-level nasomaxillary fracture occurs on the side of impact versus a lower-level piriform rim fracture on the opposite side, which results from the diminished transmission of forces. The greatest frequency of maxillary fractures results from assaults and motor vehicle collisions, with sports accounting for 5% to 8% of such fractures (Table 13-4).[23,26,32,65]

Zygoma Fractures. The zygoma is a separate bone of the facial region that becomes one of the interfaces between the skull base and the facial skeleton. Studies evaluating

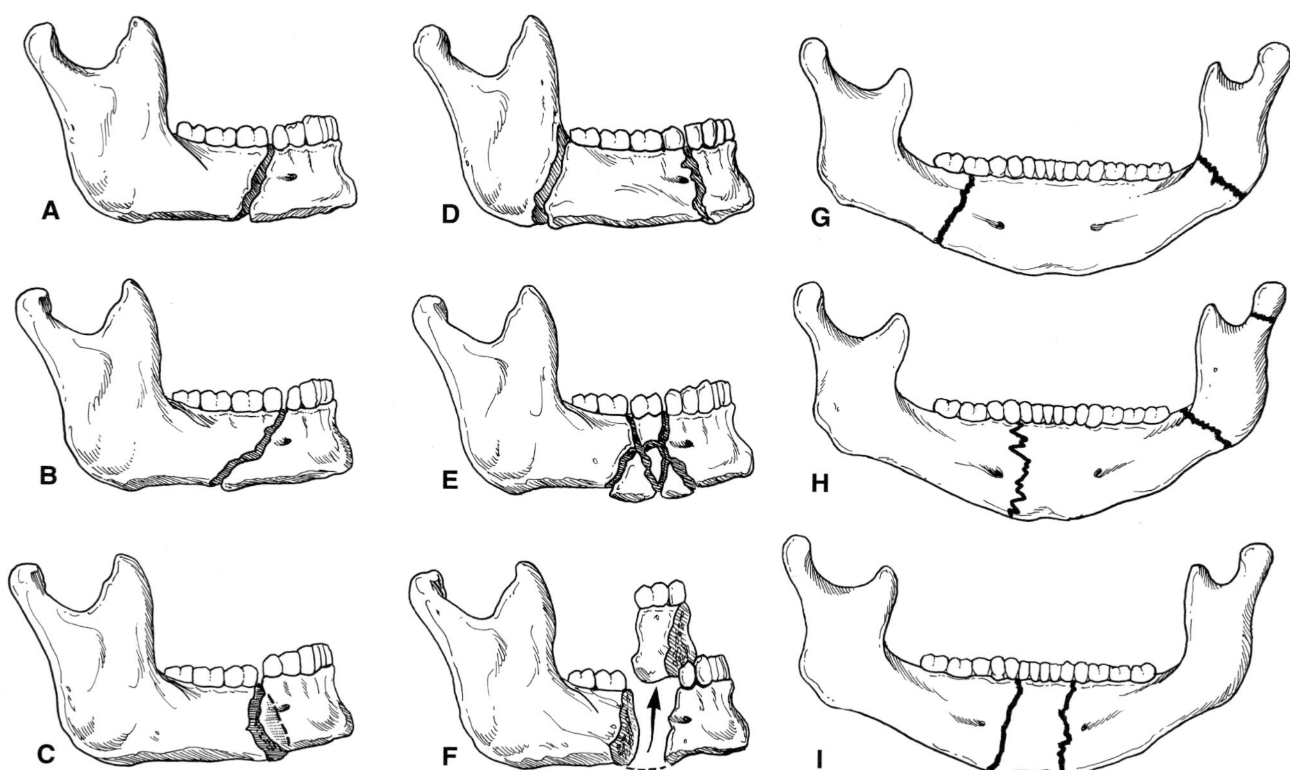

FIGURE 13-3. Categories of mandibular fractures. **A,** Single fracture (transverse fracture); **B,** Single fracture (oblique fracture); **C,** Single fracture (oblique-surface fracture); **D,** Unilateral (segmental fracture); **E,** Comminuted (fragmented) fracture; **F,** Fracture with bone defect; **G,** Multiple fracture (segmental fracture); **H,** Unilateral segmental fracture and contralateral single fracture; **I,** Bilateral segmental fracture. (From Greenberg AM [ed]: Craniomaxillofacial Fractures: Principles of Internal Fixation using the AO/ASIF Technique; New York, Springer-Verlag, 1993; and Spiessl B: Internal Fixation of the Mandible. Berlin, Springer-Verlag, 1989.)

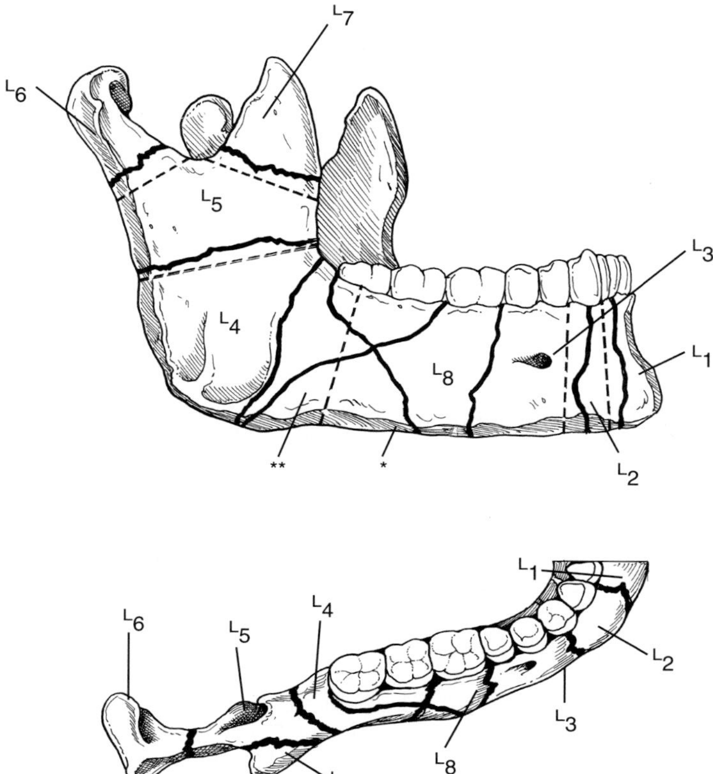

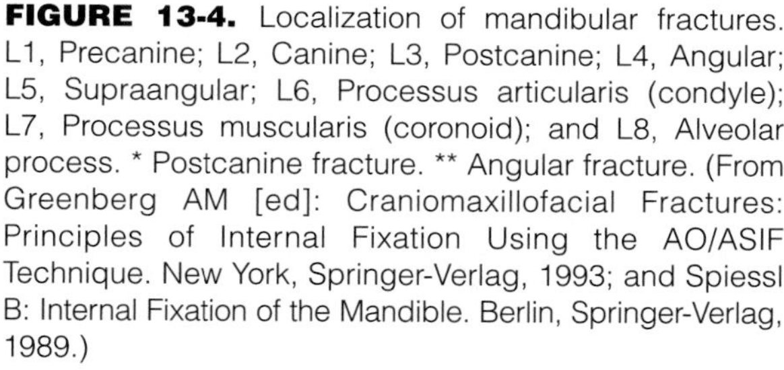

FIGURE 13-4. Localization of mandibular fractures. L1, Precanine; L2, Canine; L3, Postcanine; L4, Angular; L5, Supraangular; L6, Processus articularis (condyle); L7, Processus muscularis (coronoid); and L8, Alveolar process. * Postcanine fracture. ** Angular fracture. (From Greenberg AM [ed]: Craniomaxillofacial Fractures: Principles of Internal Fixation Using the AO/ASIF Technique. New York, Springer-Verlag, 1993; and Spiessl B: Internal Fixation of the Mandible. Berlin, Springer-Verlag, 1989.)

TABLE 13-2

Mandible Fracture Epidemiology

Study	Male/ female	Most frequent age (yr)	Cause (%)					
			MVA	Bicycle/ MCA	Assault	Occupational	Falls/ home	Sports
Rix et al. (1991)[59]	90	20–30	8	0	73	4	11	6
Haug et al. (1990)[24]	60	16–35	33	4	54	1	4	4
Bochlogyros (1985)[5]	77	20–29	41	17	19	7	13	3
Ellis et al. (1985)[13]	76	20–40	13	2	55	2	21	4
Olson et al. (1982)[48]	78	20–29	48	14	34	1	8	2

From Greenberg AM (ed): Craniomaxillofacial Fractures: Principles of Internal Fixation Using the AO/ASIF Technique, Springer-Verlag, 1993.

MVA—motor vehicle accidents; MCA—motorcycle accidents.

TABLE 13-3

Maxillary Fracture Locations (LeFort Classification)

Study	LeFort level (%)							Number of patients in study
	I	II	III	0/I	I/II	II/III	0/II	
Haug et al. (1990)[24]	38	28	17	9	2	6	0	53
Cook and Rowe (1990)[9]	32	47	21	NI	NI	NI	NI	95
Kahnberg and Göthberg (1987)[32]	29	35	13	23	—	—	—	266
Abiose (1986)[1]	47	24	24	NI	NI	NI	NI	17
Hill et al. (1984)[27]	35	61	3	NI	NI	NI	NI	31
Sofferman et al. (1983)[62]	14	33	10	0	0	43	0	21
Steidler et al. (1980)[65]	22	53	18	2	4	1	0	240
Adekeye (1980)[2]	6	34	6	20	4	0	21	212

From Greenberg AM (ed): Craniomaxillofacial Fractures: Principles of Internal Fixation Using the AO/ASIF Technique. New York, Springer-Verlag, 1993.

NI—not investigated.

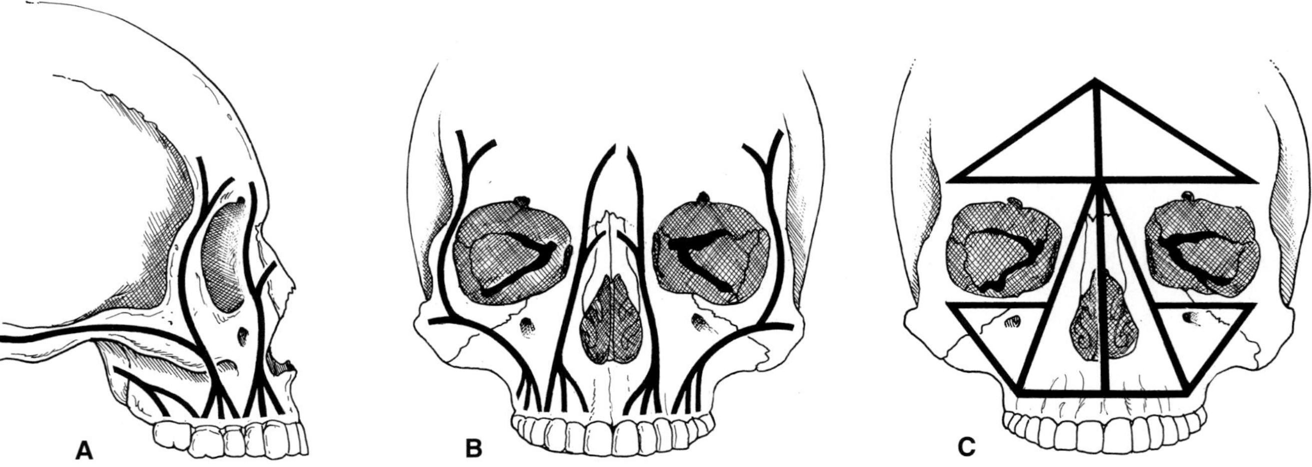

FIGURE 13-5. Traditional concept of the distribution of masticatory forces throughout the face delineating the six facial buttresses. **A,** Lateral view. **B,** Anteroposterior view. **C,** Contemporary concept of facial trusses under tension during asymmetric mastication and facial muscle pull. (Adapted from Sicher H, Tandler J: Anatomie fur Zahnartze. Wien, Verlag von Springer, 1928; and Greenberg AM [ed]: Craniomaxillofacial Fractures: Principles of Internal Fixation using the AO/ASIF Technique. New York, Springer-Verlag, 1993.)

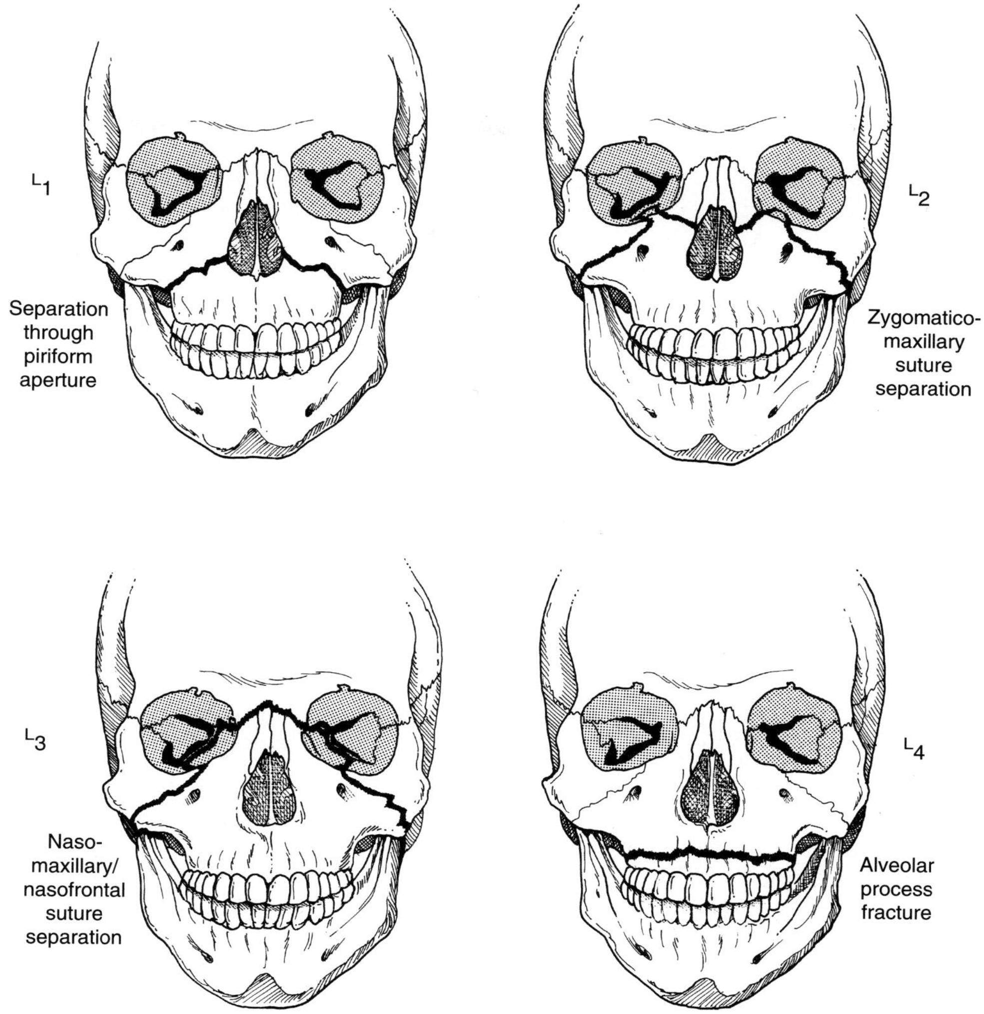

FIGURE 13-6. Localization of maxillary fractures. L1, Separation through piriform aperture; L2, Separation through zygomaticomaxillary suture; L3, Separation through nasomaxillary and nasofrontal suture; and L4, Alveolar process. (From Greenberg AM [ed]: Craniomaxillofacial Fractures: Principles of Internal Fixation using the AO/ASIF Technique. New York, Springer-Verlag, 1993.)

TABLE 13-4

Mandible Fracture Epidemiology

Study	Male/ female	Most frequent age (yr)	Cause (%)					
			MVA	Bicycle/ MCA	Assault	Occupational	Falls/ home	Sports
Haug et al. (1990)[24]	83	26–30	66	8	13	4	2	8
Kahnberg and Göthberg (1987)[32]	NI	NI	35	11	27	27	—	—
Sofferman et al. (1983)[62]	71	25	76	NI	NI	NI	NI	NI
Steidler et al. (1980)[65]	83	20–29	69	8	9	4	1	5

From Greenberg AM (ed): Craniomaxillofacial Fractures: Principles of Internal Fixation Using the AO/ASIF Technique, Springer-Verlag, 1993.
MVA—motor vehicle accidents; MCA—motorcycle accidents; NI—not investigated.

TABLE 13-5

Zygoma Fracture Location

Study	Location (%)					Number of patients in study
	Non-displaced	Arch	Body	Fragmented	Blow-out	
Haug et al. (1990)[24]	11	27	53	9	NI	98
Ellis et al. (1985)[13]	15	8	62	8	3	2067
Fisher-Brandies and Dielert (1984)[15]	8	9	80	2	NI	97

From Greenberg AM (ed): Craniomaxillofacial Fractures: Principles of Internal Fixation Using the AO/ASIF Technique. New York, Springer-Verlag, 1993.

NI—not investigated.

the incidence of isolated zygomatic fractures are infrequently reported in the literature, which is a reflection of the lack (until more recently) of an appropriate classification system. The Knight and North classification was a management-oriented classification system based on the stability of fractures managed without fixation and the unstable fractures that would require fixation.[34] Haug and Greenberg have devised a system that is oriented toward the anatomic involvement of the bone and its suture articulations, which may be involved in fractures and become sites for internal fixation.[23] Zygomatic fractures are distributed based on the particular anatomic sites of involvement (Table 13-5),[13,15,26] whether they involve the arch, supra-arch, frontozygomatic, zygomaticomaxillary, zygomaticotemporal, or orbital floor regions (Fig. 13-7).

Zygomatic fractures can be complicated by the involvement of the vital structures of the eye, and a thorough ophthalmologic examination is essential in their management, which requires consultation with an ophthalmologist (see box, Signs and Symptoms of Zygoma Fractures). Visual acuity testing, extraocular muscle evaluation, pupillary reflexes, and globe position are the most important general ophthalmologic considerations after occurrence of these injuries. Zygomatic fractures most commonly result from assaults, falls, and motor vehicle collisions, whereas 4% to 11% result from a sports injury (Table 13-6).[13,15,26]

Nasal and Nasoethmoid Fractures. Nasal and naso-orbital-ethmoid fractures are among the most frequently reported skeletal fractures because of their delicate bony structures and relative prominence in the face.[28,42] There are numerous classification systems for the nasal region that range from simple to complex,[16,21,47,67] with some systems oriented toward management approaches.[45] These systems, however, are not part of a uniform facial fracture classification system and are difficult to organize (Table 13-7).[25,73] Haug and Prather, in a survey given in 1991 to 20 patients, noted that the entire nasal bone had a higher frequency of fracture than the naso-orbital-ethmoid complex.[25] These fractures may be localized to the nasal tip; entire nasal bones; nasal bone and frontal process of the maxilla; nasal, ethmoid, frontal process of the maxilla; and nasal spine of the frontal bone (Fig. 13-8). The majority of these fractures result from assaults and motor vehicle collisions, whereas 0 to 27% result from sports injuries (Table 13-8).[8,25,73]

Frontal Bone Fractures

Frontal bone fractures are less common than other fractures of the craniomaxillofacial skeleton because of their greater thickness and biomechanical advantages. Local anatomic considerations such as the degree of pneumatization and nasofrontal duct configuration may influence the tendency of certain individuals to be predisposed to fractures. Few studies have been reported, and all have evaluated small patient groups (Table 13-9).[12,29,49,64,70] Frontal bone fractures are classified according to the involvement of the supraorbital rim, anterior table, posterior table, or sinus floor (Fig. 13-9). Motor vehicle collisions, assaults, and occupational causes are the most frequent reasons for frontal fractures, whereas 3% to 5% result from sports injuries (Table 13-10).[11,29,37,49,52,70]

Other cranial fractures and their incidence will be discussed elsewhere in this text. Various diagnostic algorithms can be developed to approach the treatment of patients who have craniomaxillofacial injuries. As with all trauma patients, the ATLS guidelines are an excellent resource that includes primary and secondary assessments to determine patient stability and basic life support (see ATLS guidelines).[3] All patients must undergo a complete history and physical examination, with particular signs guiding the clinician to order more extensive tests and laboratory or radiologic investigational studies.

FIGURE 13-7. Localization of zygoma fractures. L1, Arch; L2, Supra-arch; L3, Displacement at fronto zygomatic suture; L4, Displacement at zygomaticotemporal suture; L5, Displacement at zygomatico-maxillary suture; and L6, Orbital floor. (From Greenberg AM [ed]: Craniomaxillofacial Fractures: Principles of Internal Fixation Using the AO/ASIF Technique. New York, Springer-Verlag, 1993.)

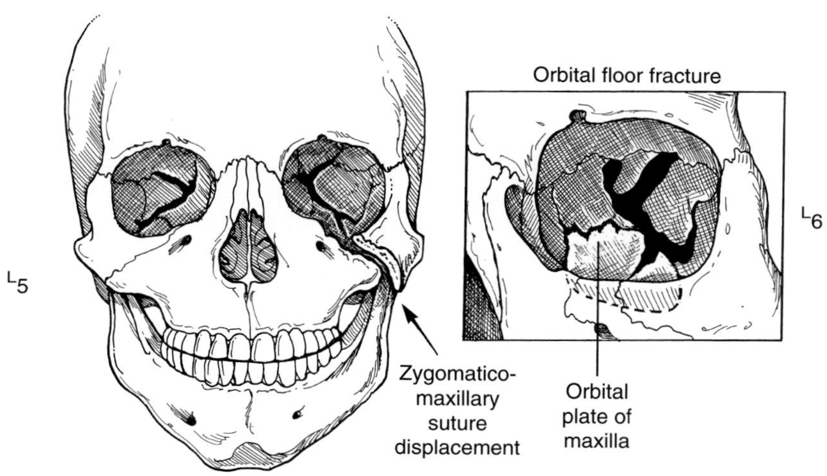

TABLE 13-6

Zygoma Fracture Epidemiology

Study	Male/ female	Most frequent age (yr)	Cause (%)					
			MVA	MCA	Assault	Home Occupational	Falls	Sports
Haug et al. (1990)[24]	60	21–35	38	5	45	1	7	4
Ellis et al. (1985)[13]	80	20–40	11	1	45	3	22	11
Fisher-Brandies and Dielert (1984)[15]	86	16–20	NI	NI	NI	NI	NI	NI

From Greenberg AM (ed): Craniomaxillofacial Fractures: Principles of Internal Fixation Using the AO/ASIF Technique. New York, Springer-Verlag, 1993.

MVA—motor vehicle accidents; MCA—motorcycle accidents; NI—not investigated.

TABLE 13-7

Nasal Fracture Location

Study	Location (%)				Number of patients in study
	Entire nasal tip	Nasal bone	Naso-orbital	Naso-orbital-ethmoid	
Haug and Prather (1991)[26]	15	40	35	10	20
Williamson et al. (1981)[73]	NI	NI	54	46	13

From Greenberg AM (ed): Craniomaxillofacial Fractures: Principles of Internal Fixation Using the AO/ASIF Technique. New York, Springer-Verlag, 1993.

NI—not investigated.

PHYSICAL EVALUATION

Primary providers who care for individuals who engage in sports and athletic competition must be well versed in disorders and injuries of the craniomaxillofacial region. Having reviewed the types of traumatically induced soft- and hard-tissue injuries common to the head and neck region, the practitioner must apply this knowledge in a systematic manner when caring for patients suspected of having sustained such injuries. As with all acute care, the ABCs of life support are always a place to start. The ATLS protocols for treatment of the trauma patient are also an excellent methodology, and the craniomaxillofacial aspects of the primary survey and the more detail-oriented examination of the secondary survey (American College of Surgeons) will be reviewed.[3] Given the wide range of sports played today, accidents may occur in a variety of unfavorable locations, such as swimming pools, fresh and salt water, and at high altitudes (alpine skiing, mountaineering, rock climbing, etc.).

Ensuring that the patient's airway is intact is the examiner's first responsibility, and because the oral cavity and the dentition are often primary trauma sites, care must be taken to remove nonpermanent dentures, mouthguards, loosened bridges, and avulsed teeth and to establish hemostasis if the tongue or oral mucosa are lacerated and profuse hemorrhage is present. If a cervical injury is suspected, a cervical collar should be placed on the patient until radiographs can establish the integrity of the spinal column. This limits the ability to position the head for opening or ensuring patency of the airway.

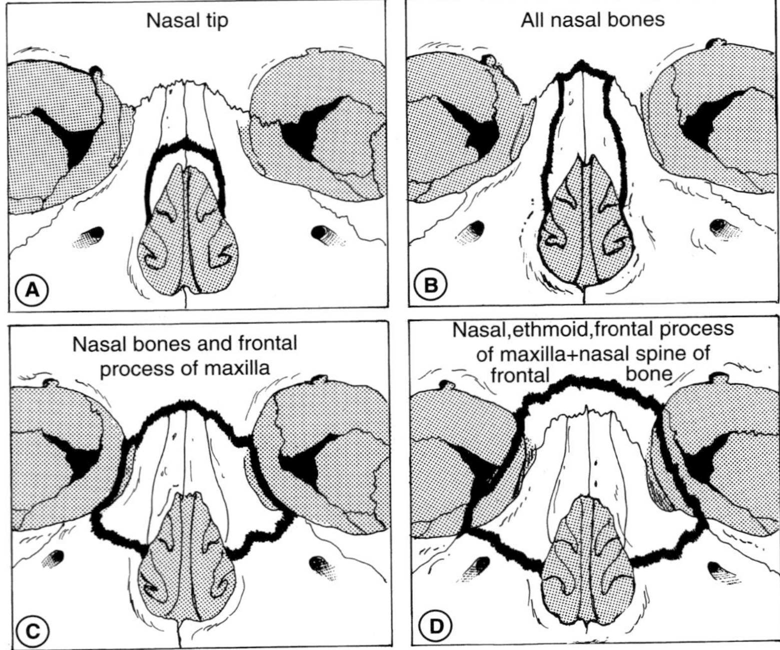

FIGURE 13-8. Localization of nasal and naso-orbital-ethmoid fractures. **A,** Nasal tip; **B,** Entire nasal bones; **C,** Nasal bone and frontal process of maxilla; and **D,** Nasal, ethmoid, frontal process of maxilla, nasal spine of frontal bone. (From Greenberg AM [ed]: Craniomaxillofacial Fractures: Principles of internal Fixation Using the AO/ASIF Technique. New York, Springer-Verlag, 1993.)

TABLE 13-8

Nasal Fracture Epidemiology

Study	Male/ female	Most common age (yr)	Cause (%)				
			MVA/ MCA	Assault	Occupa- tional	Falls/ home	Sports
Haug and Prather (1991)[26]	80	20–30	50	45	0	5	0
Clayton and Lesser (1986)[8]	73	23	27	46	0	0	27
Williamson et al. (1981)[73]	100	27	54	46	0	0	0

From Greenberg AM (ed): Craniomaxillofacial Fractures: Principles of Internal Fixation Using the AO/ASIF Technique. New York, Springer-Verlag, 1993.
MVA/MCA—motor vehicle accident/motorcycle accident.

Jaw thrust may be necessary as an initial maneuver until further measures are taken, such as intubation, cricothyrotomy, or tracheostomy. Breathing may be maintained or reestablished by manual or mechanical types of support, depending on the location of the patient (in the hospital or otherwise). A cursory neurologic examination should be performed, and control of any excessive hemorrhage should be obtained.

Clinical examination should begin with a thorough history of the trauma because details regarding the mechanism, magnitude and site of impact, and symptomatology will be important. If the patient is unconscious, it is important to ascertain the events from a witness. Past medical and surgical history, including pertinent medications and allergies, are required.

When cervical injuries are suspected, the head and neck examination should begin with the cervical collar in place on the patient. Radiographs may be taken first if a cervical injury is strongly suspected, and should consist of a minimum of a lateral, posteroanterior (with all seven cervical vertebrae observed), and an open-mouth Waters' view of the dens. If these initial radiographs are insufficient, a swimmer's view, CT, or MRI may be necessary to complete the radiologic examination. Once radiography has established skeletal integrity of the spinal column, the cervical collar may be removed to permit physical examination of the neck. The soft tissues of the neck should be observed for the presence of ecchymosis, edema, and lacerations, and manual palpation should proceed along the lateral vertebral processes first, followed by the posterior processes from caudad to cephalad to assess pain or tenderness and irregularities such as step defects or abnormal contours. Examination of the head should begin with the scalp, which should be inspected for lacerations, ecchymosis, edema, and Battle's signs around the ears, which may indicate a skull base fracture. Palpation of the cranium is performed, and care should be taken to elicit complaints of pain or tenderness, crepitus, or contour irregularities of bone, with special attention directed toward the presence of depressed skull fractures.

TABLE 13-9

Frontal Bone Fracture Locations

Study	Location (%)				Number of patients in study
	Supra- orbital rim	Anterior table	Anterior/ posterior table	Floor	
Onishi et al. (1989)[49]	77	61	19	12	42
Wallis and Donald (1988)[70]	NI	54	39	3	72
Stanley and Becker (1987)[64]	NI	44	56	64	50
Duval et al. (1987)[12]	NI	65	35	NI	112
Ioannides et al. (1984)[29]	48	43	13	NI	23

From Greenberg AM (ed): Craniomaxillofacial Fractures: Principles of Internal Fixation Using the AO/ASIF Technique. New York, Springer-Verlag, 1993.
NI—not investigated.

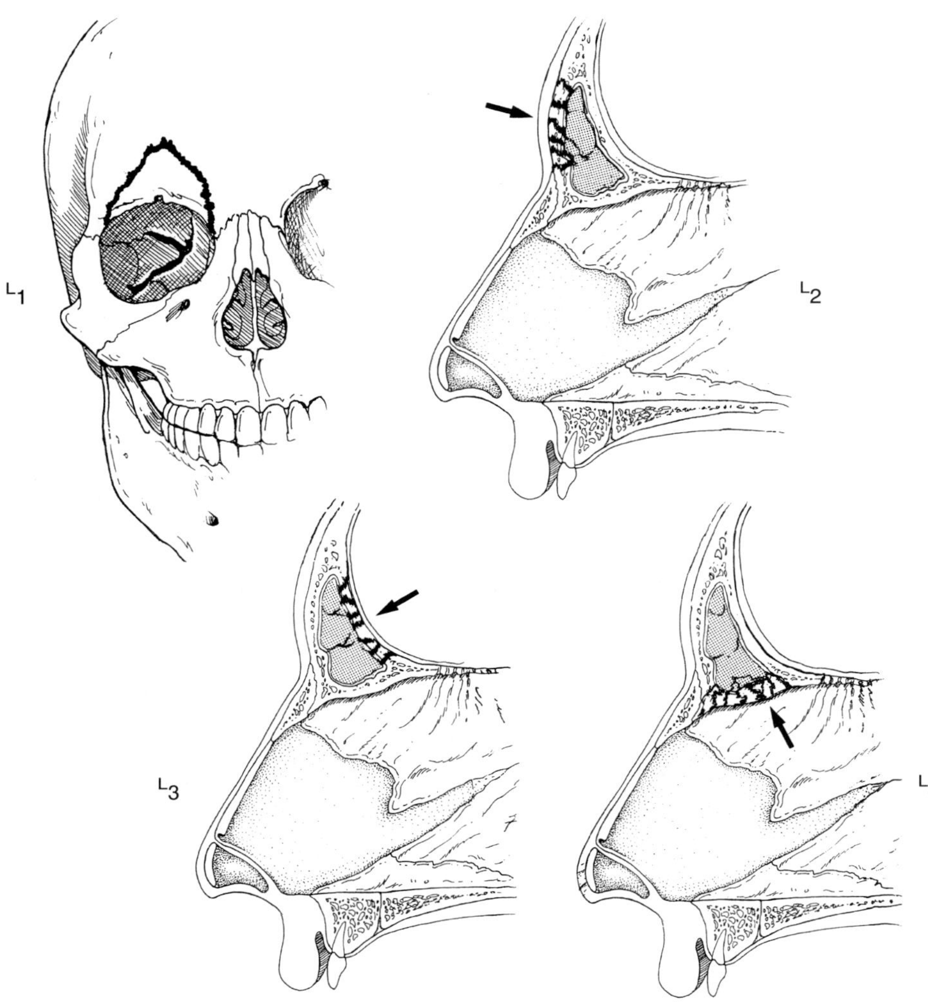

FIGURE 13-9. Localization of frontal fractures. L1, Supraorbital rim; L2, Anterior table; L3, Posterior table; and L4, Sinus floor. (From Greenberg AM, [ed]: Craniomaxillofacial Fractures: Principles of Internal Fixation Using the AO/ASIF Technique. New York, Springer-Verlag, 1993.)

TABLE 13-10 Frontal Bone Fracture Epidemiology

Study	Male/ female	Most frequent age (yr)	Cause (%)				
			MVA/ MCA	Suicide and Assault	Occupa- tional	Falls/ home	Sports
Onishi et al. (1989)[49]	84	NI	84	0	5	5	5
Wallis and Donald (1988)[70]	85	32.0	71	17	7	0	6
Ioannides et al. (1984)[29]	83	33.5	70	4	17	9	0
Donald (1982)[11]	66	34.3	71	24	0	5	0
Peri et al. (1981)[52]	80	20–30	85	0	12	—	3
Larrabee et al. (1980)[37]	91	24.0	44	28	28	—	—

From Greenberg AM (ed): Craniomaxillofacial Fractures: Principles of Internal Fixation Using the AO/ASIF Technique. New York, Springer-Verlag, 1993.
MVA/MCA—motor vehicle accidents/motorcycle accidents; NI—not investigated.

Neurologic Injuries

The neurologic examination should establish the patient's level of consciousness, orientation toward intellectual function, emotional stability, and cognition. Given the high incidence of brain injury in contact sports, this aspect of the examination should be thorough because initial signs of severe head trauma can be subtle. If the patient demonstrates progressive cerebral dysfunction, the possibility of evolving intracranial injury, hypoxia, or hypotension is indicated. Drug abuse must also be considered as an etiology of these symptoms.

Cranial nerves need to be examined in a systematic manner because they may indicate the presence of injuries to the brain, cranium, eyes, ears, or facial skeleton. Cranial nerve I (olfaction) is not easily tested. Cranial nerve II should be evaluated for visual acuity and with penlight testing for the light reflex, which, when combined in an alternating manner between eyes, permits evaluation of the cranial nerve III consensual light reflex. Unreactive dilated pupils or a lack of the consensual reflex is indicative of severe CNS injury. Cranial nerve III, IV, and VI provide extraocular movement, which is easily evaluated by directional testing. Inability to move the eye in all directions may indicate extraocular muscle entrapment secondary to orbital fractures, severe edema, or a brain stem injury in the absence of gross structural orbital deformities. Cranial nerve V provides sensory innervation to the face, and the presence of altered sensation may indicate underlying facial bone fractures. Cranial nerve VII provides innervation to the muscles of facial expression, which when partially injured is reflective of a severed nerve trunk or its more peripheral branches, whereas complete loss of function indicates a skull base fracture or temporal bone involvement. Cranial nerve VIII is easily examined by hearing tests. Cranial nerve IX, X, and XII provide mobility and sensation to the soft palate, uvula, tongue, and pharynx. Altered taste sensation may indicate injury to the chorda tympani, which travels from the lingual branch of cranial nerve V to cranial nerve IX, and can indicate trauma to the glenoid fossa or temporomandibular joint (an occasional complaint of boxers). Cranial nerve XI will be intact if shoulder lifting is possible.

Cerebellar function is established by testing for the ability to touch the nose with a forefinger with the eyes opened or closed, and walking heel to toe in a straight line with eyes opened or closed. Additional general motor examination can include testing for reflexes and observing muscle tone and overall posture. Decerebrate or decorticate postures indicate serious brain injuries. The sensory system can be readily evaluated by pin testing, directional testing, and temperature sensitivity. Altered sensation posterior to the ears in the coronal plane is suggestive of cervical spine or skull base injuries. The presence of significant brain, spinal cord, cervical spine, or cranial injuries requires consultation with a neurosurgeon.

Soft Tissue Injuries (Integument and Oral Mucosa)

The skin of the scalp, neck, and face and oral and oropharyngeal mucosa should be examined thoroughly for the presence of lacerations, abrasions, contusions, edema, ecchymosis, emphysema, burns, or avulsive defects. Skin injuries may reflect more severe underlying skeletal or other vital structure problems. Deep lacerations need to be explored for the presence of debris, especially in the case of lip lacerations in which dental fragments may be embedded. Periapical dental radiographs are often helpful. Other deep, vital soft-tissue structures must be considered, such as the major salivary gland ducts (submandibular duct under the tongue, parotid duct across the midface), function of which can be confirmed by dye studies (sialography). Hemorrhage from arterial sources often must be ligated to achieve hemostasis and can often be significant, such as in scalp injuries and in deep neck and facial vessels. Underlying fractures of the cranium and facial bones can be a source of severe hemorrhage and often require reduction to achieve control of hemorrhage. Nerve injuries associated with lacerations often require repair, although because of their presence anterior to a line perpendicular to the Frankfort horizontal plane through the lateral canthus of the eye, they are often untreated because the nerve diameter is too small.

Ophthalmologic Injuries

Ophthalmologic injuries frequently result from sports trauma,[51,69] and they can consist of the full range of extraocular, intraocular, orbital bone, and neurologic problems—individually and in combination. These injuries may be as acute as penetrating globe injuries, globe avulsion, optic nerve compression or severence (with total blindness), retinal detachment, or orbital roof and floor blowout. Ocular injuries require immediate diagnosis and management in consultation with an ophthalmologist.

Examination of the eye should begin with visual acuity because this is potentially the most important problem, followed by the neurologic examination of light and consensual reflexes. These signs will determine the extent of injuries to the optic nerve, orbital apex contents, and the superior orbital fissure contents. Fundoscopic examination will detect the presence of hemorrhages, lens dislocation, and retinal disorders. The external eye and the sclera, subconjunctiva, cornea, eyelids, and lacrimal apparatus need to be examined for lacerations, abrasions, penetration, ecchymosis, and emphysema. Certain sports have greater rates of eye injuries because of the high degree of contact, explosive nature, and use of accessory equipment, such as hockey pucks and sticks, and baseball bats and balls.

Mandible Fractures

Mandibular fractures should be suspected in individuals with intraoral or extraoral ecchymosis, lacerations, edema, inferior facial asymmetry, lip and chin altered sensation, jaw hypomobility, altered dental occlusion, and other signs and symptoms (see box, Signs and Symptoms of Mandibular Fractures). Patients may complain of the teeth not meeting correctly and the inability to bite appropriately. Clinical evaluation should begin with inspection of the skin, oral mucosa, dentition, alveolar bone, and dental prostheses, followed by bimanual palpation. It is necessary to first establish the status of the dentoalveolar region and the presence of fractured, luxated, avulsed, or displaced teeth and prostheses. The mandible should then be grasped with the thumbs along the incisal edges (cusps) of the teeth and the forefingers along the inferior border, moving around the dental arch to determine the presence of pain, tenderness (Fig. 13-10), or mobile segments. The finger positions are changed for the posterior mandibular body and ramus so that the forefingers grasp the mandibular body and ramus with the thumbs along the inferior border, looking for similar signs of pain, tenderness, or segment mobility. Palpate the preauricular region while asking the patient to open and close the jaw to search for the presence of pain, tenderness, or unusual protruding masses (indicative of condylar segment displacement). Otoscopic examination of the tympanic membrane is important to detect the presence of external auditory canal lacerations or hemotympanum, which are indicative of condylar fractures. When mandibular fractures are suspected, evaluation by radiographic examination should follow. The most important radiograph for mandibular evaluation is the panoramic radiograph.

CHECKLIST

Signs and Symptoms of Mandibular Fractures

- Trismus
- Edema
- Laceration or abrasion
- Ecchymosis
- Malocclusion
- Mental nerve paresthesia
- Crepitus
- Deviation upon opening
- Asymmetry
- Step defect along inferior border

From Greenberg AM (ed): Craniomaxillofacial Fractures: Principles of Internal Fixation Using the AO/ASIF Technique. New York, Springer-Verlag, 1993.

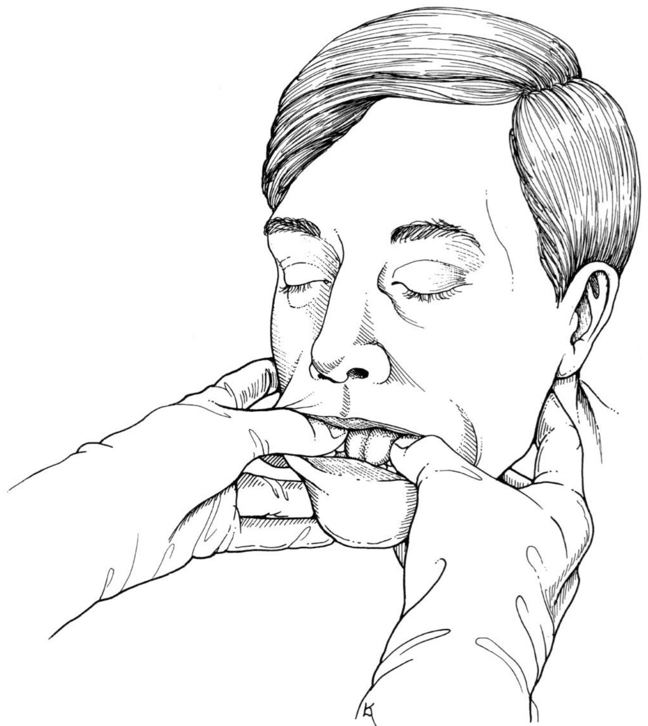

FIGURE 13-10. Examination of a suspected mandibular fracture. Thumbs on occlusal surface edges and forefingers on inferior border of mandible. (From Greenberg AM [ed]: Craniomaxillofacial Fractures: Principles of internal Fixation Using the AO/ASIF Technique. New York, Springer-Verlag, 1993.)

Maxillary Fractures

Like mandibular fractures, suspected maxillary fractures may be present in patients with intraoral or extraoral ecchymosis, lacerations, edema, midfacial retrusion, upper lip altered sensation, jaw hypomobility, altered dental occlusion, and other signs and symptoms (see box, Signs and Symptoms of Maxillary Fractures). Patients may complain of the teeth not meeting correctly and the inability to bite appropriately. These patients often present with an "open bite" deformity and flattened midface.

Clinical evaluation should begin with inspection of the skin, oral mucosa, dentition, and alveolar bone, dental prostheses, followed by bimanual palpation. It is necessary to establish the status of the dentoalveolar region and the presence of fractured, luxated, avulsed, or displaced teeth and prostheses. Because maxillary fractures occur at various levels of the midface, they may involve only the dental portion or more superiorly include the orbital, zygomatic, and nasal regions. Periorbital symptomatology includes ecchymosis, subconjunctival hemorrhage, and nasal hemorrhage, and if there is associated anterior cranial fossa involvement, there may be a dural tear with cerebrospinal rhinorrhea with its classical tramline appearance. Nasal involvement may be noted as a widened intercanthal distance or traumatic telecanthus. Standard measurements are

CHECKLIST

Signs and Symptoms of Maxillary Fractures

- Tenderness
- Flattened face
- Lengthened face
- Periorbital ecchymosis
- Air emphysema
- Paresthesia of cheek or nose
- Malocclusion
- Crepitus
- Edema
- Ecchymosis of vestibule
- Subconjunctival hemorrhage
- Cerebrospinal fluid leak
- Step defect at zygomatic or nasomaxillary buttress

From Greenberg AM (ed): Craniomaxillofacial Fractures: Principles of Internal Fixation Using the AO/ASIF Technique. New York, Springer-Verlag, 1993.

available for the intercanthal distance and may be useful for the diagnosis of nasoethmoid involvement (28.6–33.0 mm in women and 28.9–34.5 in men).[24] Commonly, the skin overlying the midface may have a crackling sensation on palpation, which indicates subcutaneous emphysema associated with the disrupted maxillary and paranasal sinuses.

LeFort II (level II) maxillary fractures will be clinically evident by grasping the maxillary incisors with the dominant hand and palpating the nasal bridge with the less dominant hand, and upon manipulation attempting to detect the presence of movement at the nasal bridge (Fig. 13-11). LeFort III (level III) maxillary fractures are detected by a similar maneuver: the less dominant hand will grasp the bilateral frontozygomatic sites to detect mobility upon manipulation (Fig. 13-12). If fractures are suspected, radiographic imaging of this region should be obtained and may range from plain radiographs to CT. In children, these fractures are less common, but because of the presence of tooth buds in the pediatric facial skeleton, CT scanning should be performed.[31,55]

Zygoma Fractures

Patients with zygomatic fractures typically present with periorbital edema, ecchymosis, subconjunctival hemorrhage, malar flattening, difficulty with mandibular movement, and altered sensation of the posterior dental quadrant or overlying cutaneous region. Globe position may be altered with the presence of exophthalmus or enophthalmus, based on the degree of orbital floor or wall involvement and the disruption of the suspensory ligament. Other signs and symptoms (see box, Signs and Symptoms of Zygoma Fractures) must be fully determined, and radiography is especially helpful because of the extensive edema that may be present.

Examination for zygomatic fractures should begin with palpation of the supraorbital region, moving from a

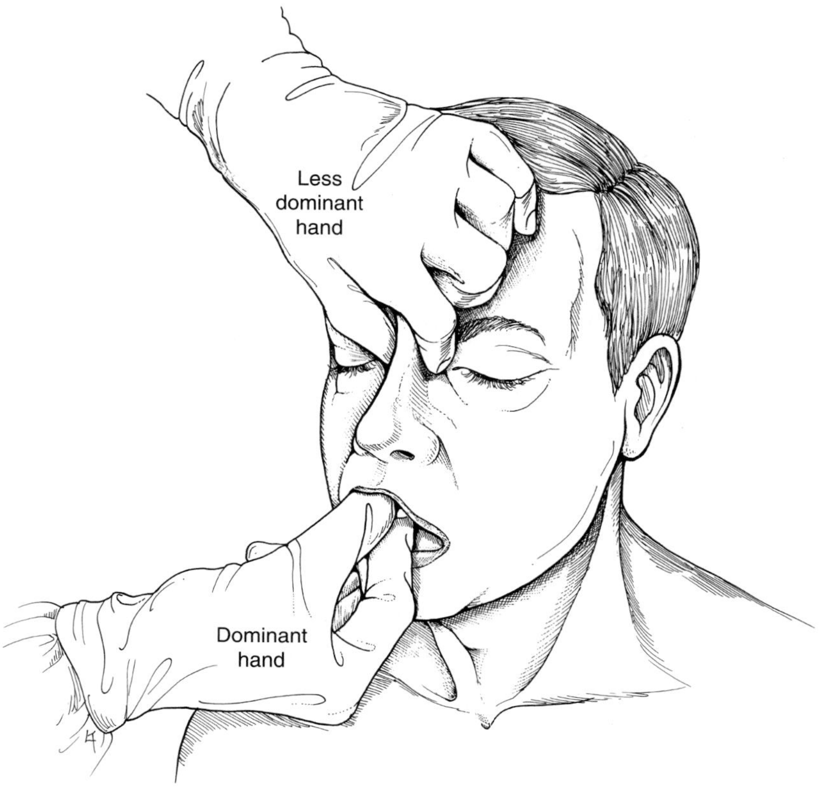

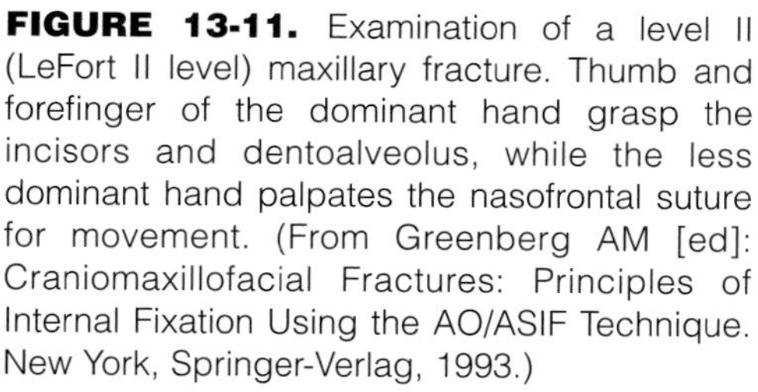
FIGURE 13-11. Examination of a level II (LeFort II level) maxillary fracture. Thumb and forefinger of the dominant hand grasp the incisors and dentoalveolus, while the less dominant hand palpates the nasofrontal suture for movement. (From Greenberg AM [ed]: Craniomaxillofacial Fractures: Principles of Internal Fixation Using the AO/ASIF Technique. New York, Springer-Verlag, 1993.)

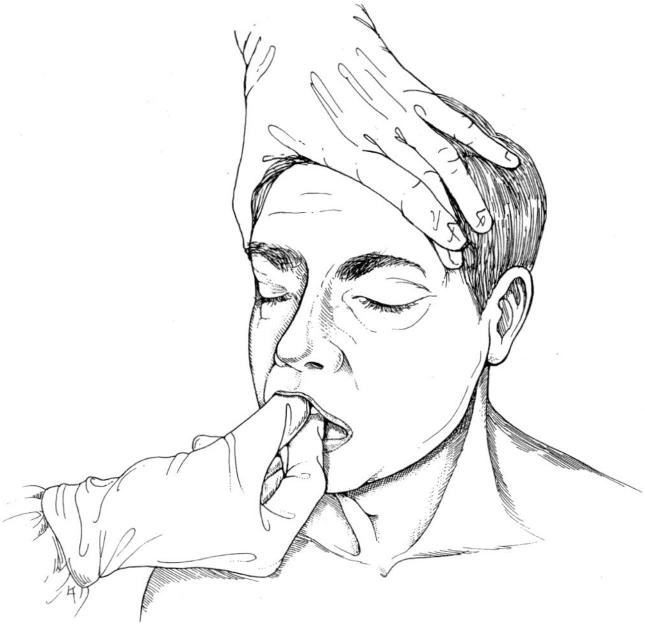

FIGURE 13-12. Examination of a level III (LeFort III level) maxillary fracture. Thumb and forefinger of the dominant hand grasp the incisors and dentoalveolus, while the less dominant hand palpates the frontozygomatic suture for movement. (From Greenberg AM [ed]: Craniomaxillofacial Fractures: Principles of internal Fixation Using the AO/ASIF Technique. New York, Springer-Verlag, 1993.)

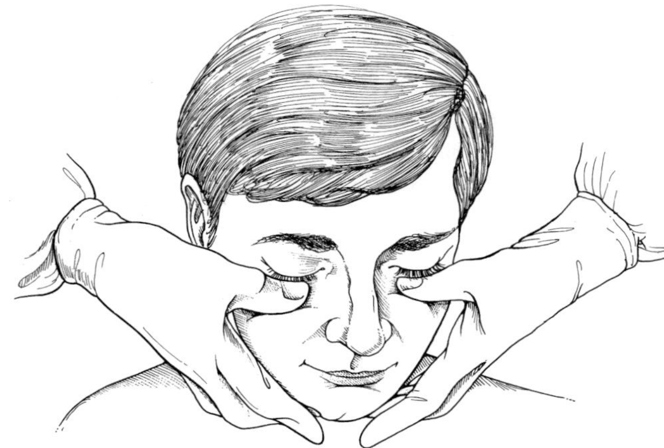

FIGURE 13-13. Clinical examination of the infraorbital rims in a patient with a suspected zygoma fracture. (From Greenberg AM [ed]: Craniomaxillofacial Fractures: Principles of Internal Fixation Using the AO/ASIF Technique. New York, Springer-Verlag, 1993.)

lateral to medial direction and with care to observe for tenderness over the frontozygomatic region. The infraorbital rim should then be palpated, with simultaneous palpation of the contralateral side as a reference. Stepping may be noted over the infraorbital region because the zygomatic body is often medially and inferiorly displaced (Fig. 13-13). The zygomatic arch should be palpated to determine the presence of stepping or tenderness. Finally, intraoral examination is performed, which should include palpation of the zygomaticomaxillary buttress. Ophthalmologic examination should be thorough because there may be extraocular muscle entrapment with limitation of gaze, diplopia, enophthalmus, exophthalmus, and globe injury (see box, Ophthalmologic Sequelae of Complex Injuries). Radiographic examination should consist of a minimum of a Waters' view and submentovertex with panoramic radiography, and CT axial and coronal examination are useful.

CHECKLIST

Signs and Symptoms of Zygoma Fractures

Periorbital ecchymosis
Lateral subconjunctival hemorrhage
Paresthesia of nose and cheek
Unequal pupil height
Downward slope of lateral canthus
Flattening of cheek contours
Trismus
Edema
Air emphysema
Diplopia
Exophthalmus/enophthalmus
Ecchymosis of buccal vestibule
Crepitus
Limited extraocular movements
Step defects at zygomaticomaxillary, frontozygomatic, or zygomaticotemporal sutures

From Greenberg AM (ed): Craniomaxillofacial Fractures: Principles of Internal Fixation Using the AO/ASIF Technique. New York, Springer-Verlag, 1993.

CHECKLIST

Ophthalmologic Sequelae of Complex Injuries

Hyphema
Lens dislocation
Retinal detachment
Optic nerve compression
Vitreous hemorrhages
Superior orbital fissure syndrome
Orbital apex syndrome
Ophthalmoplegia
Carotid-cavernous fistula
Globe avulsion
Chemosis
Epiphora
Enophthalmus
Exophthalmus
Telecanthus

From Greenberg AM (ed): Craniomaxillofacial Fractures: Principles of Internal Fixation Using the AO/ASIF Technique. New York, Springer-Verlag, 1993.

Nasoethmoid Fractures

Nasoethmoid fractures vary from simple nasal tip fractures to fracture dislocation of the nasoethmoid complex into the base of the skull. Simple nasal fractures may be limited to the nasal bridge and displacement of the nasal septum. There are many symptoms of nasoethmoid fractures that are seen in fractures of the maxilla and zygoma (see box, Signs and Symptoms of Nasoethmoid Fractures). When nasal fractures involve more than the nasal tip and are complex naso-orbital-ethmoid fractures, severe problems, such as traumatic telecanthus, loss of nasal projection, and cerebrospinal rhinorrhea may result. The medial canthal attachments may be disrupted with loss of the medial canthal angle.

Examination should proceed with inspection for edema, ecchymosis, and lacerations of the overlying skin and associated periorbital region. Palpation of the nasal bridge can determine whether the nasal bones are intact or displaced. Nasal speculum examination of the intranasal mucosa can determine the presence of septal displacement, septal hematoma, or mucosal lacerations. If nasal fractures are suspected, imaging should be obtained, which may include plain radiographs (simple fractures) or CT scanning (complex fractures).

CHECKLIST

Signs and Symptoms of Nasoethmoid Fractures

Periorbital ecchymosis
Medial subconjunctival hemorrhage
Bilateral epistaxis
Traumatic telecanthus
Nasal contour deformity
Cerebrospinal fluid leak
Crepitus
Diplopia
Tenderness
Edema
Laceration

From Greenberg AM (ed): Craniomaxillofacial Fractures: Principles of Internal Fixation Using the AO/ASIF Technique. New York, Springer-Verlag, 1993.

Supraorbital Rim and Frontal Sinus Fractures

Periorbital ecchymosis is the most frequently noted sign in supraorbital rim and frontal sinus fractures, followed by soft-tissue lacerations, and many other signs and symptoms (see box, Signs and Symptoms of Supraorbital Rim and Frontal Sinus Fractures). Soft-tissue edema may obscure the underlying frontal bone fracture. These injuries range from simple to severe, from minor nondisplaced supraorbital rim or outer table fractures to displaced inner table fractures with dural tears, brain injury, and cerebrospinal rhinorrhea. Other clinical complaints may include altered sensation of the brow and forehead, visual complaints, and headache. Examination of the patient should proceed from inspection to palpation, with the detection of crepitus suggestive of soft-tissue emphysema. If a deep laceration is present, bone fragments and foreign bodies may be palpable or directly visualized by exploration. If a frontal fracture is suspected, imaging is necessary and should include plain radiographs at a minimum, with CT scanning obtained if a penetrating injury or neurologic damage is suspected. Surgical exploration is often necessary to determine whether the posterior table is involved and the nasofrontal ducts are patent.

CHECKLIST

Signs and Symptoms of Supraorbital Rim and Frontal Sinus Fractures

Periorbital ecchymosis
Subconjunctival hemorrhage
Laceration
Flatness of forehead
Edema
Tenderness
Crepitus
Exposed bony fragments
Cerebrospinal fluid leak
Exophthalmus
Paresthesia of forehead
Step defect of supraorbital rim

From Greenberg AM (ed): Craniomaxillofacial Fractures: Principles of Internal Fixation Using the AO/ASIF Technique. New York, Springer-Verlag, 1993.

REFERENCES

1. Abiose PO: Maxillofacial skeleton injuries in the western states of Nigeria. Br J Oral Maxillofac Surg 24:31–39, 1986.
2. Adekeye EO: The pattern of fractures of the facial skeleton in Kaduna, Nigeria. Oral Surg Oral Med Oral Pathol 49:491–495, 1980.
3. American College of Surgeons: Initial assessment and management. In Advanced Trauma Life Support Course for Physicians. Chicago, American College of Surgeons, 1989.
4. Andreaseon JO: Traumatic Injuries of the Teeth. Philadelphia, WB Saunders, 1981.
5. Bochlogyros PN: A retrospective study of 1,521 mandibular fractures. J Oral Maxillofac Surg 43: 597–599, 1985.
6. Castaldi CR: Prevention of craniofacial injuries in ice hockey. Dent Clin North Am 35:647–656, 1991.
7. Cerulli G, Carboni A, Mercurio A, Perugini M, Becelli R: Soccer related craniomaxillofacial injuries. J Craniofac Surg 13: 627–630, 2002.

8. Clayton MI, Lesser THS: The role of radiography in the management of nasal fractures. J Laryngol Otol 100:797–801, 1986.
9. Cook HE, Rowe M: A retrospective study of 356 midfacial fractures occurring in 225 patients. J Oral Maxillofac Surg 48:574–578, 1990.
10. Crow RW: Diagnosis and management of sports-related injuries to the face, in sports dentistry. Dental Clin North Am 35:719–732, 1991.
11. Donald PJ: Frontal sinus ablation by cranialization. Arch Otolaryngol 108:142–146, 1982.
12. Duval AJ, Porto DP, Lyons D, et al: Frontal sinus fractures. Arch Otolaryngol Head Neck Surg 113: 933–935, 1987.
13. Ellis E, El Attar, Moos KF: An analysis of 2067 cases of zygomatico-orbital fracture. J Oral Maxillofac Surg 43:417–428, 1985.
14. Ellis E, Moos KF, El-Attar A: Ten years of mandibular fractures: An analysis of 2,137 cases. Oral Surg Oral Med Oral Pathol 59:120–129, 1985.
15. Fisher-Brandies E, Dielert E: Treatment of isolated lateral midface fractures. J Maxillofac Surg 12: 103–106, 1984.
16. Giles HD, Kilner TP: The treatment of the broken nose. Lancet i:147–149, 1929.
17. Greenberg AM: Basics of AO/ASIF principles and stable internal fixation of mandibular fractures. In Greenberg AM (ed): Craniomaxillofacial Fractures: Principles of Internal Fixation Using the AO/ASIF Technique. New York, Springer Verlag, 1993.
18. Greenberg AM: Management of facial fractures. NYSDJ 42–47, 1998.
19. Gruss JS, Babak PJ, Egbert MA: Craniofacial fractures, an algorithim to optimize results. Clin Plast Surg 19:195–206, 1992.
20. Gruss JS, Mackinnon SE: Complex maxillary fractures: Role of buttress reconstruction and immediate bone grafts. Plast Reconstr Surg 85:9–22, 1986.
21. Harrison DH: Nasal injuries: Their pathogenesis and treatment. Br J Plast Surg 32:57–64, 1979.
22. Haug RH: Basics of stable internal fixation of maxillary fractures. In Greenberg AM (ed): Craniomaxillofacial Fractures: Principles of Internal Fixation Using the AO/ASIF Technique. New York, Springer Verlag, 1993.
23. Haug RH, Greenberg AM: Etiology, distribution, and classification of fractures. In Greenberg AM (ed): Craniomaxillofacial Fractures: Principles of Internal Fixation Using the AO/ASIF Technique. New York, Springer-Verlag, 1993.
24. Haug RH, Likavec MJ: Evaluation of the craniomaxillofacial trauma patient. In Greenberg AM (ed): Craniomaxillofacial Fractures: Principles of Internal Fixation Using the AO/ASIF Technique. New York, Springer-Verlag, 1993.
25. Haugh RH, Prather JL: The closed reduction of nasal fractures: An evaluation of two techniques. J Oral Maxillofac Surg 49:1288–1292, 1991.
26. Haug RH, Prather J, Inderesano AT: An epidemiologic survey of facial fractures and concomittant injuries. J Oral Maxillofac Surg 48:926–932, 1990.
27. Hill CM, Crosher RF, Carroll MJ, et al: Facial fractures—the results of a prospective four year study. J Oral Maxillofac Surg 12:267–270, 1984.
28. Illum P, Kristenson C, Jorgenson K, et al: The role of fixation in the treatment of nasal fractures. Clin Otolaryngol 8:191–195, 1983.
29. Ioannides C, Freihofer HPM, Bruaset I: Trauma of the upper third of the face. J Maxillofac Surg 12: 255–261, 1984.
30. James RB, Frederickson C, Kent JN: Prospective study of mandible fractures. J Oral Surgery 39: 275–281, 1981.
31. Kaban CLB: Diagnosis and treatment of fractures of the facial bones in children 1943–1993. J Oral Maxillofac Surg 51:722–729, 1993.
32. Kahnberg KE, Gothberg KAT: LeFort fractures: A study of frequency, etiology, and treatment. Int J Oral Maxillofac Surg 16:154–159, 1987.
33. Khalil AF, Shaladi OA: Fractures of the facial bones in the eastern region of Libya. Br J Oral Surg 19: 300–304, 1981.
34. Knight JS, North JF: The classification of malar fractures: An analysis of displacement as a guide to treatment. Br J Plast Surg 13:325–339, 1961.
35. Lahti H, Sane J, Ylipaavalniemi P: Dental injuries in ice hockey games and training. Med Sci Sports Exerc: Preventive measures for sports medicine. Sports Med 32: 400–402, 2002.
36. Landry GL: Sports injuries in childhood. Pediatric Annals 165–168, 1992.
37. Larrabee WF, Travis LW, Tabb HG: Frontal sinus fractures: Their suppurative complications and surgical management. Laryngoscope 90:1810–1813, 1980.
38. LeFort R: Etude experimentale sur les fractures de la machoire superieure. Rev Chir 23:208–227, 1901.
39. LeFort R: Etude experimentale sur les fractures de la machoire superieure. Rev Chir 23:360–379, 1901.
40. LeFort R: Etude experimentale sur les fractures de la machoire superieure. Rev Chir 23:479–507, 1901.
41. Lephart SM, Fu FH: Emergency treatment of athletic injuries. Dent Clin North Am 35:707–717, 1991.
42. Lundun K, Ridell A, Sandberg N, et al: One thousand maxillofacial and related fractures at the ENT clinic in Gothberg. Acta Otolaryngol 75:359–361, 1973.
43. Maladiere E, Bado F, Meningaudi JP, et al: Aetiology and incidence of facial fractures sustained during sports: a prospective study of 140 patients. Int J Oral Maxillofac Surg 30: 291–295, 2001.

44. Manson PN, Hoopes JE, Su CT: Structural pillars of the facial skeleton: An approach to the management of LeFort fractures. Plast Reconstr Surg 66:54–61, 1980.
45. Markowitz BL, Manson PN, Sargent L, et al: Management of the medial canthal tendon in nasoethmoid orbital fractures: The importance of the central fragment in classification and treatment. Plast Reconstr Surg 87:843–853, 1991.
46. McGraw BL, Cole RR: Pediatric maxillofacial trauma, age related variations in injury. Arch Otolaryngol Head Neck Surg 116:41, 1990.
47. Murray JA, Maran AGD, Butsuttil A, et al: A pathological classification of nasal fractures. Injury 17:338–344, 1986.
48. Olson RA, Fonseca RJ, Zeitler DL, et al: Fractures of the mandible: review of 580 cases. J Oral Maxillofac Surg 40:23–28, 1982.
49. Onishi K, Nakajima T, Yoshimura Y: Treatment and therapeutic devices in the management of frontal sinus fractures. J Craniomaxillofac Surg 17:58–63, 1989.
50. Overview of Sports Related Injuries to Persons 5–14 Years of Age. Washington, US Consumer Product Safety Commission, 1981.
51. Pashby TJ: Eye injuries in hockey. In Vinger PF (ed): Ocular Sports Injuries (International Opthalmology Clinics). Boston, Little, Brown, 1981.
52. Peri G, Chabannes S, Menes R, et al: Fractures of the frontal sinus. J Maxillofac Surg 9:73–80, 1981.
53. Perkins SW, Dayan SH, Sklarew EC, et al: The incidence of sports-related facial trauma in children. Ear Nose Throat J 79: 62–64, 636, 638, 2000.
54. Pinkham JR, Kohn DW: Epidemiology and prediction of sports-related traumatic injuries. Dent Clin North Am 35:609–625, 1991.
55. Posnick JC, Wells M, Pron GE: Pediatric facial fractures: Evolving patterns of treatment. J Oral Maxillofac Surg 51:836–844, 1993.
56. Prein J, Hammer B: Stable internal fixation of midfacial fractures. Facial Plast Surg 5:221–230, 1988.
57. Ranalli DN: Prevention of craniofacial injuries in football. Dent Clin North Am 35:627–643, 1991.
58. Ranalli DN, Demas PN: Orofacial injuries from sports: preventive measures for sports medicine. Sports Med 32: 400–402, 2002.
59. Rix L, Stevenson ARL, Punnia-Moorthy: An analysis of 80 cases of mandibular fracture treated with miniplate osteosynthesis. Int J Oral Maxillofac Surg 20:337–341, 1991.
60. Rowe NL: Fractures of the facial skeleton in children. J Oral Surg 26:505, 1968.
61. Rowe NL, Williams JL: Maxillofacial Injuries. Edinburgh, Churchill Livingstone, 1985.
62. Sofferman RA, Danielson PA, Quatela V, et al: Retrospective analysis of surgically treated LeFort fractures. Arch Otolaryngol 109:446–448, 1983.
63. Spiessl B: Internal Fixation of the Mandible: A manual of AO/ASIF Principles. New York, Springer Verlag, 1989.
64. Stanley RB, Becker TS: Injuries of the nasofrontal orifices in frontal sinus fractures. Laryngoscope 97: 728–731, 1987.
65. Steidler NE, Cook RM, Reade PC: Incidence and management of major middle third facial fractures at the Royal Melbourne Hospital. Int J Oral Surg 9: 92–98, 1980.
66. Stoll P, Schilli W: Primary reconstruction with AO miniplates after severe craniomaxillofacial trauma. J Craniomaxillofac Surg 16:18–21, 1988.
67. Stranc MF, Robertson GA: A classification of injuries of the nasal skeleton. Ann Plast Surg 32:57–64, 1979.
68. Torg JS, Vesgo JJ, Sennett B, Das M: The national football head and neck injury registry: 14 year report on cervical quadriplegia, 1971–1984. JAMA 254:3439–3443, 1985.
69. Vinger PF: The incidence of eye injuries in sports. In Vinger PF (ed): Ocular Sports Injuries (International Opthalmology Clinics). Boston, Little, Brown, 1981.
70. Wallis A, Donald PJ: Frontal sinus fracture: A review of 72 cases. Laryngoscope 98:593–598, 1988.
71. Watson AWS: Incidence and nature of sports injuries in Ireland: Analysis of four types of sport. Am J Sports Med 21:137–143, 1993.
72. William RJ 3rd, Marx RG, Barnes R, et al: Fractures about the orbit in professional American football players. Am J Sports Med 29: 55–57, 2001.
73. Williamson LK, Miller RH, Sessions RB: The treatment of nasofrontal ethmoidal complex fractures. Otolaryngol Head Neck Surg 89:587–593, 1981.

14 Dental Injuries

Michael D. Kurtz, Joe H. Camp, and Jens O. Andreasen

Preseason dental and oral screening should be the first step in the prevention of sports-related dental injuries.[81] The more information available before an injury occurs, the better from a management and medicolegal standpoint.[90] Experienced trainers, team physicians, and dentists know that logistically this may not always be convenient or possible, especially in the case of visiting team players. Even if the information is incomplete, the more information gathered in advance the better. This information may include medical and dental histories, clinical examination and dental charting, radiographic survey, and customary photos and models.

Much of this information, especially radiographs, will serve as a baseline for comparison should an injury occur. Radiographs can also help identify problems that have the potential to remove the athlete from competition during the season. Such problems include impacted wisdom teeth, periapical radiolucencies, and teeth with deep decay. Panorex radiographs may be considered efficacious because they require less time to take than a full mouth series, do not subject the athlete to gagging, and show more of the maxillary and mandibular jaw bones.

Study models are important records. They can be used to fabricate a valuable piece of protective equipment—a custom mouthguard. Use of custom-made mouthguards has proven to reduce the number and severity of sports-related dental and orofacial traumatic injuries and possibly cerebral concussions.

Sports participants are at risk for unique and distinct kinds of injuries. In turn, different diagnostic and treatment needs may be necessary.[87] For example, avid use of smokeless tobacco among baseball players would suggest greater significance for an oral cancer examination. Babe Ruth is said to have died from this. In one study, smokeless tobacco was found to have a detrimental effect on visuo-motor performance, particularly on movement smoothness.[28] College appears to be a time when many students are trying a range of tobacco products, including smokeless tobacco, and are in danger of developing lifelong nicotine dependence.[96,110]

Gender equity issues have lead us to focus attention on emerging issues in women's oral health. A comprehensive discussion of dental and orofacial injuries, fads and habits such as tongue-piercing, smokeless tobacco, eating disorders, and performance-enhancing drugs is covered in *Dental Clinics of North America*.[95]

The exact mechanisms of injury to teeth are mostly unknown and not investigated. Direct trauma from a high-velocity object, such as a baseball that takes a bad hop and strikes the maxillary incisors, is likely to cause a fracture (Fig. 14-1). Alternatively, good lip coverage will diffuse the force of the blow, lower the velocity of the ground ball, and distribute the energy of impact over a wider area, causing greater surrounding hard- and soft-tissue damage (e.g., an avulsion). In other words, low-velocity trauma causes greatest damage to the hard and soft tissues that surround the teeth, whereas high-velocity trauma is more likely to fracture the teeth.[9,10,46]

Another mechanism, indirect trauma, occurs when the mandible whiplashes into collision with the maxilla. This trauma can occur from a blow to the chin, such as an uppercut in boxing, a football tackle, or a hockey stick. The concussion is capable of shattering posterior teeth (Fig. 14-2).[9,46]

Any traumatic dental injury has the potential to challenge pulp vitality even if not apparent initially. Electrical and thermal pulp tests on freshly traumatized teeth are unreliable, and their results should not be relied on heavily. Pain, palpation, percussion, and radiography

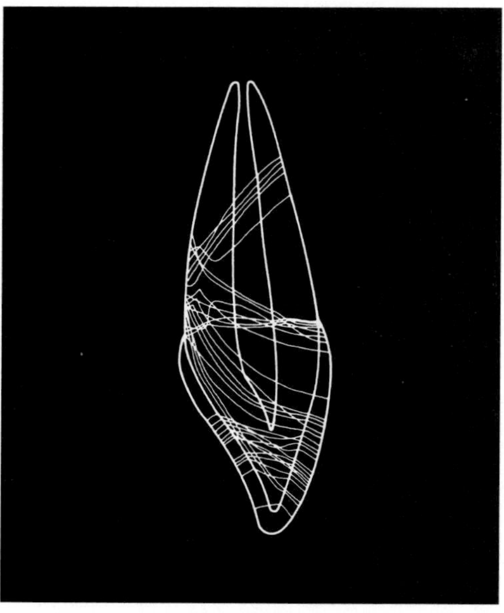

FIGURE 14-1. Facio-lingual directions of 33 fracture lines caused by frontal impacts. (From Andreasen J: Traumatic Injuries of the Teeth, 2nd ed. Philadelphia, WB Saunders, 1981.)

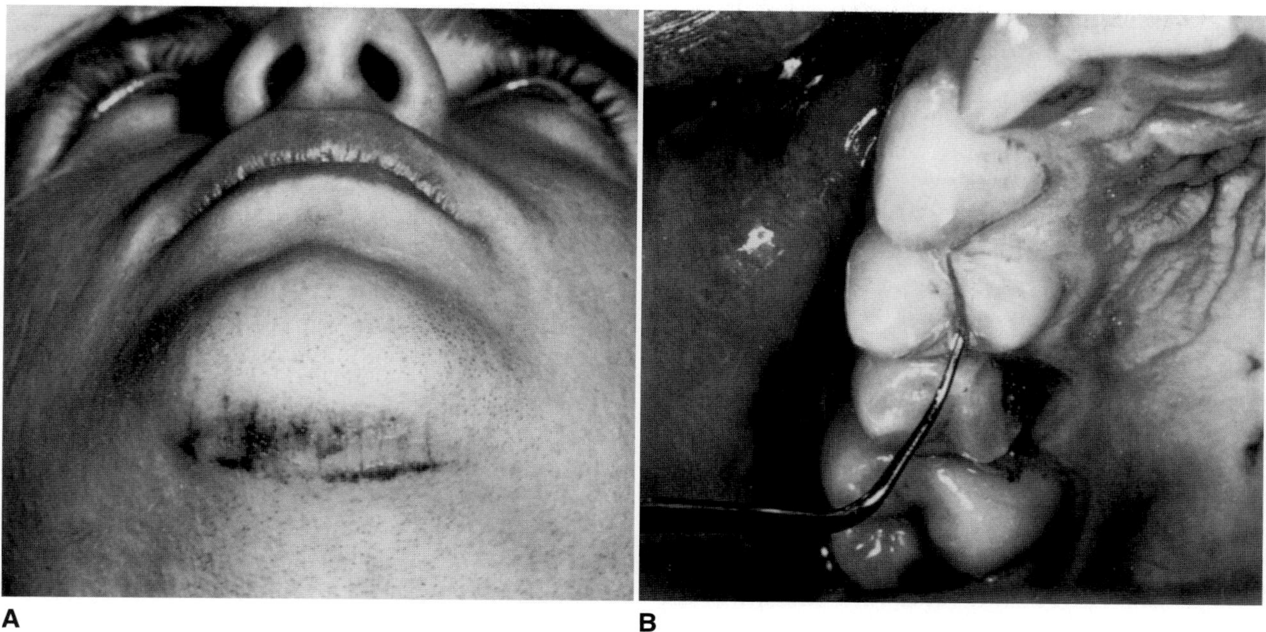

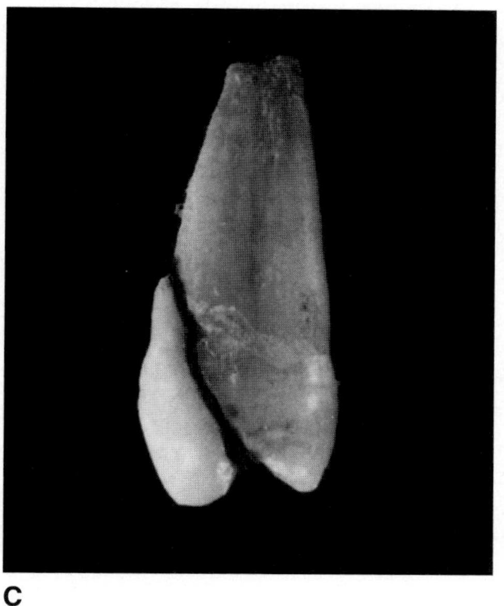

FIGURE 14-2. Complicated crown–root fractures of posterior teeth. **A,** Trauma to the chin. **B,** Complicated crown–root fractures of both right first and second premolars. **C,** Lateral view of extracted first premolar. (From Andreasen J, Andreasen F: Textbook and Color Atlas of Traumatic Injuries to the Teeth, 2nd ed. St Louis, Mosby–Year Book, 1994.)

are more indicative. Patients should be recalled to monitor pulp vitality at 1, 3, and 6 months after trauma. Thereafter, it is recommended pulp vitality be evaluated at 6-month intervals for several years.[37] A similar recall regimen may be instituted for teeth that have been displaced and are at risk of developing external root resorption or ankylosis.

The classification of dental sports injuries varies from author to author. The application of general standards for traumatic injuries to teeth is helpful especially when compiling or comparing statistics. Four basic categories of traumatic injuries to the oral cavity will be discussed: teeth, periodontal tissues, supporting bone, and gingival and oral mucosa.[9]

TEETH

Crown Fractures

Crown fractures are most likely to result from high-velocity trauma. Pulpal vitality has a better chance of being maintained than with low-velocity trauma, which is customarily associated with displacement injuries. Crown fractures occur more frequently in permanent teeth, whereas primary teeth are more likely to be displaced. Severe overjet will predispose a maxillary incisor to fracture, especially if there is lack of lip coverage (Fig. 14-3).[59] Early interceptive orthodontics helps reduce this risk.[73]

Crown Fractures Involving Enamel. Enamel infraction is a crack in the enamel without loss of tooth substance.

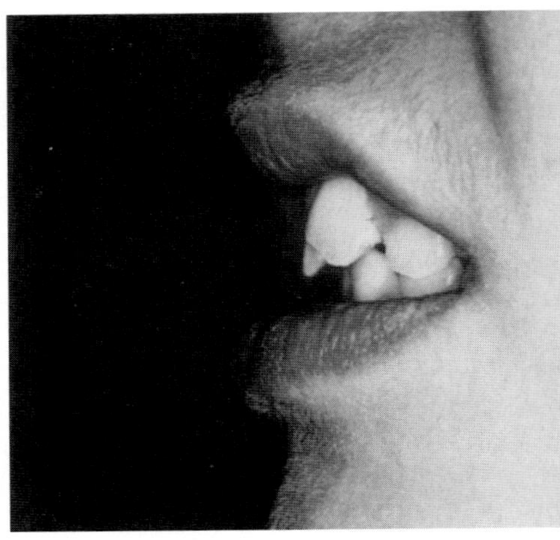

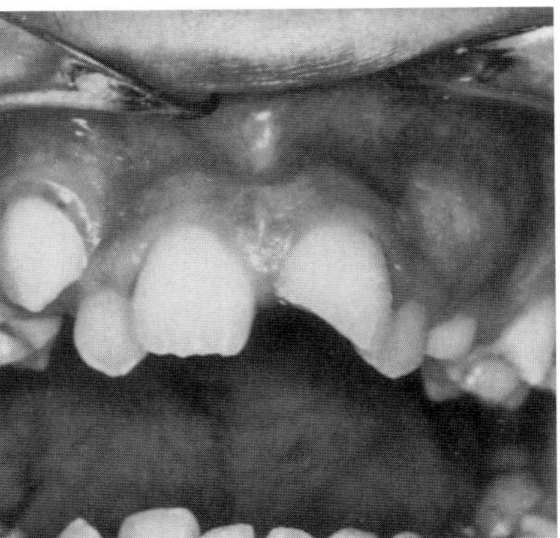

FIGURE 14-3. Predisposition to crown fracture. **A,** Protruding central incisors with incomplete lip coverage. **B,** Crown fracture of a left central incisor. (From Andreasen J, Andreasen F: Textbook and Color Atlas of Traumatic Injuries to the Teeth, 3rd ed. St Louis, Mosby–Year Book, 1994.)

The crack usually runs parallel to the direction of the enamel prisms. The resulting craze line extends to the dentin–enamel junction and may lead to subsequent chipping of the tooth. Cracked tooth syndrome can be difficult to diagnose. Sensitivity to hot, cold, sweets, or biting pressure may result. Enamel infraction can be caused by acute or chronic trauma such as grinding (bruxism) or clenching (e.g., weightlifting). Bonded restorations such as Belleglass or porcelain onlays can be useful in arresting the progression of enamel infraction.[20,40]

Enamel fracture is a loss of tooth substance confined to the enamel. The attending dentist may need to round sharp edges or consider acid-etch bonding of composite to prevent further injury to soft tissues or for aesthetics (Fig. 14-4).

Crown Fractures Involving Enamel and Dentin. Fractures involving dentin and exposing dentinal tubules often result in thermal sensitivity. The reduction of this sensitivity, usually taking 6 to 8 weeks, correlates to the formation of reparative dentin.[102] Restoration of the tooth can usually be accomplished by acid-etch composite bonding with adequate pulpal protection (Fig. 14-5).

Crown Fractures Involving Enamel, Dentin, and Pulp. This complicated crown fracture exposes the pulp to bacterial infection and directly challenges tooth vitality. If left untreated, the fracture will usually lead to either a proliferative (pulpal hyperplasia) (Fig. 14-6) or destructive response (pulpal necrosis) (Fig. 14-7). Bacterial infection will necessitate pulpectomy and root canal therapy.[30] This may require a more significant restorative procedure, such as a post and crown. Whenever maintenance of vitality is important, the exposed pulp should be isolated and covered as soon as possible to prevent microorganisms from establishing an infection. Studies have demonstrated that injured pulpal tissues in germ-free animals usually heal, irrespective of the severity of

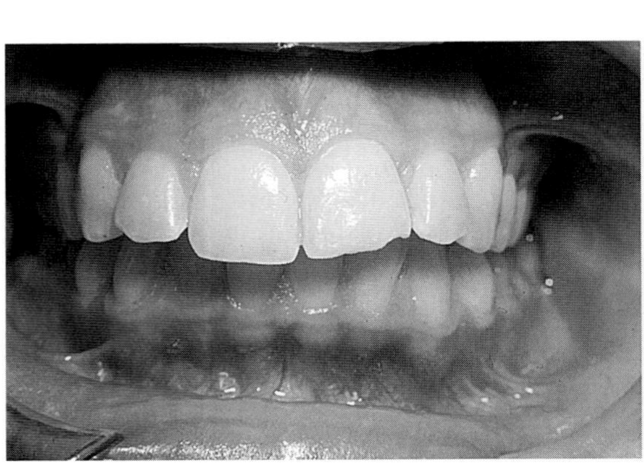

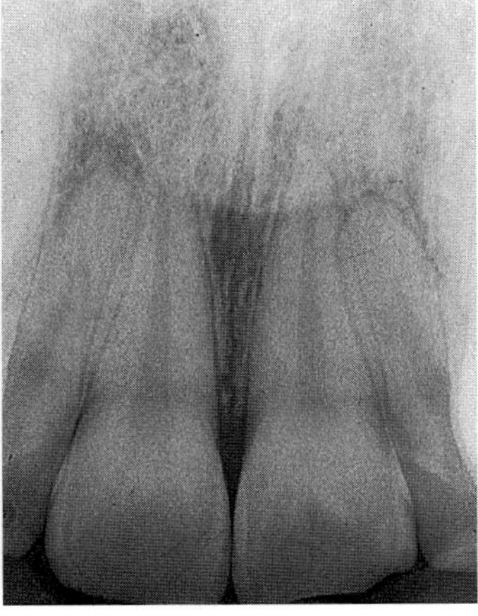

FIGURE 14-4. Enamel fracture of the maxillary left central incisor involving the distoincisal angle. **A,** Photograph and **B,** radiograph of fracture.

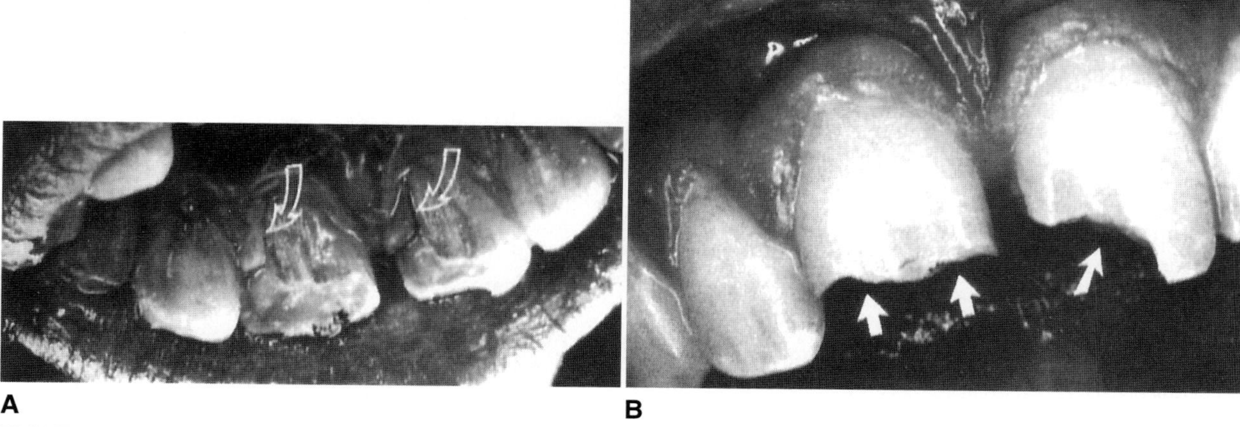

FIGURE 14-5. Crown fractures involving enamel and dentin. **A,** Mirror view of palatal "chisel" type fractures. **B,** Direct facial view of incisal edge and mesio-incisal angle fractures. (From Bakland L: Traumatic injuries. In Ingle J, Taintor J: Endodontics, 2nd ed. Philadelphia, Lea & Febiger, 1985.)

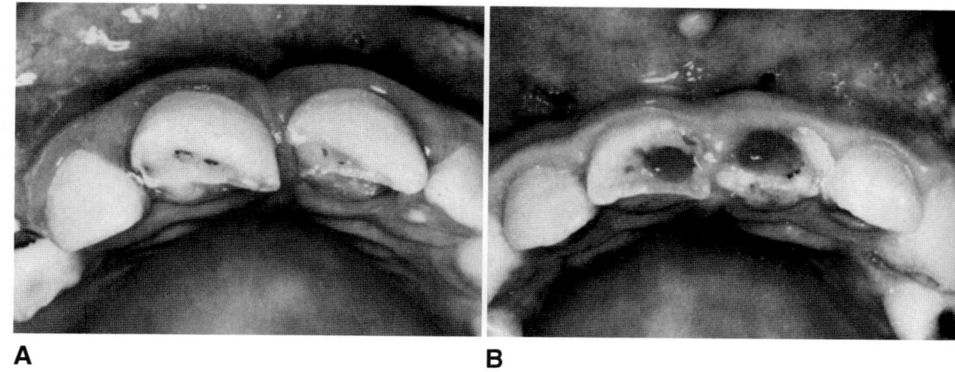

FIGURE 14-6. Complicated crown fractures of central incisors. **A,** Small traumatic pulp exposures. **B,** Pulp proliferation in complicated crown fractures left untreated for 21 days. (From Andreasen J, Andreasen F: Textbook and Color Atlas of Traumatic Injuries to the Teeth, 3rd ed. St Louis, Mosby, 1994.)

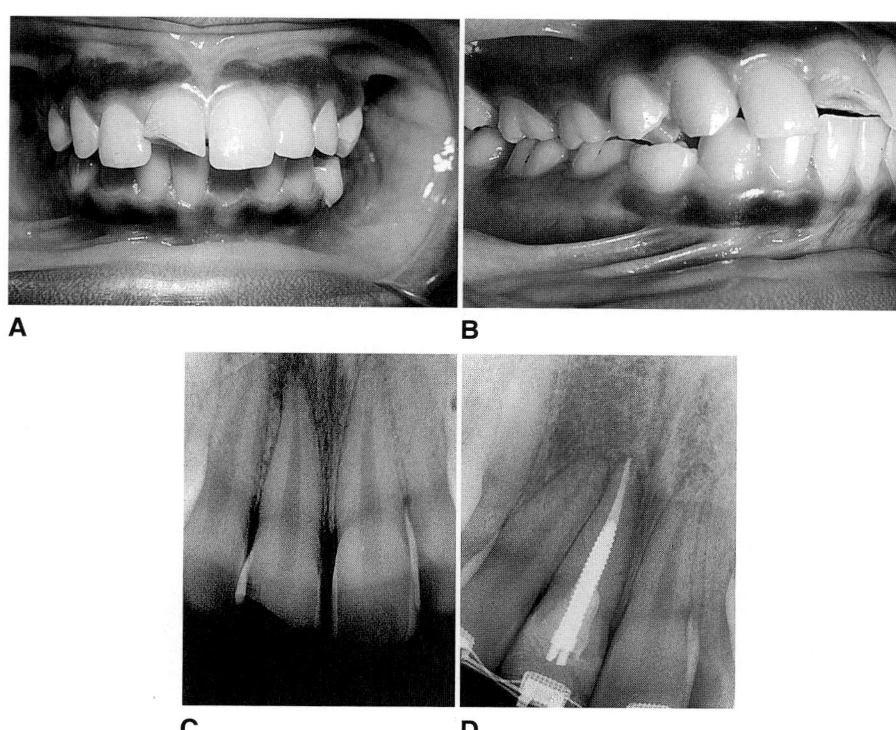

FIGURE 14-7. Pulp necrosis in an untreated anterior tooth with a crown fracture involving enamel, dentin, and pulp. **A,** Fractured maxillary right central incisor. **B,** Untreated pulp exposure that has developed a necrotic response. Note staining where dentinal tubules have aspirated blood. **C,** Periapical radiolucency. **D,** Radiograph showing resolution of periapical pathology five years after root canal therapy. Note Dentatus screw post (distributed by Dentatus—Dentatus USA, New York, NY) and concurrent orthodontic treatment.

the pulp exposure.[60,85] When possible, these procedures should be performed under rubber dam isolation. According to the Centers for Disease Control and Prevention in Atlanta, Georgia, dental rubber dam isolation also helps limit the transmission of all blood-borne pathogens, including HIV and HBV, by minimizing spatter of blood and blood-contaminated saliva.[105]

When immature teeth are injured, it is essential that pulpal vitality be maintained to allow completion of root development. This will permit better canal obturation should vitality be compromised and pulpectomy become necessary in the future. Afterward, a permanent restoration could be placed. One of the following two procedures should be selected as appropriate:

1. Pulp capping is used for small traumatic exposures free of inflammation and treated within hours of injury. A hard-setting calcium hydroxide material (e.g., Life–Kerr Corporation, Orange, CA; Dycal—Dentsply International Inc., L.D. Caulk Division, Milford, DE) is used to dress the exposure before placement of a temporary restoration.
2. Pulpotomy uses a sterile diamond bur[43] at high speed with copious cooling water to remove sufficient inflamed tissue, usually 2 to 3 mm, to expose healthy uninflamed tissue. Damp cotton pellets are used to achieve hemostasis. Life or Dycal is then applied or $Ca(OH)_2$ United States Pharmacopia (USP) powder mixed with saline is carried to the pulp, and a hard-setting base can be placed over it.

Signs of successful pulp capping and pulpotomy are (Fig. 14-8)[37] absence of pain, negative percussion, normal thermal sensitivity, negative palpation, and absence of radiographic periapical pathosis; radiographic dentin bridging; and radiographic evidence of continued root development. Possible complications include canal calcification, internal resorption, and pulp necrosis.

Crown–Root Fractures

There are two categories of crown–root fractures:

1. Uncomplicated—involving enamel, dentin, and cementum only. Missing tooth structure can be restored by bonding, 3/4 crown, or full crown as appropriate (Fig. 14-9).
2. Complicated—involving enamel, dentin, cementum, and pulp (Fig. 14-10), usually requiring prompt root canal therapy (RCT) so that a post and crown may be fabricated (see Fig. 14-2).

Pulpal considerations are essentially the same as those for crown fractures. After fragment removal, the remaining portion of the tooth can be surgically exposed, provided the fracture site is less than 2 mm below the level of the alveolar bone. Otherwise, orthodontic or surgical extrusion to about 2 mm coronal to the alveolar crest must be considered. Extrusion will expose enough tooth structure to rebuild the tooth prosthetically, provided there is sufficient root length (Fig. 14-11). If the coronal fragment comprises more than one third of the clinical root length, the tooth is indicated for removal.[9] Extraction is also indicated for vertical fractures when the fracture line follows the long axis of the tooth.

Root Fractures

Root fractures involve dentin, cementum, and pulp and account for 7% or fewer of injuries to permanent teeth.[7] Surprisingly, most teeth with radicular fractures remain vital, and only 20% to 40% become nonvital.[4] The patient's main complaint is sensitivity to biting pressure. Mobility of the tooth may be indicative of root fracture. Percussion with a mouth-mirror handle will assist in confirming the diagnosis. Fracture location can be determined by gentle digital palpation over the facial aspect of

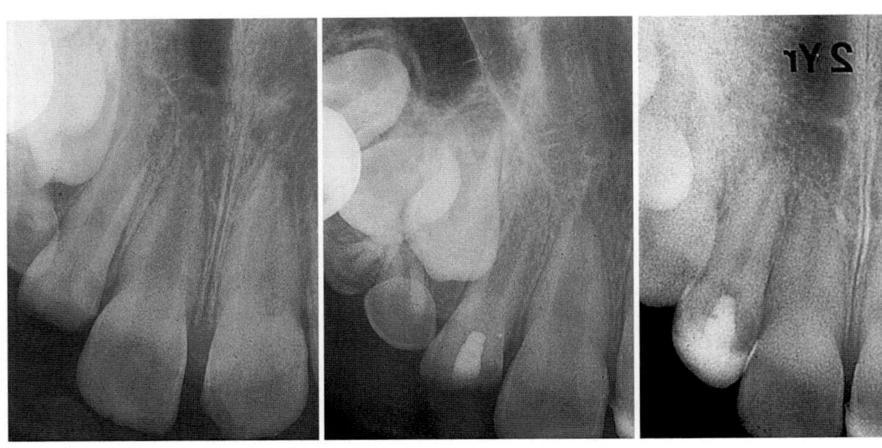

FIGURE 14-8. Radiographs of continued root development following a pulpotomy. **A,** Maxillary lateral incisor with incomplete root development and a pulp exposure. **B,** Effects of calcium hydroxide following a pulpotomy. **C,** Two-year follow-up: root formation is completed and the pulp remains vital. Note the dentinal bridge just superior to the calcium hydroxide.

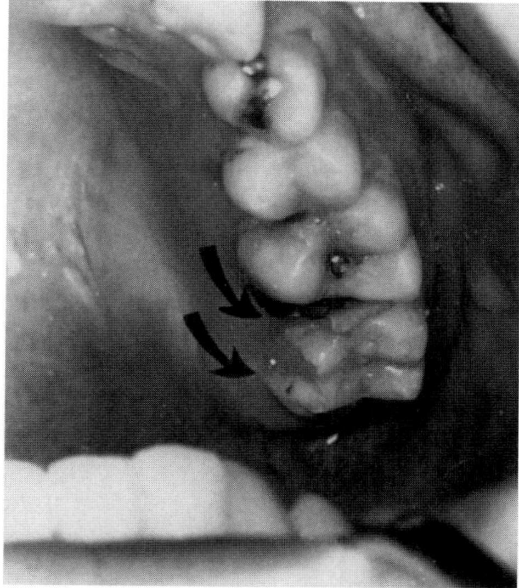

A

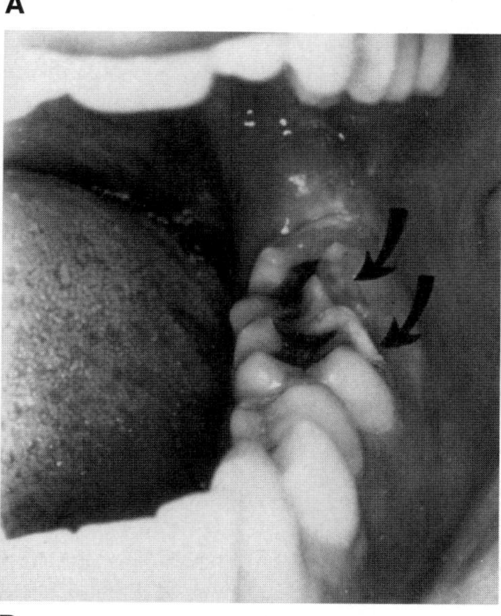

B

FIGURE 14-9. Uncomplicated crown–root fractures (not exposing the pulp) resulting from a blow to the chin. The fractures of the lingual cusps in the maxillary arch correspond to the fractures of the buccal cusps in the mandibular arch. **A,** Maxillary arch. **B,** Mandibular arch. (From Andreasen J, Andreasen F: Textbook and Color Atlas of Traumatic Injuries to the Teeth, 3rd ed. St Louis, Mosby, 1994.)

the suspected root fracture. This examination is done while holding and delicately rocking the crown of the suspect tooth between the thumb and forefinger of the clinician's other hand.

Prompt reduction and fixation with a rigid acid-etched splint will promote healing by calcific callus formation internally (on the root canal wall) and externally (on the root surface) (Fig. 14-12). Experience has shown the farther coronally a radicular fracture is located, the longer a splint should be left in place. This period can vary from 3 to 6 months. A far coronal fracture may need to be left in place for 1 year or exchanged for a permanent-type splint, such as a Maryland bridge. If reduction is insufficient, edema has caused some separation, or if fixation is deficient, which allows too much mobility, then fibrous connective tissue healing similar to periodontal ligament may result. If these conditions are somewhat exaggerated, new alveolar bone may actually form between the fracture segments. With severe dislocation, there will be nonunion (Fig. 14-13). Usually, the apical segment will remain vital, and the incisal segment will undergo necrosis with granulation tissue formation between the two segments. RCT can be confined to the incisal (coronal) segment. If evidence of resorption is present, the canal is initially filled with $Ca(OH)_2$. Once the resorption is healed, the canal is obturated with gutta percha. This is also true if the root is sufficiently immature and wide open so as to interfere with the creation of a positive stop to prevent overfilling and extrusion of gutta percha or cement sealer.

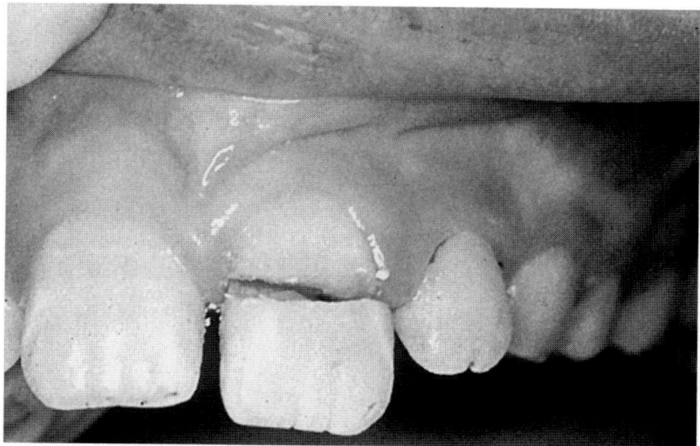

FIGURE 14-10. Complicated crown–root fracture of an anterior tooth. (Courtesy of the International Academy for Sports Dentistry.)

PERIODONTAL TISSUES

Nondisplacement Injuries

Nondisplacement injuries are characterized by edema, bleeding, and trauma to periodontal ligament (PDL) fibers. These PDL fibers can be damaged by tearing, stretching, or compression. Clinically, there is sensitivity to percussion and palpation. Relief of the occlusion by selective grinding of the opposing teeth and a soft diet for several weeks are generally recommended. Radiographic follow-up evaluation for 1 year is advisable to rule out the need for endodontic therapy.

Concussion. Concussion is an injury to the PDL with no visible loosening or displacement of the tooth from its alveolus. The chief complaint is tenderness to touch or biting pressure (Fig. 14-14).

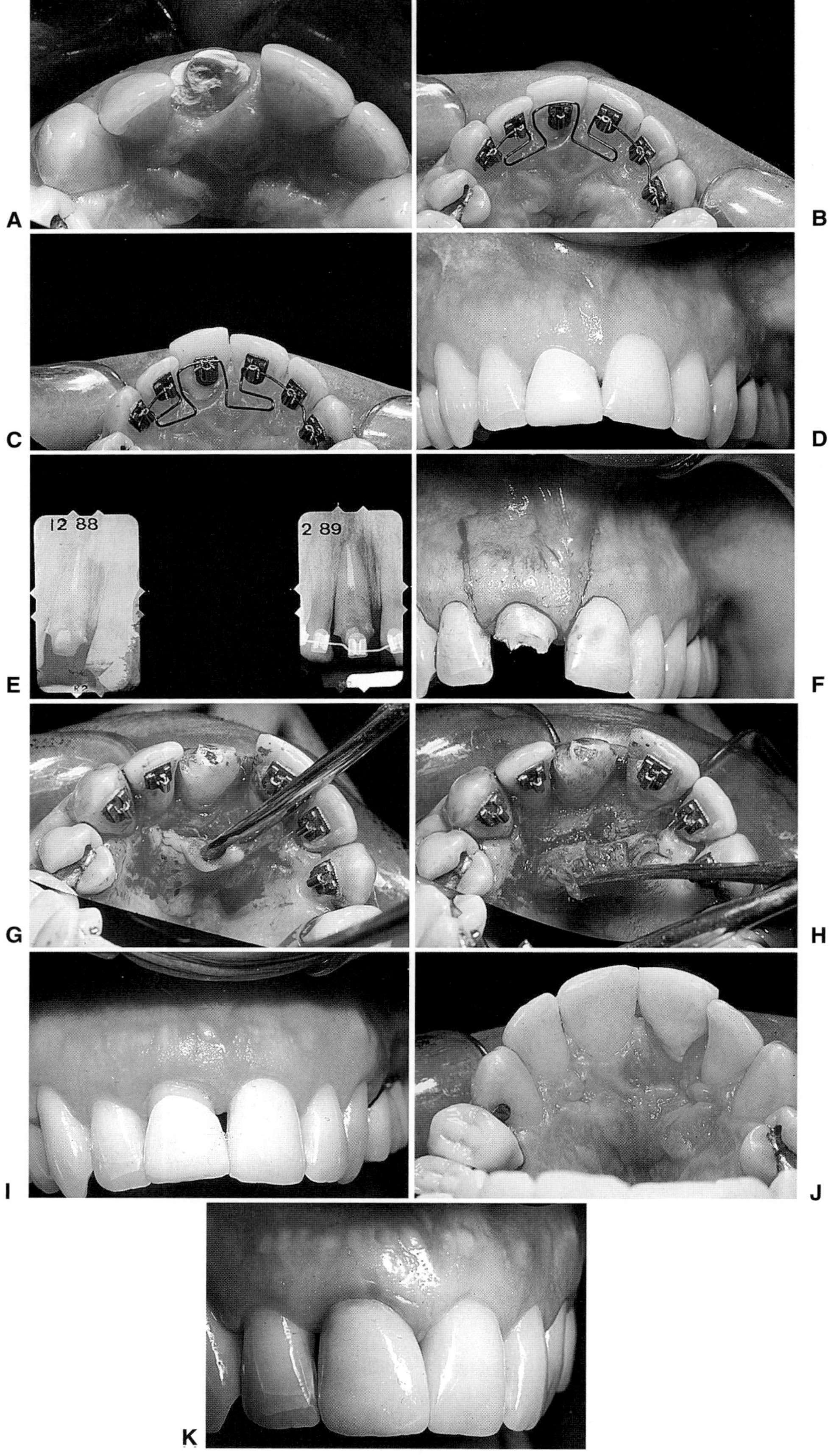

FIGURE 14-11. Multidisciplinary extrusion of a complicated crown–root fracture involving an anterior tooth using lingual braces and periodontal surgery. **A,** Traumatically fractured maxillary right central incisor. **B,** Provisional restoration following cementation and placement of an orthodontic appliance. **C,** Activation of orthodontic appliance. **D,** Alterations of gingival margins immediately following eruption. **E,** Pre- and posteruption radiographs. **F,** A very conservative labial periodontal flap design. **G,** Palatal view demonstrating depth of fracture. **H,** Postosseous resection. **I,** Labial view, healed. Note the amount of crown length gained without losing papillae, the lack of root exposure of neighboring teeth, and the gingival margins of central incisors. **J,** Palatal view showing amount of crown length gained. **K,** Final result. Restorative dentistry by Dr. Daniel Budasoff, NY, NY. (All photographs courtesy of Frank Celenza Jr., DDS, New York, NY.)

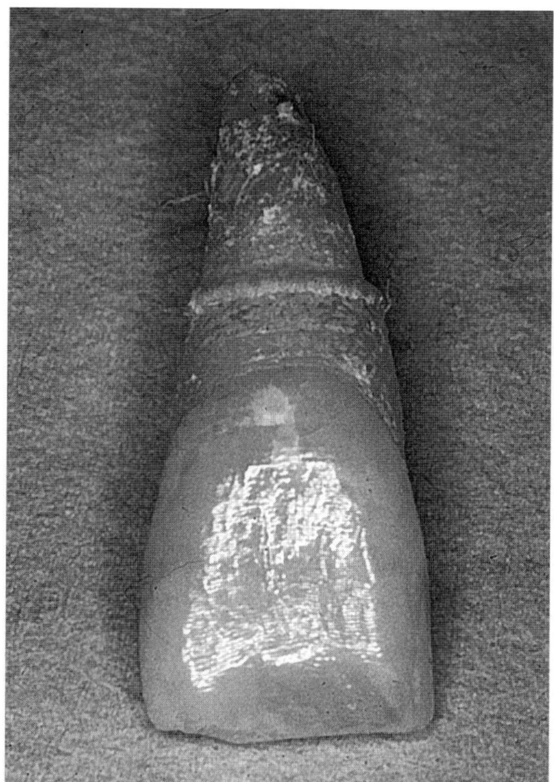

FIGURE 14-12. Extracted tooth with a previous root fracture healed with a calcific callus. (From Fountain SB, Camp JH: Pathways of the Pulp, 6th ed. St Louis, Mosby–Year Book, 1994.)

Subluxation. Subluxation is characterized by discernable loosening of the tooth in the horizontal direction without demonstrable clinical or radiographic displacement. It may be sufficient to cause bleeding in the periodontal ligament, with hemorrhage visible in the gingival crevice (see Fig. 14-14). If several teeth are involved and if there is significant mobility, short-term splinting may be used.

Displacement Injuries

Displacement injuries are most likely to occur as the result of low-velocity trauma.[9] Moderate overjet of the maxillary incisors with good lip coverage would predispose them to displacement rather than fracture. Early orthodontics might help to intercept this problem. Patients with displacement injuries may complain of discomfort, swelling, discoloration of the crown of the tooth, mobility, or a change in their occlusion. Primary teeth are more apt to be displaced than permanent teeth. About 50% of permanent teeth with displacement injuries will require RCT.[97]

Pulpal necrosis, root resorption, pulp calcification and obliteration, and loss of alveolar crestal bone height are the major complications of displacement injuries. $Ca(OH)_2$ can be used to fill the root canal of teeth exhibiting root resorption. This will help arrest the process before future filling with gutta percha.[32] $Ca(OH)_2$ should be retained between 6 to 12 months for intruded teeth and about 12 months for avulsed teeth, depending on whether resorption is ongoing. $Ca(OH)_2$ powder is mixed with a liquid and delivered as a paste. Anesthetic carpule solution or physiologic saline can be used as a carrier solvent. Premixed pastes are available from commercial vendors. Some examples are Tempcanal (Pulpdent Corp., Watertown, MA), Hypo-Cal (Ellman International, Hewlett, NY), and Calasept (distributed by J. S. Dental Manufacturing Inc., Ridgefield, CT). Because it is absorbable, the paste should be removed and refreshed every 3 to 4 months as needed and cannot be used as a permanent root canal filler.[23]

Displacement injuries may need splinting to limit mobility and promote healing. Splints that cause gingival inflammation or subject teeth or alveolar bone to active pressures or tensions will cause PDL inflammation, external root resorption, or ankylosis. Emdogain for periodontal healing following light to moderate trauma-related replacement resorption associated with replantation has been proposed to prevent or delay recurrance of ankylosis in some cases.[34] Oral surgical wire ligatures and arch bars should not be used in managing traumatized teeth (Fig. 14-15).[37] An arch wire between 0.015″ and 0.030″, about the size of paperclips, can be shaped and bonded passively using acid-etch resin. According to Andreasen,[12] prolonged rigid splinting of avulsed teeth for more than 7 to 10 days may lead to external root resorption and ankylosis. Splinting time for luxated teeth can range between 2 to 3 weeks, depending on the severity of the injury and the patient's healing abilities.

Extrusion. Extrusion is a partial avulsion of the tooth out of the alveolar socket. It is accompanied by radiographic evidence of increased width of the PDL space (Fig. 14-16).

Lateral Luxation. Lateral displacement is a sideways dislocation of the tooth accompanied by comminution or fracture of the alveolar socket. Usually the coronal portion of the tooth is driven palatally or lingually, and the apical portion is driven in a facial direction. To free an apically locked tooth from a fenestration through buccal plate, coronally directed finger pressure over the apex of the root may be helpful (Fig. 14-17).[10]

Intrusion. Intrusion is a displacement of the tooth in the direction of the alveolar bone caused by axially directed forces accompanied by comminution or fracture of the alveolar socket. The highest incidence of pulpal necrosis in teeth with displacement injuries occurs with intrusions. About 96% of intruded permanent teeth will undergo pulpal necrosis.[5,9] In mature teeth, after 7 to 10 days to allow some PDL healing, pulpectomy and

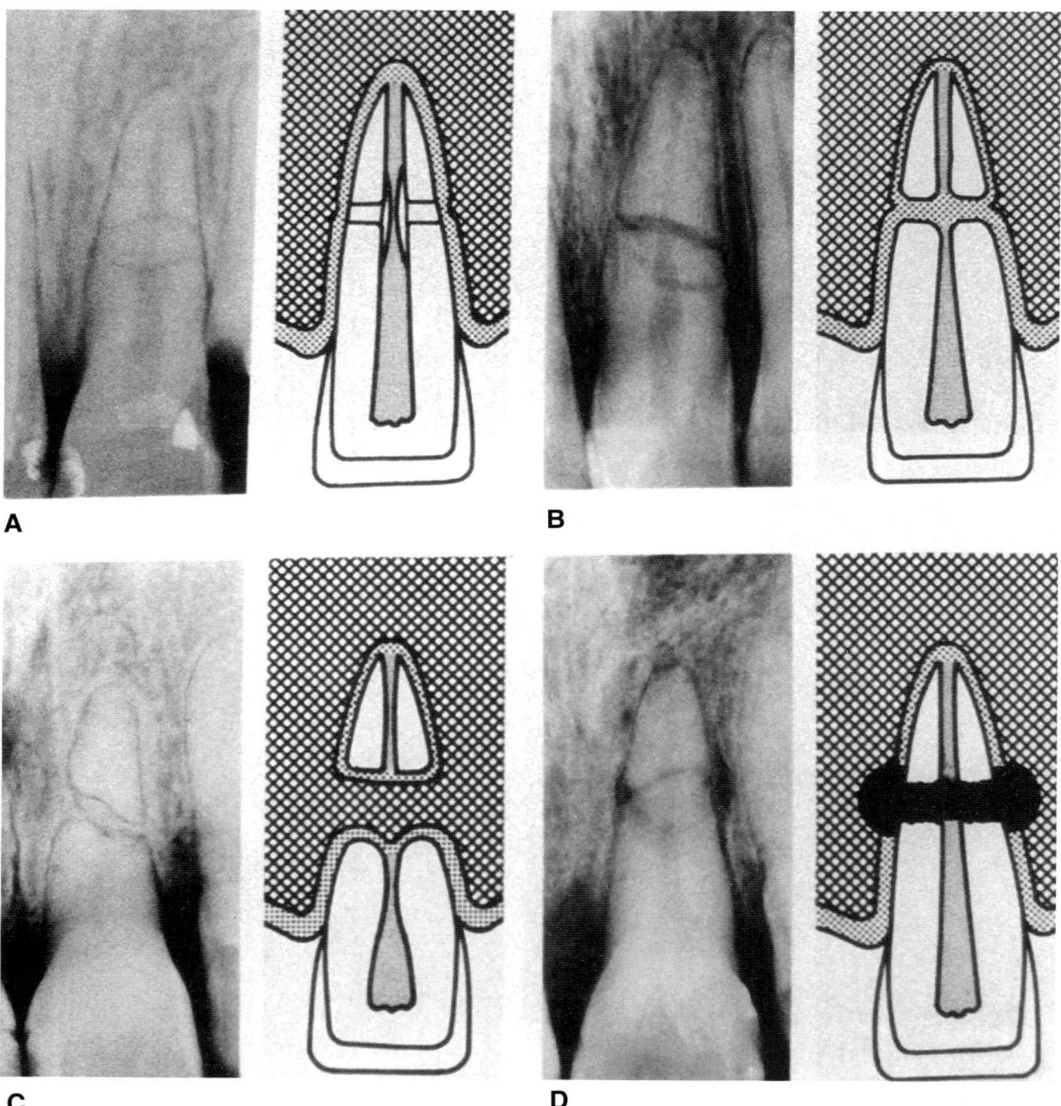

FIGURE 14-13. Radiographs and diagrams illustrating various modalities of healing after root fracture. **A,** Calcified tissue. **B,** Interposition of connective tissue. **C,** Interposition of bone and connective tissue. **D,** Interposition of granulation tissue. (From Andreasen J: Traumatic Injuries of the Teeth, 2nd ed. Philadelphia, WB Saunders, 1981.)

$Ca(OH)_2$ therapy are necessary to decrease the likelihood of accompanying root resorption.[9,31] An intruded tooth with incomplete root formation will sometimes spontaneously reerupt. Mature teeth are best treated by prompt orthodontic extrusion back into position (Fig. 14-18). This extrusion will help reduce the complications of loss of alveolar crestal bone height and external root resorption or ankylosis. Severe intrusions may require surgical repositioning and splinting. Any intruded tooth that extends into the nasal cavity must also be surgically repositioned.

Avulsion. Avulsion is the complete displacement of the tooth from its socket. The maxillary central incisors are the most frequently avulsed teeth (Fig. 14-19). Avulsion is not an uncommon occurance in sports.[66] The sooner an avulsed tooth is replanted, the better its chances of survival.[47] Immature teeth with incomplete root formation have a potential to revitalize and survive. In a sports setting, immediate replantation might be accomplished by the team trainer, physician, or dentist. Maintenance of periodontal ligament integrity is critical, therefore no attempt to scrub, treat chemically, or sterilize the tooth should be made. The tooth should be handled by its crown rather than by its root. Any clot may be dislodged by gentle rinsing with saline or aspiration without damaging the socket. If an avulsed tooth cannot be replanted to its original position without force, it is probably safer

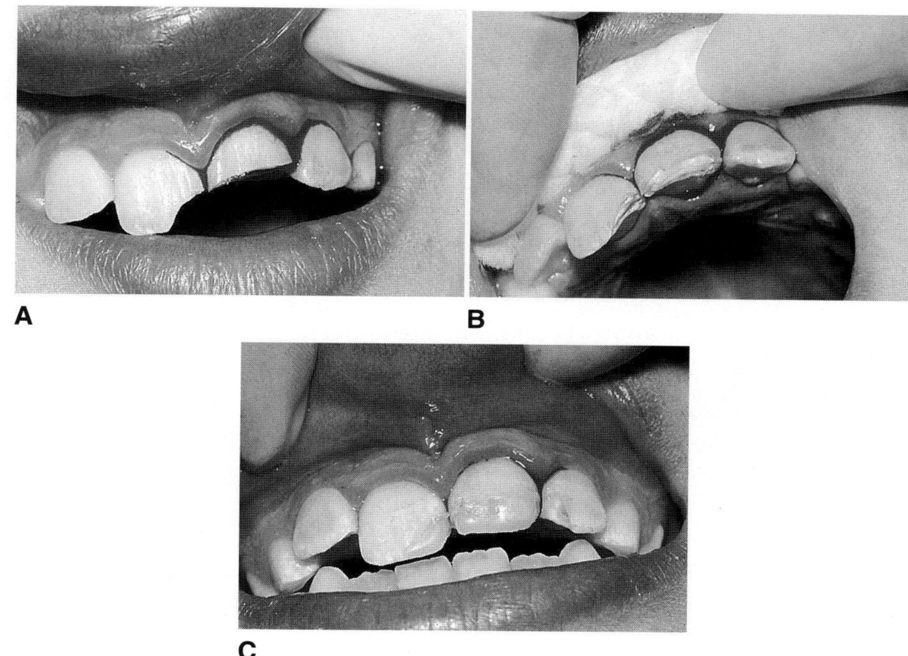

FIGURE 14-14. Concussion and subluxation with accompanying crown fractures. **A,** The maxillary incisor fractured at the angle has suffered a concussion and is very sensitive to touch but exhibits neither mobility nor displacement. The horizontally fractured incisor has been subluxated, is bleeding from the periodontal ligament, and has a concomitant pulp exposure. **B,** Fracture after Dycal has been applied over the pulp exposure and the exposed dentin. **C,** Acid-etch composite has been placed to retain the Dycal dressing. No attempt is made at this phase to restore esthetics because of danger of further injury from manipulation of the teeth. Esthetics are addressed after periodontal healing.

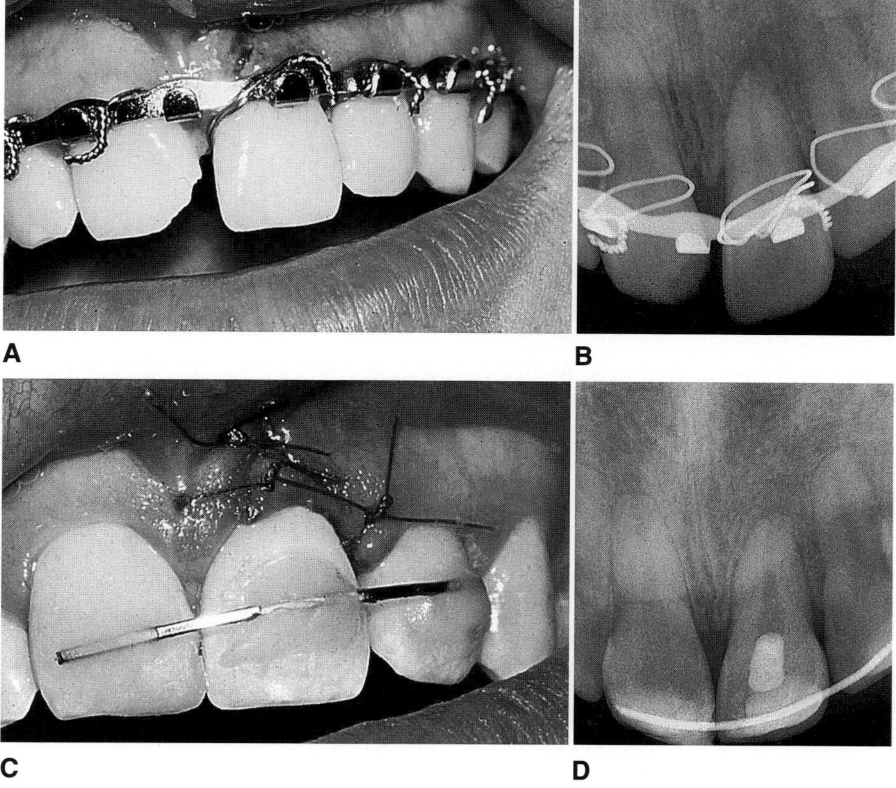

FIGURE 14-15. An improperly treated avulsed central incisor. **A,** The maxillary left central incisor was avulsed and replanted, and an arch bar splint was placed. The replanted tooth has extruded either because of the force of the ligature wire on the root or because the tooth was not properly repositioned. The arch bar and wires are a gingival irritant. Note that the maxillary left central incisor has a crown fracture and that no sutures were placed in the torn gingival tissues. **B,** Corresponding radiograph showing the improper position of the replanted incisor. Note the degree of displacement of the tooth from its socket. **C,** The maxillary left central incisor following proper reposition and resplinting several hours following the mistreatment. The fractured left incisor has been restored with a Dycal base and composite restoration. The gingival tissues have been sutured. **D,** Corresponding radiograph showing the tooth back in its socket.

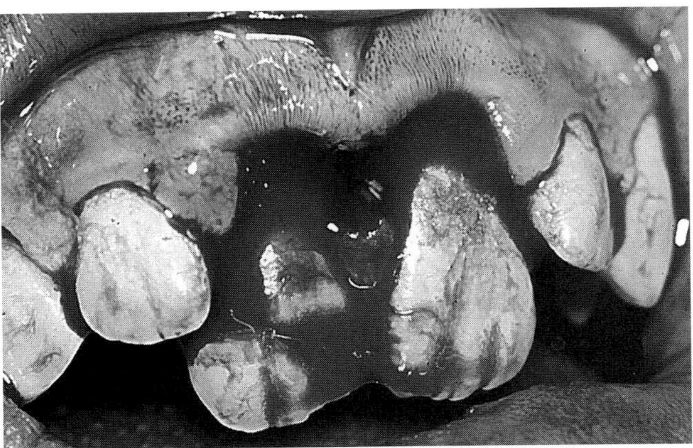

FIGURE 14-16. Extrusion of the maxillary left central incisor. The tooth has partially left its alveolus and there is bleeding from the gingival sulcus. (From Kruger E, Schilli W: Oral and Maxillofacial Traumatology. Chicago, Quintessence, 1982.)

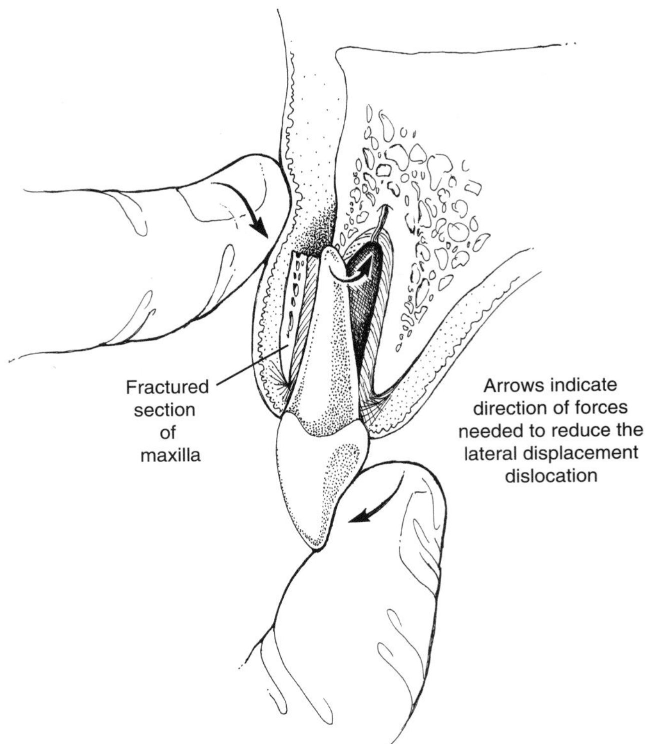
Fractured section of maxilla
Arrows indicate direction of forces needed to reduce the lateral displacement dislocation

FIGURE 14-17. Repositioning a lateral displacement. (Illustration by Lydia Kibiuk. Adapted from Andreasen J, Andreasen F: Textbook and Color Atlas of Traumatic Injuries to the Teeth, 3rd ed. St Louis, Mosby–Year Book, 1994.)

to move it into correct position after healing using orthodontics. Avoid wrapping the tooth in tissue paper or gauze, which will encourage desiccation. Debris can be flushed with a transport media (i.e., Hank's Balanced Salt Solution), normal saline, or cold water according to availability in an emergency. Cotton pliers or a wet sponge can be used to gently remove persistent debris. Immediate systemic antibiotic therapy helps prevent infection of the pulp and PDL to promote healing. Precautions against *Clostridia tetani* as outlined in the section on lacerations should be considered within 48 hours.

In situations where replantation is delayed more than 20 minutes, the type of storage media and the method of

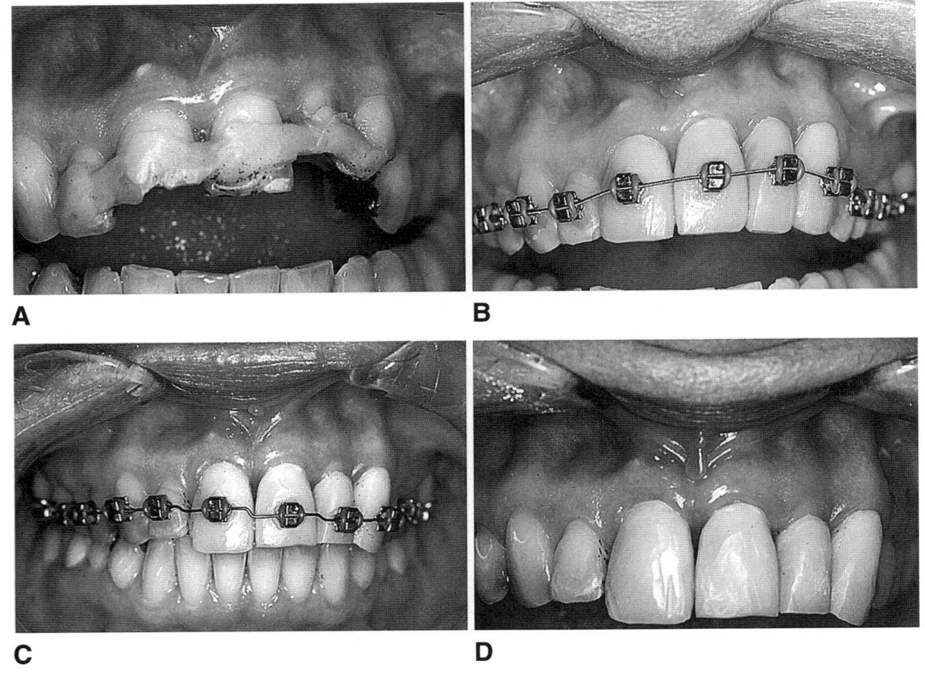
A
B
C
D

FIGURE 14-18. Intrusive displacement of maxillary anteriors. **A,** Four maxillary teeth (#8 to #11) that have been traumatically intruded and splinted in a hospital emergency room. **B,** Later provisional restorations were placed and an orthodontic appliance activated to erupt the teeth back towards normal position. **C,** Post-eruption. Note favorable alteration to free gingival margin architecture. **D,** Removal of orthodontic appliance. Provisional restorations will be removed and permanent restorations will be fabricated. (Courtesy of Frank Celenza Jr., DDS, New York, NY.)

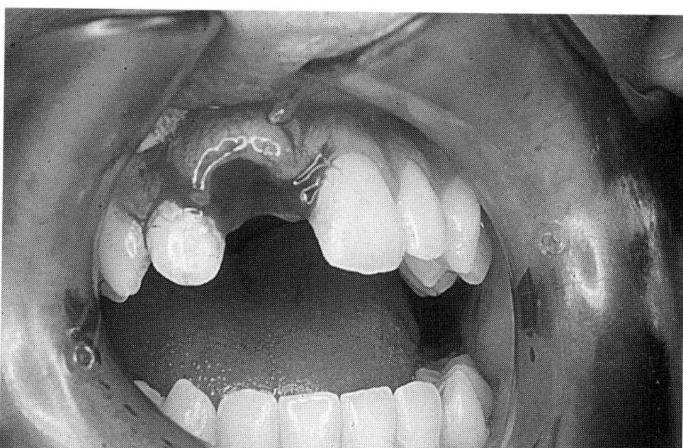

FIGURE 14-19. Avulsed maxillary right central incisor. (Courtesy of Ray R. Padilla, DDS, West Covina, CA.)

handling become important issues. A tooth allowed to air dry will lead to PDL necrosis with replacement resorption (ankylosis) or inflammatory resorption (external root resorption). In ankylosis, the body attempts to repair the resorption by laying down new alveolar bone in direct apposition to the tooth. The PDL space is obliterated and becomes absent radiographically.[12] This clinically immobilizes the tooth and leads to loss of PDL proprioception. External (inflammatory) root resorption is the body's attempt to eliminate infected calcified tissue, bacteria, and their toxic lytic by-products. It is characterized histologically by granulation tissue in the PDL adjacent to large areas of root resorption. External root resorption can be prevented by pulpectomy before a bacterial infection is established.[2,3,8] Infection prevention is also a good reason to initiate immediate antibiotic therapy after replantation.[49]

Revascularization is a possibility in replanted immature teeth with open apices. Conversely, untreated avulsed teeth with mature roots always develop pulpal necrosis and external root resorption.[11] For this reason, RCT using $Ca(OH)_2$ to fill should routinely be done to replanted teeth with complete root development 1 to 2 weeks after replantation as a preventive measure. This time period corresponds with the time when the splint needs to be removed. Pulpectomy and RCT are not initiated in immature teeth unless signs of pulpal necrosis are observed. Mineral Trioxide Aggregate (MTA) has been proposed as a potential material to create an apical plug at the end of the root canal system to allow apexification.[41] These teeth must be monitored closely for signs of degeneration. Replanted immature teeth that lose their vitality have a poor prognosis.

For avulsed teeth, Hank's Balanced Salt Solution is an older media that has been used to maintain mammalian cells in tissue culture. Viaspan, a newer media, has been used for organ-transplant storage. Sterile solutions of Hank's Balanced Salt Solution or Viaspan, which have compatible physiologic osmolalities, qualify as superior storage media.[64,107] A packaged commercial transport media called EMT Toothsaver (SmartPractice, Phoenix, AZ) should be available in any training room, emergency field kit, gym, or sports complex[37] (Fig. 14-20). EMT Toothsaver has been marketed in Europe for a number of years under the label Dentosafe and has a shelf-life of up to two years from the date of manufacture. Each bottle has a color-coded sterility monitor. The efficacy of EMT Toothsaver is supported by studies.[88,89] Milk,[17] saliva for intraoral or extraoral transport, normal saline,[6] and polyethylene wrap[2] have been used with some success. Cold milk is a better storage medium than saliva because it has fewer bacteria and a more compatible physiologic osmolality.[17,57,74]

Replanted teeth undergo gradual ankylosis but are capable of functioning for many years. An excellent update on the clinical management of avulsed teeth has been provided by M. Trope in *Dental Traumatology*.[106] *Dental Traumatology* is the combined official publication of the International Association for Dental Traumatology and the International Academy for Sports Dentistry.[94]

SUPPORTING BONE

Comminution of the Alveolar Socket

This is a shattering into a number of small fragments and crushing of the alveolus resulting from compressive trauma, such as that found with intrusions and lateral displacements.

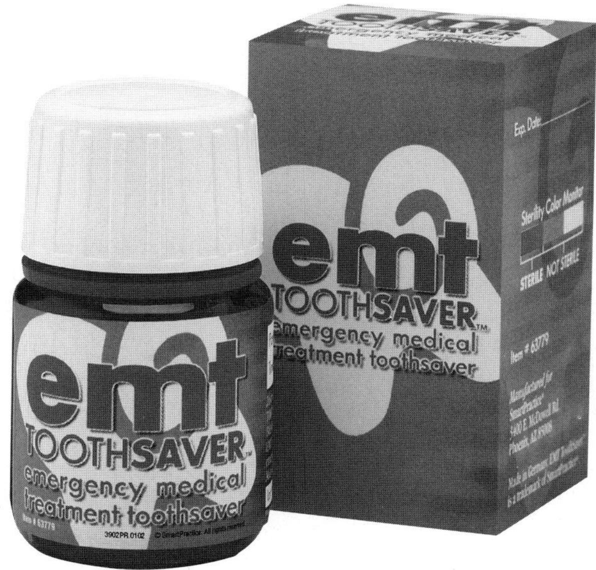

FIGURE 14-20. EMT Toothsaver tooth preserving system. (Courtesy of SmartPractice, Phoenix, AZ.)

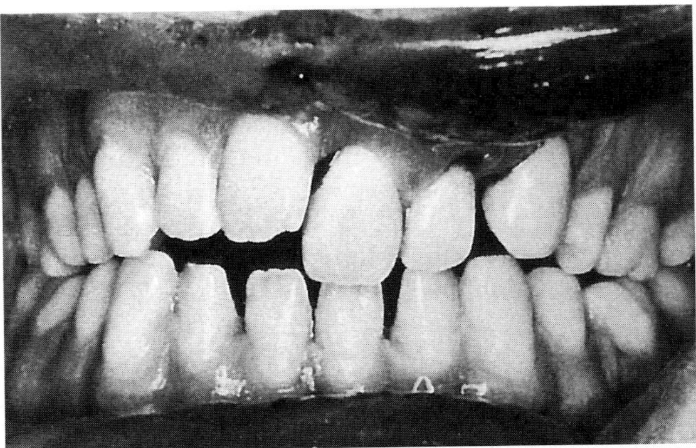

FIGURE 14-21. Fracture of the alveolar process involving the maxillary left central and lateral incisors. (From Kruger E, Schilli W: Oral and Maxillofacial Traumatology. Chicago, Quintessence, 1982.)

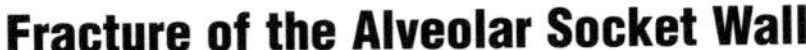

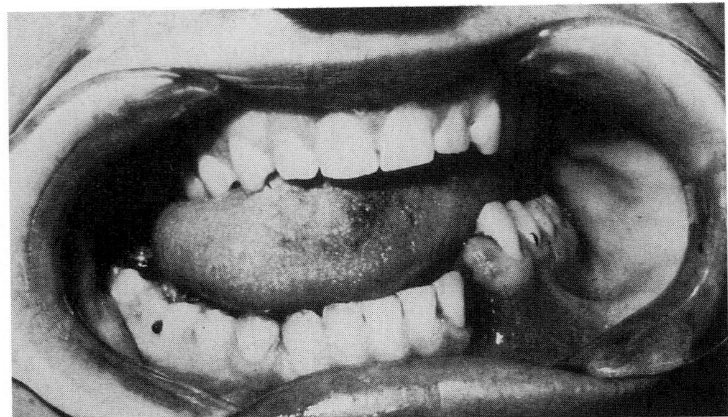

FIGURE 14-22. Mandibular fracture that is displaced and unstable following facial trauma. Note the change in the occlusion. (From Ranalli DN: Dent Clin North Am 35(4):711, 1991.)

Fracture of the Alveolar Socket Wall

This is a fracture limited to the facial or lingual (palatal) wall of the alveolar socket. These fractures are most often associated with lateral displacements.

Fracture of the Alveolar Process

When two or more neighboring teeth are able to be moved jointly as a block, a clinical diagnosis of fracture of the alveolar bone can be made (Fig. 14-21). This injury is common in ice hockey where sticks, frozen pucks, and fists abound. A fracture of the alveolar process may involve the alveolar socket.

Fracture of the Jaw

The patient should be examined clinically and appropriate radiographs ordered.[54] If a patient complains of having difficulty putting his or her teeth together, a fracture of the jaw should be ruled out. Conversely, some fractures do not exhibit occlusal disharmony.

Fracture of the Mandible. Airway management is the most important aspect of emergent treatment with mandibular fractures. Fast-traveling frozen hockey pucks routinely deliver sufficient force to fracture a mandible (Fig. 14-22).

A mandible may be evaluated for fracture by having the patient open his or her mouth gently. Slight bilateral pressure is applied at the angles of the mandible. If there is a fracture, the patient will usually point to the area of discomfort.[54] As with a fracture of the alveolar process, a fracture of the mandible may or may not involve the alveolar socket.

It is believed that athletes may be predisposed to certain kinds of injuries based on existing anatomic conditions. For instance, impacted wisdom teeth may predispose the athlete to fracture of the mandible at the angle.[113] Systemic or dental conditions yielding localized weakness, such as mandibular cysts or semierupted mandibular wisdom teeth with accompanying pericoronitis, can also be contributory. Periodontal bony defects may also be related to the location of a fracture line.[65]

According to Haug and Greenberg,[44] mandibular fractures are the most frequently, completely, and consistently investigated facial fractures. The rank order of occurrence by anatomic location in the general population may be deduced from the total of studies cited and extrapolated to sports injuries (Table 14-1 and Fig. 14-23).

Fracture of the Maxilla. This is an uncommon sports injury. To evaluate a fracture of the maxilla, hold the bridge of the nose with one hand while the other hand grasps the anterior maxilla and palate. If there is mobility of the maxilla without movement of the bridge of the nose, a horizontal fracture of the maxilla or a LeFort I injury is suspected. If mobility is felt at the bridge of the nose, a LeFort II or LeFort III fracture is possible.[54] Panoramic and Waters' view radiographs are useful in evaluating LeFort fractures. Fractures of the maxillary

TABLE 14-1 Occurrence of Mandibular Fractures

Rank Order of Occurrence	Anatomic Location of Fracture
1	Corpus (body)
2	Angle
3	Condylar process
4	Symphysis
5	Ramus
6	Coronoid process

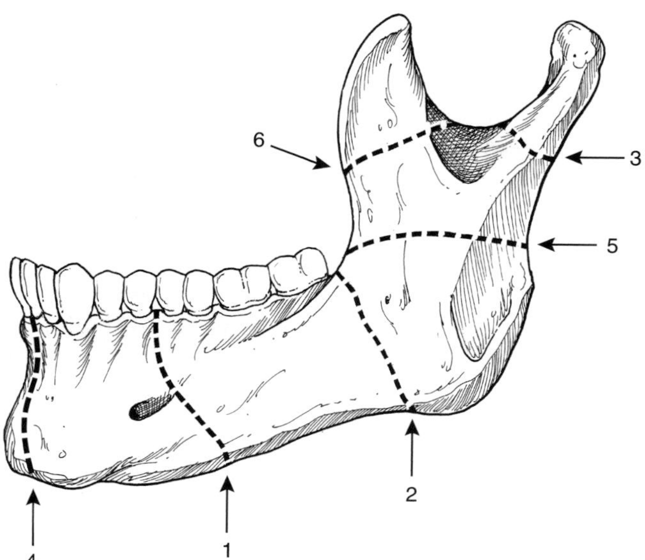

FIGURE 14-23. Fractures of the mandible by rank order of occurrence. (Illustration by Lydia Kibiuk. Adapted from Spiessl B: Internal Fixation of the Mandible.New York, Springer-Verlag, 1989. Reproduced with permission.)

sinus walls are best seen on Waters', Caldwell, or lateral plate views of the face.[86]

GINGIVAL AND ORAL MUCOSA

Lacerations

A laceration is a tearing wound usually produced by a sharp object. These wounds must be explored for foreign matter and debrided before suturing (Fig. 14-24). Radiographic examination of a laceration will help locate radioopaque foreign objects such as tooth fragments and orthodontic brackets. Careful inspection and cleansing of the wound are required to rule out contamination with nonradioopaque materials such as plastic and wood. The need for antibiotic coverage and precautions against tetanus should be considered. Penicillin, amoxicillin, or erythromycin seem to have the appropriate spectra and work well on nonallergic individuals for intraoral infections.

Irregular Lacerations. Irregular lacerations can occur anywhere intraorally, including the gingiva, oral mucosa, lips, tongue, palate, and pharynx. A through-and-through laceration of the lip with blunt trauma (e.g., a punch) is probably the most common maxillofacial injury and should be routinely examined for tooth fragments. Approximation of the vermillion border is crucial when suturing.[54]

The tongue is very vascular and its location strategic. Direct pressure may be necessary to control profuse bleeding and keep the airway patent. Injuries to the tongue can cause post-traumatic swelling leading to dysphagia, dysmasesis, drooling, dysgeusia, and dysphonia.

Regular Lacerations. Incisions and punctures are special kinds of lacerations containing geometric symmetry. Incisions are prevalent in hockey in which ice skate blades can cut lips and tongues (Fig. 14-25). These types of wounds may bleed profusely and can be a challenge to suture and achieve good approximation of the borders of the tissue.

Punctures are potentially dangerous. Commonly, baseball cleats have been known to cause puncture wounds when a player attempts to steal a base by sliding. *C. tetani* is an anaerobic spore-forming gram positive bacillus found in soil and feces. It causes the infectious disease tetanus characterized by intermittent tonic spasms of voluntary muscles. Trismus of the masseter muscles accounts for the name *lockjaw*. Its pathogenicity stems from the effects of its neurotoxin, *tetanospasmin*, produced by the introduction and germination of spores in host tissue. Toxin is released upon cell lysis. In clean wounds in which the blood supply is good and O_2 tension is high, germination of the spores rarely occurs. This emphasizes the importance of prompt, thorough debridement. Generally, whenever a previously immunized patient sustains a wound, a booster of toxoid should be injected to produce protective antibodies within a couple of weeks. Patients who have not been immunized previously should receive human tetanus immune globulin (250 U) because the antibody response to an initial dose is too slow to be useful. Full-blown tetanus has a mortality rate of 50%, and should be managed by an infectious disease physician.

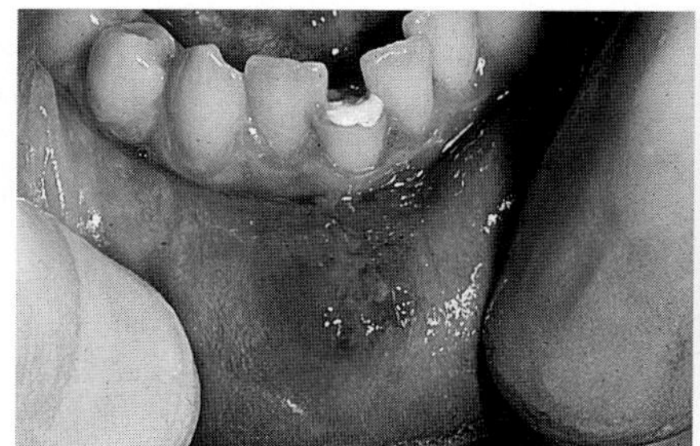
A

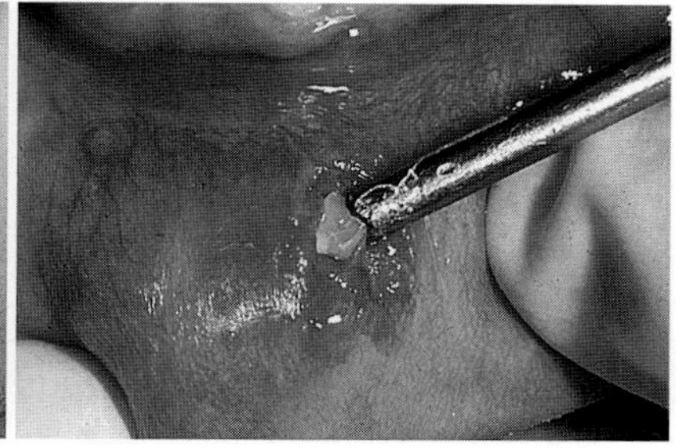
B

FIGURE 14-24. Foreign object in the lip. **A,** The patient was seen in the emergency room after an injury. The lip was sutured and a dressing placed on the fractured mandibular incisor. The sutures were removed the following day because of patient complaints. **B,** A fractured tooth segment was found in the lower lip. (Courtesy of Dr. Dan Kolzet, Durham, NC.)

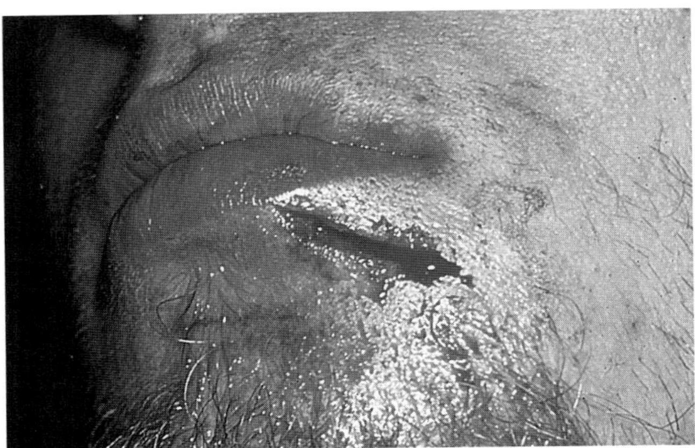

FIGURE 14-25. Incision laceration inferior to vermillion border of left lower lip caused by an accident involving a skate blade during an ice hockey game. (Courtesy of Ray R. Padilla, DDS, West Covina, CA.)

Contusions

A contusion is a bruise usually produced by blunt trauma that causes subgingival or submucosal hemorrhage with accompanying swelling, pain, and discoloration (i.e., hematoma). The majority of hematomas will resorb with no treatment. On rare occasions, a hematoma may become encapsulated. Proteolytic enzymes like papain given systemically are ineffective.[99] As liquefaction proceeds, aspiration with a large-bore needle (at least 18-gauge) is helpful.

Abrasions

An abrasion is an excoriation of the superficial epithelial layer of gingiva or mucosa resulting from shearing trauma such as rubbing or scraping. This friction wound generally leaves a raw, bleeding surface, sometimes with foreign bodies encapsulated. Management usually consists of appropriate antibiotic coverage and removal of foreign bodies.

MOUTH PROTECTOR CONSIDERATIONS

Objectives

Protection from hard- and soft-tissue injuries, jaw fractures, and temporomandibular joint (TMJ) and miniscular injuries are obvious goals of mouth protection. More than half of all facial sports injuries involve either fractures of the alveolar process or luxation of teeth.[75] What are some of the other objectives that the ideal mouth protector needs to offer?

Retention, protection, and durability have been used as yardsticks to measure the efficacy of mouthguards. As an indication of the protection mouthguards provide, hardness, penetration, rebound, and dynamic resilience have been studied.[26,42] Mouthguards are exposed to high compressive stresses when in use. As an indication of durability, the tensile strength, tear strength, elongation, and moduli of elasticity have also been measured.[26,42] Generally, thickness of material correlates with impact energy absorption.[83] One study concluded the optimal thickness for EVA mouthguard material with a Shore A hardness of 80 is around 4 mm. Increased thickness may slightly improve performance but significantly reduce wearer comfort and acceptance.[111]

Epidemiologic evidence exists suggesting that wearing a mouthguard will prevent dental and oral injuries.[52,72] This applies to contact and noncontact sports.[51] In 1973, the National Collegiate Athletic Association (NCAA) football rules committee adopted the mouth-protector rule. The following year, professional football followed suit by embracing a similar requirement.[19] In 1990, the NCAA mandated the use of brightly colored mouthguards to promote their use and facilitate the ability of officials to observe player compliance. More than half of officials surveyed believed this rule had resulted in more frequent use by athletes and a decrease in dental injuries.[92,93] To this day, compliance and utilization of mouthguards remains a significant problem despite advances in fabrication.[33,71] It is important to note that coaches generally have the most direct control over participants in their respective sports. They can be the targets of lawsuits when injuries occur. The basis for liability is generally negligence.[68] Athletes should be advised that custom-made mouthguards offer the greatest comfort, fit, durability, and protection against dental injuries.[15] Other than fluoridation, mouthguards rank as one of the most important contributions that dentistry has made to preventive medicine.

Unlike football, ice hockey, and boxing, which are collision sports, basketball is considered a light contact sport. Jumping, dunking, and flying elbows asserting possession after a rebound are characteristic. Basketball, lacrosse, and wrestling are sports with a very high incidence of dental injuries.[72] The substantial rate of orofacial injuries among high school athletes participating in basketball and wrestling needs to be minimized.[69] This can be inferred from the nature of these sports and because most players are inattentive to mouthguard use. One can speculate that this occurs because there are no regulations requiring the use of mouthguards.[24,72] Mandatory mouth protection education in these sports may be useful.[77]

A mouthguard needs to be comfortable for an athlete and minimize sore spots and gagging. It should have almost no effect on breathing.[56] The more oxygen an athlete is able to deliver to muscle tissue, the less lactic acid build-up and the less fatigue. The mouthguard should interfere little with speech and be time- and cost-effective to fabricate. The device needs to be able to negotiate orthodontic brackets, missing or erupting teeth, and tori. When not in use, a mouthguard should be

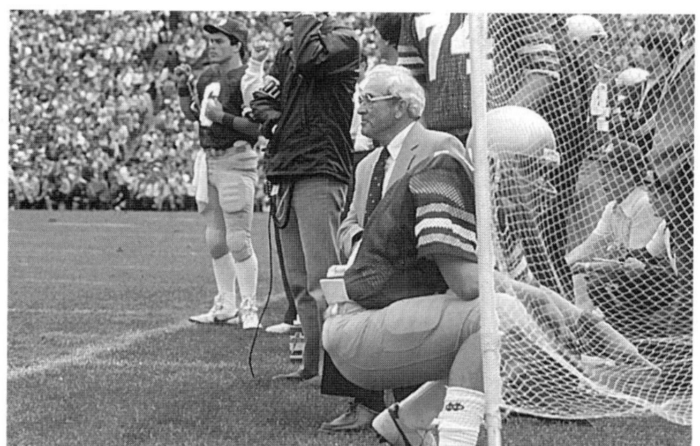

FIGURE 14-26. Dr. John Stenger kneels at the sidelines watching his Notre Dame boys, mouthguards inserted, power their way to victory. (Courtesy of John Stenger, DDS, South Bend, IN.)

soaked in mouthwash to keep it odor-free and tasting fresh. It should be rinsed in cold water before and after each insertion.

Cervical Injuries

Dr. John Stenger's classic 5-year clinical study on Notre Dame football players began in 1958 and was published in 1964 (Fig. 14-26).[104] Dr. Stenger, the initiator of the concept of physiologic dentistry, based much of his work on that of James B. Costen, MD, a Washington University otolaryngologist.[29] By means of before and after cephalometric radiographic tracings, Stenger demonstrated differences in the position of the mandibular condyle, the hyoid bone, and the cervical vertebrae (C2–C4) when the teeth were in centric occlusion versus when the bite was opened by a custom-made mouthguard to the vertical dimension of the freeway space (Fig. 14-27).

In the spring of 1963, with the encouragement of then trainer Gene Paszkiet, a decision was made to equip the entire Notre Dame football team with a new model ethylene vinyl acetate (EVA) mouthguard. As expected, the number of injuries to the teeth and jaws declined. There was also an impressive reduction in cerebral concussions. A serendipitous correlation between wearing the mouthguards and a decrease in neck injuries was an important finding.[103,104] "A reduction in the number of neck injuries was an unexpected result of wearing the mouthguards. Neck injuries had increased since the use of the face bar had become mandatory. During the 1962 season at Notre Dame, six or seven players had chronic neck problems, and four of them wore cervical collars. Cervical traction was routine therapy for these players. An automatic traction device was ordered by the athletic department and delivered during the summer to replace the manual one in use. Fortunately, because of the mouthguards worn by the players prone to neck injuries, the new machine, ordered in anticipation of more injuries, has never been unpacked. Furthermore, not a single Notre Dame player who faithfully wore his mouthguard during the 1963 season found it necessary to wear a cervical collar."[104]

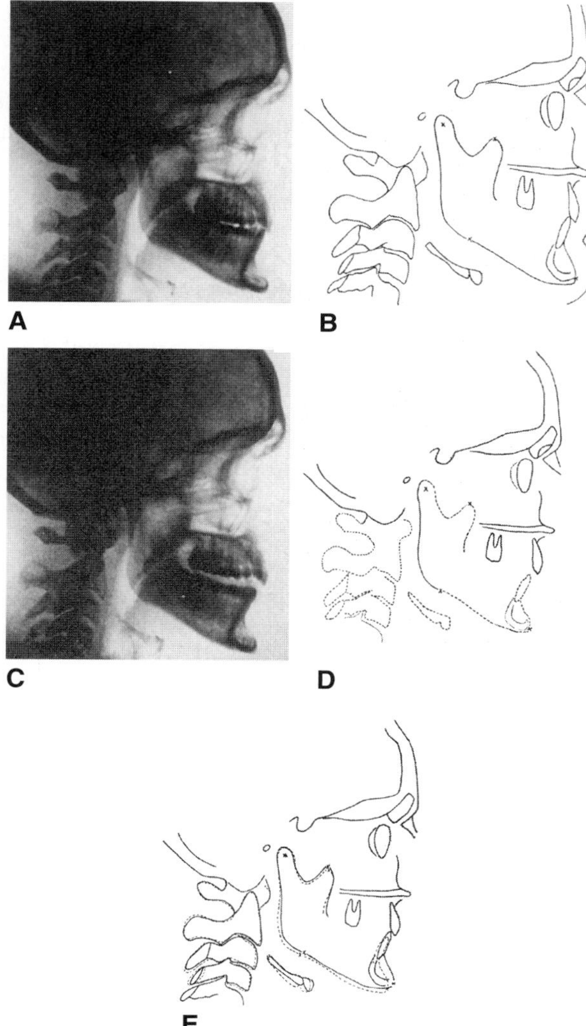

FIGURE 14-27. Changes in position of the mandible, hyoid bone, and cervical vertebrae. **A,** Cephalometric radiograph with teeth in occlusion. **B,** Solid line tracing of A. **C,** Cephalometric radiograph showing mouthguard inserted. This film was taken 30 seconds after the first film while the patient's position remained unchanged in the headholder. **D,** Dashed line tracing of C. **E,** Composite tracing of B (solid line) and D (dashed line). (From Stenger JM, et al: Mouthguards: Protection against shock to head, neck and teeth. JADA 69:273–281, 1964.)

Cerebral Concussions

In a 1967 study, Hickey et al.[53] of the University of Kentucky used a cadaver to measure changes in intracranial pressure and bone deformation. The mandible was struck from below by a device designed to deliver a uniform repeatable force. Changes in intracranial pressure were measured by tubing inserted through a hole drilled in the cranium and secured by acrylic resin. Changes in intracranial pressure were ascertained first without a mouth protector inserted, second with a natural rubber mouthguard in place, and lastly using a vacuum-formed mouth protector (Fig. 14-28). The results clearly demonstrated that mouthguards reduce intracranial shock wave propagation. Further, intracranial pressure differences between natural rubber and vacuum-formed vinyl mouth protectors were not significant.[53] Caution should be exercised concerning proprietary claims of mouthguard superiority regarding degree of shock absorbency. Winters and Leahy examined the possible correlation between the frequency of cerebral concussion and the type of mouthguard used by football players in 17 NCAA Division III teams. They concluded that incomplete or poorly maintained mouthguards may increase the risk for mild concussion during common, head-to-head impact.[13] In another study of 50 men's Division I college basketball programs, an Internet Web site was used to submit weekly reports of the number of athlete exposures, mouthguard users, concussions, oral soft tissue injuries, dental injuries, and dentist referrals. This basketball study accounted for 70,936 athlete exposures. The study concluded that custom-fitted mouthguards did not significantly affect the rates of concussions or oral soft tissue injuries, but did significantly reduce the morbidity and expense resulting from dental injuries in men's Division I college basketball.[70] It should be pointed out that basketball is considered a contact and not a collision sport like boxing, football, and ice hockey. In ice hockey, full face shields reduce the risk of facial and dental injuries without increasing the risk of neck injuries, concussions, or other injuries.[16]

Performance Enhancement

In 1977, a controversial article by Dr. Stenger[103] triggered an avalanche of clinical and experimental studies. He proposed that a lack of posterior bite support and malocclusion were factors that limited athletic performance. The first published study to test this hypothesis appeared in 1978.[101] Its author, Stephen D. Smith, DMD, Director of the TMJ Clinic at the Philadelphia College of Osteopathic Medicine, obtained permission from head coach Dick Vermeil to study 25 Philadelphia Eagles football players.

Using wax bites to reposition the mandible, Smith used a kinesiologic muscle challenge known as the isometric deltoid press to determine the ideal three-dimensional occlusal position at which to construct a Mandibular Orthopedic Repositioning Appliance (MORA), which would mimic mouthguard design. A MORA similarly repositions the mandible anteriorly, increases the vertical dimension, and changes the head posture relationship.[38] Smith believed he demonstrated a positive correlation between the posture of the jaw and the ability of the arm musculature to give strong contraction. His critics denounced his applied kinesiologic methods, calling them unscientific, and dubbed his results statistically insignificant.

Since Smith's initial report, there have been numerous studies that have produced apparently conflicting results. An excellent review and critique of the salient studies has been presented by Forgione et al.[35] They charged

> "one commentator,[58] a reviewer,[27] and three authors of original studies[45,98,114] with having made emphatic general statements critical of the original results and later studies supporting Stenger's proposed relationship despite the following: (1) Most of these experiments used subjects with no apparent malocclusions or lack of posterior support[14,21,50,80,84,109,114] and others, mixed occlusions.[22,98,100,101,112] (2) Most researchers[1,14,21,22,45,50,78,80,84,98,108,109,112] set bite appliances by techniques other

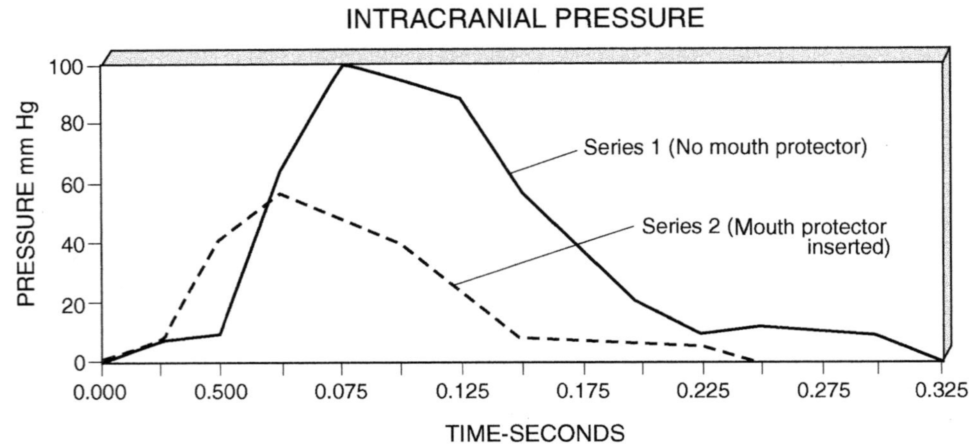

FIGURE 14-28. Intracranial pressure changes. Series 1, without mouth protector; Series 2, with mouth protector inserted. Notice the significant decrease in both shock wave amplitude and period. (Adapted from Hickey JC, et al: The relation of mouth protectors to cranial pressure and deformation. JADA 74(4): 735–740, 1967.)

than kinesiologic guidance, a functional technique, assuming or implying that all MORAs are equivalent. (3) Researchers used data showing no increase in isokinetic tests of strength to criticize studies of isometric strength[1,21,22,45,50,84,98,108] while commenting on strength unqualifiedly. (4) Some researchers used either questionable statistics, experimental design or both.[21,22,50,98] (5) Some authors[22,27,45,98] and a commentator[58] have invoked placebo as a criticism of evidence that supports Stenger's proposal even though the placebo effect has not been demonstrated in any of the studies that have employed a placebo control condition. The belief that the placebo effect is omnipresent has even fostered an explanation for its lack of appearance."[78]

For the most part, criticism of performance enhancement has been aimed at study designs, controls, period (long-term vs. short-term), double blindness, and the placebo effect.[63]

There is almost universal agreement that designing one indisputable study is not an easy task. It would be very difficult to satisfy all investigators, scientists, and clinicians. At one point, Joseph J. Marbach, DDS, former director of the world's first TMJ Clinic[67] at Columbia University's School of Dental and Oral Surgery stated, "There is no way that true double-blind studies can be done to measure any changes that occur as a result of repositioning because the researcher will know if he is testing a functional occlusal splint and the patient will know that the splint is in and something is supposed to change as a result."[79]

So, if you cannot prove something scientifically, how do you know it works? It is the opinion of this author that the kinesiologically adjusted mouthguards made by selected clinicians do work. Brainchild of Dr. Richard Kaufman of Oceanside, New York,[61] the Mouthpiece of Champions is a kinesiologically adjusted mouthguard that has gained tremendous patient acceptance. At this point, they are prized and sought after repeatedly by many prominent professional athletes who have had long experience with a variety of other mouthguards.

Mouth Protector Construction

External Mouth Protectors. Youth ice hockey is the rage in Canada. An external mouthguard has been designed into the helmet strap. It is reminiscent of a miniature baseball catcher's mask for the oral cavity (Fig. 14-29). Dr. Arthur Wood of Toronto received the Canada Medal for promoting its use as a cost-effective way to decrease dental injuries among Canadian youth.[25]

Internal Mouth Protectors. The maxillary central incisors are the most frequently traumatized teeth, and consequently, a mouthguard is usually constructed for the maxillary arch. However, in cases of mandibular prognathism, it may be desirable to reverse this or construct a bimaxillary appliance.

Stock mouthguards are inexpensive, can be purchased over-the-counter, and are ready for immediate use. They are often ill-fitting and may interfere with breathing and speech because they must be held in position by keeping the teeth together. However, they are occasionally convenient to have available in case of loss or damage to an athlete's custom mouthguard during an event.

Mouth-formed mouthguards are a compromise between stock and custom-made. They are adapted by the direct method intraorally. The most popular is commonly referred to as "boil and bite." Often it is made of a thermoplastic material, usually EVA copolymer. It is softened by boiling water and adapted intraorally while warm by literally biting into the material. Another variety comes with a shell, usually of ethylene vinyl chloride. It is lined with soft, chemically setting ethyl methacrylate. It is the opinion of this author that

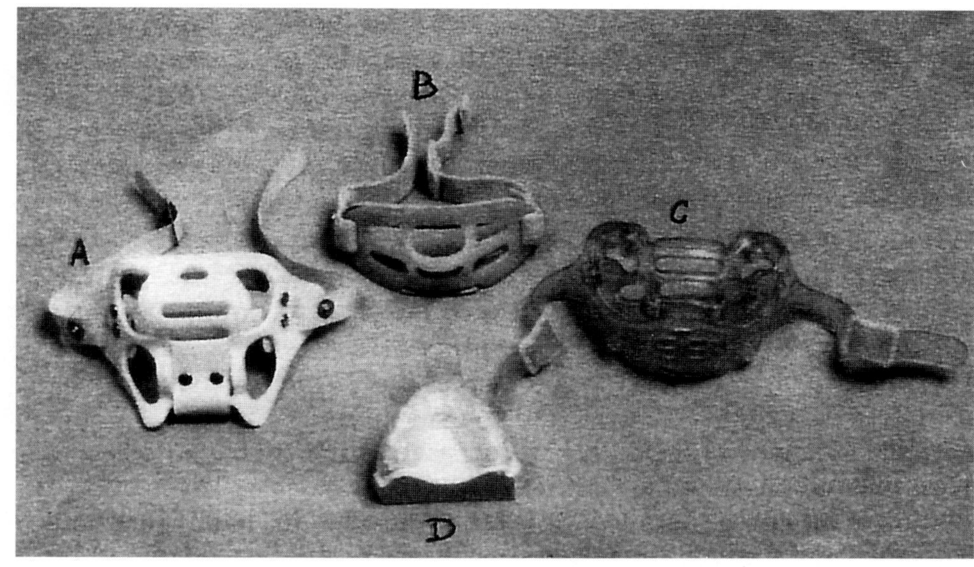

FIGURE 14-29. Types of mouthguards: *A, B,* and *C,* are external mouthguards widely used from 1970 to 1980 in Sweden *(A)*, Canada *(B)*, and the United States *(C)*. *D,* Custom-made mouthguard formed on a model of the player's maxillary teeth. (From Castaldi C, et al: The Sports Mouthguard: Its Use and Misuse in Ice Hockey. In Safety in Ice Hockey, ASTM STP 1050. Philadelphia, 1989.)

the public should be informed that stock and mouth-formed mouthguards, including the "boil and bite" kind, bought at sporting good stores do not provide the optimal level of care and protection. Ill-fitting mouthguards may leave players at risk unexpectedly. Serious athletes merit the superior comfort, fit, and performance of properly-fitted custom-made mouthguards. However, the best mouthguard is the one that is worn at the time trauma is encountered.

Custom-made mouthguards are fabricated indirectly on a stone model of the athlete's dentition.[48] This is made from a dental impression, usually alginate. Custom mouthguards are the most expensive but are superior in virtually every aspect. Smart athletes make a point to have spares in case of loss or damage.

The majority of custom mouthguards are vacuum custom-made. They are fashioned by first heating a 3 to 5 mm thick sheet of EVA held in a frame on a vacuum-forming machine until it exhibits a specific amount of droop or sag (Fig. 14-30). The sheet is then vacuum-formed over a stone model or cast that has been prepared from the dental impression and sprayed with separating medium, usually silicone. For best results, the model or cast is poured in die stone and trimmed to just greater than the size and shape of the anticipated design of the final mouthguard. Die stone is preferable because the model is less likely to fracture during forming and when the mouthguard material is separated from the model. If the palate is eliminated in advance from the model, greater suction and closer adaptation will be achievable. The use of dry models that have been soaped rather than wet models will yield closer adaptation.[115] This is because EVA material is hydrophobic (Fig. 14-31). If a strap is needed to attach the mouthguard to a football or ice hockey facemask this is best accomplished before cooling. The EVA can be reheated with a torch and/or flameless heat gun to spot weld an EVA strap. Otherwise, it is best to allow the material to cool to room temperature undistrubed on the model for at least 20 minutes before separation. This reduces separation deformation.

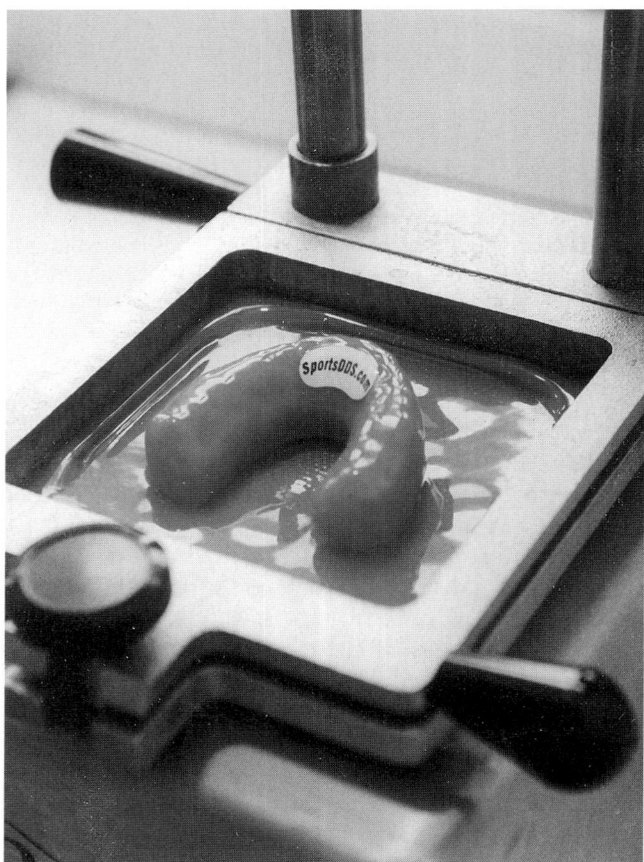

FIGURE 14-31. Frame holding EVA material has been lowered and vacuumed over model on vacuum platform. (Courtesy of SportsDDS.com, Hollis Park Gardens, NY.)

After the mouthguard is separated from the model it is trimmed and polished (Fig. 14-32). This can be facilitated

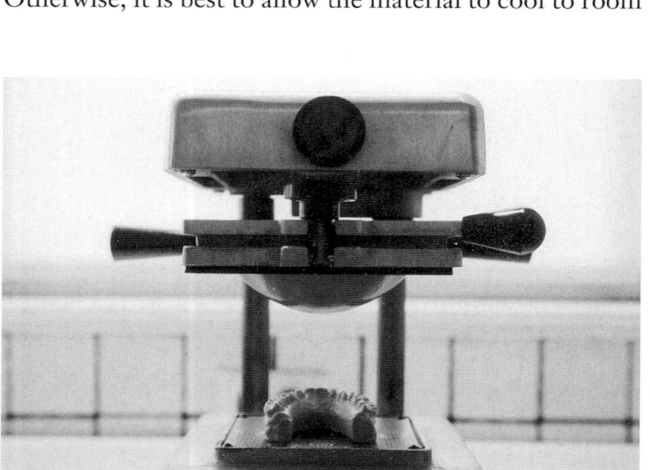

FIGURE 14-30. Ethylene vinyl acetate heated and beginning to droop while model sits ready on vacuum platform. (Courtesy of SportsDDS.com, Hollis Park Gardens, NY.)

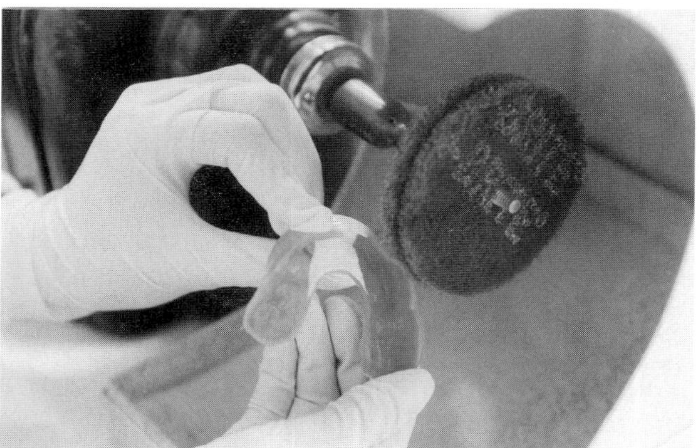

FIGURE 14-32. Mouthguard being trimmed and polished after separation from model. (Courtesy of SportsDDS.com, Hollis Park Gardens, NY.)

by chilling the mouthguard in icewater and using a Scotch-Brite nylon wheel available through E.C. Moore Company Inc. of Dearborn, Michigan. Also, if desired, an identification label can be placed anywhere. To accomplish this, the location for the label is selected, the mouthguard chilled, and channeled with a heatless stone. The label is placed inside the trough, and just enough clear EVA copolymer is added to cover the label. Applying heat will melt and seal the EVA. Finger pressure using a moistened cloth can be applied to smooth the area over the label. Gentle flaming can be used to establish a glossy finish. Gentle heating of the occlusal surface of the mouthguard immediately followed by having the athlete bite down with it in place will equilibrate the occlusal contact. This will yield a superior, balanced occlusion.[76]

Heated EVA can be formed in other ways. One method uses positive pressure rather than a vacuum to adapt the same EVA sheet material. Positive pressure yields a much more accurately adapted mouthguard than the vacuum fabricated custom method. This is because it operates off a dental compressor at about 90 psi which is several atmospheres of pressure. Second, heat laminating thinner 2 mm sheets of EVA rather than thicker 3 to 5 mm sheets yields improved adaptation and conformity to the model. Pressure laminating has an added bonus in that placement of decals and identification labels is simplified. A wonderful outline of the pressure-laminating technique is covered in the *Journal of the California Dental Association*.[82] Three of the major manufacturers of the pressure-laminating equipment are located in Germany. Great Lakes Orthodontics of Tonawanda, New York, imports the Biostar and Ministar from Scheu Dental (Fig. 14-33A and B). The Drufomat from Dreve Dental (Fig. 14-33C) and the Erkopress from Erich Kopp GmgH (Fig. 14-33D) are each reliable machines. All of these machines are capable of producing admirably adaptated custom mouthguards using the pressure-laminating technique.

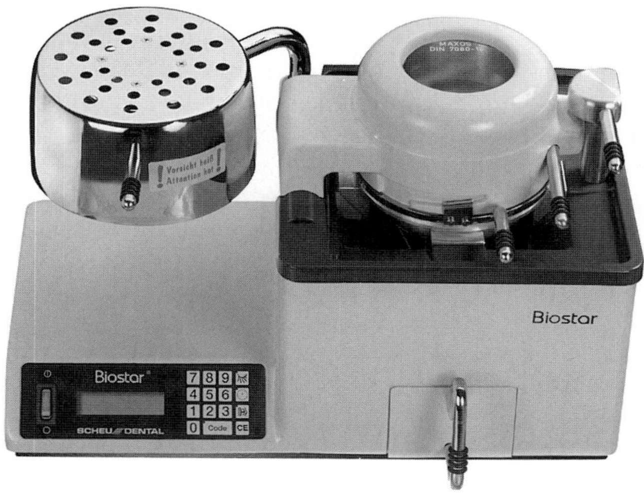

FIGURE 14-33A. Biostar positive pressure machine. The Biostar is capable of fabricating many orthodontic appliances. (Courtesy of Great Lakes Orthodontics, Tonawanda, NY.)

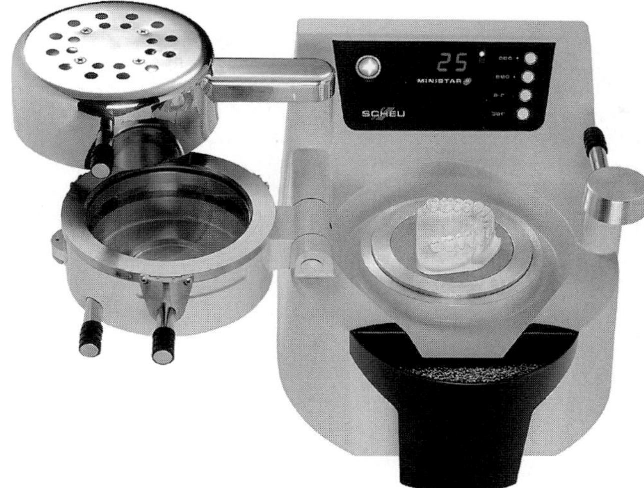

FIGURE 14-33B. Ministar positive pressure machine. (Courtesy of Great Lakes Orthodontics, Tonawanda, NY.)

A hybrid of the vacuum custom-made and pressure-laminating techniques is available from Dental Resources Inc. in Delano, Minnesota. A pressure dome assembly fits over the vacuum table of their Proform vacuum machines (Fig. 14-33E). It operates off the dental compressor. The Erkoform-RVE is a digitally controlled, self-contained thermoforming system that does not require compressed air. The RVE contains its own vacuum pump and

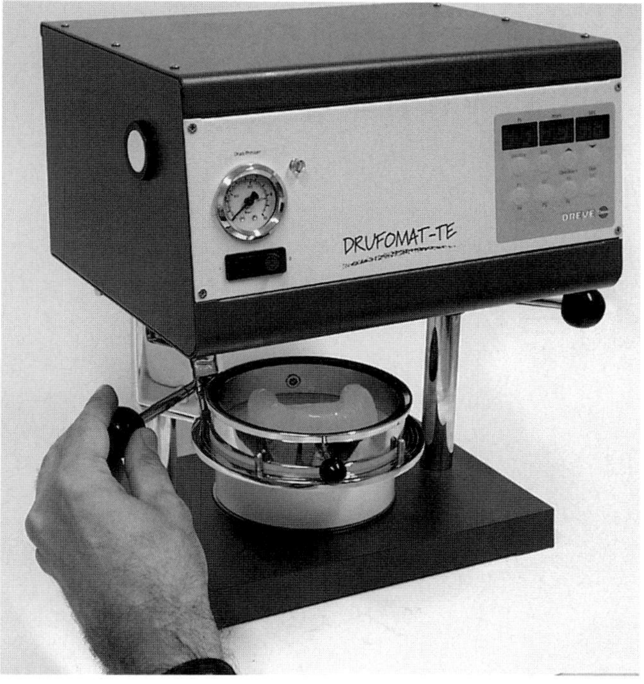

FIGURE 14-33C. Drufomat positive pressure machine. (Courtesy of Exacta Dental Products, Auburn Hills, MI.)

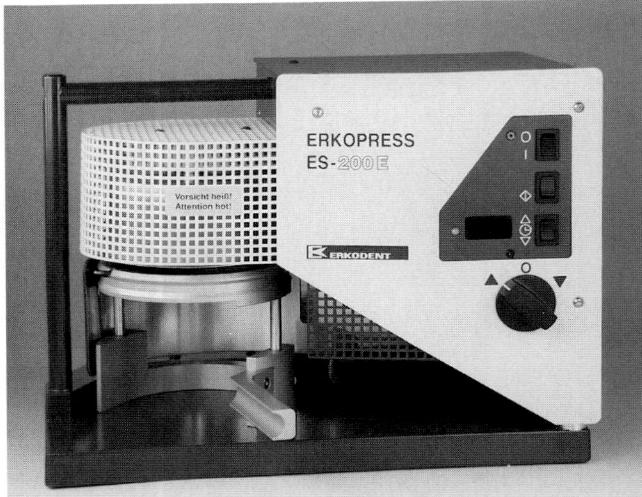

FIGURE 14-33D. Erkopress ES-200E positive pressure machine. (Courtesy of Glidewell Laboratories, Newport Beach, CA.)

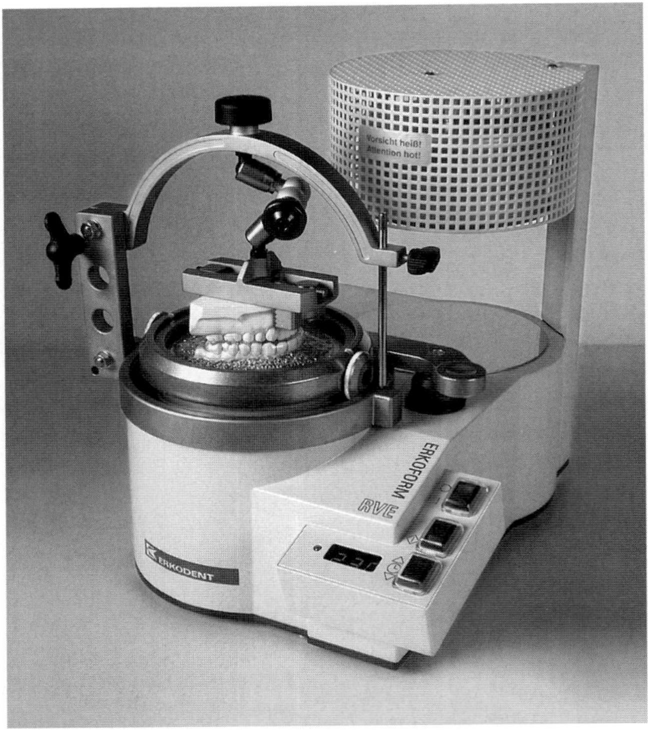

FIGURE 14-33F. Erkoform-RVE sudden vacuum machine with Occluform. (Courtesy of Glidewell Laboratories, Newport Beach, CA.)

precharge feature that produces a sudden vacuum for more precise adaptation (Fig. 14-33F).

Another technique used to fabricate superior custom mouthguards involves heat flasking. These are bimaxillary guards resembling orthodontic positioners. They are used in situations in which it is important to maintain a precise jaw relationship indexed by a dentist. The flasking procedure is roughly the same whether the material is (nonsheet) EVA or vulcanized natural rubber (Fig. 14-34).

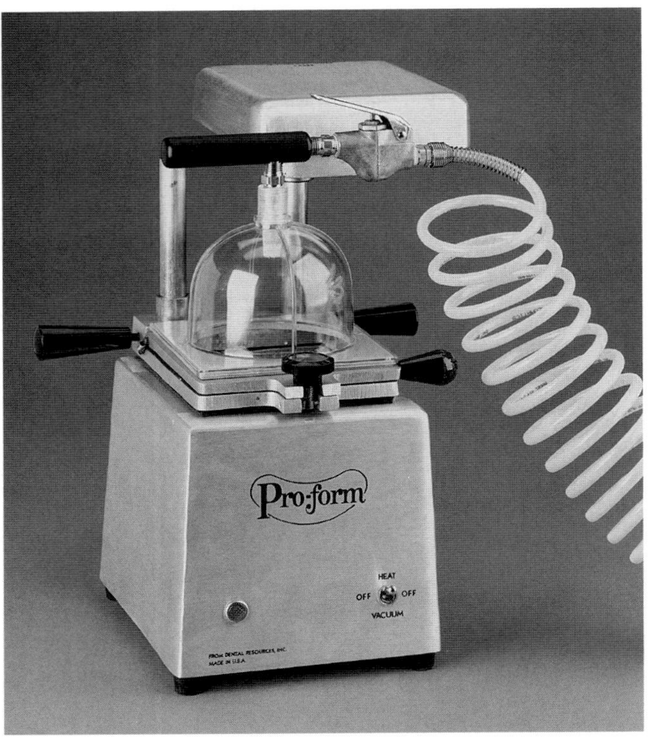

FIGURE 14-33E. Proform vacuum machine with pressure dome. (Courtesy of Dental Resources, Delano, MN.)

Boxing and martial arts mouthguards need to provide an extra degree of protection to both dental arches, especially against TMJ injuries and cerebral concussions. Some believe that the posterior vertical dimension should be increased beyond rest to yield a larger mandibular condylar separation from the glenoid fossa.[55] These mouthguards need to be made of a firmer material to resist bite-through and change in "power bite" position that heavy clenching might produce. In one study, it was found that power athletes clench their teeth and that this allows an athlete to brace and experience a rise or burst in muscle power.[18]

Boxing and martial arts mouthguards need to be engineered with provisos for maximum oxygen exchange. Maintaining an adequate airway in the event of nasal obstruction from a blow is an important consideration.[55] One way to accomplish this is by eliminating the flange on the lower portion of the mouthguard, which uncovers the mandibular incisors and creates space for breathing. Barring allergy, its elasticity, resistance to deformation during clenching, and historic use since the beginning of the century give natural rubber a certain appeal to some professional boxers.

EVA copolymer has become the material of choice. When manufactured, the physical properties of a polymer

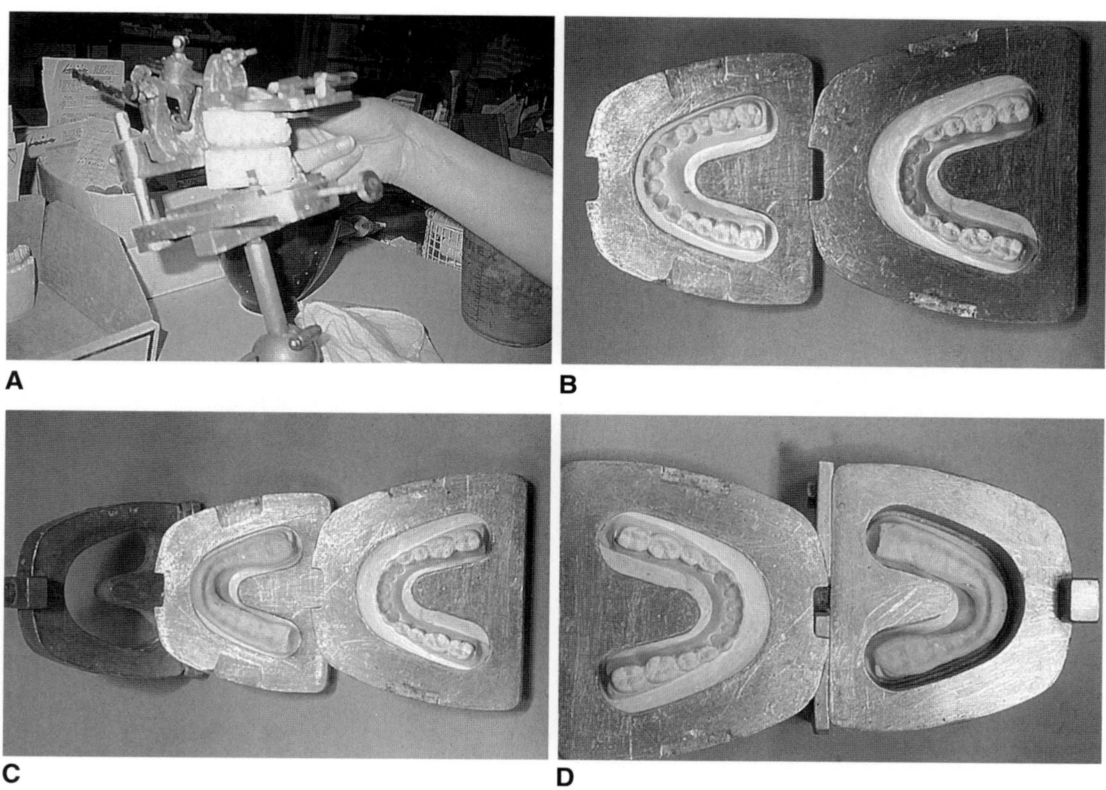

FIGURE 14-34. Heat flasked mouthguard fabrication. **A,** Models mounted in three-dimensional articulator similar to Galletti. **B,** Individual models mounted into flask. **C,** Cavity unit prepared for mounting (note mouthguard material). **D,** Cavity unit mounted into flask. *Continued*

can be varied by such additives as antioxidants and stabilizers, fillers, plasticizers, lubricants, coloring, and flavoring agents.[26] The thermoplastic abilities of EVA make it an attractive material with which to work. Commercial glue gun material is EVA to which a tackisizer has been added. Some orthodontic laboratories use a commercial glue gun to help maxillary and mandibular EVA mouthguards stick together to form a bimaxillary guard like those used in boxing and martial arts. The firmness of EVA can be controlled by adjusting the proportion of ethylene to acetate during copolymerization. This is because the number of cross-links in the polymer chain can be manipulated. Also, the amount of plastisizer incorporated can be varied. Allesee Orthodontic Appliances of Sturtevant, Wisconsin, has a selection of colored, flavored, and scented EVAs. They report that by allowing athletes to personalize their appliances, there is a noticeable improvement in athlete compliance.

DENTAL SPORTS TRAUMA READINESS

Dental Injury Assessment

Studying sports injuries including dental injuries has been made easier through the use of the International Sports Injury System (ISIS). Dr. Nicola Biasca, Chair of Orthopedic Surgery at Spital Oberengadin, Samedin, Switzerland, states, "The database is an Internet-based database system that makes it possible to early detect any changes in injury pattern through the years…. The ISIS system is a valid and reliable way of documenting injuries and if used worldwide it can give very important information concerning injuries, epidemiology, and treatment." More details can be found by visiting www.SportsDDS.com/ISIS.htm. Dr. Biasca is listed in the Sports Dentistry Directory under Switzerland. The Directory serves as a virtual Who's Who in Sports Dentistry; go to www.SportsDentistry.com. Another excellent computer-based application is the Sports Related Dental Injuries Risk Assessment. It has three components: data gathering, data analysis, and reporting of results of the assessment.[36]

Dental injuries are seldom life-threatening and should be triaged only after more serious medical injuries. Naturally, a team physician, dentist, or trainer must first consider "ABC" injuries (airway, breathing, or circulatory), neurologic signs and symptoms, and the overall well-being of the athlete. A history furnishes important information regarding the nature and severity of an injury.[91] Where and what kind of dental or oral injury has been incurred should be determined. This would include how,

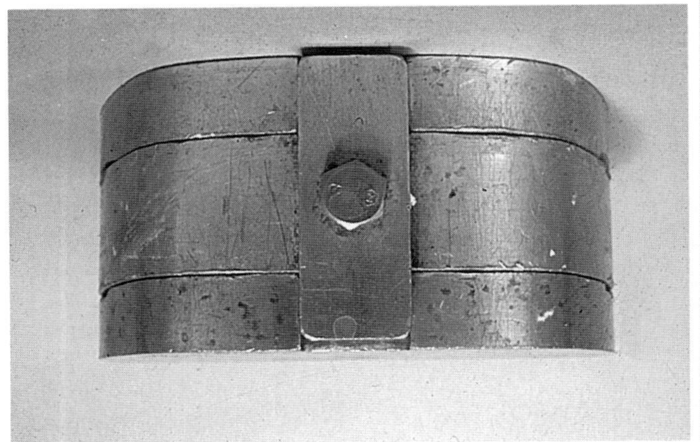

E

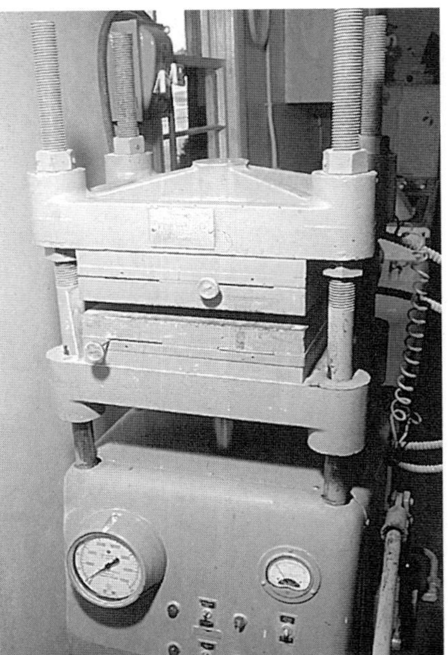

F

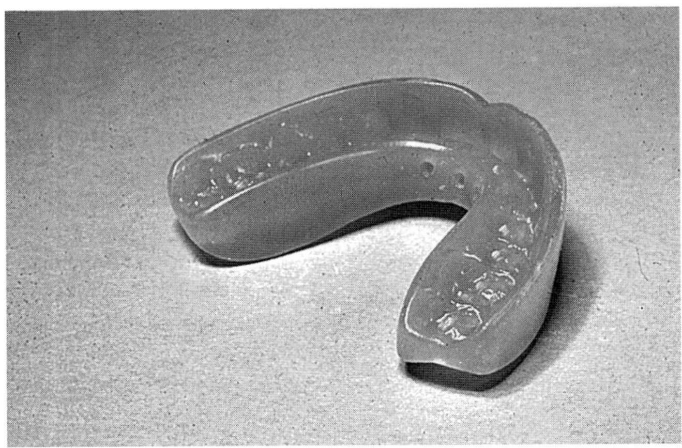

G

FIGURE 14-34, cont'd. E, Mouthguard material inserted into closed flask. **F,** Flask inserted into hydraulic press. **G,** Bimaxillary mouthguard after finishing and polishing. (Courtesy of Allesee Orthodontic Appliances, Sturtevant, WI.)

when, and where did the injury occur? Was the injury witnessed? Can the athlete put his or her teeth together normally? Is there sensitivity to hot, cold, or biting pressure? When did the athlete receive a tetanus shot? Are antibiotics necessary?

If there is bleeding, an attempt to discover its source can be made in the field. A sterile 4″ × 4″ gauze sponge can be used to wipe away the blood. With repeated blotting and careful observation, the general source of bleeding may be identified.[24] Soft-tissue injuries are usually conspicuous. If the source of bleeding is apparently a tooth, digital palpation from a gloved hand can be used to explore and compare mobility, pain, and numbness, and detect sharp edges. Any fracture that involves more than just enamel will render the tooth sensitive to orally inhaled air. This is particularly noticeable in winter sports such as ice hockey and football.[24]

The TMJ should be examined for capsular or miniscular injuries. Direct and indirect trauma to the TMJ may cause fibrous adhesion, ankylosis, and/or fracture.[116] Limitations on jaw movement and discomfort should be explored. Deviations when opening and closing, tenderness, or swelling of the affected joint should be noted. Crepitus and abnormalities of the head of the condyle can be detected by palpating externally with the index fingers over the area of the TMJ. Pinkie fingers inserted into the external auditory meati are also a good test. The patient is instructed to open, close, and go into excursions. Fractured mandibular condyles can sometimes be detected in this fashion.

TMJ traumatic injuries can be managed with cold compresses for the first 24 hours, soft diet, nonsteroidal anti-inflammatory medications, and aspirin. Trismus, ankylosis, fracture, or dislocation of the condyle must also be considered.[46] Later, vigorous physical therapy to maintain the normal range of mandibular motion and prevent ankylosis is recommended.[62] For more information, refer to the textbook written by Dr. Harold Gelb.[39]

After clinical examination, all areas of possible traumatic injuries should be radiographed for immediate diagnostic purposes and to establish a baseline against which to compare at follow-up appointments.[23]

Dental and Oral First-Aid

The contents of a dental field emergency kit will vary depending on the idiosyncrasies of the attending coach, trainer, dentist, or physician, the particular sport, and the availability and sophistication of a nearby treatment facility. Contents should be planned in advance, and those items with limited shelf lives should be replaced at regular intervals to sustain trauma readiness. For example, EMT Toothsaver has a shelf life of about 2 years (see Fig. 14-20).

The principles of dental and oral first-aid follow generally established guidelines for trauma. Direct pressure on an oral wound using sterile 2″ × 2″ or 4″ × 4″ gauze sponges is useful to achieve hemostasis and prevent the development of a hematoma. Elevation of the head is helpful. Rinsing, spitting, nose blowing, or sucking through a straw, creating a negative intraoral pressure, can sometimes exacerbate bleeding. If the episode continues, a decision may have to be made concerning the athlete's continued competition. Cold packs help reduce swelling, pain, and subsequent ecchymosis. Immobilization of loose or broken teeth can sometimes be achieved by gentle biting with or without a mouthguard in place. A Barton bandage is a circumferential head dressing that secures the mandible to the maxilla (Fig. 14-35). This dressing reduces movement and eases pain and suffering during transport of the patient with a suspected mandibular fracture. Caution should be exercised and the potential for emitus and airway obstruction considered. Medications for pain and prevention of infection may need to be prescribed in some patients.

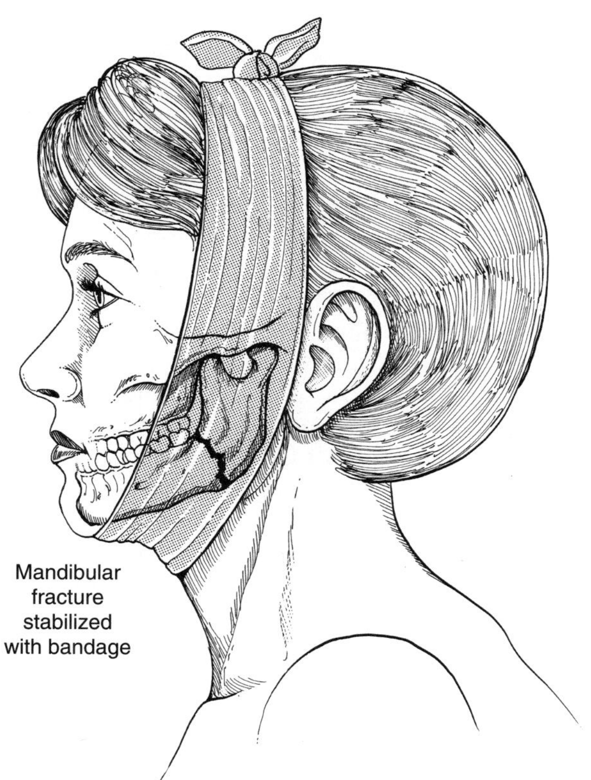

FIGURE 14-35. Barton bandage supporting the mandible for athlete transport. (Illustration by Kibiuk.)

REFERENCES

1. Allen M, et al: Occlusal splints (MORA) vs. placebos show no difference in strength in symptomatic subjects: Double blind cross-over study. Can J Appl Sport Sci 9(3):148–152, 1984.
2. Andersson L: Dentoalveolar ankylosis and associated root resorption in replanted teeth: Experimental and clinical studies in monkeys and man. Swed Dent J Supp 56:1, 1988.
3. Andersson L, et al: Progression of root resorption following replantation of human teeth after extended extra-oral storage. Endo Dental Traumatol 5:38, 1989.
4. Andreasen FM, Andreasen JO, Bayer T: Prognosis of root fractured permanent incisors: Prediction of healing modalities. Endod Dent Traumatol, 5:11–22, 1989.
5. Andreasen FM, Vestergaard Pedersen B: Prognosis of luxated permanent teeth: The development of pulp necrosis. Endod Dent Traumatol 1:207–220, 1985.
6. Andreasen J: Effect of extra-alveolar period and storage media upon periodontal and pulpal healing after replantation of mature permanent incisors in monkeys. Int J Oral Surg 10:43, 1981.
7. Andreasen J: Etiology and pathogenesis of traumatic dental injuries: A clinical study of 1298 cases. Scand J Dent Res 78:329, 1970.
8. Andreasen J: External root resorption: Its implication in dental traumatology, paedodontics, periodontics, orthodontics and endodontics. Int Endo J 18:109, 1985.
9. Andreasen J, Andreasen F: Textbook and Color Atlas of Traumatic Injuries to the Teeth, 3rd ed. St. Louis, Mosby, 1994.

10. Andreasen JO, Borum M, Jacobsen HL, Andreasen FM: Replantation of 400 traumatically avulsed permanent incisors. I. Diagnosis of healing complications. Endod Dent Traumatol 11:51–58, 1995.
11. Andreasen JO, Borum M, Jacobsen HL, Andreasen FM: Replantation of 400 avulsed permanent incisors. II. Factors related to pulp healing. Endod Dent Traumatol 11:59–68, 1995.
12. Andreasen JO, Borum M, Jacobsen HL, Andreasen FM: Replantation of 400 avulsed permanent incisors. IV. Factors related to periodontal ligament healing. Endod Dent Traumatol 11:76–89, 1995.
13. Barth, J, Freeman J, Winters, J: Management of sports-related concussions. Dent Clin North Am 44(1):67–83, 2000.
14. Bates R, Atkinson W: The effects of maxillary MORA's on strength and muscle efficiency tests. J Craniomandib Pract 1(4):37–42, 1983.
15. Bemelmanns P, Pfeiffer P: Incidence of dental, mouth, and jaw injuries and the efficacy of mouthguards in top ranking athletes. Sportverletz Sportschaden 14(4):139–143, 2000.
16. Benson BW, Mohtadi NG, Rose MS, Meeuwisse WH: Head and neck injuries among ice hockey players wearing full face shields vs half face shields. JAMA 282(24):2328–2332, 1999.
17. Blomlof L, et al: Storage of experimentally avulsed teeth in milk prior to replantation. J Dent Res 62:912, 1983.
18. Boroojerdi B, Battaglia F, Muellbacher W, Cohen LG: Voluntary teeth clenching facilitates human motor system excitability. Clin Neurophysiol 111(6):988–993, 2000.
19. Brotman I, Rothschild H: Report of a breakthrough in preventive dental care for a national football league team. JADA 88:553, 1974.
20. Brunton PA, Cattell P, Trevor Burke FJ, Wilson NH: Fracture resistance of teeth restored with onlays of three contemporary tooth-colored resin-bonded restorative materials. J Prosthet Dent 82(2):167–171, 1999.
21. Burkett L, Bernstein A: Strength testing after jaw repositioning with a mandibular orthopedic appliance. Physician Sports Med 10(2):101–107, 1982.
22. Burkett L, Bernstein A: The effect of mandibular position on strength, reaction time and movement time on a randomly selected population. NY State Dent J 49(5):281–285, 1983.
23. Camp J: Diagnosis and management of sports-related injuries to the teeth. Dent Clin North Am 35(4):733–756, 1991.
24. Castaldi C: First aid for sports-related dental injuries. Physician Sports Med 15(9):81–89, 1987.
25. Castaldi C: The Sports Mouthguard: Its Use and Misuse in Ice Hockey, Safety in Ice Hockey, vol 3. Philadelphia, ASTM STP, 1993.
26. Chaconas S, et al: A comparison of athletic mouthguard materials. Am J Sports Med 13(3): 193–197, 1985.
27. Chiodo G, Rosenstein D: Mandibular athletic repositioning appliance and athletic performance. JODA Winter:31–33, 1986.
28. Contreras-Vidal JL, Van den Heuvel CE, Teulings HL, Stelmach GE: Visuo-motor adaptation in smokeless tobacco users. Nicotine Tob Res 1(3):219–227, 1999.
29. Costen J: Neuralgias and ear symptoms involved in general diagnosis due to mandibular joint pathology. J Kansas Med Soc 315–321, 1935.
30. Cvek M: A clinical report on partial pulpotomy and capping with calcium hydroxide in permanent incisors with complicated crown fractures. J Endo 4:232, 1978.
31. Cvek M: Endodontic treatment of traumatized teeth. In Andreasen J: Traumatic Injuries of the Teeth, 2nd ed. Philadelphia, WB Saunders, 1981.
32. Cvek M, et al: Treatment of non-vital permanent incisors with calcium hydroxide. Odontol Rev 25:43, 1974.
33. Ferrari CH, Ferreira de Medeiros JM: Dental trauma and level of information: Mouthguard use in different contact sports. Dent Traumatol 18(3): 144–147, 2002.
34. Filippi A, Pohl Y, von Arx T: Treatment of replacement resorption with Emdogain: A prospective clinical study. Dent Traumatol 18(3):138–143, 2002.
35. Forgione A: Strength and bite, Part I: An analytical review. J Craniomandib Prac 9(4):305–315, 1991.
36. Fos, P, Pinkham, J, Ranalli, D: Prediction of sports-related dental traumatic injuries. Dent Clin North Am 44(1):19–33, 2000.
37. Fountain SB, Camp JH: Traumatic Injuries in Pathways of the Pulp, 6th ed. St. Louis, CV Mosby Co., 1994.
38. Gelb H: A too-polite silence about shoddy science: Dynamic strength testing and beyond. J Craniomandib Prac 10(1):75–79, 1992.
39. Gelb H: New Concepts in Craniomandibular and Chronic Pain Management. London, Mosby-Wolfe, 1994.
40. Geurtsen W, Garcia-Godoy F: Bonded restorations for the prevention and treatment of the cracked-tooth syndrome. Am J Dent 12(6):266–270, 1999.
41. Giuliani V, Baccetti T, Pace R, Pagavino G: The use of MTA in teeth with necrotic pulps and open apices. Dent Traumatol 18(4):217–221, 2002.
42. Going R, Loehman R, Chan M: Mouthguard materials: Their physical and mechanical properties. JADA 89:132–138, 1974.
43. Granath L, Hagman G: Experimental pulpotomy in human bicuspids with reference to cutting technique. Acta Odontol Scand 29:155, 1971.
44. Greenberg AM, Haug RH: Etiology, Distribution, and Classification of Fractures. New York, Springer-Verlag, 1993.

45. Greenberg M, Cohen S, Springer P, et al: Mandibular position and upper body strength: A controlled clinical trial. JADA 103:576–579, 1981.
46. Greenberg M, Springer P: Diagnosis and management of oral injuries. In Torg J (ed): Athletic Injuries to the Head, Neck and Face, 2nd ed. St Louis, Mosby–Year Book, 1991.
47. Grossman L, Ship I: Survival rate of replanted teeth. Oral Surg 29:899, 1970.
48. Guevara P, Ranalli P: Techniques for mouthguard fabrication. Dent Clin North Am 35:627–645, 1991.
49. Hammarstrom L, et al: Replantation of teeth & antibiotic treatment. Endo Dental Traumatol 2:51, 1986.
50. Hart D, et al: The effect of vertical dimension on muscular strength. J Orthop Sports Phys Ther 3(2):57–61, 1981.
51. Heintz W: Mouth protection for athletics today. In Godwin W, Long B, Cartwright C (eds): The Relationship of internal Protection Devices to Athletic Injuries and Athletic Performance. Ann Arbor, University of Michigan, 1982.
52. Heintz W: Mouth protectors: A progress report. JADA 77:632, 1968.
53. Hickey J, et al: The relation of mouth protectors to cranial pressure and deformation. JADA 74: 735–740, 1967.
54. Hildebrandt J: Dental and maxillofacial injuries. Clin Sports Med 1(3):449–468, 1982.
55. Hildebrandt JR, Garner-Nelson J: Mouthguard Protection for Boxing. US Olympic Committee, Colorado Springs, CO, 1990.
56. Holland GJ, et al: Custom vs. commercial mouth guard use: Effect on exercise metabolic-ventilatory response of trained distance runners. NCSA J Applied Sports Sci Res 3: 1989.
57. Huang SC, Remeikis NA, Daniel JC: Effects of long-term exposure of human periodontal ligament cells to milk and other solutions. J Endod 22(1): 30–33, 1996.
58. Jakush J: Divergent views: Can dental therapy enhance athletic performance? JADA 104(3):292–298, 1982.
59. Jarvinen S: Incisal overjet and traumatic injuries to upper permanent incisors. A retrospective study. Acta Odontal Scand 36:359, 1978.
60. Kakehashi S, et al: The effects of surgical exposures of dental pulps in germ-free and conventional laboratory rats. Oral Surg 20:340, 1965.
61. Kaufman R, Kaufman A: An experimental study on the effects of the MORA on football players. Basal Facts 6(4): 119–126, 1984.
62. Keith D, Orden A: Orofacial athletic injuries and involvement of the temporomandibular joint. J Mass Dental Soc 43(4):11–15, 1994.
63. Kerr I, Lawrence: Mouth guards for the prevention of injuries in contact sports. Sports Med 415–427, 1986.
64. Krasner P, Person P: Preserving avulsed teeth for replantation. JADA 123:80, 1992.
65. Krekeler G, Petsch K, Flesch-Gorlas M: Der Frakturverlauf in parodontalen Bereich. Dtsch Zahnärztl Z 38:355–357, 1983.
66. Kumamoto DP, Winters J, Novickas D, Mesa K: Tooth avulsions resulting from basketball net entanglement. J Am Dent Assoc 128(9):1273–1275, 1997.
67. Kurtz M: Columbia University and those that made it the Mecca of dental education. Bull Hist Dent 26(2):86–103, 1978.
68. Kurtz M, Breitweiser RF, Protect yourself and your athletes by requiring properly fitted mouthguards as standard equipment, The Redwoods Group, http://www.redwoodsgroup.com/articles-8.asp, Morrisville, NC, April, 2000.
69. Kvittem B, Hardie NA, Roettger M, Conry J: Incidence of orofacial injuries in high school sports. J Public Health Dent 58(4):288–293, 1998.
70. Labella CR, Smith BW, Sigurdsson A: Effect of mouthguards on dental injuries and concussions in college basketball. Med Sci Sports Exerc 34(1): 41–44, 2002.
71. Lang B, Pohl Y, Filippi A: Knowledge and prevention of dental trauma in team handball in Switzerland and Germany. Dent Traumatol 18(6):329–334, 2002.
72. Lee-Knight C, et al: Dental injuries at the 1989 Canada Games: An epidemiological study. JCDA 58(10):810–815, 1992.
73. Lewis T: Incidence of fractured anterior teeth as related to their protrusion. Angle Orthop 29:128, 1959.
74. Lindskog S, et al: Mitosis and microorganisms in the periodontal membrane after storage in milk or saliva. Scand J Dent Res 91:465, 1983.
75. Linn E: Facial injuries sustained during sports and games. J Max Fac Surg 14:83–88, 1986.
76. Maeda Y, et al: Mouthguard and occlusal force distribution. J Osaka Univ Dent Sch 30:125–130, 1990.
77. Maestrello-deMoya M: Orofacial trauma and mouth-protector wear among high school varsity basketball players. J Dent Child 56(1):36–39, 1989.
78. McArdle W, et al: Temperomandibular joint repositioning and exercise performance: A double blind study. Med Sci Sports Exerc 16(3):228–233, 1984.
79. Moore M: Corrective mouth guards: Performance aids or expensive placebos? Phys Sports Med 9(3):130, 1981.
80. Novich M, Schwartz R: The athletes mouthpiece. Clin Proc Dent 7(3):18–21, 1985.
81. Padilla R, Balikov S: Sports dentistry: Coming of age in the '90s. JCDA 21:27–37, 1993.
82. Padilla RR, Lee TK: Pressure-laminated athletic mouthguards: A step-by-step process. J Calif Dent Assoc 27(3):200–209, 1999.

83. Park J: Methods to improved mouthguards. First International Symposium on Biomaterials, Korea Research Institute of Chem Tech, Daedeog-Danji, Taejon, Korea, Aug 12–13, 1993:1–18.
84. Parker M, et al: Muscle strength related to use of inter-occlusal splints. Gen Dent 32(2):105–109, 1984.
85. Paterson R, Watts A: Further studies on the exposed germ-free dental pulp. Int Endo J 20:112, 1987.
86. Pavlov H: Radiographic evaluation of the skull and facial bones. In Torg J: Athletic Injuries to the Head, Neck, and Face, 2nd ed. St Louis, Mosby–Year Book, 1991.
87. Pinkham J, Kohn D: Epidemiology and prediction of sports-related traumatic injuries. Dent Clin North Am 35(4):609–626, 1991.
88. Pohl Y, Filippi A, Kirschner H: Auto-alloplastic transplantation of a primary canine after traumatic loss of a permanent central incisor. Dent Traumatol 17(4):188–193, 2001.
89. Pohl Y, Tekin U, Boll M, Filippi A, Kirschner H: Investigations on a cell culture medium for storage and transportation of avulsed teeth. Aust Endod J 25(2):70–75, 1999.
90. Pollack B: Legal considerations in sports dentistry. Dent Clin North Am 35(4):809–829, 1991.
91. Powers M: Diagnosis and management of dentoalveolar inuries. In Fonseca R, Walker R: Oral and Maxillofacial Trauma. Philadelphia, WB Saunders, 1991.
92. Ranalli D, Lancaster D: Attitudes of college football officials regarding NCAA mouthguard regulations and player compliance. Public Health Dent 53(2):96–100, 1993.
93. Ranalli D, Lancaster D: Comparative evaluation of college football officials' attitude toward NCAA mouthguard regulations and player compliance. Pediatr Dent 15(6):398–402, 1993.
94. Ranalli DN: Sports dentistry and dental traumatology. Dent Traumatol 18(5):231–235, 2002.
95. Ranalli DN, Rye LA: Oral health issues for women athletes. Dent Clin North Am 45(3):523–539, vi–vii, 2001.
96. Rigotti NA, Lee JE, Wechsler H: US college students' use of tobacco products: Results of a national survey. JAMA 284(6):699–705, 2000.
97. Rock W, Grundy M: The effect of luxation and subluxation upon the prognosis of traumatized incisor teeth. J Dent 9:224, 1981.
98. Schubert M, et al: Changes in shoulder and leg strength in athletes wearing mandibular orthopedic repositioning appliances. JADA 108(3):334–337, 1984.
99. Schultz R: Facial Injuries, 3rd ed. Chicago, Year Book Medical Publishers, 1988.
100. Smith S: Adjusting mouthguards kinesiologically in professional football players. NY State Dent J 48(5):298–301, 1982.
101. Smith S: Muscular strength correlated to jaw posture and the TMJ. NY State Dent J 44(7): 278–283, 1978.
102. Stanley H, et al: The rate of tertiary (reparative) dentin formation in the human tooth. Oral Surg 21:180, 1966.
103. Stenger J: Physiologic dentistry with Notre Dame athletes. Basal Facts 2(1):8–18, 1977.
104. Stenger J, et al: Mouthguards: Protection against shock to head, neck and teeth. JADA 69:273–281, 1964.
105. Summers C: In personal communication to Department of Health and Human Services, Centers For Disease Control, Atlanta, GA, October 15, 1991.
106. Trope M: Clinical management of the avulsed tooth: Present strategies and future directions. Dent Traumatol 18(1):1–11, 2002.
107. Trope M, Friedman S: Periodontal healing of replanted dog teeth stored in Viaspan, milk, and Hanks Balanced Salt Solution. Endo Dent Traumatol 8:183, 1992.
108. Vegso J, et al: The effect of an orthopaedic intraoral mandibular appliance on upper body strength. Med Sci Sports Exer 13(2):115–116, 1981.
109. Verban E, et al: The effects of mandibular orthopedic repositioning appliance on shoulder strength. J Craniomandib Pract 2(3):232–237, 1984.
110. Walsh MM, et al: Smokeless tobacco cessation intervention for college athletes: Results after 1 year. Am J Public Health 89(2):228–234, 1999.
111. Westerman B, Stringfellow P, Eccleston J: EVA mouthguards: How thick should they be? Dental Traumatology, 18(1):24-27, 2002.
112. Williams M, Chaconas S, Bader P: The effect of mandibular position on appendage muscle strength. J Prosthet Dent 49(4):560–567, 1983.
113. Yamada T, et al: A study of sports-related mandibular angle fracture: Relation to the position of the third molars. Scand J Med Sci Sports 8(2):116–119, 1998.
114. Yates J, et al: Effect of a mandibular orthopedic repositioning appliance on muscular strength. JADA 108(2):331–333, 1984.
115. Yonehata Y, Maeda Y, Machi H, Sakaguchi RL: The influence of working cast residual moisture and temperature on the fit of vacuum-forming athletic mouth guards. J Prosthet Dent 89(1):23–27, 2003.
116. Yucel E, Borkan U, Mollaoglu N, Gunhan O: Histological evaluation of changes in the temporomandibular joint after direct and indirect trauma: An experimental study. Dent Traumatol 18(4): 212–216, 2002.

15 Otorhinolaryngology

Gwen S. Korovin and
Andrew G. Sikora

Otorhinolaryngology is a vital area of sports medicine. The ear, nose, and face are prominent structures poorly shielded from injury, and thus frequently involved in sports-related trauma. The head and neck encompass the organs of speech and hearing, and the upper aerodigestive tract. These structures are essential for communication, respiration, and awareness of one's surroundings. Thus, injuries or illnesses affecting these areas have obvious potential to compromise athletic performance. Although the head and neck area are common sites of sports-related trauma, it is important to remember that these injuries may be associated with injuries to other parts of the body. Physicians who care for a patient who has sustained a sports-related injury must be aware of the possibility for multiple injuries, and be prepared to provide appropriate emergency treatment and refer appropriately for definitive care.

Certain sports such as shooting, swimming, and self-contained underwater breathing apparatus (SCUBA) and skin diving are associated with unique ear, nose, and throat problems unrelated to trauma. In addition to managing acute illness, the otorhinolaryngologist may be called on to medically clear participants for these activities, and may follow patients over time to manage chronic conditions and prevent disability.

Even recreational athletes often subject themselves to the demands of competition or rigorous training schedules and expect their bodies to operate at high performance levels. Managing the unique needs and concerns of these highly motivated individuals can be a rewarding aspect of otorhinolaryngologic practice.

GENERAL PRINCIPLES

Injuries

Sports injuries to the head and neck area are common. In managing these injuries, it is important to get the athlete back to playing the sport as soon as possible; however, management should not be compromised because of these pressures. Once treatment is given, the athlete must be informed of the risks of reinjury in this very vulnerable area of the body.

Fortunately, there has been a great decrease in the number and severity of sports-related head and neck traumas, resulting from the wearing of face masks and guards, ear protectors, nose guards, and neck protection. Practitioners should emphasize the use of protective gear by all athletes, be they children or adults, professionals or amateurs.

Ear, Nose, and Throat Problems

The athlete being treated for medical problems in the head and neck area may be prescribed a number of medications. These medications can have side effects, such as sedation or increased adrenergic tone, with the potential to alter athletic performance. The physician prescribing these medications must be aware of the special demands of the sports in which his or her patient may engage. The treatment of the professional athlete may add a further dimension, as certain medications may need to be approved by the sport and others may be banned.

Since the upper aerodigestive tract is a portal into the body, infections of the upper respiratory system can lead to more widespread infections, locally and systemically. The physician managing a sports-related problem in another part of the body must be aware of this. This is especially important if a surgical procedure is being planned, since infections should be treated or given adequate time to resolve prior to any elective surgery. If emergency or urgent care is necessary, preoperative antibiotic prophylaxis may be required.

EAR PROBLEMS

Trauma to the ear may occur at various sites. Figure 15-1 shows the anatomy of the external, middle, and inner ear, any of which may be injured. The auricle, or the outer ear or pinna, is easily injured because of its prominent location on the head. An abrasion to this area must be cleansed well. Any foreign material in the wound must be removed. Antibiotic ointment may be useful to prevent local infection.

Lacerations of the auricle must be inspected carefully and repaired as soon as possible. If the injury only involves the skin, it must be carefully cleansed, and the skin can be reapproximated using 5-0 or 6-0 nylon. If the injury also involves cartilage, the edges of the cartilage must be carefully approximated in a separate layer using 4-0 or 5-0 chromic. It is important to reapproximate the edges well for proper healing and good cosmetic results. If the laceration involves the external auditory canal, it may require packing to prevent stenosis.[24,40]

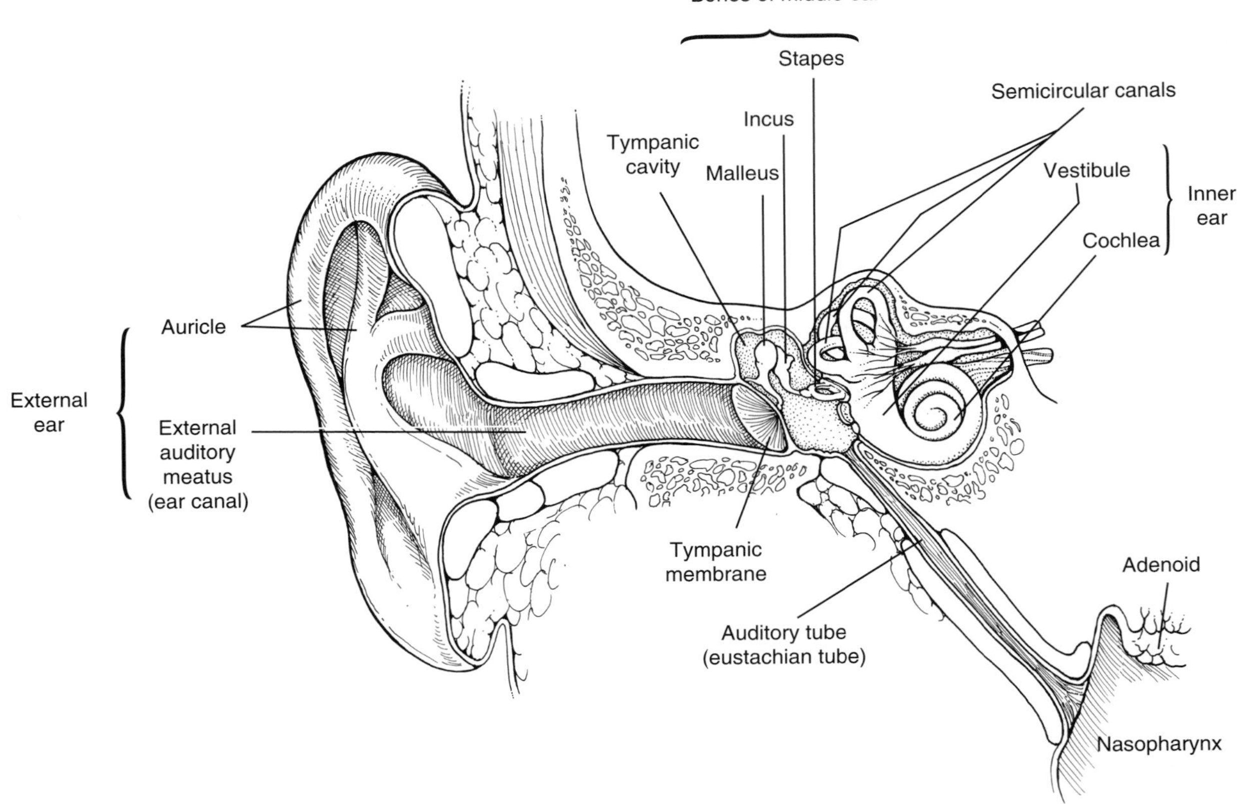

FIGURE 15-1. Anatomic drawing of the external, middle, and inner ear.

Partial or total avulsion of the ear may also occur. If a partial avulsion is found, it can be reattached. The outcome depends on the extent of the avulsion and the available blood supply. Total avulsion, which is rare, most often results in severe deformity. The best chance for successful outcome may occur if the cartilage is buried in the postauricular region or superficial abdominal wall for use in a delayed reconstruction. Figure 15-2 shows a healed partial avulsion that was not reattached.

Contusions of the auricle may also occur. If it is minor, the injury can be observed. If there is an area of ecchymosis, cold compresses and analgesia may be needed. If the injury is more severe, a hematoma may occur. More severe injury usually results from blunt trauma and results in sudden, painless swelling. It is a very common injury in wrestling. An auricular hematoma is seen in Figure 15-3.

The bleeding associated with hematoma occurs only on the anterior surface of the auricle where the skin is closely adherent to the perichondrium and cartilage. Posteriorly, there is a cushion of subcutaneous fat, which acts as protection. The bleeding has been shown by Ohlsen et al. to occur between the perichondrium and the cartilage.[33] If the hematoma is not drained, the blood is replaced by fibrous tissue. A cauliflower ear or perichondritis can result.

There are many types of management published in the literature.[16] The most conservative management is

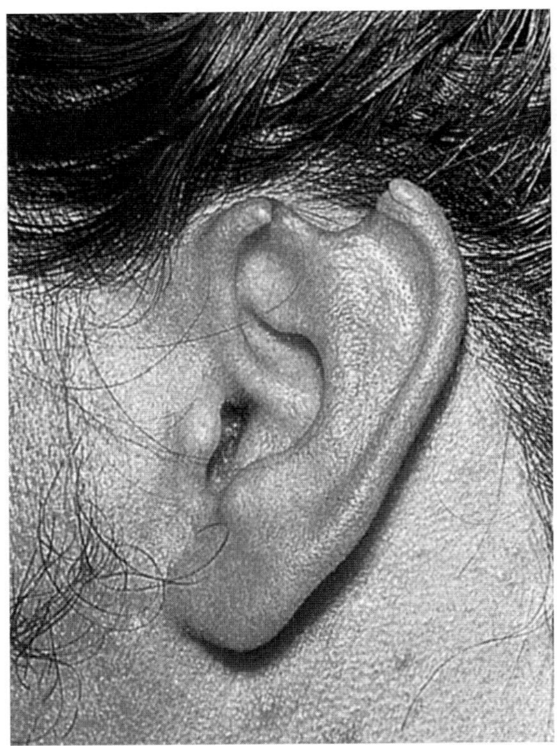

FIGURE 15-2. Healed area of partial avulsion injury to the auricle without reattachment. (From Bull TR: A Color Atlas of E.N.T. Diagnosis, 2nd ed. London, Mosby-Wolfe, 1987.)

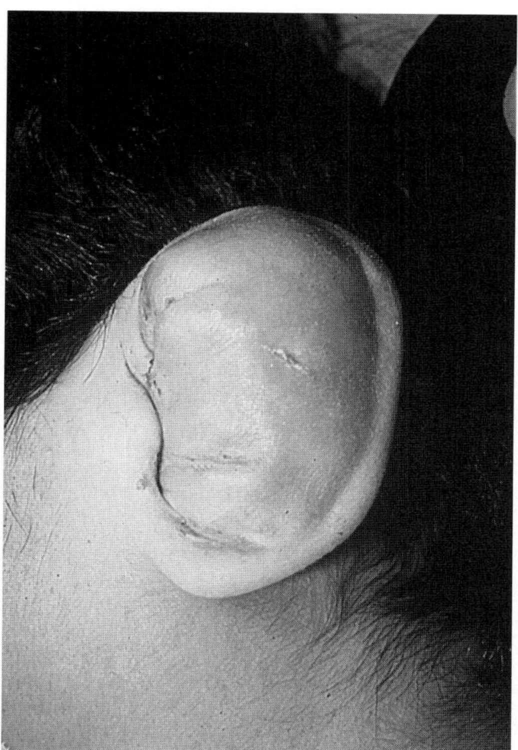

FIGURE 15-3. An auricular hematoma involving the entire anterior auricle.

needle aspiration of the hematoma. This procedure is demonstrated in Figure 15-4. However, in cases of recurrent or persistent hematoma, and when the blood has already formed an organized clot, incision and drainage are often necessary. Figure 15-5 shows a hematoma that has been incised and drained. A bolster dressing of some type is usually needed. Various bolsters have been described, including cotton bolsters, dental rolls, and plaster molds. Occasionally a drain is left in place to prevent reaccumulation. Management of an established cauliflower ear requires excising and thinning of the deformed cartilage. An example of a cauliflower ear is seen in Figure 15-6.

Perichondritis or chondritis may also occur, as seen in Figure 15-7. The symptoms include pain, fever, and erythema and fluctuation of the affected part of the auricle. Management may include intravenous antibiotics. Chondritis can cause necrotic cartilage to develop, which must be debrided.

Thermal injury to the auricle may also occur. The pinna has a prominent, exposed position on the head. It is vulnerable because of its poor insulation, its minimal subcutaneous tissue, and its tenuous distal blood supply. Frostbite can occur rapidly with wind and cold exposure during winter sports.[24]

In its early stages, frostbite causes numbness of the pinna. Pallor and edema may occur with thawing, and vesicles and bullae may form. Cellular destruction and small vessel injury may cause necrosis and infection to occur in the more severe cases.

Management involves quick, but gentle rewarming. Analgesics may be needed. Blebs require sterile aspiration. If necrosis occurs, surgical debridement or antibiotic treatment may be necessary.

Sunburn may also cause significant problems. The superior portion of the pinna is exposed to direct sunlight and mild to severe burns may occur. Mild burns can be managed with cool compresses and emollients. More severe burns may result in erythema, pain, edema, and blistering. Infection can ensue. Management may include corticosteroids and possibly antibiotics.

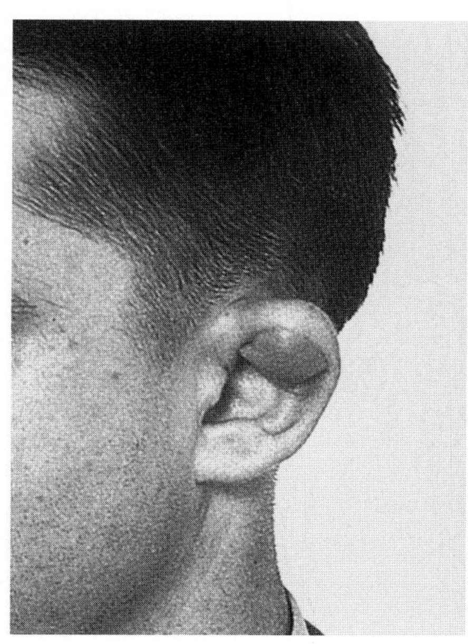

A

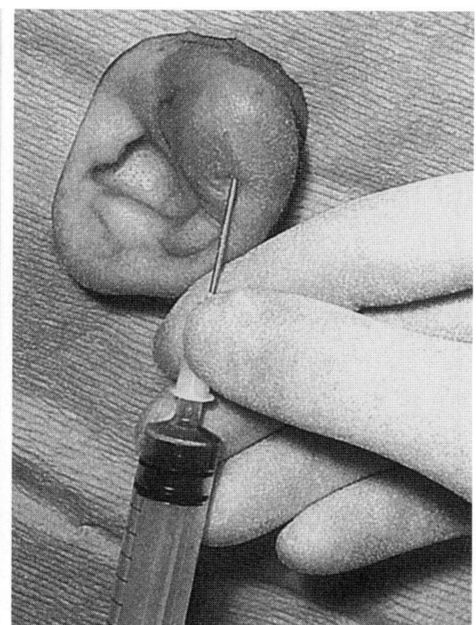

B

FIGURE 15-4. A, Auricular hematoma of the upper auricle. **B,** Needle aspiration of the hematoma for drainage. (From Bull TR: A Color Atlas of E.N.T. Diagnosis, 2nd ed. London, Mosby-Wolfe, 1987.)

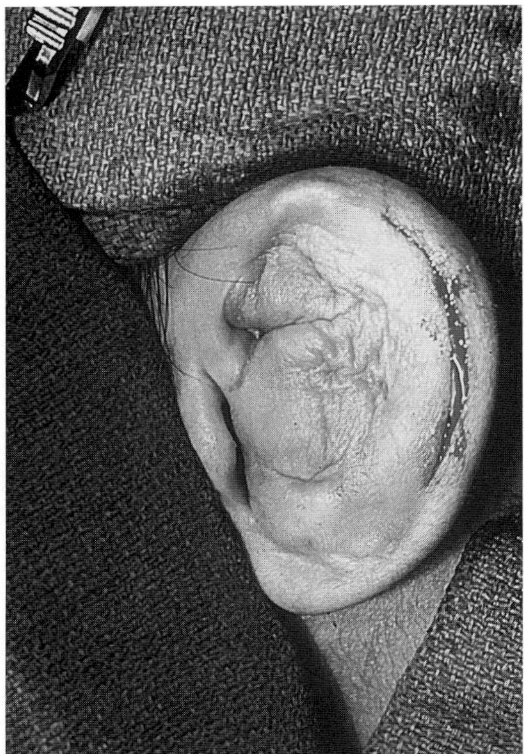

FIGURE 15-5. Surgical incision and drainage of an auricular hematoma.

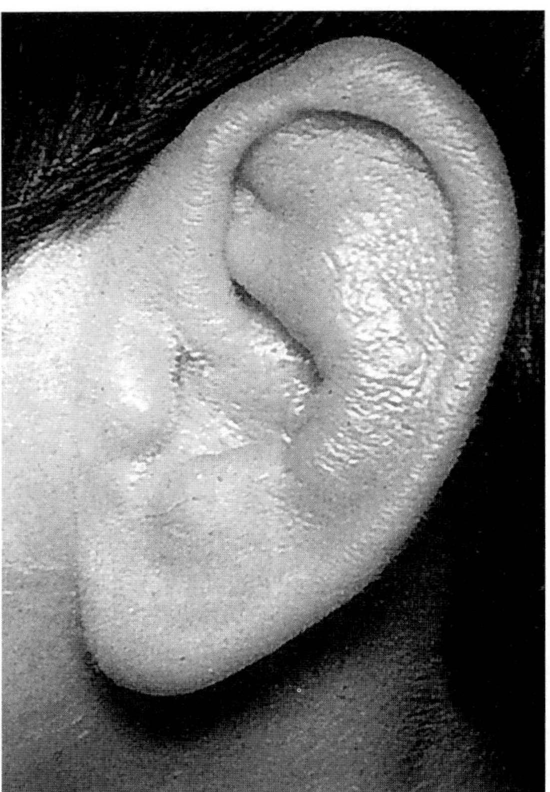

FIGURE 15-7. Perichondritis of the auricle. (From Bull TR: A Color Atlas of E.N.T. Diagnosis, 2nd ed. London, Mosby-Wolfe, 1987.)

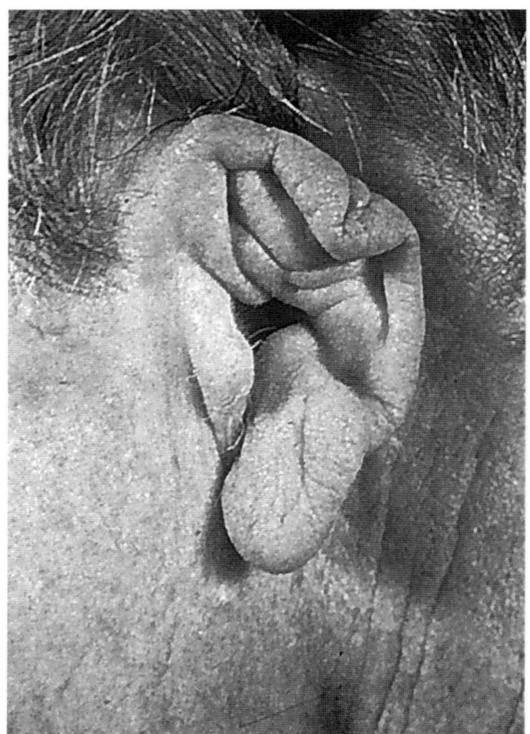

FIGURE 15-6. Cauliflower ear after repeated septal hematomas that were untreated. (From Bull TR: A Color Atlas of E.N.T. Diagnosis, 2nd ed. London, Mosby-Wolfe, 1987.)

In addition to trauma of the external ear, trauma may also have significant effects on the middle and inner ear. Blast injuries to the ear often occur during sports activities. Of 91 cases of blast injuries to the ear studied in Israel, 31 resulted from sports-related activities.[5] Sports accidents and ball games accounted for 13 of these cases, and swimming and water sport activities accounted for the other 18. The swimming accidents represent a special group because these injuries are often associated with water contamination of the ear. Problems that occurred in these 31 cases included hearing loss, earaches, tinnitus, vertigo, and purulent otorrhea.

The most common middle ear injury is perforation of the tympanic membrane, which can result from penetrating injuries, blast injuries, or blunt trauma. A sudden blow that seals the external auditory meatus may cause a significant increase of ear pressure in the canal and cause the tympanic membrane to rupture. Figure 15-8 shows a perforation of a tympanic membrane and Figure 15-9 shows a perforation with an associated hematoma.

Injury to the tympanic membrane may cause pain, hearing loss, bleeding, and possibly dizziness. An otoscopic examination is necessary, and audiogram should be performed. The ear must be kept dry. Antibiotics are often used prophylactically. Most traumatic perforations heal

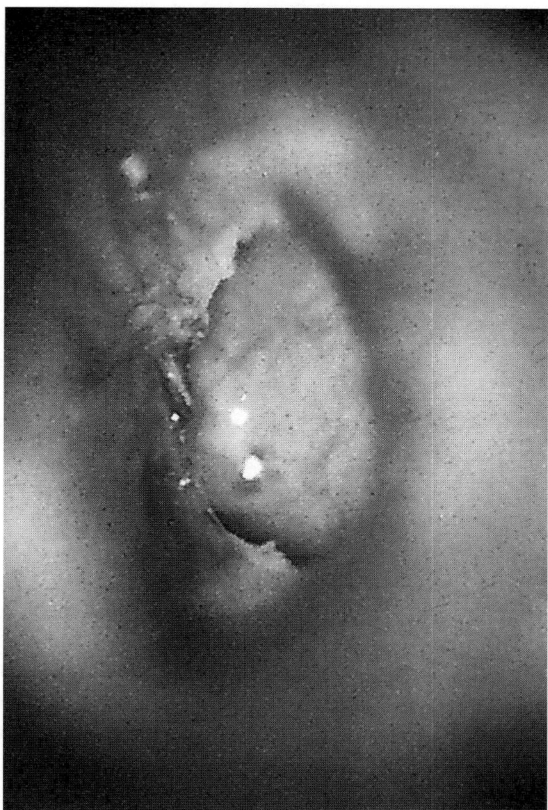

FIGURE 15-8. Large tympanic membrane perforation with underlying middle ear cavity seen. (From Bull TR: A Color Atlas of E.N.T. Diagnosis, 2nd ed. London, Mosby-Wolfe, 1987.)

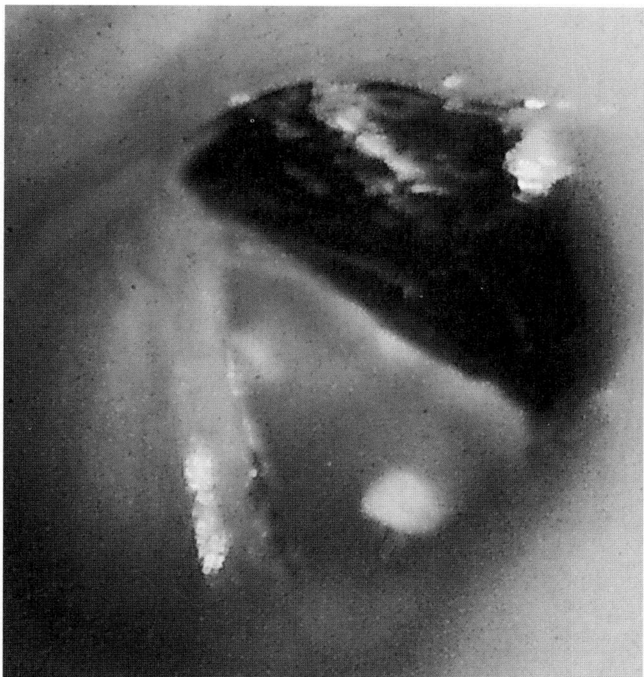

FIGURE 15-9. Tympanic membrane perforation with associated hematoma. (From Bull TR: A Color Atlas of E.N.T. Diagnosis, 2nd ed. London, Mosby-Wolfe, 1987.)

spontaneously. There is a positive correlation between the size of the tympanic membrane perforation and the time to resolution. If the perforation does not close, a tympanoplasty may be performed to improve hearing and prevent infection.

Trauma may result in injury to the ossicular chain, causing a permanent conductive hearing loss. This hearing loss can occur in conjunction with a tympanic membrane perforation. An audiogram is needed for the evaluation. Middle ear exploration and repair may be necessary for this type of injury.

Trauma to the inner ear may be caused by blast or penetrating injuries. A labyrinth concussion may result from a severe blow to the head, causing either temporary or permanent dysfunction of either the cochlea or vestibular labyrinth or both.[10] This concussion can result in sensorineural hearing loss or in mild to severe vertigo. Evaluation includes audiogram and possibly electronystagmogram (ENG). Management may include observation, antivertiginous medications, and avoidance of positions that induce the vertigo. Exercises designed specifically for the inner ear balance mechanism may be helpful in chronic cases.

Trauma may result in a perilymphatic fistula, which is a fistula between the middle and inner ear, resulting in a leakage of perilymphatic fluid.[18,25] Symptoms may include the sudden onset of vertigo, nystagmus, or sensorineural hearing loss. Diagnosis is made by symptoms and an audiologic evaluation. Treatment is primarily observation, strict bedrest, and use of laxatives and cough suppressants to avoid transient increases in intracranial pressure. The condition may require exploration of the middle ear and closure of the leak if it does not close spontaneously. Although some otologic surgeons do advocate immediate exploration, others believe this exploration may be of questionable long-term value.

Noise-induced trauma is another risk of certain sports activities. Rifle shooting is one example. The trauma may be temporary or permanent. Tinnitus can also occur. Management includes observation and subsequent ear protection to prevent further injury.

Severe blows to the head during sports activities can result in temporal bone fractures.[1,32] This injury is often associated with other neurologic injuries. Fractures may result in conductive hearing loss caused by tympanic membrane perforation, hemotympanum, or ossicular chain disruption. There can also be an associated sensorineural hearing loss, facial nerve injuries, or cerebrospinal fluid (CSF) otorrhea or rhinorrhea. They may also be associated with vertigo caused by labyrinth concussion or more severe damage to the labyrinth. Physical findings may include postauricular hematoma, hemotympanum if the drum is intact, and the leakage of blood or CSF from the external auditory canal if the drum has been perforated. Diagnosis is made by clinical exam, computed tomography scans, and magnetic resonance imaging. Management depends on the extent of the injuries, but is usually conservative initially unless the injury is associated with immediate facial paralysis.

Infections in the ear may result from sports activities or may affect the ability to participate in the sport. External otitis or "swimmer's ear" is an infection of the external ear canal.[26,31] It may occur when there is local trauma to the skin of the external canal or the ear is in a hot and humid environment. Water can be a source of bacteria.

Symptoms of an otitis externa include mild to severe pain in the canal, which often seems to worsen when pulling on the auricle; itching; a feeling of fullness; hearing loss; and enlarged lymph nodes in the periauricular region. Examination of the ear reveals erythema and edema of the external ear canal with a varying amount of white, yellow, green, or black debris. The external canal may swell shut. The infection can be caused by different types of bacteria, including *Pseudomonas aeruginosa* and *Staphylococcus aureus*, and various fungi. Otitis externa with fungal debris is seen in Figure 15-10. Management includes suctioning of debris and topical application of drops. Systemic antibiotics may be needed. A wick may be placed in the external canal if swelling is so severe that the drops cannot penetrate.

Otitis media, or middle ear infection, can occur independently or in association with an otitis externa. Otitis media is an inflammation of the tympanic membrane and middle ear mucosa. Symptoms include pain, hearing loss, possible otorrhea, and possible vertigo. Examination may show erythema and bulging of the tympanic membrane. Purulent drainage may be seen in the external canal. Management includes antibiotics and analgesia.

Serous otitis media can also occur. Serous otitis media is a collection of fluid behind the tympanic membrane.

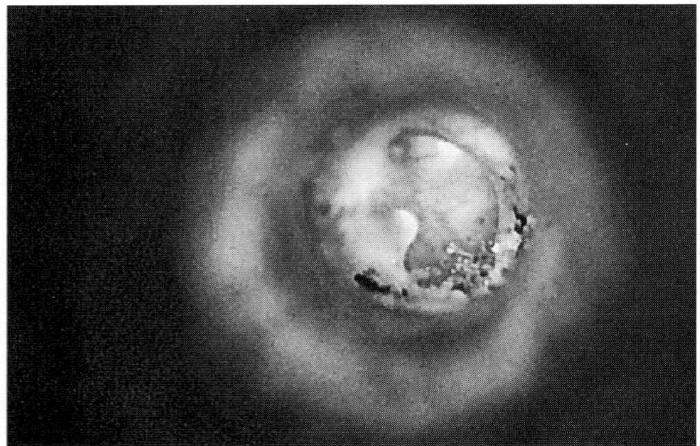

FIGURE 15-10. Otitis externa showing black fungal spores in the external auditory canal. (From Bull TR: A Color Atlas of E.N.T. Diagnosis, 2nd ed. London, Mosby-Wolfe, 1987.)

It is seen with or after acute otitis media and it is often seen with barotuma.

Labyrinthitis may result from infection of the inner ear. It is usually caused by a virus, but rarely it is caused by a bacterial infection. The condition causes vertigo in most patients, and it is almost always self-limited. Management includes antivertiginous medications, such as meclizine and valium, and supportive care.

Another swimming-related otologic problem is the development of external auditory canal exostoses, or bony swellings of the canal.[7,49] These are particularly associated with cold-water swimming, and are seen in swimmers, surfers, and skin and SCUBA divers. Usually asymptomatic, they can grow to the point where they occlude the canal sufficiently to cause a conductive hearing loss or predispose to external otitis. Treatment is surgical, and patients often require multiple procedures over time.

NASAL PROBLEMS

Like the external ear, the nose occupies a prominent, vulnerable position on the head and is the site of some common sports-related problems. External trauma to the nose often results in epistaxis.[11] Figures 15-11 and 15-12 illustrate nose anatomy and vascularity.

Most cases of bleeding cease spontaneously. Initial management is firm digital compression of the soft part of the nose for 5 to 10 minutes. Ice applied externally may be helpful for vasoconstriction. Topical vasoconstrictors such as phenylephrine-containing nasal sprays may be helpful. If bleeding occurs, the patient should lean forward to avoid swallowing the blood.

If bleeding continues, the nasal cavity must be examined to determine if the site of the bleeding is anterior or posterior. A majority of nose bleeds occur on the anterior septum from a group of vessels known as Kiesselbach's plexus. Anatomic deformities of the anterior septum, including septal deviation and spurs, may predispose to this problem. Allergies or upper respiratory infections may also be contributory. Nasal cautery using silver nitrate or electrocautery can control bleeding if the site is identified. Figure 15-13 shows an area of the septum cauterized with silver nitrate.

If the bleeding site is either not controlled well with cautery, is too posterior, or is not identifiable, nasal packing may be necessary. Different types of packing include Vaseline gauze strips, merocel packs, oxycel, and gelfoam. Significant bleeding may require the use of an inflatable pack. Posterior bleeds will require a posterior pack and hospitalization. Rarely, surgical ligation of the bleeding vessels is necessary. An algorithm to help guide the management of epistaxis is seen in Figure 15-14.

Nasal fractures are a common sports injury, and probably have been since ancient times.[23] Diagnosis is made by the occurrence of epistaxis, observed external

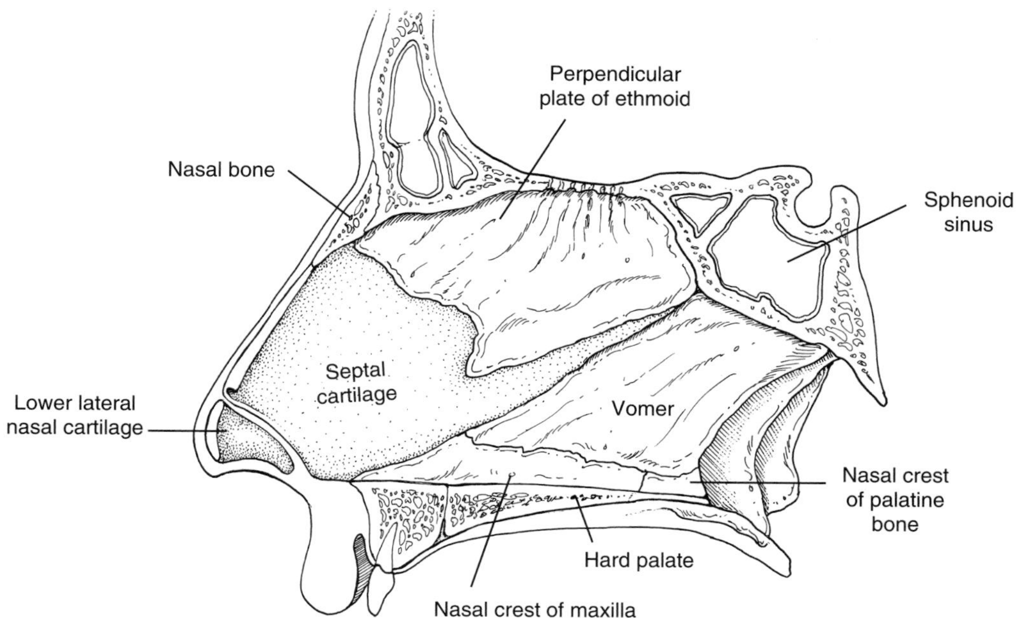

FIGURE 15-11. Anatomy of the nose.

displacement of the nasal bones, localized bone tenderness, obstruction of the nasal airway, deformity, or swelling of the septum. Figure 15-15 shows a fracture of the nasal bone.

Early treatment of the fracture is most important.[38] Ice should be applied immediately. The epistaxis must be controlled. Simple reduction of the fracture can be performed in the first 1 to 2 hours. After several hours, increased swelling occurs. To then perform an adequate reduction, a wait of 3 to 5 days until the swelling subsides is necessary. A closed reduction is possible within 7 to 10 days of the injury. After this time, healing has occurred, and a wait of at least 1 month is needed to do an open reduction of the fracture. Nasal fractures in children should be reduced within 4 days. A displaced nasal fracture has the best chance of healing if a closed

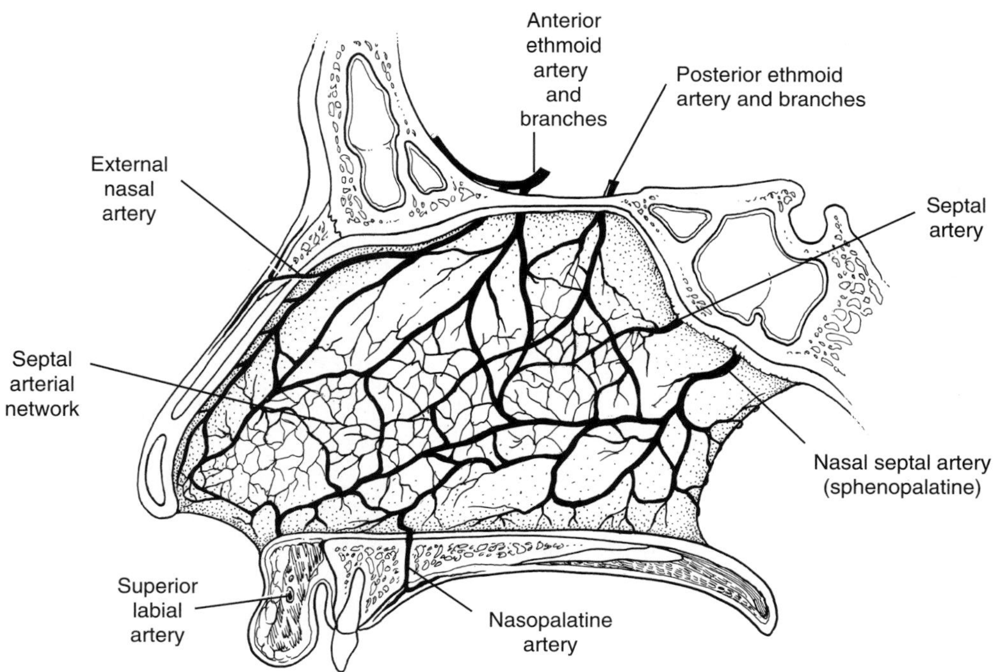

FIGURE 15-12. Vascularity of the nose.

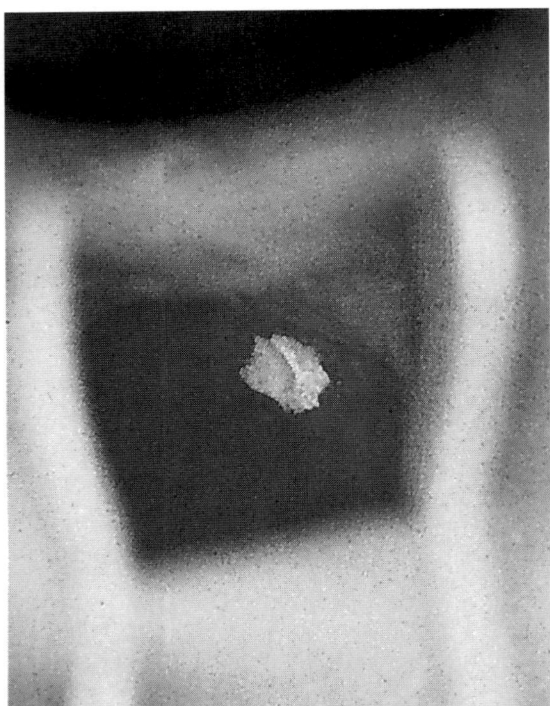

FIGURE 15-13. Nasal septum viewed after application of silver nitrate to a bleeding spot. (From Bull TR: A Color Atlas of E.N.T. Diagnosis, 2nd ed. London, Mosby-Wolfe, 1987.)

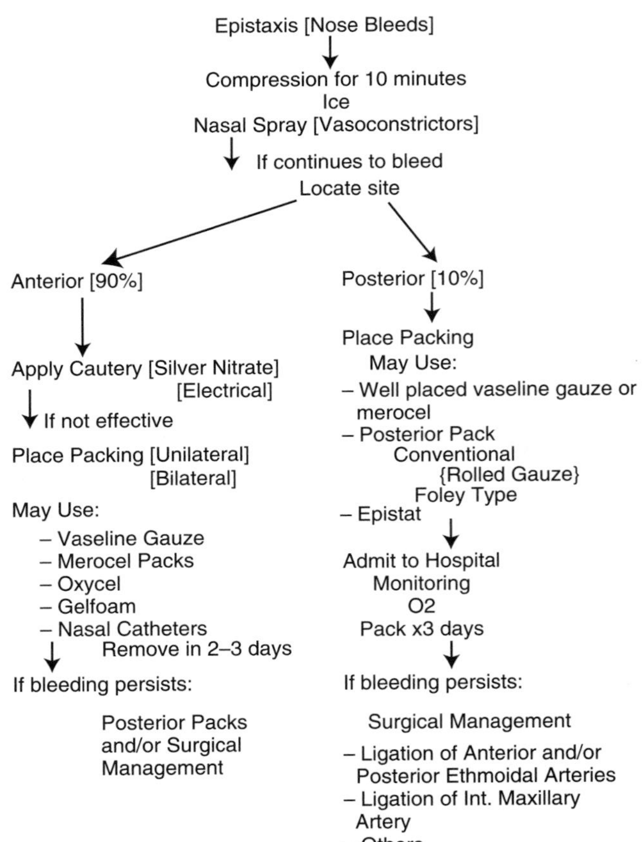

FIGURE 15-14. Algorithm for the management of nose bleeds.

reduction is performed. The reduction may be done under a local anesthesia or a general anesthesia. Children usually require a general anesthetic. Once the bones are realigned, it may be necessary to place external tape, a splint, or packing. In the case of a comminuted or compound fracture, an open reduction may be necessary in the early stages after the injury. Open techniques in children should be conservative.

If the force of impact is greatest over the nasal bridge, injury to the mid-nasal bone may occur. There is no effective way to perform a closed reduction on this type of injury. Callous formation may occur, and this would require open reduction, if so desired.

More extensive injury to the nasal region may cause fracture of the ethmoid bone or medial orbital wall.[13,39] Injury to the roof of the ethmoid or cribriform plate could potentially cause a cerebrospinal fluid leak or anosmia. One case of pneumocephalus has been reported after a water jet injury to the nose resulting from a water skiing fall.[8] Injury may occur to the nasolacrimal apparatus, leading to persistent tearing of the eye, or to the medial canthal tendon, leading to pseudohypertelorism.

In addition to nasal fractures, trauma to the nose may cause soft-tissue injuries. Contusions and abrasions require gentle cleansing. Band-Aid or Steri Strip application may be needed, with possible application of antibiotic ointment. Ice compresses may be useful to minimize swelling.

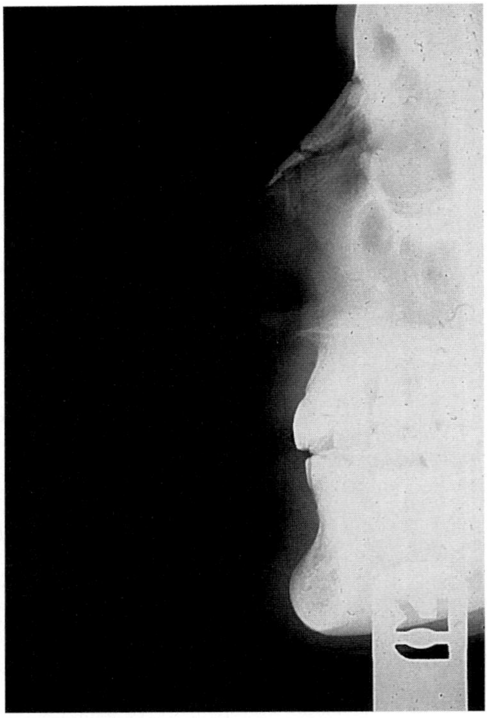

FIGURE 15-15. Nasal fracture of the mid-nasal bone with minimal displacement.

Laceration and avulsion injuries may occur. These must be inspected for underlying nasal skeletal injury, and careful cleansing and suturing may be necessary.

A study performed in Oxford, England, evaluating 50 consecutive children with nasal injuries revealed that 34% resulted from sports trauma.[9] Many of these injuries were abrasions or lacerations; however, 19 children did have skeletal injuries. Many of the fractures were of the greenstick variety and easily could have escaped diagnosis. In other fractures, there was little external deformity and a large disruption to the internal architecture. The study states the need for careful examination in children and adults when nasal injuries result from sports-related activities.

Another serious type of nasal injury is a septal hematoma, which may occur in conjunction with fractures or independently.[17] In this injury, blood collects between the septal cartilage or bone and their mucosal covering. The hematoma deprives the cartilage of the blood supply.

Examination of the nose if a hematoma is present may reveal edema and ecchymosis of the septum with narrowing of the airway, and bulging into the nasal cavity may be seen. There is usually no bleeding externally. Nasal obstruction is noted. The presence of septal hematoma requires emergency treatment. Prompt drainage should be performed by either needle aspiration or by an open procedure. Placement of a drain may be necessary, and packing may be placed, dependent on the extent of the condition. If the hematoma is not drained, a septal abscess may result, which can lead to necrosis of the septal cartilage and a subsequent saddle nose deformity.

Although septal hematomas are uncommon in children, when they do occur, they can cause devascularization of large segments of cartilage, on which the structural support and future nasal growth depend. Therefore, nasal injuries in children must be carefully examined to rule out this condition. Additionally, untreated septal abscess can provide an infectious focus which can progress to meningitis or cavernous sinus thrombosis.

Besides trauma, rhinitis is a very common nasal problem in sports and athletic events. Different types of nasal inflammation may be present and cause difficulties for the athlete. Rhinitis resulting from infection can cause nasal obstruction, nasal drainage, epistaxis, and headache. Allergic rhinitis may also cause these problems.

Vasomotor rhinitis can lead to persisting nasal drainage in the absence of infections or allergic symptoms. It can be controlled by ipatropium bromide (anticholinergic) nasal spray. Rhinitis medicamentosa, or rebound nasal congestion caused by topical decongestant abuse, causes nasal obstruction, dryness, and epistaxis. Nasal polyposis can cause obstruction of nasal breathing and predispose to infection. Mucosal atrophy caused by endocrinologic abnormalities or hormonal or drug effects can also cause nasal obstruction and dryness.

Changes in nasal anatomy and physiology caused by inflammation, infection, or other medical conditions may lead to difficulties in breathing, with a detrimental effect on the athlete's ability to perform.

In addition to the athlete's own anatomy and physiology, the environment in which he or she performs the sport may have a significant effect on the nose. Cold air, polluted air, and extreme temperature or weather changes may affect the nasal airway. Sulfates, ozone, and particulate matter can also cause irritation. Exposure to formaldehydes, glues, paints, cleaner, and vinyls such as may be found in gymnasiums may have detrimental effects. The athlete could subsequently develop a variety of problems, including rhinitis, sinusitis, nasal polyposis, eustachian tube dysfunction, and epistaxis.

Management of various forms of rhinitis may include the use of antihistamines, decongestants, cromolyn nasal sprays, steroid nasal sprays, and immunotherapy. Potential side effects must be considered when prescribing to the athlete.

Because nasal airflow in many individuals is limited by anatomic factors, one approach to improving athletic performance is the use of external nasal dilators, such as Breathe Right strips (CNS, Inc., Minneapolis, MN). Breathe Right is a rigid, drug-free strip that resembles an elongated butterfly-type bandage, and is illustrated in Figure 15-16. It is said to gently pull open the nasal passages, increasing the flow of oxygen to the lungs. The company claims that Breathe Right reduces nasal airway

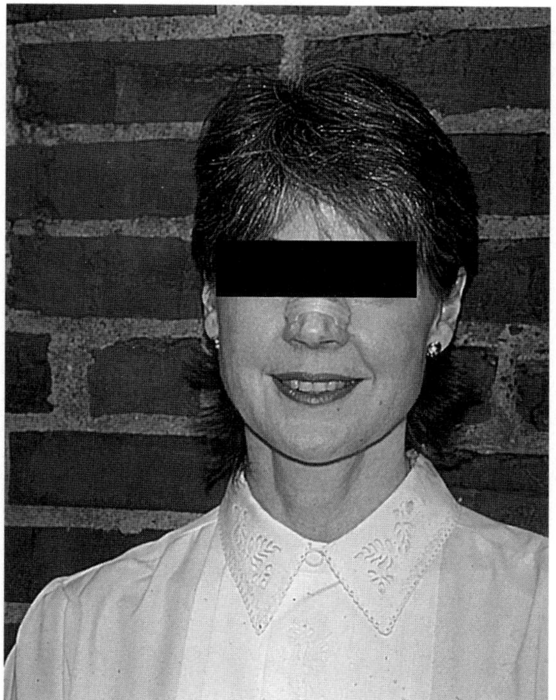

FIGURE 15-16. Photograph of a Breathe Right strip placed across the nasal dorsum.

resistance by up to 31%. Despite numerous studies, the efficacy of external nasal dilators remains controversial. Most studies demonstrate widening of the nasal valve and improved nasal airflow in at least some subjects, but fewer studies demonstrate reproducible decreases in exercise-related effort or objective physiologic improvements.[14,19,34,35,47,48]

THROAT AND LARYNX PROBLEMS

Although the throat is rarely involved in sports-related injuries, infection of the throat or tonsils, with its accompanying pain and fever, can be detrimental to an athlete's performance. Laryngitis can impair communication with teammates or peers.

However, the larynx, due to its anterior and somewhat prominent location, is vulnerable to sports-related injuries. The shield-like effect of the thyroid cartilage, which protects the larynx, can be overcome with application of enough force, resulting in blunt or penetrating laryngeal injuries. The evaluation and treatment of suspected laryngeal trauma must be expeditious because these injuries are associated with a high incidence of airway instability.[12,20,41]

Blunt trauma to the larynx occurs most frequently in high-velocity sports such as hockey, bicycling, and motorcycling. Direct trauma can actually crush the larynx and upper trachea, causing neck pain, odynophagia, and dyspnea. Even in a simpler laryngeal fracture, pain, tenderness, and swelling over the anterior neck can occur. Figure 15-17 shows a tracheal cartilage fracture. In a simple fracture or a crush injury, hemoptysis, hoarseness, aphonia, or odynophonia (pain with speaking) may occur. Examination of the neck may reveal ecchymosis or crepitus of the neck. There may be absence or blunting of the laryngeal prominence (Adam's apple) with injury of the thyroid cartilage or underlying structures.

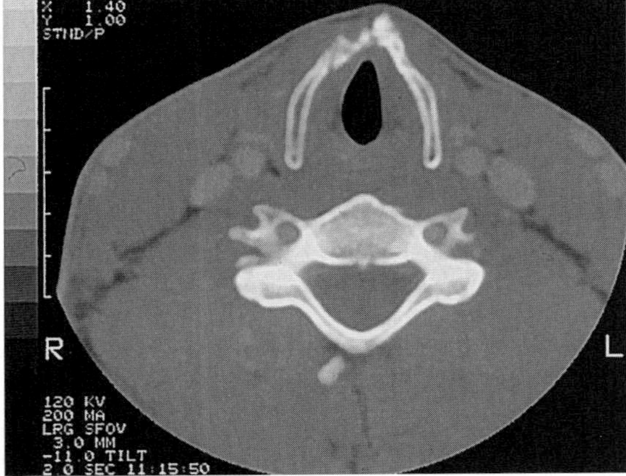

FIGURE 15-17. Comminuted fracture of the tracheal cartilage. This patient also suffered a hemorrhage of his underlying vocal cord.

Any injury to this area requires immediate examination. Initial evaluation must rule out airway obstruction. It may be necessary to intubate or perform a tracheostomy, with tracheostomy preferred in the case of severe or potentially unstable injury. Even an initially stable-appearing airway can be lost rapidly, so injuries suspicious for laryngeal injury should be expeditiously transferred to a medical facility. Radiographs can help evaluate the extent of the injury. Plain films may give some useful information, but computed tomography scans will be needed for more detail and surgical road mapping. The throat and larynx must be visualized by fiberoptic laryngoscopy to look for mucosal tears, bleeding, and submucosal contusions or hematomas. Patients must be closely observed for development of airway obstruction of gradual onset.

Management of a nondisplaced fracture is observation. More severe injuries may require thorough endoscopy and open repair of the laryngeal framework.

Penetrating trauma to the larynx falls under the category of "freak accidents" in sport events. The trauma may be accompanied by neck pain, dysphagia, dyspnea, crepitus, hemoptysis, or a change in the voice. Immediate management includes a careful check of the airway, clearing the airway of secretions, and performing lateral neck radiographs. Additional management may involve observation, endoscopy, CT evaluation, angiography, or surgical exploration and subsequent repair, as in the management of blunt laryngeal trauma. An algorithm for the management of airway obstruction from either blunt or penetrating trauma is seen in Figure 15-18.

Laryngeal trauma can cause a vocal fold hematoma/hemorrhage or vocal fold tear. This could also occur from excessive yelling. Examination would include flexible and/or rigid laryngoscopy with possible stroboscopy. Management may include the need for vocal rest until the abnormal condition resolves.

An unusual but potentially significant problem that can limit athletic performance is exercise-induced laryngomalacia.[2,45] During vigorous exercise, the speed and force of airflow through the glottis is increased to allow respiration to keep up with metabolic demands. In some children and young adults, laryngeal tissues may deform excessively during strenuous exercise, causing airway obstruction and exercise limitation. Inability to recognize this condition may result in the diagnosis of exercise-induced asthma in patients without reactive airway disease. Endoscopic laryngeal surgery to ablate redundant tissues may increase exercise tolerance.[4]

NECK INJURIES

Sports-related injuries to the neck range from superficial ones to those that are potentially life-threatening. Minor abrasions or lacerations may result from blunt trauma, requiring simple local first-aid. A hematoma can occur,

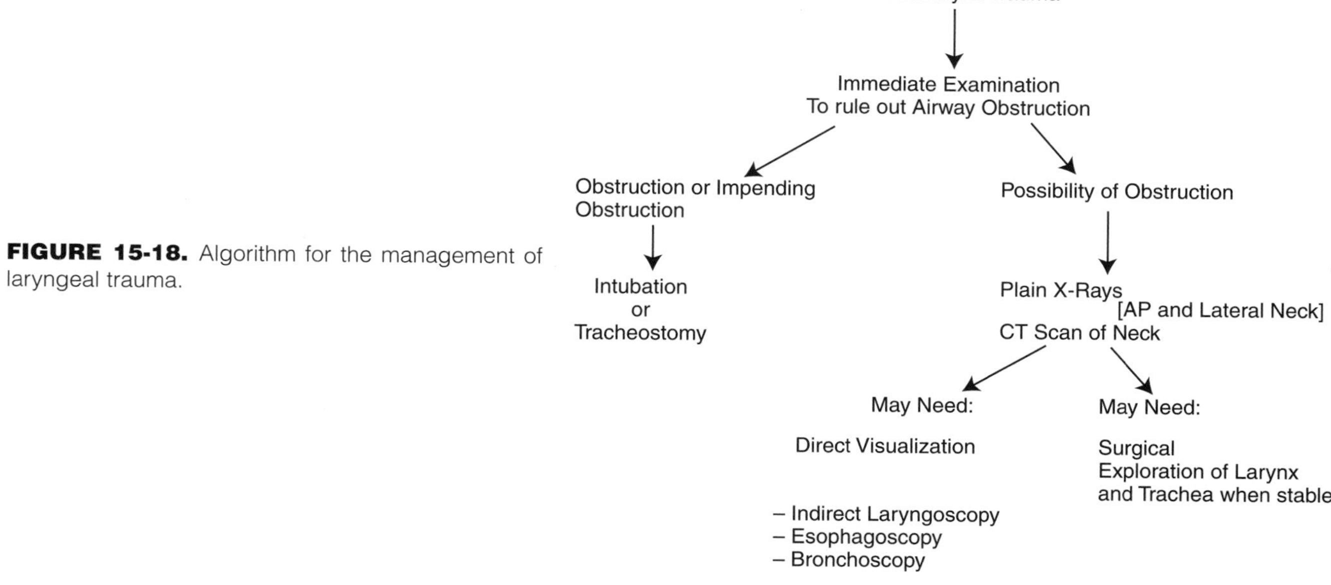

FIGURE 15-18. Algorithm for the management of laryngeal trauma.

causing pain, swelling, and ecchymoses. Although most of these are self-limited, some may enlarge progressively. Persistent hemorrhage resulting from bleeding from a large vessel can cause progressive airway obstruction or vascular compression, and intubation or tracheotomy may be needed to protect the airway. Severe or expanding hematomas may require angiography to localize a bleeding source, and control may require interventional radiology consultation, or surgical exploration and vessel ligation. Potential complications include cranial nerve deficits and the formation of arteriovenous fistulas.

Penetrating trauma to the neck during sports injuries is very rare. Immediate evaluation of the airway is mandatory, and neurologic evaluation is important.[22,30,46] If there is significant injury to the vasculature of the neck, excessive hemorrhage, absent pulses, and an expanding neck mass may be seen. Management includes pressure to the bleeding site, an angiogram, and probable surgical exploration. Although traditionally any penetrating injury of the neck that extends deep to the platysma muscle is explored surgically, selective observation of some injuries is an emerging management strategy.

SPECIAL PROBLEMS ASSOCIATED WITH SCUBA AND SKIN DIVING

Most health problems arising during skin and SCUBA diving are directly or indirectly caused by the elevation in water pressure that occurs with increasing depth below the water's surface. Since air is compressible but solid and liquid tissue are not, it is the air-containing spaces of the body—particularly the ear and paranasal sinuses—that are most commonly subject to diving-related injury.

The majority of injuries involve the ear, which contains a large air-filled space (the middle ear and mastoid) and fragile moving parts. Under normal conditions, pressure differences between the middle ear and the ambient environment are equalized through the eustachian tube. However, when eustachian function is impaired, or when divers fail to actively utilize the eustachian tube to equalize pressure during descent, barotrauma may result. The most common barotrauma-related complaint is "middle ear squeeze" caused by relative negative pressure in the middle ear when pressure is not adequately equalized during descent.[36] Although pain will cause many divers to abort their dive within a few feet of the water's surface, continued descent can result in severe otalgia, conductive hearing loss, sensation of aural fullness, and dizziness, and can progress to perforation of the tympanic membrane. These symptoms can usually be avoided by actively equalizing middle ear pressure through periodic autoinsufflation during descent, and by not diving when suffering from an upper respiratory infection or uncontrolled allergies. Some prophylactic benefit may be obtained by judicious use of topical nasal (oxymetazolin) or systemic (pseudoephedrine) decongestants, but all new medicines should receive an initial trial on nondiving days.[6] Some dive masters advise against ever using a systemic medication.

If the eustachian tube remains blocked, symptoms can persist after diving, although they are usually mild if the tympanic membrane has not ruptured. On physical exam, the eardrum may appear retracted and hyperemic if intact, and hemotympanum may be observed due to hemorrhage within the middle ear space. Most cases will resolve spontaneously, or respond to topical nasal or systemic decongestants and gentle autoinsufflation (accomplished by pinching the nose shut and gently performing a Valsalva maneuver). Refractory cases, or those associated with persistent serous effusion of the middle ear, may require myringotomy with or without pressure equalization tubes. Small perforations will usually resolve spontaneously if the patient keeps the ear dry and refrains from diving; they infrequently require surgical repair.

Even in the presence of a functioning eustachian tube, impacted cerumen or the use of earplugs may cause "canal squeeze" when air trapped in the external auditory canal between the plug and the intact eardrum fails to equalize pressure while diving. This creates a relative negative pressure in the external auditory canal, causing edema and bullae formation of the external canal skin and tympanic membrane. This may progress to hemorrhage of the external canal, and may infrequently cause tympanic membrane rupture. Usually no treatment is required except to refrain from swimming and diving until the canal skin has had time to heal, to avoid opportunistic external otitis. The condition is easily avoided by refraining from using earplugs, and removing impacted cerumen prior to diving.

A more serious problem is barotrauma to the delicate inner ear, which may be caused by implosive or explosive forces acting on the oval or round windows during descent or during forceful attempts to equalize middle ear pressure.[36,42,43] Acute injury may cause a perilymph fistula, with associated hearing loss, vertigo (often associated with nausea and vomiting), and tinnitus. Inner ear barotrauma may be distinguished from middle ear or external canal injury by featuring vertigo as a prominent symptom and a sensorineural pattern of hearing loss on audiogram. Otoscopic appearance of the tympanic membrane can be normal if concomitant damage to the middle ear or external canal has not occurred. Inner ear decompression sickness also may present as sensorineural hearing loss, vertigo, and tinnitus (see the following paragraphs). Since the systemic complications of decompression sickness may be life-threatening, these symptoms should be treated as initial signs of decompression sickness when they occur after dives deep enough to require staged decompression (see the following paragraphs). Treatment of traumatic perilymphatic fistula is described above in the section on injuries to the ear. Although many fistulas will close with 7 to 10 days of conservative treatment, those that do not may require surgery. In addition to acute injury to the inner ear, a number of studies, mostly of professional divers, suggest that repeated diving may be a risk factor for insidious high-frequency sensorineural hearing loss.[21,27,44]

Decompression sickness is not caused by barotrauma, but by the increased solubility of nitrogen gas in blood and tissue as water pressure increases during descent. During ascent, depressurization reverses this phenomenon, allowing nitrogen gas to leave supersaturated tissues and form bubbles in tissue and blood. These bubbles can occlude the microvasculature and cause injury to the joints, lungs, central nervous system, and inner ear.[29,43] Symptoms of decompression sickness may be mild or severe, and can occur at variable times after surfacing, although they will usually occur within several hours of diving. Symptoms can include arthralgias, headache, staggering gate, change in mental status, parasthesias, lumbar and abdominal pain, and stroke-like neurologic deficits. Less frequently, pulmonary involvement can cause chest pain, dyspnea, and catastrophic cardiopulmonary collapse. Inner ear manifestations of decompression sickness are as described in the preceding paragraphs, and may be reversible or may leave the diver with residual deficits after recovery. Inner ear decompression sickness may be significantly more common in divers with a patent foramen ovale.[15] The cornerstone of treatment of decompression sickness is cardiopulmonary support as needed, provision of fluids and oxygen, and expeditious transportation to a hyperbaric oxygen chamber.[28] Decompression sickness is observed only after SCUBA, never after skin diving.

Alternobaric vertigo is caused by unequal pressure within the right and left middle ear spaces during ascent or descent, and results in vertigo (usually lasting less than 10 minutes) without tinnitus or hearing loss. A similar syndrome may be seen in those diving in cold water while wearing a hood that allows unequal amounts of cold water to reach the left and right external auditory canal, causing caloric vertigo and nystagmus. Both these types of vertigo usually resolve spontaneously—their primary significance is that dizziness of any cause underwater may be disorienting and dangerous.

Diving-related injury to the paranasal sinuses is much less common than otologic injury.[3,37] A condition analogous to middle ear squeeze, known as *sinus squeeze*, may occur when a sinus ostium becomes totally occluded, preventing equalization of pressure within the sinus lumen. Relative negative pressure then causes edema and hemorrhage of the sinus mucosa. Symptoms include sensation of facial pain and pressure, and may include numbness of the face or upper teeth; they will generally resolve after the dive is terminated. Conditions predisposing to blockage of the sinus ostia include upper respiratory infection, allergies, nasal polyps, preexisting sinus disease or structural abnormality, and nasal septal deviation. Medical or surgical treatment of these conditions may be required before diving can be resumed.

Epistaxis during diving is common and is thought to be due to pressure differences which traumatize fragile vessels in the nasal septum. It usually resolves spontaneously, or with external compression of the nose, and is rarely serious.[36]

An excellent synopsis of otorhinolaryngology pertinent to skin and SCUBA diving is provided by Reuter.[36] Diving-related medical information, including the location of the nearest decompression chamber, can be obtained from the Divers Alert Network provided by the Duke University Medical Center (919-684-8111).

SUMMARY

Otorhinolaryngology is an important area in the vast field of sports medicine. Injuries and illnesses of the ears, nose, throat, and neck can significantly impair athletic performance. The relative prominence of these structures makes them common sites of sports-related trauma. Primary care physicians, otorhinolaryngologists, orthopedists, and others who care for these athletes must work together to provide comprehensive medical care.

REFERENCES

1. Alvi A, Bereliani AT: Trauma to the temporal bone: Diagnosis and management of complications. J Craniomaxillofac Trauma 2(3):36–48, 1996.
2. Beaty MM, Wilson JS, Smith RJ: Laryngeal motion during exercise. Laryngoscope 109(1):136–139, 1999.
3. Becker GD, Parell GJ: Barotrauma of the ears and sinuses after scuba diving. Eur Arch Otorhinolaryngol 258(4):159–163, 2001.
4. Bent JP 3rd, et al: Pediatric exercise-induced laryngomalacia. Ann Otol Rhinol Laryngol 105(3): 169–175, 1996.
5. Berger G, Finkelstein Y, Harell M: Non-explosive blast injury of the ear. J Laryngol Otol 108(5): 395–398, 1994.
6. Brown M, Jones J, Krohmer J: Pseudoephedrine for the prevention of barotitis media: a controlled clinical trial in underwater divers. Ann Emer Med 21(7):849–852, 1992.
7. Chaplin JM, Stewart IA: The prevalence of exostoses in the external auditory meatus of surfers. Clin Otolaryngol 23(4):326–330, 1998.
8. David, SK Jr, Guarisco JL, Coulon RA Jr: Pneumocephalus secondary to a high-pressure water injury to the nose. Arch Otolaryngol Head Neck Surg 116(12):1435–1436, 1990.
9. East CA O'Donaghue G: Acute nasal trauma in children. J Pediatr Surg 22(4):308–310, 1987.
10. Fitzgerald DC: Head trauma: Hearing loss and dizziness. J Trauma 40(3):488–496, 1996.
11. Frazee TA, Hauser MS: Nonsurgical management of epistaxis. J Oral Maxillofac Surg 58(4):419–424, 2000.
12. Fuhrman GM, Stieg FH 3rd, Buerk CA: Blunt laryngeal trauma: Classification and management protocol. J Trauma 30(1):87–92, 1990.
13. Gaboriau HP, McDonald WD: Management of orbital fractures. J La State Med Soc 148(6): 241–243, 1996.
14. Gehring JM, et al: Nasal resistance and flow resistive work of nasal breathing during exercise: Effects of a nasal dilator strip. J Appl Physiol 89(3):1114–1122, 2000.
15. Germonpre P, et al: Patent foramen ovale and decompression sickness in sports divers. J Appl Physiol 84(5):1622–1626, 1998.
16. Giffin CS: Wrestler's ear: Pathophysiology and treatment. Ann Plast Surg 28(2):131–139, 1992.
17. Ginsburg CM: Nasal septal hematoma. Pediatr Rev 19(4):142–143, 1998.
18. Glasscock ME 3rd, et al: Traumatic perilymphatic fistula: How long can symptoms persist? A follow-up report. Am J Otol 13(4):333–338, 1992.
19. Griffin JW, et al: Physiologic effects of an external nasal dilator. Laryngoscope 107(9):1235–1238, 1997.
20. Hanft K, et al: Diagnosis and management of laryngeal trauma in sports. South Med J 89(6):631–633, 1996.
21. Haraguchi H, et al: Progressive sensorineural hearing impairment in professional fishery divers. Ann Otol Rhinol Laryngol 108(12):1165–1169, 1999.
22. Hersman G, et al: The management of penetrating neck injuries. Int Surg 86(2):82–89, 2001.
23. Lascaratos JG, et al: From the roots of rhinology: The reconstruction of nasal injuries by Hippocrates. Ann Otol Rhinol Laryngol 112(2):159–162, 2003.
24. Lee D, Sperling N: Initial management of auricular trauma. Am Fam Physician 53(7): 2339–2344, 1996.
25. Maitland CG: Perilymphatic fistula. Curr Neurol Neurosci Rep 1(5):486–491, 2001.
26. Mirza N: Otitis externa. Management in the primary care office. Postgrad Med 99(5):153–154, 157–158, 1996.
27. Molvaer OI, Lehmann EH: Hearing acuity in professional divers. Undersea Biomed Res 12(3): 333–349, 1985.
28. Moon RE: Treatment of diving emergencies. Critical Care Clinics 15(2):429–456, 1999.
29. Nachum Z, et al: Inner ear decompression sickness in sport compressed-air diving. Laryngoscope 111(5):851–856, 2001.
30. Nason RW, et al: Penetrating neck injuries: Analysis of experience from a Canadian trauma centre. Can J Surg 44(2):122–126, 2001.
31. Nichols AW: Nonorthopaedic problems in the aquatic athlete. Clin Sports Med 18(2):395–411, viii, 1999.
32. Nosan DK, Benecke JE Jr, Murr AH: Current perspective on temporal bone trauma. Otolaryngol Head Neck Surg 117(1):67–71, 1997.
33. Ohlsen L, Skoog T, Sohn SA: The pathogenesis of cauliflower ear. An experimental study in rabbits. Scand J Plast Reconstr Surg 9(1):34–39, 1975.
34. O'Kroy JA, et al: Effects of an external nasal dilator on the work of breathing during exercise. Med Sci Sports Exerc 33(3):454–458, 2001.

35. O'Kroy JA: Oxygen uptake and ventilatory effects of an external nasal dilator during ergometry. Med Sci Sports Exerc 32(8):1491–1495, 2000.
36. Reuter SH: Underwater medicine: Otolaryngologic considerations of the skin and scuba diver. In Paparella, MM (ed): Philadelphia, Saunders, pp 3231–3257.
37. Roydhouse N: 1001 disorders of the ear, nose and sinuses in scuba divers. Can J Appl Sport Sci 10(2):99–103, 1985.
38. Rubinstein B, Strong EB: Management of nasal fractures. Arch Fam Med 9(8):738–742, 2000.
39. Sargent LA Rogers GF: Nasoethmoid orbital fractures: Diagnosis and management. J Craniomaxillofac Trauma 5(1):19–27, 1999.
40. Sarti EL, Lucenti FE: Ear trauma. In Lucente FE, Sotol SM (eds): Essential Otolaryngology. New York, Raven Press, 1988.
41. Schaefer SD: The acute management of external laryngeal trauma. A 27-year experience. Arch Otolaryngol Head Neck Surg 118(6):598–604, 1992.
42. Sheridan MF, Hetherington HH, Hull JJ: Inner ear barotrauma from scuba diving. Ear, Nose & Throat J 78(3):181, 184, 186–187, 1999.
43. Shupak A, et al: Diving-related inner ear injuries. Laryngoscope 101(2):173, 1991.
44. Skogstad M, Haldorsen T, Arnesen AR: Auditory function among young occupational divers: a 3-year follow-up study. Scand Audiol 29(4):245–252, 2000.
45. Smith RJ, et al: Exercise-induced laryngomalacia. Ann Otol Rhinol Laryngol 104(7):537–541, 1995.
46. Tariq M, et al: Penetrating neck injury: Case report and evaluation of management. J Laryngol Otol 114(7):554–556, 2000.
47. Tong TK, Fu FH, Chow BC: Effect of nostril dilatation on prolonged all-out intermittent exercise performance. J Sports Med Phys Fitness 41(2):189–195, 2001.
48. Tong TK, Fu FH, Chow BC: Nostril dilatation increases capacity to sustain moderate exercise under nasal breathing condition. J Sports Med Phys Fitness 41(4):470–478, 2001.
49. Whitaker SR, et al: Treatment of external auditory canal exostoses. Laryngoscope 108(2):195–199, 1998.

16 The Cervical Spine, Spinal Cord, and Brachial Plexus

Joseph S. Torg

This chapter will present clear, concise guidelines for the classification, evaluation, and management of athletic injuries that occur to the cervical spine, spinal cord, and brachial plexus. Although all athletic injuries require careful attention, evaluation and management of these injuries require particular caution. The actual or potential involvement of the nervous system creates a potentially high-risk situation in which the margin for error is low. An accurate diagnosis is imperative because the clinical picture is not always representative of the potential seriousness of the problem. In general, athletic injuries to the cervical spine, spinal cord, and brachial plexus can be classified into two major groups: 1) catastrophic and potentially catastrophic, or those injuries in which permanent neurologic sequelae is a major factor; and 2) noncatastrophic, or those in which the major problem is the potential for chronic nonneurologic disability.

EMERGENCY MANAGEMENT

There are several principles that should be considered by those responsible for athletes who may sustain injuries to cervical spine and spinal cord.

1. The team physician or trainer should be designated as the person responsible for supervising on-the-field management of a potentially serious injury. This person is the "captain" of the medical team.
2. Planning must ensure the availability of all necessary emergency equipment at the site of potential injury. At a minimum, a spineboard, stretcher, and equipment necessary for the initiation and maintenance of cardiopulmonary resuscitation should be included.
3. Planning must ensure the availability of a properly equipped ambulance and a hospital equipped and staffed to handle emergency neurologic problems.
4. Planning must ensure immediate availability of a telephone for communicating with the hospital emergency room, ambulance, and other responsible individuals in case of an emergency.

Treating the spine-injured athlete is a process that should not be done hastily or haphazardly. Being prepared to handle this situation is the best way to prevent actions that could convert a repairable injury into a catastrophe. The necessary equipment should be readily accessible, in good operating condition, and all assisting personnel should be trained to use it properly. On-the-job training in an emergency situation is inefficient. Everyone should know what must be done beforehand, so that on a signal the "game plan" can be put into effect.

A means of transporting the athlete must be immediately available in a high-risk sport such as football and on call in other sports. The medical facility must be alerted to the athlete's condition and estimated time of arrival so that adequate preparation can be made.

Having the proper equipment is essential. A spineboard is necessary and is the best means of supporting the body in a rigid position. It is essentially a full-body splint. By splinting the body, the risk of aggravating a spinal cord injury, which must always be suspected in the unconscious athlete, is reduced. In football, bolt cutters and a sharp knife or scalpel are also essential in case it becomes necessary to remove the face mask. A telephone must be available to call for assistance and to notify the medical facility. Oxygen should be available and is usually carried by ambulance and rescue squads, although it is rarely required in an athletic setting. Rigid cervical collars and other external immobilization devices can be helpful if properly used. Manual stabilization of the head and neck is recommended if other means are not available.

Properly trained personnel must know who is in charge. Everyone should know how to perform cardiopulmonary resuscitation and how to move and transport the athlete. Personnel should know where emergency equipment is located, how to use it, and the procedure for activating the emergency support system. Individuals should be assigned specific tasks beforehand so that duplication of effort is eliminated. Being well prepared helps to alleviate indecisiveness and second-guessing.

Prevention of further injury is the single most important objective. Any action that could possibly cause further injury should not be taken. The first step should be to immobilize the head and neck by supporting them in a stable position, and then, in the following order, check for breathing, pulse, and level of consciousness (Fig. 16-1).

If the victim is breathing, the mouthguard should be removed, if present, and the airway maintained. It is necessary to remove the face mask only if the respiratory situation is threatened or unstable or if the athlete remains unconscious for a prolonged period. The chin strap should be left on.

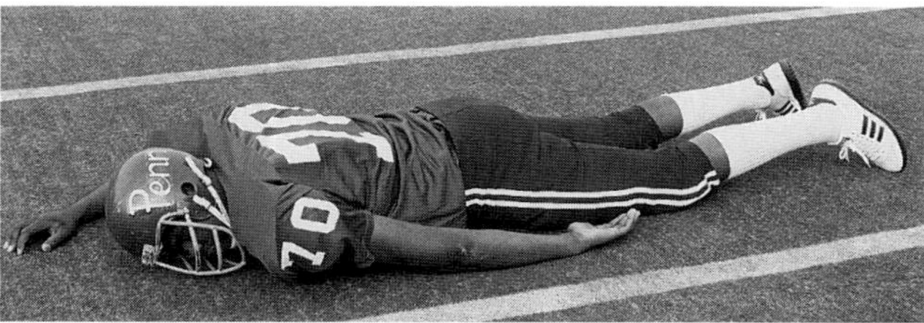

A

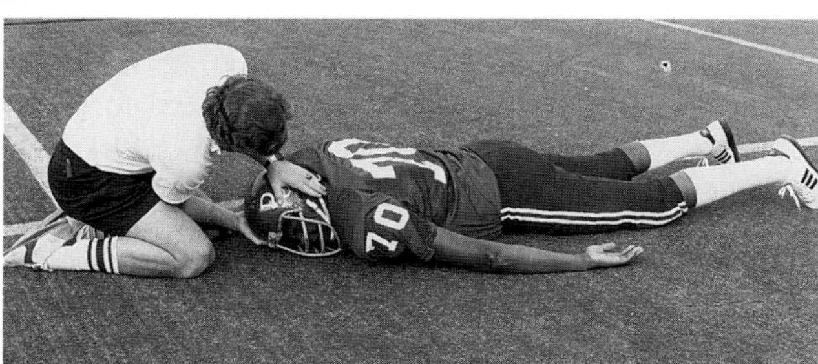

B

FIGURE 16-1. A, Athlete with suspected cervical spine injury may or may not be unconscious. However, those who are unconscious should be treated as though they had a significant neck injury. **B,** Immediate manual immobilization of the head and neck unit. First, check for breathing. (From Torg JS [ed]: Athletic Injuries to the Head, Neck and Face. Philadelphia, Mosby–Year Book, 1991.)

Once it is established that the athlete is breathing and has a pulse, neurologic status should be evaluated. The level of consciousness, response to pain, pupillary response, and unusual posturing, flaccidity, rigidity, or weakness should be noted.

At this point, the situation should be maintained until transportation is available. If the athlete is face down, change his or her position to face up by logrolling him or her onto a spineboard (Fig. 16-2). Gentle longitudinal traction should be exerted to support the head without attempting to correct alignment, and no attempt should be made to remove the helmet. There is controversy between emergency medicine physicians and technicians on one hand and team physicians and athletic trainers on the other; existing emergency medical services guidelines mandate removal of protective headgear before transport of an individual suspected of having a cervical spine injury. These guidelines were implemented with full-face motorcycle helmets in mind to facilitate airway accessibility and application of cervical spine–immobilizing devices. Such a procedure contradicts the long-standing principle adhered to by team physicians and athletic trainers of leaving the helmet in place on the football player suspected of having a cervical spine injury until he or she is transported to a definitive medical facility. It must be emphasized that this particular problem is of more than academic interest. Specifically, there have been occasions when emergency medical technicians

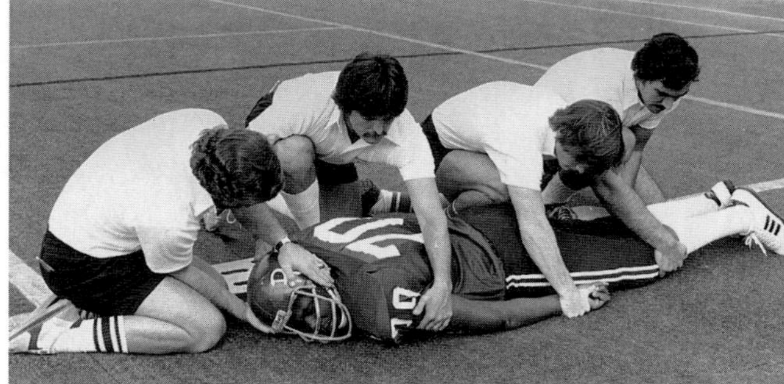

A

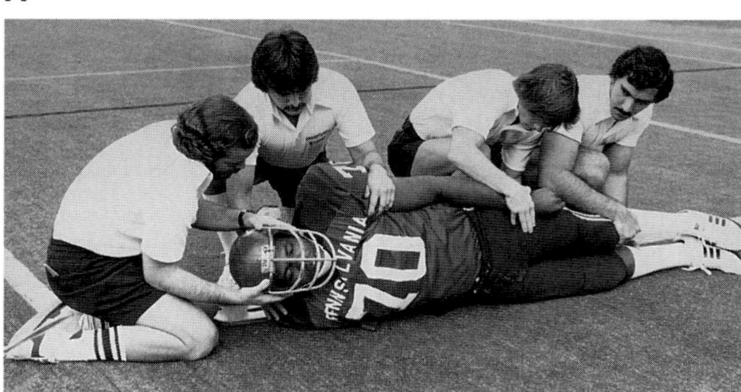

B

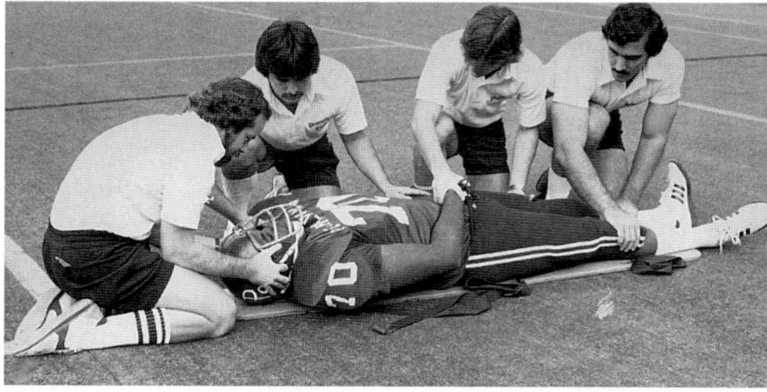

C

FIGURE 16-2. Logroll to a spine board. **A,** This maneuver requires four individuals: the leader to immobilize the head and neck and to command the medical support team, and three individuals who are positioned at the shoulders, hips, and lower legs. **B,** The leader uses the crossed-arm technique to immobilize the head. This technique allows the leader's arms to "unwind" as the three assistants roll the athlete onto the spine board. **C,** The three assistants maintain body alignment during the roll. (From Torg JS [ed]: Athletic Injuries to the Head, Neck and Face. Philadelphia, Mosby–Year Book, 1991.)

under the direction of the emergency room physicians unfamiliar with the nuances of the relationship between helmet, shoulder pads, and the injured cervical spine have precipitated on-site turf battles by refusing to move the injured player before helmet removal. Such episodes represent more than an honest difference of opinion and are clearly detrimental to the well-being of the injured player. It is the view of this author that removal of the football helmet and shoulder pads on-site exposes the potentially injured spine to unnecessary and awkward manipulation and disruption of the immobilizing capacity of the helmet and shoulder pads. Also, removal of the helmet subjects a potentially unstable spine to a hyperlordotic deformity. If there are no problems with respiration, the helmet of a football player suspected of having a cervical spine injury should remain on until he or she reaches a definitive medical facility.

If the athlete is not breathing or stops breathing, the airway must be established. If face down, he or she must be brought to a face-up position. The safest and easiest way to accomplish this is to logroll the athlete into a face-up position. In an ideal situation, the medical support team has five members: the leader, who controls the head and gives the commands only; three members to roll; and one to help lift and carry when necessary. If time permits and the spineboard is on the scene, the athlete should be rolled directly onto it. However, breathing and circulation are more important at this point.

With all medical support team members in position, the athlete is rolled toward the assistants—one at the shoulders, one at the hips, and one at the knees. They must maintain the body in line with the head and spine during the roll. The leader maintains immobilization of the head by applying slight traction and by using the crossed-arm technique. This technique allows the arms to unwind during the roll (see Fig. 16-2).

The face mask must be removed from the helmet before rescue breathing can be initiated. The type of mask that is attached to the helmet determines the method of removal. Bolt cutters are used with the older single- and double-bar masks. The newer masks that are attached with plastic loops should be removed by cutting the loops with a sharp knife or scalpel, and the entire mask should be removed so that it does not interfere with further rescue efforts.

Once the athlete has been moved to a face-up position, breathing and pulse should be evaluated quickly. If there is still no breathing or if breathing has stopped, the airway must be established. The jaw-thrust technique is the safest first approach to open the airway of a victim who has a suspected neck injury because, in most cases, it can be accomplished by the rescuer grasping the angles of the victim's lower jaw and lifting with both hands, one on each side, displacing the mandible forward while tilting the head backward. The rescuer's elbows should rest on the surface on which the victim is lying.

If the jaw-thrust is not adequate, the head tilt–jaw lift should be substituted. Care must be exercised not to overextend the neck. The fingers of one hand are placed under the lower jaw on the bony part near the chin and lifted to bring the chin forward, which supports the jaw and helps to tilt the head back. The fingers must not compress the soft tissue under the chin, which might obstruct the airway. The other hand presses on the victim's forehead to tilt the head back.

The transportation team should be familiar with handling a victim with a cervical spine injury, and they should be receptive to taking orders from the team physician or trainer. It is extremely important not to lose control of the athlete's care; therefore, the team physician or trainer should be familiar with the transportation crew that is used. In an athletic situation, arrangements with an ambulance service should be made before the event.

Lifting and carrying the athlete requires five individuals: four to lift, and the leader to maintain immobilization of the head. The leader initiates all actions with clear, loud, verbal commands (Fig. 16-3).

The same guidelines apply to the choice of a medical facility as to the choice of an ambulance; it should be equipped and staffed to handle an emergency head or neck injury. There should be a neurosurgeon and an orthopedic surgeon to meet the athlete on arrival. Radiographic facilities should be standing by.

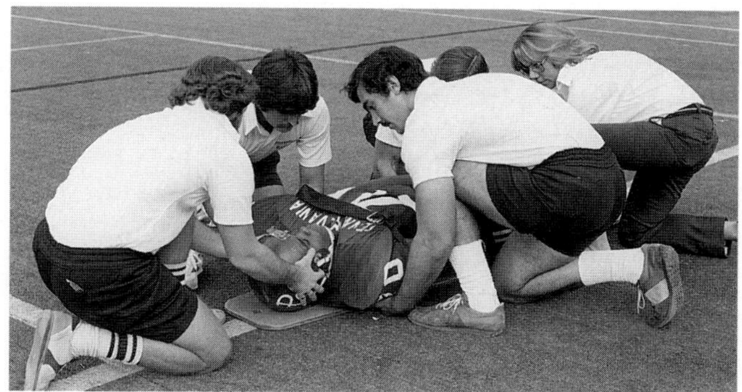

A

B

FIGURE 16-3. A and **B,** Four members of the medical support team lift the athlete on the command of the leader. The leader maintains manual immobilization of the head. The spineboard is not recommended as a stretcher. An additional stretcher should be used for transporting over long distances. (From Torg JS [ed]: Athletic Injuries to the Head, Neck and Face. Philadelphia, Mosby–Year Book, 1991.)

Once the athlete is in a medical facility and permanent immobilization measures are instituted, the helmet is removed. The chin strap may be unfastened and discarded. The athlete's head is supported at the occiput by one person while the leader spreads the earflaps and pulls the helmet off in a straight line with the spine (Fig. 16-4).

Despite the advent of such high-tech imaging modalities as computed axial tomography and magnetic resonance imaging, the initial radiographic examination of a patient with suspected or actual cervical spine trauma remains routine. The preliminary study, while immobilization of the head, neck, and trunk are maintained, includes an anteroposterior and lateral examination of C1–C7. If a major fracture, subluxation, dislocation, or evidence of instability is not evident, the remainder of the routine examination, including open mouth and oblique views, should be obtained. Depending on the neurologic and comfort status of the patient, lateral flexion and extension views should be obtained at some point. Computed tomography and magnetic resonance imaging may provide more detailed information, although horizontally oriented fractures and subtle subluxation are best identified on the routine radiographs. The choice of imaging technique will depend on the results of routine examination, neurologic status of the patient, preference of the responsible physician, and availability of the imaging modalities.

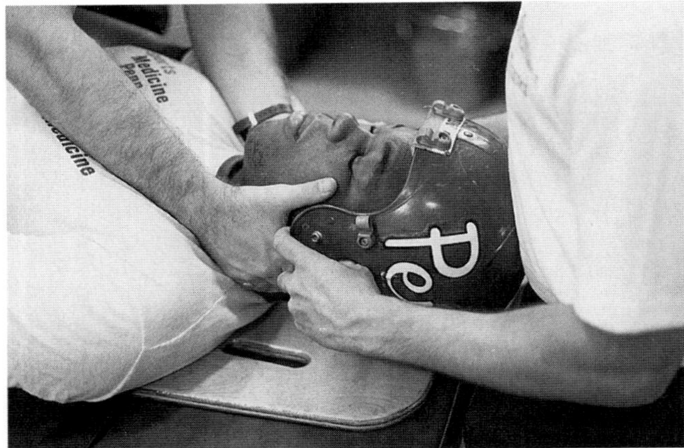

A

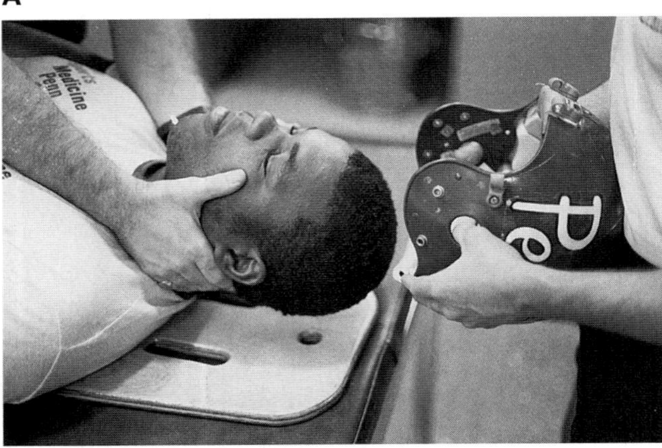

B

FIGURE 16-4. A, The helmet should be removed only when permanent immobilization can be instituted. The helmet may be removed by detaching the chin strap, spreading the earflaps and gently pulling the helmet off in a straight line with the cervical spine. **B,** The head must be supported under the occiput during and after removing the helmet. (From Torg JS [ed]: Athletic Injuries to the Head, Neck and Face. Philadelphia, Mosby–Year Book, 1991.)

PREVENTION

Athletic injuries to the cervical spine resulting in injury to the spinal cord are infrequent but catastrophic events. Accurate descriptions of the mechanism or mechanisms responsible for a particular injury transcend academic interest. Before preventative measures can be developed and implemented, identification of the mechanisms involved in the production of the particular injury is necessary.

Injuries resulting in spinal cord injury have been associated with football, water sports, wrestling, rugby, trampolining, and ice hockey. The use of epidemiologic data, biomechanical evidence, and cinematographic analysis has: 1) defined and supported the involvement of axial load forces in cervical spine injuries, 2) demonstrated the success of appropriate football rule changes in the prevention of these injuries, and 3) emphasized the need for use of epidemiologic methods to prevent cervical spine and similar severe injuries in other high-risk athletic activities.

Data on cervical spine injuries resulting from participation in football have been compiled by a national registry since 1971.[11–13] Analysis of epidemiologic data and cinematographic documentation clearly demonstrate that the majority of cervical fractures and dislocations resulted from axial loading. On the basis of this observation, rule changes banning deliberate "spearing" and the use of the top of the helmet as the initial point of contact in making a tackle were implemented at the high school and college levels. Subsequently, a marked decrease in cervical spine injury rates has occurred. The occurrence of permanent cervical quadriplegia decreased from 34 instances in the 1976 season to one in the 1991 season (Fig. 16-5).

Identifying the cause and prevention of cervical quadriplegia resulting from football involves four areas: 1) the role of the helmet–face mask protective system; 2) the concept of the axial-loading mechanism of injury; 3) the effect of the 1976 rule changes banning spearing and the use of the top of the helmet as the initial point of contact in tackling; and 4) the necessity for continued research, education, and rules enforcement.

Classically, the role of hyperflexion had been emphasized in cervical spine trauma whether the injury resulted

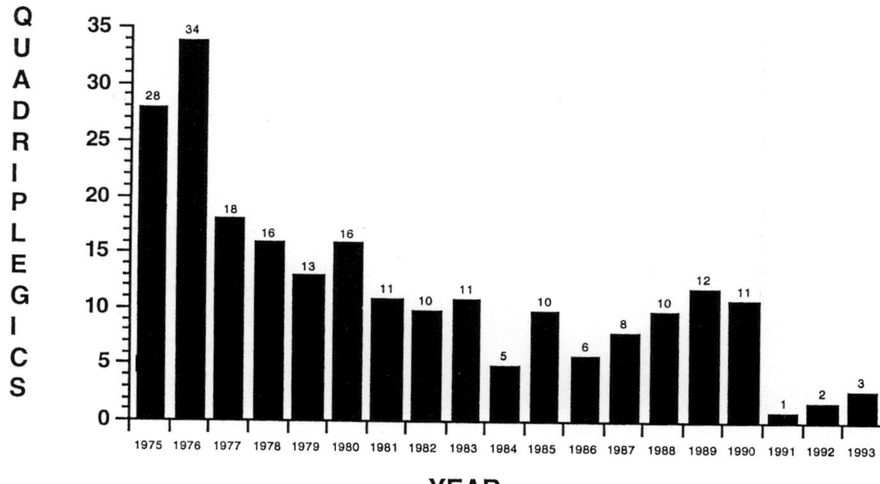

FIGURE 16-5. Yearly incidence of permanent cervical quadriplegia.

from a diving accident, trampolining, rugby, or American football. Epidemiologic and cinematographic analyses have established that most cases of cervical spine quadriplegia that occur in football resulted from axial loading. The protective capabilities provided by the modern football helmet resulted in the advent of playing techniques that have placed the cervical spine at risk of injury with associated catastrophic neurologic sequelae. Rather than an accidental event, techniques have been deliberately used that place the cervical spine at risk of catastrophic injury. Recent laboratory observations also indicate that athletically induced cervical spine trauma results from axial loading.

In the course of a collision activity such as tackle football, most energy inputs to the cervical spine are effectively dissipated by the energy-absorbing capabilities of the cervical musculature through controlled lateral bending, flexion, and extension motion. However, the vertebrae, discs, and ligamentous structures can be injured when contact occurs on the top of the helmet with the head, neck, and trunk positioned in such a way that forces are transmitted along the longitudinal axis of the cervical spine.

With the neck in this anatomic position, the cervical spine is extended because of normal cervical lordosis. When the neck is flexed to 30°, the cervical spine straightens. In axial-loading injuries, the neck is slightly flexed, and normal cervical lordosis eliminated, thereby converting the spine into a straight, segmented column. Assuming the head, neck, and trunk components to be in motion, rapid deceleration of the head occurs when it strikes another object, such as another player, trampoline bed, or lake bottom. This results in the cervical spine being compressed between the rapidly decelerated head and the force of the oncoming trunk. When the maximum vertical compression is reached, the straightened cervical spine fails in a flexion mode, and fracture, subluxation, or unilateral or bilateral facet dislocation can occur.

Refutation of the "freak accident" concept with the more logical principle of cause and effect has been most rewarding in dealing with problems of football-induced cervical quadriplegia. Definition of the axial-loading mechanism in which a football player, usually a defensive back, makes a tackle by striking an opponent with the top of the helmet was key in this process (Fig. 16-6). Implementation of rule changes and coaching techniques eliminating the use of the head as a battering ram have resulted in a dramatic reduction in the incidence of quadriplegia since 1976 (see Fig. 16-5). The author believes that the majority of, if not all, athletic injuries to the cervical spine also result from axial loading.

Tator et al.[9] identified 38 acute spinal cord injuries resulting from diving accidents and observed that "in most cases, the cervical spine was fractured and the spinal cord crushed. The top of the head struck the bottom of the lake or pool." Scher,[6] reporting on vertex impact and cervical dislocation in rugby players, observed that "when the neck is slightly flexed, the spine is straight. If significant force is applied to the vertex when the spine is straight, the force is transmitted down the long axis of the spine. When the force exceeds the energy-absorbing capacity of the structures involved, cervical spine flexion and dislocation will result." Tator and Edmonds[8] have reported on the results of a national questionnaire survey done by the Canadian Committee on the Prevention of Spinal Injuries Due to Hockey, which recorded 28 injuries involving the spinal cord,

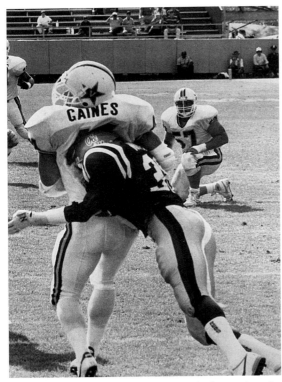

FIGURE 16-6. With the advent of the polycarbonate helmet–face mask protective device, use of the top or crown of the helmet as the initial point of contact in blocking and tackling became prevalent. Contact is made; the head abruptly stops; the momentum of the body continues; and the cervical spine is literally crushed between the two. In this instance, the fracture–dislocation injured the spinal cord. The injured player collapses, having been rendered quadriplegic.

17 of which resulted in complete paralysis. They noted that in this series, axial loading was found to be the most common mechanism of cervical spine and spinal cord injury resulting from head impact into the boards, with the most frequent inciting event being a push or check from behind.

CLASSIFICATION

Catastrophic and Potentially Catastrophic Injuries

Catastrophic and potentially catastrophic injuries to the cervical spine and cord are classified as follows.

1. Cervical subluxation
2. Unilateral and bilateral facet dislocation
3. Unstable cervical fractures—axial-load teardrop fracture
4. Spear tackler's spine

Cervical Subluxation. Athletic injuries to the cervical spine resulting in either translatory or angulatory instability are uncommon. It is generally accepted that up to 2 mm of translatory displacement is normal. White et al.[17] have defined clinical instability and established 3.5 mm translation and 11° of rotation as two factors to be used in determining indications for surgical stabilization. There are no data regarding the degree of risk presented by 2.0 to 3.5 mm of translation.

Unilateral and Bilateral Facet Dislocation. Experience with unilateral and bilateral facet dislocations has been reported recently.[16] More favorable results of immediate reduction of unilateral and bilateral facet dislocations have been observed and deserve emphasis. Three cases of unilateral facet dislocation reduced within 3 hours of the injury and subsequently fused experienced significant neurologic recovery. Four other patients, two who were treated expectantly and eventually underwent an open reduction and laminectomy and two treated with closed reduction with skeletal traction, have had no neurologic recovery. In four injuries of bilateral facet dislocation in which reduction was achieved by either open or closed method, although there was no neurologic recovery, all four survived their injuries. However, three children whose dislocations were not successfully reduced all died. Prompt reduction of cervical dislocations to relieve cord deformation is recommended.

Unstable Cervical Fractures—Axial-Load Teardrop Fracture. The most frequently occurring cervical spine fracture associated with instability, cord compromise, and major neurologic sequelae is the three-part, two-plane, axial-load teardrop fracture.[10] The fracture pattern, in addition to the anterior inferior vertebral body teardrop fracture, is associated with sagittal vertebral body and posterior neural element fractures (Fig. 16-7). In those sustaining this injury as a result of tackle football, 85% were rendered and remained quadriplegic.

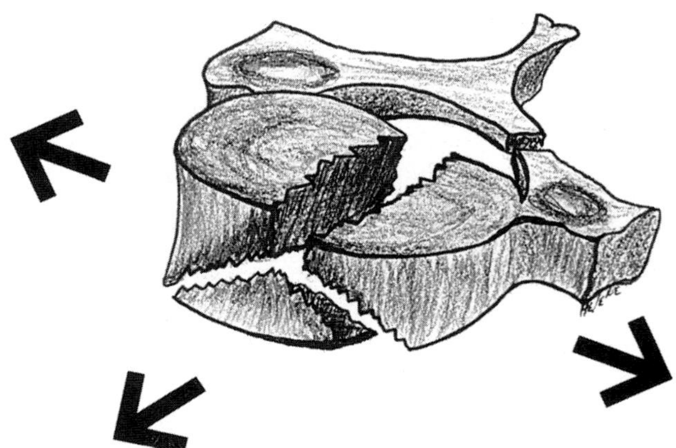

FIGURE 16-7. Diagrammatic representation of the three part–two plane vertebral body compression fracture demonstrates the anteroinferior teardrop and the sagittal vertebral body fractures and associated fracture through the lamina. (From Torg JS [ed]: Athletic Injuries to the Head, Neck and Face. Philadelphia, Mosby–Year Book, 1991.)

Spear Tackler's Spine. A subset of football players has been identified who demonstrated: 1) developmental narrowing (stenosis) of the cervical spinal canal, 2) persistent straightening or reversal of the normal cervical lordotic curve on erect lateral radiographs obtained in the neutral position, 3) concomitant preexisting post-traumatic radiographic abnormalities of the cervical spine, and 4) documentation of having used the spear-tackling technique.[15]

Of 15 patients evaluated because of complaints referable to the cervical spine or brachial plexus, four resulted in permanent neurologic deficit: 1) two with quadriplegia, 2) one with incomplete hemiplegia, and 3) one with residual long-track signs.

Although anecdotal, it is proposed that the permanent neurologic injury resulted from axial loading of a persistently straightened cervical spine from use of head-impact playing techniques. It is recommended that individuals who possess the characteristics of spear-tackler's spine be precluded from participation in collision activities that expose the cervical spine to axial energy inputs.

Spinal Cord Resuscitation. Research obtained during the past 20 years has established the principles of brain resuscitation in the management of closed head injuries. It is recognized that regarding resulting morbidity, the same pathophysiologic and mechanistic phenomena occur in acute spinal cord trauma. Specifically, it is secondary spinal cord injury phenomena caused by hypoxia, edema, and aberration of cell membrane potential that are largely responsible for resulting neurologic deficits. The principles of spinal cord resuscitation are proposed as an attempt to reverse secondary changes that occur to obtain maximal neurologic recovery. These measures include the following:

1. Management of any aberrations and neurovascular function with particular regard to maintaining blood pressure and spiratory function
2. Prompt initiation of measures to affect reduction of spinal deformity to relieve cord deformation
3. Prompt disabilization of the injured cervical segment
4. Administration of corticosteroid intravenously in doses recommended by Bracken et al.[2] This measurement involves the administration within 8 hours of injury of methylprednisolone, 30 mg/kg, given as a bolus followed by an infusion of 5.4 mg/kg/hr for 23 hours. Patients who receive methylprednisolone within 8 hours of injury improved significantly after 6 months compared with those who received a placebo. It is believed that the steroid acts by suppressing the breakdown of the cell membrane by inhibiting lipid peroxidation and hydrolysis at the injury site. When lipid peroxidation is inhibited, the vascoreactive products of arachidonic acid metabolism reduce the blood flow at the site of injury.
5. Administration of cerebroganglosides, such as Sygen, in an attempt to facilitate a neurologic recovery

Noncatastrophic Injuries

Noncatastrophic injuries to the cervical spine, cord, and brachial plexus are those in which residual neurologic sequelae are not a problem. Rather, the major factor is whether nonneurologic disability will result, particularly if the individual returns to collision activities. Common injuries in this group are as follows:

1. Nerve root–brachial plexus injury
2. Cervical sprain and strains
3. Intervertebral disc injury
4. Cervical cord neurapraxia-transient quadriplegia
5. Stable fractures

Nerve Root and Brachial Plexus. Injury to the cervical spine, cervical discs, brachial plexus, and peripheral nerves can result in neurologic signs and symptoms involving the upper extremities. The most common are the cervical pinch–stretch neurapraxias of the nerve roots and brachial plexus. Often called "burners" or "stingers" by players and trainers, these injuries often go unreported and untreated. Injury to the cervical nerve roots and brachial plexus most frequently occurs in contact sports, particularly football, rugby, wrestling, and soccer. In football, burners are usually diagnosed in defensive players and in offensive linemen. Clancy et al.[3] reported that 49% of the football players at the University of Wisconsin had experienced at least one burner at some time during their playing career.

These injuries result from two distinct injury mechanisms: 1) traction to the brachial plexus, and 2) compression of the cervical nerve roots. Plexus traction neurapraxia occurs in younger athletes and results from ipsilateral shoulder depression and contralateral neck and head deviation. Cervical root injuries result from compression of the dorsal root ganglion in the intervertebral foramen and are the result of hyperextension and ipsilateral deviation of the cervical spine. They are often associated with degenerative changes and may be seen combined with developmental cervical stenosis.

Typically, burners occur after head and shoulder contact; the player often leaves the playing field complaining of pain and numbness and inability to move the involved upper extremity. Pain is usually experienced radiating from the base of the neck into the shoulder and down the arm, including the hand. Burning paresthesias and numbness may accompany the pain and also radiate into the arm and hand. Most often these symptoms are not dermatomal in distribution. Weakness may occur, and characteristically the deltoid, spinati, and biceps are affected; motor weakness is often not initially apparent and may not manifest until a few days after the injury. Repeated neurologic evaluation therefore is mandatory. Characteristically, the signs and symptoms are transient and resolve within minutes. In those athletes in whom pain and paresthesia abate, a normal neurologic examination is required, and, most important, a full pain-free range of cervical motion is needed before the athletes' return to contact activity. Also, players must demonstrate normal strength on clinical examination before they return to participation. Those who have recurrent symptoms without weakness require careful follow-up evaluation; continued symptoms associated with weakness preclude further athletic participation.

Clancy et al.[3] recommended classifying these injuries based on the staging system of Seddon. Neurapraxia, the mildest form of injury, represents a reversible aberration in axonal function. Focal demyelinization can occur, producing an electrophysiologic conduction block or conduction slowing. Complete recovery usually occurs immediately or within a maximum of 2 weeks. Axonotmesis is an injury in which the axon and myelin sheath are disrupted, but the epineurium remains intact. Wallerian degeneration occurs distal to the point of injury; functional recovery may occur, but it can be incomplete and unpredictable. The most severe injury, neurotmesis, is rarely seen in athletes and results in complete disruption of the nerve. Prognosis is poor, and generally the patient does not recover.

Brachial plexus injuries are more likely to occur in younger patients with less well-developed neck musculature. Usually, these are traction injuries resulting from lateral neck flexion away from the involved area and shoulder depression to the side of involvement. Neck pain can be present, but it is usually not a prominent feature; when present, cervical spine radiographs are indicated. Typically, pain and paresthesias involving the arm and shoulder are transient. On examination, a Spurling test result is negative. Weakness typically involves the deltoid, spinati, and biceps and might not be evident initially on clinical examination, and a follow-up evaluation becomes necessary.

Root lesions result from compression of the nerve root or dorsal root ganglion in the intervertebral foramen and are generally associated with radiologic evidence of cervical disc disease and developmental stenosis. In football players, these injuries usually occur when the player reaches the college or professional level. Hyperextension with ipsilateral neck flexion is the common mechanism of injury. Neck pain and a decreased cervical range of motion may be present, and the Spurling test is positive. Plain radiographs may be normal or demonstrate loss of normal cervical lordosis and degenerative disc changes. Magnetic resonance imaging is indicated in patients with a persistent neurologic deficit and prolonged or recurrent symptoms and will demonstrate either acute disc herniation or degenerative disc disease with asymmetric disc bulging. In the author's experience, patients often have developmental spinal stenosis, degenerative disc disease, and asymmetric disc bulging that results in root irritation with cervical hyperextension.

Initial management must be directed toward evaluation of the cervical spine, shoulder girdle, affected upper extremity, and peripheral nervous system. The first obligation of the physician is to rule out serious cervical spine injury. A history of bilateral symptoms or symptoms including the lower extremities should alert the physician to the possibility of cord neurapraxia, cervical spine fracture, or ligamentous injury. In this instance, the spine should be immobilized until the possibility of severe injury is ruled out. If a player complains of neck pain, a complete cervical spine evaluation is mandatory, including radiographic examination.

In brachial plexus injuries, prevention is based on an aggressive neck and shoulder strengthening program. Neck rolls, or devices such as the cowboy collar and high-profile shoulder pads also help prevent injuries by limiting the extent of lateral flexion and extension (Fig. 16-8).

Electrodiagnostic studies may be helpful but are not mandatory in the management of burners secondary to brachial plexus injury. Speer[7] demonstrated that although there was no correlation between initial physical findings and the results of electrodiagnostic testing, evidence of muscular weakness at 72 hours after the injury did correlate with a positive electromyogram. Bergfeld[1]

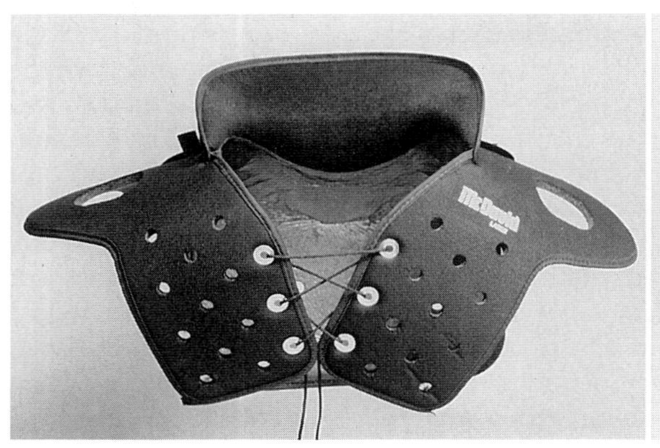
A

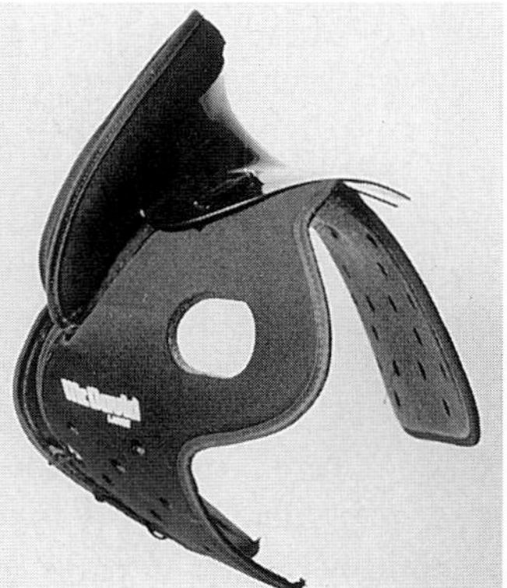
B

FIGURE 16-8. Frontal **(A)** and lateral **(B)** views of the cowboy collar. This device, which is worn under the shoulder pads of an athlete, effectively limits the extremes of extension and lateral bending of the cervical spine.

reported that electromyography findings continue to appear long after weakness has appeared resolved in clinical examinations, and therefore abnormal electromyography findings should not be used as a criterion for exclusion from athletic participation.

In individuals with cervical disc disease, the criteria for the return to sports activities is identical as for those with brachial plexus injuries. Neck and shoulder strengthening is the key to prevention. A neck roll or cowboy collar will help control recurrences by limiting extension. Athletes with large acute herniations or with large central disc components should refrain from participation in sports activities. Players with chronic symptoms and degenerative disc disease should be counseled as to the likelihood of recurrent symptoms with athletic participation. In those patients with subjective symptoms but who have normal strength, participation is not contraindicated if the player understands the possible implications of repetitive root trauma. In rare instances, discectomy and fusion may be considered if symptoms persist. A one-level fusion is not an absolute contraindication to athletic participation.The following list summarizes nerve root and brachial plexus injuries.

1. The burner pain syndrome results from either of two distinct injury patterns: traction to the brachial plexus and compression of the cervical nerve roots.
2. Brachial plexus injuries are typically traction neurapraxias occurring in younger athletes resulting from shoulder depression and lateral neck flexion away from the side of injury.
3. Cervical root injuries typically occur in older players; they are hyperextension injuries, and they are associated with degenerative disc changes and often combined with developmental cervical stenosis.
4. Criteria for return to athletics include the absence of symptoms, normal strength, and painless, full range of motion of the cervical spine.
5. Players who experience one or more burners should wear appropriate neck rolls or a cowboy collar to prevent extreme hyperextension and lateral bend of the cervical spine (see Figs. 16-8 and 16-9).
6. A year-round neck and shoulder muscle strengthening program will aid in the prevention of the burner syndrome.

Acute Cervical Sprain Syndrome. An acute cervical sprain is a collision injury frequently seen in contact sports. The patient complains of having "jammed" his or her neck, with subsequent pain localized to the cervical area. Characteristically, the patient presents with limitation of cervical spine motion but without radiation of pain or paresthesia. Neurologic examination is negative, and radiographs are normal.

Stable cervical sprains and strains eventually resolve with or without treatment. Initially, the presence of a serious injury should be ruled out by thorough neurologic examination and determination of the range of cervical motion. Range of motion is evaluated by having the athlete: actively nod his or her head, touch his or her chin to his or her chest, extend his or her neck maximally, touch his or her chin to the left shoulder, touch his or her chin to the right shoulder, touch his or her left ear to the left shoulder, and touch his or her right ear to the right shoulder. If the patient is unwilling or unable to perform these maneuvers actively while standing erect, the evaluation should not proceed. The athlete with less than a full, pain-free range of cervical motion, persistent paresthesia, or weakness should be protected and excluded from activity. Subsequent evaluation should include appropriate radiographic studies, including flexion and extension views to demonstrate fractures or instability. If the patient has pain and muscle spasm of the cervical spine, hospitalization and head-halter traction may be indicated.

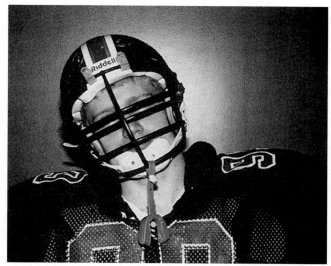

FIGURE 16-9. The combined action of the football helmet, cowboy collar, and shoulder pads effectively limits the extremes of lateral bend of the neck. (From Torg JS [ed]: Athletic Injuries to the Head, Neck and Face. Philadelphia, Mosby–Year Book, 1991.)

In general, management of athletes with cervical sprains should be tailored to the degree of severity. Immobilizing the neck in a soft collar and using analgesics and anti-inflammatory agents until there is a full, spasm-free range of neck motion is appropriate. It should be emphasized that individuals with a history of collision injury, pain, and limited cervical motion should have routine cervical spine radiographs. Also, lateral flexion and extension radiographs are indicated after the acute symptoms subside. Marked limitation of cervical motion, persistent pain, or radicular symptoms or findings may require a magnetic resonance imaging scan to rule out intervertebral disc injury.

Cervical Cord Neurapraxia with Transient Quadriplegia. The author has previously described the distinct clinical entity of the syndrome of neurapraxia of the cervical spinal cord with transient quadriplegia.[14] Sensory changes include burning pain, numbness, tingling, and loss of sensation, whereas motor changes range from weakness to complete paralysis involving upper and lower extremities. The episodes are transient, and complete sensory and motor recovery usually occurs in 10 to 15 minutes, although in some patients, gradual resolution may occur in 24 to 36 hours. Except for burning paresthesias, pain in the cervical area is not present at the time of injury, and there is complete return of motor function and full, pain-free motion of the cervical spine. This is a spinal cord phenomenon, not root or plexus, as evident by its bilaterally.

Routine radiographs of the cervical spine are characteristically negative for fracture, subluxation, or dislocation. However, radiographic findings include developmental cervical spinal narrowing, either as an isolated finding or associated with congenital fusions; ligamentous instability; or intervertebral disc disease (Fig. 16-10). Pavlov et al.[4] devised the ratio method for determining the sagittal spinal canal diameter (Fig. 16-11). The author compared the standard measurement of the canal with the anteroposterior width of the vertebral body at the midpoint of the corresponding vertebral body.

The ratio method of determining cervical spinal canal narrowing is independent of magnification factors caused by differences in target distance, object-to-film distance, or body type because the sagittal diameter of the spinal canal and that of the vertebral body are in the same anatomic plane and are similarly affected by magnification. There is normally a one-to-one relationship between the sagittal diameter of the spinal canal and that of the vertebral body, regardless of sex. A spinal canal-to-vertebral body ratio of less than 0.82 was recorded at one or more levels in all patients who experienced cervical cord neurapraxia.

The author's experience clearly indicates that those individuals who experience an episode of cervical cord neurapraxia manifested by sensory or motor symptoms have, with very few exceptions, a spinal canal-to-vertebral body ratio of 0.80 or less at one or more levels. The sensitivity of the ratio (i.e., the probability of getting a positive result in a symptomatic individual) was 100% in the author's series.[14]

The author's initial report was based solely on radiographic findings—all of the patients were evaluated before magnetic resonance imaging was widely available. The importance of the radiographic ratio determination, in addition to standardizing the films that were taken by various techniques, was to explain the pathophysiologic basis for the occurrence of cord neurapraxia. Developmental narrowing of the spinal canal in the anteroposterior plane associated with extreme flexion or extension of the spine can result in a transient compression of the cord. Penning[5] described this effect as the

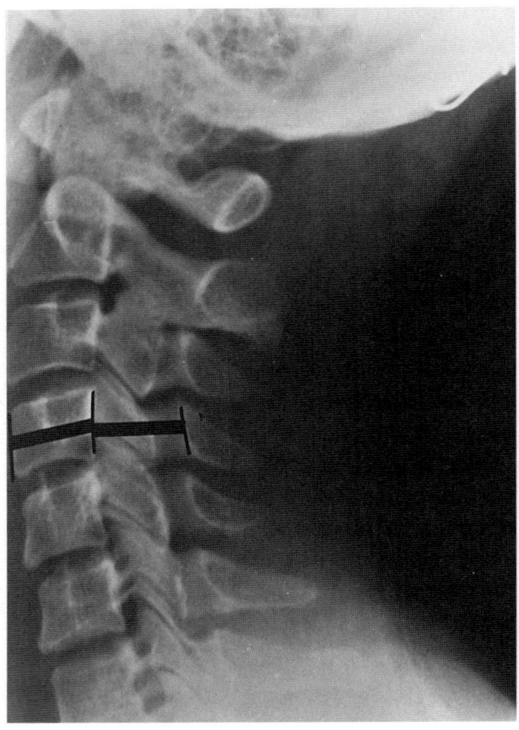

A

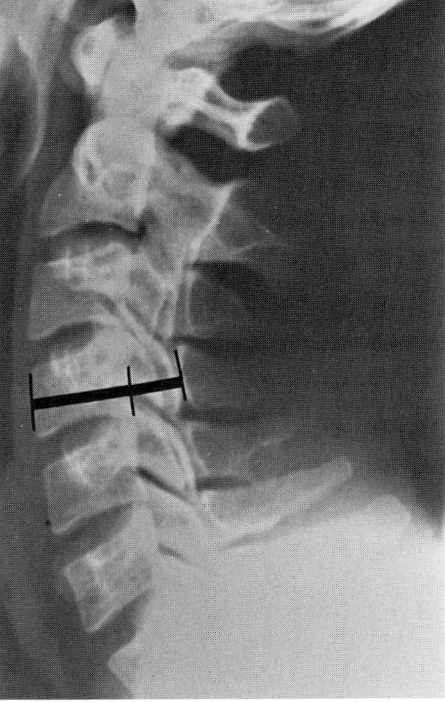

B

FIGURE 16-10. Comparison between the ratio of the spinal canal to the vertebral body of a healthy control subject with that of a stenotic patient demonstrated on lateral view radiographs of the cervical spine. Pavlov's ratio is 1:1 (1.00) in the control subject **(A)** compared with 1:2 (0.50) in the stenotic patient **(B)**. (From Torg JS, Pavlov H, Genuario S, et al: Neurapraxia of the cervical spinal cord with transient quadriplegia. J Bone Joint Surg 68A: 1354–1370, 1987.)

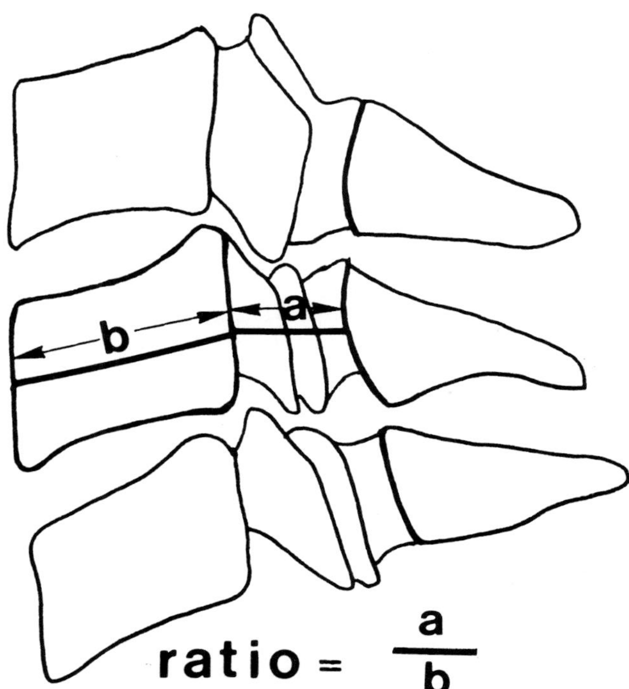

FIGURE 16-11. The spinal canal-to-vertebral body ratio is the distance from the midpoint of the posterior aspect of the vertebral body to the nearest point on the corresponding spinolaminar line *(a)* divided by the anteroposterior width of the vertebral body *(b)*. Pavlov's ratio is A/B. (From Torg JS, Pavlov H, Genuario S, et al: Neuraplaxia of the cervical spinal cord with transient quadriplegia. J Bone Joint Surg 68A:1354–1370, 1986.)

"pincer mechanism." Specifically, with hyperextension of the cervical spine, the posteroinferior aspect of the superior vertebral body and the anterosuperior aspect of the lamina of the subjacent vertebra decrease; conversely, in flexion, the lamina of the superior vertebra and the posterosuperior aspect of the subjacent vertebral body approximate with a sudden decrease in the anteroposterior diameter of the canal at that point, resulting in compression of the spinal cord (Fig. 16-12). In every instance of symptomatic developmental narrowing uncomplicated by instability or disc herniation, the neurologic manifestations are transient and completely reversible.

The low specificity of the ratio method in college and professional players results from anthropomorphic differences. Specifically, the cervical spines in these two groups are characterized by relatively larger vertebral bodies with subsequent lower ratios.

Permanent neurologic loss resulting from cervical spine injuries sustained in tackle football is a function of playing technique in which the cervical spine is axial loaded, resulting in unstable fractures or dislocations and irreversible neurologic compromise. The question of whether individuals who have experienced an episode of cord neurapraxia are predisposed to injury with permanent neurologic residua has been answered. None of the 117 known quadriplegics in the National Football Head and Neck Injuries Registry experienced previous episodes of cord neurapraxia, and none of the 110 patients in the transient cohort remained quadriplegic after an episode of cervical cord neurapraxia. Based on the random distribution of ratio determinations and the lack of correlation between the occurrence of permanent quadriplegia and prodromal episodes of cord neurapraxia, it is clear that the occurrence of cord neurapraxia does not predispose an individual to an injury associated with permanent catastrophic neurologic sequelae. There was no correlation between occurrence of permanent quadriplegia and prodromal episodes of cord neurapraxia in a tackle football population. Therefore, the author believes that the presence of uncomplicated developmental narrowing of the stable cervical spine is neither a harbinger of nor does it predispose for permanent neurologic injury.

Cervical cord neurapraxia is a transient, totally reversible phenomenon that results from compressive deformation of the spinal cord. The syndrome is caused by developmental narrowing of the cervical canal either as an isolated entity or combined with degenerative changes, instability, or congenital abnormalities. Uncomplicated stenosis of the cervical canal in a patient with a stable spine does not predispose to permanent neurologic injury. The present data do not indicate that there is a correlation between developmental narrowing and permanent neurologic sequelae in a spine rendered unstable by football-induced trauma. Data also indicate that an episode of cervical cord neurapraxia is not a harbinger or indicator of susceptibility to permanent neurologic sequelae. However, the author has in the past recommended that continued participation in collision activities be restricted in those individuals who have had a documented episode of cervical cord neurapraxia associated with: 1) ligamentous instability, 2) intervertebral disc disease with cord compression, 3) significant degenerative changes, 4) magnetic resonance imaging evidence of cord defect or swelling, 5) symptoms of positive neurologic findings lasting more than 36 hours, and 6) more than one recurrence.

As stated previously, the author described cervical cord neurapraxia using radiographic measurements and identified narrowing of the anteroposterior diameter of the cervical canal as the etiologic factor. A more recent report classifies the various clinical manifestations, measures cord and canal diameters on magnetic resonance imaging with a newly developed computer technique, and delineates management guidelines.

A retrospective review was performed of 110 cases of cervical cord neurapraxia seen in consultation by the author. Radiographs were measured as described previously, and a new technique with an MS-DOS–based system was developed to measure cord and canal diameters from the magnetic resonance imaging scans.

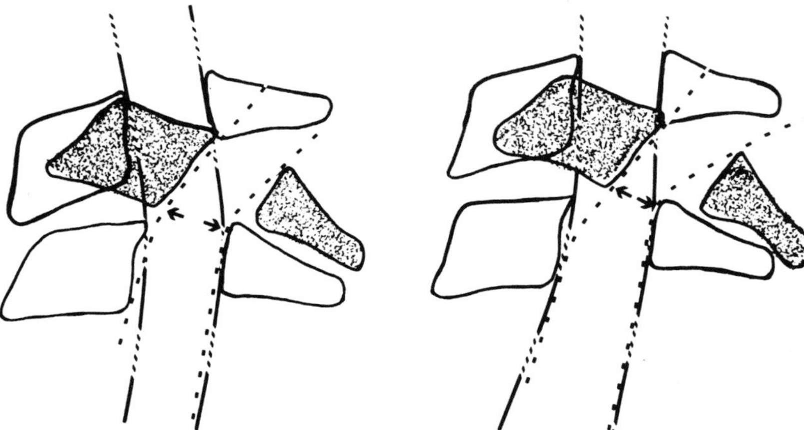

FIGURE 16-12. The pincers mechanism, as described by Penning, occurs when the distance between the posteroinferior margin of the superior vertebral body and the anterosuperior aspect of the spinolaminar line of the subjacent vertebra decreases with hyperextension, resulting in compression of the cord. With hyperflexion, the anterosuperior aspect of the spinolaminar line of the superior vertebra and the posterosuperior margin of the inferior vertebra would be the "pincers."

All injuries were sports related, and 86% occurred during football participation. Follow-up evaluation was available for 93 (85%) of the patients after an average of 22 months. Results of this study indicated that clinical manifestations (cervical cord neurapraxia type) were paralysis in 36%, weakness in 26%, and sensory changes alone in 38%. Duration of the symptoms (cervical cord neurapraxia grade) were: I—less than 15 minutes in 73%; II—more than 15 minutes but less than 24 hours in 16%; and III—more than 24 hours in 10%. The averages for the sagittal radiologic indices were: 1) Pavlov ratio, 0.69 (standard deviation [SD] = 0.11); 2) minimal magnetic resonance imaging canal diameter, 9.6 mm (SD = 1.8); 3) cord diameter, 8.1 mm (SD = 0.8); and 4) space available for the cord, 1.6 mm (SD = 1.4). There was no relationship between the various clinical manifestations and the radiologic indices. Overall, 65% of the patients returned to contact sports, with 56% of these patients having at least one recurrence of cervical cord neurapraxia. Patients with recurrence had smaller Pavlov ratios ($P < 0.05$), smaller absolute canal diameters ($P < 0.01$), and less space available for the cord ($P < 0.05$).

Based on this statistically significant data, it was concluded that: 1) individuals with uncomplicated cervical cord neurapraxia can be advised to return to play without greater risk of permanent neurologic injury; 2) the various clinical manifestations (cervical cord neurapraxia type and grade) are not related to the radiologic indices; and 3) there is a 56% recurrence rate that is correlated with the pathoanatomy (i.e., the smaller the canal, the greater the risk of recurrence).

Intervertebral Disc Injury. Acute cervical intervertebral disc herniation is exceedingly rare in high school, intercollegiate, and professional athletes. However, an acute central disc deforming the cord or the lateral disc associated with pain, limitation of full cervical motion, or neurologic symptoms is an absolute contraindication to athletic participation.

A problem seen with an increasing frequency in older collegiate and professional players is degenerative disc changes associated with repetitive microtrauma. Common radiographic findings include disc space narrowing, anterior bony ridging, and loss of normal cervical lordosis. If the individual is symptomatic and has associated loss of normal cervical motion, treatment consists of rest, including a cervical collar, heat, and analgesics until the individual is symptom-free and has full range of cervical motion.

To be noted is the association of chronic, recurrent cervical nerve root neurapraxia (burner syndrome) resulting from cervical nerve root compression in the intervertebral foramina secondary to cervical disc disease. Whereas burners have been identified to result from brachial plexus stretch injury in high school and college football players presenting with symptoms, nerve root compression in the intervertebral foramina secondary to disc disease is a more common etiology in older collegiate and professional football players with chronic, recurrent burners.

Stable Fractures. An acute fracture of either the vertebral body or posterior elements with or without associated-ligamentous laxity constitutes an absolute contraindication to participation.

The following healed, stable fractures in an asymptomatic patient who is neurologically normal and has a full range of cervical motion can be considered to present no contraindication to participation in contact activities.

1. Stable compression fractures of the vertebral body without a sagittal component on anteroposterior radiographs and without involvement of either the ligamentous or posterior bony structures
2. Healed, stable endplate fractures without a sagittal component on anteroposterior radiographs or involvement of the posterior or bony ligamentous structure
3. Healed, spinous process "clay shoveler" fractures

Relative contraindications apply to the following healed stable fractures in individuals who are asymptomatic, neurologically normal, and have a full pain-free range of cervical motion.

1. Healed, stable displaced vertebral body compression fractures without a sagittal component on anteroposterior radiographs; the propensity for these fractures to settle with increased deformity must be considered and carefully followed
2. Healed, stable fractures involving the elements of the posterior neural ring in individuals who are asymptomatic, neurologically normal, and have a full pain-free range of cervical motion In evaluating radiographic and imaging studies to find the location and subsequent healing of posterior neural arch fractures, it is important to understand that, as pointed out by Steel (personal communication), a rigid ring cannot break in one location; thus, healing of paired fractures of the ring must be demonstrated.

An absolute contraindication to further participation in contact activities exists in the presence of the following fractures.

1. Vertebral body fracture with a sagittal component
2. Fracture of the vertebral body with or without displacement with associated posterior arch fractures or ligamentous laxity
3. Comminuted fractures of the vertebral body with displacement into the spinal canal
4. Any healed fracture of either the vertebral body or posterior components with associated pain, neurologic findings, and limitation of normal cervical motion

REFERENCES

1. Bergfeld JA: Brachial plexus injury in sports: A five year follow-up. Orthop Clin North Am 23:743–744, 1988.
2. Bracken MB, Shepard MS, Collins WF, et al: A randomized, controlled trial of methylprednisolone or naloxone with treatment of acute spinal-cord injury. N Engl J Med 320:1405–1411, 1990.
3. Clancy WG, Brand RL, Bergfeld J: Upper trunk brachial plexus injuries in contact sports. Am J Sports Med 5:209–214, 1977.
4. Pavlov H, Torg JS, Robie B, Jahre C: Cervical spinal stenosis: Determination with vertebral body ratio method. Radiology 164:771–775, 1987.
5. Penning L: Some aspects of plain radiography of the cervical spine in chronic myelopathy. Neurology 12:513–519, 1962.
6. Scher AT: Vertex impact and cervical dislocation in rugby players. South Afr Med J 59:227–228, 1981.
7. Speer KP: The prolonged burner syndrome. Am J Sports Med 18:591–594, 1990.
8. Tator CH, Edmonds VE: National survey of spinal injuries in hockey players. Can Med Assoc J 130:875–880, 1984.
9. Tator CH, Edmonds VE, New ML: Diving: A frequent and potentially preventable cause of spinal cord injury. Can Med Assoc J 124:1323–1324, 1981.
10. Torg JS, Pavlov H, O'Neill MJ, et al: The axial load teardrop fracture: The isolated fracture and the three part–two plane fracture of the cervical spine… the clinical and roentgen analysis of 55 cervical spines. Am J Sports Med 19:355–364, 1991.
11. Torg JS, Vegso JJ, O'Neill J, Sennett B: The epidemiologic, pathologic, biomechanical and cinematographic analysis of football-induced cervical spine trauma. Am J Sports Med 18:50–57, 1990.
12. Torg JS, Vegso JJ, Sennett B: The national football head and neck injury registry: 14 year report on cervical quadriplegia, 1971 through 1985. JAMA 254:3439–3441, 1985.
13. Torg JS, Truex R, Quedenfeld TC: The national football head & neck injury registry: Report and conclusions. JAMA 241:1477–1479, 1979.
14. Torg JS, Pavlov H, Genuario SE, et al: Neurapraxia of the cervical spinal cord with transient quadriplegia. J Bone Joint Surg 68A:1354–1370, 1986.
15. Torg JS, Sennett B, Pavlov H: Spear tackler's spine: An entity precluding participation in tackle football and collision activities that expose the cervical spine to axial energy inputs. Am J Sports Med 21:640–649, 1993.
16. Torg JS, Sennett B, Vegso JJ, et al: Axial loading injuries to the middle cervical spine segment. Am J Sports Med 19:6–20, 1991.
17. White AA, Johnson RM, Pajobi MM, et al: Biomechanical analysis of clinical stability in the cervical spine. Clin Orthop 109:85–93, 1975.

17 The Thoracic and Lumbar Spine

Stefano M. Sinicropi,
Mark Weidenbaum, and
Jeffrey E. Deckey

More than 30 million Americans are involved in organized sports, and countless others are engaged in recreational sporting activities that place significant stress on the spinal column.[65] Few studies have comprehensively documented spine injury rates in sports overall, but limited data estimates that up to 15% of these individuals may experience a sports-related spinal injury.[14,39] The overwhelming majority of these injuries are minor and self-limiting; however, significant disability can result, with neurologic involvement in up to 1% of those affected.[39] As the number of adults, adolescents, and children participating in organized sport continues to blossom, thoracic and lumbar spine injuries will continue to receive increased attention because they affect athletes at all levels of competition. Therefore, the sports physician should be familiar with the most common thoracic and lumbar injuries to facilitate treatment, rehabilitation, and prevention. Once a diagnosis has been made and treatment initiated, the physician must evaluate the athlete to determine when and if he or she may return to sports participation. This decision is one of the most difficult tasks faced by the sports physician.

BACK PAIN AND INJURY IN SPORTS

Each sport has very specific injury patterns and rates of injury. Keene[32] noted that "surveillance and prevention of back injuries in athletes should be predicated upon studies that document the incidence and types of injuries that occur in each sport." Therefore the sports physician can somewhat tailor the clinical examination to suit the individual sport. Participants in high-contact and high-velocity sports are more likely to present with more significant spinal pathology than runners or joggers.

Participation in competitive tennis, volleyball, and cycling correlated significantly with increased back pain in children aged 8 to 16 years.[4] As noted by Hresko,[26] the most common mechanism of injury is through repetitive microtrauma, resulting in fatigue injuries. This applies to contact and noncontact sports, including gymnastics, ballet, figure skating, hockey, football, weightlifting, rowing, and diving.[28,32,34,48]

Because the growth plate is the weakest tensile link in the axial skeleton, physeal injuries may accompany disc injury in children. Annular protrusion produces traction on the ring apophysis and may avulse bony endplate fragments.[5] Traumatic vertebral ring apophyseal injury may be followed by disc prolapse and degeneration.[56]

A recent study on competitive wrestlers, gymnasts, and soccer and tennis players found unusually high frequencies of and a significant relationship between back pain (50% to 85%) and radiologic abnormalities (36% to 55%).[57] Radiologic findings indicated direct traumatic changes and disturbed vertebral growth. These findings emphasize the vulnerability of the spine during the growth period and raise significant questions about when vigorous athletic training should begin, what loads are acceptable, and who takes responsibility to prevent and detect injury in the young athlete. Approximately 80% of male weightlifters and 60% of females have degenerative disc disease by age 40.[41] In an MRI study of back injuries in young gymnasts, Goldstein et al. reported that girls who trained more than 16 hours a week in gymnastics had a significantly increased risk of back pain.[20]

Most serious cases of spinal injury occur in high-velocity or contact sports. A 5-year review of 129 wrestlers identified only three back sprains, an incidence of only 2.3% for back injury.[51] In contrast, review of 70 female gymnasts revealed nine injuries to the thoracic and lumbar spine, including two spinal fractures, two spondylolyses, and five back strains.[50] Incidence of back injury was 12.8%, more than five times higher than that of the wrestlers. Only 50% of adolescent gymnasts sustaining herniated lumbar discs were able to return to their previous level after conservative therapy without experiencing further back pain.[40] Furthermore, interspinous osteoarthrosis and spondylolysis were more common among gymnasts.[21]

Keene[31] found a 7% incidence of back injuries sustained by 4,700 varsity collegiate athletes over a 10-year period. Eighty-one percent of these injuries were to the lumbar spine. Notably, 80% of these injuries occurred during practice, and 14% occurred during preseason conditioning. Only 6% of these injuries occurred during competition. An acute injury occurred in 59% of cases, overuse in 12%, and aggravation of a preexisting condition in 29%. Football and gymnastics demonstrated the highest incidence of injury, 17% and 11%, respectively. Sixty percent of all back injuries were diagnosed as muscle strains, particularly common in football players.

Other studies have documented increased frequency of back injury in oarsmen, presumably because of the high physical demands of the sport.[25,53] Up to 82% of elite female rowers have significant low back pain.[23] Williams reported that 15% of all athletic injuries in England occur to the spine.[65] These injuries are most prevalent in automobile racing, horseback riding, parachuting, mountaineering, and weightlifting.

Certain sports appear to contribute to an increased incidence of disc degeneration. In particular, a study on retired world-class gymnasts in their second and third decades of life demonstrated an increased incidence of disc degeneration on MRI that correlated with increased incidence of back pain (Fig. 17-1).[58] Signs of disc degeneration on MRI were present in 75% of gymnasts in the study. A similar study performed on younger participants (mean age, 12 years) demonstrated no signs of increased disc degeneration in the gymnasts.[59]

The sport of golf has increasingly been associated with the development of low back pain in the professional and amateur ranks.[24] Both PGA golfers and amateur golfers report that the lower back is the most common source of injury and pain (second most common for LPGA professionals).[36,37] In one review, 90% of tournament level golfers reported previous cervical or lumbar injury. Golf injuries are generally secondary to repetitive shear, compression, and torsional forces which are magnified by overuse and incorrect swing techniques. Although golfers are usually afflicted by mechanical or discogenic back pain, Hosea and Gatt caution that, as in all other patients, all the possible etiologies for back pain should still be considered.[24] Stretching, a proper warm-up, correct swing mechanics, and the avoiding overuse are critical for prevention.

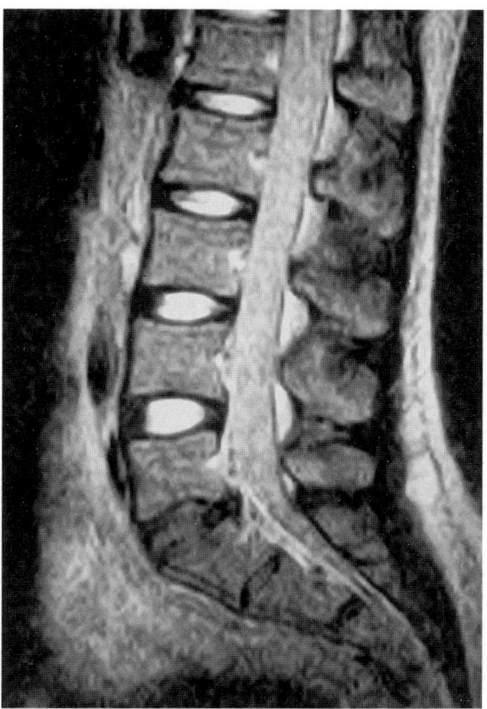

FIGURE 17-1. Magnetic resonance imaging showing disc degeneration at L5–S1. Note loss of bright white signal at L5–S1 compared with other discs, suggestive of loss of water content and degeneration.

ANATOMY

The spine and surrounding musculature is a complex biomechanical structure. Sporting activities can subject the spine to rapid and repetitive loading resulting in acute and chronic injuries to the thoraco-lumbar spine. Knowledge of pertinent spinal anatomy and spinal mechanics is central to understanding mechanisms of injury and principles of management.[10] The vertebral column involves a delicate balance between osseous and soft-tissue structures, with alternating bony vertebrae and fibrocartilaginous discs. The osseous component of the spine is divided into 7 cervical (neck), 12 thoracic (chest), 5 lumbar (lower back), and multiple fused sacral vertebrae.

The vertebrae increase in size and in their ability to support load as one descends caudally (toward the tail) to the sacrum. Vertebral connections with each other occur through the discs and through posterior articulations called facets. Intervertebral discs are not simply uniform soft-tissue structures, but are very complex in their anatomy, biomechanics, and physiology. The discs also increase in size as one moves from cervical to lumbar. Despite great regional anatomic differences, the spine always functions to provide structural support, harmonious movement, and neural protection. Changes in one region may affect other regions and the spine as a whole. The cervical spine is discussed elsewhere in this text.

Thoracic and Lumbar Vertebrae

The thoracic pedicles originate from the superior aspect of the vertebral body. Thoracic laminae are short, relatively thick, and overlap slightly. Thoracic spinous processes are long and are directed posteriorly and inferiorly. Thoracic facets generally face posteriorly and slightly outward, although orientation changes from frontal to sagittal with caudal progression. The inferior facet originates at the anterior part of the lamina and faces anteriorly and slightly inward. This facet configuration permits increased rotation in the thoracic spine. However, rotation is limited, in part, by the intact rib cage and sternum.

Thoracic vertebrae are unique because of their articulation with the ribs. The second through ninth ribs articulate with the corresponding superior and inferior vertebrae at the intervertebral disc. The head of the rib articulates with the superior costal facet of the adjacent vertebral body and the inferior costal facet of the vertebra above. The rib tubercle articulates with the corresponding transverse process costal facet. The first, tenth, eleventh, and twelfth ribs have complete facets for articulation with their respective vertebra. The eleventh and twelfth ribs do not articulate with the transverse processes.

Viewed in the horizontal plane, lumbar vertebrae are kidney-shaped. Their pedicles are thick, originating from the superior posterolateral aspect of the vertebral body. They give rise to short, broad laminae that meet to form wide horizontal spinous processes. Unlike the thoracic laminae, the lumbar laminae do not overlap, and there is a space between each lamina, which is spanned by the ligamentum flavum. The articular facets project vertically. The superior facet faces postero-medially and articulates with the inferior facet of the vertebrae above in a reciprocal fashion (Fig. 17-2). The sagittal alignment of the facets allows increased flexion and extension compared with the thoracic spine.

Intervertebral Disc

Interposed between the vertebral bodies are fibrocartilaginous intervertebral discs that become progressively

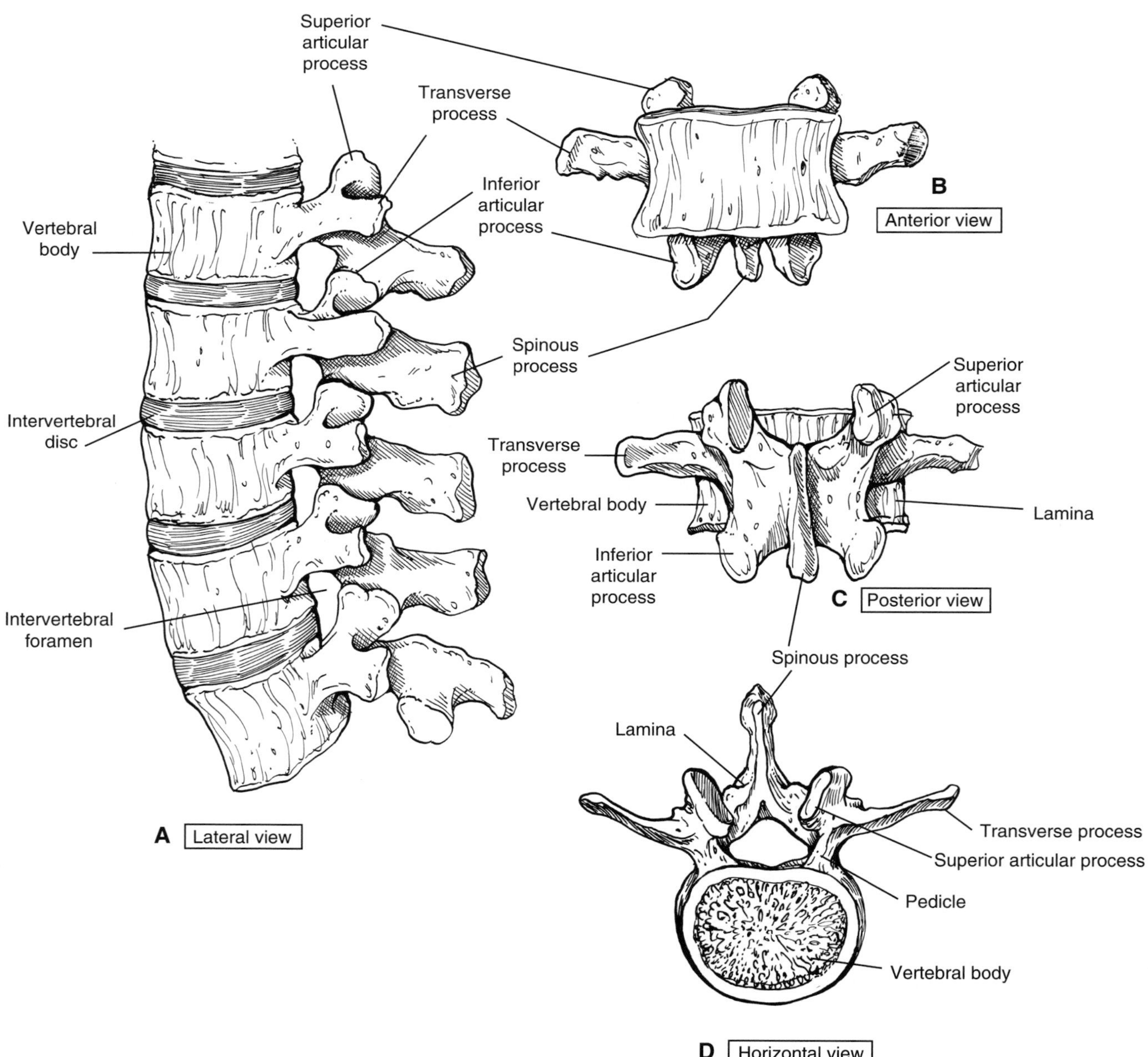

FIGURE 17-2. Views of the lumbar spine. **A,** Lateral (sagittal plane); **B,** Anterior (frontal plane); **C,** Posterior (frontal plane); **D,** Horizontal (axial plane).

larger and thicker as one descends the vertebral column, accounting for 20% to 30% of vertebral column height.[43] The discs connect the vertebrae, allow limited motion, and facilitate force distribution. The increased percentage of disc per unit area in the lumbar spine results in increased flexibility in this area.

The disc includes an outer fibrocartilaginous ring, the annulus fibrosus, surrounding the inner gelatinous nucleus pulposus. The annulus fibrosus is composed of a series of concentric lamellae with alternating fiber orientations that function to contain the nucleus pulposus and to provide increased torsional strength. The nucleus pulposus assumes an eccentric position within the disc space as determined in part by the sagittal contour at each anatomic level of the spine. The outer portion of the annulus fibrosus attaches to the vertebrae above and below via Sharpey's fibers.[11] The inner portion of the annulus, the transition zone, blends with the nucleus pulposus. The annulus fibrosus and nucleus pulposus are contained above and below by cartilaginous vertebral endplates. Outer layers of the annulus fibrosus are vascularized, whereas the remainder of the disc receives its nutrition via diffusion through the endplates.

The annulus fibrosus contains approximately 60% to 70% water, and this figure remains relatively constant with age.[45] Collagen is the other major component of the annulus fibrosus, giving it tensile strength. Although the nucleus pulposus is approximately 80% water, much of its dry weight comes from proteoglycans. These proteoglycans are huge molecules with high concentrations of negative fixed charge, giving them a strong affinity for water (hydrophilic). Thus, water is pulled into the disc as a result of the electrochemical effect of the proteoglycans in the nucleus pulposus. Because external osmotic, hydrostatic, and mechanical forces tend to push water out of the disc, the proteoglycan hydrophilic effect is an essential part of the equilibrium necessary to maintain disc hydration. Water and proteoglycan content decrease with age and degeneration.

Injury to the intervertebral disc results in abnormal load sharing and motion in the affected and adjacent neuromotion segments.

Ligaments

Numerous ligamentous structures support the thoracic and lumbar spine. The anterior longitudinal ligament (ALL) runs along the ventral surface of the vertebral bodies. The posterior longitudinal ligament (PLL) lies along the posterior aspect of the vertebral body within the spinal canal. Posteriorly, the ligamentum flavum (yellow ligament) at each level extends from the anterior surface of the proximal laminae to the lamina below. The facets are diarthrodial joints surrounded by capsules that provide stability, limit motion, and help to maintain the joint. The costovertebral joints are reinforced by ligamentous structures, including the radiate and the costotransverse ligaments. The supraspinous and interspinous ligaments connect the spinous processes posteriorly.

The ligamentous structures are more pronounced in the lumbar spine, which may result from the relative lack of bony stability present in the lumbar spine compared with the thoracic spine, which is reinforced by the rib cage. The ligamentum flavum, also thicker in the lumbar spine, serves as a barrier to the spinal canal between adjacent lumbar laminae (Fig. 17-3).

Muscles

The muscles of the spine are aligned longitudinally from the skull to the pelvis and provide support and motion to the axial skeleton. Unlike the ligaments that provide passive restraint only, muscles provide both passive and active restraints. They provide the critical support necessary to resist the forces to which the spine is subjected. The musculature can be divided into flexors and extensors and intrinsic and extrinsic. Understanding how these muscle groups contribute to spinal stability is critical to prevention and rehabilitation of sports-related injuries.

The flexors can be divided into two layers: intrinsic and extrinsic. The psoas muscle (intrinsic) originates from the anterior aspect of the spine, has a very short moment arm, and is an important stabilizer of the spine. The abdominal muscles (extrinsics) are the second layer, have a mechanical advantage as flexors with their longer moment arm. The rectus abdominus is most active in midline flexion, and the oblique muscles (internal and external) are most active in flexion out of the midline plane.

The extensors of the back may be divided into two layers: deep and superficial. The superficial muscles, which are associated with the shoulder girdle and upper limb, must not be overlooked when evaluating back injuries. The deep muscles of the spine consist of five major groups, including the splenius, the erector spinae, the transversospinalis, the interspinalis, and the intertransversarial.

The splenius consists of the splenius cervicis and splenius capitis and is located in the cervical spine.

The erector spinae is a massive group of muscles that occupy the vertebrocostal groove. It consists of the spinalis, longissimus, and the iliocostalis. It lies directly under the thoracic and lumbar fascia. It originates from the posterior aspect of the sacrum, iliac crest, and lumbar spinous processes. The muscle splits into three groups, consisting of the midline spinalis, the longissimus, and the iliocostalis. The erector spinae extends along the entire spine; however, it consists of short fasicles that span 6 to 8 segments.

The iliocostalis lumborum begins at the iliac crest and inserts on the angles of the lower six ribs. The next portion, the iliocostalis thoracis, originates from the

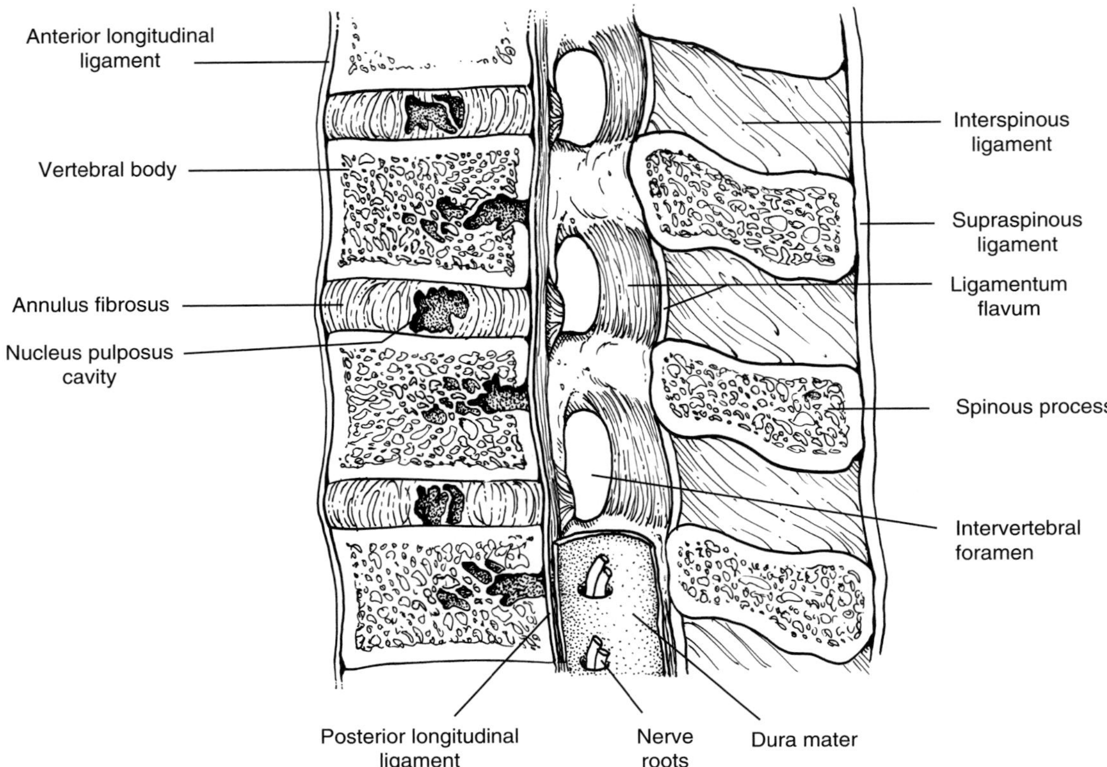

FIGURE 17-3. Midline sagittal view illustrating important soft tissues in the lumbar spine.

upper border of the lower six ribs and attaches to the upper six ribs. Finally, the iliocostalis cervicis originates from the angles of the upper six ribs and inserts on the transverse processes of C4 to C6.

The longissimus consists of thoracic, cervical, and capital portions. The longissimus thoracis inserts onto the lower nine or ten ribs and their corresponding transverse processes. The longissimus cervicis originates from the upper four to six ribs and inserts onto the transverse processes of C2 through C6. The longissimus capitis bridges the articular processes of the lower four cervical vertebrae with the posterior margin of the mastoid process.

The spinalis muscle is the most medial and least defined of the erector spinae musculature. The spinalis capitis, cervicis, and thoracis originate and insert onto the spinous processes.

The erector spinae are actively involved in extension and lateral bending of the spine. The capitis portion of the longissimus muscle may also bend the neck laterally and rotate the head to the ipsilateral side. The erector spinae serves as an antagonist, controlling the extent and rate of flexion.

The next group of spinal musculature is the transversospinalis. This group lies deep to the erector spinae. The muscles originate on the transverse processes and insert onto the spinous processes four to six levels cephalad. They act as primary rotators of the spine and also participate in extension.

The final two groups of muscles, the interspinalis and intertransversarial, are less defined. In the lumbar and cervical regions, they consist of pairs of muscles running between the spinous and transverse spines. In the thorax, they exist as the levatores costarum, which originate from the transverse process and insert onto the rib below. They act to elevate the ribs during respiration.

The deep muscles of the thoracic and lumbar spine are enveloped by the thoracic and lumbar fascia. In the thorax, there is a thin, transparent layer covering the thoracic musculature that becomes thicker inferiorly as it enters the lumbar spine. This fascia attaches to the iliac crest and posterior sacrum.

Other extrinsic muscle groups that factor into spinal mechanics are the gluteals and the hamstrings.

Neural Structures

Neural structures include the spinal cord and nerve roots and all related entities. A detailed discussion of these is beyond the scope of this chapter, but a brief overview is presented here.

The spinal cord lies within the spinal canal, extending down from the cervical spine, through the thoracic spine, to the upper lumbar spine. The cord tapers to a terminal region called the conus medullaris, which usually lies at L1–L2. Below this level, the neural elements in the spinal canal continue as spinal nerve roots, collectively called the cauda equina (Fig. 17-4). The conus medullaris is anchored by the filum terminale, a tough structure that inserts into the top of the sacrum. The cord and the cauda equina are contained within a protective sac and are bathed in cerebrospinal fluid (CSF). The outer layer of this sac is the dura mater.

Each spinal nerve exits the spinal canal through an opening called the intervertebral foramen. The nerve courses out through the foramen, under the pedicle of the vertebra forming the roof of the foramen. The floor of the foramen is formed by the pedicle of the vertebra below.

The spinal nerves contain mixed fibers (motor, sensory, and visceral). They are composed of ventral and dorsal rootlets that unite and form the spinal nerve in the intervertebral foramen. The spinal nerve divides into a dorsal and ventral ramus as it exits the intervertebral foramen.

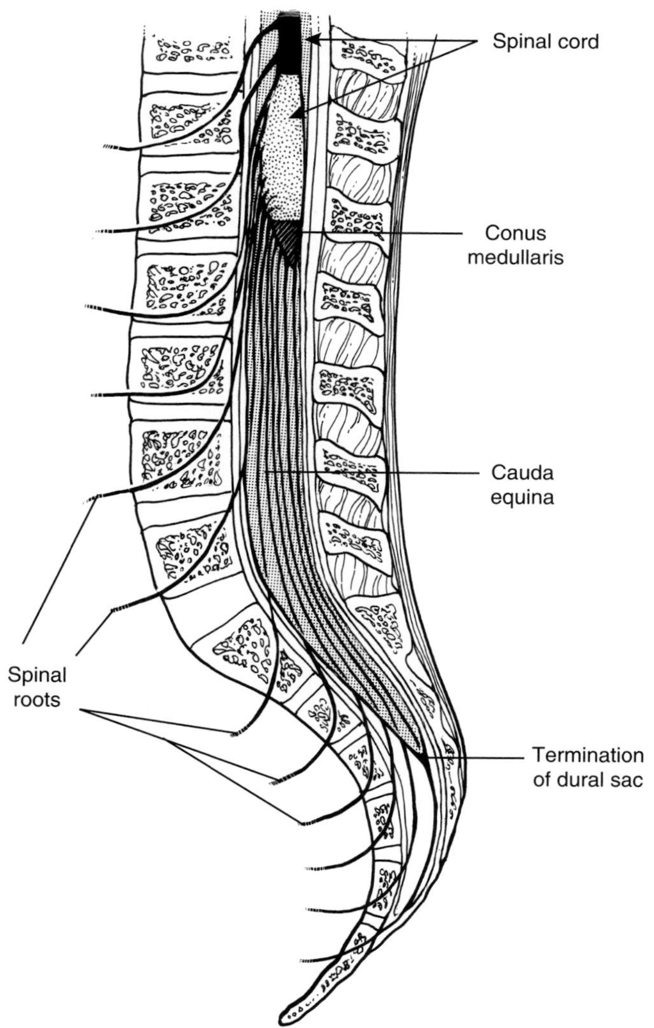

FIGURE 17-4. Illustration of the spinal cord, conus medullaris, and cauda equina.

The ventral rami supply a larger distribution, including the lumbosacral and coccygeal plexi. They also supply the intercostal nerves, which run in the groove along the inferior aspect of the rib.

The dorsal rami serve a limited distribution, consisting of the musculocutaneous innervation of the back. This area includes the spinous process to the angle of the rib in the thorax and to the lateral aspect of the paravertebral fascia in the lumbar spine. The dorsal rami enter the deep musculature of the back immediately after their exit from the intervertebral foramen. They divide into medial and lateral branches. In the lumbar region, the dorsal rami of L1, L2, and L3 provide cutaneous innervation via the superior cluneal nerves that exit over the posterior iliac crest. Branches of the dorsal rami may innervate the facet capsules and parts of the posterior annulus fibrosus. The dorsal rami of S1, S2, and S3 provide sensation via the middle cluneal nerves, and the dorsal rami of S4 and S5 provide sensation over the coccyx.

The L4, L5, S1, and S2 roots contribute to the sciatic nerve, a cable-like structure that includes the common peroneal and tibial nerves, which pass through the greater sciatic foramen, inferior to the piriformis muscle, lateral to the ischial tuberosity, and under the gluteus maximus muscle.

Vascular Supply

The blood supply to the thoracic and lumbar spine is predominantly from segmental arteries that originate directly from the aorta. These segmental arteries divide to form ventral and dorsal branches that supply the vertebral body. The dorsal branches provide the major blood supply to the dorsal musculature. A branch enters the intervertebral foramen and further divides, supplying blood to the nerve roots and spinal cord. The segmental arteries contain anastamosing branches that provide flow from segment to segment. There is significant variation in segmental arterial supply to the spinal cord.

The venous drainage parallels the arterial vasculature. An intervertebral plexus surrounds the spinal cord, which feeds into the segmental veins and drains directly into the vena cava.

BIOMECHANICS

Insight into the biomechanics of the spine requires knowledge of the forces applied in relation to the normal shape of each spine segment. The vertebral column must resist axial, torque or rotational, and shear forces while allowing motion in the sagittal plane (flexion, extension), the frontal plane (left and right lateral bend), and the horizontal plane (axial rotation). This controlled motion is facilitated via the combined effects through the three-joint complex (i.e., the disc and two facet joints at each level). Some motions, such as lateral bend, are coupled, which means they involve rotation in several planes (i.e., axial rotation and sagittal extension). Repetitive and/or supraphysiologic axial compression, torsion, tensile forces, and combinations of these forces can all lead to injury. Spinal biomechanics are extremely complex and are mentioned here primarily to alert the reader to review these matters in detail.

Although the spine is straight in the frontal plane, there are four curves in the sagittal plane. The cervical and lumbar regions are lordotic, whereas the thoracic and sacral regions are kyphotic. These balanced curves maintain the center of gravity over the pelvis and increase the load-carrying capacity of the spine. There is increased stress and susceptibility to injury at the junctions between the thoracolumbar and lumbosacral regions.

The motions of flexion and extension are best accomplished in the lumbar region where the facets are oriented in a sagittal plane. The posterior musculature and ligamentous structures primarily limit this motion. Forward flexion, initiated by the anterior musculature, results in compression of the anterior disc, bulging of the annulus, and separation (distraction) of the facets and their associated capsules. Flexion in the lumbar spine increases the size of the intervertebral canal and foramina. Flexion also increases nerve root tension. Therefore, in compressive conditions (i.e., spinal stenosis) flexion relieves compression of the neurologic structures and improves pain. Conversely, in situations of increased root tension (i.e., disc herniation) flexion precipitates increased tension and pain.

Active extension, initiated by the posterior musculature, produces compression of the posterior vertebral disc and overlapping of the facet joints. It is limited by the ALL and the posterior osseous structures. Extension in the lumbar spine decreases the size of the intervertebral canal and foramina. Extension also decreases nerve root tension. Therefore, in compressive conditions (i.e., spinal stenosis) extension exacerbates compression of the neurologic structures and worsens pain. Conversely in situations of increased root tension (i.e., disc herniation) extension relieves tension and improves pain.

The coronally oriented thoracic facets allow for maximum rotation, but the presence of the rib cage limits all motion and adds stability to these segments. Lateral bending combines flexion and rotation. Rotation is primarily limited by facet joint orientation and by disc thickness and integrity.

The disc must resist compressive, shear, and tensile forces. Axial forces are transmitted to the nucleus pulposus, which spans out radially against the annulus and creates a hoop stress.[27] The annulus is best suited to resist tensile and shear forces. Injury to the intervertebral disc occurs primarily through torque and shear forces which can result in radial and circumferential tears.

The soft tissue supports of the lumbar spine function like guide wires. The abdominal muscles provide nearly 30% of lumbar support via hydrostatic column effects.[64] Accordingly, weakness in these structures results in abnormal increase in lordosis with higher stress on soft-tissue supports.

CLINICAL HISTORY IN THE EVALUATION OF THE ATHLETE'S SPINE

The concepts outlined previously must be kept in mind when clinically evaluating athletes. With each patient, the examiner must attempt to correlate mechanism of injury with pertinent anatomy.

The history is perhaps the most important aspect of the clinical evaluation. The patient's chief complaint enables the clinician to remain focused while obtaining information concerning the mechanism, timing, quantity, quality, and location of symptoms.

Mechanism of Injury

If the patient is able to recall an exact cause of injury, it is extremely important to obtain a detailed description. For example, pain in the back after a direct blow from a football helmet is likely to be secondary to a contusion or posterior element injury. A description of the event may require the assistance of an observer present at the time of injury.

Timing

Did the pain occur immediately after an injury or did it gradually occur hours later? These answers help to differentiate between a break or contusion versus a muscular strain, which may not present in such an acute manner. Did the patient have pain before the injury? Is the pain constant, or is it intermittent? Is the pain associated with a certain activity? Does the pain occur at night? Pain that exists before the injury may be a chronic process possibly aggravated by the injury. Pain associated with upright activity may be a mechanical problem. Night pain should invoke concern about an infection or neoplasm. Pain radiating into the buttocks may result from spinal stenosis. Spondylolisthesis often presents during this age group as radiating pain. Groin pain is often pathognomonic of hip pathology.

Quantity

It is important to use a value scale to quantitate the amount of pain to help judge injury severity. Simple pain scales such as a 1–10 pain rating can be very useful in diagnosis and management.

Quality

The description of pain quality is very important. Is the pain a dull ache, or is it a sharp, stabbing pain? Is there "electricity, tingling, or numbness" shooting down the patient's leg? Is there any associated weakness? Does anything make the pain better or worse? Ask the patient to describe the condition in his or her own words. Does forward flexion relieve the symptoms (spinal stenosis)?

Location

Localization of pain provides critical support for a specific diagnosis. Is the pain isolated to a certain site in the back? Is it midline, or does it include the paraspinal areas? What about the sciatic notch and the sacroiliac joints? Does the pain radiate into the buttocks or lower extremities? This information should be obtained carefully but without "leading" the patient.

It is fundamentally important to separate back pain from leg pain. Back pain is usually synonymous with a structural problem (posterior structures). It may also result from irritation of the posterior primary ramus, the small branch coming posteriorly off the nerve root immediately after its exit from the foramen. This branch supplies the facet capsules, posterior annulus, and some of the local musculature.

In contrast, leg pain is usually synonymous with neurologic problem. Pain radiating to the leg, particularly below the knee, suggests irritation of the large ventral portion of the root exiting from the canal via the foramen and continuing distally into the leg. The term *sciatica* is often used to refer loosely to pain radiating down the leg for whatever reason, although it specifically refers to nerve root compression (most commonly L5 or S1) by a herniated nucleus pulposus. Pain radiating down the leg as a result of nerve root irritation is referred to as *radiculopathy.* Determining the dermatomal distribution of these symptoms within the leg is essential in identifying the specific nerve root involved.

After obtaining the history of the present illness, carefully review the medical, surgical, family, and social history. When evaluating athletes with back complaints, it is important to realize that their symptoms may not be related to their athletic endeavors. It is important to investigate what psychosocial factors may be involved in pain causation and pain perception. The potential economic and legal ramifications of the injury, especially in high-level athletes, must be investigated to complete the work-up.

PHYSICAL EXAMINATION OF THE ATHLETE'S SPINE

Having completed the history, the clinician should have formulated a working differential diagnosis, which will be further refined through physical examination of the spine by inspection, palpation, neurologic evaluation, and testing of range of motion. It is important to have the patient fully disrobe (down to underwear) before the examination.

Inspection

Inspection should begin with the patient standing in the upright position (if possible). Initially, one should observe the skin by looking for ecchymosis, swelling, old scars, cafe au lait spots (associated with neurofibromatosis), lipomata, and tufts of hair (associated with congenital defects).

Alignment

Curvature of the spine can be best appreciated from behind with the patient leaning forward. Often, rotation of the vertebral column will accompany a scoliotic curve, resulting in a unilateral prominence of the rib cage known as a rib hump. Asymmetry of the shoulder or pelvis may also result from scoliosis, and a discrepancy in leg length may be another cause of pelvic tilt leading to back pain. Viewing the patient from the side will allow evaluation of the spine in the sagittal plane. Look for changes in thoracic kyphosis or lumbar lordosis. Muscle spasm secondary to acute injury often leads to loss of lumbar lordosis.

Observation

The patient should be asked to perform several routine tasks, which will provide a quick assessment of his or her overall condition. For example, having the patient walk on his or her toes and heels provides information as to the general strength of the lower extremities. Having the patient walk (preferably without knowing he or she is being observed) may reveal a spinal radiculopathy with associated leg pain and weakness or Trendelenburg signs suggestive of hip abnormality.

Flexion in the lower spine leads to the reversal of lumbar lordosis and rotation of the pelvis. Commonly with lower spine injuries, muscle spasm will prevent motion in the lumbar spine, and, thus, flexion will be performed solely through rotation of the pelvis while maintaining lumbar lordosis. Limitation of forward flexion may also result from hamstring tightness.

Evaluation of extension should be performed in the standing position. Extension places stress on the posterior elements, including the pars interarticularis and facet joints, and it will decrease the opening of the intervertebral foramen. Symptoms secondary to abnormality in these regions may be exacerbated by this motion. A step off in the lower back may represent spondylolisthesis. Rotation and lateral bending can be best evaluated with the patient sitting on a chair that secures the pelvis and lower extremities. Rotation and lateral bending should be symmetric. Lateral bending may compress the intervertebral foramen on the ipsilateral side, aggravating impingement of the spinal nerve in patients with radicular symptoms.

Palpation

The spine should be palpated in a systematic fashion to identify areas of tenderness. It is often helpful to begin palpating in a pain-free area. Touching the patient without causing pain will gain his or her confidence, reduce anxiety, and allow him or her to define more accurately areas of tenderness. The top of the iliac crests are a rough reference for L4–L5. Focal areas of tenderness, called *point tenderness*, usually represent acute trauma, such as a contusion, strain, musculoligamentous tear, or fracture.

The deep and superficial musculature of the back should be carefully palpated. The paraspinal muscles may demonstrate tenderness and rigidity, indicating spasm with loss of range of motion. The range of motion of the spine may be difficult to evaluate because, unlike the extremities, there is no matched control to serve as a reference. Furthermore, the segments act with the pelvis and hips to provide overall motion and may be difficult to isolate.

As noted previously, careful examination is essential to localize abnormalities involving the sacroiliac joints, iliac crests, and the greater sciatic notch. Often, conditions affecting these areas may present with complaints of "back pain" that is not really coming from the back. Because injury to these structures can also result in limited radiation of pain to the leg, it is particularly important to physically localize them.

Further distally in the pelvis lies the coccyx, which is injured frequently. Pain in the area of the coccyx is called *coccydynia* and is characterized by exquisite local tenderness. This pain may be better appreciated by palpating the anterior and posterior aspects of the coccyx during a rectal examination.

Physical examination should also include palpation of the costovertebral angles and the abdomen. Although kidney infections, stones, or contusions are not usually considered sports injuries, these may present with back pain. Intraabdominal abnormalities, such as a dissecting aortic aneurysm, may also refer pain to the back. Although rare, this condition should be kept in mind, particularly when examining older athletes.

Neurologic Examination

This portion of the examination should routinely focus on motor, sensory, and reflex evaluation of the thoracic and lumbar regions. Sensory testing should be conducted with attention to individual dermatomes. Motor testing should also be performed according to known segmental innervation patterns (see box, Lower Extremity Innervation).[20] Of note, manual strength testing by the examiner may fail to reveal relative weakness of an athlete's trunk or legs because an examiner's hands and arms may not be strong enough to overcome these muscle groups, even when partially weakened. Therefore, when possible, heel and toe walking and squatting and rising from full squat are important motor tests. Evaluation of deep tendon reflexes will also assist in identifying the level of neurologic involvement (see box, Lower Extremity Deep Tendon Reflexes).

Multiple maneuvers have been described that place tension on the sciatic and femoral nerves to elicit radicular findings. Straight leg raising places tension on the sciatic nerve.[47] The test result is considered positive if radicular symptoms are reproduced when the straight leg is raised above 30° with the patient supine. Dorsiflexion of the ankle will place greater tension on the nerve and should exacerbate the patient's symptoms. The Lasègue test,[52] performed in the supine position, also places tension on the sciatic nerve. With the hip and knee initially flexed to 90°, the knee is slowly extended to elicit the radicular symptoms. Like the Valsalva maneuver, the Milgram test[19] is designed to increase the intrathecal pressure. In the supine position, the patient is asked to maintain both extended legs approximately three inches off the table for 30 seconds. If there is root impingement, the increase in intrathecal pressure will exacerbate radicular symptoms.

The Patrick (FABER) test is used to detect hip or sacroiliac abnormality. The patient lies supine on the examining table with the foot of the involved side placed on the opposite knee, which positions the hip in flexion, abduction, and external rotation (i.e., FABER). Downward force applied to the knee with the pelvis secure produces pressure on the sacroiliac joint. Pain radiating to the groin is suggestive of hip abnormality.

Additional physical exam findings that would confirm sacro-illiitis would include pain on direct palpation of the joint and the development of pain and pressure with a reverse straight-leg raise on that side. This condition is usually treatable with a combination of physical therapy and non-steroidal anti-inflammatory medications. Selective steroid injections of the sacroiliac joint

CHECKLIST

Lower Extremity Innervation

- ☐ Hip flexion: T12, L1, L2, L3
- ☐ Knee extension: L2, L3, L4 femoral nerve
- ☐ Hip adduction: L2, L3, L4 obturator nerve
- ☐ Ankle dorsiflexion: L4 deep peroneal nerve
- ☐ Toe dorsiflexion: L5 deep peroneal nerve
- ☐ Ankle eversion: S1 superficial peroneal nerve
- ☐ Ankle plantar flexion: S1 posterior tibial nerve

CHECKLIST

Lower Extremity Deep Tendon Reflexes

- ☐ Patellar reflex: L4
- ☐ Posterior tibialis reflex: L5 (difficult to elicit)
- ☐ Achilles tendon reflex: S1

can also be performed for diagnostic and therapeutic purposes.

Acute Neurologic Deficits

When there is a possibility of acute neurologic deficit with spinal cord injury, precaution must be taken regarding immobilization, oxygenation, and medical management. Protocols exist for this and must be strictly followed to minimize risk of neurologic deterioration. Neurologic status is determined by evaluation of the sensorium and the central nervous system and the cervical, thoracic, lumbar, and sacral spinal segments.

Injury to the spinal cord may be classified as complete or incomplete. Early documentation of completeness of cord injury is essential because prognosis and management are vastly different for complete versus incomplete spinal cord injuries. Incomplete spinal cord injury refers to any situation where some but not all neurologic function is lost in the spinal cord or conus medullaris. Neurologic function remains normal proximal to the area of injury but is lost distally. Neurologic loss may be minimal as manifested by slight numbness or slight weakness in a limited area. Conversely, it may be near total, with apparent total loss of all sensory, motor, and reflex activity, including bowel and bladder function. In this setting, careful examination is crucial to identify any remaining function, no matter how limited. It is important to assess the integrity of sacral innervation while conducting the neurologic examination. The S2, S3, S4, and S5 dermatomes provide sensation around the anus. Because the sacral plexus also supplies the intrinsic muscles of the foot and the sphincters of the bowel and the bladder, even a flicker of intrinsic foot function (toe motion) may indicate residual cord function and, therefore, incomplete cord injury. This condition is referred to as *sacral sparing.*

With sudden and complete neurologic injury (paraplegia or quadriplegia), there is no hope for neurologic recovery. In contrast, if the injury is incomplete, there may be potential for some neurologic recovery, although the specific scope of return cannot be predicted. Numerous grading schemes (Frankel classification, Motor Index Score, etc.) have been developed to assess the scope of neurologic dysfunction. Of note, the Babinski reflex is a pathologic reflex, which, if present, indicates upper motor neuron injury.

The presence of spinal shock may confuse initial assessment of completeness of neurologic injury. *Spinal shock* refers to a physiologic state of paralysis, hypotonia, and areflexia after an acute spinal cord injury. This state may be reversible and often lasts 24 to 72 hours. The return of the bulbocavernosus reflex indicates the end of spinal shock. This reflex is evaluated by noting anal sphincter contraction in response to squeezing the glans penis in men or pulling gently on the Foley catheter in women. If the reflex is not present, the cord is in a state of spinal shock, indicating the possibility of future neurologic recovery.

Fortunately, spinal cord injury is very rare, particularly to the thoracic and lumbar regions. In part, this is because of the excellent protection and limited mobility of the thoracic region. In the more mobile lumbar region, there is no spinal cord because the conus terminates at L1–L2, with the cauda equina continuing distally. The conus is susceptible to injury, in part because of its location near the thoracolumbar junction, the area most often associated with vertebral fracture. Compression of the cauda equina may be caused by acute disc herniation, osseous fragments, hematoma, and a host of other entities. When this condition is acute, it is a surgical emergency known as *cauda equina syndrome.* This situation presents with bowel and bladder dysfunction (usually urinary retention), saddle anesthesia in the perineal area, and varying degrees of lower extremity weakness and loss of sensation. Failure to immediately decompress the involved neural elements results in permanent functional loss. These acute neurologic conditions are rare, however.

Evaluation of the Injured Spine on the Playing Field

When injured on the field, the athlete should not be moved before examination. This precaution also applies to the athlete's equipment, which should not be removed until a targeted history and physical examination have been performed. Any suspicion of potential spinal injury should be managed with great caution, and the patient should be immobilized on a backboard. Complaints of numbness, tingling, or weakness in the legs, significant back pain after a high-velocity injury, or significant muscle spasm limiting movement should be managed with immobilization.[14] Off the field, the clinician has the luxury of being able to obtain a detailed history, perform an exhaustive examination, and request diagnostic testing.

RADIOGRAPHIC ASSESSMENT OF THE THORACO-LUMBAR SPINE

On or off the field, the clinician should have a working differential diagnosis after completing the history and physical examination. When necessary, radiographic examinations should be performed to confirm this clinical diagnosis. In a classic article, Hirsh and Nachemson reported that objective neurologic signs (not including SLR) obtained on physical examination have a 55% positive predictive value in predicting the presence of a disc herniation.[22] Radiologic exams combined with the physical examination greatly improve diagnostic accuracy. These tests should not be ordered in a "shotgun" manner, wherein the test is being ordered to make the diagnosis. Rather, each test requested should be designed to answer a specific question. Diagnostic tests should be reviewed with the radiologist, providing him or her with the pertinent history and physical findings. Test results must be clinically correlated, so the entire picture makes sense. When used correctly, these tests are invaluable. Some radiographic studies are particularly sensitive and may produce false-positive results, which have virtually no connection with the issue at hand. Clinical judgment is essential in directing management.

Plain radiographs are routinely used as the first step in the radiographic evaluation of the spine. They allow assessment of the alignment and integrity of the osseous structures within the vertebral column. Radiographs are commonly obtained in the anteroposterior, lateral, and oblique planes. Spinal curvature in the frontal plane (scoliosis) may be assessed on the anteroposterior view. In addition, the status of the transverse processes may be determined. Widening of the interpedicular distance associated with loss of vertebral height may represent a burst fracture with possible involvement of the spinal canal. The lateral projection clearly demonstrates the vertebral bodies, intervertebral disc spaces, posterior structures, and the overall alignment of the spine in the sagittal plane. This view is especially helpful in evaluating compression fractures, dislocations, and degenerative changes within the spine. The oblique projection permits identification of defects within the pars interarticularis and evaluation of the intervertebral foramina. In this view, the pars is known as the "neck" of the "Scottie dog." Occasionally, lateral flexion and extension views are obtained to assess segmental instability demonstrated by increased angulation or translation of the vertebral bodies.

Computed tomography (CT) enables direct visualization of osseous and the soft tissues of the spine. Axial cuts permit assessment of the spinal canal for evidence of encroachment by herniated discs or retropulsed bony fragments from vertebral body fractures. Multiple sections in various planes may be performed, making this technique especially useful in evaluating fractures. Using computerized software, two- and three-dimensional views of the spine may be reconstructed, facilitating three-dimensional evaluation. The accuracy of CT imaging can be somewhat improved with the addition of water-soluble contrast agents in the diagnosis of disc herniation.[29,30]

Magnetic resonance imaging (MRI) has greatly advanced the ability to evaluate the soft tissues of the spine, including the intervertebral discs, neural structures, and musculoligamentous components. It is especially valuable in demonstrating degeneration and herniation of the intervertebral discs. T-2 weighted images are quite sensitive in characterizing degenerative changes within the disc, as well as being able to depict annular tears. Vertebral body marrow adjacent to end plates of degenerated discs often will show changes on both T-1 and T-2 weighted imaging. The MRI is also able to evaluate surrounding soft tissues for evidence of trauma, including edema and hematoma formation, epidural abscesses, neoplasms, epidural fibrosis, and intrinsic cord abnormalities such as syringomyelia. Most data suggests equivalent ability of MRI and CT to accurately diagnose herniated discs, although MRI more accurately detects a host of other soft tissue abnormalities.[29,30,60] The addition of contrast material (gadolinium) that highlights vascularized areas can help to differentiate scar (epidural fibrosis) from disc.[27]

Myelography, in conjunction with computed tomography, remains an excellent but invasive diagnostic technique for evaluating the contents of the spinal canal and exiting nerve roots. Myelography helps to diagnose extradural neural compression indirectly by observing changes in the normally contrast-filled structures of the spinal canal. With the continued improvement of MRI, the use of myelography (despite the advent of water-soluble agents) has declined because of related side effects such as headache, nausea, vomiting, and other systemic problems. It still remains a powerful and accurate diagnostic tool in certain settings, such as severe deformity and revision surgery.

Nuclear imaging, such as the technetium bone scan, is an extremely sensitive modality that is invaluable for detection of increased osteoblastic activity and vascularity throughout the skeleton. Such increase in activity may reveal occult stress fractures, healing fractures, response to infection or tumor, metabolic bone disease, and a host of other conditions. For example, a bone scan may assist in evaluating patients in whom there is a high suspicion of spondylolysis, even though plain radiographs appear normal. Similarly, a bone scan may be used to screen the skeleton for metastatic lesions and infection. Unfortunately, the bone scan is limited by its lack of specificity and therefore is not very useful in evaluating degenerative conditions.

Single proton emission computed tomography (SPECT) is felt to have a significant and growing role in evaluating adolescents and children with a history of back pain. It is strongly recommended that any athlete with longer than 1 month of clinically significant back pain should have a lumbar bone scan and a SPECT scan.[61] In a recent study of athletes with prolonged back pain and normal radiographs, bone scan showed stress fractures in 17 of 33 patients and SPECT was positive in 16 of 24 patients.[19] Numerous others have also reported that SPECT can detect a stress fracture when conventional x-rays and/or bone scan are normal.[1,13] In a study of 34 patients with a SPECT scan positive for spondylolysis, Anderson et al. found that radiographs and bone scan failed to demonstrate the pars lesion in 53% and 19% of the patients respectively.[1] Therefore in cases of a normal bone scan and radiographs, a stress fracture of the pars cannot be ruled out without a SPECT scan.[19] Subsequently, CT scans and MRI can help to further delineate pathology.

INJURIES

Soft-Tissue Injuries

The majority of injuries to the thoracic and lumbar spine are self-limiting and do not come to the attention of a clinician. Many of these injuries are contusions, musculotendinous strains, and ligamentous sprains. Contusions result from blunt trauma sustained by a direct blow. Often, the athlete is able to recollect an incident responsible for the injury. On physical examination, a contusion will present as a relatively discrete area of point tenderness with occasional overlying ecchymosis. Given a history of blunt trauma to the spine and point tenderness over the posterior elements on physical examination, the examiner should consider conventional radiographs to rule out the possibility of a fracture. A contusion may result in paraspinal muscle spasm that limits range of motion of the spine. Management of this injury includes an initial period of icing followed by stretching and strengthening of the supporting structures. The athlete should not be permitted to return to competition until normal ranges of motion and strength have been restored. If these criteria are not met, the spine's ability to withstand trauma may be limited, and the athlete will be susceptible to further injury.

Muscular or ligamentous injury affecting the spine may result from an acute event or from repetitive stress producing a chronic, insidious process. In the latter case, injury may be subtle, and the athlete may not be able to recall a particular incident. Further probing may expose need for altering the training regimen.

Acute musculoligamentous strains and sprains of the thoracic and, more commonly, lumbar and lumbosacral spine are the most common injuries to these regions. These injuries are characterized by nonradiating back pain of an unclear etiology. Common causes include change in level of activity, overuse activity, inadequate conditioning, poor posture, and improper lifting. Initially, a radiograph is not needed, particularly in young patients, but one should be taken if symptoms persist 2 to 3 weeks. Management consists of rest, icing for the first 72 hours, nonsteroidal anti-inflammatory drugs (NSAIDs), and muscle relaxants, followed by physical modalities and controlled exercise with focus on strength and endurance, heat, transcutaneous electrical nerve stimulation, and education. Ninety percent of injuries resolve within 2 months.[44]

Chronic muscular or ligamentous injuries often present with vague symptoms of back discomfort. The origin of these symptoms is difficult to localize on examination. Movement placing stress on the injured structure may reproduce symptoms. As mentioned previously, an initial period of icing followed by stretching and strengthening is required. The chronicity of this condition must be reinforced to the patient. The athlete may need to stop or alter the training regimen possibly responsible for the injury. NSAIDs may be considered as adjuncts to rehabilitation.

Because the intervertebral disc is susceptible to herniation and degeneration, this area has an important potential for pathology. With age, there is a decrease in the proteoglycan content of the nucleus pulposus, leading to loss of hydration. The nucleus loses its ability to absorb stress and increases the demands placed on the annulus fibrosus and other supporting structures. Repetitive axial and torsional stresses applied to the disc lead to tears of the annulus and subsequent herniation of the nucleus pulposus.[16]

Tears of the annulus can produce disabling pain without herniation. The patient can present with intense pain, spasms, and referred leg pain. Symptoms are exacerbated by any increases in intrathecal pressure such as flexion, sitting, coughing, and sneezing. Management is conservative and includes rest, NSAIDs and antispasmodic medications, and physical therapy.

The majority of disc herniations occur in the lumbar spine. Symptoms of disc herniation may present acutely after a traumatic insult or may develop gradually without an inciting event, especially in the middle-aged or older athlete. Lumbar disc herniation is most common in the third and fourth decades, but it may occur at any age, including adolescence. The chief complaint is usually pain, often described as radiating from the back or buttock into the leg, which may be accompanied by numbness and weakness involving the lower extremity. It is important to obtain the exact distribution of the patient's symptoms. Complaints of bilateral leg pain or bowel and bladder symptoms should alert the clinician to the possibility of cauda equina compression syndrome. Pain is exacerbated with coughing or Valsalva maneuver because this increases intrathecal pressure and may increase contact between the irritated nerve root and its surrounding structures. Symptoms are often exacerbated in the sitting position, particularly with driving. Sitting reduces lumbar lordosis. As a result of the three-joint complex, this position unloads the facets but increases load on the disc, increases intradiscal pressure, and, therefore, symptoms, at the affected level.

On inspection, the patient may lean toward or away from the involved side, depending on the location of the herniation (Fig. 17-5). This leaning relieves pressure on the compressed nerve root by opening the intervertebral foramen. Midline tenderness in the lower back is common and is often accompanied by paraspinal spasm. Radicular symptoms may be reproduced by performing femoral or sciatic nerve tension tests or by performing a Valsalva maneuver. The nerve tension tests must reproduce the patient's radicular symptoms to be considered significant. Straight leg testing in the sitting position (along with a host of other clinical examinations) may help differentiate real abnormality from malingering. A careful neurologic examination, noting a specific dermatomal sensory deficit, corresponding segmental motor weakness, and decreased deep tendon reflexes, may

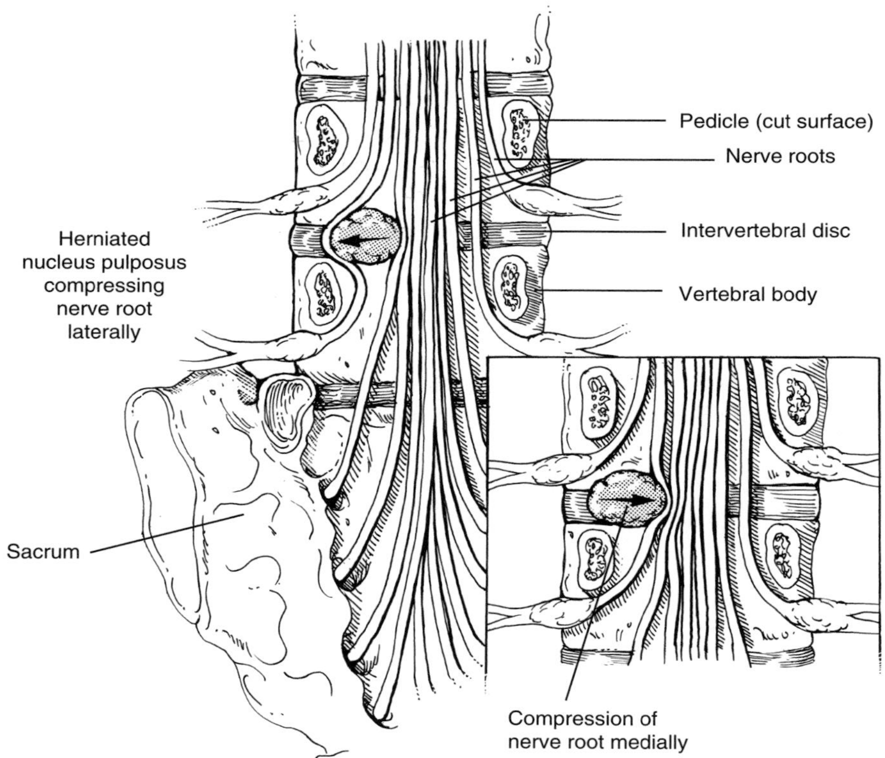

FIGURE 17-5. Herniated disc material impinging on adjacent nerve roots. Patients will involuntarily position themselves to minimize pressure on nerve roots.

identify the compressed nerve root. If there is concern of cauda equina compression syndrome, evaluation of sacral innervation is imperative. This evaluation should include sensory testing around the anus and rectal tone evaluation. Of note, adolescent athletes with disc herniations may present with back pain and hamstring tightness and minimal neurologic or radicular symptoms.

Plain radiographs may demonstrate indirect evidence of disc degeneration, such as decreased or irregular disc spaces. However, plain radiographs do not directly demonstrate disc herniations. MRI is the initial radiographic evaluation of choice for delineating disc abnormality. Other techniques (computed tomography, myelography) can also help to delineate pathology.

In the absence of an acute neurologic deficit, the mainstays of managing annular tears and herniated discs include rest, NSAIDs and antispasmodic medications, and physical therapy. Bedrest should be kept to less than 2 to 7 days, and controlled activity (therapy, rehabilitation) is initiated as soon as it is tolerable. If the pain is extreme, narcotics may be necessary. Many patients will markedly improve within 10 days, but conservative treatment should continue for 6 weeks before other measures are attempted. If leg pain persists beyond this period, a series of epidural steroid injections may be considered. Maximum benefit is usually within 2 weeks, with a maximum of three injections given per year. Responses vary greatly, with short-term improvement seen in roughly 40% of patients, but no significant long-term results have been demonstrated.[63] Rehabilitation must include stretching, strengthening, and modalities. Abdominal strengthening and lumbar extension exercises are beneficial. Therapy should be started early to prevent deconditioning. Return to athletic competition must be considered on an individual basis. Patients with significant pain relief, no neurologic sequelae, and normal range of motion may resume unrestricted activities. Education and lifestyle changes may be necessary to prevent recurrence.

Absolute surgical indications include cauda equina compression syndrome and progressive neurologic impairment. Patients without neurologic deficit who have not responded to conservative therapy may also be considered as elective candidates for surgical intervention if there is clear correlation between symptoms, physical findings, imaging, and electrodiagnostic (electromyography, somatosensory-evoked potential) testing. Successful return to vigorous athletic activity may be possible after surgery. More than 80% of athletes returned to sports after percutaneous or open discectomy, usually 8 weeks after surgery.[38] After surgical decompression, careful evaluation is necessary before return to athletics because functional impairment increases risk for further injury.

Degeneration of the intervertebral disc without annular tears or herniation may be another source of low back pain. With disc degeneration, more stress is transferred to the ligamentous and osseous structures of the spine, which may lead to arthrosis of the facet joints and hypertrophy of the supporting ligaments.

The presentation of degenerative disc disease varies. Symptoms may consist of pain isolated to the back or pain radiating into the buttocks and lower extremities. These symptoms are usually aggravated with increased activity, especially forward flexion. On physical examination, findings may include midline tenderness and paraspinal muscle spasm, resulting in a limited range of motion. Disc degeneration is extremely common in the older population, regardless of symptoms. It is important to consider other possible etiologies responsible for the patient's complaints before making the diagnosis of degenerative disc disease. Management of a symptomatic degenerative disc includes NSAIDs, exercises, and modalities. Exercises should concentrate on strengthening abdominal and paraspinal musculature to relieve stress on the vertebral column.

Although rare, thoracic disc herniations exist and are most common in the fourth decade of life.[2] Signs and symptoms of thoracic disc herniation vary widely and often may be subtle and associated with mild, but persistent, back pain. With a postero-lateral herniation, impingement of a thoracic nerve root may lead to chest wall pain that follows a dermatomal distribution. Often the neurological symptoms are absent or subtle, with mild changes in trunk sensation and lower extremity weakness. An athlete with a central herniation leading to direct impingement of the cord may demonstrate long track signs on examination, including the Babinski sign and clonus. The most important feature in establishing the diagnosis is a high degree of suspicion. The diagnosis is best confirmed by MRI or myelography. Management is usually conservative, including bedrest and NSAIDs followed by rehabilitation consisting of stretching and strengthening. Epidural injection with steroids may provide some relief if symptoms persist. Surgery is indicated if there is significant neurologic involvement. Anterior approaches are safest.

Sprains of the sacroiliac joint are another common source of back pain. This important joint within the pelvis is subject to large stresses and has strong restraining ligaments. Sudden and repetitive low-grade movements may result in injury. These injuries are often overlooked and are characterized by unilateral pain over the sacroiliac joint that may radiate to the buttock, leg, and groin. Symptoms may be exacerbated with standing and sitting as these impart shear and rotational forces across the joint. Stabilizing the pelvis by maintaining the opposite hip extended while flexing the hip on the affected side will usually reproduce the symptoms, as will the FABER maneuver. Result of straight leg raising is normal, as is neurologic examination. Management consists of NSAIDs, sacroiliac mobilization and manipulation, modalities, heat, sacroiliac and trochanteric belts, stretches, and sacroiliac injections. Many patients are relieved to learn that their problem is "not their back" and will resume activity despite residual pain.

The facet syndrome is another painful condition, primarily of the lumbar spine, characterized by local back pain with para-lumbar tenderness. Pain may be exacerbated with lumbar extension, whereas straight leg raising leads to hip, buttock, and back pain, but rarely referred leg pain. Typically, the patient will complain of pain when rising from the seated flexed position. Management is limitation of activity, NSAIDs, modalities, and manipulation. Facet injections do not exceed placebo effects.

"Kissing spines," commonly found in female gymnasts, refers to interspinous bursitis wherein the interspinous ligament develops a pseudobursa and there is chronic inflammation and even osteophyte formation on the adjacent spinous processes.[21] Injections of local anesthetic and steroids have been described to manage this condition.

The piriformis syndrome is another pain syndrome wherein the sciatic nerve is irritated as it passes near the piriformis muscle. This often-vague condition leads to deep pain along the posterior aspect of the hip that often radiates down into the leg. Unlike disc disease, there is no correlation of radicular pain with Valsalva maneuver. The condition occurs six times more frequently in women than men. It is suspected pain is triggered on active hip external rotation and with passive internal rotation of the hip. Management is with rest, NSAIDs, stretching, local injections, and, rarely, partial surgical release of the piriformis.

Osseous Conditions

Fractures. Fractures of the thoracic and lumbar spine occur infrequently in athletics and are usually associated with high-velocity or contact sports. The stability of the spinal column must be evaluated after each injury. Denis[12] described an anatomic classification of fractures according to a three-column system. The anterior column is composed of the ALL and the anterior two thirds of the vertebral body and annulus. The middle column consists of the PLL and the posterior third of the vertebral body and annulus. The posterior column includes the facets and spinous processes and the posterior ligamentous structures, including the ligamentum flavum, facet capsules, and interspinous and supraspinous ligaments. This classification has been modified to highlight the importance of bone soft-tissue components in each of the three columns.[15,62]

Trauma to the vertebral column results from excessive application of compression, distraction, rotation, or shear forces. The resulting injuries include compression fractures, burst fractures, flexion–distraction fractures, and fracture dislocations. Instability is unusual with anterior column involvement only but becomes an issue with disruption of the middle column. Fractures of the anterior column followed by posterior ligamentous disruption may also lead to spinal instability.

Compression fractures are the most common type of fracture in the thoracic spine. In these injuries, flexion or axial loading leads to failure of the anterior cortex of the vertebral body. The amount of trauma necessary to produce this injury depends on the quality of the bone within the vertebral body. Skydiving has a high incidence of spine compression fractures, and these injuries account for 17% of skeletal injuries in this sport.[44] Axial loading while seated, such as in falls in alpine or cross-country skiing, commonly leads to compression fractures.[22]

In healthy athletes, a great deal of energy is required to produce a compression fracture. In individuals with osteoporosis, the amount of force necessary for compression fracture may be trivial. This issue is of increasing concern as more older patients with decreased bone mass pursue sports.[18] If the fracture occurs in a young individual with minimal trauma, the possibility of an abnormal fracture should be investigated.

Compression fractures may be classified according to the amount of anterior compression. Most compression fractures do not have associated neurologic conditions and are relatively stable. Plain radiographs, especially the lateral view, will allow evaluation of the anterior and posterior cortices, and the amount of compression and angulation can be determined. Most fractures involve less than 25% loss of anterior body height (Fig. 17-6). As compression approaches 50%, there are concerns of instability caused by posterior ligamentous failure.[17]

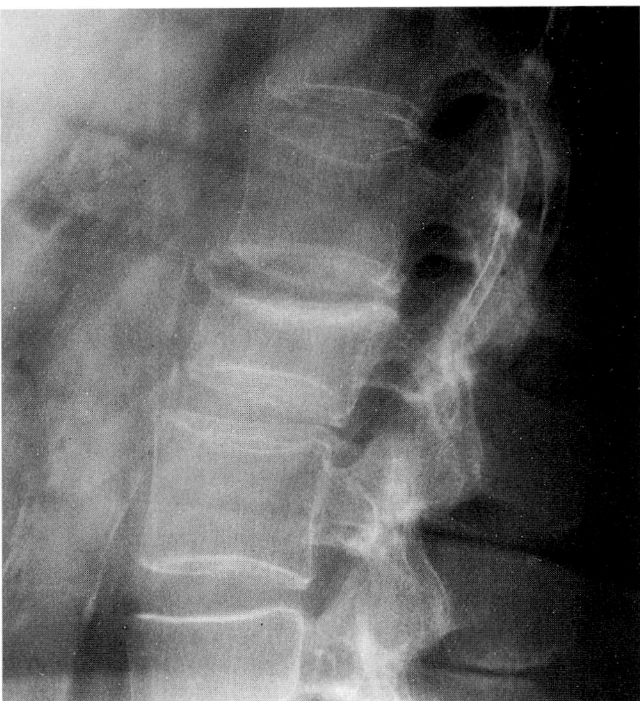

FIGURE 17-6. Compression fracture at L2. Note mild loss of anterior vertebral body height.

Compression fractures are extremely painful, resulting in paraspinal muscle spasm and limited range of motion. On physical examination, the patient will exhibit diffuse tenderness surrounding the fractured vertebra. A thorough neurologic examination should be conducted. It is important to document any neurologic symptoms after the injury, even if transient. Any signs of neurologic involvement require further evaluation for possible spinal injury.

Initial management of compression fractures includes pain control and bedrest. Management of stable fractures involves bracing in a rigid hyperextension orthosis. Stabilization will provide pain relief and will also prevent progression of kyphosis during fracture healing. The length of bracing depends on the patient's bone quality and healing potential, although 8 to 12 weeks are usually needed. Progression of kyphosis must be monitored in patients with severe compression fractures or multiple compression fractures. After bracing and resolution of pain, the patient is started on a rehabilitation regimen including strengthening and stretching to regain range of motion. Fractures with more than 50% compression or 20° of angulation are potentially unstable and must be observed closely for progression. Surgical decompression and stabilization are indicated for instability and progressive neurologic involvement.

Burst fractures involving the posterior vertebral body cortex have serious implications. Disruption of the middle column leads to mechanical instability and the possibility of neurologic injury resulting from retropulsed fragments within the spinal canal. On the anteroposterior view, an increased distance between the pedicles may represent disruption of the posterior cortex, indicating a possible burst fracture. Computed tomography is most effective in demonstrating the fracture configuration and integrity of the spinal canal. Surgical decompression and stabilization are often necessary for burst fractures.

Flexion–distraction (seat-belt injuries) and fracture–dislocation injuries rarely occur in sports and are usually related to high-velocity activities, such as high-diving, automobile racing, and skydiving. These injuries have a high incidence of spinal cord trauma and usually require surgical decompression and stabilization. It is the responsibility of the clinician on the field to recognize the seriousness of the injury and to immobilize the patient properly before evacuation. Neurologic evaluation is crucial, and evidence of progression requires emergency decompression. Plain radiographs and computed tomography are standard for evaluating the osseous integrity of the vertebral column. MRI is extremely helpful in assessing trauma to the surrounding soft tissues, including the ligamentous structures, intervertebral disc, and spinal cord.

Transverse process fractures generally result from a direct blow. Frequently, the athlete is able to recall an incident responsible for the injury, and pain is localized to the fracture site. Overlying tissues may be contused.

Diagnosis of a fracture is confirmed by plain radiographs. This fracture pattern is stable, and management is aimed at pain relief and followed by restoration of range of motion. When these goals are achieved, the patient may return to athletic participation. Cold therapy for the first 48 to 72 hours is followed by heat, rest, and immobilization until the patient is nearly asymptomatic. Stretching and strengthening exercises can then begin. Protection with a flak jacket may be necessary if contact sports are resumed before complete resolution of symptoms.

Participation in noncontact sports may begin after an appropriate period of immobilization and rehabilitation from a spinal fracture. Involvement in contact sports must be considered on an individual basis. In a young athlete without surgical intervention, contact sports may be considered after proper discussion regarding potential risks involved.

In children, vertebral apophysitis resulting from microfractures may present with point tenderness or with vague pain. Management is rest followed by stretching and strengthening rehabilitation. Similarly, anterior ring apophyseal fracture caused by recurrent flexion results in wedging of thoracolumbar or lumbar vertebral bodies.[48] Management is semirigid bracing to unload anterior elements until symptoms abate.

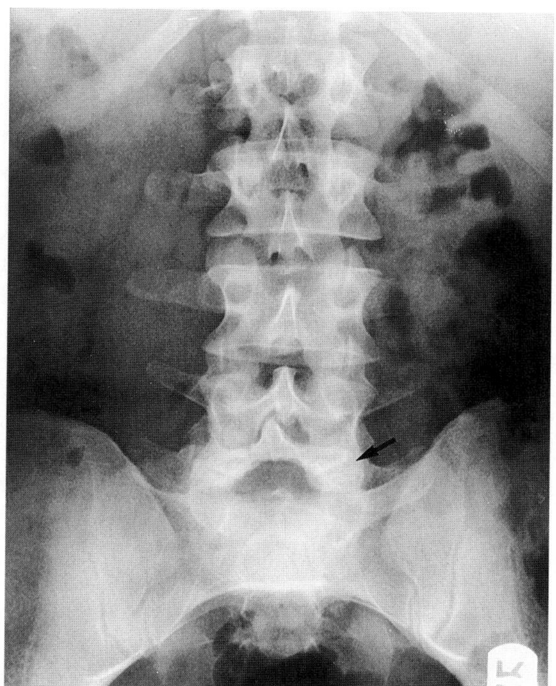

FIGURE 17-7. Anteroposterior radiograph of spondylolysis with pars defect seen at L5 *(arrow)*.

Spondylolysis and Spondylolisthesis. Athletes of all ages commonly complain of mild lumbar symptoms after strenuous workouts, but these symptoms generally resolve quickly without affecting the training schedule and requiring medical evaluation. In contrast, recurrent complaints of vague, but persistent, back pain, buttock ache, and hamstring tightness associated with activity should alert the clinician to an underlying spondylolysis or spondylolisthesis.[33]

Spondylolysis refers to a defect in the pars interarticularis (Fig. 17-7). The defect is believed to be a fatigue fracture secondary to repetitive stresses placed on the pars during hyperextension.[66] A pars interarticularis that is genetically predisposed to weakness may be the underlying cause of failure.[35] Repetitive stress on the pars from impingement by the inferior facet of the cephalad vertebra may result in microfractures, with continued stress leading to overt fracture. As a result, the disc bears excessive shear loads, and spondylolisthesis (slippage) may occur if excessive loading continues.[34] The incidence of spondylolysis in the general population is approximately 5%.[2] Studies demonstrate a hereditary predisposition,[3] with Eskimo populations having an incidence as high as 50%.[55] Spondylolysis is believed to be the most common cause of back pain in children and adolescents, although many people with spondylolysis are asymptomatic. The presence of spondylolysis does not necessarily implicate it as the pain source. Clinical correlation is essential to establish a causal relationship.

Certain athletic activities, including gymnastics, diving, wrestling, weightlifting, and football, are associated with an increased incidence of spondylolysis.[17] Certain features of these sports, such as upright weightlifting, dismounts from gymnastics, three-point stance contact in football, hard tennis overhead serve, and competitive diving, result in repetitive axial loading with the spine in extension.[9,64] Often, a single event responsible for the symptoms cannot be recalled. The pain is often unilateral, nonradiating, increased with activity (especially on extension), and relieved with rest. Physical examination may reveal decreased lumbar motion and hamstring tightness, a slight list caused by spasm, and exacerbation of pain with rotation and extension. Result of neurologic testing is normal, and result of straight leg raising is negative.

Diagnosis can be established radiographically using plain films, bone scanning, and single photon emission computer tomography imaging. Oblique radiographs may demonstrate the defect in the pars interarticularis (i.e., the "neck" of the "Scottie dog"). During the first several weeks, radiographs may appear normal. A bone scan may help in establishing an early diagnosis. Diagnostic bone scanning can be used when plain films are negative for determining defect acuteness and to rule out other conditions.

Management of spondylolysis remains controversial and ranges from benign neglect to surgical stabilization.[7] Management may vary depending on when the diagnosis is first established. Early on, the lesion in the pars represents a stress reaction with an increased potential for healing. Radiographs may appear normal, but a bone scan will demonstrate increased activity within the pars. Some clinicians recommend limiting activity, wearing a soft corset, and beginning flexion exercises.[67] Many others achieve excellent results with cessation of all extension exercises and immobilization in a rigid polypropylene orthosis. In the acute setting, patients need 8 to 12 weeks of rest and corset wear, with a brace or cast if full relief does not occur within 2 to 3 weeks of initial rest. Casting or bracing in an antilordotic position has been recommended.[40] Eighty-eight percent of athletes with low back pain from spondylolysis became symptom-free and were able to return to full athletic participation after rigid bracing.[54] In contrast, Blanda et al.[6] reported an 82% success rate using bracing with maintenance of lumbar lordosis for 3.5 months to approximate the fragments. They also emphasized the importance of abdominal exercises, hamstring stretching, and pelvic tilt once patients had become asymptomatic. Premature return to activity resulted in continued pain with activities of daily living. Early aggressive nonoperative management was essential to prevent long-term effects.

The patient must be fully asymptomatic before returning to activity. As a note of caution, some enthusiastic patients may not complete bracewear for the recommended period. Permanent avoidance of upright overhead weightlifting is prudent because fusion may be needed if symptoms become chronic. Education and reassurance are essential.

A visible pars defect on plain radiographs in conjunction with a normal bone scan most likely represents a chronic spondylolysis with limited healing potential. This defect should be managed conservatively with limitation of extension activities, lightweight corset for comfort, and abdominal muscle strengthening until symptoms resolve. Surgical intervention is rarely necessary for spondylolysis, although symptoms persisting at least 6 months despite bracing may warrant surgical stabilization.

Spondylolisthesis is an anterior displacement of one vertebral body over another. The most common type in childhood is isthmic spondylolisthesis secondary to elongation or fracture of the pars interarticularis (Fig. 17-8).[66] This type is believed to be a continuum of bilateral spondylolysis with loss of soft-tissue integrity leading to slippage, usually of L5 on S1. The severity of the slip is based on the amount of displacement compared with the width of the vertebral body below. Grades I to IV refer to slippage of 25%, 50%, 75%, or 100%. Grade V, where L5 is completely off, is called spondyloptosis.

The patient will usually present with low back pain. Occasionally, particularly with high-grade slips, patients will experience radicular symptoms, hamstring spasm, and symptoms of stenosis (Fig. 17-9). Physical examination may reveal flattening at the lumbosacral articulation because this is a kyphotic deformity of L5–S1. There

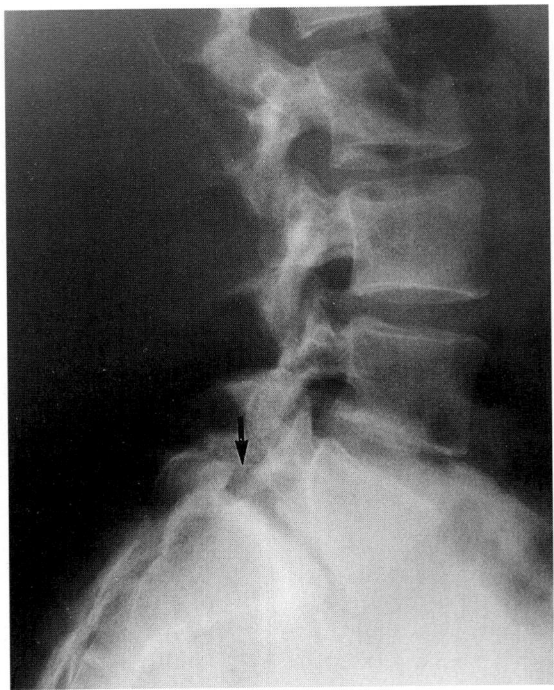

FIGURE 17-8. Lateral radiograph of Grade I spondylolisthesis of L5 on S1, with clear pars interarticularis defect (arrow).

may be compensatory lumbar hyperlordosis above the spondylolisthesis. A palpable step off may exist, along with a transverse abdominal crease, limited forward flexion, and trunk shortening. Results of neurologic examination and straight leg raising are generally negative, but subtle L5 radicular signs should be specifically pursued.

The anteroposterior radiograph may reveal the classic "Napoleon's hat" caused by superimposition of the body of L5 over the sacrum. Diagnosis is confirmed by lateral radiographs.

The most critical question to ask as a clinician is whether continuing competitive sports will result in the progression of spondylolisthesis. Grade I spondylolisthesis is managed similarly to spondylolysis. Symptoms must resolve prior to allowing return to contact sports even in the mildest cases. In a recent study of 86 young, asymptomatic, competitive athletes with spondylolisthesis (mostly Grade I), radiologic tests showed a 10.5% progression in 33 of 86 athletes while in 46 the displacement either did not change or decreased. They concluded "there is no justification for generally advising children and adolescents with spondolytic spondylolisthesis not to partake in competitive sports." [42] Grade II lesions are also managed conservatively, but return to contact or hyperextension sports, such as gymnastics, is somewhat controversial. Progression of low-grade slips is uncommon, but additional risk factors, including young age at presentation, female sex, dome-shaped sacrum, and high slip angle, must be factored into the decision to allow

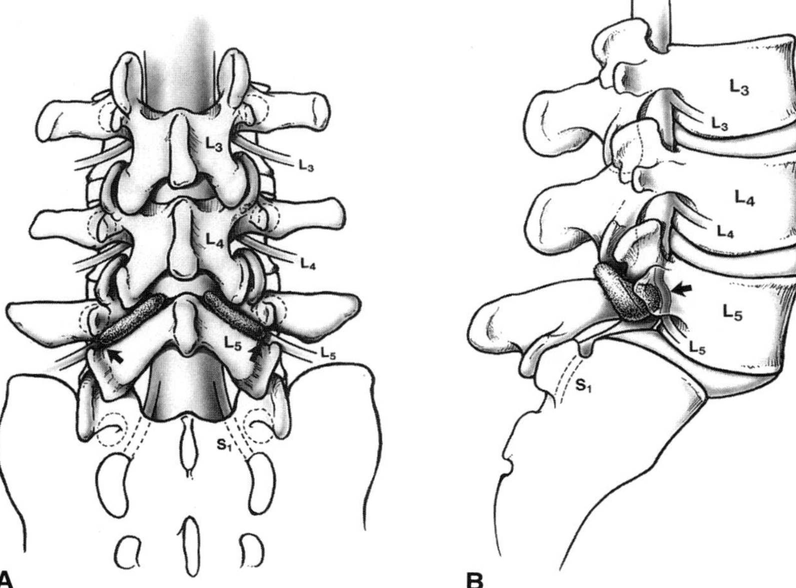

FIGURE 17-9. Posterior (**A**) and lateral (**B**) views of spondylolisthesis, illustrating how a defect in the pars interarticularis may lead to L5 nerve root compression, resulting in back and leg pain.

return to sport. Symptomatic patients with Grade I or II slips after 6 to 12 months of conservative treatment may be considered for fusion.

It is imperative that all children with high-grade slips be followed for possible progression regardless of symptoms. Grade III and IV lesions are likely to progress, and surgery is likely indicated.[6] Spondylolysis and spondylolisthesis are complex conditions, and their management is under constant review. The reader is encouraged to pursue this topic more fully in the literature.

Deformity. Many children and adults wonder if their spinal deformity will affect sports participation. The majority of spinal deformities do not require bracing or surgery and have virtually no effect on the athlete (Fig. 17-10). When bracing is required, activity should be promoted to prevent deconditioning, stiffness, and weakness resulting from bracewear disuse. Clinical outcomes regarding scoliosis progression at cessation of management were similar when bracewear was liberalized to include 3 to 4 hours of aggressive sports participation each day compared with conventional 23-hour per day bracing.[49]

In the absence of structural defects, the major limitation related to spinal deformity results from chest wall deformity and reduction in vital capacity.[8] In the presence of a structural alteration (congenital scoliosis or kyphosis), contact sports should be avoided because structural effects may result in abnormal ranges of motion and decreased mechanical strength.

Deformity in the sagittal plane (kyphosis) may present as postural roundback. This flexible, smooth curvature is reducible with supine hyperextension and may be

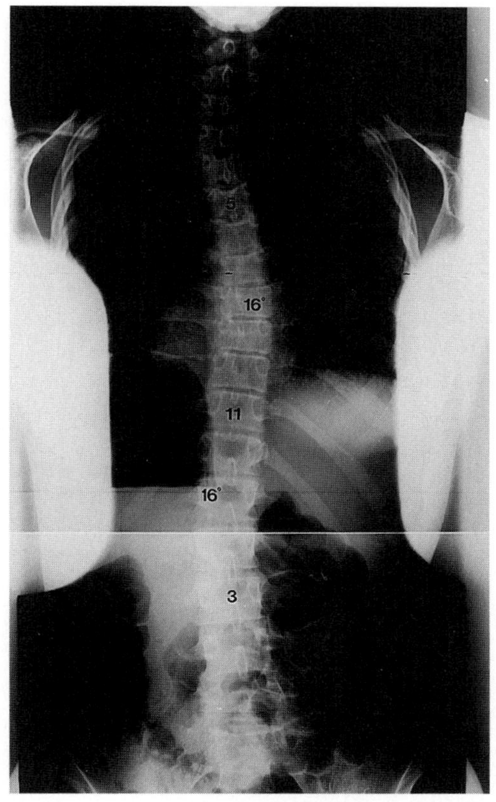

FIGURE 17-10. Posteroanterior radiograph showing balanced 16° scoliotic curves in a skeletally mature 15-year-old girl 2 years past onset of menses. This minimal deformity does not require any management and does not affect athletic activity.

accompanied by pain. Reassurance and an exercise program to strengthen the posterior musculature are appropriate. Alternatively, kyphosis may present as Sheuerman's disease, a condition of unclear etiology characterized by short and sharp curvature that is stiffer, often accompanied by pain, and characterized by radiographic changes in the vertebral endplates and ring apophyses. Activity should be restricted, followed by a posterior strengthening program. Whether or not bracing is required, the patient should be instructed to avoid overhead weightlifting. If pain recurs, activity should be restricted again. Optimum bracing is with a Milwaukee brace. Surgery is indicated for stiff, progressive, large curves (Fig. 17-11).

Lumbar hyperlordosis (sway back) may present with lumbar pain and tight hamstrings. If the curve is flexible, antilordosis exercises and abdominal strengthening are adequate. Antilordosis bracing is necessary for more rigid curves.

Patients are very concerned about returning to sports and exercise after spinal surgery. There are no established guidelines for surgeons regarding either appropriate sports or the appropriate time to resume sports after spinal surgery. A survey of 278 members of the Scoliosis Research Society revealed that most patients were returned to gym class (noncontact sports) between 6 months and 1 year after surgery. Of those surveyed, 55% suggested or required that patients never return to collision sports.[46] Care must be individualized, although, in general, patients undergoing short fusions may return to more vigorous activity than those undergoing longer fusions. A return 1 year after surgery with radiographically proven solid fusion and absence of symptoms is reasonable for short fusions. If long metal implants have been used, contact sports must be eliminated because of the risks of stress at the ends of the fusion. In a study of 59 patients with idiopathic scoliosis, both conservatively treated and surgically treated patients suffered an impairment of sports activities compared with age-matched controls. The study found that sports activity is not more restricted after extended spinal fusion than it is after nonoperative treatment.[45]

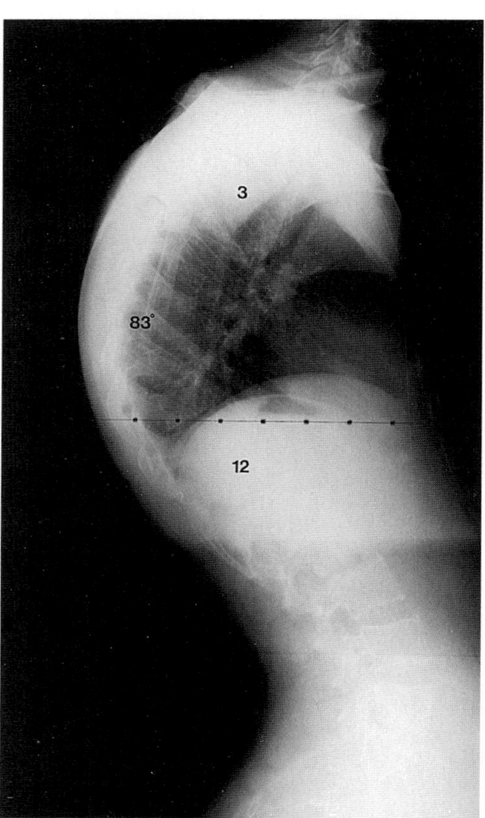

FIGURE 17-11. Lateral radiograph showing severe kyphosis in 14-year-old boy. A deformity of this magnitude requires surgical correction.

Patients with ankylosing spondylitis should attempt to maintain normal posture, and activity should be encouraged, along with judicious use of NSAIDs.

General Caution

Young athletes are at the age typical for the initial presentation of musculoskeletal tumors, such as osteoid osteoma and osteoblastoma, aneurysmal bone cysts, and osteogenic sarcoma. Disc space infection (discitis) is another possibility. Although these entities are rare, they must be kept in mind, particularly if symptoms persist.

In all patients, persistent fever is worrisome, possibly suggestive of disc space infection or vertebral osteomyelitis. Has there been recent surgery or an invasive procedure? Elevation of erythrocyte sedimentation rate and leukocytes, positive bone scanning, or disc space narrowing with endplate irregularity are suspicious. Weight loss, anorexia, or pain at rest raise concern for malignancy.

Finally, there are a host of conditions resulting in back pain that have nothing to do with the back. Pain referred to the back may originate from vascular, abdominal, and pelvic disorders, genitourinary and renal disorders, and others. Compulsive physical examination, including abdominal, rectal, and pelvic examination when necessary, and appropriate blood, urine, and radiographic testing, will minimize the chance of missing these potentially elusive disorders.

REFERENCES

1. Anderson K, et al: Quantitative assessment with SPECT imaging of stress injuries of the pars interarticularis and response to bracing. J Pediatr Orthop 20(1):28–33, 2000.
2. Arce CA, Dohrmann GJ: Herniated thoracic discs. Neurol Clin 3:383, 1985.

3. Baker DR, McHollic W: Spondyloschisis and spondylolisthesis in children. J Bone Joint Surg [Am] 32:933, 1956.
4. Balague F, et al: Non-specific LBP among schoolchildren: A field survey with analysis of some associated factors. J Spinal Disord 7:374–379, 1994.
5. Banks GM, Transfeldt EE: Biomechanics: Clinical applications. In Weinstein S (ed): The Pediatric Spine: Principles and Practice. New York, Raven Press, 1994.
6. Blanda J, Bethem D, Moats W, Lew M: Defects of pars interarticularis in athletes: A protocol for nonoperative treatment. J Spinal Disord 6:406–411, 1993.
7. Bradford DS, Iza J: Repair of the defect in spondylolysis or minimal degrees of spondylolisthesis by segmental wire fixation and bone grafting. Spine 10:673–679, 1985.
8. Chong KC, Letts RM, Cumming GR: Influence of spinal curvature on exercise capacity. J Pediatr Orthop 1:251–254, 1981.
9. Ciullo JV, Jackson DW: Pars interarticularis stress reaction, spondylolysis and spondylolisthesis in gymnasts. Clin Sports Med 4:95–110, 1985.
10. Clemente CD: Anatomy: A Regional Atlas of the Human Body. Philadelphia, Lea and Febiger, 1975.
11. Coventry MB: The intervertebral disc: Its microscopic anatomy and pathology. J Bone Joint Surg [Am] 27:105–112, 1945.
12. Denis F: The three column spine and its significance in the classification of acute thoracic and lumbar spinal injuries. Spine 8:817–831, 1983.
13. Dutton JA, Hughes SP, Peters AM: SPECT in the management of patients with back pain and spondylolysis. Clin Nucl Med 25(2):93–96, 2000.
14. Eismont FJ, Kitchel SH: Orthopaedic Sports Medicine. Principles and Practice, vol 2. Philadelphia, WB Saunders, 1994.
15. Farcy JPC, Weidenbaum M: A preliminary review of the use of Cotrel-Dubousset instrumentation for spinal injuries. Bull Hosp Jt Dis Orthop Inst 48:44, 1988.
16. Farfan HF, et al: The effects of torsion on the lumbar intervertebral joints: The role of torsion in the production of disc degeneration. J Bone Joint Surg [Am] 52:468–497, 1970.
17. Flemming JE: Spondylolysis and spondylolisthesis in the athlete. Spine 4:339–345, 1990.
18. Frymoyer JW, Pope MH, Kristiansen T: Skiing and spinal trauma. Clin Sports Med 1:309–318, 1982.
19. Garces GL, Gonzalez-Montoro I, Rasines JL, Santonja F: Early diagnosis of stress fracture of the lumbar spine in athletes. Int Orthop 23(4):213–215, 1999.
20. Goldstein JD, Berger PE, Windler GE, Jackson DW: Spine injuries in gymnasts and swimmers. An epidemiologic investigation. Am J Sports Med 19(5):463–468, 1991.
21. Hazlett J: Kissing spines. J Bone Joint Surg [Am] 46:1368–1369, 1964.
22. Hirsh L, Nachemson A: The reliability of lumbar disc surgery. Clin Orthop 29:189–195, 1963.
23. Hoppenfeld S: Physical Examination of the Spine and Extremities. New York, Appleton-Century-Crofts, 1976.
24. Hosea TM, Gatt CJ Jr: Back pain in golf. Clin Sports Med 15(1):37–53, 1996.
25. Howell DW: Musculoskeletal profile and incidence of musculoskeletal injuries in lightweight women rowers. Am J Sports Med 12:278–282, 1984.
26. Hresko MT, Micheli LJ: Sports medicine and the lumbar spine. In Floman Y (ed): Disorders of the Lumbar Spine. Rockville, MD, Aspen, 1990.
27. Hueftle MG, et al: Lumbar spine: postoperative MR imaging with Gd-DTPA. Radiology 167(3): 817–824, 1988.
28. Jackson DW, Wiltse LL, Circncoine RJ: Spondylolysis in the female gymnast. Clin Orthop 177:68–73, 1976.
29. Jackson RP, et al: The neuroradiographic diagnosis of lumbar herniated nucleus pulposus: I. Spine 12:1356–1361, 1989.
30. Jackson RP, et al: The neuroradiographic diagnosis of lumbar herniated nucleus pulposus: II. Spine 14:1362–1367, 1989.
31. Keene JS, et al: Back injuries in college athletes. J Spinal Disord 2:190–195, 1989.
32. Keene JS: Thoracic and lumbar fractures in winter sports. Am J Sports Med 216:39, 1987.
33. King H: Back pain in children. In Weinstein S (ed): The Pediatric Spine: Principles and Practice. New York, Raven Press, 1994.
34. Letts M, Smallman T, Afanasie R, Gouw G: Fracture of the pars interarticularis in adolescent athletes: A clinical-biomechanical analysis. J Pediatr Orthop 6:40–46, 1986.
35. Lindholm TS, Ragni P, Ylikoski M, Poussa M: Lumbar isthmic spondylolisthesis in children and adolescents. Radiologic evaluation and results of operative treatment. Spine 15(12):1350–1355, 1990.
36. McCarroll JR, Retting AC, Shelbourne KD: Injuries in amateur golfers. Physician and Sports Medicine 18(3):122–126, 1990.
37. McCarroll JR, Gioe TS: Professional golfers and the price they pay. Physician and Sports Medicine 10(7): 64–70, 1982.
38. Matsunaga S, Sakou T, Taketomi E, Iijiri K: Comparison of operative results of lumbar disc herniation in manual laborers and athletes. Spine 18:2222–2226, 1993.
39. Maxwell C, Spiegal A: The rehabilitation of the athelete following spinal injuries. In Hochschuler

SH (ed): The Spine in Sports. Philadelphia, Hanley and Belfus, 1990, pp 281–292.
40. Micheli LJ: Low back pain in the adolescent: Differential diagnosis. Am J Sports Med 7:362–364, 1979.
41. Micheli LJ: Back injuries in gymnastics. Clin Sports Med 4:85–93, 1985.
42. Muschik M, et al: Competitive sports and the progression of spondylolisthesis. J Pediatr Orthop 16(3):364–369, 1996.
43. Panjabi MM, White III AA: Clinical Biomechanics of the Spine, 2nd ed. Philadelphia, JB Lippincott, 1990.
44. Parsch D, et al: Sports activity of patients with idiopathic scoliosis at long-term follow-up. Clin J Sport Med 12(2):95–98, 2002.
45. Petras AF, Hoffman EP: Roentgenographic skeletal injury patterns in parachute jumping. Am J Sports Med 11:325–328, 1983.
46. Rubery PT, Bradford DS: Athletic activity after spine surgery in children and adolescents: results of a survey. Spine 27(4):423–427, 2002.
47. Schamm S, Taylor T: Tension signs in lumbar disc prolapse. Clin Orthop 75:195–204, 1971.
48. Semon RL, Spengler D: Significance of lumbar spondylolysis in college football players. Spine 16:172–174, 1981.
49. Shelokov AP, Herring JA: Spinal deformities and participation in sports. In Hochschuler SH (ed): The Spine in Sports. Philadelphia, Hanley & Belfus, 1990.
50. Snook GA: Injuries in women's gymnastics—A 5 year study. Am J Sports Med 7:242–244, 1979.
51. Snook GA: Injuries in intercollegiate wrestling—A 5 year study. Am J Sports Med 10:140–144, 1982.
52. Spangfert E: Lasegue's sign in patients with lumbar disc herniation. Acta Orthop Scand 42:459, 1971.
53. Stallard MC: Backache in oarsmen. Br J Sports Med 14:105–108, 1980.
54. Steiner EM, Micheli LJ: The use of a modified Boston brace to treat symptomatic spondylolysis. Orthop Trans 7:20, 1983.
55. Stewart TD: The age incidence of neural arch defects in Alaskan natives considered from the standpoint of etiology. J Bone Joint Surg [Am] 35:937–950, 1953.
56. Sward L, et al: Acute injury of the vertebral ring apophysis and intervertebral disc in adolescent gymnasts. Spine 15:144–148, 1990.
57. Sward L, Hellstrom M, Jacobsson B, Peterson L: Back pain and radiologic changes in the thoraco-lumbar spine of athletes. Spine 15:124–129, 1990.
58. Sward L, et al: Disc degeneration and associated abnormalities of the spine in elite gymnasts: A magnetic resonance imaging study. Spine 16:437–443, 1991.
59. Tertti M, et al: Disc degeneration in young gymnasts: A magnetic resonance imaging study. Am J Sports Med 18:206–208, 1990.
60. Thornbury JR, et al: Disk-caused nerve compression in patients with acute low-back pain: Diagnosis with MR, CT myelography, and plain CT. Radiology 186(3):731–738, 1993.
61. Watkins RG. Lumbar disc injury in the athlete. Clin Sports Med 21(1):147–165, 2002.
62. Weidenbaum M, Farcy JPC: Surgical management of thoracic and lumbar burst fractures. In Bridwell KH, DeWald RL (eds): The Textbook of Spinal Surgery. Philadelphia, JB Lippincott, 1991.
63. Wiesel SW, Boden SD: Diagnosis and management of cervical and lumbar disease. In Weinstein JN, Rydevik BL, Sonntag VKH (eds): Essentials of the Spine. New York, Raven Press, 1995.
64. Wilhite J, Huurman WW: Thoracic and lumbosacral spine. In Mellon MM, Walsh WM, Shelton GL (eds): The Team Physicians Handbook. Philadelphia, Hanley & Belfus, 1990.
65. Williams JG: Biomechanical factors in spinal injuries. Br J Sports Med 14:14–17, 1980.
66. Wiltse LL, Widell EH, Jackson DW: Fatigue fracture—the basic lesion in isthmic spondylolisthesis. J Bone Joint Surg [Am] 57:17–22, 1975.
67. Wiltse LL, Jackson DW: Treatment of spondylolisthesis and spondylolysis in children. Clin Orthop 117:92–100, 1976.

18 The Shoulder

Christopher S. Ahmad, Ken Yamaguchi, Ira Wolfe, and Louis U. Bigliani

Recent gains in the understanding and awareness of sports-related shoulder pathology and dysfunction have led to a greater interest in optimal management of sports-related shoulder injuries in athletes. The shoulder is now recognized as a primary source of functional disability in a large variety of sports, particularly those with repetitive overhead motions. Most athletes will experience disabling shoulder pain at some time in their careers requiring, at the minimum, a period of rest or inactivity.

In addition to overuse-acquired problems, traumatic injuries of the shoulder such as dislocations, fractures, or acromioclavicular separations have been observed with increasing frequency with the involvement of larger and more physical athletes. Both nontraumatic and traumatic injuries require early recognition and management to provide a better functional result and faster return to activities.

In this chapter, a systematic approach to the evaluation and treatment of the athlete's shoulder is presented. Relevant anatomy and biomechanics will provide the necessary foundation for understanding the different shoulder injuries. A discussion on general shoulder evaluation including a detailed history and physical examination for the initial, acute stages and in the recurrent or chronic stages will follow. Focused evaluation and management for specific injuries divided into nontraumatic and traumatic categories will be presented. Specific guidelines for acute and conservative management and indications for orthopedic referral will be discussed.

ANATOMIC AND BIOMECHANICAL CONCERNS

Bony Anatomy

The shoulder comprises three bones: the clavicle, the scapula, and the proximal humerus. Each is uniquely shaped to articulate with the others, allowing large degrees of motion. The clavicle, when viewed anteriorly, appears relatively straight but is actually an S-shaped bone that spans from the sternum medially to the acromial portion of the scapula laterally. It serves as a frame for muscle attachment, a shield for underlying major arteries and nerves, and an osseous strut preventing the shoulder girdle from medial and inferior displacement.[15] This laterally directed strut is important to shoulder motion because it allows major muscular actions to be directed toward humeral or scapular motion rather than medial humeral displacement.

Functionally, the clavicle can be divided into three parts: the medial third, which is important for neck strap muscle attachments and articulation with the sternum; the central third, which is more tubular and relatively muscle-free; and the distal third, which is important for the acromioclavicular articulation and scapular–clavicular stability.

The scapula is a complex, triangular-shaped bone that serves as a base for seventeen muscle attachments that allow for mobility and stability for the otherwise inherently unstable shoulder joint. The scapulothoracic position is connected to the axial skeleton through the clavicle and axioscapular muscles: the trapezius, serratus anterior, rhomboid major, rhomboid minor, and levator scapulae. The normal resting position is over the posterior–lateral aspect of the thorax between the second and seventh spinal segments. Because of its articulation with the rounded thorax, the scapula rests 30° anterior to the coronal plane.

In addition to the axioscapular muscular attachments, the scapula serves as the origin for the rotator cuff, which is formed by the confluence of the subscapularis, supraspinatus, infraspinatus, and teres minor muscles.

There are three important bony processes of the scapula: the coracoid, acromion, and glenoid. The coracoid serves as an anterior point for muscular and ligamentous attachment between the axial and appendicular portions of the body. The coracobrachialis and short head of the biceps originate from the coracoid and insert distally in the arm, and the pectoralis minor inserts in the chest wall. Additionally, there are important ligamentous attachments to the clavicle, proximal humerus, and intrascapular to the acromial process.

The acromion is a flat, lateral expansion of the scapular spine that projects superiorly over the humeral head. The acromion forms from two or three ossification centers that fuse at approximately 22 years of age. An unfused epiphysis can be mistaken for a fracture in the younger athletic population. In older individuals, a nonunion of one or more of the ossification centers, known as os acromiale, can also be mistaken for a fracture. Os acromiale occurs 1.6% of the time and is bilateral 60% of the time.[29,39]

The acromion, scapular spine, and distal clavicle serve as the point of origin for the deltoid. The acromion also articulates with the distal clavicle and is attached to the corocoid via the coracoacromial ligament. The acromion together with the coracoacromial ligament forms the coracoacromial arch, which creates the roof of the subacromial space through which the posterior rotator cuff, primarily the supraspinatus, passes. Because pathology in this location has been implicated in the mechanical abutment and impingement of the supraspinatus tendon, the coracoacromial arch has been thoroughly investigated.[10,21,39,41] Bigliani and Morrison described a simple, clinically relevant classification of acromial morphology divided into three types: Type I, flat; Type II, curved; and Type III, hooked, with an anterior–inferior facing spur. Type III, hooked, acromions have been associated with a significantly higher incidence of rotator cuff tears.[10]

Articular Anatomy

Different from most other articulations in the body, the glenohumeral joint is inherently unstable. It is more similar to a ball and plate articulation in contrast to the ball and socket articulation of the stable hip joint. The articular glenoid is relatively shallow, with a disproportionately small surface area, ranging from 25% to 33% of the humeral head surface.[29,39,44,45] The lack of bony contribution to joint contact allows for a less constrained and more mobile joint. Therefore, stability is inherently compromised and depends on static capsular restraints and dynamic muscular contribution from the rotator cuff.

The capsular restraints have been well characterized.[9,18,29,39,47] There are three glenohumeral ligaments that are thickenings of the capsule and are divided into superior, middle, and inferior bands. The ligaments contain mechanoreceptors that contribute to proprioceptive feedback for the glenohumeral joint. The inferior glenohumeral ligament is further divided into superior and posterior components and is commonly thought of as a sling on the inferior portion of the joint. This ligament is considered to be the most important capsular restraint to anterior and posterior glenohumeral subluxation. Glenohumeral dislocations usually occur in the upper elevations of arm position where these ligaments become taut, acting as checkreins to dislocation at the extremes of motion. Laxity in the ligaments, either as part of an avulsion from the glenoid rim or acquired intrasubstance stretching from repetitive micro- or macrotrauma, can cause clinically significant instability from several mechanisms: loss of checkrein function in sudden shifts of motion where muscular activity cannot compensate, loss of appropriate proprioceptive feedback for coordinated muscular contraction, and loss of checkrein function causing repeated stresses on surrounding musculature and fatigue failure. All of these mechanisms are commonly seen in disorders of the athlete's shoulder.

The glenoid labrum contributes to glenohumeral stability by deepening the socket by as much as 50%.[44,45] This increase in glenohumeral conformity provided by the labrum may also contribute to a suction effect of negative intraarticular pressure, further increasing stability. Avulsion of the anterior-inferior labrum from an anterior-inferior glenohumeral dislocation has been termed a *Bankart lesion.*

The coracohumeral ligament functions to resist humeral external rotation and inferior translation. The ligament spans from the anterior portion of the greater tuberosity to the coracoid. Significant pathologic contraction in this ligament results in loss of external rotation, which is a characteristic finding in frozen shoulder or adhesive capsulitis.

Muscular Anatomy

The proximal humerus is enveloped by a thick muscular sleeve responsible not only for gross movement of the extremity but also stabilization of the glenohumeral joint during motion. The muscles can be divided into three groups:

1. Primary glenohumeral muscles, which are the deltoid, subscapularis, supraspinatus, infraspinatus, teres minor, and teres major
2. Scapulothoracic musculature, which includes the trapezius, rhomboids, levator scapulas, serratus anterior, and pectoralis minor
3. Multiple joint muscles, which include the pectoralis major, latissimus dorsi, biceps brachia, and triceps brachia

The deltoid is the prime mover of the shoulder and is functionally divided into three parts: the anterior deltoid, responsible for flexion; the middle deltoid, responsible for scapular plane abduction (elevation); and the posterior deltoid, responsible for extension. Additionally, the anterior and posterior portions of the deltoid can work together for abduction. Among the three parts of the deltoid, loss of the anterior deltoid is most devastating because its function cannot be replaced.

The rotator cuff, which comprises the supraspinatus, infraspinatus, teres minor, and subscapularis, works in concert with the deltoid to provide arm elevation. The primary vector of muscle pull through the deltoid is vertical, which leads to superior translation of the humerus and impingement of the rotator cuff against the coracoacromial arch, if not properly controlled. The rotator cuff protects itself from this impingement by dynamically stabilizing the humeral head in the glenoid socket during arm elevation. The posterior rotator cuff is important in external rotation and prevention of anterior subluxation of the humerus. The subscapularis is important in internal rotation and humeral head stabilization.

The teres major also is an internal rotator of the humerus.

Because muscular contraction of the rotator cuff is important for glenohumeral stability in the superior, anterior, and posterior directions, subluxation in these directions may indicate existing rotator cuff dysfunction or, conversely, could cause rotator cuff disease.

Radiographic Anatomy

As with other parts of the body, radiographic evaluation of the shoulder should include a minimum of two views taken perpendicular to each other. Because of the relative difficulty of obtaining a good lateral view of the shoulder, this basic principle is often neglected, especially in the trauma setting where it is most important.

The standard trauma views are recommended for initial evaluation and consist of a scapular plane anteroposterior, Y-scapulolateral, and axillary views. The scapular plane anteroposterior view is taken at 45° from the anteroposterior plane of the thorax to account for scapular inclination. This allows for a true profile projection of the glenohumeral joint with superimposition of the anterior and posterior glenoid rims, minimizing overlap by the humeral head.

The Y-scapulolateral and axillary views provide right-angle projections to the anteroposterior view. The Y-scapulolateral view taken from posteromedial to anterolateral along the spine of the scapula is a true lateral view of the scapula. The "Y" is formed by the coracoid anteriorly, scapular spine posteriorly, and the scapular body inferiorly; the glenoid and humeral head is found at the center of the "Y." The axillary view is a true lateral view of the glenohumeral joint and is taken with arm abduction and neutral rotation in a cranially directed fashion through the axilla. Because this view requires some abduction, it is often not done in the acute, trauma setting. It is important to note that only 30° to 40° of abduction is required, which is generally well tolerated. In the rare circumstance in which a true axillary view cannot be obtained, a velpeau axillary view can suffice. The velpeau axillary view is taken from superior to inferior by having the patient lean backward over the film while the injured extremity remains in its immobilizer.

In addition to the standard trauma series, several specialized views can be helpful, depending on the clinical situation. The 10° cephalic tilt view highlights the acromioclavicular joint. The scapular outlet view is helpful for evaluating acromial morphology. Magnetic resonance imaging can give a highly accurate representation of the rotator cuff tendons and muscles.

Relevant Biomechanics

Glenohumeral motion is generally considered to have three axes of rotation: flexion and extension, abduction and adduction, and internal and external rotation. This glenohumeral motion is amplified and augmented by a coordinated contribution of scapulothoracic motion. Without coordinated scapulothoracic motion, glenohumeral motion would be limited to about 80° to 90° from the mechanical abutment of the greater tuberosity against the acromion. Generally, glenohumeral motion is accompanied by scapulothoracic motion at a 2:1 ratio, although the exact relationship varies depending on the relative position during abduction.

Overhead throwing is divided into five distinct phases: 1) wind-up, during which the rhythm and momentum for throwing is initiated; 2) cocking, in which the shoulder is abducted and at extreme external rotation and the lower extremity is beginning rotation toward the target; 3) acceleration, in which the arm begins horizontal adduction and internal rotation to accelerate the arm toward ball release (remember that the hand is moving as fast as the ball at this point); 4) ball release, in which the arm is forward to the body and elbow extension occurs to generate the last portion of velocity; and 5) follow-through, during which tremendous rotator cuff and biceps exertion strain is developed to decelerate the arm and stabilize the shoulder.[14] Although described primarily for the baseball pitcher, all sports-related overhead activities are generally variations of this theme.[5,23,29,39]

EVALUATION OF THE PAINFUL SHOULDER

Acute Assessment and First Aid

When working as the sports medicine provider for athletic events, ability to acutely assess shoulder injuries is required. Prompt initial evaluation should begin with a brief, directed history to identify mechanism of injury, presence of neurologic symptoms, and preexisting medical conditions. Following the history, a careful neurovascular assessment should be made of the upper extremity. This cannot be overemphasized because most injuries in the athletic setting can lead to some short-term disability or inconvenience, and missed vascular compromise can lead to loss of the limb. The radial and ulnar arterial pulses should be palpated, and capillary refill, coloration, and warmth should be assessed. Careful documentation of the vascular status will not only ensure prompt recognition, but will also allow for serial observations when subtle injuries are present.

Additionally, gross neurologic status should be determined by assessing strength and subjective sensation throughout the upper extremities. Neurologic injuries are not uncommon because of the proximity of the brachial plexus to the shoulder girdle. This is especially relevant to glenohumeral dislocations. Early recognition can lead to prompt reduction and decrease the severity of neurologic injury.

Once the neurovascular status is confirmed to be intact, an examination for more subacute problems can be performed. Any interfering athletic clothing or equipment should be removed to carefully observe the shoulder for gross deformities, lacerations, swelling, or bruising. Palpation can pinpoint possible injuries. If the examination does not indicate obvious dislocation or fractures, active range of motion can be attempted. Any significant pain preventing range of motion should be an indication to stop and immobilize the extremity in a sling and swathe for transport of the athlete to an emergency facility where radiographs can be taken.

The acute management of a witnessed anterior dislocation of the shoulder is controversial. With appropriate experience and training, a physician can accurately diagnose a dislocation and perform a relatively atraumatic relocation in the acute setting before muscle spasm takes place. However, in rare circumstances in which fracture accompanies dislocation, an inappropriate reduction maneuver can cause either displacement or propagation—a very serious complication.

Office Assessment

As with any other medical evaluation, obtaining an accurate history is essential in the overall clinical assessment of shoulder dysfunction.[6] Shoulder pain typically has a specific traumatic etiology that assists in correct diagnosis. A thorough history and physical examination supported with appropriate diagnostic tests will allow the diagnosis of the majority of shoulder disorders. Conditions such as cervical radiculopathy, tumors, acromioclavicular joint disorders, and systemic rheumatologic diseases must be carefully considered.

HISTORY

A thorough history systematically obtained will avoid missing information that the patient may feel is unimportant but is relevant to the shoulder problem (see box, History). Hand dominance, occupation, and athletic activities should be recorded to appreciate functional demands and future expectations. The dominant shoulder of a throwing athlete is a different challenge from the nondominant shoulder of a sedentary executive. In addition, certain activities may contribute to the pathology: the relationships between weightlifting and osteolysis of the distal clavicle,[13,40] and between repetitive minor injury (e.g., gymnastics or butterfly swimming) and shoulder instability[7] are well established.

A general medical history should be obtained, with special attention to symptoms suggestive of a systemic or rheumatologic disorder. Underlying conditions such as diabetes mellitus and metastatic cancer can cause a frozen shoulder. Furthermore, a family history may often be helpful (e.g., generalized ligamentous laxity in a patient with shoulder instability).

The precise nature of the patient's chief complaint, usually pain, weakness, stiffness, or instability, should be well understood. It is important to document the duration, provocation, severity, and timing of symptoms, especially pain. Rest pain and night pain are especially common in patients with shoulder pathology. Anatomic and mechanical conditions, such as impingement and glenohumeral arthritis, usually cause these symptoms, but infection and tumor must also be considered.

The mechanism of any injury and the nature of exacerbating activities should be documented. An accident or trauma may initiate a shoulder problem, but often there is no history of injury. Frequently, a patient may have had shoulder symptoms before an injury that exacerbated them, as in a patient who suffers an acute extension of an impingement rotator cuff tear. The pattern of pain should be recorded. An episodic history of severe pain and inflammation may suggest calcium, whereas recurrent pain with the arm in abduction and external rotation after

CHECKLIST

History

Patient
- ☐ Hand dominance
- ☐ Occupation
- ☐ Athletics
- ☐ Sports
- ☐ Level of competition
- ☐ Relation to shoulder problem (e.g., weightlifting and osteolysis of the distal clavicle)
- ☐ Other medical disorders (e.g., diabetes, genetic disorders, cancer)
- ☐ Family history (e.g., arthritis, ligamentous laxity)

Shoulder Disorder
- ☐ Chief complaint
- ☐ Pain
- ☐ Weakness
- ☐ Stiffness
- ☐ Instability
- ☐ Symptom pattern
- ☐ Duration
- ☐ Provocation
- ☐ Severity
- ☐ Location
- ☐ Injury
- ☐ Traumatic
- ☐ Atraumatic
- ☐ Repetitive microtrauma
- ☐ Preexisting condition
- ☐ Level of disability
- ☐ Athletics
- ☐ Occupation
- ☐ Daily tasks

Related Symptoms
- ☐ Cervical pain
- ☐ Neurologic
- ☐ Cervical radiculopathy
- ☐ Brachial plexus
- ☐ Peripheral nerve
- ☐ Chest (e.g., cardiac, lung, herpes zoster)

a hard injury in the same position may implicate anterior instability.

It is important to elicit complaints of other adjacent regions such as the neck, chest, heart, upper back, and arm. Cervical disease can be difficult to separate from intrinsic mechanical shoulder disorders, and the two frequently coexist. Nevertheless, neck pain is often referred to the posterior shoulder and trapezius and may be felt into the hand. Shoulder disorders more frequently hurt deep inside or down the front of the upper arm, and do not usually extend beyond the elbow. Furthermore, neck pain is often related to the position of the cervical spine and becomes more severe after driving or long periods of sitting.

Numbness or tingling in the hand may indicate cervical disease or peripheral nerve entrapment. However, shoulder instability, especially when a significant inferior component is present, can produce episodic brachial plexus stretch symptoms. Similarly, conditions that result in loss of shoulder suspension, such as acromioclavicular dislocation and trapezius palsy,[28] can cause brachial plexus traction.

CHECKLIST

Examination

Inspection
- ☐ Muscle atrophy
- ☐ Bone prominences
- ☐ Deformity (e.g., biceps long-head rupture)
- ☐ Generalized laxity (e.g., thumb, elbow)

Palpation
- ☐ Sternoclavicular joint
- ☐ Acromioclavicular joint
- ☐ Rotator cuff and tuberosities (e.g., calcium deposits)
- ☐ Glenohumeral joint line
- ☐ Trapezius muscle spasm

Cervical Spine
- ☐ Rotation
- ☐ Flexion–extension
- ☐ Pain with motion

Range of Motion
- ☐ Elevation
- ☐ Active
- ☐ Passive
- ☐ External rotation
- ☐ Internal rotation

Strength
- ☐ External rotation
- ☐ "Lift-off" test (internal rotation)

Provocative Tests
- ☐ Subacromial impingement sign
- ☐ Anterior apprehension
- ☐ Posterior stress test
- ☐ Horizontal adduction

Shoulder Laxity
- ☐ Sulcus
- ☐ "Drawer"

PHYSICAL EXAMINATION

Physical examination is also performed systematically, and includes inspection, palpation, range of motion, strength testing, stability, and provocative tests (see box, Examination). The patient should be examined with both shoulders fully exposed: men disrobe above the waist, and women are given gowns that are tied under the shoulder in the axilla so that they are "strapless" (Fig. 18-1). Inspection is performed from in front and behind, assessing muscle atrophy and contour, bone prominences, and deformity. Atrophy of the spinati is best evaluated from behind (Fig. 18-2).

Palpation is performed, checking for areas of localized tenderness and crepitus (Fig. 18-3). The acromioclavicular joint should always be carefully palpated because it is a frequently overlooked source of symptoms. Localized tenderness over the rotator cuff may result from calcific tendinitis and should be correlated with rotational radiographs of the humerus (Fig. 18-4). Anterior and posterior joint-line tenderness may be present with glenohumeral instability, and posterior joint-line tenderness is commonly noted in glenohumeral arthritis. The cervical spine should be gently rotated, flexed, and extended. If this maneuver reproduces the patient's "shoulder" pain, consideration should be given to a cervical etiology.

Range of motion is evaluated and recorded (Fig. 18-5). Elevation is measured in the scapular plane. Passive elevation is more accurately measured while the patient is supine, to avoid arching of the back. No effort is made to isolate glenohumeral motion; total elevation, consisting of glenohumeral and scapulothoracic motion, is more reproducibly measured and more functionally relevant. Active elevation is measured while the patient is erect. External rotation, with the arm at the side, is measured supine to eliminate trunk rotation. Internal rotation is measured erect by the highest vertebral level to which the thumb may be brought up the patient's back.

Manual strength may be reduced because of pain, precluding quantitative assessment. External rotation weakness can be present in long-standing rotator cuff tears, but may be secondary to pain, cervical radiculopathy, or suprascapular nerve palsy. It is best to test external rotation strength with the elbow flexed and the arm at the side to avoid a contribution from the deltoid muscle (Fig. 18-6). Gerber and Krushell[16] have noted that to fully internally rotate the extended arm, an intact and functioning subscapularis is required. A "lift off" test to assess the subscapularis is positive (and loose subscapularis function demonstrated) when there is a lag between passive and active internal rotation: the patient cannot lift the hand posteriorly off the lumbar region of the back (Fig. 18-7). Recently, the role of rupture or incompetence

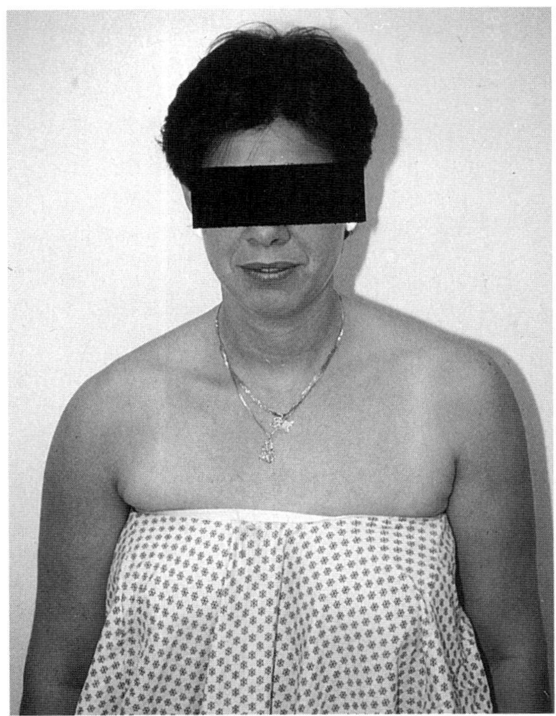

FIGURE 18-1. The arms are not placed through the sleeves of the gown. Rather, the gown is tied under the arms to be "strapless." This allows full inspection throughout the examination.

of the subscapularis muscle has been described.[16] A careful neurologic assessment is mandatory when there is significant weakness of the muscle groups, and electromyography may be indicated.

Specific "provocative" tests assist accurate diagnosis. The subacromial impingement sign will elicit pain in patients with subacromial impingement syndrome (Fig. 18-8). The examiner stabilizes the scapula with one hand and brings the arm up into forced elevation with the other. A positive test elicits pain as the greater tuberosity is forced against the coracoacromial arch. It is important to realize that a frozen shoulder will invalidate this test because there will be restricted motion in all directions, not just elevation, with pain at the extremes. The subacromial injection test is positive when a subacromial injection of local anesthetic eliminates pain from the

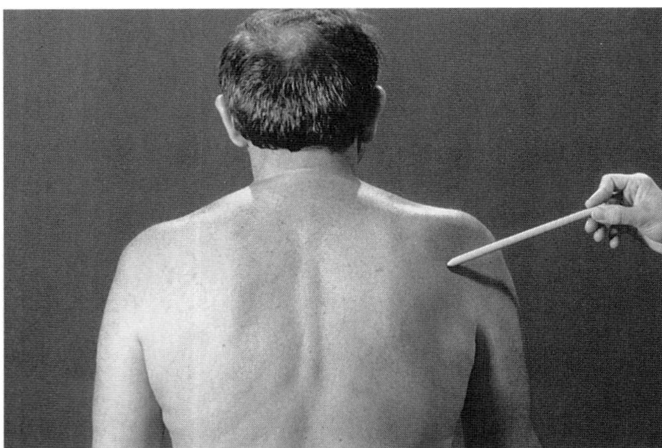

FIGURE 18-2. Spinati atrophy is best appreciated from the back. The scapular spine becomes prominent relative to the adjacent hollowed-out supraspinatus and infraspinatus. This patient had spinati atrophy from a massive rotator cuff tear.

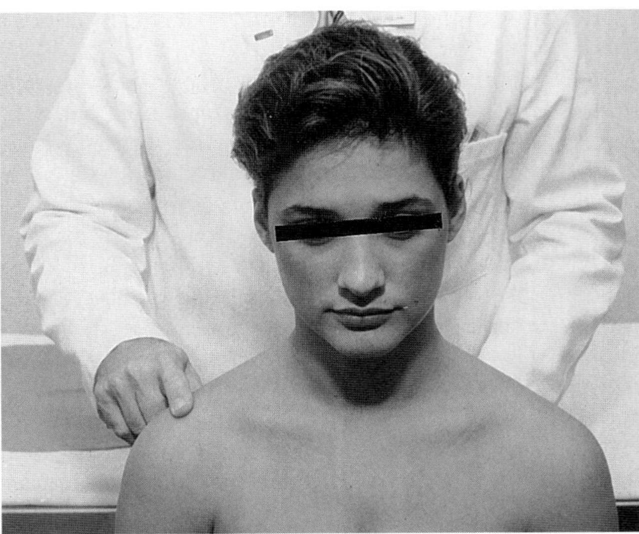

FIGURE 18-3. Palpation is carefully performed to elicit any areas of localized tenderness. Here the acromioclavicular joint is being palpated.

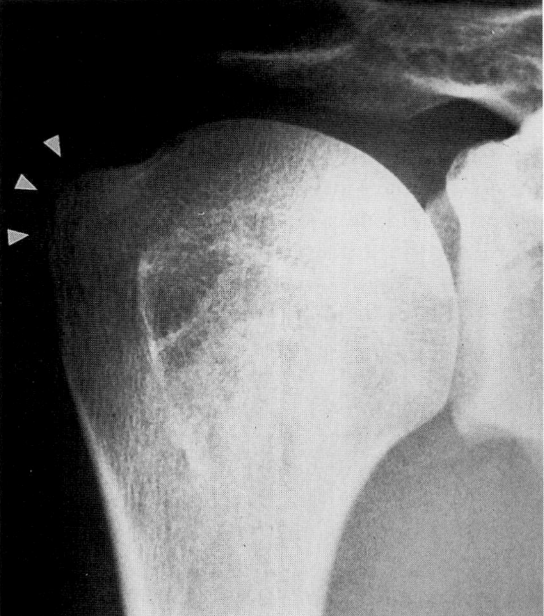

FIGURE 18-4. This patient was referred because of shoulder pain unresponsive to arthroscopic labral debridement. Only one of three rotation views brought the calcium deposit (arrows) into view. A steroid injection completely relieved the symptoms, and the patient continues pain-free 1 year after the injection.

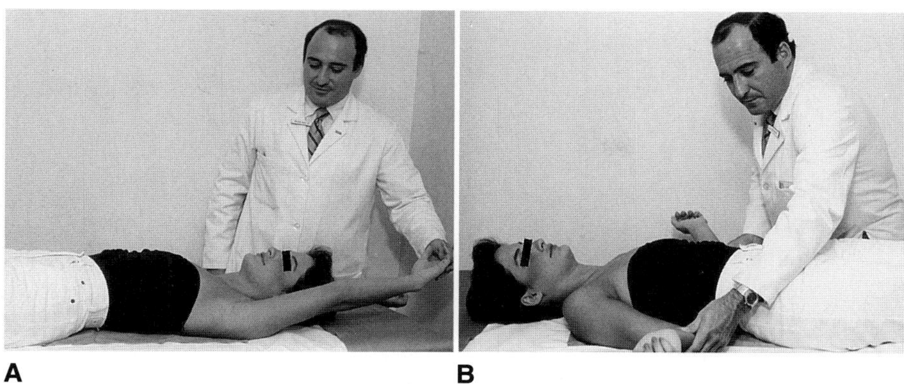

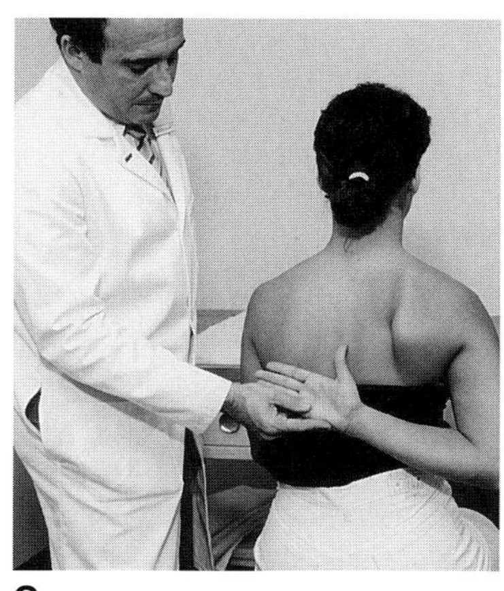

FIGURE 18-5. A, Passive total elevation is measured supine in the scapular plane and is a combination of glenohumeral and scapulothoracic motion. **B,** Passive external rotation is measured supine, which minimizes trunk rotation. **C,** Passive internal rotation is measured by the highest vertebral level to which the thumb may be brought up the patient's back. This technique may be invalidated if there is a significant restriction of elbow motion.

impingement sign. Pain from the acromioclavicular joint may be elicited with horizontal adduction of the arm across the chest and internal rotation of the arm up the back, but this sign is not specific for the acromioclavicular joint. A local anesthetic injection into the acromioclavicular joint can be of diagnostic value. Because of the frequent overlap of acromioclavicular arthritis and impingement syndrome, especially in older patients, a "differential" injection test is often helpful. The most symptomatic element is generally injected first.

The anterior apprehension sign is the classic provocative test for anterior instability. The arm is brought up into a position of extension, abduction, and external rotation, and anterior pressure is placed on the proximal humerus (Fig. 18-9). Patients with instability will generally guard against this position because of fear of shifting or dislocating anteriorly. Patients with subluxations may only have pain. Posterior instability is tested with the "posterior stress test" checking for apprehension or, more commonly, pain with the arm in 90° forward flexion and

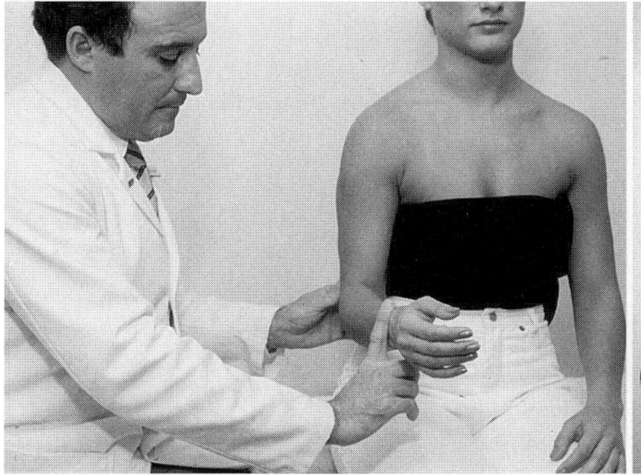

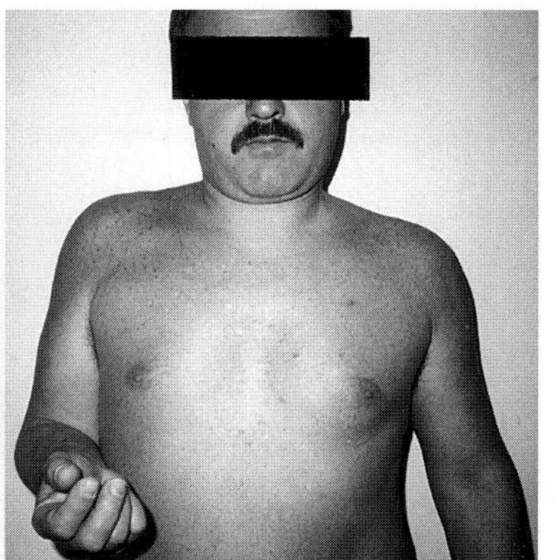

FIGURE 18-6. A, External rotation strength is evaluated with the arms at the side. Weakness may be mimicked by pain and in some cases may be more reliably measured after a subacromial injection of local anesthetic.[7] **B,** Patients with massive rotator cuff tears may have severe weakness of external rotation. This patient had 11 passive external rotation supine, but in the standing position, his arm "drops off" to internal rotation despite his efforts to actively externally rotate.

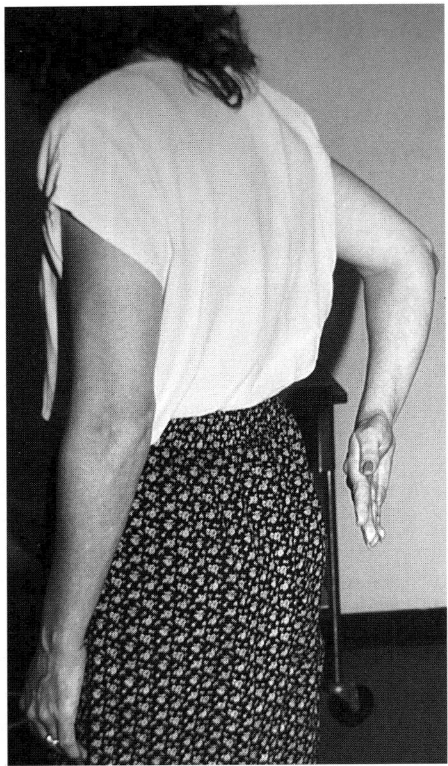

FIGURE 18-7. The lift-off test is performed by having the patient lift his or her hand from the resting position on the lumbar region of the back. Alternatively, the examiner may place the patient's arm in internal rotation with the hand elevated above the back and buttocks and ask the patient to maintain this position. A patient with subscapularis pathology will be unable to perform this maneuver.

internal rotation while applying posterior pressure to the elbow (Fig. 18-10).[11,35] The scapula must be stabilized. Posterior inferior instability is checked by elevating the arm to 120°. Inferior laxity is assessed by pulling downward on the arm to create a sulcus sign (Fig. 18-11), which is a separation of the superior humerus from the acromion.

Generalized ligamentous laxity (Fig. 18-12) may be present in patients with multidirectional instability, but may be absent in those with acquired shoulder laxity after repetitive microtrauma (e.g., butterfly swimming).

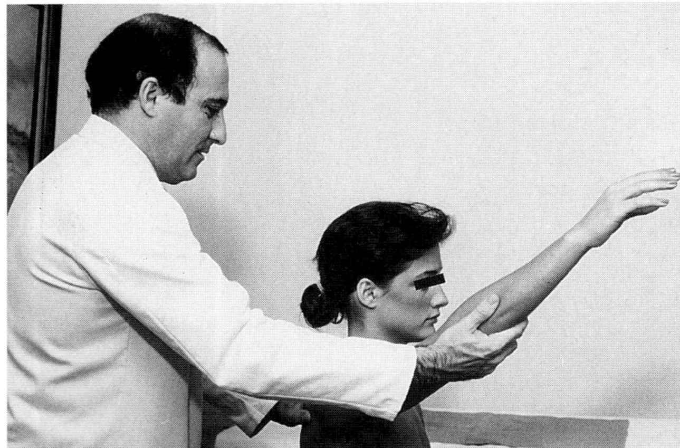

FIGURE 18-8. The impingement sign is elicited by stabilizing the scapula with one hand and bringing the arm up into forced elevation with the other. This will elicit pain in a patient with subacromial impingement syndrome.

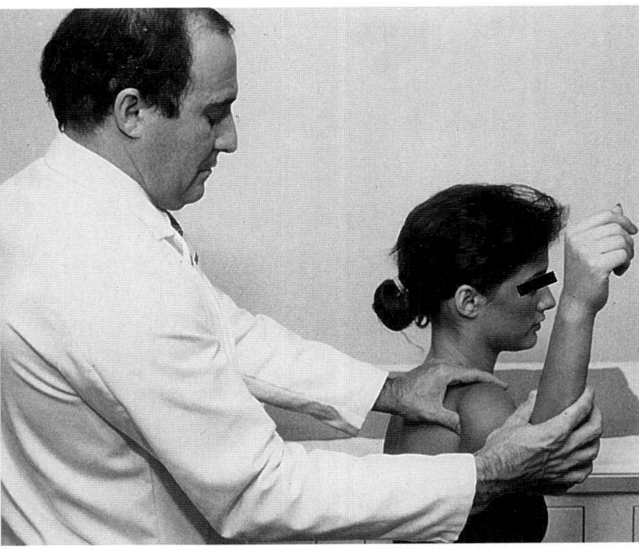

FIGURE 18-9. The anterior apprehension maneuver is performed by bringing the arm up into a position of extension, abduction, and external rotation and by placing forward pressure on the proximal humerus. A patient with instability will generally be apprehensive and guard against this position for fear of shifting or dislocating anteriorly. A patient with subluxations may only have pain.

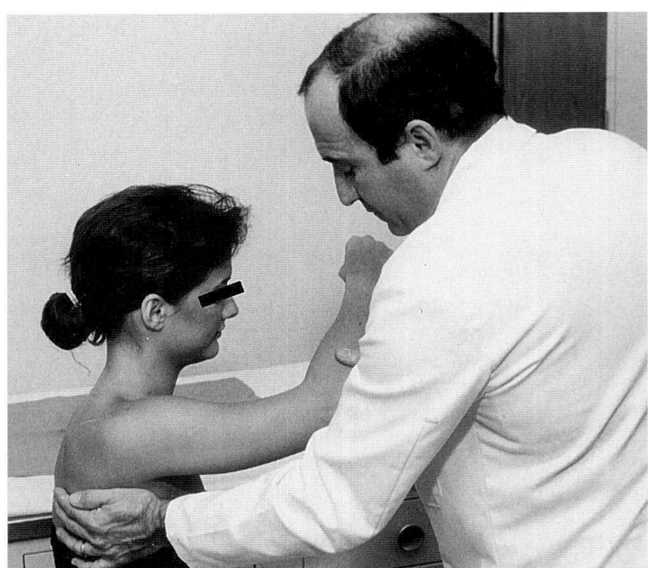

FIGURE 18-10. The posterior stress test is performed with the arm in 90° forward flexion and internal rotation while applying posterior pressure to the elbow with the scapula stabilized.

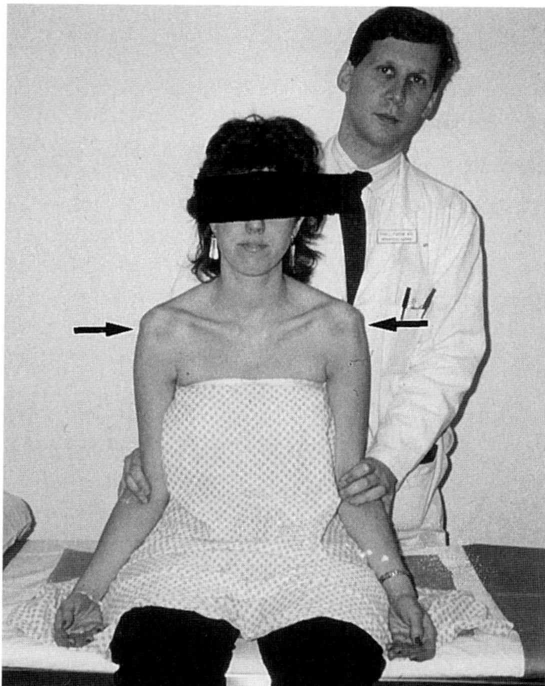

FIGURE 18-11. This patient with multidirectional instability has bilateral sulcus signs (arrows) elicited by placing downward traction on the arms. A sulcus is formed between the acromion and the inferiorly translating humerus.

Both shoulders should be assessed for anteroposterior translation, a shoulder "drawer" sign (Fig. 18-13).

CHECKLIST

Diagnostic Modalities

Routine Blood Studies
- ☐ CBC, ESR, SMAC, latex fixation
- ☐ Others as indicated

Radiographs, Routine
- ☐ Anteroposterior in internal rotation, external rotation, neutral
- ☐ "Outlet" view
- ☐ Axillary

Radiographs, Special
- ☐ Anteroposterior and cephalic tilt anteroposterior views with soft-tissue technique to demonstrate AC joint
- ☐ Special views (e.g., Stryker, Hermodssen) to demonstrate Hill-Sachs defect
- ☐ Modified axillary views (e.g., "velpeau axillary")
- ☐ Cervical spine

Special Diagnostic Modalities
- ☐ Arthro–computed tomography scan
- ☐ Labral pathology
- ☐ Glenoid bone changes
- ☐ Three-dimensional computed tomography reconstruction
- ☐ Arthrogram
- ☐ Ultrasonography
- ☐ Magnetic resonance imaging
- ☐ Arthro–MRI
- ☐ Electrodiagnostic studies (e.g., EMG, SSEP)
- ☐ Isokinetic muscle testing

DIAGNOSTIC MODALITIES

Routine blood tests may be obtained to check for conditions such as systemic rheumatologic disorders, infections, and tumors, which may cause shoulder symptoms (see box, Diagnostic Modalities).

All patients should have routine radiographs taken to assist in the diagnosis of tumors, fractures, or dislocations. This should include anteroposterior views of the scapular plane in neutral, internal, and external rotations, a lateral view in the scapular plane, and an axillary view. Rotational views are of value in detecting calcium deposits. The internal rotation anteroposterior view will generally demonstrate a Hill-Sachs defect, which is an impression

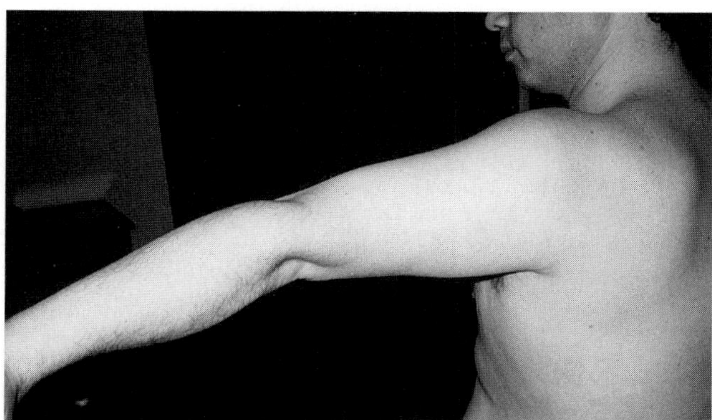

FIGURE 18-12. Another common finding with generalized laxity is the ability to hyperextend the elbow.

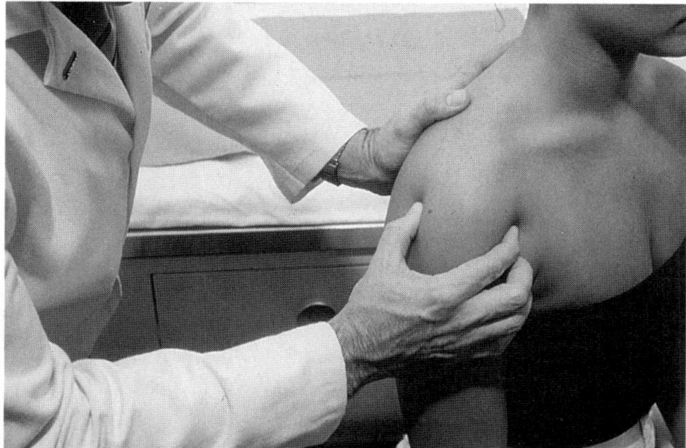

FIGURE 18-13. Anteroposterior laxity may be assessed by stabilizing the scapula and by attempting to translate the humerus forward and backward in the glenoid, a shoulder "drawer sign."

fracture caused during anterior dislocations (see Fig. 18-11). The external rotation anteroposterior view shows the greater tuberosity in profile, and patients with impingement may have sclerosis, cysts, or excrescences of the greater tuberosity. Spurs and sclerosis of the anterior acromion may be apparent on anteroposterior views, but acromial morphology may be best appreciated on a lateral view, especially if taken with slight caudal tilt. Such an "outlet view" can also be helpful in assessing the technical success of arthroscopic acromioplasty.

The axillary view will demonstrate posterior dislocations, which may be missed on anteroposterior views, and glenoid reactive changes or fractures associated with instability.

The acromioclavicular joints are frequently overpenetrated on standard views, and acromioclavicular films with soft-tissue technique, anteroposterior and cephalic tilt anteroposterior views, may pick up subtle arthritis, fractures, or osteolysis.

Additional views are occasionally necessary, and include special views to demonstrate the Hills-Sachs defect such as the Stryker notch view (Fig. 18-14), modified axillary views that do not require removing an acutely injured arm from the sling, weighted acromioclavicular views to check for an acromioclavicular separation, and other views. Cervical spine radiographs are often obtained because of associated neck pain, especially in older patients.

Magnetic resonance imaging scans have become increasingly reliable in detecting rotator cuff tears, degree of retraction, and atrophy of the muscle bellies (Fig. 18-15).[19]

Ultrasonography has been reported to be an inexpensive, noninvasive imaging modality for the rotator cuff that can detect partial tears. However, reliability has varied with investigators and criteria for cuff pathology.

Electromyograms and nerve conduction studies are useful in differentiating peripheral nerve injuries and entrapments, brachial plexus disorders, and cervical radiculopathies. Somatosensory-evoked potential testing may also be useful, especially when the predominant symptoms are sensory. Cybex testing can document functional deficits and serve as a baseline for the evaluation of rehabilitation protocols.

SPECIFIC NONTRAUMATIC INJURIES

Rotator Cuff Disorders

Sports Commonly Involved. Rotator cuff disease occurs in participants of virtually all sports but should be especially suspected in athletes involved in sports with repetitive overhead motions. These include baseball, football (quarterbacks), swimming, tennis (racket sports), volleyball, field events (javelin), gymnastics, and weightlifting.

Background. Commonly referred to as *impingement syndrome*, rotator cuff–associated pain can be primary bursitis, tendinitis from overuse, impingement from mechanical abutment, or secondary from glenohumeral instability all resulting in pain, weakness, and diminished athletic performance.[4,12,20,22,23,26,27,30,31,37,39,48] Whatever the primary etiology, there is a staged progression of pathology. In Stage I, age is less than 24 years and there is reversible edema and hemorrhage of the tendon. In Stage II, age is 25 to 40 years and there is tendinitis and fibrosis, which can become chronic. In Stage III, age is greater than 40 years and there is full-thickness rotator cuff tearing, often requiring operative repair. This age-related characterization of rotator cuff disease is accelerated in athletes involved in sports with overhead motions secondary to increased forces on the cuff tendons and the repetitive aggravating motions.

Pathomechanics. Many factors have been implicated in rotator cuff pathology, including extrinsic tendon injury from compression against an abnormal coracoacromial arch, internal abutment against the glenoid rim, tendon and bursal swelling in a confined space, tensile overload from glenohumeral instability, and intrinsic tendon injury from tendon inflammation.[3,10,23,27,29,30,39]

Whether a primary or secondary effect, subacromial impingement is thought to be an ongoing cause of tendon injury by the time surgical intervention is considered.

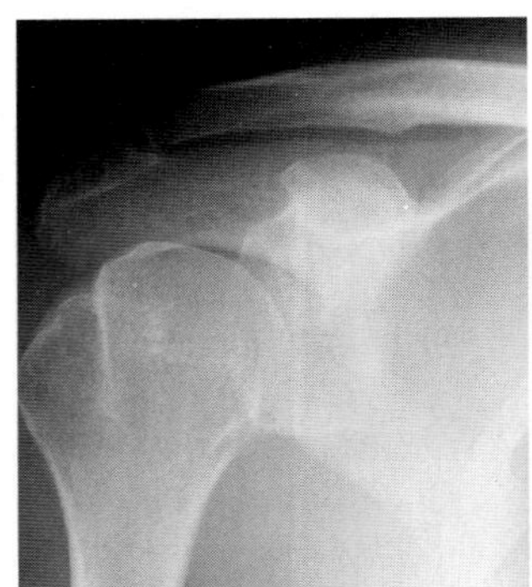

A

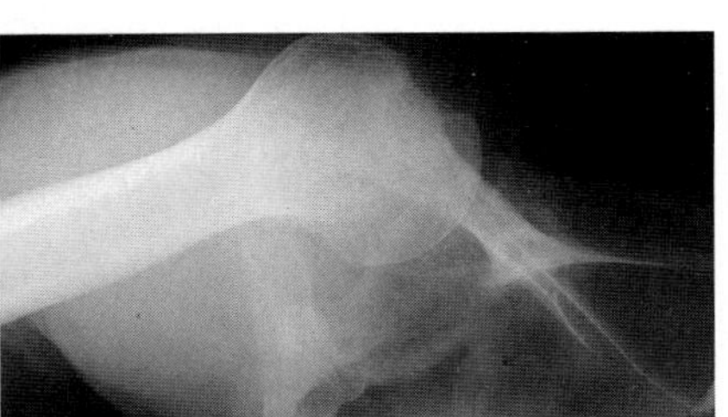

B

FIGURE 18-14. The posterolateral humeral head impression fracture (Hill-Sachs defect) associated with recurrent anterior dislocations is usually well demonstrated on the internal rotation anteroposterior view. Occasionally, other views are helpful in assessing its extent. **A,** Internal rotation anteroposterior view. **B,** Stryker notch view.

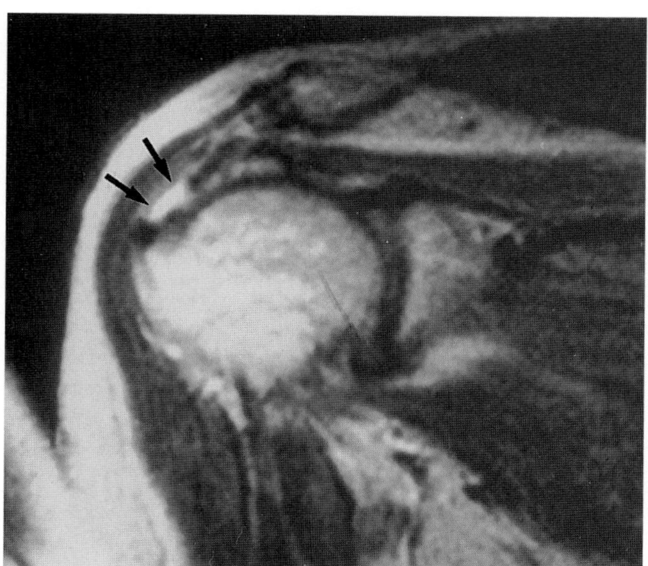

FIGURE 18-15. T2-weighted magnetic resonance imaging shows a bright signal (arrows) consistent with fluid in a supraspinatus tear. This was confirmed at surgery.

The supraspinatus insertion on the greater tuberosity must repeatedly pass under the coracoacromial arch when the arm is used for vigorous overhead activity. As described in the anatomy section, the rotator cuff passes between the coracoacromial arch above and the humeral head below. Narrowing of the outlet from spur formation on the anterior acromion, coracoacromial ligament thickening, or hypertrophy of the AC joint can mechanically irritate the rotator cuff. Conversely, alterations in rotator cuff function from stress overload or tendinitis seen with instability can decrease humeral head stabilization, leading to superior migration and secondary impingement. Bigliani et al. have demonstrated a relationship between acromial morphology and rotator cuff tears in cadavers,[10] and contact studies on the subacromial space at the Columbia-Presbyterian Orthopaedic Research Laboratory have found that contact is centered on the supraspinatus insertion where cuff tears generally originate, supporting an impingement etiology to rotator cuff disease.

Recently, an internal impingement mechanism has also been implicated in select patients with glenohumeral instability who are involved in overhead sports.[23] In this proposed mechanism, anterior translation of the humeral head with arm abduction and external rotation (seen during cocking for throwing) can cause abutment of the articular side of the rotator cuff against the posterior–superior glenoid rim.

Calcific tendinitis is a variety of rotator cuff disease unrelated to impingement. Acute pain is thought to be caused by the intermittent release of calcium from the tendon, irritating the bursa. Calcific tendinitis usually responds well to steroid injection.

Specifics of History and Examination. The majority of rotator cuff disorders can be accurately diagnosed with history, physical examination, and appropriate imaging studies. These patients usually present with insidious onset of pain with overhead activities. The pain is located most often in the anterior deltoid, and may be referred over the deltoid and down to mid-arm. With disease progression the pain is often felt at night and can awaken patients from sleep.

On examination, the typical pain can be reproduced with forward flexion in internal rotation known as the impingement sign. This pain is often reduced with a subacromial injection of lidocaine (impingement test). Three specific manual muscle tests are performed to assess the possibility of a rotator cuff tear. The lift-off test assesses the subscapularis. Supraspinatus involvement is tested by determining strength with thumb-down abduction at 70° in the scapular plane and infraspinatous and teres minor by testing external rotation strength at the side. Complete posterior rotator cuff tears result in inability to maintain external rotation, which is called the *external rotation lag sign.*

In the young athlete, the examination should also focus on possible instability as the primary etiology for rotator cuff disease. In contrast to primary impingement, pain is often posterior and the patient may complain of a "dead arm" with overhead activities. Apprehension and relocation tests and sulcus and range of motion examinations should be performed. Impingement signs and tests will also be positive from the secondary bursitis.

Routine radiographs, including supraspinatus outlet films, should be obtained on the initial visit. Additional studies such as magnetic resonance imaging should generally be reserved until conservative therapy has failed and operative intervention is being considered. High-performance athletes who require immediate rotator cuff evaluation for prognosticating return to sports should undergo immediate MRI.

Conservative Management. Initial management consists of rest, avoidance of overhead activity, and anti-inflammatory medication to reduce the acute inflammation. Physical therapy first focuses on stretching exercises to regain complete range of motion and then on strengthening of the rotator cuff. Care should be taken not to overstretch the shoulder. If pain persists, a subacromial injection of lidocaine and steroid preparation is often helpful to break the inflammation. However, there are no long-term benefits from either the oral or injected anti-inflammatory medication without a directed physical therapy regimen.

Indications for Orthopedic Referral. Patients should be considered for orthopedic referral when conservative treatment has failed to provide satisfactory improvement or if the care provider is uncomfortable with conservative measures such as subacromial injections.

Operative Management. Operative management involves bursectomy and decompression of the subacromial arch by coracoacromial ligament excision and resection of the anterior–inferior acromion (Fig. 18-16). Specific operative management is predicated on the presence or absence of a significant rotator cuff tear. When a rotator cuff tear is absent or small, surgery is performed arthroscopically. If a significant tear is present, formal open repair is preferred.

Glenohumeral Instability

Sports Commonly Involved. Glenohumeral instability is seen in athletes involved in high-energy sports in which traumatic unidirectional dislocations are common and in repetitive overhead motion sports in which microtrauma is prevalent. These sports include football, basketball, baseball, hockey, swimming, tennis (racket sports), volleyball, field events (javelin), gymnastics, and weightlifting.

Background. Multidirectional or unidirectional instability of the shoulder is more common than was previously realized.[3,17,18,25,29,31,34,39,42,47] These patients have symptomatic glenohumeral instability in one or more than one direction: anterior, inferior, and posterior. There is a common misconception that multidirectional instability is limited to young, sedentary patients with generalized ligamentous laxity who often present with bilateral symptoms and signs as opposed to unidirectional patients, who are thought to have a unilateral traumatic etiology. Multidirectional instability is usually acquired from repetitive microtrauma as seen in butterfly swimming or gymnastics.

In the authors' experience, patients with shoulder instability do not always easily fall into distinct categories (unidirectional versus multidirectional) (Fig. 18-17). This is especially true of athletes, often lax to begin with, who subject their shoulders to repetitive microtrauma on a daily basis but may also suffer a superimposed injury. The authors have found that athletes with anterior instability constitute a spectrum from unidirectional anterior instability to frank multidirectional instability with pronounced inferior capsular laxity rather than falling into simple discrete groups.

Pathomechanics. The primary pathology in shoulders with acquired instability (without a specific traumatic event) is capsular laxity and redundancy, with instability possible in anterior, inferior, or posterior directions. In addition to capsular laxity, avulsion of the capsular ligaments from the anterior glenoid rim may occur, further destabilizing the joint.

Specifics of History and Examination. Patients with acquired instability may present in a variety of ways. A previous dislocation may have occurred without significant injury and spontaneously reduced. An extremely hypermobile shoulder can become symptomatic with minimal trauma or even routine activities of daily living. Symptoms can be vague and complex, but certain complaints may suggest the directions of instability involved. Inferior instability is suggested by pain associated with carrying heavy suitcases or shopping bags. Occasionally, these symptoms are accompanied by traction paresthesias. Pain associated with weight training (bench press), pushing open heavy or revolving doors, or use of the arm in a forward flexed and internally rotated position usually suggests a component of posterior instability.

The physical examination may demonstrate evidence of generalized ligamentous laxity, such as hyperextension at the elbows, the ability to approximate the thumbs to the forearms, hyperextension of the metacarpophalangeal joints, or patellofemoral subluxation. In some

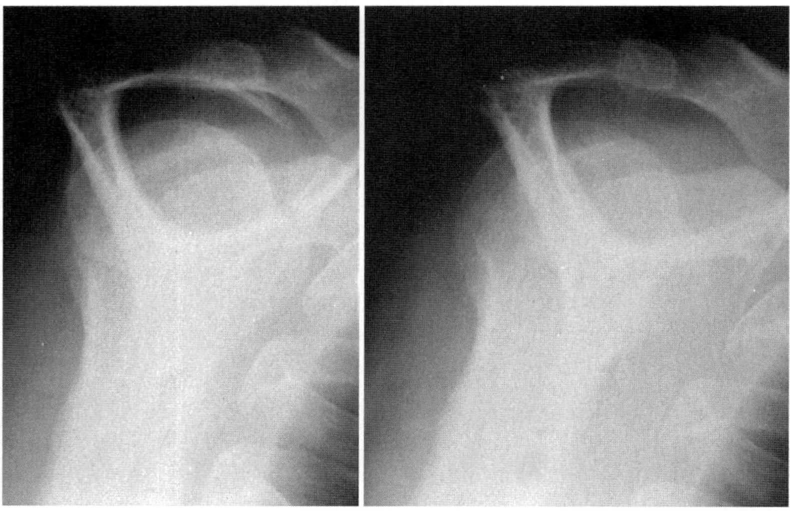

FIGURE 18-16. A, Preoperative outlet view (left) demonstrates a large anterior acromial spur extending into the coracoacromial ligament. The spur was removed arthroscopically as confirmed by a postoperative view (right). **B,** This patient had a prominent, curved anterior acromion (left), which was converted to a flat acromion (right) arthroscopically.

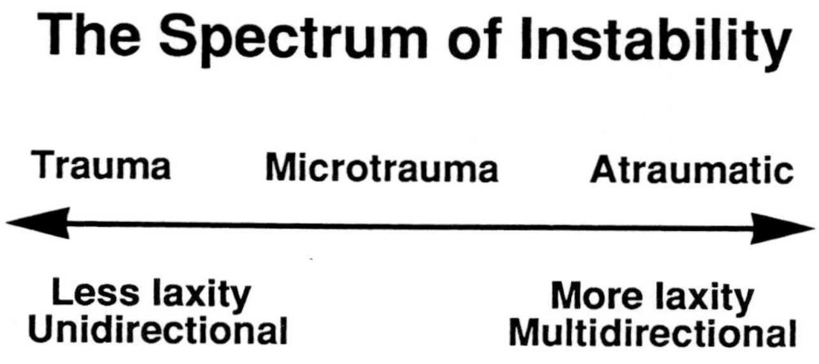

The Spectrum of Instability

Trauma — **Microtrauma** — **Atraumatic**

←——————————————→

Less laxity
Unidirectional

More laxity
Multidirectional

FIGURE 18-17. The spectrum of instability.

of these patients, hypermobile acromioclavicular and sternoclavicular joints can be sources of symptoms. It is important, therefore, to examine these joints for tenderness, inferior humeral subluxation with stress on the arm in neutral (sulcus sign) (Fig. 18-8), or abduction, which suggests inferior laxity. Additionally, close inspection of the scapulothoracic articulation should be performed because concomitant scapulothoracic instability may occasionally be present. There may be multiple positive findings using the following maneuvers: anterior and posterior load and shift tests, anterior and posterior apprehension tests, relocation test, and the push–pull test. The aim is to produce humeral translations either anteriorly, posteriorly, or inferiorly (relative to the glenoid), and to document that these translations reliably elicit the patient's usual pain and discomfort.

Determining the primary direction of instability on physical examination is often challenging. The shoulder may move from a dislocated to a reduced position or from a reduced to a dislocated position. Maintaining the fingers of one hand on the coracoid anteriorly and on the posterolateral acromion can aid in this determination. Multiple physical examinations are helpful in assessing these patients.

Symptoms must be reproduced with provocative maneuvers because increased laxity itself may be normal for an individual and is not an indication for surgical stabilization procedures. Asymptomatic shoulders may show substantial translation on clinical testing. In addition, joint laxity may be remarkable enough to distract the examiner from the primary source of pain, such as a painful acromioclavicular joint or a cervical radiculopathy. Conversely, laxity may be hard to demonstrate even in a shoulder with multidirectional instability if pain, muscle spasm, and guarding prevent subluxation. It is helpful to examine the contralateral, asymptomatic shoulder for laxity. If it is extremely loose, it may be a clue to the multidirectional nature of the affected side.

Plain radiographs are generally normal but should be evaluated for the presence of humeral head defects or glenoid lesions, such as osseous Bankart fragments, reactive bone, or wear. An arthro CT scan is invasive and can detect capsular and labral lesions. Magnetic resonance imaging is noninvasive and can demonstrate the redundant capsule and labral lesions.

Conservative Management. Once the diagnosis of instability has been established, a prolonged course of rehabilitation is instituted with emphasis on strengthening the rotator cuff, deltoid, and scapulothoracic stabilizing

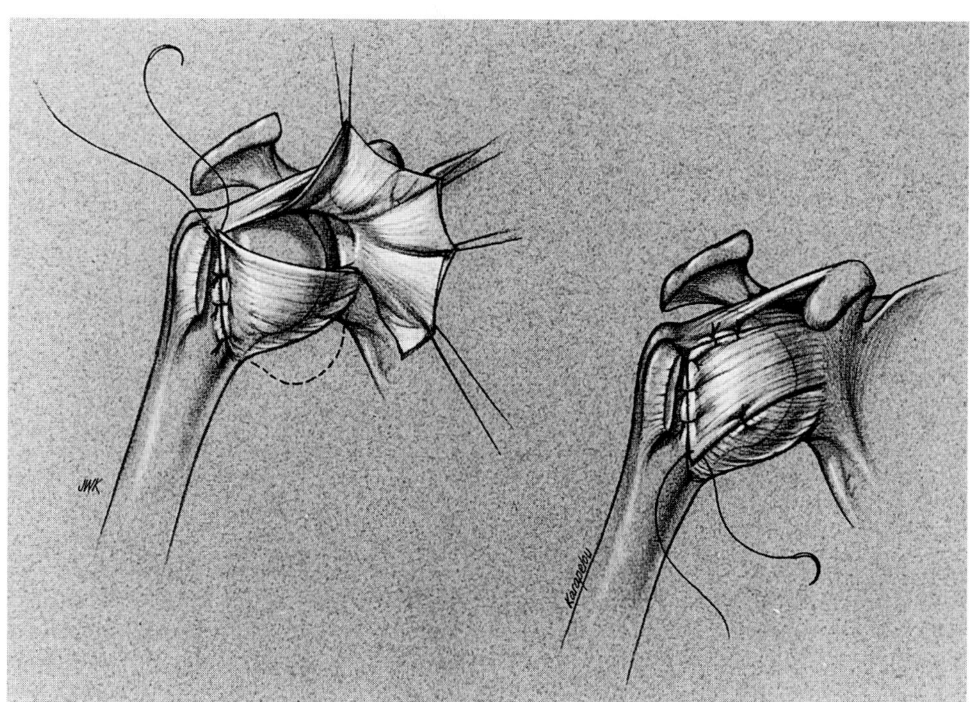

FIGURE 18-18. Schematic of anterior–inferior capsular shift.

muscles with the arm below the shoulder. Patients with multidirectional instability may occasionally develop a secondary impingement syndrome and a subacromial steroid injection may provide relief sufficient for the patient to resume therapy.

During the rehabilitation program, motivation should be monitored to ensure the patient is mature enough to cooperate in the rehabilitation effort required after surgery and to screen out those patients seeking secondary gain.

Patients with acquired instability may develop the ability to dislocate the shoulder at will. This is especially true if certain positions will reliably result in a dislocation (e.g., the humeral head falls out posteriorly whenever the arm is raised in the forward plane in internal rotation). Such "positional dislocators" may demonstrate this for the examiner, if requested, but otherwise patients should do their best to avoid such positions. Although positional dislocators can demonstrate instability on command, they do not necessarily have accompanying psychiatric disorders and are amenable to surgical correction.

These patients must be differentiated, however, from true voluntary dislocators who have underlying psychiatric problems and who use asymmetric muscle pull to dislocate the shoulder, or even to hold it out, for dramatic effect. To complicate matters, there is a small group of patients who have developed a habitual initiation of improper muscle firing patterns, which also produce dislocations by asymmetric muscle pull. These patients can be unaware of this pattern and may be without psychiatric disturbance. Nevertheless, both groups of "muscular dislocators" are poor candidates for stabilization procedures. Those with psychiatric disturbances need counseling and, with respect to the shoulder, skillful neglect. The group with habitually improper muscle use may be treated successfully with muscle retraining and biofeedback.

Indications for Orthopedic Referral. Any patient sustaining a traumatic dislocation should be immediately referred for orthopedic consultation. A patient may have a subtle fracture or be a candidate for early operative intervention. Additionally, a patient with episodes of multiple, recurrent dislocations should be referred because conservative treatment is unlikely to help. If the patient has prolonged symptoms of subluxation or pain, without dislocation, and has not responded to conservative management, including an exercise regimen, surgery may be indicated, and the patient should be referred.

Operative Management. Operative management involves imbrication or "tightening" of the redundant inferior joint capsule coupled with repair of any capsular–labral avulsion from the anterior glenoid rim (Fig. 18-18). Presently, a relatively higher rate of failures associated with arthroscopic repairs has narrowed indications for this approach to those patients who have had less than five dislocations, who cannot self-reduce, do not participate in contact sports, and do not have signs of generalized ligamentous laxity. For either open or arthroscopic techniques, the surgery goal is to restore anatomy by correcting capsular laxity or labral avulsion.

Adhesive Capsulitis

Sports Commonly Involved. Adhesive capsulitis is rare in active, healthy people involved in athletics. It is not generally associated with any particular sport, but it can be seen in older athletes or in those with diabetes in whom concomitant tendinitis can lead to periods of immobility and subsequent stiffness.

Background. Adhesive capsulitis, also known as frozen shoulder, is a primary shoulder disorder of unknown etiology characterized by progressive pain and restriction of glenohumeral motion. The condition can occur after any injury or inflammation around the shoulder joint that requires a period of immobilization. Other associated factors include diabetes, trauma, breast surgery, and hypothyroidism.[29,39] Because missed dislocations, osteoarthritis, and impingement can lead to a loss of range of motion, frozen shoulder is a diagnosis of exclusion, and other factors should be carefully ruled out.

Pathomechanics. Frozen shoulder is characterized by chronic inflammation and fibrosis of the glenohumeral capsule, leading to marked restriction of joint volume and later adhesions from articulating surfaces to the capsule. The inflammatory process also extends to the subacromial bursa and coracohumeral ligament. The disease has been categorized into three clinical stages: I, early diffuse pain with range of motion largely intact; II, adhesive stage where there is progressive loss of range of motion; and III, gradual resolution of motion.

Specifics of History and Examination. A patient with adhesive capsulitis initially has diffuse pain, often indistinguishable from impingement. The pain is accompanied by a reduction in passive and active range of motion. The loss of motion is generally global but always involves reduction in external rotation. Classically, a patient with frozen shoulder has pain at the end of the range of motion. He or she can be comfortable within the restricted range of motion but have pain—often severe—when inadvertently extending past his or her range. Because painful splinting can cause a loss of motion, selective lidocaine injections are often helpful.

Conservative Management. Nonoperative management with physical therapy emphasizing stretching for the range of motion is successful in the majority of patients. The physical therapy is augmented with symptomatic support, such as nonsteroidal and injected steroid medication. Improvement can be slow, with recovery taking up to 1 year.

Indications for Orthopedic Referral. Because many conditions, some severe, can cause loss of motion, referral should probably be made early to confirm the diagnosis of adhesive capsulitis. The advent of scalene block catheters and relatively less-invasive arthroscopic procedures has provided for more aggressive management of refractory cases.[36]

Distal Clavicle Osteolysis

Sports Commonly Involved. Distal clavicle osteolysis is classically seen in the power weightlifter but can also be found in athletes prone to blunt trauma to the shoulder in sports such as hockey, football, rugby, wrestling, skiing, skating, and bicycling.

Background. This condition is characterized by pain and osteolysis of the distal clavicle and is seen in athletes who undergo repetitive stress on the acromioclavicular joint or have had an acute injury, such as acromioclavicular separation.[13,40] It is most commonly associated with power weightlifters who perform bench press and military press.

Pathomechanics. The pathomechanics of osteolysis are poorly understood. Characteristic radiographic changes include osteoporosis, osteolysis, or osteophyte formation of the distal clavicle without acromial changes. Usually, the condition is unilateral and self-limiting with respect to symptoms. Bony reconstitution is uncommon.

Specifics of History and Examination. A patient will present with a dull ache centered over the acromioclavicular joint. Often, there is an accompanying trapezius spasm. Pain is also exacerbated by flexion and cross-body adduction. Clavicular view radiographs with a 35° cephalic tilt are helpful in making the diagnosis.

Conservative Management. Successful conservative management includes rest and activity modification. Activity modification in the weightlifter includes weight reduction, increased repetitions, and substitution of exercises. If rest does not help, acromioclavicular joint steroid injections can be helpful.

Indications for Orthopedic Referral. Orthopedic referral can be sought after a trial of conservative therapy has failed to achieve satisfactory improvement.

Operative Management. Operative management consists of distal clavicle excision of 4 to 5 mm from an arthroscopic approach if the joint is stable.[8,49] If the acromioclavicular joint is unstable, an open excision with transfer of the coracoacromial ligament may be indicated.

SPECIFIC TRAUMATIC INJURIES: BONY

Bony injuries or fractures of the shoulder can be difficult clinical entities that would require an extensive discussion beyond the scope of this section.[2,5] This section is necessarily abbreviated and tailored to athletic concerns. Because of the complex nature of shoulder fractures, these injuries should be referred for at least an initial orthopedic evaluation.

Proximal Humerus Fractures

Sports Commonly Involved. Proximal humerus fractures are generally rare in the athletic population but can occur in any high-energy contact sports such as football, hockey, rugby, skiing, and wrestling. In the skeletally immature population, growth-plate stress fractures can occur in baseball pitchers from repetitive overhead throwing. Additionally, proximal humerus fractures should be suspected in the context of glenohumeral dislocations, especially in patients aged more than 40 years.

Background. Proximal humerus fractures are generally rare in the young athletic population with maintained bone strength. However, in high-energy contact sports or in those with repetitive overhead motions, fractures can occur. Mechanism of injury usually involves a fall on the outstretched hand, causing an axial load transferred to the humeral head. In skeletally immature athletes, surgical neck stress fractures can occur through the growth plate from repetitive overhead motion. Less commonly, a direct blow to the lateral shoulder can cause a fracture. Two of the most common patterns involve a physial fracture of the surgical neck and greater tuberosity fractures associated with an anterior dislocation. The surgical neck physis of the proximal humerus does not fuse until the age of 20, and a younger athlete can fracture this relatively weak area. Known as a "little league shoulder," these stress fractures heal quickly with rest if recognized early.

Pathomechanics. Fractures of the proximal humerus occur in predictable patterns based on old physial scars. These injuries can include some combination of fractures involving the lesser tuberosity, greater tuberosity, anatomic neck, and surgical neck. As stated previously, in the athletic population, surgical neck and greater tuberosity fractures predominate. The surgical neck fracture can tolerate a relatively large degree of angulation and displacement and is usually managed nonoperatively. The greater tuberosity fracture, in contrast, will not tolerate much displacement and is often surgically reduced and repaired in the younger population. Because the rotator cuff is attached to the greater tuberosity, any significant displacement implies a tear, which also may require surgical repair.

Specifics of History and Examination. Significant trauma or dislocation of the shoulder is accompanied by immediate pain located around the upper arm and is exacerbated by any movement. On examination, there often is ecchymosis and swelling around the shoulder.

A mandatory careful neurovascular examination must be performed because of the significant incidence of associated injuries.

Antecedent trauma may not be present in a younger child with physial stress fractures. Adolescents with little league shoulder can have a history of repetitive overhead throwing and associated nondisplaced physial fractures.

Conservative Management. If a fracture is suspected, the extremity should be immobilized in a sling and swathe, and appropriate radiographs should be obtained.

Operative Management. Operative management of proximal humerus fractures can take numerous forms. Surgical goals are to anatomically reduce the displaced fracture fragments followed by fixation using heavy, nonabsorbable sutures or wires that incorporate the rotator cuff for strength. Alternatively, percutaneous pin fixation can be used in select surgical neck fractures. More severe fractures require more extensive fixation methods or even prosthetic replacement.

Clavicle Fractures

Sports Commonly Involved. Clavicle fractures are the most common bony injuries seen about the shoulder. They occur in high-energy, contact sports, most notably football and hockey, or in bicycling and skiing resulting from falls.

Background. The most common mechanism for fracture of the clavicle is a fall on an outstretched arm or a direct blow with an object, as can occur in hockey or lacrosse. The fractures predominate in the shaft (80%), followed by distal (15%), and medial (5%) aspects.[29,39] Associated neurovascular injuries are rare despite their close anatomic proximity, and most fractures heal uneventfully within 8 weeks.

Pathomechanics. Because the primary function of the clavicle is to strut the shoulder girdle away from the thorax, fractures result in inferior and anterior displacement with gravity as the major deforming factor.

Fracture characteristics depend on location relative to ligamentous insertions. Distal clavicle fractures occur in the lateral third of the shaft where the coracoclavicular ligaments originate. These fractures usually involve a tear or bony avulsion of the coracoclavicular ligaments and functionally simulate acromioclavicular joint separations (see the section on acromioclavicular separations). Because the small distal fragment displaces inferiorly and anteriorly away from the proximal shaft, these fractures have a high incidence of painful nonunions when not surgically stabilized. In contrast, fractures of the midshaft reduce relatively well and heal well with conservative management. Medial third fractures are rare and displace little. These fractures heal well with symptomatic management. The medial growth plate of the clavicle fuses as late as age 22 years and, therefore, a fracture before this age is often through the epiphysis and is commonly a Salter II–type. These injuries are also managed conservatively.

Specifics of History and Examination. Displaced clavicle fractures are easily apparent on inspection secondary to the subcutaneous location. Nondisplaced fractures demonstrate swelling and palpable pain. Associated problems such as skin compromise or neurovascular injury should be carefully evaluated because they can easily be missed, leading to serious complications.

Although standard anteroposterior radiographs are commonly sufficient, cephalic tilt clavicle views show the fracture more clearly.

Conservative Management. Midshaft fractures are managed conservatively with a figure-eight strap or simple sling. The figure-eight strap must be fitted properly with a snug fit, which can be uncomfortable. Because the arm sling has been shown to be equally effective, it is generally preferred. When using the sling, it is important to adequately support the weight of the arm to counteract the anterior and inferior displacement.

Operative Management. Operative management of acute clavicle fractures historically has been reserved for distal third fractures. These fractures are generally managed with operative reduction and fixation with circlage wires or sutures and screws. Additional fixation is secured to the coracoid process, depending on the relative integrity of the ligaments.

Acromial, Glenoid, and Scapular Body Fractures

Sports Commonly Involved. Acromial and scapular body fractures are rare but can be seen in athletes who participate in high-energy contact sports such as football, skiing, or bicycling. Glenoid fractures are relatively more common and in the athletic population are seen in the context of glenohumeral dislocations.

Background. Acromial fractures can result from either a direct blow or a fall on the point of the shoulder. More typically, this will result in either an acromioclavicular separation or clavicle fracture. Because these fractures are rare, the clinician should not mistake an unfused growth plate for fracture. Previously discussed in the anatomy section, fusion of the growth plates takes place around the age of 22 years. In older individuals, an os acromiale, which is a nonunion of the growth plate, may also be present. Os acromiale occurs approximately 1.6% of the time and is bilateral 60% of the time.[29,39] The growth plates occur in a characteristic location at the junction between the anterior and middle third of the acromion. Fractures, in contrast, generally occur near the scapular spine base.

Scapular fractures represent high-energy injuries to the posterior thorax and are usually undisplaced in the context of athletics. These fractures are stable and heal well because of the abundant surrounding musculature. An athlete sustaining this fracture should have a careful work-up for associated blunt thorax injuries, such as pneumothorax.

Pathomechanics. Acromial fractures must be watched carefully. Because the lateral deltoid originates here, these fractures tend to angulate inferiorly, closing down the coracoacromial arch. A small reduction of the subacromial space is poorly tolerated, and these fractures often require operative fixation.

Scapular fractures, as stated previously, usually heal well because of the abundant investing musculature. However, secondary problems such as adhesions or fibrosis of the subscapular bursa can occur, causing pain and alteration of scapulothoracic mechanics.

In the athletic population, glenoid fractures occur usually in the context of glenohumeral dislocations. These fractures are seen on the anterior–inferior glenoid rim and, when significant in size, can severely affect glenohumeral stability. Also referred to as bony Bankart fractures, these fractures represent a combination axial load and bony avulsion injury from pull of the inferior glenohumeral ligaments.

Specifics of History and Examination. A patient with an acromial fracture will have sustained injury directly to the point of the shoulder. Pain will be palpable directly on the acromial base with associated ecchymosis. This contrasts with os acromiale or growth plate injuries, which show less evidence of trauma and have more anterior acromial pain. Specific radiographic studies that should be taken include the West Point and axillary views.

Scapular fractures are diagnosed with true anteroposterior radiographs of the shoulder. They are often seen as incidental findings on athletes who have sustained significant thorax trauma. In the context of athletics, these fractures are usually nondisplaced and difficult to detect. Palpable tenderness on the scapula should direct clinical suspicion on radiographic interpretation. The clinical examination should include evaluation for associated injuries such as rib fractures, pneumothorax, kidney contusions, and aortic dissections.

Glenoid fractures seen in athletics most commonly are associated with anterior, traumatic dislocations; it is very rare to see more complex fractures. Careful evaluation of standard anteroposterior and axillary radiographs will often show the displaced fragment of glenoid rim displaced in an anterior and inferior direction. When necessary, special views, such as the West Point or computed tomography scan images, help visualize the presence and extent of these fractures.

Conservative Management. All the previously discussed fractures should be acutely immobilized with a sling and swathe for further evaluation. If nonoperative management is elected, the sling is continued. For acromial fractures, 4 to 6 weeks of arm support is required with careful follow-up evaluation for any displacement. For nondisplaced scapular fractures, motion is encouraged as soon as tolerated to prevent scapulothoracic adhesions. Larger glenoid fractures associated with instability are usually managed oppressively.

Operative Management. Displaced or angulated acromial fractures are managed with operative reduction and fixation using parallel screws or figure-eight wires. Glenoid displacement is the main indication for surgical reduction and fixation of scapular body fractures. Anterior rim glenoid fractures are managed usually with operative reduction and fixation with screws. Rarely, small or severely comminuted fragments are excised and a coracoid transfer performed. These procedures are achieved through a standard instability repair approach, using some elements of capsular repair.

SPECIFIC TRAUMATIC INJURIES: SOFT TISSUE

Rotator Cuff Tear

Sports Commonly Involved. Traumatic tears of the rotator cuff are rare in younger athletes. In older athletes who have been involved for many years in repetitive overhead sports such as baseball, tennis, swimming, or football (quarterback), these partial tears usually represent acute extensions of chronic tendinitis or partial tears. In younger athletes, traumatic tears may occur when playing in football or wrestling.

Background. Traumatic rotator cuff tears are seen with violent internal rotation of the arm against resistance or in falls on the outstretched arm. Rarely, they are seen when an attempt is made to throw heavy objects. Because the rotator cuff tends to be thick and robust, these traumatic avulsion injuries are rare in the younger, athletic population.

Pathomechanics. Because the rotator cuff functions in external rotation and stabilization of the humeral head, violent rotation or luxation can cause avulsion. These acute injuries are different clinical entities from chronic, attrition rotator cuff disease. The tendons tend to comprise healthy, well-vascularized tissue with muscle atrophy or scaring. When repaired in a timely fashion, a patient tends to have excellent functional recovery. For an older athlete with acute extension of a chronic process, the same principles outlined previously for nontraumatic rotator cuff disease still apply.

Specifics of History and Examination. The patient will generally complain of sudden, intense pain after one of the previously mentioned injury mechanisms. Pain is accompanied by significant weakness in shoulder motion. When an acute tear is suspected, early imaging with magnetic resonance imaging is appropriate to confirm the diagnosis. Other specifics of history and examination were outlined previously for nontraumatic rotator cuff disease.

Conservative Management. Initial conservative management is usually a sling for symptomatic relief. However, once a diagnosis of acute, full-thickness tear is confirmed, early operative repair provides the best chance for functional recovery. Partial tears can be managed with early symptomatic management followed by a directed physical therapy program.

Indications for Orthopedic Referral. Acute tears diagnosed by magnetic resonance imaging should be referred early for surgery. A patient with partial-thickness tears can be referred after failure to progress with conservative treatment.

Operative Management. Because acute tears tend to be mobile without chronic scarring, they often can be repaired in an arthroscopically assisted fashion through small incisions with excellent results.[33] Larger chronic tears require open repair.

Glenohumeral Dislocation

Sports Commonly Involved. Initial, traumatic dislocations are seen in participants of high-energy impact sports or result from significant falls. The sports most often involved include football, rugby, hockey, wrestling, boxing, skiing, skating, or bicycling.

Background. Dislocations most often occur anteriorly, involving an abducted and externally rotated arm position such as bracing for a fall or when the arm is violently caught by another player. Uncommonly, a direct blow to the shoulder can cause a dislocation.

In the young, athletic population, these dislocations tend to recur. Recurrence rates vary from 50% to 90% after initial, traumatic dislocation, with higher rates associated with athletes who participate in sports with repetitive overhead motion and younger individuals.[18,29,38,46]

Pathomechanics. Anterior glenohumeral dislocations always involve some element of anterior–inferior capsular attenuation.[9,24] The greater duration of symptoms and number of dislocations result in greater anterior capsular redundancy.[1] Additionally, frequently there is an avulsion of the anterior–inferior glenoid labrum with attached anteroinferior glenohumeral ligament. In the younger population, this acute capsular damage does not incite a vigorous inflammatory response with subsequent scarring and joint retraction. Rather, the capsule remains lax and can no longer serve as an adequate checkrein to extremes of motion. Recently, an alteration in capsular, proprioceptive feedback has been suggested as a mechanism for recurrent instability. In this model, the attenuated capsule cannot relay adequate proprioceptive feedback to initiate contraction of stabilizing, surrounding musculature.

Specifics of History and Examination. Diagnosis of an acutely dislocated shoulder is usually obvious by examination and history. The athlete will usually relate a history of significant trauma involving external rotation and abduction of the shoulder. Rarely, insignificant trauma can cause a first-time dislocation. The dislocated shoulder will show deformity with a subacromial sulcus and palpable fullness anterior and inferior from the humeral head. The arm is generally held in some external rotation and abduction. A careful neurovascular examination should be performed, especially for axillary nerve injury.

On radiographs, anteroposterior and axillary views should be inspected carefully for any fractures. This inspection is especially important on prereduction radiographs because a missed, nondisplaced fracture can be propagated or displaced by an inappropriate reduction maneuver.

Conservative Management. Once anatomic reduction is achieved, nonoperative management is preferred. The arm is immobilized in a sling. Although the exact length of time is controversial, 4 to 6 weeks of wearing the sling is generally accepted. After 4 to 6 weeks, a directed physical therapy program that stresses rotation strengthening internally is prescribed. However, strengthening exercises should begin as soon as the patient is comfortable. These exercises should strengthen the internal and external rotation, deltoid, and scapular muscles so there is a balanced approach.

Indications for Orthopedic Referral. Because of the possibility of subtle fractures, acute traumatic dislocation should generally be referred for initial evaluation.

Operative Management. Arthroscopic or open operative management may be performed for an acute dislocation in the dominant arm in throwing athletes and in individuals who will return to repetitive, stressful, overhead activity.

Acromioclavicular Separations

Sports Commonly Involved. Acromioclavicular separations are relatively common injuries seen in participants of contact sports, especially hockey, and in victims of significant falls. Those sports most often involved include hockey, football, rugby, wrestling, skiing, skating, and bicycling.

Background. These injuries generally result from a blow or a fall directly on the shoulder. The separations are graded as follows: Grade I, pain and swelling at the acromioclavicular joint without radiographic subluxation; Grade II, subluxation without complete dislocation; and Grade III, complete dislocation of the joint.[39] Grade I and II injuries heal well with conservative, symptomatic management. Management of Grade III injuries is somewhat controversial. Although most of these injuries heal without significant functional limitations, conservative management will result in a persistently dislocated joint that may be at higher risk for painful arthrosis. Most physicians prefer nonoperative management; however, in the high-performance athlete engaging in overhead motion there may be a role for acute stabilization. Other commonly accepted indications for operative fixation include herniation of the distal clavicle through the trapezius and locking of the clavicle posterior to the acromion.

Pathomechanics. The distal clavicle is stabilized to the acromion primarily through three ligaments: the superior acromioclavicular joint capsule and ligament and two coracoclavicular ligaments. Under normal, physiologic loads, the superior acromioclavicular ligament is most important for stabilizing the joint-form luxation. With higher loads, the coracoclavicular ligament becomes more important for stabilizing against superior displacement, and the superior acromioclavicular ligament remains the primary restraint against anterior–superior–posterior displacement.

With Grade I injuries, there is an isolated sprain of the acromioclavicular ligaments and no tear. In Grade II separations, there is a tear of the acromioclavicular ligaments, leaving the coracoclavicular ligaments as the primary restraint. In Grade III separations, the acromioclavicular and coracoclavicular ligaments are torn, with no remaining ligamentous restraints.

Specifics of History and Examination. Patients with acromioclavicular separations relate a history of fall or force directly on the shoulder. With Grade I separations, there is tenderness and edema at the joint. Grade II and III separations will also show deformity from a more prominent distal clavicle. These separations should be checked for reducibility. If a partial reduction cannot be obtained, herniation through the trapezius should be suspected.

Distal clavicle anteroposterior radiographs with the arm in the dependent position should be obtained. Bilateral views help make the diagnosis when subtle luxation is present. Because the clavicle displaces posterior and anterior views, an axillary radiograph is also necessary.

Conservative Management. Nonoperative management consists of a snug-arm sling to support the weight of the arm. Special slings are available to hold the distal clavicle in the reduced position, but they are ineffective and have lead to skin breakdown at the top of the acromioclavicular joint.

Indications for Surgical Referral. Surgical fixation of a separated acromioclavicular joint is achieved by open reduction and stabilization of the distal clavicle with sutures secured to the coracoid. The coracoacromial ligament is then transferred from the acromion to the distal clavicle to reconstruct the torn coracoclavicular ligaments.

SLAP Lesions

Sports Commonly Involved. Superior labrum anterior posterior (SLAP) lesions are common in sports with repetitive throwing or trauma to the shoulder from falls, such as baseball, basketball, and football.

Background. SLAP tears of the glenoid labrum represent tears unique to the superior labrum.

Pathoanatomy. Four types of tears have been described.[43] Type 1 involves labral fraying, type 2 involves separation of the labrum from the glenoid, type 3 involves a bucket-handle tear of the superior labrum with central displacement of the tear into the joint, and type 4 involves a bucket-handle tear that extends into the biceps tendon.

Specifics of History and Examination. SLAP lesions are usually caused by a traumatic mechanism such as falling on an abducted, forward-flexed arm or from repetitive violent throwing activities. Patients complain of pain associated with overhead movement in abduction, external rotation, and extension. Examination reveals tenderness of the biceps tendon within the bicipital groove and a positive active compression test as described by O'Brien.[32] Conventional MRI may not demonstrate the torn labrum and MRI enhanced with gadolinium may be required.

Conservative Management. Suspected SLAP lesions are initially treated with a trial of rest, activity modification, and rotator cuff and peri-scapular muscle strengthening.[43]

Indications for Orthopedic Referral. Patients who fail to achieve satisfactory relief with conservative treatment should be referred to the orthopedic surgeon.

Operative Management. Type 1 and 3 lesions are treated with arthroscopic debridement of the frayed labum or excision of the torn labrum. Type 2 and 4 lesions are treated with debridement and stabilization.[43]

Peripheral Nerve Injuries

Sports Commonly Involved. Peripheral nerve injuries to the suprascapular, axillary, long thoracic, and spinal accessory nerves are rare. Suprascapular nerve injury is seen in athletes who participate in activities with repetitive overhead motion, especially baseball pitchers and volleyball players. Other nerve injuries are seen in those who participate in contact sports in which there is blunt trauma to the shoulder girdle.

Background. All of these peripheral nerve injuries are uncommon but should always be considered in the differential diagnosis for atrophy, diffuse tenderness, and weakness about the shoulder.[28] These injuries can occur from seemingly insignificant injury, but more often are associated with significant injuries or overuse episodes.

Suprascapular nerve deficits can occur as isolated nerve compression syndromes from entrapment at the suprascapular or spinoglenoid notch or from ganglia. These syndromes often occur with insidious onset. Conversely, they can result from a blow to the shoulder or from repetitive overhead and cross-body motions. Conservative management of rest and nonsteroidal medication is often helpful. Surgical management of exploration and decompression, if necessary, has a good prognosis if significant muscle atrophy has not occurred.

Axillary nerve injuries are the most common and are often associated with dislocations or fractures of the proximal humerus. Rarely, a direct blow to the lateral shoulder can result in axillary nerve injury. These injuries are almost always neurapraxias, and there is a good prognosis for recovery with conservative management.

Long thoracic and spinal accessory nerve injuries associated with blunt trauma, in contrast to axillary and suprascapular injuries, have a more guarded prognosis. Nerve explorations and decompressions are usually not successful, and prolonged observation is generally used. Conservative management involves strengthening of the periscapular, adjunctive musculature. Long thoracic nerve palsies can be idiopathic, usually in throwers, and have a good prognosis for recovery. A 1-year observation period is recommended for the long thoracic nerve, and a 3-month period is recommended for the spinal accessory nerve.

Pathoanatomy. The suprascapular nerve is formed from C5 and C6 spinal roots and branches from the upper trunk of the brachial plexus. The nerve enters the superior border of the scapula through the scapular notch, which is bridged by a thick, transverse ligament. The nerve gives off branches to the supraspinatus and courses around the scapular spine laterally to enter the infraspinatus fossa where it terminates into a number of muscular branches. In 50% of patients, the nerve passes the spinoglenoid ligament—an aponeurotic band separating the spinati. Compression of the nerve usually occurs at the notch or spinoglenoid ligament.[39]

The axillary nerve is responsible for innervation of the important deltoid muscle, teres minor, and overlying skin. The nerve also forms from C5 and C6, but it branches distally from the posterior cord. It courses anterior to the subscapularis muscle until it travels posterior directly under the glenohumeral joint to give off a circumflex branch, which innervates the deltoid. The close proximity of the nerve to the anterior–inferior glenohumeral joint results in susceptibility to concomitant injury with dislocations and fractures.

The long thoracic nerve originates directly from the confluence of the C5, C6, and C7 spinal roots, after which it courses down the anterolateral chest wall to innervate the serratus anterior muscle. Injury to this nerve can occur with blunt chest wall trauma or through several poorly understood mechanisms, including viral illness, prolonged recumbency, or overhead throwing.

The spinal accessory nerve is a cranial nerve that enters the neck from the jugular foramen to descend through the posterior triangle to innervate the trapezius muscle. Injuries can result from traction from a blow to the point of the shoulder or from direct blows.

Specifics of History and Examination. Each of the previously discussed nerve injuries is characterized by specific muscle atrophy or dysfunction and diffuse pain. Thus, suprascapular nerve injuries result in weakness to external rotation; axillary nerve injuries result in weakness to elevation; long thoracic nerve injuries result in scapular winging seen best when pushing forward against a wall; and spinal accessory nerve injuries result in weakness to elevation and shoulder shrug. When suspected, electromyographic studies, in conjunction with a clinical examination, will confirm the diagnosis.

Conservative Management. Nonoperative management consists of supportive, symptomatic care during observation. Range of motion and strengthening of adjacent, overlapping musculature is used. Serial electromyography can be helpful for following recovery or determining prognosis.

Indications for Orthopedic Referral. Confirmed nerve injuries or documented muscle dysfunction, especially in the presence of significant atrophy, indicate orthopedic referral.

Operative Management. Operative management of peripheral nerve injuries to the suprascapular and axillary nerve are directed toward exploration, neurolysis, repair, or grafting because good muscle transfers are unavailable. In contrast, there are good muscle transfers for reconstituting serratus anterior and trapezius palsies, and they are generally preferred.

REFERENCES

1. Ahmad CS, et al: Anteromedial capsular redundancy and labral deficiency in shoulder instability. Am J Sports Med 31:247–252, 2003.
2. Anderson T: Difficult sports-related shoulder fractures. Clin Sports Med 9:31–37, 1990.

3. Andrews JR, Kupferman SP, Dillman CJ: Labral tears in throwing and racquet sports. Clin Sports Med 10:901–911, 1991.
4. Bigiliani LU, Kimmel J, McCann PD, Wolfe I: Repair of rotator cuff tears in tennis players. Am J Sports Med 20:112–117, 1992.
5. Bigliani LU, Flatow EL, Pollock RG: Fractures about the shoulder. In Rockwood CRJ, Green DP (eds): Fractures in Adults. vol 1. Philadelphia, Lippincott, 1996, pp 1055–1107.
6. Bigliani LU, Flatow EL: History, physical examination, and diagnostic modalities. In McGinty JB (ed): Operative Arthroscopy. New York, Raven Press, 1991.
7. Bigliani LU, et al: Inferior capsular shift procedure for anterior-inferior shoulder instability in athletes. Am J Sports Med 22:578–584, 1994.
8. Bigliani LU, Nicholson GP, Flatow EL: Arthroscopic resection of the distal clavicle. Orthop Clin North Am 24:133–141, 1993.
9. Bigliani LU, et al: Tensile properties of the inferior glenohumeral ligament. J Orthop Res 10:187–197, 1992.
10. Bigliani LU, et al: The relationship of acromial architecture to rotator cuff disease. Clin Sports Med 10:823–838, 1991.
11. Bloom MH, Obata WG: Diagnosis of posterior dislocation of the shoulder with use of Velpeau axillary and angle-up roentgenographic views. J Bone Joint Surg Am 49:943–949, 1967.
12. Burnham RS, et al: Shoulder pain in wheelchair athletes. The role of muscle imbalance. Am J Sports Med 21:238–242, 1993.
13. Cahill BR: Osteolysis of the distal part of the clavicle in male athletes. J Bone Joint Surg Am 64:1053–1058, 1982.
14. Dillman CJ, Fleisig GS, Andrews JR: Biomechanics of pitching with emphasis upon shoulder kinematics. J Orthop Sports Phys Ther 18:402–408, 1993.
15. Flatow EL: The biomechanics of the acromioclavicular, sternoclavicular, and scapulothoracic joints. Instr Course Lect 42:237–245, 1993.
16. Gerber C, Krushell RJ: Isolated rupture of the tendon of the subscapularis muscle. Clinical features in 16 cases. J Bone Joint Surg Br 73:389–394, 1991.
17. Gross ML, Brenner SL, Esformes I, Sonzogni JJ: Anterior shoulder instability in weight lifters. Am J Sports Med 21:599–603, 1993.
18. Higgs GB, Weinstein D, Flatow EL: Evaluation and treatment of acute anterior glenohumeral dislocations. Sports Med Arthroscopy Rev 1:190–201, 1993.
19. Iannotti JP, et al: Magnetic resonance imaging of the shoulder. Sensitivity, specificity, and predictive value. J Bone Joint Surg Am 73:17–29, 1991.
20. Ireland ML, Andrews JR: Shoulder and elbow injuries in the young athlete. Clin Sports Med 7:473–494, 1988.
21. Janda DH, Loubert P: Basic science and clinical application in the athlete's shoulder. A preventative program focusing on the glenohumeral joint. Clin Sports Med 10:955–971, 1991.
22. Jobe FW, Moynes DR, Antonelli DJ: Rotator cuff function during a golf swing. Am J Sports Med 14:388–392, 1986.
23. Jobe FW, Pink M: Classification and treatment of shoulder dysfunction in the overhead athlete. J Orthop Sports Phys Ther 18:427–432, 1993.
24. Kuriyama S, Fujimaki E, Katagiri T, Uemura S: Anterior dislocation of the shoulder joint sustained through skiing. Arthrographic findings and prognosis. Am J Sports Med 12:339–346, 1984.
25. Lo YP, Hsu YC, Chan KM: Epidemiology of shoulder impingement in upper arm sports events. Br J Sports Med 24:173–177, 1990.
26. McMaster WC, Troup J: A survey of interfering shoulder pain in United States competitive swimmers. Am J Sports Med 21:67–70, 1993.
27. Meister K, Andrews JR: Classification and treatment of rotator cuff injuries in the overhand athlete. J Orthop Sports Phys Ther 18:413–421, 1993.
28. Mendoza FX, Main WK, Main K: Peripheral nerve injuries of the shoulder in the athlete. Clin Sports Med 9:331–342, 1990.
29. Miller MD, Cooper DE, Warner JP: The Shoulder: Review of Sports Medicine and Arthroscopy. Philadelphia, WB Saunders, 1995.
30. Miniaci A, Fowler PJ: Impingement in the athlete. Clin Sports Med 12:91–110, 1993.
31. Neviaser TJ. Weight lifting: Risks and injuries to the shoulder. Clin Sports Med 10:615–621, 1991.
32. O'Brien SJ, et al: The active compression test: A new and effective test for diagnosing labral tears and acromioclavicular joint abnormality. Am J Sports Med 26:610–613, 1998.
33. Park JY, et al: Portal-extension approach for the repair of small and medium rotator cuff tears. Am J Sports Med 28:312–316, 2000.
34. Pforringer W, Smasal V: Aspects of traumatology in ice hockey. J Sports Sci 5:327–336, 1987.
35. Pollock RG, Bigliani LU: Recurrent posterior shoulder instability. Diagnosis and treatment. Clin Orthop 291:85–96, 1993.
36. Pollock RG, Duralde XA, Flatow EL, Bigliani LU: The use of arthroscopy in the treatment of resistant frozen shoulder. Clin Orthop 304:30–36, 1994.
37. Richardson AB, Jobe FW, Collins HR: The shoulder in competitive swimming. Am J Sports Med 8: 159–163, 1980.
38. Richmond DR: Handlebar problems in bicycling. Clin Sports Med 13:165–173, 1994.
39. Rockwood CR, Matsen FA (eds): The Shoulder. Philadelphia, WB Saunders, 1990.

40. Scavenius M, Iversen BF: Nontraumatic clavicular osteolysis in weight lifters. Am J Sports Med 20:463–467, 1992.
41. Silliman JF, Hawkins RJ: Current concepts and recent advances in the athlete's shoulder. Clin Sports Med 10:693–705, 1991.
42. Smasal V, Pforringer W: [Ice hockey injuries. Studies of the highest West German league]. Sportverletz Sportschaden 1:181–184, 1987.
43. Snyder SJ, et al: SLAP lesions of the shoulder. Arthroscopy 6:274–279, 1990.
44. Soslowsky LJ, Flatow EL, Bigliani LU, Mow VC: Articular geometry of the glenohumeral joint. Clin Orthop 181–190, 1992.
45. Soslowsky LJ, et al: Quantitation of in situ contact areas at the glenohumeral joint: A biomechanical study. J Orthop Res 10:524–534, 1992.
46. Tsai L, et al: Shoulder function in patients with unoperated anterior shoulder instability. Am J Sports Med 19:469–473, 1991.
47. Warren RF: Instability of shoulder in throwing sports. Instr Course Lect 34:337–348, 1985.
48. Wilk KE, Arrigo C: Current concepts in the rehabilitation of the athletic shoulder. J Orthop Sports Phys Ther 18:365–378, 1993.
49. Zawadsky M, Marra G, Wiater JM, et al. Osteolysis of the distal clavicle: Long-term results of arthroscopic resection. Arthroscopy 16:600–605, 2000.

19 The Elbow and Forearm

Robert T. Goldman and Peter D. McCann

Elbow and forearm injuries are becoming more common as more people participate in throwing and racquet sports. Injuries may involve the bony articulations, muscles, ligaments, tendons, capsule, or nerves, all of which may impair elbow function. The majority of injuries to the elbow and forearm in the athlete are chronic, overuse injuries. These injuries result from repetitive intrinsic and extrinsic overload causing cumulative trauma. In adults, soft tissues such as ligaments and tendons become attenuated. In children, apophyses—the weakest link in the immature musculoskeletal system—are susceptible to stress injuries. Early management should be directed toward decreasing pain and inflammation, followed by strengthening and conditioning of the structures surrounding the elbow. Appropriate rehabilitation remains the cornerstone of successful management of overuse injuries of the elbow, facilitating patients' return to activity. Acute injuries to the elbow and forearm, although less common than chronic injuries, also plague the athlete. To fully understand the significance of injuries to the elbow and forearm, functional anatomy, patterns of injury, and current management options will be reviewed.

ELBOW ANATOMY

The elbow is a hinged joint composed of three distinct articulations: the radiocapitellar joint, the ulnohumeral joint, and the proximal radioulnar joint (Fig. 19-1). This unique articulation provides for flexion–extension and forearm rotation (pronation–supination). The normal arc of elbow flexion is 0° to 145°, with considerable individual variation allowing hyperextension or hyperflexion.[14] Forearm pronation averages 80°, and supination averages 85°.[14] The functional elbow range of motion that permits nearly all activities of daily living is 30° to 130° of flexion, 50° of pronation, and 50° of supination.[85]

The *carrying angle* is defined as the orientation of the forearm in reference to the humerus when the elbow is in full extension. The carrying angle varies as a function of age (smaller in children than adults) and sex (females averaging 3° to 4° more than males). The normal distribution of this angle varies greatly and averages 10° valgus in male subjects and 13° valgus in female subjects.[2]

Elbow stability is composed of three elements: the bony articulations, the capsular and ligamentous structures, and the dynamic contribution of the muscles. Unlike the shoulder, the dynamic contribution of the musculature to elbow stability under normal circumstances is minimal. The articular configuration is the primary stabilizer of the elbow against varus and valgus stress at less than 20° and more than 120° of flexion.[114] Between these extremes, stability is mainly provided by the fibrous and synovial capsule, which is thickened medially and laterally to form the collateral ligament complexes.

The ulnar or medial collateral ligament complex consists of three distinct structures: the anterior oblique, posterior oblique, and transverse ligaments (Fig. 19-2). The anterior oblique ligament is a thick, discrete band with parallel fibers originating from the medial epicondyle and inserting onto the medial aspect of the coronoid process. The results of various sectioning studies have shown that the anterior oblique ligament is the primary stabilizer of the elbow against valgus stress.[84,110] The posterior oblique ligament is a fan-shaped thickening of the capsule best defined with the elbow flexed at 90°. This ligament originates from the medial epicondyle and inserts onto the medial margin of the semilunar notch. The transverse ligament, which does not appear to have any effect on elbow stability, originates from the medial olecranon and inserts onto the inferior medial aspect of the coronoid process.

The radial or lateral collateral ligament complex provides varus stability to the elbow joint and is composed of four structures. The *radial collateral ligament* originates from the lateral epicondyle and inserts into the annular ligament. The *lateral ulnar collateral ligament* originates from the lateral epicondyle and inserts onto the crista supinatoris of the ulna. Rupture of this ligament has been determined to be the primary lesion in posterolateral rotatory instability of the elbow.[96] The *annular ligament* and the *accessory collateral ligament* ensure the proper articulation of the proximal radioulnar joint but contribute little to varus stability of the elbow.[79]

Although providing minimal stability in the static situation, the flexor–pronator muscle group of the forearm functions as a secondary dynamic stabilizer of the elbow against valgus stress. Likewise, the anconeus muscle provides secondary dynamic stability against varus stress.[107]

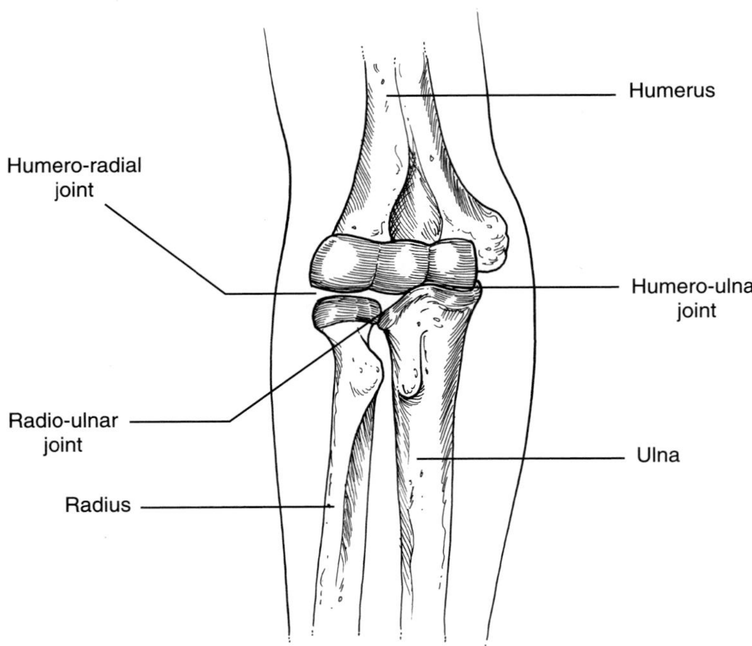

FIGURE 19-1. Bony anatomy of the elbow.

OVERUSE INJURIES

Overuse injuries are caused by repetitive intrinsic or extrinsic overload, or both, resulting in microtrauma to soft tissues such as ligaments or tendons (Table 19-1). Intrinsic overload is the force from muscular contraction, concentric or eccentric, that can lead to tendinitis or muscular injury. Extrinsic overload is a tensile overload caused by excessive joint torque forces stressing the soft tissue and resulting in stretching and eventual disruption. Extrinsic overload also may be attributed to compression causing abrasion or impingement. Microrupture of soft tissues results in compromise by an imperfect healing process. In children, as apophyses undergo ossification, they are susceptible to stress injuries, resulting in local inflammation, irregular ossification patterns, overgrowth, and pain.

Management of overuse injuries should always start with prevention. Prevention should include education, overall flexibility, strengthening and endurance, proper warm-up and stretching, and avoidance of fatigue. Proper mechanics and equipment are also important.

Once an athlete develops an overuse injury, an aggressive nonoperative program should be started. The acronym PRICEMM[107] can be used to remember the modalities. First, **p**rotect the elbow from further injury. **R**est the elbow from the offending event, but allow the

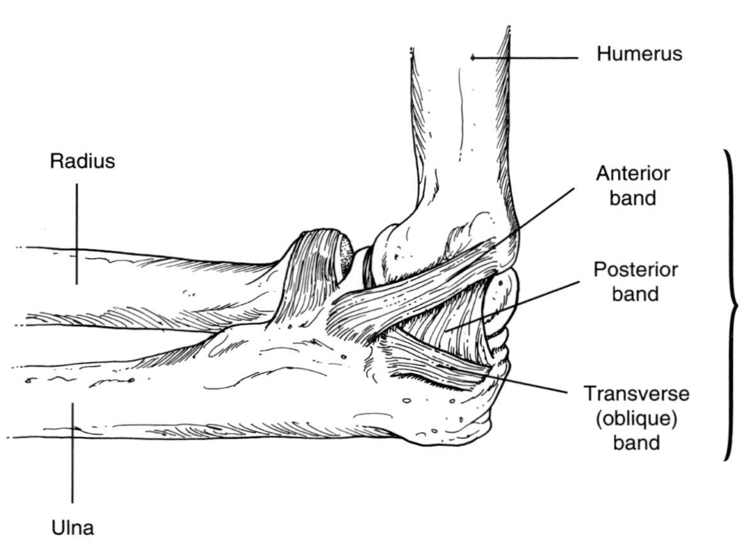

FIGURE 19-2. Medial collateral ligament complex of the elbow.

TABLE 19-1

Sports that Commonly Produce Elbow Injuries

Sport	Common injury
Racquet sports	Lateral epicondylitis with backhand
Golf	Medial epicondylitis on down-swing with trailing arm
	Lateral epicondylitis at impact with leading arm
Basketball	Posterior compartment with follow-through on jump shot
Waterskiing	Valgus extension overload of posterior compartment with trick skiing
Bowling	Flexor–pronator soreness
Baseball	Valgus stress of pitching medial traction, lateral compression, posterior abutment
Volleyball	Valgus stress at impact of spiking
Football	Valgus stress with throwing a pass; hyperextension and dislocation, and olecranon bursitis with direct trauma
Gymnastics	Radiocapitellar overload and posterior impingement with weight-bearing on extended elbow
Weight training	Ulnar collateral ligament sprain, ulnar nerve irritation
Field events	
Shotput	Posterior impingement with follow-through
Javelin	Valgus–extension overload of throwing; medial traction posterior abutment, lateral compression
Canoeing, kayaking	Distal bicipital tendinitis
Archery	Extensor muscle fatigue, lateral epicondylitis of bow arm
Rock climbing	Brachialis or distal biceps tendinitis

From Safran MR: Elbow injuries in athletes: A review. Clin Orthop 310:257–277, 1995.

athlete to continue, maintaining cardiovascular fitness. **I**ce, **c**ompression with an elastic bandage, and **e**levation are mainstays of nonoperative management. Nonsteroidal anti-inflammatory **m**edications are successful at relieving the pain and inflammation. Several **m**odalities, such as transcutaneous electrical stimulation and ultrasound, also have proven helpful.[88] A rehabilitation program should be instituted after the acute symptoms have resolved, with a gradual return to activity.

If a quality rehabilitation program is not successful and the patient has constant pain or persistent pain that affects activity, surgery may be indicated. The common features of the many surgical techniques used to manage overuse injuries include identification and excision of the pathologic tissue and reconstruction using normal tissue to close the defect. Healthy scar tissue can form that can withstand the repetitive stresses that the weakened, abnormal tissue could not. After the surgery, the repaired tissue is protected, and gradual postoperative rehabilitation is performed before the patient returns to sports activity.

TENDINOPATHIES

Lateral Epicondylitis: Tennis Elbow

Lateral epicondylitis is arguably the most common source of elbow pain in the general population. It occurs 7 to 20 times more frequently than medial epicondylitis.[28] It was first described more than 100 years ago in a tennis player,[73] but has since been described in association with many other athletic and nonathletic endeavors. The typical patient is a recreational tennis player aged 35 to 50 years who plays three to four times a week. They are usually inadequately conditioned and often use poor technique. Advanced tennis players who warm up, use good technique, and are well conditioned rarely suffer from lateral epicondylitis.[92]

Lateral epicondylitis is a chronic tendinitis of the extensor muscles, primarily the extensor carpi radialis brevis, caused by overuse in intensity and duration. It has been shown that 50% of club tennis players older than 30 years have experienced symptoms characteristic of lateral epicondylitis at least once.[91] One half of these players noted minor symptoms with a duration of less than 6 months, whereas the other half had major symptoms lasting an average of 2.5 years. Several factors have been associated with this problem: heavier, stiffer, more tightly strung racquets; incorrect grip size; inexperience; and poor backhand technique.

Lateral epicondylitis presents as lateral elbow pain that has an insidious onset beginning with pain after vigorous activity and progressing to pain during the activity. On examination, there is pain with passive wrist flexion and with active wrist extension. There often is point tenderness 1 to 2 cm distal to the lateral epicondyle. Grasping or pinching with the wrist extended (coffee cup test) usually reproduces pain at the point of tenderness.[28] Radiographic results are frequently normal, although 22% of patients will have evidence of a spur at the lateral epicondyle or calcification of the common extensor tendon.[88] The differential diagnosis of lateral epicondylitis includes radial tunnel syndrome (compression neuropathy of the posterior interosseous nerve), localized intraarticular pathology, or subtle instability of the radiocapitellar joint.

Surgical pathology reveals that the extensor carpi radialis brevis tendon is implicated as the source of pain and pathologic change.[92] Surrounding extensor tendons may be involved as well. Initial management is nonoperative (PRICEMM) and is often successful. Proper technique and equipment modifications, such as reduced racquet string tension and a cushioned grip, are useful adjuncts.[29] A counterforce brace has also been useful in managing tennis elbow. These braces are 5- to 6-cm wide nonelastic bands that are applied to encircle the forearm just below the elbow. A number of theories have been presented to explain how the brace works. Essentially, the brace causes a change in the sequence and direction of muscle pull, which decreases the force of muscle contraction by shortening the effective length of the muscle.[45]

If the initial nonoperative management is ineffective after 3 to 4 weeks, injection with xylocaine, 1%, with methylprednisolone just below the extensor carpi radialis brevis origin may be indicated. Some authors recommend no more than three injections in this area per year because they may cause further degeneration of the tendon and subsequent rupture.[87]

If nonoperative management fails to return the athlete to his or her usual activities by 3 to 4 months, which occurs in approximately 10% of patients, Nirschl[90] recommends surgical intervention. Others wait up to 1 year before considering surgical treatment.[87] Many surgical procedures have been described for management of refractory lateral epicondylitis. The procedure of choice is surgical excision of the torn, scarred portion of the tendon and any granulation tissue.[92] One may elect to repair the remaining tendon back to the lateral epicondyle after first drilling the bone to enhance the local blood supply. Once full range of motion is achieved after surgery, a graduated exercise program is initiated. Tennis can usually be resumed after 3 months when adequate strength has returned and little or no pain remains. Of those patients who underwent surgical management for refractory tennis elbow, 85% returned to full activities without pain, 12% improved but still had residual pain with vigorous activities, and 3% showed no improvement.[92]

Medial Epicondylitis

Medial epicondylitis is a tendinitis of the flexor–pronator muscle group. This condition primarily involves the pronator teres and flexor carpi radialis muscles, with occasional involvement of the flexor carpi ulnaris.[67] These two muscles are susceptible to inflammation and injury because they span two joints (wrist and elbow). Excessive valgus forces combined with repetitive flexor forearm muscle pull can produce an overuse syndrome in the common flexor origin. Athletic activities producing this condition include baseball, golf, and racquet sports.

Patients complaining of medial epicondylitis describe aching pain in the medial forearm musculature, originating from the medial epicondyle. These patients occasionally note swelling of the medial elbow and weakness of grip strength related to pain. The pain usually worsens with throwing, serving, or hitting with a forearm stroke. On examination, patients have pain slightly distal and lateral to the medial epicondyle, which increases with resisted wrist flexion and forearm pronation. Conditions that may be mistaken for medial epicondylitis include acute injuries, such as disruption of the common flexor muscle origin with a throwing injury, or rupture of the medial collateral ligament.[107] These entities usually can be differentiated by careful physical examination. Varying degrees of ulnar neuropathy can be seen either separate from or together with medial epicondylitis.[88] This may result from local inflammation or edema from the injured flexor–pronator muscle group, causing a compression neuropathy in the region of the cubital tunnel. Electromyography may be used to distinguish ulnar neuropathy from medial epicondylitis. Radiographs of patients with medial epicondylitis usually appear normal, although medial ulnar traction spurs may be present.

Management of medial epicondylitis is similar to that of lateral epicondylitis. The basic principles (PRICEMM) act to relieve the acute and chronic inflammatory symptoms. After the initial symptoms resolve, a therapy program aimed at gradually increasing flexibility, strength, and endurance is initiated. A counterforce brace has been used in the management of medial epicondylitis, but it has not proved to be as successful as in lateral epicondylitis.[87] A gradual resumption in play is recommended when symptoms have subsided, generally 6 to 12 weeks after injury. For refractory cases, after 4 to 6 weeks of treatment, a local corticosteroid injection may be helpful. Care must be taken not to inject directly into the tendon or ulnar nerve because of risk of damage to these structures.

Indication for surgical management of medial epicondylitis is persistent pain at the medial elbow, unresponsive to a well-managed rehabilitation program for 6 to 12 months.[54] Intraarticular pathology and neurologic dysfunction must be ruled out. Various surgical techniques have been described to manage medial epicondylitis, but most result in significant flexor–pronator strength deficits that may be debilitating to an athlete. In performing any procedure for medial epicondylitis, care must be taken to prevent injury to the ulnar nerve and medial collateral ligament. The recommended technique[115] involves incising the common flexor tendon off the epicondyle, debriding the abnormal tissue from the undersurface of the flexor–pronator mass, and then suturing the tendon back to the epicondyle, which should be abraded to provide an adequate blood supply for healing.

The patient is usually splinted for 7 to 10 days, after which gentle active elbow, wrist, and hand range of motion exercises are begun. At 4 to 6 weeks, a progressive strengthening program begins with return to activity generally attained 4 months after surgery. In a review of 35 patients treated surgically, a successful result was obtained in 97% of patients, with all athletically active patients returning to their sport.[115] It should be emphasized that over 90% of patients obtain complete relief of their symptoms with a structured nonoperative treatment regimen.[54]

Distal Biceps Tendon Avulsion

Avulsion of the distal biceps tendon is an uncommon injury, with 97% of biceps tendon ruptures occurring proximally.[5] Almost all cases in the literature have been in men with an average age at rupture being 50 years. Approximately 80% of ruptures occur in the dominant extremity, with bilateral cases being extremely rare.[10]

The mechanism of injury is sudden or prolonged contracture of the biceps against high-load resistance.[86] The elbow is usually flexed at 90°. The onset is sudden, although there may be a history of prodromal symptoms resulting from degenerative changes within the tendon. The tear usually occurs at the tendoosseous junction and notably leaves no stump tendon at the bicipital tuberosity.[93]

When rupture occurs, the patient usually experiences a popping or tearing sensation and presents with acute pain in the antecubital fossa. Clinical findings include tenderness, swelling, and mild-to-moderate ecchymosis in the antecubital region. The distal biceps tendon retracts proximally and is not palpable after a complete rupture. There is usually marked weakness of forearm supination and elbow flexion, although sometimes weakness may be mild because of the intact supinator and brachialis muscles. It is unusual to see radiographic evidence of avulsion fragments from the bicipital tuberosity. Partial distal biceps tendon ruptures are very rare and usually go on to complete rupture if not managed.[15]

Management of a ruptured distal biceps tendon in the athlete is surgical. The goal is to restore supination and flexion power to the elbow and forearm through anatomic repair of the tendon to the radial tuberosity. Nonoperative management can be expected to yield strength deficits of 30% in flexion and 40% in supination, whereas immediate repairs result in near normal strength.[82] Traditionally, the distal biceps tendon rupture is repaired primarily using the two-incision Boyd-Anderson technique.[16] This technique reduces the risk of radial nerve palsy. Others have reported successful repair through a single anterior extensile incision.[71,93]

After repair of the avulsed distal biceps tendon, the elbow is immobilized in 90° of flexion with a neutral or supinated forearm. A gradual range of motion and strengthening program is initiated 6 to 8 weeks after surgery. Unprotected heavy lifting should not be allowed for 6 months. Morrey has reported 97% flexion strength and 95% supination strength in patients with repairs performed within 2 weeks of injury.[86] The results of repair of chronic ruptures are not as satisfactory.

Distal Triceps Tendon Avulsion

Triceps tendon avulsion is a rare injury, perhaps the least common of all tendon ruptures.[5] Nearly 75% of the ruptures reported in the literature occurred in male subjects. The mean age at injury is 25 years, with a range of 7 to 72 years.[8] Dominant and nondominant extremities appear to be injured with equal frequency.

Most avulsions of the distal triceps tendon result from indirect trauma, usually a fall onto the outstretched upper extremity. This imparts a deceleration stress on an already contracted triceps, resulting in distal avulsion at the tendoosseous insertion.[40] The same mechanism of injury may result in olecranon fractures. The avulsed tendon usually retracts with or without a piece of bone from the proximal olecranon. Some of these injuries may result from a direct blow to the elbow. Additionally, spontaneous avulsion of the distal triceps tendon has been reported in patients with hyperparathyroidism, Marfan syndrome, systemic lupus erythematosus, and in those prescribed systemic steroids.[82]

On clinical examination, patients with a distal triceps tendon avulsion have pain and swelling at the posterior aspect of the elbow. A palpable depression just proximal to the olecranon may be noted. Ecchymosis is usually present several days after injury. Testing of elbow extension strength is important to determine whether the tear is partial or complete. Loss of active extension of the elbow signifies a complete tear of the triceps tendon.[40] Radiographs should be performed in all suspected cases. Avulsed flecks of bone from the olecranon have been demonstrated in approximately 83% of patients.[8,40,111]

Management of distal triceps tendon avulsion is surgical repair to restore extension strength. If full active elbow extension is demonstrated on physical examination, the injury is partial and can be followed without surgical repair.[40] For complete tears, the accepted method of repair is reattachment of the avulsed triceps tendon to the olecranon with nonabsorbable sutures through drill holes in bone.[40,111] If a large fragment of the olecranon is avulsed, open reduction and internal fixation are indicated. In cases of delayed reconstruction, an inverted tongue of triceps fascia can be used as a turned-down flap for repair.[49]

After surgery, the elbow is immobilized in 30° to 45° of flexion for 2 to 4 weeks before a graduated range of motion and strengthening program is begun. An extension night splint is used for the first 3 months after repair.

Patients may return to active contact sports when maximum motion and extension strength have been obtained, usually at 6 months after surgery. Generally, excellent extension strength is restored after surgical repair.

OLECRANON BURSITIS

The function of the olecranon bursa is to allow the skin to glide freely over the bony prominence of the olecranon. It is a closed sac, lined by synovium, that is interposed between the skin and triceps tendon and olecranon process. The bursa does not communicate with the elbow joint, except in patients with rheumatoid arthritis.[108] The olecranon bursa is not present at birth and is first seen in children aged 7 to 10 years.[25] The size of the bursa increases with age until adulthood.

Traumatic olecranon bursitis is the most common condition affecting the olecranon bursa.[108] In the athlete, traumatic episodes may result in an acute inflammatory response. The bursal walls become thickened and edematous, and the bursal-lining cells produce excess fluid. If the trauma is severe enough to disrupt vessels, the bursa will contain frank blood. Repeated episodes of lesser trauma give rise to a chronic inflammatory process with persistent effusions.

Septic olecranon bursitis commonly occurs in athletes.[48] The source of infection may be from superficial skin breaks, which may seem innocuous. Other sources include coexisting dermatitis, acne lesions colonized with bacteria, or hematogenous sources. Trauma is the most frequently implicated predisposing factor. Steroid injections have also been found to precipitate septic bursitis. By far the most common infecting organism is *Staphylococcus aureus*, with β-hemolytic *Streptococcus* and other *Staphylococcus* species also seen.[109]

The most common cause of olecranon bursitis is trauma, with the history of a single event or multiple lesser traumas to the tip of the elbow frequently found. Soft-tissue swelling is always present, and careful examination can determine whether the swelling is the thickened bursa, fluid within the bursa, or both. If the process is chronic, nodules consisting of fibrin can be felt within the bursa.[108] Radiographic evaluation may show soft-tissue swelling. Olecranon spurs or calcium deposits may be seen in older patients (Fig. 19-3).

The problem with evaluating olecranon bursitis occurs in the athlete who has a history of either acute or repetitive trauma with a tender, swollen olecranon bursa and overlying skin that is red, warm, and edematous. This is a common presentation in athletes such as football players who play on artificial surfaces without elbow pads[66] or wrestlers who have mat trauma. The physician must determine whether this is an infectious process. Whenever septic bursitis is a possible diagnosis, sterile aspiration of the bursal fluid for analysis by gram stain and culture is essential.

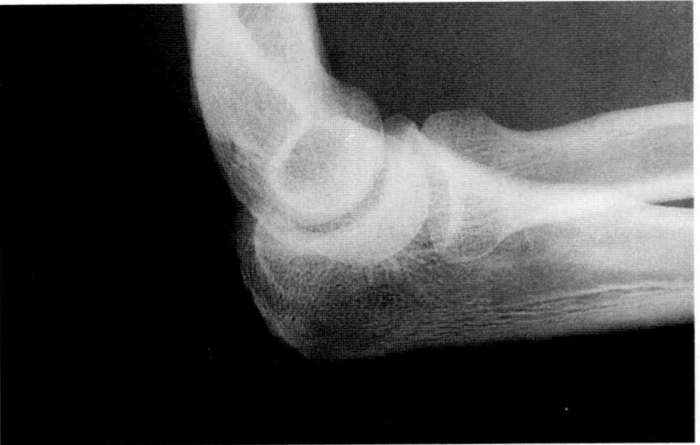

FIGURE 19-3. Olecranon spur causing olecranon bursitis.

In most instances of traumatic olecranon bursitis, the bursa is enlarged, minimally tender, and nontense. Management is symptomatic with rest, ice, and compression. Nonsteroidal anti-inflammatory drugs may be of some benefit. If there is fluid in the bursa, it may be aspirated and a compression dressing applied. It is not necessary to interrupt athletic participation. It is probably best to protect the bursa with an elbow pad.

In the acute traumatic event in which there is blood in the bursa and limited elbow range of motion, sterile aspiration to evacuate the blood followed by a compression dressing and frequent icing may decrease the chances of progression to chronic bursitis.[108] Blood or fluid may continue to reaccumulate, necessitating additional aspirations. Occasionally, instilling a small amount of corticosteroid after aspiration may minimize the inflammatory process.[66]

When the bursitis is chronic and disabling with inclusion bodies present, it is unlikely that resolution will occur without surgery. Surgery usually consists of complete bursal excision with a small portion of the underlying bone at the tip of the olecranon.[108] It is important to keep the skin flap as thick as possible and to avoid injuring the ulnar nerve. The elbow should be splinted in 45° to 60° of flexion for 10 days to allow wound healing. Range of motion exercises are begun, combined with bicep and tricep-strengthening exercises. Athletic participation can resume in 4 to 6 weeks. Elbow pads should be used until all tenderness has subsided.

When septic bursitis is suspected, fluid should be aspirated and cultures obtained. The elbow should be splinted, and frequent heat treatments instituted. If there are no systemic signs of infection and little cellulitis, oral broad-spectrum antibiotics are administered. If significant clinical improvement ensues over the next 2 to 3 days, the treatment is continued; if not, the bursa should be opened and drained, and intravenous antibiotics used.[48] The duration of antibiotic therapy has not been clearly delineated and is usually based on the clinical response of the patient. Return to athletics is attempted only after there is full resolution of all symptoms from the septic bursitis. If there is a recurrence, the bursa should be excised completely.

THROWING INJURIES

Biomechanics and Pathophysiology

The pitching motion, which is seen in many sports, can be broken down into different phases to facilitate a better understanding of the motion (Fig. 19-4). The terms *wind-up*, *early cocking*, *late cocking*, *arm acceleration*, *arm deceleration*, and *follow-through* are used to delineate the phases in the analysis of throwing. With the use of video and electromyography analysis, the kinetics and kinematics of throwing can be determined. The elbow is flexed at about 85° during the wind-up and cocking phases. It is then rapidly extended during early acceleration until ball release. Forces acting on the elbow include valgus torque and tensioning of the medial elbow structures, reaching a maximum at late cocking; extension torque during acceleration; and flexion and varus torque after ball release.[35]

Injury to the elbow usually occurs during the acceleration phase of throwing. At late cocking, a large forward force is generated by the shoulder musculature to bring the upper arm forward and create acceleration. Because the forearm and hand lag behind, a considerable valgus force is generated at the elbow, with peak angular velocities reaching more than 4500° per second.[98] These large forces are absorbed by the supporting structures on the medial side of the elbow. If the forces generated exceed the tensile strength of the ulnar collateral ligament, microtears will occur. If throwing continues in the presence of injury, attenuation and eventual rupture of the ligament will result. At the same time, considerable compression forces are placed on the lateral side of the elbow. This force is primarily absorbed by the cartilaginous surfaces of the radial head and the capitellum, leading to microfractures, osteochondritis dissecans, and loose body formation.[30]

As acceleration of the arm continues, the triceps forcefully contract and the elbow rapidly extends as the thrown object is released. Normally, this force is absorbed by the anterior capsular structures and bicep and brachialis muscles. If the elbow is slightly subluxated in a valgus position, because of insufficiency of the ulnar collateral ligament, impaction of the posterior medial olecranon in the olecranon fossa results as extension occurs.[117] Over time, this impaction can lead to chondromalacia and osteophyte formation, producing pain during the follow-through phase of throwing. Pitching-related injuries to the elbow can be classified as medial tension overload, lateral compression, and extensor overload.

Medial Tension Injuries

Medial tension injuries result from repetitive dynamic stress during the late cocking and acceleration phases of throwing, with injury to the ulnar collateral ligament, flexor–pronator muscle group, and the ulnar nerve most common.[43] Symptoms occur predominantly in baseball pitchers but are also observed in other sports. Pain is usually observed during forced extension and valgus strain during the acceleration phase. The pitcher is usually effective for two or three innings and then suffers a gradual loss of control, especially early release, which causes him or her to throw high. Often, a pitcher compensates by snapping the elbow in an attempt to gain speed, but this snapping usually causes further loss of control.

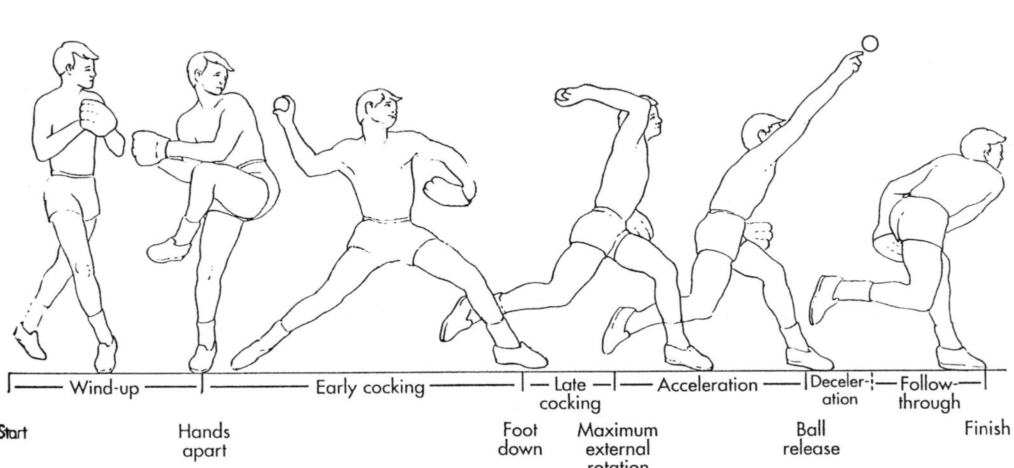

FIGURE 19-4. Illustration of the six phases of pitching. (From DiGiovine NM, Jobe FW, Pink M, et al: An electromyographic analysis of the upper extremity in pitching. J Should Elbow Surg 1:15–25, 1992.)

Pain is localized to the medial aspect of the elbow and the olecranon process. In addition to examining the elbow, careful attention should be paid to the flexibility of the shoulder. Restricted shoulder range of motion alters the normal throwing mechanics and places increased valgus stress on the elbow, resulting in medial elbow pain.[79]

Valgus stress testing of the elbow is performed by placing the patient's hand against the side of the examiner's body, with the elbow held at 30° of flexion to relax the bony restraints. The examiner uses one hand to apply valgus stress to the patient's elbow while the other hand palpates the medial side of the elbow. The examination is done with the patient supine and repeated with the patient prone to allow direct visualization of the medial side of the elbow.

Routine anteroposterior and lateral radiographs of the elbow should be obtained to check for evidence of loose bodies, bone spurs, or calcification of the ulnar collateral ligament. Valgus stress radiographs can be obtained to further document valgus subluxation, but a normal stress view does not rule out the diagnosis. Magnetic resonance imaging and computed tomography also have been used in the evaluation of medial tension injuries, but their application in this setting is not yet defined.

The anterior oblique band of the ulnar collateral ligament is the most important stabilizing structure of the elbow-resisting valgus force, absorbing up to 55% of the valgus load to the flexed elbow.[83] Patients who present with problems referable to the ulnar collateral ligament often have had recurrent pain and tenderness for months along the medial aspect of the elbow. In some patients, a sudden valgus stress that exceeds the tensile strength of the ligament can cause an acute rupture of the ligament. This rupture is associated with sharp pain, swelling, and ecchymosis at the medial aspect of the elbow. More commonly, a slow deterioration in function of the elbow occurs, accompanied by increasing pain and loss of control. Instability to valgus stress testing is present in all patients. Radiographs are used to rule out loose bodies and other bony pathology. Occasionally, a calcified ulnar collateral ligament is seen in patients with chronic symptoms.[56]

Management for most patients with ulnar collateral ligament injuries is nonoperative (PRICEMM). After the acute symptoms resolve, range of motion exercises are begun. The athlete may resume a throwing program after complete resolution of pain and restoration of motion. Progressive velocity and endurance are allowed with careful supervision. Patients who continue to have ongoing pain or who cannot throw effectively after 6 months of this management are candidates for operative intervention. Options include ligament repair or reconstruction.

For acute ligament ruptures, direct repair may be considered by suturing the torn ligament directly to the bone or through drill holes.[94] Patients are then splinted for 10 days and placed in a single-axis elbow brace, allowing flexion and extension but preventing valgus stress. Results of this management indicate that 50% of patients can return to their previous level of athletic participation.

Ulnar collateral ligament reconstruction has been recommended in the acute and chronic setting. Jobe[56] advocates use of a free tendon graft of palmaris longus, plantaris, or lateral Achilles tendon. In this technique, the free tendon graft is passed through drill holes in the medial epicondyle and ulna at the anatomic sites of ligament attachment. This provides a functional substitute for the anterior bundle of the ulnar collateral ligament. The ulnar nerve is protected during this procedure and transposed anteriorly at closure. After initial immobilization, patients are begun on active range of motion exercises with a hinged brace. Strengthening begins within 4 to 6 weeks, and a throwing program is initiated after 4 months. In Jobe's initial experience, 11 of the 16 major league baseball players who had a reconstruction returned to play major league baseball.

A recent report by Altchek and colleagues describes a modification of the original Jobe technique. The "docking technique" of medial collateral ligament reconstruction may provide better tensioning of the palmaris graft.[106] In this report, 33 of 36 patients (92%) returned to their previous level of competition.

Ulnar collateral ligament reconstruction is the current recommended procedure for athletes who wish to remain at a highly competitive level of participation.[56] For less-competitive athletes, reconstruction may not be indicated because valgus instability of the elbow appears to cause little disability in activities of daily living.[64] Good functional results have been reported in patients treated nonoperatively.[58]

The flexor–pronator musculature provides dynamic support for the static stabilizing structures on the medial side of the elbow. This muscle group also flexes the wrist and pronates the forearm during throwing. Continued activity beyond the limits of fatigue can result in injury to the muscle and ulnar collateral ligament complex. Rupture of the flexor–pronator group has been reported in throwing athletes.[94]

Injury to the flexor–pronator muscle group is associated with pain and swelling along the medial aspect of the elbow and is exacerbated by extending the wrist and elbow. Minor injuries usually persist for 24 to 48 hours and may be relieved by ice, rest, and nonsteroidal anti-inflammatory medications. More severe injuries can lead to scarring and fibrosis, with resultant loss of elbow or wrist extension.

Occasionally, patients with ulnar collateral ligament insufficiency demonstrate ulnar neuritis. Ulnar neuritis may result from three etiologic factors: traction, friction, or compression.[42] Traction injuries are believed to occur secondary to valgus stress loading during pitching. Compression injuries result from impingement secondary to adhesions, calcification in the soft tissues, osteophytes, or hypertrophy of the flexor muscles of the forearm. Friction injury may occur in the subluxating nerve, which is abraded across the medial epicondyle as the elbow is rapidly flexed and extended during the normal act of pitching. A Tinel sign may be present as 40% of patients with ulnar collateral ligament insufficiency develop ulnar neuritis. Examination usually reveals tenderness along the course of the nerve at the elbow and motor and sensory changes along the distribution of the nerve. Electromyography may be helpful in confirmation of the diagnosis. Submuscular transposition of the nerve is recommended if nonoperative management fails to alleviate the symptoms.

Lateral Compression Injuries: Osteochondritis Dissecans

Lateral compression injuries occur in the throwing elbow as a result of the compression forces in the lateral compartment during the late cocking and acceleration phases and as a result of shearing forces during the deceleration phase of throwing.[62] This condition is usually seen in adolescents as traumatic osteochondritis dissecans of the radiohumeral joint. Osteochondritis dissecans may lead to debilitating osteoarthritis of the lateral elbow in the adult.

In the adult thrower, significant lateral compartment changes are rarely seen because of the debilitating nature of osteochondritis dissecans. Significant injuries of this type usually end careers before the onset of adulthood. Although the exact etiology of osteochondritis dissecans is unknown, the current theory is that it is a lesion resulting from vascular insufficiency caused by repetitive trauma.[12] The capitellar epiphyseal blood supply is tenuous, with end arterioles terminating at the subchondral plate. Repetitive valgus overload results in trauma to this vulnerable epiphysis, causing differing degrees of disruption of the vascular supply and resultant bone death and fragmentation. This lesion also has been found in a young gymnast.[7]

The typical clinical scenario of osteochondritis dissecans is a throwing athlete in the second decade of life, complaining of insidious onset of lateral elbow pain, reduced throwing effectiveness and distance, a flexion contracture of more than 15°, and occasional swelling, catching, or locking. Results of early radiographs may be normal, although, with time, islands of subchondral bone demarcated by a surrounding rarefied zone can be seen, and frequently loose bodies will be present. Computed tomography and magnetic resonance imaging are often helpful in defining the extent of the lesion.

Management of osteochondritis dissecans of the radiocapitellar joint is based on whether the overlying cartilage is intact.[12] This can be determined by arthrotomy, computed tomography arthrography, or arthroscopy if plain films do not show free fragments. If the overlying cartilage is intact, management is immobilization until most pain has resolved and then beginning active range of motion exercises without applying any forceful stresses across the elbow. Although symptoms will usually subside with rest alone, throwing is contraindicated for at least 6 months because the healing process is slow. Once full range of motion, strength, and endurance have been achieved, gradual return to throwing is allowed if the patient remains asymptomatic. Sequential radiographs are used to follow the evolution of the lesion, although in many instances radiographic abnormalities persist.

If pain and flexion contracture persist for more than 6 weeks after immobilization or if loose bodies and fragmentation are present, surgery is recommended. O'Driscoll[95] has reported excellent results using arthroscopy to remove loose bodies caused by osteochondritis dissecans and to debride flaps of articular cartilage. Indelicato[53] recommends reattaching large fragments with screws, wires, or biodegradable pins after drilling the bed to enhance vascularity. Smaller fragments are removed. Although patients reported subjective improvement, normal motion was rare.

In the adult, valgus stresses in the face of an incompetent ulnar collateral ligament result in a radiocapitellar overload syndrome.[107] This repetitive increased force leads to radial head abutment against the capitellum, resulting in chondromalacia and eventual degeneration. Osteochondral fractures and loose body formation eventually result. Patients complain of pain, catching, clicking, or locking of the elbow. Patients may have palpable loose bodies and crepitus with motion. Management consists of removal of loose bodies, either arthroscopically or open. Loose bodies usually recur if the athlete resumes throwing, especially if valgus laxity persists.

Extension Overload Injuries

A combination of valgus and extension forces in the acceleration and deceleration phases of throwing results in chronic changes of the posterior compartment of the elbow.[79] Loose bodies causing catching, locking, and restricted range of motion are the most common lesions of the posterior compartment of the elbow. Inflammatory lesions resulting from triceps tendinitis are also seen. The valgus–extension overload syndrome is a common final pathway for most posterior elbow problems.

As repetitive valgus forces lead to attenuation of the ulnar collateral ligament, posteromedial olecranon impingement occurs within the olecranon fossa.[117] The tip of the olecranon abuts against the olecranon fossa and causes local inflammation, and if inflammation persists, eventually chondromalacia, osteophytes, and loose bodies form (Fig. 19-5). Pain is typically experienced in the posterior compartment during the acceleration phase of throwing. Loss of control and early ball release

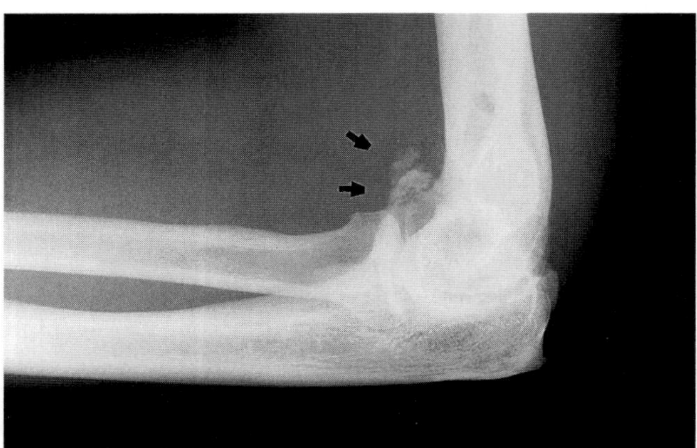

FIGURE 19-5. Loose bodies in the elbow joint.

secondary to pain usually occur after two to three innings. Symptoms are reproduced with forced extension and valgus strain to the elbow. An axial radiographic view with the elbow flexed may reveal posteromedial osteophytes on the olecranon.

Management for the early phases of the valgus–extension overload syndrome include nonsteroidal anti-inflammatory drugs and strengthening of the flexor–pronator muscle group to protect the joint. When posteromedial osteophytes or loose bodies are present, physical therapy is not curative.[117]

Recently, arthroscopy has been described to remove loose bodies and burr down osteophytes in the posterior compartment of the elbow, refered to as posterior elbow impingement.[24,88] Arthrotomy has traditionally been used with good results.[53] Open excision of the tip and medial aspect of the olecranon is performed and any loose bodies are removed. This will allow most throwers to return to their previous level of activity. The problem may recur because of the associated laxity of the ulnar collateral ligament, but the osteophytes usually take years to reform.

Stress fracture of the olecranon is an uncommon source of pain in the throwing athlete. It usually occurs at the tip of the olecranon and results from the repetitive snap of full extension.[113] If symptoms do not resolve with nonoperative treatment (PRICEMM), management should consist of excising the tip fragment or internally fixing the olecranon if the fragment is large.

NEUROPATHIES

Entrapment neuropathies of the elbow and forearm involve three major nerves (median, radial, and ulnar) that cross the elbow to innervate the musculature and provide sensation to the forearm and hand. In the athlete, most of these conditions follow direct contusion of the tissues that overlie peripheral nerves in vulnerable anatomic areas. Vigorous, repetitive athletic activity that produces inflammation and tissue swelling can also lead to nerve compression, especially in closed passages or tunnels. The pathophysiology of entrapment neuropathy involves ionic, mechanical, and vascular injury. Obstruction of venous return from the nerve secondary to inflammation initially may cause venous congestion in the vascular plexuses, resulting in anoxia and dilatation of the small vessels in the nerve.[101] Endoneurial edema ensues, increasing the effect of the initial compression, which further slows venous return. With anoxia, fibroblasts proliferate within the nerve, resulting in permanent scarring, which further inhibits nerve circulation.

When a portion of the axon is rendered ischemic, the axioplasmic transport system is also affected.[38] The integrity of the cell membrane is disrupted, and the efficiency of the sodium pump decreases. This decrease eventually leads to a loss of conduction and transmission along the nerve fiber. The segment of the axon rendered ischemic through local external or internal compression reacts by vascular mechanisms and by ionic disruption to further deteriorate nerve function. Although most entrapment neuropathies partially, if not completely, resolve after decompression, in some chronic situations, nerve dysfunction may be irreversible.

Median Nerve Entrapment: Pronator Syndrome

In the arm, the median nerve is intimately related to the brachial artery, first lying lateral to it. At the elbow, the median nerve crosses the artery anteriorly and comes to lie medially in the antecubital fossa. At the elbow, the median nerve leaves the brachial artery to pass between the two heads of the pronator teres muscle and beneath the tendinous arch of the flexor digitorum superficialis. The nerve passes distally into the forearm between the flexor digitorum superficialis and the flexor digitorum profundus muscles.

There are four sites of potential compression (Fig. 19-6), all of which may produce signs and symptoms of pronator syndrome.[38] The first of these is compression of the median nerve at the distal third of the humerus beneath the supracondyloid process at the ligament of Struthers. A second site of potential compression occurs at the lacertus fibrosis, which passes from the bicipital tendon to the flexor muscle mass and courses across the median nerve at the level of the elbow joint. A third site of potential compression is within the hypertrophied pronator teres muscle or between its two heads. Finally, the median nerve can be compressed at the tendinous arch of the flexor digitorum superficialis muscle, which is a firm and sharp-free border beneath which the nerve passes. Occasionally, an abnormal fibrous band may extend from either head of the pronator teres to the tendinous arch and become an additional source of compression.

Pronator syndrome presents with pain in the proximal volar surface of the forearm that generally increases

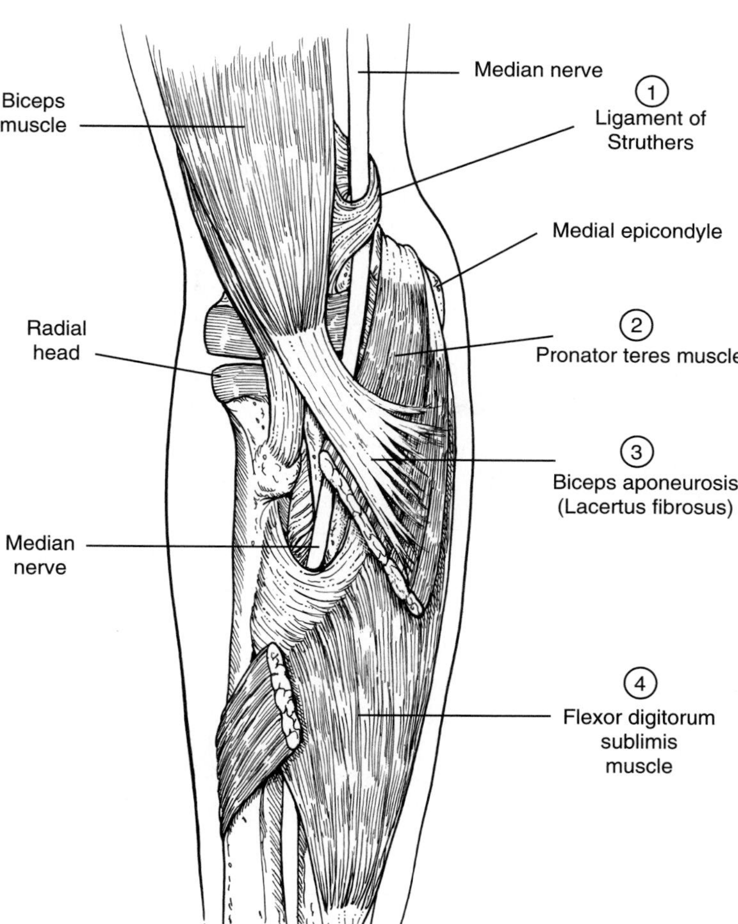

FIGURE 19-6. Four sites of potential compression of the median nerve that may produce median nerve entrapment in the elbow and forearm.

with activity. The symptoms are often vague, with a fatigue-like pain described by many patients. Repetitive, strenuous motions often provoke the symptoms, which usually develop insidiously. In addition, there may be reduced sensibility or paresthesias in the radial three and a half digits of the hand. The absence of these neurologic findings does not preclude this condition.[21]

On examination, patients with pronator syndrome have aggravation of their symptoms with resisted pronation of the forearm.[101] Direct pressure over the proximal portion of the pronator teres, approximately 4 cm distal to the antebrachial crease, while exerting moderate resistance to pronation may be a more reliable test. If the ligament of Struthers is the site of compression, flexion of the elbow against resistance between 120° and 135° of flexion may aggravate the symptoms. If the arch of the flexor digitorum superficialis is involved in compression, resisted flexion of the superficialis muscle of the middle finger or passive stretching of the finger and wrist flexors may elicit symptoms. A Tinel sign is usually present at the site of compression.

Distal neurovascular function is generally intact, although a careful motor examination is important to distinguish pronator syndrome from anterior interosseous nerve compression. This branch of the median nerve is exclusively motor and controls the flexor digitorum profundus of the index finger, the flexor pollicis longus, and the pronator quadratus muscles. A characteristic posture of pinch is noted with compression of the anterior interosseous branch of the median nerve.[101] This posture consists of hyperextension of the distal interphalangeal joint of the index finger and hyperextension of the interphalangeal joint of the thumb as one attempts a pinch. Electromyography and nerve conduction studies have had disappointing results in diagnosing pronator syndrome and in differentiating the various sites of compression of the median nerve.[21] Therefore, clinical history and physical examination are the mainstays for accurate diagnosis.

Management of median nerve entrapment should be nonoperative for at least 6 weeks. The regimen should consist of splinting and nonsteroidal anti-inflammatory drugs with curtailment of all weight-lifting activities. Surgical decompression is reserved for severe or refractory cases. The operative management for pronator syndrome consists of a detailed exploration of the median nerve in the proximal forearm.[38] If a supracondyloid process (found in 1% of the general population) is present, it should be explored, and the ligament of Struthers released. The median nerve is then followed distally to the lacertus fibrosis, which should be routinely divided. The nerve is then traced as it enters the forearm between the two heads of the pronator teres muscle. The superficial head is elevated and divided along the course of its fibers to decompress and explore the median nerve. The flexor digitorum superficialis arch is incised, completing the distal extent of exploration for pronator syndrome. Further dissection distally may be necessary to decompress the anterior interosseous branch of the nerve. After surgery, the patient is splinted in neutral rotation for a few days. Active range of motion exercises are begun within 1 week, with restricted pronation for 3 weeks.

Radial Nerve Entrapment: Radial Tunnel Syndrome

Compression neuropathies of the radial nerve occur in predictable areas along the course of the nerve.[39] The radial nerve pierces the lateral intermuscular septum to proceed from the posterior to anterior compartment of the humerus. The septum is a common cause of nerve compression, especially during open reduction and internal fixation of humerus fractures. As the nerve proceeds to the level of the radiocapitellar joint, it divides into its major branches: the posterior interosseous and superficial radial nerves. At this level, the nerve enters the radial tunnel, which is situated between the brachioradialis and brachialis in the distal arm to the distal edge of the supinator in the forearm. In the radial tunnel, the posterior interosseous nerve passes between the two heads of the supinator muscle, the proximal edge of which is called the arcade of Frohse. The superficial radial nerve passes superficial to the supinator muscle and is covered anteriorly by the brachioradialis muscle.

There are four sites of compression within the radial tunnel (Fig. 19-7). The first site consists of fibrous bands lying anterior to the radial head at the entrance to the radial tunnel. The second site occurs at a fan-shaped group of vessels called the leash of Henry, which lies across the radial nerve and supplies the brachioradialis and extensor carpi radialis longus muscles. The third site of potential compression occurs at the tendinous margin of the extensor carpi radialis brevis near the supinator muscle. The fourth site of compression is the most common and occurs as the radial nerve enters the supinator muscle through the arcade of Frohse.

Athletes presenting with radial tunnel syndrome have often performed repetitive rotatory movements of the forearm in conjunction with their sport, such as tennis.[70]

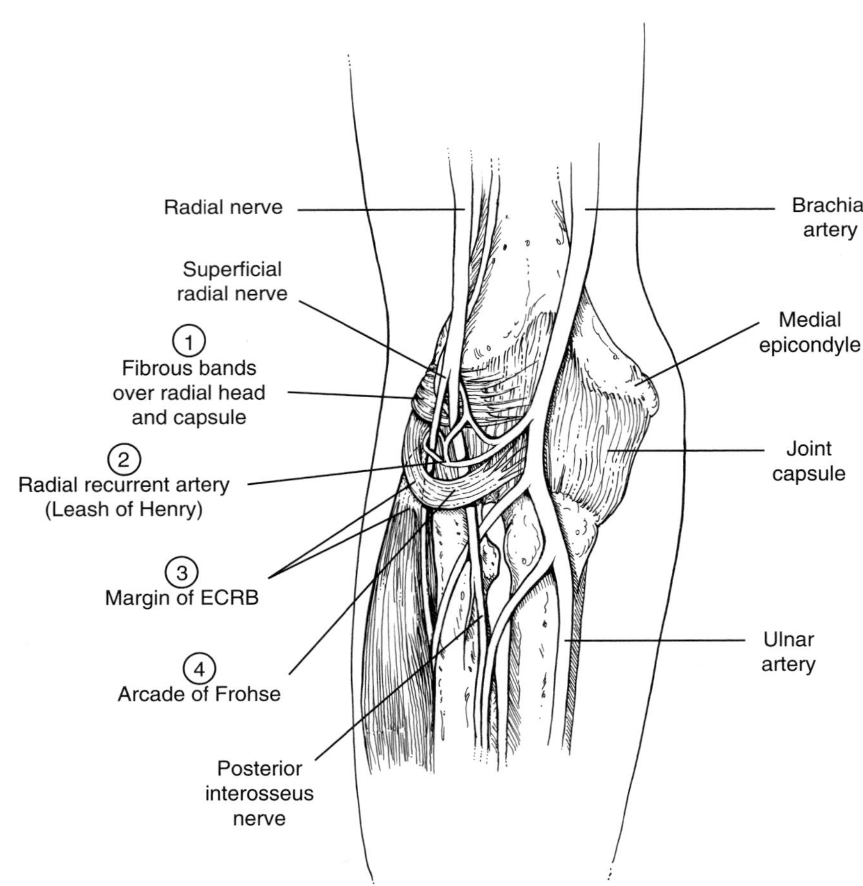

FIGURE 19-7. Four sites of potential compression of the radial nerve at the elbow causing radial nerve entrapment.

Most people with this syndrome are manual laborers performing pronation and supination movements. The patient usually complains of pain well localized to the extensor mass just below the elbow and that is aching in character. Forearm pronation, often with wrist flexion, intensifies the pain. Night pain and pain after physical exertion are also seen. Differentiation between radial tunnel syndrome and lateral epicondylitis may be difficult but can be determined by careful physical examination.[70]

Examination of the patient with radial tunnel syndrome reveals three pathognomonic signs.[104] First, tenderness to palpation is most severe over the radial nerve palpated through the mobile wad muscle mass just distal to the radial head. Pain can occasionally be localized down into the forearm. Second, resisted extension of the middle finger with the elbow extended produces pain at the site of tenderness. This pain results from compression by a fascial extension from the extensor carpi radialis brevis. The third sign is pain on resisted supination of the extended forearm. This pain is distinguished from pain localized to the lateral epicondyle. Electromyography findings are unreliable, and a normal electrophysiologic finding does not exclude the diagnosis of radial tunnel syndrome.[101] In the athlete suspected of having radial tunnel syndrome, diagnostic blocks with small amounts of lidocaine, 1%, can be administered at various points along the radial nerve. If pain is relieved and accompanied by a deep radial nerve palsy and a complementary injection more proximal in the region of the lateral epicondyle does not relieve the patient's symptoms, the diagnosis of radial tunnel syndrome is made.

In the acute stage, radial tunnel syndrome should be managed with rest, splinting, and nonsteroidal anti-inflammatory drugs for at least 2 months. Surgery is reserved for refractory cases not responding to conservative management. The radial tunnel can be decompressed through an anterolateral approach.[101] In this way, the radial nerve can be evaluated from above the elbow through the radial tunnel to the distal end of the supinator. The leash of vessels are ligated, and the fibrous margin of the extensor carpi radialis brevis over the radial nerve should be incised. The dissection continues to the arcade of Frohse, where the deep branch of the radial nerve dives into the substance of the supinator muscle. Division of the supinator muscle allows visualization of the radial nerve to its point of arborization. After surgery, the patient is immobilized for 1 week and then begun on range of motion exercises. A strengthening program is begun after restoration of motion. If the nerve has been damaged, recovery may take 3 to 4 months.

Ulnar Nerve Entrapment: Cubital Tunnel Syndrome

Ulnar neuropathy at the elbow can be related to a number of etiologic factors. Most commonly in the athlete, the ulnar nerve is compressed or stretched at the elbow or proximal forearm.[101] The nerve is particularly vulnerable as it passes subcutaneously under a thick band of fascia around the medial epicondyle and in the area where it passes between the two heads of the flexor carpi ulnaris muscle. The majority of athletic events that result in cubital tunnel syndrome involve throwing or racquet sports.[55]

The ulnar nerve passes from the anterior to posterior compartment of the arm by penetrating through a fibrous thickening called the ligament of Struthers, located approximately 8 cm above the medial epicondyle (Fig. 19-8). The ligament of Struthers is the most proximal source of ulnar nerve entrapment. The ulnar nerve then courses posteriorly to the medial epicondyle and enters the cubital tunnel. The roof of the tunnel is formed by a ligament that extends from the medial epicondyle to the medial border of the olecranon process. The remaining boundaries of the tunnel are the ulnar collateral ligament, the medial edge of the trochlea, and the medial epicondylar groove. After exiting the cubital tunnel, the ulnar nerve continues into the forearm between the two heads of the flexor carpi ulnaris muscle.

The ulnar nerve is a mobile structure, elongating and moving medially during elbow flexion.[6] Therefore, tethering of the nerve by scar tissue interferes with its mobility and adversely affects its function. Additionally, during flexion, the volume of the cubital tunnel is reduced because of changes in surrounding ligaments.[116]

The pathophysiology of ulnar neuritis in the throwing athlete usually involves a traction injury caused by a cubitus valgus deformity.[55] The considerable tension forces generated on the medial side of the elbow increase the possibility of a traction neuritis. Hypermobility of the ulnar nerve, secondary to either congenital or developmental laxity of soft tissue constraints, may cause subluxation or dislocation of the nerve anterior to the medial epicondyle.[26] This subluxation or dislocation will result in a friction neuritis, which appears to affect baseball pitchers more than any other athlete. Compression secondary to hypertrophy of the confluence of the flexor carpi ulnaris heads can also occur in baseball pitchers.[46] Ischemic changes may occur in the ulnar nerve with marked elbow flexion and wrist extension. Intraneural pressure may increase up to six times by causing physiologic stretch of the nerve and additional external compression.[99]

The clinical findings of ulnar neuritis at the elbow involve pain at the medial side of the proximal forearm, which may radiate proximally or distally. This pain may be accompanied by paresthesias, dysesthesias, or anesthesia in the ring and middle fingers. These findings usually precede any detectable motor weakness of the hand.[101] Muscle wasting of the ulnar intrinsic muscles of the hand is a late finding, but not uncommon. Clumsiness or heaviness of the hand and fingers, especially after pitching a few innings, may be a primary complaint. The athlete

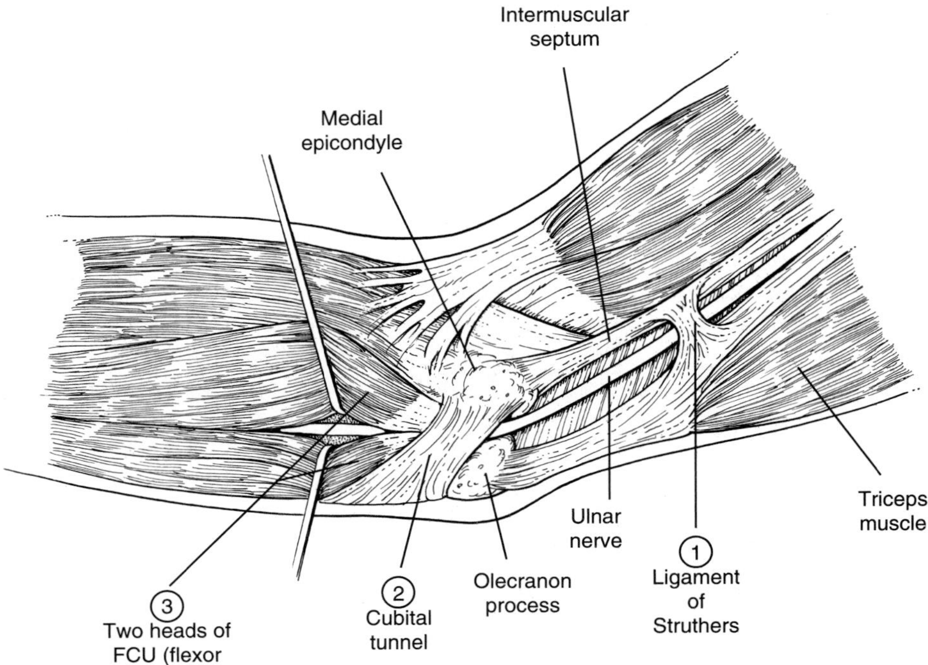

FIGURE 19-8. Three sites of potential ulnar nerve entrapment at the elbow.

with a subluxating or dislocating ulnar nerve may complain of a painful snapping or popping sensation when the elbow is rapidly flexed and extended, with sharp pain radiating into the forearm and hand.[26]

An important localizing physical finding on examination is a positive Tinel sign on percussion of the nerve at the elbow.[39] The ulnar nerve may also be manually subluxated or dislocated from the ulnar groove.[26] The nerve may feel thickened and be tender to palpation. The elbow flexion test may increase or incite symptoms of ulnar nerve compression at the elbow.[22] Both elbows are fully flexed with full extension of the wrists to maximize compressive and tensile forces on the nerve. Patients note numbness and tingling throughout the distribution of the ulnar nerve. The rapid onset and resolution of symptoms make this a useful and reliable test for cubital tunnel syndrome.

Radiographs should be taken to rule out bone spurs or intraarticular abnormality, which may cause impingement of the ulnar nerve. Electrodiagnostic studies may aid in diagnosis; nerve conduction velocities reduced by more than 33% across the elbow suggest cubital tunnel syndrome.[101] Other anatomic areas of ulnar nerve compression, such as cervical ribs and Guyon's canal, must also be ruled out by careful history and examination.[55]

Nonoperative management of ulnar neuritis consists of minimizing the pressure increases that occur about the ulnar nerve with elbow flexion or direct contact.[33] The pressure is minimized by the use of elbow pads and splinting the elbow at 90°. Icing the area may prevent edema and subsequent inflammation that may result in scarring. Approximately 50% of patients with mild ulnar neuritis can expect to recover with this management. In patients whose symptoms are unrelieved after 4 to 6 weeks or who have evidence of motor weakness, intrinsic atrophy, or significant loss of sensation, surgical decompression of the ulnar nerve may be necessary.

There are four basic operative procedures that are performed for ulnar neuropathy at the elbow. They are simple decompression, subcutaneous anterior transposition, submuscular anterior transposition, and medial epicondylectomy.

Decompression of the ulnar nerve is a simple procedure applicable only if there is localized compression of the nerve by the aponeurosis between the heads of the flexor carpi ulnaris.[41] This compression can be seen at surgery by an indentation in the nerve and prestenotic swelling at the site of compression. If any other abnormality is noted, one of the other procedures should be performed.

Anterior transposition of the nerve is the most common procedure performed for cubital tunnel syndrome.[68] The advantage of this procedure is that all pathology is correctable because the nerve is transposed anterior to the medial epicondyle. The nerve is first identified proximally at the level of the ligament of Struthers. Any nerve entrapment is identified and decompressed. The ulnar nerve is traced distally behind the medial epicondyle, where it is released from its tunnel. The aponeurosis and heads of the flexor carpi ulnaris are divided to complete the decompression. The nerve is then elevated from its bed and transposed anteriorly.

The nerve can be left in a subcutaneous position or placed in a submuscular position after elevating the flexor muscles from the medial epicondyle. The flexor origin is next reattached to the epicondyle. After surgery, patients are placed in a splint for 7 to 10 days, after which they are gently mobilized. When the nerve is transposed submuscularly, strengthening is begun after 3 to 4 weeks to allow for adequate tissue healing. The submuscular position affords greater protection of the nerve, and excellent results are achieved with this technique in more than 80% of patients.[33] This technique also has the lowest recurrence rate.

Medial epicondylectomy has been used in the past with fair results.[63] The ulnar nerve is not exposed and, therefore, is at minimal risk of damage. The theory behind this technique is that tension on the nerve as it passes behind the medial epicondyle is removed after excision. This removal of tension will allow the nerve to slide forward and seek its optimum position and tension. Potential disadvantages include missing additional sites of compression, creating new sources of compression as the nerve slides anteriorly, and disrupting the origin of the flexor muscle mass. This procedure is rarely performed today for ulnar neuritis.

ELBOW DISLOCATION

Elbow dislocation in the athlete is not a common injury, having an incidence of 0.1% of all athletic injuries.[31] The mechanism of injury is usually a posterolateral rotatory directed force with a fall on the outstretched hand. O'Driscoll et al.[97] have suggested that extension and a varus stress can disrupt the lateral collateral ligament complex, allowing a perched dislocation. Further forces rotate the forearm and allow a complete dislocation. Others have suggested that with hyperextension, the olecranon impinges on the olecranon fossa, thus levering the ulna and radius from their capsular and ligamentous constraints.[89]

Elbow dislocations can be classified according to the position of the olecranon in reference to the distal humerus. Posterior dislocations (direct, medial, or lateral) are the most common (Fig. 19-9). Anterior dislocations are rare and can occur in young patients, in whom hyperextension allows the olecranon to slide under the trochlea.[13] Divergent dislocations also are rare and require tearing of the interosseous membrane, annular ligament, and distal radioulnar joint capsule.[32]

When complete elbow dislocation occurs, the medial collateral ligament complex is usually disrupted.[97] The anterior capsule and brachialis muscle are also torn or significantly stretched. Others have suggested that the lateral collateral ligament structures must also be disrupted.[58] The most common injuries associated with complete elbow dislocation include radial head and neck fractures (10%), avulsion of the medial or lateral epicondyles (12%), and coronoid fractures (10%).[80] Neurovascular injuries, although uncommon, are potentially devastating. The brachial artery can be injured during dislocation or relocation.[1] The median nerve may become entrapped in the joint after elbow reduction.[100] Injuries to the ulnar nerve and occasionally to the radial nerve may occur.

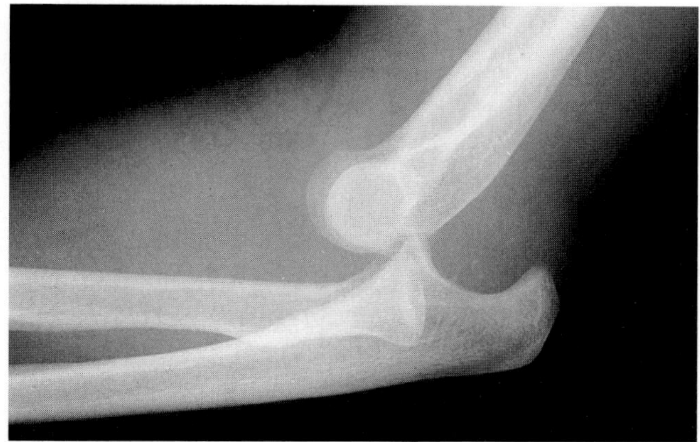

FIGURE 19-9. Radiograph of posterior elbow dislocation.

Although elbow dislocations may be diagnosed clinically, swelling often obscures the bony landmarks about the elbow. Radiographic examination is essential to make the diagnosis of elbow dislocation and to assess associated fractures. The radiographs will also define the type and direction of dislocation. Assessment of the extremity for neurovascular injury is mandatory before reduction.

The goal of management of any elbow dislocation is the restoration of articular alignment as expeditiously and atraumatically as possible. Although an elbow dislocation can often be reduced without any anesthetic, if several hours have elapsed and soft-tissue swelling and spasm have occurred, a general or regional anesthetic may be necessary to minimize the required force. Multiple attempts at reduction should be avoided because the potential to create additional soft-tissue and muscle trauma will increase, thus predisposing to ectopic bone.[112]

Several techniques have been described for reduction of the dislocated elbow. The most predictable technique is that of gentle traction applied to the extended forearm with countertraction on the humerus.[47] The olecranon is then manipulated distally and anteriorly until the coronoid clears the trochlea of the humerus. Residual medial or lateral displacement can be corrected, followed by gentle flexion of the forearm. The reduction is often appreciated by a palpable and occasionally audible "clunk." In the anterior dislocation, one has to flex the elbow to unlock the olecranon from the front of the humerus. Divergent dislocations need separate reductions of each bone. After a manuever is performed, reduction is confirmed by radiographs and clinical examination. The elbow should be ranged from full extension to full flexion to ensure that no block to motion exists and to document any instability in the plane of motion. After a posterior dislocation, instability usually occurs in extension. In addition, the elbow should be subjected to varus and valgus stress in full extension and moderate flexion to check for instability.

Irreducible elbow dislocations are uncommon. They are usually seen with associated fractures[34] or resulting from buttonholing through muscle or fascia.[44] Rarely, a bone fragment or avulsed medial epicondyle may become interposed in the joint, preventing complete reduction. Irreducible dislocations, incomplete reductions, and chronic dislocations usually require open reduction. Brachial artery and median nerve injuries after reduction attempts may require open reduction and exploration if function does not promptly return.

After reduction of simple elbow dislocations, careful evaluation of the neurovascular status is necessary for 24 to 48 hours. The elbow should be splinted in a safe zone (at least 90° of flexion) for 7 to 10 days, after which active range of motion exercises are begun. A hinged brace with a controlled extension block should be used in patients demonstrating instability on examination. This brace will protect the collateral ligaments and prevent subluxation on extension. After 3 weeks, the extension block can be decreased, and full range of motion can be obtained in 6 to 8 weeks.

In uncomplicated cases, 50% of patients will have a normal range of motion.[59] Some will develop a flexion contracture of up to 15°, especially if they are immoblized longer than 3 weeks. In dislocations with associated injuries, the results are much poorer, with flexion contractures of more than 30° being common.[59] Complications after elbow dislocation include recurrent instability, stiffness, myositis ossificans, and neurovascular dysfunction.

For the athlete, a devastating complication is recurrent elbow instability. Although uncommon, it is more likely when the initial dislocation occurs in children or adolescents.[118] Although recurrent dislocation is an obvious diagnosis, recurrent subluxation may be more subtle. O'Driscoll et al.[96] have described the examination technique, which is analogous to the pivot shift test of the knee, used to diagnose recurrent instability of the elbow. The elbow is extended with valgus stress and then supinated, causing the radial head to roll below the capitellum and the ulna to externally rotate on the trochlea. With elbow flexion and pronation, a clunk is felt as the elbow reduces. The deficiency allowing this instability is believed to result from an incompetent lateral ulnar collateral ligament.[96] Others have postulated that an attenuated medial collateral ligament or failure of the anterior capsule to heal may lead to recurrent elbow instability.[118] O'Driscoll et al.[96] recommend reconstructing the lateral ulnar collateral ligament with a tendon graft to manage recurrent elbow instability.

Residual stiffness tends to increase with associated injuries, prolonged immobilization, and formation of heterotopic ossification. Some have investigated loss of motion and correlated it with the type of dislocation. Josefsson et al.[59] thought that loss of motion was greater with lateral or posterolateral dislocations and that motion loss was greater in adults than in children. An extension turnbuckle splint is used to treat these patients, although results are unpredictable. Occasionally, open capsular releases are required to regain motion in severe cases.

Ectopic bone is frequently seen with elbow fracture–dislocations. Innocuous ectopic calcification, which occurs in ligaments or capsule, must be distinguished from true myositis ossificans, which can be a devastating complication. Myositis ossificans is associated with multiple attempts at reduction or may occur after surgical intervention.[112] It usually causes pain, swelling, and severely restricted range of motion. Seventy percent of patients with myositis ossificans show some improvement with nonoperative treatment.[112] The remainder of patients may require surgery to remove the painful, persistent mass. Surgery is performed only after the lesion is mature, at least 6 months after the injury.[105] A bone scan may be used to distinguish between the active (immature) lesion and the inactive (mature) lesion. Additionally, the sedimentation rate and alkaline phosphatase activity should be normal when the lesion is mature. Patients should be treated with indomethacin after surgery for 3 to 6 months to retard new bone formation, which recurs in two-thirds of patients.[103]

Vascular injury is uncommon after elbow dislocation. The brachial artery is vulnerable to injury and must be assessed carefully before and after reduction. A pulseless distal extremity may result from vascular disruption or spasm. An arteriogram can differentiate between disruption, intimal tear, and spasm.[1] Surgical repair is usually required for complete vascular compromise. Collateral circulation around the elbow may provide the extremity with adequate blood supply, eliminating the need for surgical intervention. Compartment syndrome after elbow dislocation has been reported within the first 24 to 48 hours and must not be overlooked after elbow reduction.[69] Neurologic injuries may occur in up to 20% of elbow dislocations.[69] These are primarily traction injuries to the ulnar nerve caused by valgus stretch or mechanical compression of the median nerve either before or after closed reduction. Rarely, the radial nerve is injured. Neurologic injuries may take 3 to 6 months to resolve completely. If the ulnar and median nerves are both injured, it is likely the brachial artery is injured.

FRACTURES OF THE ELBOW AND FOREARM

Fractures of the elbow and forearm that result from participation in sports are classified the same way as fractures in any post-traumatic injury. The majority of these fractures result from direct trauma, but occasionally may occur from indirect activities such as a fall on an outstretched arm or twisting motion to the elbow. Basic principles of management include adequate immobilization, elevation, and icing of the affected extremity. Radiographic evaluation includes anteroposterior and lateral views visualizing the joints above and below the injury, comparison views of the contralateral extremity (especially in the pediatric population), and additional tests such as oblique radiographs, tomograms, computed tomography, and magnetic resonance imaging if deemed necessary for diagnosis. It is extremely important to obtain anatomic restoration of the osseous structures involved to prevent limitation of motion and function. Stable fixation of fractures is important to allow early motion and use of the extremity. Most serious injuries about the elbow leave a residual flexion deformity, usually ranging between 5° and 15°, despite meticulous management and early range of motion. Although this is acceptable for normal activities of daily living, this limitation can be career ending for an athlete requiring full flexion and extension of the elbow. Detailed classification and management of various fractures about the elbow and forearm are covered in many orthopedic fracture textbooks. In the following section, common fractures of the elbow and forearm and their management will be briefly discussed.

Distal Humerus Fractures

Because of the complex anatomy of these fractures, they are very difficult to manage. These injuries have a propensity for post-traumatic and postoperative stiffness. One third of all fractures about the elbow involve the distal humerus and most commonly occur in children aged 5 to 10 years.[60] Many classifications exist based on anatomy and fracture pattern. Broadly, these fractures can be classified as extracapsular (epicondylar fractures), supracondylar, and intraarticular (unicondylar, bicondylar, capitellum, and trochlea fractures).

Epicondylar fractures are all extracapsular, with medial epicondyle fractures more common than lateral epicondyle fractures. These injuries are rare in adults. Medial epicondyle fractures occur in young throwing athletes, who subject their elbows to high valgus stresses.[11] The fractures can be acute (undisplaced or displaced) or chronic (Little Leaguer's elbow). In adults, these injuries may result from direct trauma.[11] Medial epicondyle fractures may occur secondary to elbow dislocation and may spontaneously reduce on relocation.[51] The acceptable amount of displacement for medial epicondyle fractures is 2 to 3 mm, with some authors recommending up to 1 cm.[51] Management for undisplaced or minimally displaced fractures is immobilization for 10 days with the elbow flexed to 90° and the forearm pronated and wrist flexed to reduce flexor pull. Displaced or incarcerated fragments can be reduced manually or managed with open reduction and internal fixation. Early motion is mandatory to avoid stiffness. There is a high incidence of ulnar nerve symptoms with medial epicondyle fractures.[20]

Fractures of the lateral epicondyle are very rare and are secondary to varus stress at the elbow or a direct blow.[20] Most are managed by immobilizing the elbow at 90° of flexion with the forearm supinated and wrist extended to minimize the extensor pull. They rarely need open reduction and internal fixation.

Supracondylar fractures are the second-most common fracture in children aged 5 to 10 years.[60] The fractures occur during a fall on the outstretched hand with a flexed elbow and, therefore, are usually of an extension pattern. These injuries can be associated with injuries to the brachial artery and median, radial, or ulnar nerves.[51] A careful neurovascular examination is mandatory before and after reduction. Management involves closed reduction if possible. This reduction is done by extending the forearm, applying traction, and then flexing the joint to lock the distal fragment onto the end of the humerus. The arm is immobilized in flexion with careful monitoring of the neurovascular status. Other modes of management include traction, closed reduction and percutaneous pinning, and open reduction and internal fixation for very unstable fractures. Complications include neurovascular injury and malalignment. Displaced supracondylar fractures in adults usually require open reduction and internal fixation.

Medial and lateral condyle fractures account for 5% of all distal humerus fractures.[20] Lateral condyle fractures are more common than medial condyle fractures. These fractures can be divided into two types based on whether the lateral wall of the trochlea remains attached to the humerus (type I) or attached to the fracture fragment (type II).[77] These fractures usually result from falling on an outstretched hand with a varus or valgus force to the elbow.[51] Collateral ligament injuries may be associated with these fractures.[60] The neurovascular status of the extremity must be evaluated before reduction. Although these injuries are intraarticular, closed management has been advocated in the past.[78] If successfully reduced, these fractures must be immobilized for 4 to 6 weeks. More recently, open reduction and internal fixation has been advocated, even for minimally displaced fractures.[20] This will allow early mobilization of the elbow and quicker return of function. In the event reduction cannot be achieved, overhead traction can be considered. Complications of these fractures and their management include malunion, nonunion, avascular necrosis, cubitus varus or valgus deformity, and restricted range of motion.

Bicondylar fractures are the most common type of distal humerus fracture in the adult.[20] The injury occurs when the olecranon acts as a wedge driven into the trochlea, forcing the fracture proximally into the humerus.[51] The elbow must be flexed more than 90° for a bicondylar fracture to be produced.[52] If the elbow is flexed less than 90°, an olecranon fracture will result instead. Up to 50% of these fractures are open injuries. Many classifications exist based on fracture pattern, separation of fragments, and comminution. Closed reduction and casting has lost popularity because of the very high incidence of stiffness.[60] Traction followed by immobilization has been advocated by some.[65] "Bag of bones" treatment has been used for highly comminuted fractures in elderly, osteopenic patients by placing the elbow in a sling and instituting early mobilization.[19] Currently, open reduction and internal fixation is ideally advocated, using either a transolecranon or triceps-splitting approach.[51] After surgery, these patients are mobilized as soon as possible. Complications include delayed union, nonunion, ankylosis, myositis ossificans, and ulnar neuritis.[20,60]

Capitellum fractures account for 6% of all distal humerus fractures.[20] They are associated with radial head fractures and posterior elbow dislocations. The mechanism of injury is a shear force in the coronal plane displacing the capitellum from the lateral condyle of the humerus.[51] These fractures are classified as two types: type I (Hahn-Steinthal) is a complete fracture of the capitellum, and type II (Kocher-Lorenz) is a shear fracture of the articular surface shell with a thin layer of subchondral bone. Diagnosis of these fractures can be difficult, with lateral radiographs being particularly helpful. Sometimes a positive fat pad sign on a radiograph is the only clue to a fracture.[20] Management of type I fractures is open reduction and internal fixation through a lateral approach if the fragment is displaced.[51] In most cases of type II fractures, excision of the fragments is necessary because fixation is difficult.[51] In all cases, early postoperative motion is necessary for successful outcome. Complications include loss of motion, especially when fragments have been excised; avascular necrosis of the capitellum; and nonunion.[20,60] Avascular necrosis and nonunion may require delayed excision.

Isolated fractures of the trochlea are rare.[51] Small fragments should be excised, and early range of motion instituted. For larger fragments, open reduction and internal fixation is necessary. Care must be taken to prevent injury to the ulnar nerve during operative exposure.

Radial Head Fractures

Approximately 20% of all elbow trauma and 33% of elbow fractures involve fractures of the radial head.[81] Ten percent are associated with elbow dislocations, and 10% of elbow dislocations have associated radial head fractures. Fifteen percent to 20% of radial head fractures involve the radial neck, especially in children. Fractures of the radial head are most frequently caused by direct longitudinal loading, usually from a fall on the outstretched hand.[51] This effect is compounded with valgus stresses. Radial head fractures may be associated with injury to the ulnar collateral ligament complex resulting from the valgus stress. Any injury that causes an elbow dislocation may also cause a radial head fracture.

The most widely used classification of radial head fractures (Fig. 19-10) is that of Mason[74]: type I are undisplaced,

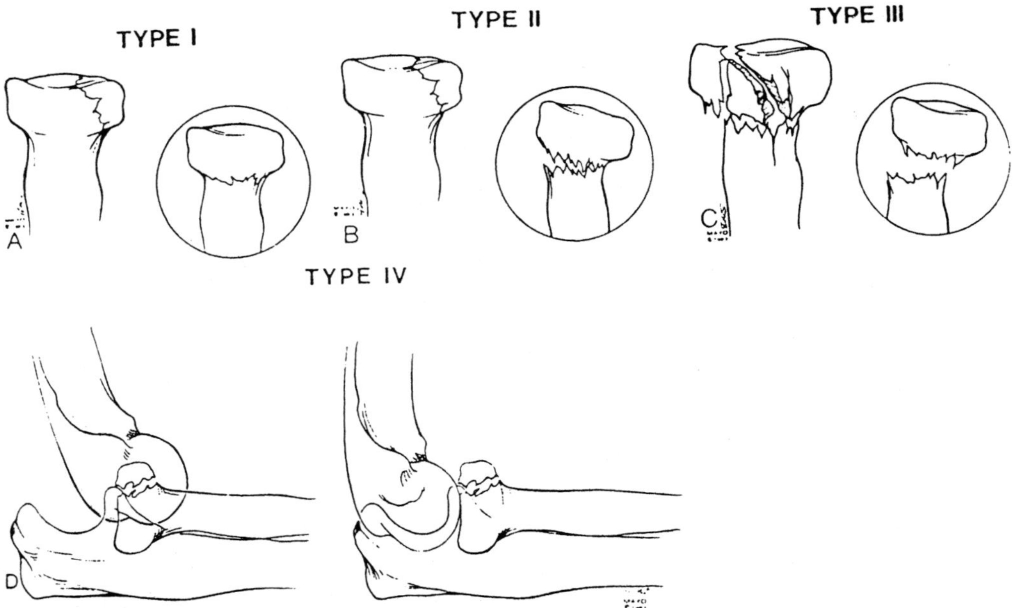

FIGURE 19-10. Mason classification of radial head fractures. (From Morrey BF: Radial head fractures. In Morrey BF (ed): The Elbow and Its Disorders. Philadelphia, WB Saunders, 1985.)

type II are displaced, type III are comminuted, and type IV[57] are any of the previous associated with an elbow dislocation. Distal radioulnar joint injuries are important to identify in association with radial head fractures because excision of the radial head may allow proximal subluxation of the radius, resulting in wrist pathology. This is called the Essex-Lopresti lesion.[37]

Anteroposterior and lateral view radiographs are usually sufficient to diagnose a radial head fracture. Occasionally, a radiocapitellar view or tomography is necessary to delineate the fracture.[51] Aspiration of the hemarthrosis and injection of lidocaine, 1%, will allow a complete examination of the elbow to assess if there is a mechanical block to motion.[60] If the patient also has pain on the medial aspect of the elbow, ulnar collateral ligament injury must be suspected. Pain at the wrist is suspicious for associated distal radioulnar joint injury.

Management options vary for the type of fracture and the associated injuries. For undisplaced type I fractures, hematoma may be aspirated to reduce the pain and swelling.[50] This is therapeutic and diagnostic to decide if there is blockage to motion. Patients are treated with a sling for comfort, and early motion is begun. Ninety percent will do well, but 10% will lose some motion, especially extension.

Management of type II fractures depends on the stability of the fracture pattern. If stable, early motion should be attempted. If unstable and surgery is not elected, immobilization should be maintained for 2 to 3 weeks. If surgery is elected and the fragment is small, excision of the fragment may be performed. If the fragment involves more than 30% of the radial head or is displaced more than 3 mm, open reduction and internal fixation or radial head excision proximal to the annular ligament may be performed.[81]

Type III fractures are usually managed with radial head excision.[81] In patients with proximal migration of the radius resulting from concomitant distal radioulnar joint injury, preservation of the radial head is important. If the radial head is excised, consideration should be given to inserting a silicone radial head prosthesis to act as a spacer, although this is not predictable in preventing proximal translation of the radius.[72]

In type IV fractures, management consists primarily of reducing the elbow dislocation and then dealing with the radial head fracture. Because the radial head is a secondary stabilizer of the elbow to valgus stress, excision may lead to gross instability of the elbow because of the injured medial collateral ligament complex.[51] If the radial head is excised, a silicone prosthesis may be inserted to act as a buttress. The elbow should be protected in a hinged orthosis with an extension stop. This orthosis allows early motion but protects against valgus stress and recurrent dislocation during capsular healing. Flexion contractures of 15° to 30° and reduced rotation of 25° to 50° are not uncommon. Delayed excision of the radial head may be performed to improve pain and motion.[18]

Olecranon Fractures

Fractures of the olecranon (Fig. 19-11) occur in response to three main types of injury.[51] Direct trauma resulting from a fall on the point of the elbow or a direct blow to the olecranon often results in a comminuted fracture. Indirect trauma such as a fall on the outstretched hand with the elbow flexed accompanied by a strong contraction of the triceps can result in an oblique or transverse fracture through the olecranon. Finally, a combination of direct and indirect forces may act to produce displaced, comminuted fractures. In cases of extreme violence, a fracture–dislocation may occur.

All fractures of the olecranon have an intraarticular component. Inability to extend the elbow actively against gravity is the most important sign to be elicited on examination. This inability indicates the discontinuity of the triceps mechanism. The presence or absence of this sign determines management for these fractures. Ulnar nerve injuries may accompany this fracture.[51] Anteroposterior and particularly lateral radiographs are necessary to evaluate the extent of these fractures.

Olecranon fractures can be classified as undisplaced (<2 mm, no separation on flexion, and able to extend against gravity) or displaced.[27] Displaced fractures can be further divided into avulsion fractures, oblique and transverse fractures, comminuted fractures, and fracture–dislocations. Management is based on this classification.

Undisplaced fractures are best managed by immobilization in a long-arm cast with the elbow in 45° to 90° of flexion.[23] The cast can be removed after 3 weeks to allow protected range of motion exercises, avoiding flexion past 90° until union is complete at 6 to 8 weeks. Displaced fractures require open reduction and internal fixation or primary excision.[51] The goals of surgery are to maintain extension power of the elbow, to avoid incongruity of the

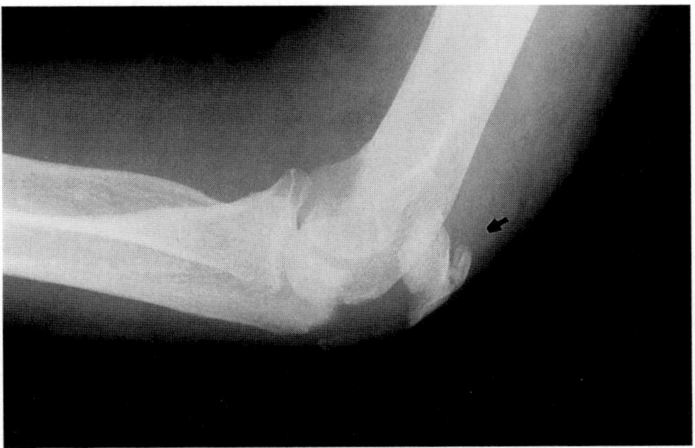

FIGURE 19-11. Displaced fracture of the olecranon.

articular surface, to restore stability of the elbow, and to prevent stiffness of the joint. For transverse and stable oblique fractures, tension band wiring or intramedullary fixation is the preferred management.[23] Comminuted and other unstable fractures can be managed with neutralization plates and screws. Excision of the proximal fragment and repair of the triceps tendon to the remaining olecranon can be used for tip avulsion fractures or comminuted fractures in osteoporotic patients.[51] Up to 80% of the olecranon can be removed without producing instability of the elbow joint.[75]

A complication after olecranon fracture is loss of motion in 50% of patients.[36] Post-traumatic arthritis develops in 20% to 30% of patients, especially in the event of articular cartilage damage and bone loss, and nonunion occurs in 5% of olecranon fractures. Treatment of young, active patients with a nonunion should be open reduction and internal fixation with bone grafting at the fracture site. Excision of the ununited proximal fragment with reattachment of the triceps is performed in older patients.[51]

Coronoid Process Fractures

Coronoid process fractures occur in 2% to 10% of elbow dislocations.[60] There are three types: type I is a tip avulsion, type II involves less than 50% of the coronoid, and type III involves more than 50% of the coronoid.[102] All may be associated with other fractures of the elbow. Management addresses the fracture and the dislocation. After the dislocation is reduced, type I fractures can be managed like a simple dislocation with early range of motion. Types II and III are similarly managed if the elbow is stable. If the elbow is unstable, type II and type III coronoid fractures may require open reduction and internal fixation.[60]

Fractures of the Shafts of the Radius and Ulna

The radius and ulna are relatively parallel bones articulating proximally and distally. The ulna acts as a fixed strut around which the bowed radius rotates in pronation and supination.[3] Between the two shafts lies the interosseous membrane that separates the two compartments of the forearm and provides for longitudinal support of the radius if the radial head is resected.[3] If satisfactory functional results are to be achieved in the management of fractures of the forearm, length, axial alignment, rotational alignment, and normal radial bow must be restored. Therefore, open reduction and internal fixation are recommended for most displaced diaphyseal fractures of the forearm in adults.[61]

Fracture of the radius and ulna, or "both bones fracture," usually results from some type of direct blow to the forearm.[3] Occasionally, a fall on the outstretched arm will cause a fracture to both bones. These fractures are almost always displaced because of the extreme force necessary to break both bones. Patients with this injury have pain, deformity, and loss of function of the forearm and hand. Soft-tissue damage and swelling always accompany this fracture. Compartment syndrome and neurovascular damage is occasionally seen and should be ruled out in all cases.[3] Anteroposterior and lateral radiographs will show the pattern of fracture and the degree of comminution. Elbow and wrist films are necessary to assess associated injuries. Management of undisplaced fractures of the radius and ulna, although rare, is cast immobilization with frequent radiographic follow-up evaluations to check for displacement.[3] Displaced fractures in children can be treated with closed reduction and casting, but this injury in adults is usually managed by open reduction and internal fixation with plates and screws or intramedullary nails. Bone grafting may be necessary in cases with significant comminution. Most studies examining compression plating of "both bones" forearm fractures report union rates of more than 95%, with excellent functional results.[4] Plates may be removed 18 months after healing, but the extremity should be protected for 6 weeks with a splint to prevent fracture through a screw hole. Complications of open reduction and internal fixation of forearm fractures include nonunion, malunion, neurovascular injury, compartment syndrome, and synostosis.

Fracture of the ulna alone, or "nightstick fracture," is fairly common and results from a direct blow to the ulna.[3] Injury to the proximal and distal radioulnar joints must be ruled out. Undisplaced fractures can be managed with a long-arm cast or functional brace with frequent radiographic evaluation to assess displacement. Displaced fractures (>10° of angulation or more than 50% translation) should be managed with open reduction and internal fixation with compression plating.[61]

A Monteggia fracture is a fracture of the proximal third of the ulna, with an associated dislocation of the radial head.[3] The most common type is anterior dislocation, but posterior and lateral dislocations are also seen. The mechanism of injury varies depending on the type of lesion and direction of dislocation. A fall on the outstretched hand with the forearm in pronation or a direct blow to the posterior aspect of the elbow may result in a Monteggia fracture.[3] The forearm externally rotates, and the ulna acts as a fulcrum to dislocate the radial head anteriorly. A posterior radial head dislocation may be caused by supination rotational forces, and a lateral dislocation may result from a direct blow to the inner aspect of the elbow.[3] Frequently, the posterior interosseous nerve is injured in a Monteggia fracture.[17] Anteroposterior and lateral radiographs are mandatory to avoid missing the radial head injury. Treatment differs depending on the patient's age. In children, Monteggia fractures can successfully be managed by closed reduction and cast immobilization.[9] In adults, closed reduction of the radial head and open reduction and internal fixation of the ulna fracture is the management of choice.[3] Positioning of the elbow and forearm is important after surgery. In cases of anterior and lateral radial head dislocations, the elbow should be held in 110° of flexion with the forearm in supination for 6 weeks to prevent redislocation of the radial head.[3] When the radial head has dislocated posteriorly, the elbow should be maintained in 70° of flexion with the forearm pronated for 6 weeks.[3] Complications of Monteggia fractures include nonunion, malunion, posterior interosseous nerve palsy, and redislocation of the radial head.[3]

Isolated fractures of the radius usually occur in the proximal two-thirds of the shaft and are not common. Most injuries severe enough to fracture the radius at this level will also fracture the ulna.[3] When this fracture is undisplaced, the forearm should be immobilized in a long-arm cast in supination. Radiographs should be taken frequently because this fracture tends to displace. Displaced fractures can be managed with compression plating or intramedullary nail fixation with care to maintain the normal radial bow.

A Galeazzi fracture (Fig. 19-12) is a solitary fracture of the radius at the junction of the middle and distal thirds and is associated with a dislocation or subluxation of the distal radioulnar joint.[61] The injury to the radioulnar joint may be purely ligamentous, or the ulnar styloid may be avulsed. The mechanism of injury is a direct blow to the dorsolateral side of the wrist or a fall on the outstretched hand combined with pronation of the forearm.[76] There is usually prominence of the head of the ulna, with tenderness over the distal radioulnar joint. Neurovascular damage is rare. Optimal results are obtained by compression plating of the radius fracture anteriorly.[61] Anatomic fixation of the radius will usually result in reduction of the distal radioulnar joint. If this joint is still subluxed, closed reduction and percutaneous pinning may be performed. After surgery, patients should be splinted in supination for 6 weeks. The most common complication of a Galeazzi fracture is angulation of the fracture and subluxation or dislocation of the distal radioulnar joint.[3]

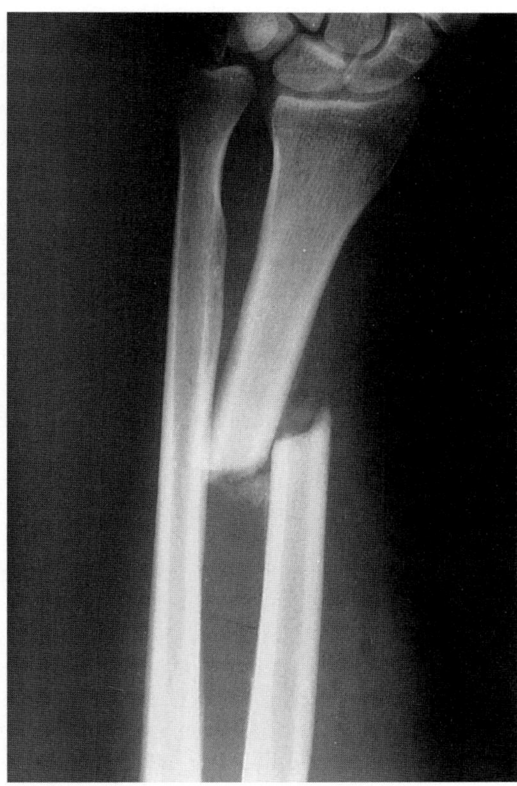

FIGURE 19-12. Radiograph of a fracture at the junction of the middle and distal thirds of the radius associated with subluxation of the distal radioulnar joint. (Galeazzi fracture).

REFERENCES

1. Amsallem JL, Blankstein A, Bass A, Horoszowski H: Brachial artery injury: A complication of posterior elbow dislocation. Orthop Rev 15:61–64, 1986.
2. An KN, Morrey BF, Chao EYS: Carrying angle of the human elbow joint. J Orthop Res 1:369–378, 1984.
3. Anderson LD, Meyer FN: Fractures of the shafts of the radius and ulna. In Rockwood CA, Green DP, Bucholz RW (eds): Fractures in Adults. New York, JB Lippincott, 1991.
4. Anderson LD, Sisk TD, Tooms RE, Park WI: Compression plate fixation in acute diaphyseal fractures of the radius and ulna. J Bone Joint Surg 57A:287–297, 1975.
5. Anzel SH, Covey KW, Weiner AD, Lipscomb PR: Disruption of muscles and tendons: An analysis of 1014 cases. Surgery 45:406–412, 1959.
6. Apfelberg PB, Larson SJ: Dynamic anatomy of the ulnar nerve at the elbow. Plast Reconstr Surg 51:76–81, 1973.
7. Aronen JG: Problems of the upper extremity in gymnastics. Clin Sports Med 4:61–71, 1985.
8. Bach BR, Warren RF, Wickiewicz TL: Triceps rupture: A case report and literature review. Am J Sports Med 15:285–289, 1987.
9. Bado JL: The Monteggia lesion. Clin Orthop 50:71–86, 1967.
10. Baker BE, Bierwagen D: Rupture of the distal tendon of the biceps bracchii: Operative vs. non-operative treatment. J Bone Joint Surg 67A:414–417, 1985.
11. Bernstein SM, King JD, Sanderson RA: Fractures of the medial epicondyles of the humerus. Contemp Orthop 3:637–642, 1981.
12. Bianco AJ: Osteochondritis dissecans. In Morrey BF (ed): The Elbow and Its Disorders. Philadelphia, WB Saunders, 1985.

13. Blatz DJ: Anterior dislocation of the elbow. Findings in a case of Ehlers–Danlos syndrome. Orthop Rev 10:129, 1981.
14. Boone DC, Azen SP: Normal range of motion of joints in male subjects. J Bone Joint Surg 61A:756–759, 1979.
15. Bourne MH, Morrey BF: Partial rupture of the distal biceps tendon. Clin Orthop 271:143–148, 1991.
16. Boyd HB, Anderson LD: A method for reinsertion of the distal biceps bracchii tendon. J Bone Joint Surg 43A:1041–1043, 1961.
17. Boyd HB, Boals JC: The Monteggia lesion. A review of 159 cases. Clin Orthop 66:94–100, 1969.
18. Broberg MA, Morrey BF: Results of delayed excision of the radial head after fracture. J Bone Joint Surg 68A:669–674, 1986.
19. Brown RF, Morgan RG: Intercondylar T–shaped fractures of the humerus. J Bone Joint Surg 53B:425–428, 1971.
20. Bryan RS, Morrey BF: Fractures of the distal humerus. In Morrey BF (ed): The Elbow and Its Disorders. Philadelphia, WB Saunders, 1985.
21. Buchthal F, Rosenfalck A, Trojaborg W: Electrophysiological findings in entrapment of the median nerve to wrist and elbow. J Neurol Neurosurg Psychiatry 37:340, 1974.
22. Buehler MJ, Thayer DT: The elbow flexion test—a clinical test for cubital tunnel syndrome. Clin Orthop 233:213, 1988.
23. Cabanela ME: Fractures of the proximal ulna and olecranon. In Morrey BF (ed): The Elbow and Its Disorders. Philadelphia, WB Saunders, 1985.
24. Cain EL, Andrews JR: Arthroscopic management of posterior elbow impingement in throwers. Tech Shoulder and Elbow Surg 2:118–130, 2001.
25. Chen J, Alk D, Eventov I, Weintroub S: Development of the olecranon bursa: An anatomic cadaveric study. Acta Orthop Scand 58:408–409, 1987.
26. Childress HM: Recurrent ulnar nerve dislocation at the elbow. Clin Orthop 180:168–173, 1975.
27. Colton CL: Fractures of the olecranon in adults: Classification and management. Injury 5:121–129, 1973.
28. Coonrad RW: Tendinopathies at the elbow. Instruct Course Lect 40:25–32, 1991.
29. Coonrad RW: Tennis elbow. Instruct Course Lect 35:94–101, 1986.
30. DeHaven KE, Evarts CM: Throwing injuries of the elbow in athletes. Orthop Clin North Am 4: 801–808, 1973.
31. DeHaven KE, Lintner DM: Athletic injuries: Comparison by age, sport, and gender. Am J Sports Med 14:218–224, 1986.
32. DeLee JC: Transverse divergent dislocation of the elbow in a child. J Bone Joint Surg 63A:322, 1981.
33. Dellon AL: Review of treatment results for ulnar nerve entrapment at the elbow. J Hand Surg 11:199–205, 1986.
34. Devadoss A: Irreducible posterior dislocation of the elbow. Br Med J 3:659, 1967.
35. DiGiovine NM, Jobe FW, Pink M, Perry J: An electromyographic analysis of the upper extremity in pitching. J Should Elbow Surg 1:15–25, 1992.
36. Eriksson E, Sahlen O, Sandahl U: Late results of conservative and surgical treatment of fracture of the olecranon. Acta Chir Scand 113:153–166, 1957.
37. Essex–Lopresti P: Fractures of the radial head with distal radial–ulnar dislocations. J Bone Joint Surg 33B:244–247, 1951.
38. Eversmann WW: Compression entrapment neuropathies of the upper extremity. J Hand Surg 8:759–766, 1983.
39. Eversmann WW: Entrapment and compression neuropathies. In Green DP (ed): Operative Hand Surgery. New York, Churchill Livingstone, 1988.
40. Farrar EC, Lippert FG: Avulsion of the triceps tendon. Clin Orthop 161:242–246, 1981.
41. Feindel W, Stratford J: The role of the cubital tunnel in tardy ulnar nerve palsy. Can J Surg 1:287–300, 1958.
42. Glousman RE: Ulnar nerve problems in the athlete's elbow. Clin Sports Med 9:365–377, 1990.
43. Glousman RE, Barron J, Jobe FW, et al: An electromyographic analysis of the elbow in normal and injured pitchers with medial collateral ligament insufficiency. Am J Sports Med 20:311–317, 1992.
44. Greiss M, Messias R: Irreducible posterolateral elbow dislocation: A case report. Acta Orthop Scand 58:421–422, 1987.
45. Groppel JL, Nirschl RP: A mechanical and electromyographical analysis of the effects of various joint counter-force braces on the tennis player. Am J Sports Med 14:195–200, 1986.
46. Hang Y: Tardy ulnar neuritis in a Little League baseball pitcher. Am J Sports Med 9:244–246, 1981.
47. Hankin FM: Posterior dislocation of the elbow: A simplified method of closed reduction. Clin Orthop 190:254–256, 1985.
48. Ho G, Tice AD, Kaplan SR: Septic bursitis in the prepatellar and olecranon bursae. Ann Intern Med 89:21–27, 1978.
49. Holder SF, Grana WA: Complete triceps tendon avulsion. Orthopedics 9:1581–1582, 1986.
50. Holdsworth BJ, Clement DA, Rothwell PN: Fractures of the radial head—the benefit of aspiration: A prospective controlled trial. Injury 18:44–47, 1987.
51. Hotchkiss RN, Green DP: Fractures and dislocations of the elbow. In Rockwood CA, Green DP, Bucholz RW (eds): Fractures in Adults. New York, Lippincott, 1991.

52. Hurley JA: Complicated elbow fractures in athletes. Clin Sports Med 9:39–57, 1990.
53. Indelicato PA, Jobe FW, Kerlan RK, et al: Correctable elbow lesions in professional baseball players. Am J Sports Med 7:72, 1979.
54. Jobe FW, Ciccotti MG: Lateral and medial epicondylitis of the elbow. J Am Acad Orthop Surg 2:1–8, 1994.
55. Jobe FW, Fanton GS: Nerve injuries. In Morrey BF (ed): The Elbow and Its Disorders. Philadelphia, WB Saunders, 1985.
56. Jobe FW, Stark H, Lombardo SJ: Reconstruction of the ulnar collateral ligament in athletes. J Bone Joint Surg 68A: 1158–1163, 1986.
57. Johnston GW: A follow-up of one hundred cases of fracture of the radial head with a review of the literature. Ulster Med J 31:51–56, 1962.
58. Josefsson PO, Gentz CP, Johnell O, Wendeberg B: Surgical vs. non-surgical treatment of ligamentous injuries following dislocation of the elbow joint: A prospective randomized study. J Bone Joint Surg 89A:605–608, 1987.
59. Josefsson PO, Johnell O, Gentz CP: Long-term sequelae of simple dislocation of the elbow. J Bone Joint Surg 66A:927–930, 1984.
60. Jupiter JB, Mehne DK: Trauma to the adult elbow and fractures of the distal humerus. In Browner BD, Jupiter JB, Levine AM (eds): Skeletal Trauma. Philadelphia, WB Saunders, 1992.
61. Kellam JF, Jupiter JB: Diaphyseal fractures of the forearm, In Browner BD, Jupiter JB, Levine AM (eds): Skeletal Trauma. Philadelphia, WB Saunders, 1992.
62. King JW, Brelsford HJ, Tullos HS: Analysis of the pitching arm of the professional baseball pitcher. Clin Orthop 67:116–123, 1969.
63. King T, Morgan FP: Late results of removing the medial humeral condyle for traumatic ulnar neuritis. J Bone Joint Surg 41B:51–55, 1959.
64. Kuroda S, Sakamaki K: Ulnar collateral ligament tears of the elbow joint. Clin Orthop 218:266–271, 1986.
65. Lansinger O, Mare K: Intercondylar T fractures of the humerus in adults. Acta Orthop Traumatol Surg 100:37, 1982.
66. Larson R, Osternig LR: Traumatic bursitis and artificial turf. Am J Sports Med 2:183–188, 1974.
67. Leach RE, Miller JK: Lateral and medial epicondylitis of the elbow. Clin Sports Med 6:259–272, 1987.
68. Leffert RD: Anterior submuscular transposition of the ulnar nerve by the Learmonth technique. J Hand Surg 7:147–155, 1982.
69. Linscheid RL: Elbow dislocations. In Morrey BF, ed: The Elbow and Its Disorders. Philadelphia, WB Saunders, 1985.
70. Lister GD, Belsole RB, Kleinert HE: The radial tunnel syndrome. J Hand Surg 4:52–59, 1979.
71. Louis DS, Hankin FM, Eckinrode JF, et al: Distal biceps bracchi tendon avulsion: A simplified method of operative repair. Am J Sports Med 14:234–236, 1986.
72. Mackay I, Fitzgerald B, Miller JH: Silastic replacement of the head of the radius in trauma. J Bone Joint Surg 61B:494–497, 1979.
73. Major HP: Lawn-tennis elbow. BMJ 2:557, 1883.
74. Mason ML: Some observations on fractures of the head of the radius with a review of one hundred cases. Br J Surg 42:123–132, 1954.
75. McKeever FM, Buck RM: Fracture of the olecranon process of the ulna. JAMA 135:1–5, 1947.
76. Mikic ZD: Galeazzi fracture dislocations. J Bone Joint Surg 57A:1071–1080, 1975.
77. Milch H: Fractures of the external humeral condyle. JAMA 160:529–539, 1956.
78. Milch H: Fractures and fracture dislocations of the humeral condyles. J Trauma 4:592–607, 1964.
79. Miller CD, Savoie FH: Valgus extension injuries of the elbow in the throwing athlete. J Am Acad Orthop Surg 2:261–269, 1994.
80. Morrey BF: Elbow dislocation in the athlete. In DeLee JC, Drez D (eds): Orthopaedic Sports Medicine. Philadelphia, WB Saunders, 1994.
81. Morrey BF: Radial head fracture. In Morrey BF (ed): The Elbow and Its Disorders. Philadelphia, WB Saunders, 1985.
82. Morrey BF: Tendon injuries about the elbow. In Morrey BF (ed): The Elbow and Its Disorders. Philadelphia, WB Saunders, 1985.
83. Morrey BF, An KN: Articular and ligamentous contributions to the stability of the elbow joint. Am J Sports Med 11:315–319, 1983.
84. Morrey BF, An KN: Functional anatomy of the ligaments of the elbow. Clin Orthop 201:84–90, 1985.
85. Morrey BF, Askew LJ, An KN, Chao EYS: A biomechanical study of normal elbow motion. J Bone Joint Surg 63A:872–877, 1981.
86. Morrey BF, Askew LJ, An KN, Dobyns JH: Rupture of the distal tendon of the biceps bracchii: A biomechanical study. J Bone Joint Surg 67A:418–421,1985.
87. Morrey BF, Regan WD: Tendinopathies about the elbow. In DeLee JC, Drez D (eds): Orthopaedic Sports Medicine. Philadelphia, WB Saunders, 1994.
88. Moskal MJ, Savoie FH, Field LD: Arthroscopic treatment of posterior elbow impingement. AAOS Inst Course Lect 48:399-404,1999.
89. Neviaser JS, Wickstrom JK: Dislocations of the elbow: A retrospective study of 115 patients. South Med J 70:172–173, 1977.
90. Nirschl RP: Muscle and tendon trauma: Tennis elbow. In Morrey BF (ed): The Elbow and Its Disorders. Philadelphia, WB Saunders, 1985.
91. Nirschl RP: Tennis elbow. Orthop Clin North Am 4:787–800, 1973.

92. Nirschl RP, Pettrone FA: Tennis elbow—the surgical treatment of lateral epicondylitis. J Bone Joint Surg 61A:832–839, 1979.
93. Norman WH: Repair of avulsion of insertion of biceps bracchii tendon. Clin Orthop 193:189–194, 1985.
94. Norwood LA, Shook JA, Andrews JR: Acute medial elbow ruptures. Am J Sports Med 9:16–19, 1981.
95. O'Driscoll SW: Arthroscopy of the elbow. J Bone Joint Surg 74A:84–94, 1992.
96. O'Driscoll SW, Bell DF, Morrey BF: Posterolateral rotatory instability of the elbow. J Bone Joint Surg 73A:440–446, 1991.
97. O'Driscoll SW, Morrey BF, An KN: Elbow dislocation and subluxation: A spectrum of instability. Clin Orthop 280:186, 1992.
98. Pappas AM, Zawacki RM, Sullivan TJ: Biomechanics of baseball pitching: A preliminary report. Am J Sports Med 13:216–222, 1985.
99. Pechan J, Julius I: The pressure measurement in the ulnar nerve: A contribution to the pathophysiology of the cubital tunnel syndrome. J Biomech 8:75–79, 1975.
100. Pritchard DJ, Linscheid RL, Svien HJ: Intra-articular median nerve entrapment with dislocation of the elbow. Clin Orthop 90:100–103, 1973.
101. Regan WD, Morrey BF: Entrapment neuropathies about the elbow. In DeLee JC, Drez D (eds): Orthopaedic Sports Medicine. Philadelphia, WB Saunders, 1994.
102. Regan WD, Morrey BF: Fractures of the coronoid process of the ulna. J Bone Joint Surg 71A: 1348–1354, 1989.
103. Ritter ME, Gioe TJ: The effect of indomethicin on para-articular ectopic ossification following total hip arthroplasty. Clin Orthop 167:113, 1982.
104. Ritts ED, Wood MB, Linscheid RL: Radial tunnel syndrome: A ten year surgical experience. Clin Orthop 279:201–205, 1987.
105. Roberts JB, Pankratz DG: The surgical treatment of heterotopic ossification of the elbow following long-term coma. J Bone Joint Surg 61:760–763, 1979.
106. Rohrbough JT, Altchek DW, Hyman J, et al: Medial collateral ligament reconstruction of the elbow using the docking technique. Am J Sports Med 30:541–548, 2002.
107. Safran MR: Elbow injuries in athletes: A review. Clin Orthop 310:257–277, 1995.
108. Singer KM, Butters KP: Olecranon bursitis. In DeLee JC, Drez D (eds): Orthopaedic Sports Medicine. Philadelphia, WB Saunders, 1994.
109. Soderquist B, Hedstrom SA: Predisposing factors, bacteriology, and antibiotic therapy in 35 cases of septic bursitis. Scand J Infect Dis 18:305–311, 1986.
110. Sojbjerg JO, Ovesen J, Nielsen S: Experimental elbow instability after transection of the medial collateral ligament. Clin Orthop 218:186–190, 1987.
111. Tarsney FF: Rupture and avulsion of the triceps. Clin Orthop 83:177–183, 1972.
112. Thompson HC, Garcia A: Myositis ossificans: Aftermath of elbow injuries. Clin Orthop 50:129–134, 1967.
113. Tullos HS, Erwin WD, Woods GW, et al: Unusual lesions of the pitching arm. Clin Orthop 88:169, 1972.
114. Tullos HS, Schwab G, Bennett JB, Woods GW: Factors influencing elbow instability. Instruct Course Lect 30:185–199, 1981.
115. Vangsness CT, Jobe FW: Surgical treatment of medial epicondylitis: Results in 35 elbows. J Bone Joint Surg 73B: 409–411, 1991.
116. Wadsworth TG: The external compression syndrome of the ulnar nerve at the cubital tunnel. Clin Orthop 124:189–204, 1977.
117. Wilson FD, Andrews JR, Blackburn TA, McCluskey G: Valgus extension overload in the pitching elbow. Am J Sports Med 11:83–87, 1983.
118. Zeier FG: Recurrent traumatic elbow dislocation. Clin Orthop 169:211–214, 1982.

20 The Wrist

Melvin P. Rosenwasser, Robert H. Wilson, and Jerome D. Chao

The last decade has seen great strides made toward understanding the complexities of the wrist. However, although approximately 25% of all athletic injuries occur in the hand and wrist,[1] the understanding of wrist injuries in athletes continues to lag behind other anatomic areas such as the knee and shoulder. Generally, participants in organized sports are predisposed to chronic or repetitive injury.[61] The dilemma in managing these common afflictions is the controversy regarding the criteria for normal wrist anatomy, motion, and function.[32] The bony anatomy provides structure, and there is little debate about its function. But the intricate intrinsic and extrinsic ligaments, which are responsible for stability and function, have been subject to differing interpretations.[26,78] This chapter will attempt to cover common sports injuries to the bones, soft tissue, and neurovascular structures of the wrist.

ANATOMY

Carpal Bones

The wrist consists of eight small bones that articulate tightly into a compact, mobile structure (Fig. 20-1). The carpal bones consist of the proximal row (scaphoid, lunate, and triquetrum), the distal row (trapezium, trapezoid, capitate, and hamate), and the pisiform. They possess sufficient strength to sustain enormous forces. There is very little space between them. Some are nearly completely covered by cartilage. There are no primary insertions of tendons to the carpal bones, but the distal row may receive secondary insertions.

The capitate is the largest carpal bone and the keystone of the carpus. It articulates with the long finger metacarpal, providing the longitudinal axis for the wrist. Injury to the capitate often leads to nonunion or avascular necrosis.[2,46] It is the first carpal bone to ossify in the developing child. The other carpal bones will then begin to ossify in a sequential, counterclockwise pattern with the hamate next in line.

The scaphoid is the most commonly injured bone. It has an odd shape, much like a twisted peanut shell. It has a peculiar pattern of blood supply that depends on the dorsal radial artery vessels,[2] which enter into the distal end of the bone and leave the proximal end vulnerable to osteonecrosis if that blood supply is interrupted by fracture.

One to two capsular branches of the radial artery supply blood to the lunate. Like the name, the lunate has the shape of a crescent moon when viewed laterally, and it and the scaphoid articulate with the radius to form the radiocarpal joint.

Along with the scaphoid and lunate, the triquetrum completes the proximal row. It is an infrequent site of injury, well protected by the soft tissues, pisiform, and triangular fibrocartilage. Bony and soft-tissue injury to the ulnar carpus is often misunderstood and misdiagnosed, such as pisiform fracture or pisotriquetral injury.

Although included as a carpal bone, the pisiform is actually a large sesamoid of the flexor carpi ulnaris ensheathed in tendoligamentous tissue. It rests palmarly on the triquetrum and does not bear axial weight like the rest of the carpus.

The hamate has an odd configuration with its wedge shape and palmarly projecting "hook." This structure forms a strut between the carpal tunnel and Guyon's canal and provides stable insertions for the ligaments that span these tunnels for the important neurovascular structures. The hook of the hamate is subject to injury because of its projection palmarward either from direct blow or avulsion.

The trapezium and trapezoid comprise the carpal articulations with the thumb and index fingers. Whereas the thumb carpometacarpal joint enjoys a great deal of motion (flexion, extension, adduction, abduction, pronation, and supination), the index carpometacarpal joint is allowed limited radial and ulnar deviation. The deep, opposing "saddle-shaped" surfaces at the trapeziometacarpal articulation account for its universal joint motion.

The distal radius provides the junction of the forearm and wrist. The congruous scaphoid and lunate facets give the radiocarpal joint bony stability (Fig. 20-2). Yet, slight alteration of the articular relationship (2 mm of displacement) can lead to abnormal force distribution and wear.[36] The sigmoid notch is an articular groove on the ulnar side of the distal radius that allows the radius to rotate around the ulna. Lister's tubercle is a bony projection on the dorsal radius that functions as a pulley for the extensor pollicis longus (EPL).

Injury to the carpal bones occurs less frequently in the immature skeleton. However, the active physeal growth center of the distal radius is commonly injured. It is responsible for 80% of radial longitudinal growth. There

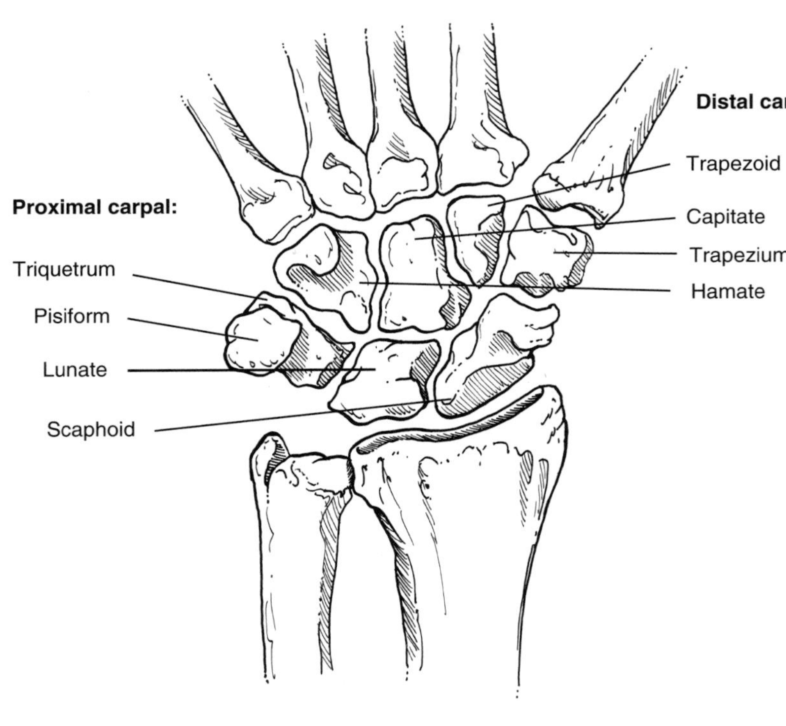

FIGURE 20-1. Wrist bones. The carpal bones consist of the proximal row (scaphoid, lunate, and triquetrum), the distal row (trapezium, trapezoid, capitate, and hamate), and the pisiform.

is substantial remodeling potential for many fractures occurring near the physis; however, there is also a significant risk of growth disturbance in displaced, crushed, or chronically injured distal radial epiphyses.[42]

Carpal Ligaments

Extrinsic. The wrist possesses a complex array of fibrous linkages or ligaments.[44,75] The ligaments control the complex motion of the carpus as an intercalated link between the forearm and hand. Most ligaments provide a connection between the carpal bones and the distal radius and ulna. These extrinsic ligaments are confluent with the wrist capsule. Collateral and dorsal ligament support is relatively weak, but the palmar ligaments are the strongest and most critical. Taleisnik[77] has described the radial palmar ligaments as the radioscaphocapitate (radiocapitate), radiolunate (long radiolunate), and radioscapholunate (short radiolunate) (Fig. 20-3). Besides being the primary stabilizer of the scaphoid proximal pole, the radioscapholunate ligament serves as a mesentery for blood supply. Lastly, the V-shaped deltoid ligament is responsible for maintaining midcarpal stability, and its components include scaphocapitate and capitotriquetral bands.

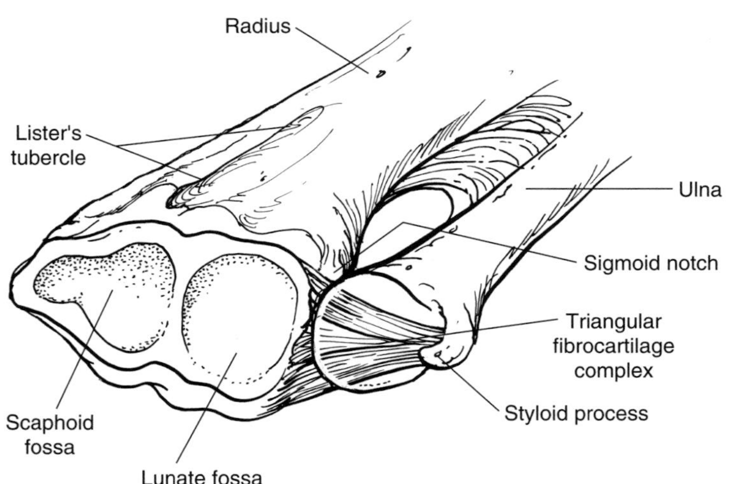

FIGURE 20-2. The distal radius articulates with the carpus through the scaphoid and lunate facets. It articulates with the distal ulna via the sigmoid notch. The triangular fibrocartilage complex inserts into ulnar border of the radial articular surface.

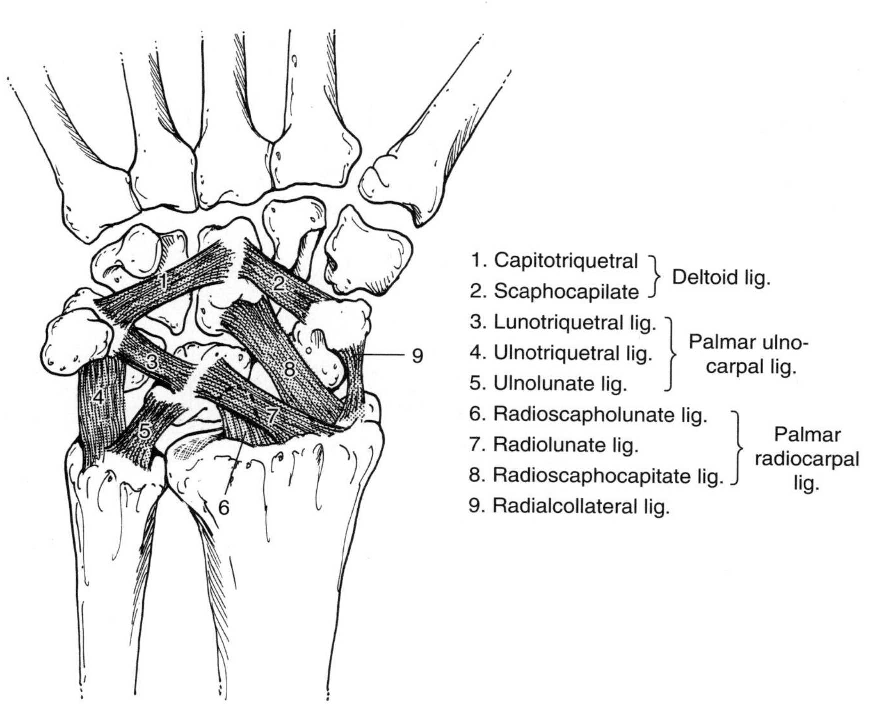

FIGURE 20-3. The palmar extrinsic ligaments of the wrist include the radiolunate, radioscapholunate, radioscaphocapitate, radial collateral, ulnolunate, lunotriquetral, and V or deltoid.

Intrinsic. The interosseous ligaments provide strong linkages between the carpal bones within the wrist capsule. The scapholunate ligament is important in maintaining proximal row stability and normal wrist kinematics, and it is the most commonly injured interosseous ligament. Of similar significance is the lunotriquetral ligament. Lunotriquetral injuries are less common and may be difficult to detect, particularly if there is no radiographic evidence of instability.

Triangular Fibrocartilage Complex

Although the ulnar articular surface area is small, the ulnar carpus is supported by the triangular fibrocartilage complex (TFCC) (Fig. 20-4).[54] The TFCC consists of the triangular fibrocartilage (TFC) with palmar and dorsal radioulnar ligaments, which provide strong ligamentous support for the distal radioulnar joint and a stable articular surface for the ulnocarpal joint. This structure experiences significant stress in rotation and deviation of the wrist. The substantial palmar ulnocarpal ligament completes the TFCC; it provides stability with power grip. There is a fibrocartilaginous meniscal homologue in a minority of patients that may have some load-bearing function.

Dorsal Soft Tissue

Tendons. The dorsal tendons that cross the wrist originate from extensor muscles of the forearm that animate the wrist and hand. At the distal radius, the extensor retinaculum protects the tendons while ensheathing them in a complex pulley system that prevents bowstringing. The extensor retinaculum divides the traversing tendons into six compartments (Fig. 20-5). The first and most radial compartment connects the abductor pollicis longus (APL) and extensor pollicis brevis (EPB) tendons to the thumb. The extensor carpi radialis longus and brevis (ECRL, ECRB) are in the second compartment. They are powerful wrist extensors. Lister's tubercle forms the radial border of the third compartment, serving as a pulley for the EPL as it courses radially toward the thumb. The EPL dorsally and the APB and EPB palmarly serve as the border for the anatomic "snuff-box" (Fig. 20-6). The scaphoid and radial artery are palpable in this area. The large fourth compartment includes the extensor indicis proprius (EIP) and the extensor digitorum communis (EDC) tendons, and compartments five and six contain the extensor digiti minimi (EDM) and extensor carpi ulnaris (ECU), respectively. The ECU is confined within the dorsal distal ulnar groove by strong ligamentous attachments.

Palmar Soft Tissue

Tendons. The flexor carpi radialis (FCR) and flexor carpi ulnaris (FCU) are the primary wrist flexors. The FCR travels within the confined space of its long fibro-osseous sheath.[7] It inserts into the index metacarpal primarily, with secondary slips to the long finger metacarpal and the trapezium. The stronger FCU inserts proximally onto the pisiform and has no fibrous sheath. The palmaris longus

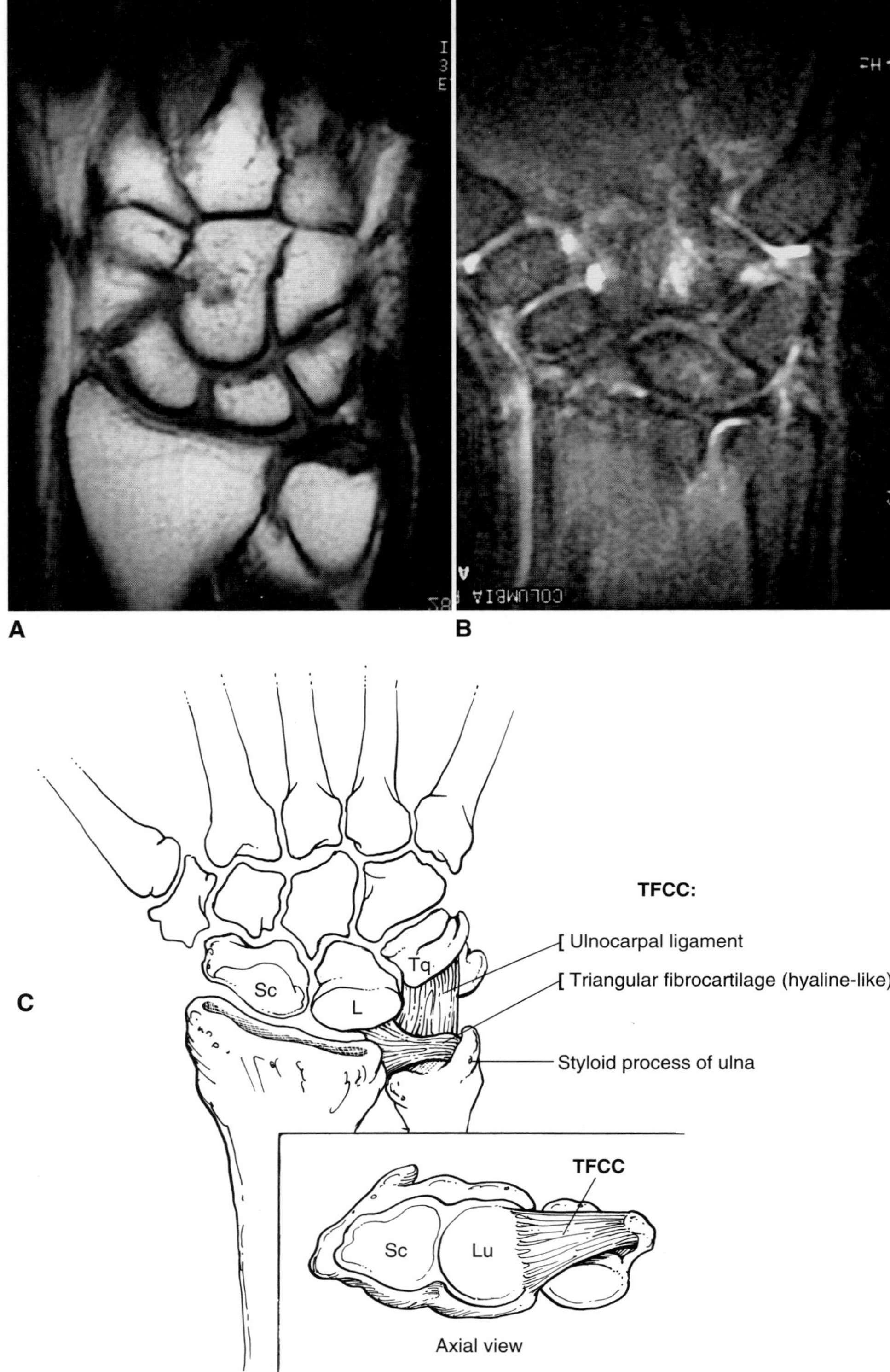

FIGURE 20-4. The triangular fibrocartilage complex consists of the ulnocarpal ligament and triangular fibrocartilage primarily. These structures are very important for the stability of the ulnar side of the wrist. **A** and **B,** Coronal MRI of ligamentous anatomy of the ulnar wrist. **C,** Coronal and axial diagrams of TFCC components.

becomes confluent with the palmar fascia. This vestigial structure may help cup the palm. It is absent in 12% to 15% of the population, and it is valuable as a donor for tendon grafting and reconstructive procedures. The finger and thumb flexors also cross palmarly and are discussed below.

Neurovascular

Dorsal Nerves. Sensory innervation to the dorsal hand is provided by branches from the superficial radial nerve and the dorsal sensory branch of the ulnar nerve, and innervating the wrist capsule are the terminal fibers of the posterior interosseous nerve.

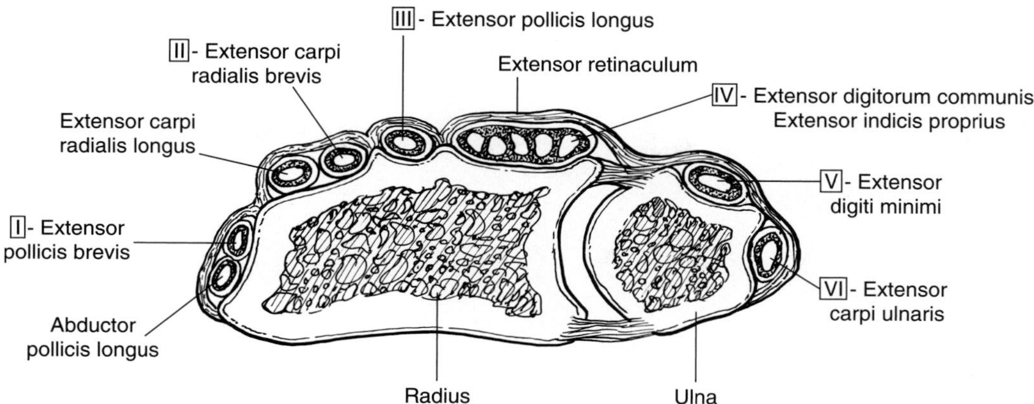

FIGURE 20-5. This axial section near the articular level of the distal radius demonstrates the six retinacular compartments that house the extensor tendons: I—abductor pollicis longus and extensor pollicis brevis, II—extensor carpi radialis longus and extensor carpi radialis brevis, III—extensor pollicis longus, IV—extensor digitorum communis and extensor indicis proprius, V—extensor digit minimi, and VI—extensor carpi ulnaris.

Carpal Tunnel. The carpal tunnel is the passageway for the median nerve and nine digital flexors. It protects the median nerve and functions as a pulley for the flexor digitorum profundus (FDP), flexor digitorum superficialis (FDS), and flexor pollicis longus (FPL) tendons. The superficial boundary is the thick, fibrous transverse carpal ligament spanning from the scaphoid tubercle to the hamate hook. The carpal bones form an arc to create its floor and sides. The tendons are covered with a synovial bursa at this level, which aids in tendon lubrication and nutrition. The median nerve is located superficially and slightly radial (Fig. 20-7). It provides sensation for most of the palm and radial three and one-half fingers. Motor branches innervate the two radial lumbricals and all of the thenar muscles with the exception of the deep head of the flexor pollicis brevis, which receives its innervation from the ulnar nerve. Eight to 10 centimeters proximal to the carpal tunnel, the median nerve gives off a palmar cutaneous branch that supplies sensation to the thenar eminence.

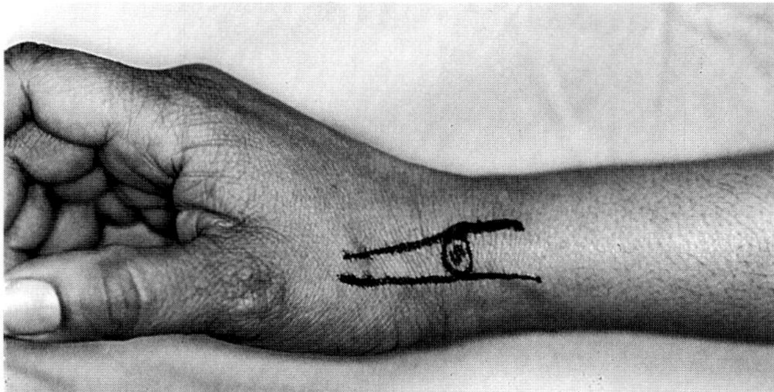

FIGURE 20-6. The "anatomic snuffbox" is easily viewed in this wrist. The dorsal boundary is the extensor pollicis longus, and the extensor pollicis brevis and abductor pollicis longus provide the palmar boundary. The proximal boundary is the radial styloid (not demarcated). The scaphoid (*S*) can be palpated in this region.

Guyon's Canal. The ulnar nerve and artery enter the hand through Guyon's canal. Its borders consist of the volar carpal ligament, palmarward; the hamate hook, radially; and the pisiform, ulnarly. The transverse carpal ligament makes up the floor of this structure. The ulnar nerve innervates the majority of the intrinsic muscles of the hand, excluding the thenar muscles and the two radial lumbricals. It does supply the deep head of the flexor pollicis brevis as well. Sensation to the ulnar one and one-half fingers is supplied via the ulnar nerve. Guyon's canal protects the neurovascular structures, but the ulnar side of the hand is often subject to direct trauma, which may lead to arterial injury.[24]

BIOMECHANICS

Kinematics

Normal wrist range of motion is 80° of flexion and 70° of extension. Radial and ulnar deviations are 20° and 30°, respectively (Fig. 20-8). Motion occurs at the radiocarpal joint and between the proximal and distal rows (midcarpal joint).[31] Patients may function well with little wrist motion, but this ability would not apply to athletic activities requiring flexibility of the wrist.

Kinetics

The wrist is important in transmitting forces between the hand and forearm. About 85° of the force transfers through the radius when the wrist is in neutral position.[19] The percentage decreases with wrist pronation or ulnar deviation. The strong radiocarpal ligaments must allow wrist motion and stability when it is loaded. Disruption of one or more of the ligamentous structures can lead to instability or malalignment. The altered kinematics may lead to pain, carpal collapse, and arthritis.

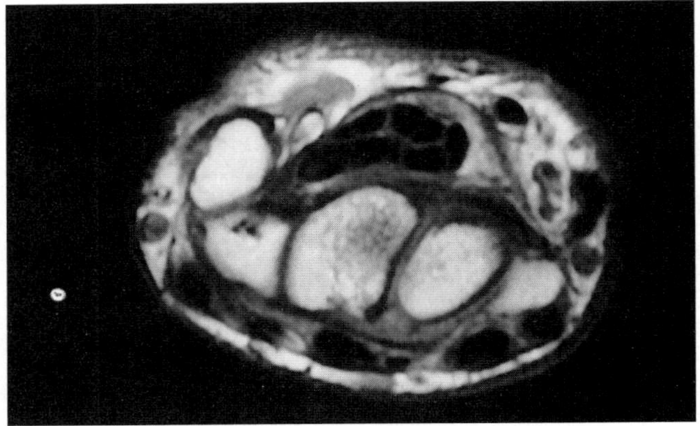

FIGURE 20-7. The axial magnetic resonance imaging section of the proximal palm shows the carpal tunnel contents. The median nerve lies radial and superficial and produces a different signal than the flexor tendons.

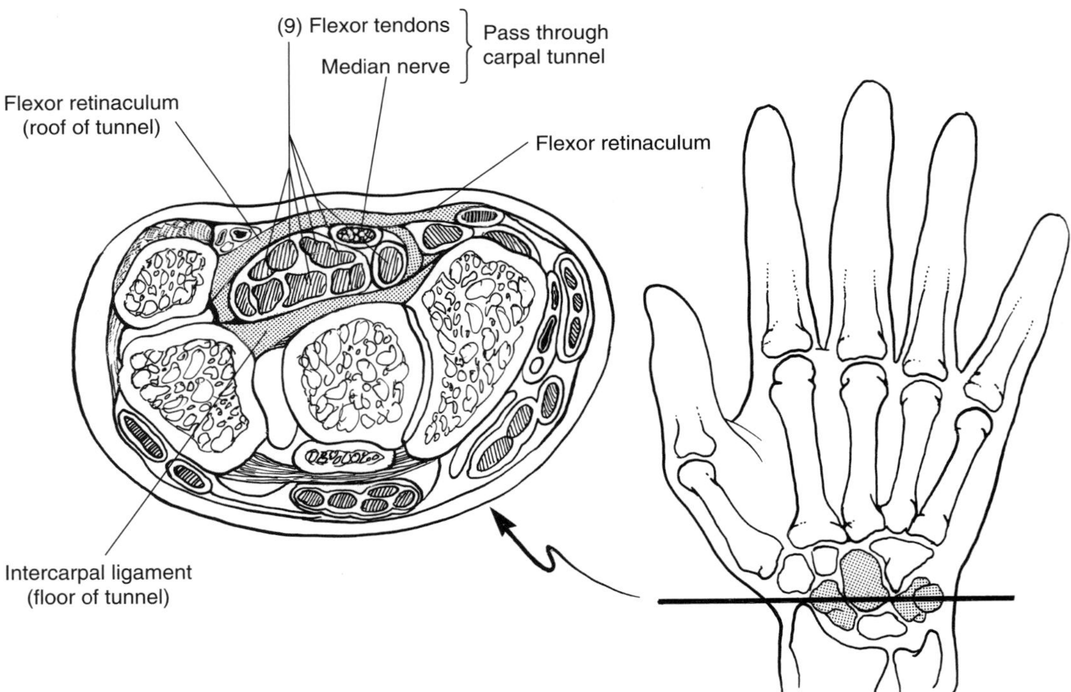

EVALUATION

History

The history of the injury and details of the chief complaint are extremely important. Obvious problems such as acute fractures, tendon ruptures, and major nerve lacerations create no diagnostic dilemmas. However, many sports injuries are categorized under the generic diagnosis of "wrist sprain."[6] Focal pain, which is reproducible, may indicate certain structural problems, therefore, it is extremely important to specify the location, severity, and chronicity of the complaint. The examiner must indicate the dominant extremity, specific sport, and energy that caused the injury. The patient should report previous injuries, provocative activities, and any confounding medical conditions or predisposing factors.

Physical Examination

On the playing field, the physical examination may be limited to inspection and palpation. The examiner should look for symmetry and alignment. A fracture or dislocation may be obvious. The examiner should check the integrity of the skin for possible lacerations, contusions, or punctures because open fractures are surgical emergencies, and any pain, swelling, alignment, and color changes should be noted. The neurologic and vascular examinations must be done completely and documented well so later examiners can assess progression. The sensory examination requires testing the autonomous zones of the median (index finger pad), ulnar (small finger pad), and radial (dorsal first webspace) nerves. Motor function may be difficult to assess because of pain, but the examiner can

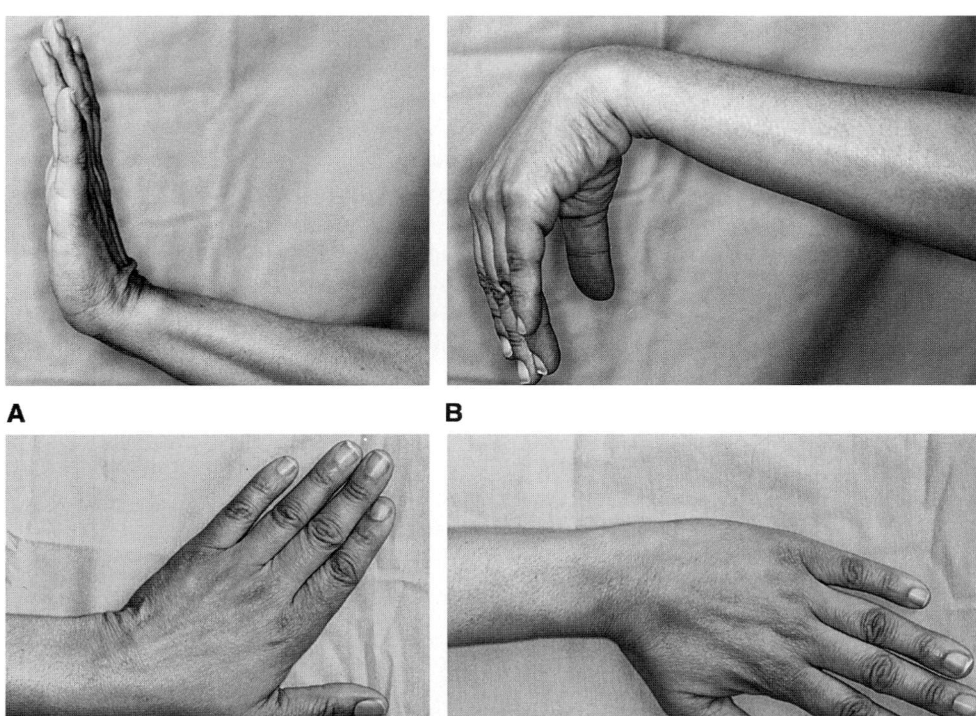

FIGURE 20-8. Wrist range of motion. **A,** Dorsiflexion. **B,** Palmar flexion. **C,** Ulnar deviation. **D,** Radial deviation.

palpate muscle group contraction in each territory. Radial and ulnar pulses should be assessed along with capillary filling. The Allen test is used to evaluate radial and ulnar artery patency and the adequacy of collateralization between the radial and ulnar circulation. The test is performed by compressing the ulnar and radial arteries and exsanguinating the hand, usually by asking the patient to make a tight fist. Upon opening the palm, the entire palmar surface of the hand should be blanched. The examiner should release the compression on one artery and check for swiftness, intensity, and area of color return and sequentially repeat to check the other vessel.

In nonacute conditions, the examiner must carefully determine the location of the complaint. The history, physical examination, plain radiographs, and more sophisticated imaging such as arthrography, computed tomography, and magnetic resonance imaging can assist in confirming a diagnosis.

Immediate Management

Immobilization plays a key role in patient comfort.[48] A firm splinting device is useful while waiting for a complete evaluation, including radiographs (Fig. 20-9). A neurovascular examination is mandatory. Elevation and ice are measures that can control swelling and reduce pain.

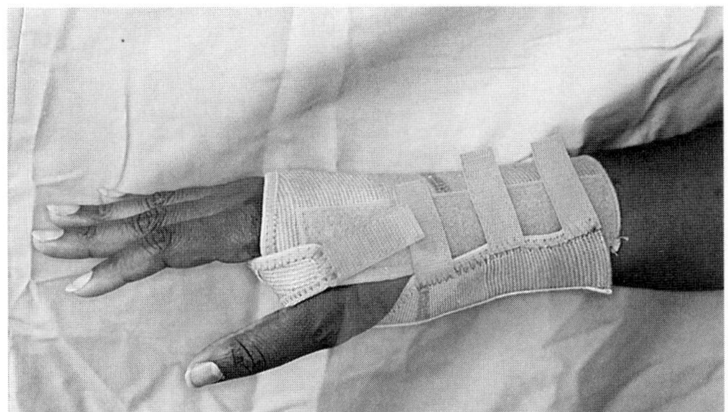

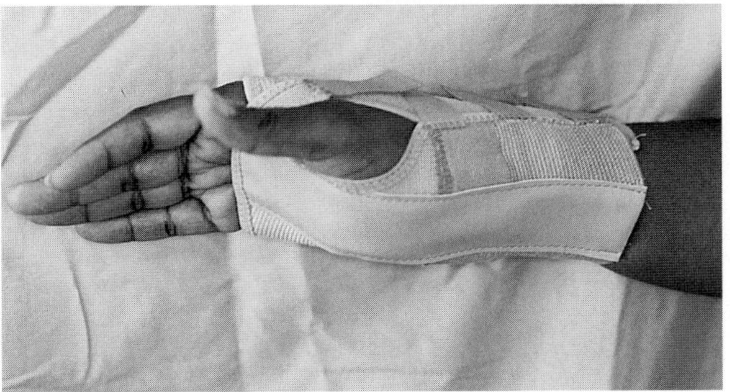

FIGURE 20-9. Wrist splint. A prefabricated device can provide some limited stability.

Imaging

Radiography remains the initial imaging modality for wrist conditions.[46] The standard series are anteroposterior, lateral, and oblique projections (Fig. 20-10).[6] Magnetic resonance imaging is ideal for evaluating bone vascularity and soft-tissue integrity. Arthrography has been useful for evaluation of the intercarpal ligaments and the TFCC. Bone scintigraphy is useful for the diagnosis of occult fractures.[74] Computed tomography has a limited role in chronic conditions, but it can be useful in assessing fracture patterns and assessing progress to bony union, particularly in scaphoid fractures.

CLASSIFICATION

Burton has classified upper extremity conditions according to tissue type and location.[10] The following description will organize wrist injuries into categories relevant to the mechanism of injury,[48] including overuse, excessive loading, trauma, and neurovascular. Additional specific disorders that are common to athletes will be described.

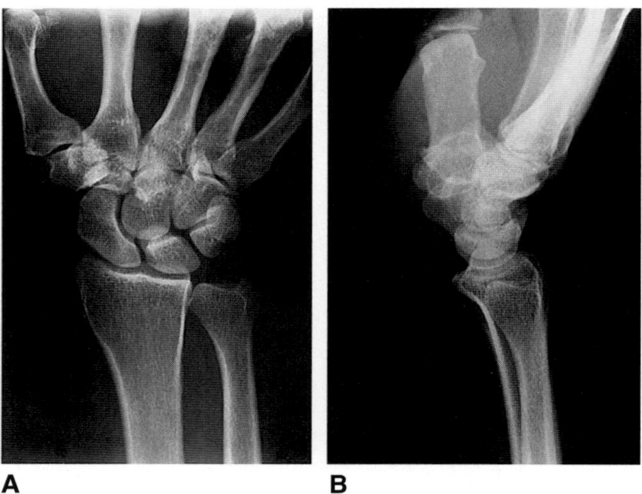

A B

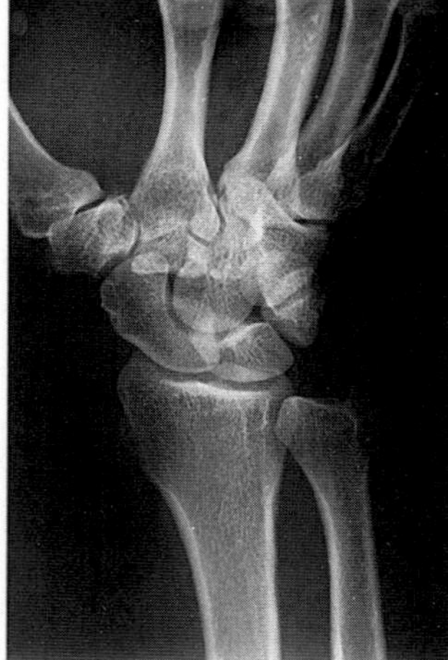

C

FIGURE 20-10. Standard screening. Radiographs of wrist. **A,** Anteroposterior view. **B,** Lateral view. **C,** Oblique view.

Overuse

Most sports injuries are the result of chronic, repetitive soft-tissue overload, fatigue, and resultant failure.[18,75] During rugged athletic activity, tendinous, ligamentous, and synovial structures suffer microscopic trauma. Collagen fibers in the tendon or ligament may fail under excessive tension. The soft-tissue healing process includes an inflammatory stage, a reparative stage, and, finally, a remodeling stage.[33,59] If the tissues are not afforded the time to completely heal, they will be even more susceptible to reinjury, leading to inflammation and pain. When a soft tissue such as synovium remains chronically in the inflammatory stage, it may undergo fibrosis and have limited potential for complete remodeling.

Most wrist overuse problems are related to tendons, especially as they pass through the limited space of a tendon sheath, under a retinaculum, or near their bony insertion. Activities that require high wrist torques cause most of the overuse injuries, including racquet sports, gymnastics, wrestling, and rowing. Conservative management allows the tissue to heal with rest while maintaining mobility and can be facilitated with oral anti-inflammatory medications, particularly some of the newer COX-2–specific inhibitors. Local peritendinous corticosteroid injection may be helpful as well. A careful, gradual return to activity will help prevent atrophy and weakness.[51] Some of these enthetic disorders do not respond to this approach and, in some cases, surgical management may be considered.

First Dorsal Compartment. Tenosynovitis of the first dorsal compartment is common in women of middle age or postpartum.[75] However, it is also seen in athletes of both sexes. The APL and EPB reside in the first dorsal compartment. Patients will complain of exquisite pain with passive wrist ulnar deviation or active thumb extension, and grip will be painful.

On examination, patients may have swelling proximal to the radial styloid. On palpation, the extensor sheath can be firm, almost nodular. A ganglion cyst may be present within the tendon sheath. Tenderness can be consistently localized proximal to the radial styloid, directly over the tendon sheath. The Finklestein test will produce marked discomfort (Fig. 20-11).[20] This test is performed by positioning the thumb fully adducted within the palm and then ulnarly deviating the wrist, which causes painful excursion of the involved tendons.

Initial management is splinting. The splint should provide firm support for the wrist and thumb, while keeping them in a functional position. The splint can be removed for periods of nonstressful exercise, and

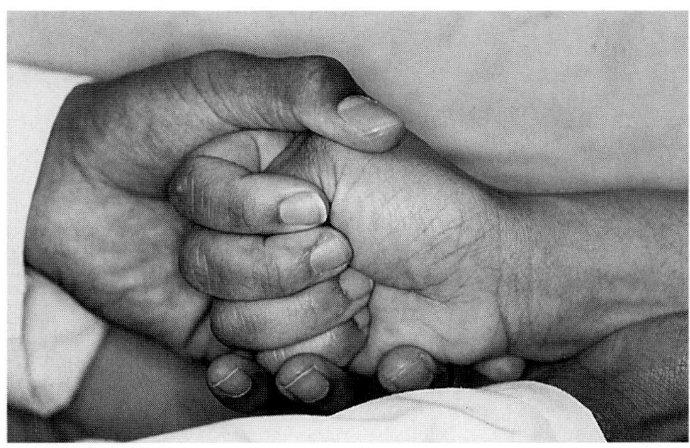

FIGURE 20-11. The Finkelstein test is performed by ulnarly deviating the wrist with the thumb in the adducted position. This test may cause significant discomfort.

nonsteroidal anti-inflammatory medication may facilitate resolution of the process. Corticosteroid injection is very useful and may effect a cure. These treatments may fail in patients with chronic injury with significant fibrosis and thickening of the sheath. Also, patients who have an anatomic variant whereby multiple slips of the APL co-exist with the EPB in the first dorsal compartment (separated by a partition or partitions within the compartment) will often fail conservative management. Those patients may be cured by surgical release.

Intersection Syndrome. Intersection syndrome is a rare condition.[28] The APL and EPB muscles cross the ECRL and ECRB tendons several centimeters proximal to the extensor retinaculum (Fig. 20-12). Patients may develop pain and swelling over this area, particularly with activity. Some patients will note audible crepitus during wrist flexion and extension. The pathophysiology is unclear but may be the result of bursitis, ECRL and ECRB tenosynovitis, or APL and EPB muscular hypertrophy or degeneration. Nevertheless, it is a problem related to excessive friction between contacting soft tissues. Intersection syndrome has been described in rowers, weight lifters, skiers,[55] and racquetball players.[70]

Initial management includes rest, splinting, and therapeutic modalities. Nonsteroidal anti-inflammatory medication and corticosteroid injection augment the conservative protocol. After the inflammatory process has resolved, reconditioning can help decrease the chances of recurrence. If there is no improvement, surgical decompression and debridement should be considered.

Extensor Pollicis Longus Tendinitis. Often, the EPL is affected by rheumatoid arthritis or distal radius fractures. The tendon is subject to late rupture in both conditions. Rarely does overuse lead to EPL tenosynovitis and rupture, but it has been reported in squash players and drummers.[33]

Initial symptoms include pain with thumb extension localized over Lister's tubercle. Pain also can radiate proximally. The history and radiographs should rule out a previous distal radius fracture. EPL muscle hypertrophy in its dorsal compartment is a postulated etiology of the condition known as "drummer boy's palsy."[52] Management consists of rest, splinting, and nonsteroidal anti-inflammatory medications. Steroid injections should be avoided for fear of hastening a rupture. Surgery includes decompression with translocation of the EPL out of Lister's canal.

Extensor Carpi Ulnaris. Athletes who heavily load the wrist, such as rowers, are prone to ECU tendinitis. Participants of racquet sports also are affected.[52] Patients describe pain on the dorsal and ulnar side of the wrist. As already noted, there are many structures tightly packed into this region, and many confounding diagnoses, such as TFCC or distal radioulnar joint injuries, must be considered. A distinctive feature of ECU tendinitis includes crepitation on wrist motion. A targeted lidocaine injection may confirm the diagnosis. Management consists of splinting and nonsteroidal anti-inflammatory medication with a gradual return to activity.

Other Extensor Tendinitis. Overuse tenosynovitis of the EDC or EDM tendon occurs uncommonly. Symptoms related to these tendons are more likely the result of direct trauma or preexisting systemic disease. However, swelling may indicate a mass effect in an enclosed space. A lesion such as a ganglion cyst, anomalous muscle,[3,35] or tumor must be ruled out.

Flexor Carpi Radialis. Flexor carpi radialis tendinitis is becoming more frequently recognized. The FCR is confined to a tight fibrous sheath as it courses across the wrist toward the index metacarpal. Chronic repetitive wrist motion can cause irritation of the synovial sheath, leading to inflammation.[22] Inflammation can also be secondary to adjacent scaphotrapezial arthritis. Pain localized over the FCR tendon is elicited with passive extension and resisted flexion. Synovitis may present as swelling just proximal to the wrist crease. Long-standing disease may cause adhesions within the fibrous sheath.

Rest, splinting, and nonsteroidal anti-inflammatory medication are the initial management protocols. Steroid injection is often required and very successful. Surgery includes release of the entire sheath.[23]

Flexor Carpi Ulnaris. The FCU may be influenced by the same activities that cause FCR tendinitis. Participants in racquet sports and golf are more commonly affected.[52] Tenderness is palpated more distally, near the insertion into the pisiform. Pisotriquetral arthritis must be ruled out either radiographically or by physical examination. Rest and splinting are usually successful in relieving symptoms.

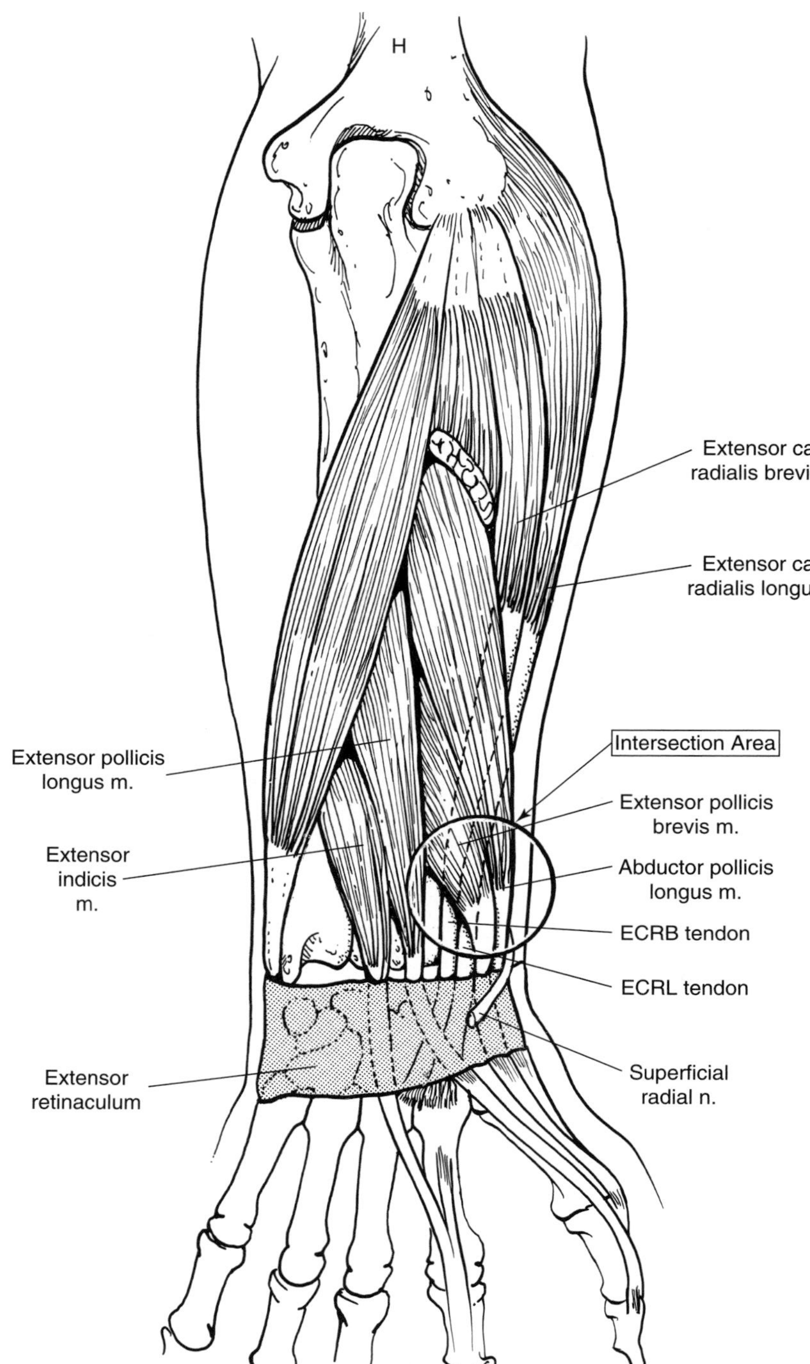

FIGURE 20-12. The affected site of the intersection syndrome is located at the crossing of the abductor pollicis longus and extensor pollicis brevis over the extensor carpi radialis longus and brevis.

Surgical management includes resection of the pisiform with possible FCU lengthening but is rarely indicated.

Ligament. Chronic ulnar-sided wrist pain should raise suspicion about a TFCC injury.[27] Complaints will range from dorsal wrist pain ("sprained wrist") to inability to hold a racquet. These patients may present with symptoms similar to ulnar-sided tendinitis. Studies have demonstrated chronic TFC perforations associated with a positive ulnar variance and with aging in asymptomatic patients (Fig. 20-13). Healthy subjects may possess asymptomatic TFC tears; however, a tear is probably abnormal in patients less than 30 years with neutral ulnar variance. Degenerative TFC injuries do not cause distal radioulnar instability.

If TFC injury is suspected, the diagnosis may be confirmed by arthrography or magnetic resonance imaging. Magnetic resonance imaging is highly sensitive in soft-tissue assessment but may not be specific.[34] Arthroscopy is useful in skilled hands because of its

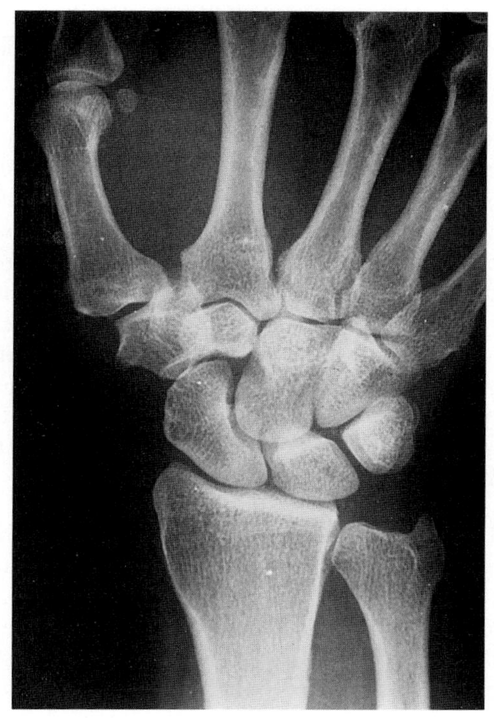

A

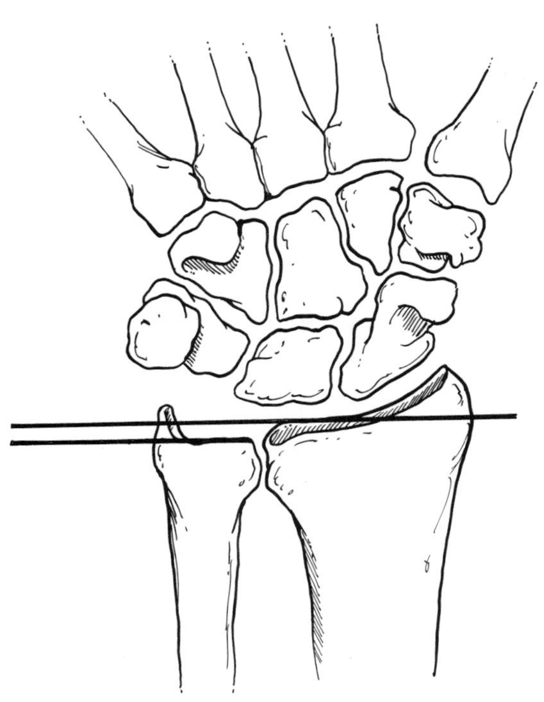

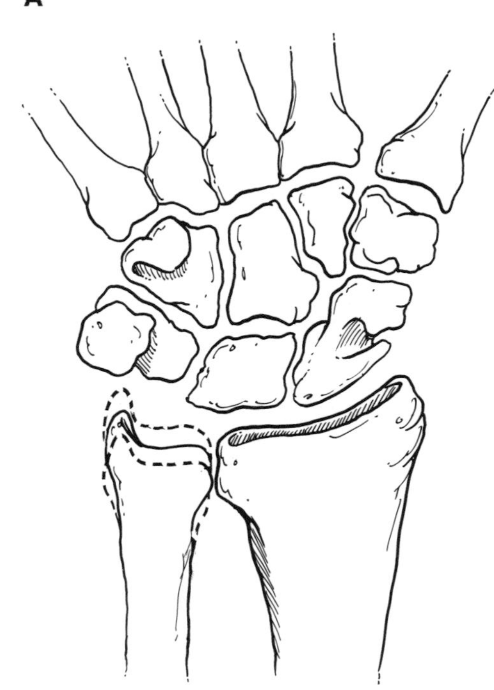

B

FIGURE 20-13. Radiograph demonstrating negative ulnar variance. **A,** Ulnar variance is measured by drawing a tangential line across the articular edge of the radius and by observing the relative level of the distal ulnar articular edge. **B,** When the line is flush with ulnar articular edge, this is considered neutral ulnar variance. If the line is distal, negative ulnar variance; and if proximal, positive ulnar variance. This measurement must be in the neutral rotation position or it may be unreliable.

diagnostic benefit and potential therapeutic indications. Tears can be visualized, and if stable, debrided with arthroscopic instruments.[81] The TFCC may require repair if there is instability of the ulnar carpus. Arthroscopy may be the most economical and efficient way to diagnose and potentially manage ulnar wrist pain that has not responded to prolonged conservative therapy.

Load-Bearing Injury

Sports requiring the use of the upper extremity as a load-bearing structure will have participants who suffer such injuries. These injuries occur primarily to gymnasts and weight lifters. These athletes place exceptional compressive and rotational forces on the wrist.[44] Most gymnasts will suffer symptoms at some point during their training and competition.[41] Their conditions usually have a chronic component, particularly if serious training and competition is begun before skeletal maturity.

Dorsal Wrist Pain. Gymnasts may complain of diffuse dorsal wrist pain with swelling and warmth. This problem is familiar to most gymnasts and has been called "wrist capsulitis" and "wrist pain syndrome"[41] in the literature. It is hypothesized that the chronically loaded dorsiflexed wrist sustains repetitive impaction trauma to the capsule or synovium, creating the diffuse inflammation and swelling.[17] Another possible cause of pain is perineural fibrosis about the posterior interosseous nerve that innervates the dorsal wrist capsule. These patients may benefit from therapeutic modalities such as ice, ultrasound, and taping, and brief periods of rest.

Distal Radial Epiphysis Stress Fracture. Previous studies have shown that young gymnasts may suffer chronic injuries to the distal radial epiphysis.[79] Patients present with symptoms of radially sided wrist pain and tenderness. Radiographs may reveal widening of the physis, cystic metaphyseal changes, and a "beaked effect" of the distal aspect of the epiphysis.[67] It is believed that these changes reflect a stress fracture or reaction. Repeated trauma may result in early physeal closure and eventual positive ulnar variance.[43] There have been reports of partial physeal closure, mimicking Madelung's deformity at the distal forearm.[80] The best treatment for these young athletes is rest with a gradual return to gymnastics once symptoms have resolved. Patients without radiographic changes may return within weeks, and those who have changes may require up to 6 months of inactivity.

Ulnar Impaction Syndrome. A published report on college gymnasts has shown a high incidence of positive ulnar variance.[41] It was postulated that this syndrome may result from a physeal injury caused by excessive compressive forces on the maturing distal radius, as noted in the preceding section. Later, patients may suffer from chronic symptoms associated with continued gymnastics, such as the pommel horse and parallel bars. This long ulna may cause tears of the TFC and chondromalacia of the lunate and triquetrum.[17] Patients with ulnocarpal abutment and degenerative changes often require a joint-leveling procedure, such as ulna shortening, to decompress this area.

Trauma

Tendon Rupture. Acute tendon rupture occurs occasionally at the tendon insertion distally more on the extensor side (mallet fingers) than the flexor side (jersey finger; FDP ring avulsion). However, intrasubstance tendon rupture at the level of the wrist is uncommon in healthy athletes. If documented, an investigation into preexisting local or systemic conditions should follow.

Extensor Carpi Ulnaris Dislocation. With forceful hypersupination and ulnar deviation, the ECU may rupture its ulnar septum and subluxate from its groove.[62] This injury has been reported in golfers, tennis players, weight lifters, basketball players, and bronco riders. Patients may present with an acute injury or with complaints of chronic painful "clicking" and "snapping" associated with wrist rotation. The diagnosis can be made by careful examination over the ECU groove. Acute cases may be managed with reduction and immobilization for several weeks, and chronic cases may require surgical reconstruction of the ECU tendon sheath.[66]

Scapholunate Ligament. Interosseous ligaments stabilize the proximal carpal row bones for normal kinematic function.[32] A high-loading force on the dorsiflexed wrist may cause ligament disruption. The scapholunate ligament is most commonly affected.[12] Some patients may be predisposed to ligament attenuation and rupture even with trivial insults. Some authors believe the radioscapholunate ligament can be ruptured along with the scapholunate, causing more severe instability.[78] This condition is called *dorsal intercalated segmental instability* and leads to an alteration in the loading pattern on the radius and scaphoid, causing accelerated cartilage wear.

Patients may present with an acute injury or chronic symptoms of pain, swelling, and crepitus. Pain is located dorsoradially over the scapholunate interval. Watson[81] has described a provocative test that consists of stabilizing and extending the distal pole of the scaphoid and then flexing and radially deviating the wrist (Fig. 20-14), which will produce a subluxation at the radioscaphoid articulation. Pain associated with a palpable "clunk" due to the subluxation constitutes a positive test result.

Normal radiographic alignment on standard views may suggest a dynamic instability.[78] Gapping and rotation between the scaphoid and lunate is consistent with a static instability. The posteroanterior clenched fist or loaded view accentuates the gap or may demonstrate a dynamic instability. The scaphoid flexes and radially deviates. This displacement is evaluated by measuring the scapholunate angle (Fig. 20-15). The normal scapholunate angle range is 30° to 60°, with an average of 47°. An angle of more than 70° is deemed abnormal. It is not uncommon that while investigating an unrelated wrist or hand problem, a relatively asymptomatic scapholunate instability may be detected. It is important to obtain comparable radiographs of the opposite wrist in those patients.

In most cases, nonsurgical management is unsatisfactory. The surgical protocol is based on the individual surgeon's training, experience, and preference. Currently, these include direct ligament reconstruction, selective fusions, fusions, capsulodeses, bone-ligament-bone constructs and the RASL procedure (Reduction and Association of the Scaphoid and Lunate).[8,15,40,76,82,83]

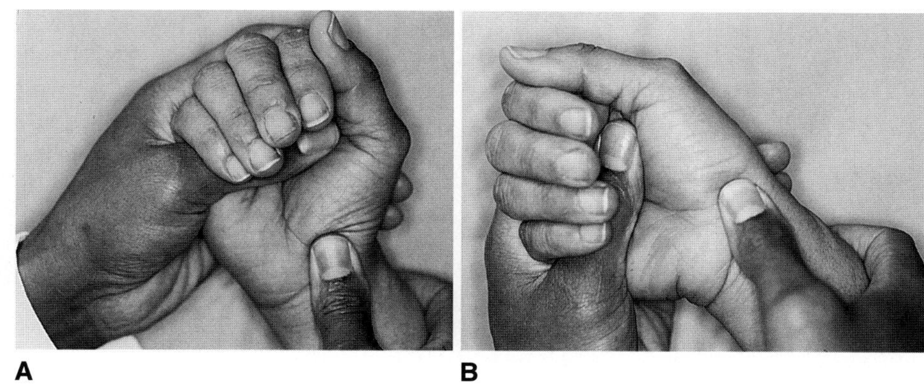

FIGURE 20-14. Scaphoid shift test. The test is performed by **(A)** stabilizing the scaphoid tubercle in the ulnarly deviated wrist, then **(B)** maintaining a dorsiflexon force while radially deviating the wrist. Scaphoid subluxation may be appreciated during the examination. Pain indicates a positive test result.

These choices are affected by chronicity and the degree of arthritis. At present, no single procedure can be confidently advocated, though wrist arthroscopy continues to play an increasing role in the management of these conditions.

Lunotriquetral Ligament. Lunotriquetral instability is less common than scapholunate instability and is difficult to confirm.[9] The mechanism of injury is often a fall with a torquing component. Patients complain of dorsoulnar wrist pain. Often, these injuries are managed as a "sprain" and do not present to the physician acutely. The provocative tests as described by Reagan et al.[63] ("ballottement") and Kleinman[26] ("shear") help to reproduce pain symptoms (Fig. 20-16). The tests are performed by stabilizing the lunate with one hand and attempting translation of

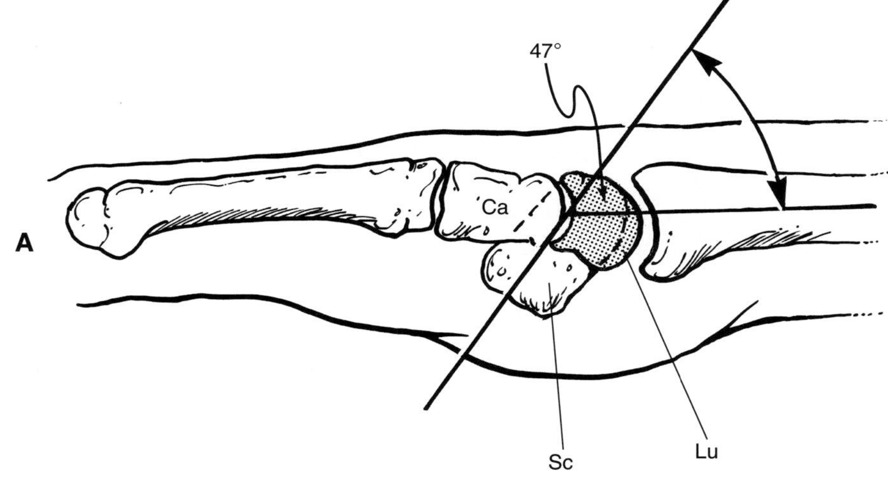

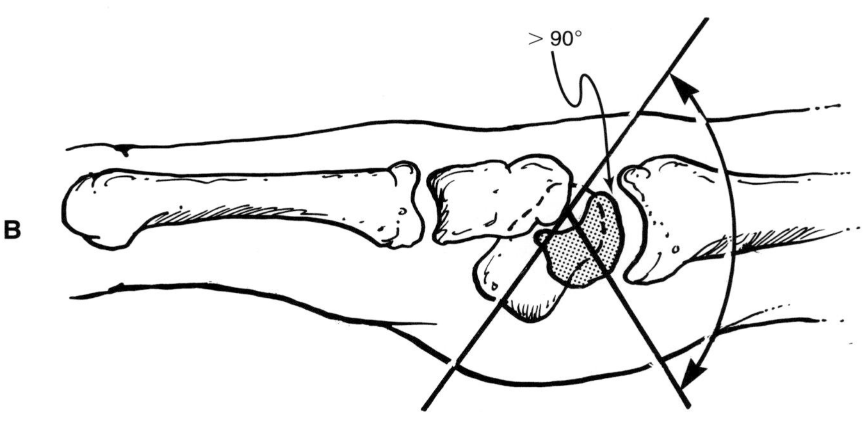

FIGURE 20-15. Scapholunate angle. **A,** Normal angle (average 47°) between scaphoid and lunate in the lateral projection. **B,** Abnormal palmar flexion of the scaphoid in relation to the dorsiflexed lunate, thereby creating an increased scapholunate angle.

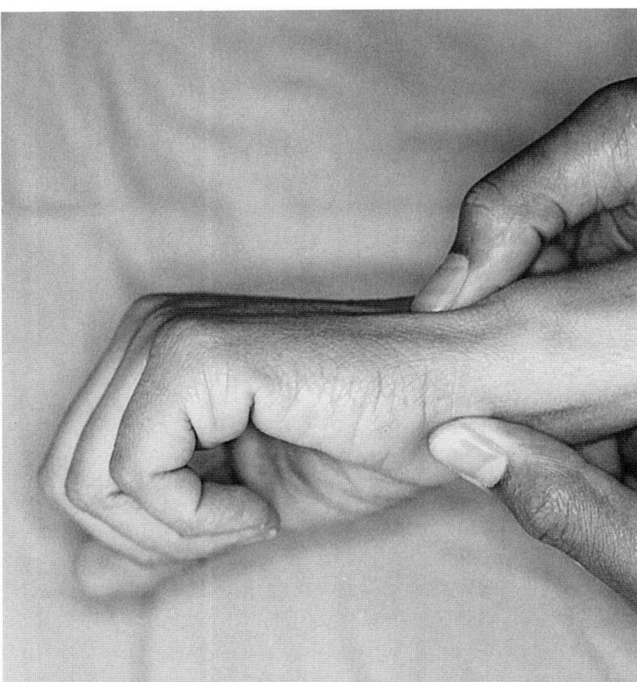

FIGURE 20-16. Ballottement test. The lunate is stabilized with one hand while dorsal and palmar translation of the triquetrum is attempted by the other by applying a dorsally directed force on the pisiform prominence. Translation or pain are positive findings of lunotriquetral abnormality.

the triquetrum palmarly and dorsally with the other. Lateral radiographs may demonstrate a scapholunate angle of less than 30°, only if there is a static deformity. An arthrogram may be nondiagnostic, but magnetic resonance imaging is becoming the most sensitive, accurate test.

Immobilization should be tried first, especially in acute cases. Chronic cases may not respond to splints, injections, or nonsteroidal anti-inflammatory medicine. Lunotriquetral arthrodesis is preferred over lunotriquetral ligament reconstruction.[26,46]

Arcuate Ligament. Patients with midcarpal instability complain of a bothersome and at times painful "click" or "clunking" wrist.[38] They may be able to demonstrate this problem voluntarily. The patient will hold the wrist in radial deviation, and with ulnar deviation, there will be an abrupt translation. This instability pattern occurs as a result of repetitive loading of the ligamentous link between the proximal and distal rows.[26,38] It can also occur with congenital ligamentous laxity. On cineradiography, the translation appears to be taking place at the triquetrohamate articulation. Painful midcarpal instability may be managed with arthrodesis, which limits motion, or ligament reconstruction, which may not provide durable stabilization for the long term. Instability at the midcarpal joint that is not painful should be managed by observation.

Triangular Fibrocartilage Complex. Many racquet, rowing, and batting sports require strong wrist action for effective performance.[52] Participants may suffer acute injuries or overuse syndromes on the ulnar side of the wrist. Wrist hyperrotation can cause tearing of the palmar or dorsal radioulnar band of the triangular fibrocartilage, leading to radioulnar instability. A fall may overload the TFC and produce intrasubstance tears or perforations of the load-bearing cushion or "disc." Patients will complain of pain that intensifies with loading and twisting. Applying compression across the ulnar side of the wrist is a good test. The "shuck" test for radioulnar translation can be performed. Also, extremes of rotation may cause crepitus or "snapping," which is indicative of instability. With instability, the distal ulna may be prominent dorsally.

Radiographs may reveal a positive ulnar variance, which is associated with TFC injuries. However, diagnosis of actual tears requires arthrography and, more recently, magnetic resonance imaging. Management of TFC injuries depends on chronicity and location, peripheral or central. An initial splinting or casting is often indicated. Failures of this approach may require arthrotomy or arthroscopy with either TFC repair or debridement.[47] Results can be predictable if the presenting complaint truly correlates with a radiographic or arthroscopic abnormality.

Scaphoid. The scaphoid is the most commonly fractured carpal bone.[39,68] The fracture typically is the result of a significant fall or blunt trauma (Fig. 20-17). Often, the injury is misinterpreted as a bad "wrist sprain." Athletes may continue to perform in their sport while the discomfort becomes tolerable. Frequently, the injury is detected late as a malaligned nonunion when the athlete suffers a second injury or develops post-traumatic wrist osteoarthritis known as scapholunate advanced collapse (or SLAC wrist). Contact sports with frequent falls like football, basketball,[13,85] and hockey will cause a high rate of scaphoid fractures.

Clinically, patients will complain of pain and tenderness localized to the anatomic snuffbox. Axial loading of the thumb provokes pain. Swelling may be mild to minimal. All injuries with localizing pain to the scaphoid area require radiographs. Serial plain radiographs and computed tomograms may demonstrate a fracture in subtle cases. Patients with a suspicious clinical examination should be treated with splinting, even if results of radiographs are negative. Often, it takes 1 to 2 weeks before the fracture line resorbs, and it can be seen with imaging. A bone scan may also confirm the diagnosis in the early post-injury period (1 to 2 weeks). There have been few reports of scaphoid stress fracture in gymnasts diagnosed by bone scan.[29,42] Magnetic resonance imaging is a highly sensitive test for fracture definition and assessment of vascularity to the vulnerable scaphoid proximal pole.

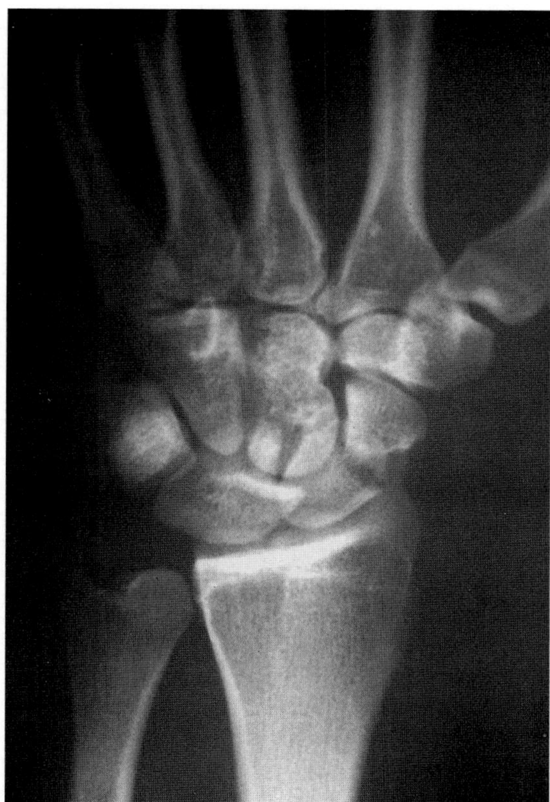

FIGURE 20-17. Transverse fracture of the scaphoid waist caused by fall onto the outstretched palm.

Scaphoid fractures, especially when displaced, may take 3 to 6 months to heal, if at all.[64] Surgery is indicated for displaced, angulated, or nonunited fractures. Anatomic reduction and stable fixation enhances function and carpal kinematics. Current concepts include the use of percutaneous internal fixation of selected scaphoid fractures including stable acute nondisplaced waist fractures with arthroscopic assistance.[71] Arguments in favor of this approach include decreasing the nonunion rate of casted fractures as well as faster return to work or sports using a less invasive approach.

Hamate. Hamate body fractures are uncommon, but the prominent hook can be injured by an avulsion of the transverse carpal ligament (Fig. 20-18). Also, direct or repetitive trauma,[57] particularly by the force of a baseball bat or tennis racquet,[73] can lead to injury. Palpation directly over the hook, which is located in the hypothenar eminence, elicits pain. Carpal tunnel radiographs may demonstrate a fracture. Plain or computed tomography shows the base of the hook in better detail. Bone scintigraphy is less specific but useful.

For acute injuries, initial management is cast immobilization to enhance healing. Frequently, the patient reports the second injury, and a nonunion is detected. Excision of the ununited fragment allows the fastest return to play. Associated complications with hamate hook nonunions include flexor digitorum profundus tendon to the small finger rupture and ulnar neuropathy.

Trapezoid. Body fracture of the trapezoid is not a reported sports injury, although osteochondral injury to the carpometacarpal joint of the index finger may occur during forceful radial and ulnar deviation in activities such as baseball batting.

Trapezium. Trapezium body fractures have been reported in cyclists,[2] but generally are rare. The mechanism is usually axial trauma while the hands rest on the handle bars. The trapezial ridge is seldom fractured, but the fracture can be easily missed. Patients will complain of pain just distal to the scaphoid tuberosity within the thenar eminence. Radiographs using the carpal tunnel view may show a fracture of the ridge. Special trapezium views are needed to examine the body appropriately.

Acute cases can be managed with protective immobilization. Chronic trapezial ridge fractures that are

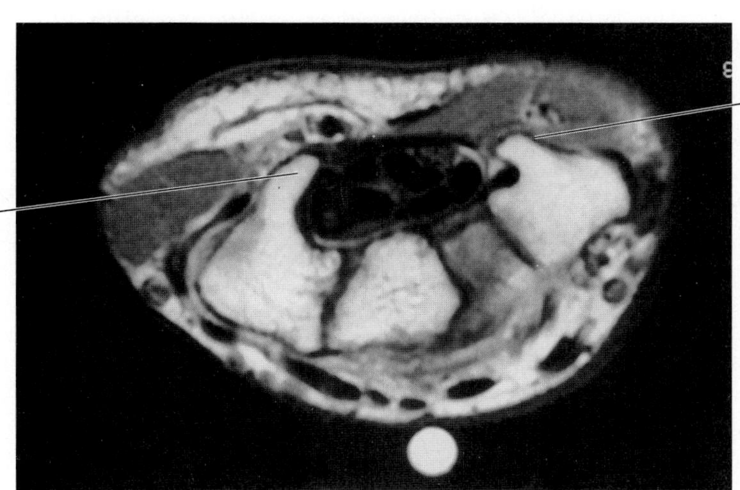

FIGURE 20-18. This computed tomography image of the distal carpal row demonstrates the palmar projections of the trapezial ridge radially and the hamate hook ulnarly.

persistently symptomatic are appropriately managed by excision of the painful ridge.

Triquetrum. The body of the triquetrum is fractured infrequently.[2] Palmarly, it is protected by the pisiform. Avulsion fractures of the dorsal surface may occur with wrist hyperextension and impingement on the hamate. Radiographically, a small fleck of bone will be seen lying dorsal to the triquetrum on the lateral projection. Patients may be treated with immobilization for a few weeks until they are comfortable. Surgery is usually not indicated, even if dorsal carpal bossing or prominence occurs.

Pisiform. Similar to the hamate, pisiform fractures result from direct trauma on the ulnar side of the palm and usually are nondisplaced. They may also result from fatigue failure. Accepted management is immobilization and protection until healing. Sometimes an osteochondral fracture will occur, resulting in chronic arthritic symptoms. Surgery is indicated if painful symptoms persist. In those cases, excision of the pisiform is curative, and return to function is routine.[56]

Capitate. Capitate fractures result from violent trauma and are most often associated with other carpal injuries. They are commonly missed fractures initially. Nondisplaced fractures can be managed by immobilization. A vulnerable blood supply to the head of the capitate may predispose to avascular necrosis and nonunion. Displaced fractures and nonunion require surgery.

Distal Radius. Distal radius fractures are most common in the elderly population but are frequently seen in younger athletes as a result of severe trauma to the wrist. The mechanism of injury is via direct or indirect high-energy forces through extremes of wrist motion. Patients will have severe pain with swelling, ecchymosis, and deformity. Radiographs will demonstrate the anatomy of the fracture (Fig. 20-19). Comminution, intraarticular extension, angulation, and shortening are criteria that help predict the success or failure of a closed reduction.[36] Displaced distal radius fractures require immediate attention with reduction and immobilization, followed by elevation and ice to control swelling. Neuromuscular assessment is essential before and after initial treatment. High kinetic energy injuries with resultant comminution may require external fixation to affect and maintain a satisfactory alignment.

Ulnar Styloid. Fractures of the ulnar styloid may accompany distal radius fractures or be seen in isolation. Distal fractures or avulsions can be followed conservatively if there is distal radioulnar stability.[16] Ulnar styloid basal fractures can be destabilizing to the ulnar carpus because the TFCC originates there. If the fracture is symptomatic and unstable, it may require open reduction and internal fixation or bony excision with reattachment of the TFC to the ulnar stump.

Cartilage. Injuries to the cartilaginous surfaces of the wrist are difficult to image even with modern techniques such as magnetic resonance imaging because of tissue resolution limitations. Arthroscopy has become the most reliable way to visualize the injury and can be used for management via debridement (Fig. 20-20).[34] It has been reported that more than 50% of patients with chronic wrist pain treated using arthroscopy will demonstrate cartilage lesions.[84]

The athlete may complain of a traumatic injury with persistent pain or recurrent locking. Symptoms consistent

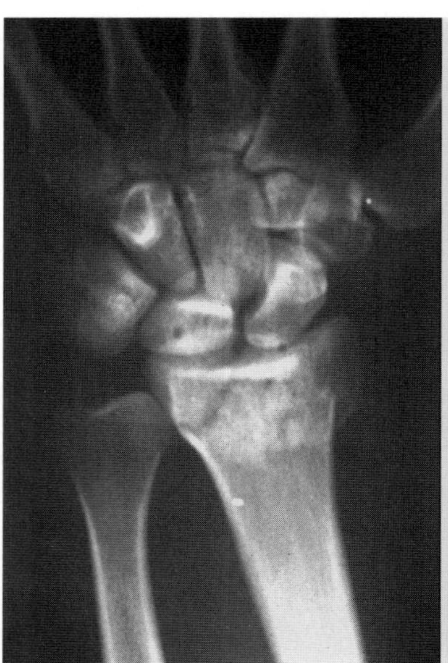

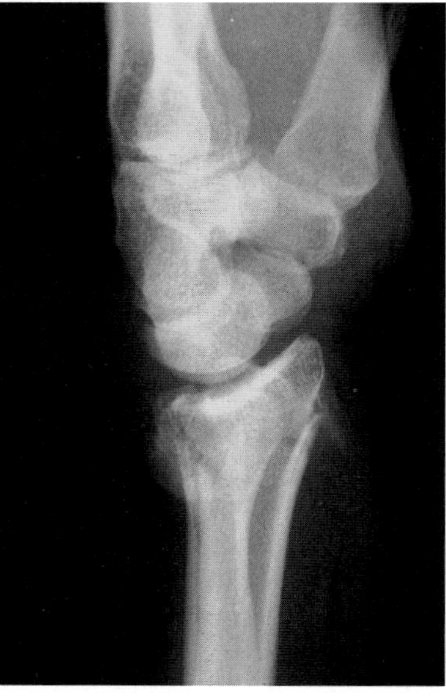

FIGURE 20-19. Intraarticular fracture of distal radius after a fall while playing basketball.

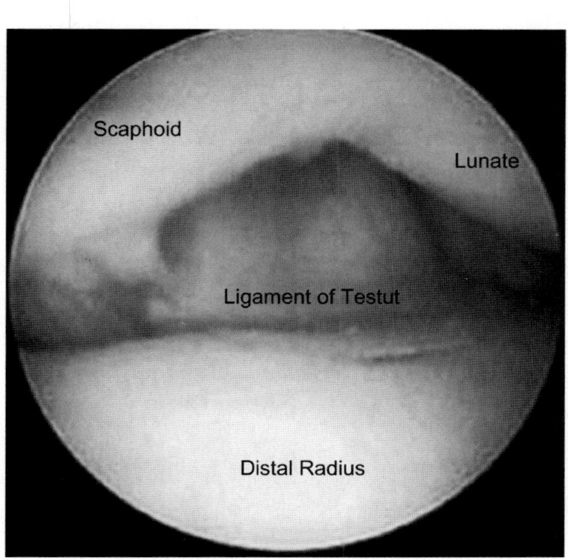

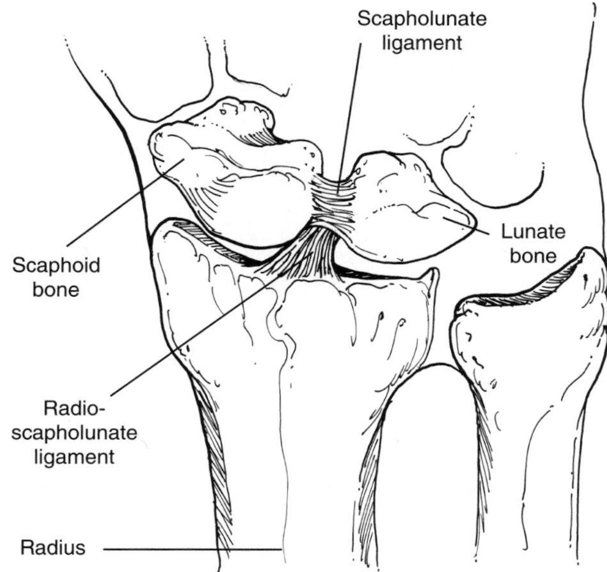

FIGURE 20-20. Arthroscopic view of radiocarpal articulation; note the intact scapholunate ligament in this patient.

with inflammation or synovitis may linger. It is important to carefully obtain a history from these patients to identify those who may have an intraarticular process consistent with an acute injury or even chronic chondromalacia.

Perilunate and Lunate Dislocation. It is important not to overlook the perilunate dislocation. Typically, a patient falls violently and sprains his or her wrist. A brief glance at the radiographs does not show a bony abnormality. But if viewed carefully, there is a dorsal dislocation of the capitate from the lunate on the lateral projection. This injury is serious, and open or closed reduction is mandatory.[2]

Hyperextension with severe loading of the wrist may cause this palmar lunate dislocation or perilunate dislocation with or without an associated scaphoid fracture (trans-scaphoid perilunate dislocation) (Fig. 20-21). These injuries should be considered as a continuum caused by the same mechanism of injury.[45] They must be addressed surgically by reduction and internal fixation.

Radioulnar. Radioulnar dislocation can result from a significant TFCC tear. This dislocation is discussed under acute ligament trauma. Proper management includes reduction and maintenance of position by immobilization or surgical repair.

Carpal Tunnel Syndrome. The carpal tunnel is a conduit for the finger flexors and median nerve. Because of its limited space, it is a common site of nerve entrapment.[4] Athletes develop carpal tunnel complaints because of repetitive wrist and hand usage. Likewise, in an anatomic variant, the lumbrical muscles may be more proximally situated in the carpal tunnel, creating a mass effect. Median nerve compression has been reported in racquetball players,[37] golfers, and rock climbers.[69] The features include intermittent numbness and paresthesias in the palmar aspect of the radial three and one-half fingers. Symptoms are exacerbated by activity and may include night pain, paresthesia, or numbness.[58] The Tinel (irritation) and Phalen (compression) signs are frequently positive. More advanced findings are persistent sensory changes and thenar weakness or atrophy. Nerve conduction studies help to quantify the degree of nerve impairment. Electromyography assists in documenting motor involvement.

It is reasonable to attempt conservative measures in mild cases. Rest, splints, and anti-inflammatory medications can be effective. Chronic or more severe disease is definitively managed with surgical release. Open carpal tunnel release may have fewer complications than endoscopic release and allows for excision of inflamed or hypertrophic synovium when indicated.

Ulnar Tunnel Syndrome. The ulnar nerve can be traumatized by direct repetitive pressure or trauma. The primary symptom is numbness and tingling on the palmar aspect of the ulnar one and one-half fingers. Cyclists may develop a "handle-bar palsy"[21,72] by chronic pressure on the ulnar nerve as it traverses Guyon's canal. Nerve conduction velocities and electromyography identify the sensory and motor components of the nerve injury. Symptoms should resolve with inactivity. Padding of the handlebars or gloves will help protect the nerve from repeated insults.[65]

Nerve Contusion. Actual nerve contusions occur primarily on the wrist dorsum. Athletes involved in contact sports

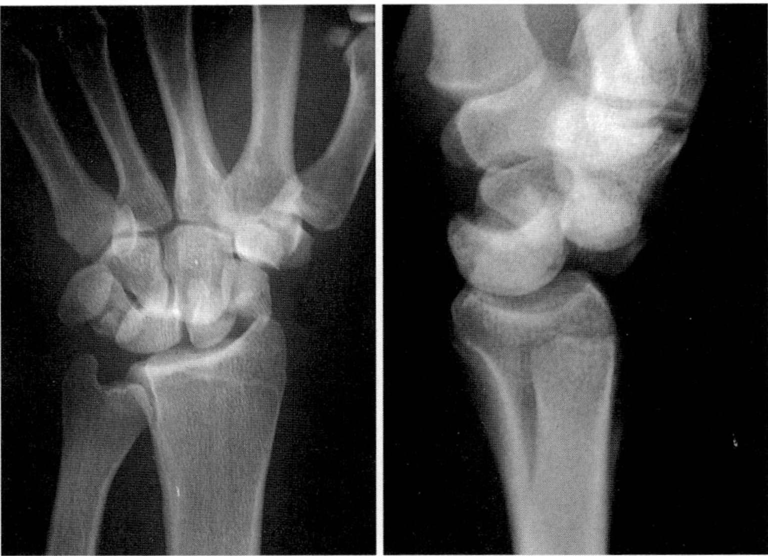

FIGURE 20-21. Severe injury of the wrist defined as having a perilunate dislocation (best viewed in the lateral projection) compounded with a scaphoid waist fracture.

suffer these injuries. Blunt trauma directed over the sensory branches of the radial or ulnar nerve causes paresthesias in their respective distributions, which is usually transient. Persistent paresthesia or pain over the dorsoradial or dorsoulnar aspect of the hand warrants immediate follow-up evaluation, with possible requirement for exploration.

Ulnar Artery. The ulnar artery is vulnerable to injury at Guyon's canal. At that level, there is very little palmar soft tissue to protect the artery (Fig. 20-22). The palmar fascia does not cover the hypothenar area, leaving the palmaris brevis, if present, as the only true protection. Cyclists, handball players, and racquet sport participants sustain significant blunt trauma directly over the artery.

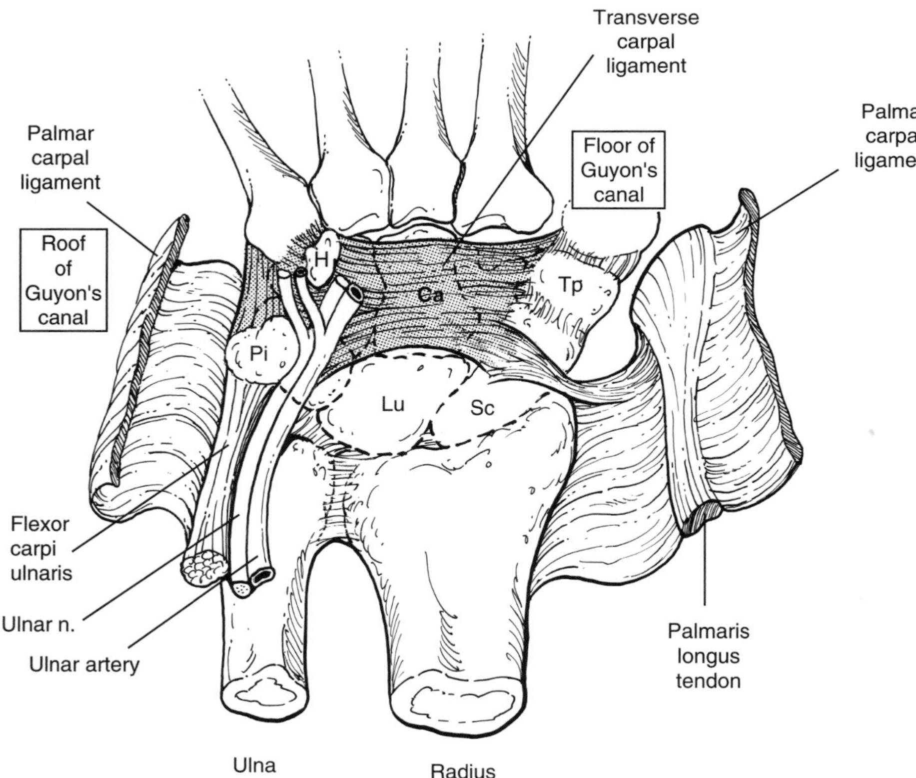

FIGURE 20-22. The ulnar nerve and artery traverse Guyon's canal. There is a bony protection on the radial (hamate) and ulnar (pisiform) aspects, but only soft-tissue protection (volar carpal ligament) palmarly.

Patients present with pain and possible ulnar nerve symptoms.[5] Raynaud's phenomenon, cold intolerance, and ischemic changes in the ulnar fingers may be documented.[11] Also, a pulsatile mass or bruit may be present if there is an aneurysm.

Thrombosis, aneurysm,[31] or vascular spasm can occur. Results of the Allen test may be positive in these patients.[60] Angiographic studies confirm the diagnosis. Suitable management is usually resection of the involved segment of artery, if hemodynamically tolerated. Otherwise, the condition demands some form of vascular reconstruction.

Ganglion Cyst. A ganglion cyst is the most common soft-tissue mass found about the wrist. It can be a source of recurrent discomfort.[86] Patients will complain of an enlarging, mobile mass on the wrist dorsum. In contact sports, it may rupture and then slowly return. Occasionally, the cyst will be less prominent but cause significant tenderness. Sometimes it will occur palmarly, adjacent to the radial artery. The cyst originates from synovial tissue and is filled with a gelatinous substance. The dorsal scapholunate ligament is the most common origin for the dorsal ganglion and the radioscaphoid joint is most common for the volar ganglion.

Management will vary according to the symptoms and size of the cyst. Extremely large or symptomatic ganglion cysts can be carefully excised. This may be performed either with a traditional open technique or with the less invasive wrist arthroscope.[53] Otherwise, they can be observed or aspirated, although there is a high recurrence rate with aspiration.

Carpometacarpal Bossing. Often seen in middle-aged women, carpometacarpal bossing is usually a painless firm mass over the hand dorsum at the base of the index metacarpal. It corresponds to osteophyte formation around the joint as a consequence of tendon insertion pull[14] or arthritis. Often, this "mass" is confused with other dorsal wrist lesions, such as the ganglion cyst, but it is more firm and immobile. Painless lesions can be observed. Painful lesions can be injected first, and then managed with excision of the spurring and joint debridement. If that fails, carpometacarpal arthrodesis should be considered.

Arthrosis and Chondromalacia. "Racquet player's pisiform" has been described[30]; it occurs in racquet sports participants. Patients complain of ulnar-sided wrist pain associated with firm grip and twisting while using the racquet. Tenderness can be localized over the pisiform bone in the hypothenar eminence. It is postulated that there is abnormal movement of the pisiform in relation to the trapezium. Cineradiography may confirm the abnormal motion. Early management is rest and administration of anti-inflammatory medications followed by surgical excision for refractory cases.[56]

Avascular Necrosis. Avascular necrosis may affect individual carpal bones. The etiology of such entities is unclear; however, repetitive trauma or loading may have a role. The scaphoid, lunate, and capitate are particularly susceptible to avascular necrosis. The blood supply to these bones is as abundant as to any other. The problem is that inflow is limited to a few vessels. Depending on the sport, the wrist is subject to significant loading, which can create stress fractures, thereby damaging the blood supply.[50]

Avascular necrosis of the lunate, or Kienböck disease, is the most common osteochondrosis seen in the general population. A slightly shortened ulna relative to the radius is a predisposing factor.[25] Avascular necrosis of the capitate is rare, although it has been reported in gymnasts.[49] Preiser's disease (scaphoid avascular necrosis) is very rare and not related to athletics.

Generally, these patients will complain of pain and stiffness, resulting from chronic synovitis. Swelling may be present, and point tenderness may be localized over the affected bone. Management for these lesions is varied and beyond the scope of this chapter. The concept is to avoid activity that will destroy the normal structure of the weakened, avascular bone and allow it to heal. Persistent pain or loss of normal architecture warrants reconstructive procedures.

SUMMARY

Clearly, wrist injury occurs in many athletic activities. When evaluating an athlete with wrist pain, it is important to understand the complex anatomy. Grasping the history and mechanism of injury will aid in classifying the problem. Most conditions result from overuse and can be managed conservatively. The key to appropriate management is the correct diagnosis. If a careful history and meticulous physical examination are complemented by specific modern imaging techniques, diagnoses that are more specific than "wrist sprain" will allow the provider and athlete to understand and treat this complex area, the wrist.

REFERENCES

1. Amadio PC: Epidemiology of hand and wrist injuries in sports. Hand Clin 6(3):379–381, 1990.
2. Amadio PC, Taleisnik J: Fractures of the carpal bones. In Green DP (ed): Operative Hand Surgery. New York, Churchill Livingstone, 1993.
3. Ambrose J, Goldstone R: Anomalous extensor digiti minimi proprius causing tunnel syndrome in the dorsal compartment. J Bone Joint Surg 57A:706–707, 1975.
4. Aulicino PL: Neurovascular injuries in the hands of athletes. Hand Clin 6(3):455–466, 1990.

5. Axe MJ, McClain EJ: Complete involvement of the ulnar nerve secondary to an ulnar artery aneurysm. Am J Sports Med 14:178–180, 1986.
6. Beckenbaugh RD: Accurate evaluation and management of the painful wrist following injury. Orthop Clin North Am 15:289–305, 1984.
7. Bishop AT, Gabel G, Carmichael SW: Flexor carpi radialis tendinitis. Part I: Operative anatomy. J Bone Joint Surg 76A(7):1009–1014, 1994.
8. Blatt G: Dorsal capsulodesis for rotary subluxation of the scaphoid. In Gelberman R (ed): Master Techniques in Orthopedic Surgery. The Wrist. New York, Raven Press, 1994.
9. Brown DE, Lichtman DM: The evaluation of chronic wrist pain. Orthop Clin North Am 15: 183–192, 1984.
10. Burton RI: Overview for athletic upper extremity injuries. AAOS Instr Course Lect 34:297–299, 1985.
11. Conn J Jr, Bergan JJ, Bell JL: Hypothenar hammer syndrome: Posttraumatic digital ischemia. Surgery 68:122–128, 1970.
12. Culver JE: Instabilities of the wrist. Clin Sports Med 5(4):725, 1986.
13. Culver JE, Anderson TE: Fractures of the hand and wrist in the athlete. Clin Sports Med 11:101, 1992.
14. Cuono CB, Watson HK: The carpal boss: Surgical treatment and etiological considerations. Plast Reconstr Surg 63:88, 1979.
15. Davis CA, Culp RW, Hume EL, Osterman AL: Reconstruction of the scapholunate ligament in a cadaver model using a bone-ligament-bone autograft from the foot. J Hand Surg 23:884, 1998.
16. Dell PC: Traumatic disorders of the distal radioulnar joint. Clin Sports Med 11:141–159, 1992.
17. Dobyns JH, Gabel GT: Gymnast's wrist. Hand Clin 6(3):493–505, 1990.
18. Dobyns JH, Sim FH, Linscheid RL: Sports stress syndromes of the hand and wrist. Am J Sports Med 6:236–253, 1978.
19. Ekenstam FW, Palmer AK, Glisson RR: The load on the radius and ulna at different positions of the wrist and forearm: A cadaver study. Acta Orthop Scand 55:363–365, 1984.
20. Finklestein H: Stenosing tendovaginitis at the radial styoid process. J Bone Joint Surg 12A:509, 1930.
21. Finelli PF: Handlebar palsy. N Engl J Med 292:702, 1975.
22. Fitton JM, Shea FW, Goldie W: Lesions of the flexor carpi radialis tendon and sheath causing pain in the wrist. J Bone Joint Surg 50:359–363, 1968.
23. Gabel G, Bishop AT, Wood MB: Flexor carpi radialis tendinitis. Part II: Results of operative treatment. J Bone Joint Surg 76A(7):1015–1018, 1994.
24. Gelberman RH, Panagis JS, Taleisnik J, et al: The arterial anatomy of the human carpus I: The extraosseous vascularity. J Hand Surg 8:367, 1983.
25. Gelberman RH, Salamon PB, Jurist JM, Posch JL: Ulnar variance in Kienböck's disease. J Hand Surg 5:272–278, 1980.
26. Kleinman W: Carpal dislocations and instabilities. In Green DP (ed): Operative Hand Surgery. New York, Churchill Livingstone, 1993.
27. Green DP: The sore wrist without a fracture. AAOS Instr Course Lect 34:300–313, 1985.
28. Grundberg AB, Reagan DS: Pathologic anatomy of the forearm: Intersection syndrome. J Hand Surg 10:299–302, 1985.
29. Hanks GA, Kalenak A, Bowman LS, Sebaestianelli WJ: Stress fractures of the carpal scaphoid: A report of four cases. J Bone Joint Surg 71A:938–941, 1989.
30. Helal B: Racquet player's pisiform. Hand 10(1): 87–90, 1978.
31. Ho PK, Dellon AL, Wilgis EFS: True aneurysms of the hand resulting from athletic injury. Am J Sports Med 13:136–137, 1985.
32. Kauer JMG: The mechanism of the carpal joint. Clin Orthop 202:16–26, 1986.
33. Kiefhaber TR, Stern PJ: Upper extremity tendinitis and overuse syndromes in the athlete. Clin Sports Med 11(1):39–55, 1992.
34. Koman LA, Mooney JF III, Poehling GG: Fractures and ligamentous injuries of the wrist. Hand Clin 6(3):477–491, 1990.
35. Kushner SH, Gellman H, Bindiger A: Extensor digitorum brevis manus—an unusual cause of exercise induced wrist pain. Am J Sports Med 17:440–441, 1989.
36. Knirk JL, Jupiter JB: Intra-articular fractures of the distal radius in young adults. J Bone Joint Surg 68A:647, 1986.
37. Layfer LF, Jones JV: Hand paresthesias after racquetball. Ill Med J 152:190, 1977.
38. Lichtman DM, Schneider JR, Swafford AR, et al: Ulnar midcarpal instability—clinical and laboratory analysis. J Hand Surg 6:515, 1981.
39. Linscheid RL, Dobyns JH: Athletic injuries of the wrist. Clin Orthop 198:141–151, 1985.
40. Lipton CB, Ugwonali OF, Sarwahi V, Chao JD, Rosenwasser MP: The treatment of chronic scapholunate dissociation with reduction and association of the scaphoid and lunate (RASL). Atlas Hand Clin 8:95, 2003.
41. Mandlebaum BR, Bartolozzi AR, Davis CA, et al: Wrist pain syndrome in the gymnast. Am J Sports Med 17(3):305–317, 1989.
42. Manzione M, Pizzutillo PD: Stress fracture of the scaphoid waist. Am J Sports Med 9:268–269, 1981.

43. Markiewitz AD, Andrish JT: Hand and wrist injuries in the preadolescent and adolescent athlete. Clin Sports Med 11(1):203–225, 1992.
44. Markoff KL, Shapiro MS, Mandlebaum BR, Teurlings L: Wrist loading patterns during pommel horse exercises. J Biomech 23:1001–1011, 1990.
45. Mayfield JK, Johnson RP, Kilcoyne RF: Carpal dislocations, pathomechanics, and progressive perilunar instability. J Hand Surg 5:226, 1980.
46. McCue FC III, Bruce JF Jr: Chapter 18. In DeLee JC, Drez Jr D (eds): The Wrist in Orthopaedic Sports Medicine. Philadelphia, WB Saunders, 1994.
47. Melone CP Jr, Nathan R: Traumatic disruption of the triangular fibrocartilage complex. Clin Orthop 275:65–73, 1992.
48. Mirabello SC, Loeb PE, Andrews JR: The wrist: Field evaluation and treatment. Clin Sports Med 11(1):1–25, 1992.
49. Murakami S, Nakajima H: Aseptic necrosis of the capitate bone. Am J Sports Med 12(2):170–173, 1984.
50. Nakamura R, Imaeda T, Suzuki K, Miura T: Sports-related Kienböck's disease. Am J Sports Med 19:88–91, 1991.
51. O'Neil DB, Micheli LJ: Overuse injuries in the young athlete. Clin Sports Med 7(3):591–610, 1988.
52. Osterman AL, Moskow L, Low DW: Soft-tissue injuries of the hand and wrist in racquet sports. Clin Sports Med 7(2):329–348, 1988.
53. Osterman AL, Raphael J: Arthroscopic resection of dorsal ganglion of the wrist. Hand Clin 11:7, 1995.
54. Palmer AK, Werner FW: The triangular fibrocartilage complex of the wrist—anatomy and function. J Hand Surg 6:153, 1981.
55. Palmer DH, Lane-Larsen CL: Helicopter skiing wrist injuries. A case report of "bugaboo forearm." Am J Sports Med 22(1):148–149, 1994.
56. Palmieri TJ: Pisiform area pain treatment by pisiform excision. J Hand Surg 7:477–480, 1982.
57. Parker RD, Berkowitz MS, Brahms MA, et al: Hook of the hamate fractures in athletes. Am J Sports Med 14:517, 1986.
58. Phalen GS: The carpal tunnel syndrome: seventeen years experience in diagnosis and treatment of 654 hands. J Bone Joint Surg 48A:211–228, 1966.
59. Pitner MA: Pathophysiology of overuse injuries in the hand and wrist. Hand Clin 6(3):355–364, 1990.
60. Porubsky GL, Brown SI, Urbaniak JR: Ulnar artery thrombosis: A sports related injury. Am J Sports Med 14:170–175, 1986.
61. Primiano GA, Lee RL: Sports related distal upper extremity injuries. Orthop Rev 13(9):61, 1984.
62. Rayan GM: Recurrent dislocation of the extensor carpi ulnaris in athletes. Am J Sports Med 11(3):183, 1983.
63. Reagan DS, Linscheid RL, Dobyns JH: Lunotriquetral sprains. J Hand Surg 9A:502–514, 1984.
64. Reister JN, Baker BE, Mosher JF, Lowe D: A review of scaphoid healing in competitive athletes. Am J Sports Med 13:159–161, 1985.
65. Rettig AC: Neurovascular injuries in the wrists and hands of athletes. Clin Sports Med 9:389–418, 1990.
66. Rowland SA: Acute traumatic subluxation of the extensor carpi ulnaris tendon at the wrist. J Hand Surg 11A:809–811, 1986.
67. Roy S, Caine D, Singer KM: Stress changes of the distal radial epiphysis in young gymnasts. Am J Sports Med 13(5):301–308, 1985.
68. Russe O: Fracture of the carpal navicular. J Bone Joint Surg 47A:759, 1960.
69. Shea KG, Shea OF, Meals RA: Manual demands and consequences of rock climbing. J Hand Surg 17A(2):200–205, 1992.
70. Silko GJ, Cullen PT: Indoor racquet sports injuries. Am Fam Phys 50(2):374–380, 383–384, 1994.
71. Slade JF 3rd, Gutow AP, Geissler WB: Percutaneous internal fixation of scaphoid fractures via an arthroscopically assisted dorsal approach. J Bone Joint Surg Am 84-A Suppl 2:21, 2002.
72. Smail DF: Handlebar palsy. N Engl J Med 292:322, 1975.
73. Stark HH, Jobe FW, Boyes JH, et al: Fracture of the hook of the hamate in athletes. J Bone Joint Surg 59A:575–582, 1977.
74. Stein F, Miale A Jr, Stein A: Enhanced diagnosis of hand and wrist disorders by triple phase radionuclide bone imaging. Bull Hosp Joint Dis 44:477, 1984.
75. Stern PJ: Tendinitis, overuse syndromes, and tendon injuries. Hand Clin 6(3):467–476, 1990.
76. Szabo RM, Slater RR Jr, Palumbo CF, Gerlach T: Dorsal intercarpal ligament capsulodesis for chronic, static scapholunate dissociation: Clinical results. J Hand Surg 27:978, 2002.
77. Taleisnik J: The ligaments of the wrist. J Hand Surg 1:110–118, 1976.
78. Taleisnik J: Wrist: Anatomy, function, and injury. AAOS Instr Course Lect 27:61–87, 1978.
79. Tolat AR, Sanderson PL, De Smet L, Stanley JK: The gymnast's wrist: Acquired positive ulnar variance following chronic epiphyseal injury. J Hand Surg 17B(6):678–681, 1992.
80. Vender MI, Watson HK: Acquired Madelung-like deformity in a gymnast. J Hand Surg 13A(1):19–21, 1988.
81. Watson HK, Ashmead DIV, Makhloof MU: Examination of the scaphoid. J Hand Surg 13A:657, 1988.

82. Watson HK, Ryn J, Akelman E: Limited triscaphoid intercarpal arthrodesis for rotary subluxation of the scaphoid. J Bone Joint Surg 68:345–349, 1986.
83. Weiss AP: Scapholunate ligament reconstruction using a bone-retinaculum-bone autograft. J Hand Surg 23(2):205, 1998.
84. Whipple TL: The role of arthroscopy in the treatment of wrist injuries in the athlete. Clin Sports Med 11:227–238, 1992.
85. Wilson RL, McGinty LD: Common hand and wrist injuries in basketball players. Clin Sports Med 12(2):265–291, 1993.
86. Wood MB, Dobyns JH: Sports-related extra-articular wrist syndromes. Clin Orthop 202:93–102, 1986.

21 The Hand

Martin A. Posner

By virtue of its dominant role in many sports activities, the hand is vulnerable to a wide variety of injuries. Most involve abrasions, contusions, and minor skin lacerations, which generally do not seriously affect the athletes' ability to continue sports participation. However, every injury should be evaluated because of the possibility of a more serious injury to underlying structures. The involvement of athletic trainers and therapists is important in this regard because they often provide the initial evaluation, particularly with injuries in organized sports at the high school and college level. This chapter will discuss the primary care of injuries to muscle–tendon units, ligaments, and bones.

MUSCLE–TENDON INJURIES

A muscle–tendon injury is a strain that results either from a single forceful contraction of the muscle against resistance (overexertion) or a sudden stretch of the muscle beyond its normal extensile range (overstretching). A muscle injury can also be caused by direct trauma, such as a sharp blow to the extremity. The muscles in the upper arm and forearm are most frequently injured in this fashion, although the intrinsic hand muscles can be similarly injured because closed trauma to the dorsal aspect of the hand is common. When trauma to the hand is severe, there may be hemorrhage within an intrinsic muscle(s), which can lead to fibrosis and contracture. Early recognition is important, and as soon as the acute swelling subsides, stretching exercises are encouraged to restore the injured muscle(s) to its normal length. To accomplish this, the joints are moved in directions opposite from the normal action of the intrinsic muscles, which flexes the metacarpophalangeal joints and extends the interphalangeal joints. The exercises are done in either of two methods: the metacarpophalangeal joint is passively held in extension and the proximal interphalangeal joint is actively and passively flexed, or both interphalangeal joints are maintained in complete flexion, usually with the aid of an elastic strap wrapped around the proximal and distal segments of the finger, and the metacarpophalangeal joint is actively and passively extended.

Regarding strains, the most frequently injured sites are the muscle belly, its musculotendinous junction, or the tendon at its bony insertion. Rarely is the tendon itself damaged unless it is diseased, as may occur when chronically inflamed. Overexertion injuries commonly affect the extrinsic muscles in the upper arm and forearm or the intrinsic muscles in the hand with activities that involve forceful and sustained gripping, such as required when playing golf or tennis. Overstretching injuries are generally confined to the extrinsic muscles. Regardless of etiology, all strains are categorized as first, second, or third degree.

A first-degree or mild strain does not compromise strength or mobility of the muscle–tendon unit. Although there may be some localized tenderness and swelling, there is rarely any ecchymoses. Management is primarily symptomatic, consisting of application of cold compresses and rest. Recovery can be expected within a few days.

A second-degree or moderate strain indicates actual damage to the muscle–tendon unit, usually a partial tear of the muscle or a partial tear of its musculotendinous junction. Generally, there is greater swelling and ecchymoses, and there is more pain with contraction of the affected muscle–tendon unit than with a first-degree injury. Differentiating between first- and second-degree strains can sometimes be difficult, and if there is any doubt about the diagnosis, it is prudent to manage the injury as the more severe second-degree injury. It is important to protect the injured muscle–tendon unit from further damage, which can best be accomplished by splint immobilization. For a sprain of a wrist muscle, tension on the muscle is relieved by splinting the wrist joint in either slight flexion or extension, depending on whether the injury is to a flexor or extensor muscle. The splint is extended to include the fingers or thumb when the injury involves the digits. Sports activities should be avoided until pain and swelling subside and strength of the injured muscle has been restored. Healing usually takes several weeks. Second-degree strains rarely leave any sequelae, provided that care is taken to prevent any additional damage to the injured muscle–tendon unit.

A third-degree or severe strain indicates rupture of some part of the muscle–tendon unit. Except for ruptures of the distal end of the biceps, third-degree strains are rare in the forearm. In the hand, however, they commonly involve the terminal extensor tendons at their insertion into the bases of the distal phalanges, the central extensor tendons over the proximal interphalangeal joints, and the flexor profundi tendons at their insertion into the distal phalanges.

Terminal Extensor Tendon

Ruptures of the terminal extensor tendons are exceedingly common injuries in sports requiring catching or hitting a ball with one's hand (i.e., football, basketball, baseball, and volleyball). Typically, the end of the finger is struck by the ball, which forces the distal interphalangeal joint into acute flexion. Most are closed injuries, and the tendon either tears or it avulses from the distal phalanx with a bony fragment. Swelling and tenderness over the dorsum of the joint may be minimal, but some loss of joint extension will usually be obvious. The flexed deformity of the distal segment is frequently referred to as a "mallet finger" or "baseball finger," although "drop finger" is probably a more accurate and descriptive term.[1] The tendon retracts and a swan-neck deformity with hyperextension at the proximal interphalangeal joint can sometimes develop, particularly in loose jointed individuals. When severe, the deformity can significantly affect function of the finger.

Although terminal extensor tendon injuries are frequently dismissed as trivial, and most are, radiographs of the injured finger are necessary because of the possibility that the distal phalanx has subluxated volarly. A subluxation can develop from two types of injuries. The first type, which is more common, occurs when the terminal extensor tendon avulses with a fracture fragment that is so large that not only is the tendon attached to it, but also most of the collateral ligaments. These ligaments not only provide lateral stability to the joint, they also provide dorsal stability. The second type of injury follows a hyperextension injury to the distal joint that causes a compression fracture to the dorsal aspect of articular surface of the distal phalanx, usually more than 50% of the articular surface. Regardless of etiology, a volar subluxation should be reduced and the distal phalanx stabilized in its correct position with a transarticular 0.032-inch Kirschner wire.[63] Failure to restore articular congruity is likely to lead to degenerative arthritis, which can be disabling. A large avulsion fracture fragment is also reduced and fixed with either a Kirschner wire or wire suture.

Because the majority of terminal extensor injuries do not result in any volar subluxation of the distal phalanx, surgery is rarely necessary, and management involves splinting the distal interphalangeal joint in extension for 6 to 8 weeks. The splint should never be applied in a manner that hyperextends the distal joint and causes the dorsal skin to blanch because it can lead to ulceration. This is most likely to occur immediately after the injury when soft-tissue swelling is most severe. Either a volar or dorsal splint can be used, although a dorsal splint is preferred because the tactile surface of the finger remains free (Fig. 21-1). A dorsal splint is also easier to change while keeping the distal joint extended. Maintaining constant extension is important because allowing the joint to flex, even for a moment, damages any tendon healing that has occurred. The athlete should be instructed in the proper technique of changing the splint without inadvertently flexing the distal joint. By pressing the fingertip down on a tabletop, the distal joint will remain extended and the proximal interphalangeal joint will be flexed, providing access to both sides of the finger. In some athletes, particularly professionals whose performance is not compromised by the injury, such as football linemen, it may be unrealistic to expect that they wear the extension splint for many weeks. In these individuals, the joint should be splinted, but only for 1 to 2 weeks, to permit some scarring to develop, which will reduce the risk that the extension lag will worsen. In selected cases, a Kirschner wire can be drilled across the joint in a percutaneous manner to hold it in extension. The proximal interphalangeal joint should never be immobilized, and active range of motion should be encouraged to prevent it from becoming stiff.

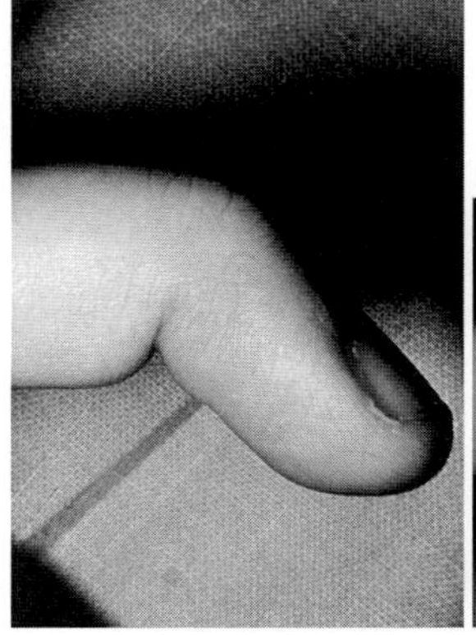

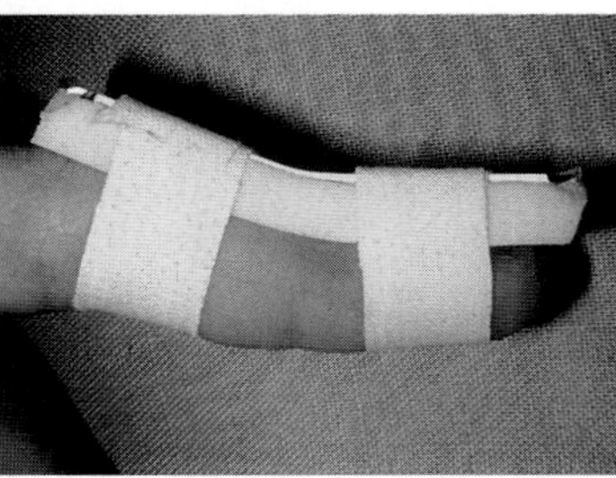

A B

FIGURE 21-1. A, Acute injury to the terminal extensor tendon resulted in a 65° "drop" finger deformity, managed **B,** with a dorsal extension splint.

Central Extensor Tendon

Injuries to the central tendon over the proximal interphalangeal joint, although not as common as injuries to the terminal extensor tendon, result in more disabling problems. They are caused either by direct trauma to the tendon or by sudden forced flexion of the joint. The central tendon tears, and the head of the proximal phalanx protrudes through the lateral bands, which slip volarly and surround the bone, similar to the edges of a buttonhole surrounding a button. This is the reason the condition is called a boutonnière deformity. (In France, it has been curiously Anglicized and is referred to as a *buttonhole deformité.*)

Initially, there may be a paucity of clinical signs, and active extension of the joint may be only minimally restricted, if at all. The diagnosis requires a careful physical examination, and an index of suspicion is often helpful. Because the entire joint is usually painful, localizing the area of maximum tenderness is important. If the examination is done in a slow and careful manner, it can usually be determined if the injury is located dorsally over the base of the middle phalanx where the central extensor tendon inserts, over the tendon itself, laterally over one of the collateral ligaments, or volarly. Although any loss of joint mobility should not be ignored, a loss of extension at the proximal interphalangeal joint is not by itself pathognomonic of a central tendon injury. It may indicate damage to the joint capsule (collateral ligament or volar plate), which is a more common injury and from which it must be differentiated. A capsular injury will affect motions limited to the proximal interphalangeal joint, but an injury to the central tendon will likely affect mobility at both interphalangeal joints. Usually, there will be some limitation of active and passive flexion at the distal joint, even if displacement of the lateral bands over the proximal interphalangeal joint is minimal.[47] Therefore, observing flexion at the distal interphalangeal joint is important in differentiating an injury confined to the capsule of the proximal interphalangeal joint, sometimes referred to as a pseudoboutonniere deformity, from an injury to the central extensor tendon, which may also involve the capsule of the joint (Fig. 21-2). Results of radiographs are usually negative unless the central tendon avulses with a fragment from the dorsal base of the middle phalanx, which is a rare occurrence.

Management in the absence of an avulsion fragment is splinting the proximal interphalangeal joint in extension. If there is no loss of extension or only a slight loss, but the dorsal aspect of the joint is tender, an extension splint should still be used. Any suspicion that the central tendon has been injured requires that the joint be splinted in extension. It is better to needlessly splint a finger, reexamine the patient in one week, and discontinue the splint if there is no tenderness or loss of mobility than to incorrectly dismiss an injury as trivial and have the athlete return weeks later with fixed joint contractures. When swelling is severe, it may be impossible to splint the proximal interphalangeal joint in full extension. In such cases, the joint is splinted in as much extension as

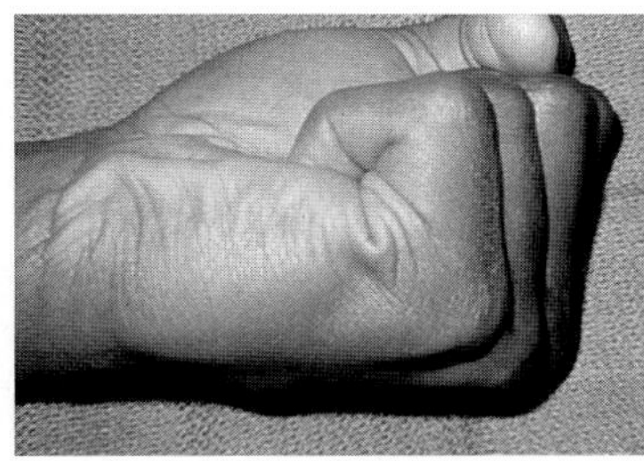

A

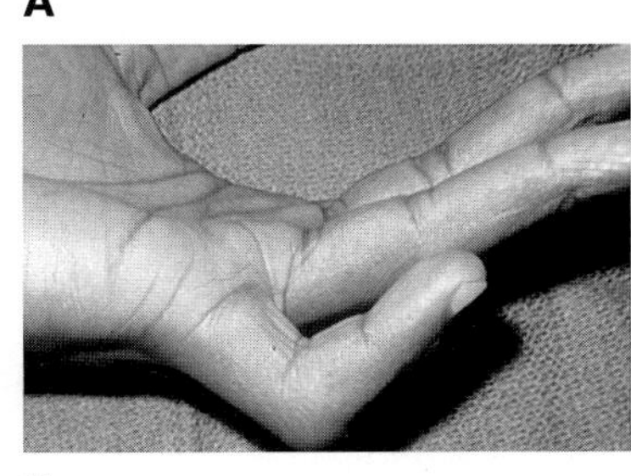

B

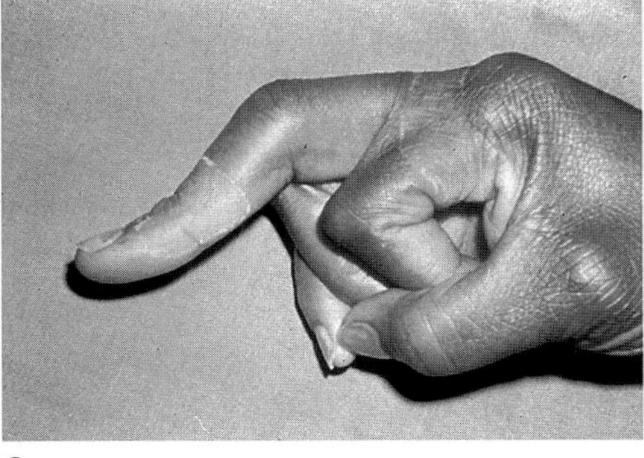

C

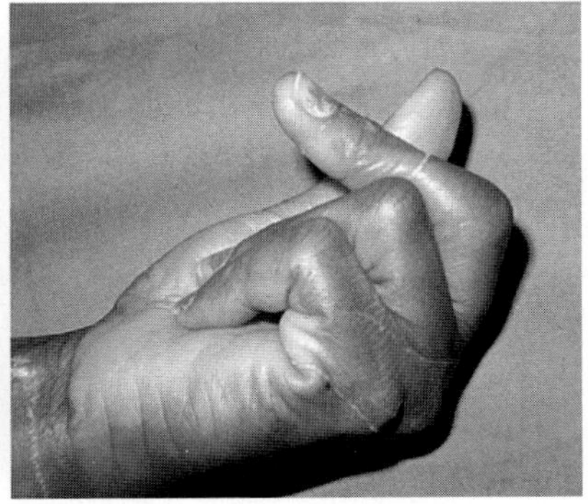

D

FIGURE 21-2. A and **B,** A pseudoboutonniere deformity resulting from scarring of the volar plate. Because there was no damage to the dorsal extensor tendon mechanism, active flexion at the distal interphalangeal joint was not affected. **C** and **D,** A boutonnière deformity. The key to the diagnosis was the position of the distal interphalangeal joint. Not only was active flexion of the joint limited, it was hyperextended in the resting position.

possible without causing the patient any undue discomfort. As swelling subsides, which may take a week, the splint is changed to achieve full joint extension. Extension splinting is maintained for 3 to 4 weeks, followed by intermittent splinting for an additional 2 to 3 weeks, during which time active range of motion exercises are encouraged. While splinted, the distal interphalangeal joint is left free to permit active and passive flexion to prevent contractures of the oblique retinacular ligaments (Fig. 21-3). In the rare case that the extensor tendon avulsed with a bone fragment, surgery is necessary to reinsert the fragment. This can best be achieved with a wire suture.

Flexor Profundus Avulsion

Avulsion of a flexor profundus tendon is a severe overstretch injury that occurs when the muscle contracts forcefully against strong resistance. It typically occurs when a sudden extension force is applied to a finger that is tightly gripping an object. Classically, these injuries are seen in the football or rugby player who, in an effort to stop or tackle an opponent, firmly grasps the opponent's jersey. The opponent struggles to pull away, and the athlete's finger gets caught in the jersey and is forcefully hyperextended. The flexor profundus tendon to the ring finger is the most commonly injured of all the profundi because the ring finger has the least amount of independent extension.[17] This lack of extension can easily be observed by placing one's palm and fingers on a flat surface and then extending each finger separately. The limited independent extension of the ring finger, which is often considered a hindrance by musicians, particularly pianists, results from the anatomic arrangement of the interconnections between the extensor tendons (the juncturae tendinae) on the dorsal aspect of the hand.[24,25] Two other theories have also been proposed to explain the propensity for rupture of the ring finger profundus: its insertion is slightly weaker than the insertions of the other profundi,[27] and when the metacarpophalangeal and proximal interphalangeal joints of the fingers are flexed with the distal interphalangeal joints extended, the ring finger is the "longest" finger and is, therefore, more exposed to be injured.[6]

Frequently, the seriousness of a profundus avulsion is not immediately apparent to the athlete because there is no obvious deformity as there is after an injury to the terminal extensor tendon. The athlete may not be aware of any inability to actively flex the distal phalanx until days or even weeks later. The clinical diagnosis of a profundus avulsion should not be difficult because it is the sole flexor of the distal interphalangeal joint. Immediately after the injury, the volar aspect of the finger is often ecchymotic, and there is tenderness at the base of the distal phalanx and over the retracted end of the tendon. The tendon can sometimes be palpated, usually in the digit and occasionally in the palm. Active flexion of the proximal interphalangeal joint may be limited if the end of the profundus retracts into the decussation of the flexor superficialis tendon. Radiographs of the injured finger are always necessary, but they can confuse an unsophisticated examiner. They may show a large avulsion fragment from the volar surface of the distal phalanx, which may distract from the more serious tendon injury, or if there is a small bony fragment that retracted with the tendon to the level of the proximal interphalangeal joint, it may be incorrectly interpreted as a chip fracture from that joint.[50]

Flexor profundus avulsions have been classified into three types.[25] In type 1 injuries, both long and short vincula have disrupted and the tendon retracts into the palm. Generally, this type of tendon avulsion is not associated with any avulsion fracture fragment. In type 2 injuries, the profundus has avulsed with a small bone

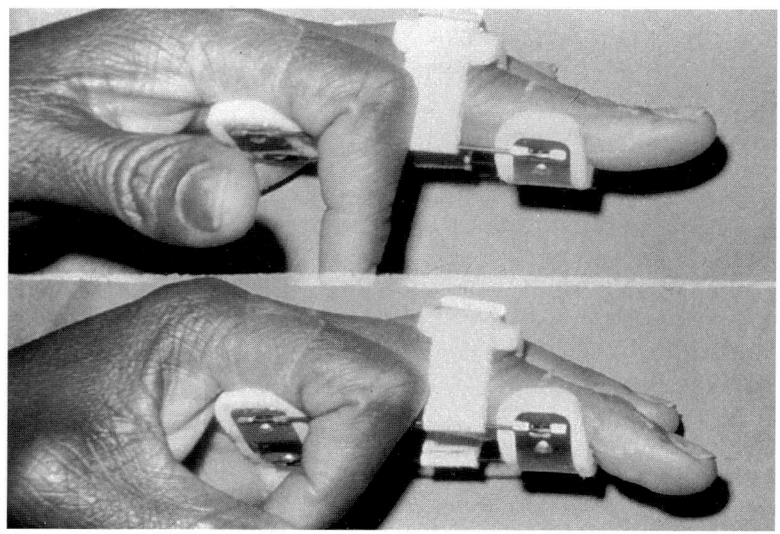

FIGURE 21-3. Proper splinting of an acute boutonnière deformity requires that the distal interphalangeal joint be left free to permit active and passive flexion. Usually, a molded splint fabricated by a hand therapist is substituted for this commercially available safety pin splint after the first week, when swelling has subsided.

fragment and retracted to the level of the proximal interphalangeal joint. The fragment, which can be easily visualized on a lateral radiograph, provides an excellent key to the location of the tendon end. A type 3 injury is associated with a large bony fragment, which is caught at the A4 pulley of the tendon sheath and is prevented from retracting further proximally. However, a profundus avulsion associated with a large bone fragment to which the tendon was no longer attached and retracted further proximally into the finger has been reported,[23] as well as a profundus avulsion combined with a comminuted fracture of the distal phalanx.[53]

Surgery is necessary for all acute flexor profundus ruptures. When swelling and ecchymosis are severe, surgery should be deferred until the soft-tissue reaction to the injury subsides, which is usually a few days. Any undue delay, which generally results from the athlete neglecting to seek immediate medical attention, can result in a secondary contracture of the muscle belly that precludes reinserting the avulsed tendon. Muscle contractures generally develop after 3 weeks, although they can occur earlier the more proximal the tendon retraction. Therefore, a type 1 injury in which the tendon has retracted into the palm should be repaired promptly, whereas a type 2 injury is not as urgent because the tendon retraction is less severe. Although surgery should still be carried out promptly for a type 2 injury, repair as late as 4 weeks after the injury may be feasible in cases when the diagnosis was delayed. For the type 3 injury, the large fracture fragment should be reduced and fixed, which will also restore function of the profundus tendon.

For a chronic profundus avulsion, surgery is necessary when function of the flexor superficialis tendon has been compromised by the retracted end of the ruptured profundus. A tendolysis is done in such cases, and the profundus tendon excised. When mobility of the proximal interphalangeal joint is complete, management of a chronic injury is either to accept the loss of flexion at the distal interphalangeal joint, which is justified if the patient has full function of the flexor superficialis tendon and the distal joint is stable (not hyperextensible), or if the distal joint is unstable, to arthrodese it in a functional position of slight flexion. Another management option for a chronic profundus avulsion is a tendon graft through the intact flexor superficialis tendon. However, this option, which may require a staged reconstruction with the preliminary insertion of a silicone rod, places the function of the intact superficialis tendon at significant risk. This risk should be understood by patient and physician. Generally, a tendon graft through an intact flexor superficialis is reserved for young patients in their teenage years or in the rare chronic rupture of a profundus to the little finger because the superficialis tendon of that finger is normally weak and usually does not provide sufficient power of flexion for many grasping activities.

LIGAMENT INJURIES

A sprain is an injury that occurs when a ligament is no longer capable of resisting a stress that is applied to it and fails. The magnitude of damage depends on the magnitude of the force and the duration of its application. Similar to muscle–tendon strains, ligament sprains are classified as first, second, or third degree.

A first-degree or mild sprain does not compromise the ligament's strength. It is generally unnecessary to protect the ligament from further damage, and only symptomatic care and rest are required. The athlete should be able to resume full sports activities within a few days. A second-degree or moderate sprain tears a portion of the ligament and may result in some functional impairment. Although the joint is stable, some laxity can usually be demonstrated when it is stressed. Management is primarily protective to avoid damage to the intact portion of the ligament. The joint is usually immobilized for several weeks, followed by active and resistive exercises to restore mobility and muscle strength. A third-degree or severe sprain is a complete tear of the ligament that usually occurs at either end of its attachments and it may be associated with an avulsion bone fragment. Ligaments that rupture within their substance are rare. Third-degree sprains indicate joint instability, and management depends on the ligament that is injured. However, there are two indications that surgery is required. The first is failure to restore articular congruity after closed reduction of a subluxation or dislocation, which would indicate that soft tissues are interposed within the joint, and the second is unstressed instability—the joint fails to remain in alignment with active motions, which indicates that there has been extensive tearing of capsular tissues.

Thumb

Carpometacarpal Joint (Trapeziometacarpal Joint). The trapeziometacarpal joint is commonly referred to as a "saddle" joint because of its unique configuration. Because of its wide range of motions in three planes (flexion–extension, abduction–adduction, and pronation–supination), it is the most important of the three thumb joints. Although the capsule of the trapeziometacarpal joint permits considerable mobility, it also provides stability, primarily by means of a short, thick ligament between the volar beak of the metacarpal and the contiguous distal portion of the ridge of the trapezium. The ligament has been called the ulnar ligament[49] and the anterior oblique ligament,[34] but a more appropriate name is the volar ligament because it accurately describes its anatomic position. In flexion and pronation (opposition), the volar beak of the metacarpal is closest to the trapezium, whereas in extension and supination, it moves away from the trapezium, a distance limited only by the volar ligament (Fig. 21-4).

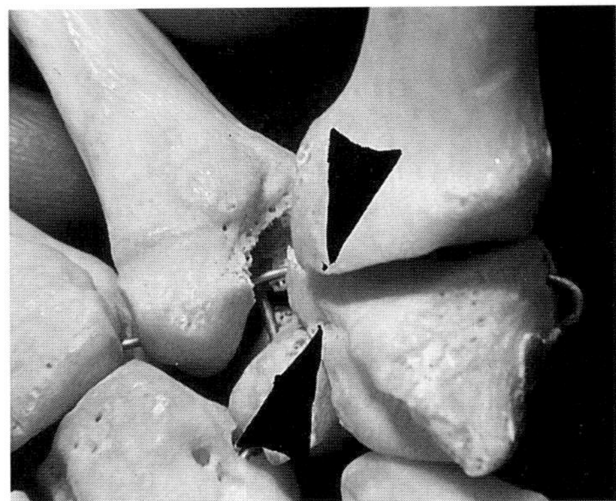
A

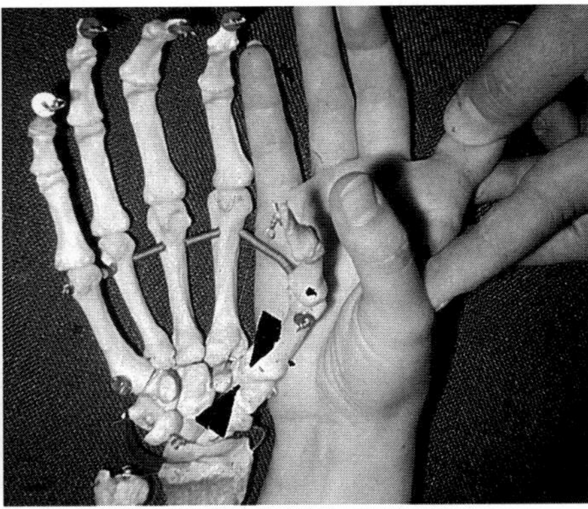
B

FIGURE 21-4. A, Anatomic view of the trapeziometacarpal joint showing the volar beak of the metacarpal to which is attached the important volar ligament. **B,** When the thumb is pronated, the volar beak of the metacarpal and corresponding surface of the trapezium are in close contact.

Although the vast majority of injuries to the trapeziometacarpal joint are fractures, isolated ligament injuries occur occasionally. An acute dislocation has been referred to as a "Bennett's fracture without a fracture."[32] However, unlike a Bennett's fracture, which is often unstable after reduction and requires internal fixation, a dislocation is usually stable after reduction, and management in a thumb spica cast for 5 to 6 weeks suffices. If the joint remains unstable after reduction, it should be pinned, which can be accomplished best by drilling a 0.032-inch Kirschner wire across the joint percutaneously. Because the volar beak of the metacarpal is closest to the trapezium in pronation and flexion, this is the position in which the metacarpal is held while the wire is drilled. The wire is maintained for a minimum of 6 weeks, by which time sufficient scarring should have developed to prevent later joint instability. Surgery for an acute dislocation is generally indicated only when reduction cannot be achieved, which indicates interposition of ligamentous tissue.[8] If surgery is required, primary repair of the volar ligament is difficult because of its short length and relative inaccessibility. A more predictable procedure is to reconstruct a new ligament using a strip of the flexor carpi radialis tendon, a technique that is more commonly used for cases of chronic nonarthritic instability.[10]

Metacarpophalangeal Joint. The metacarpophalangeal joint of the thumb is a condyloid joint like its counterpart in the fingers, but it has several important anatomic differences. The shape of the head of the first metacarpal is less spherical and its articular surface is wider and flatter with more limited cartilage on its dorsal surface than a finger metacarpal.[18] The sesamoids in the thumb are also more constant, and they are intimately connected to the intrinsics, the flexor pollicis brevis radially and the adductor pollicis ulnarly, which is not the situation in the fingers where the sesamoids are not attached to the intrinsics.[15] In addition, the insertions of the intrinsic muscles in the thumb form thicker and stronger tendinous and aponeurotic expansions on both sides of the joint than is seen in the fingers.[2] As a consequence of these differences, the flexion–extension arc of a thumb metacarpophalangeal joint is generally more limited than the metacarpophalangeal joint of a finger. Abduction and adduction motions are definitely more limited, which is consistent with the primary role of the joint, a limited hinge where stability is more important than mobility.

Anterior dislocation of the metacarpophalangeal joint is a rare injury that tears not only the dorsal capsule but also the extensor pollicis brevis tendon, which is intimately connected to the capsule and inserts with it into the base of the proximal phalanx. Usually the injury occurs in conjunction with a tear of one of the collateral ligaments because the metacarpophalangeal joint is rarely forced in a purely anterior direction. More commonly, it is forced in an anteromedial or anterolateral direction.[51] A pure flexion injury can damage both collateral ligaments, at least their dorsal portions, which normally provide dorsal stability. This injury would be evident if the proximal phalanx remained slightly volarly subluxated after a closed reduction. In such cases, surgery is indicated to repair the torn joint capsule and extensor pollicis brevis tendon. Temporary pin fixation of the joint in complete extension for 6 weeks is also necessary to counteract the normal strong flexion forces on the joint during healing.

Acute sprains of the collateral ligaments are common, with the ulnar collateral ligament (UCL) injured in about 90% of cases. Although an acute UCL sprain is frequently referred to as a "gamekeeper's thumb" (the term actually described a chronic occupational condition in Scottish gamekeepers),[7] a more appropriate term for an acute sprain is a "skier's thumb" because skiing is responsible for most of the injuries.[11,31] The mechanism of injury is a strong abduction force on the joint, whereas an acute radial collateral ligament sprain results from an adduction force, as may occur after a fall on the outstretched hand.

Regardless of which collateral ligament is injured, the diagnosis and proper classification of the sprain depends on a careful examination. The objective is to differentiate a partial sprain, in which joint stability has not been compromised, from a complete tear (third-degree sprain), which results in instability and usually requires surgery. Simply observing the thumb in its resting position provides important clues as to the severity of the injury. Ecchymoses indicate tearing of tissues that may include the collateral ligament and, if torn, the metacarpophalangeal joint may actually deviate away from the side of the injured ligament. There is tenderness over the ligament, and an effort should be made to determine if it is located proximally at the origin of the ligament's attachment to the metacarpal head or distally at its insertion into the phalanx. Stability is evaluated by stressing the joint, but before doing so, radiographs are obtained to rule out an intraarticular fracture or epiphyseal plate injury in a skeletally immature child. Ulnar collateral ligaments generally tear at their insertion (90%), and a common radiographic finding is an avulsion bone fragment at that site. Because the fragment is almost always attached to the ligament, the distance that the fragment is displaced indicates the distance that the ligament has displaced. Although a displaced fragment is generally associated with an unstable joint, instability can also exist with a nondisplaced fragment. The bone fragment in these rare cases, and usually it is associated with UCL tears, is not the result of an avulsion injury but rather a shear injury (Fig. 21-5). When the proximal phalanx realigns itself after being severely radially deviated at the moment of injury, its ulnar base strikes the metacarpal head, causing a shear fracture to the phalanx.[58] Therefore, joint stability should never be assumed to be intact solely on the basis of a radiograph that shows a nondisplaced fracture fragment.

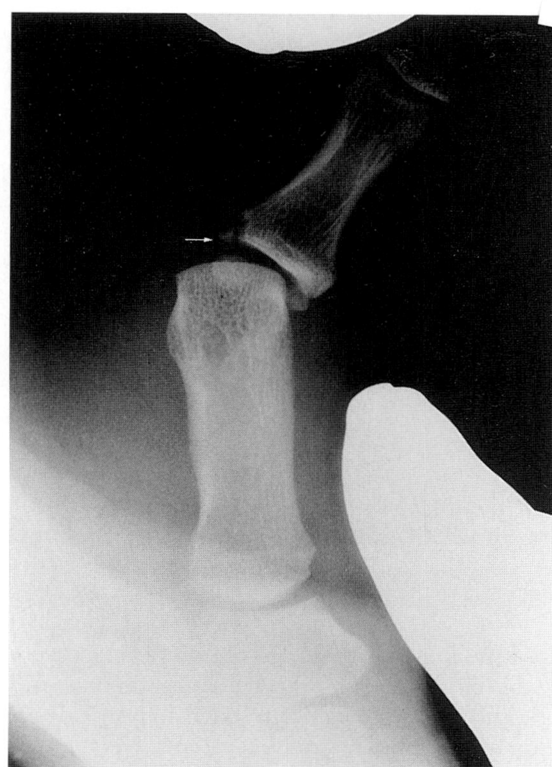

FIGURE 21-5. The small nondisplaced fracture fragment (*arrow*) in this obviously unstable thumb was not the result of an avulsion injury, but rather a shear injury.

A variety of imaging studies has been recommended to determine the severity of ligament injuries and the necessity for surgery. The objective is primarily to visualize a lesion described by Stener in 1962,[57] which occurs with some UCL ruptures, interposition of the adductor aponeurosis between the torn ligament and phalanx. Stener properly concluded that ligaments that ruptured in this fashion would never heal unless they were surgically repaired. Although imaging studies such as arthrography,[59] stress arthrography,[3] and magnetic resonance imaging[26] can demonstrate Stener lesions, they are not infallible, and a "negative" study can be misleading because most ruptures of the UCL do not result in Stener lesions yet require surgery. A Stener lesion is a reflection of the severity of the angulation of the proximal phalanx at the moment of injury (Fig. 21-6). It must have exceeded 60° because at that angle the proximal edge of the adductor aponeurosis shifts far enough distal to the base of the proximal phalanx to permit an avulsed UCL to displace outside the aponeurosis after the phalanx realigns itself.[47] Because most UCL ruptures result from injuries that cause less than 60° angulation of the metacarpophalangeal joint, imaging studies should never be the sole criterion for surgery. Rather, the decision should be based on a properly performed stress test.

Opinions vary as to the optimum position for the metacarpophalangeal joint when it is stressed. These positions vary from complete extension,[37,54] to complete flexion,[40] slight flexion,[31] and a combination of flexion and extension.[8,9,57] The rationale for stressing the joint in complete flexion is that because the collateral ligaments are maximally taut in this position, significant angulation of the joint would indicate a third-degree sprain. The problem with stressing the joint in flexion is that what may appear to be joint angulation may actually be rotation of the metacarpal at its trapeziometacarpal joint or rotation at the metacarpophalangeal joint itself resulting from laxity of the dorsal capsule, a common finding in loose-jointed individuals who have considerable metacarpophalangeal flexion (Fig. 21-7). The preferred position for stress testing is with the metacarpophalangeal joint in complete extension, and angulation of 35° or more indicates a third-degree sprain.[47] A theoretical objection to stressing the joint in complete extension is that a tear of a collateral ligament might go undetected if the accessory collateral ligament, which is normally taut in extension, remains intact. However, this situation has not been observed. Unlike the metacarpophalangeal

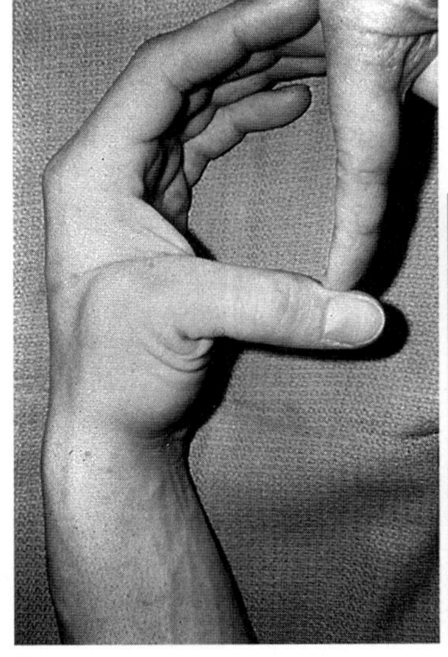

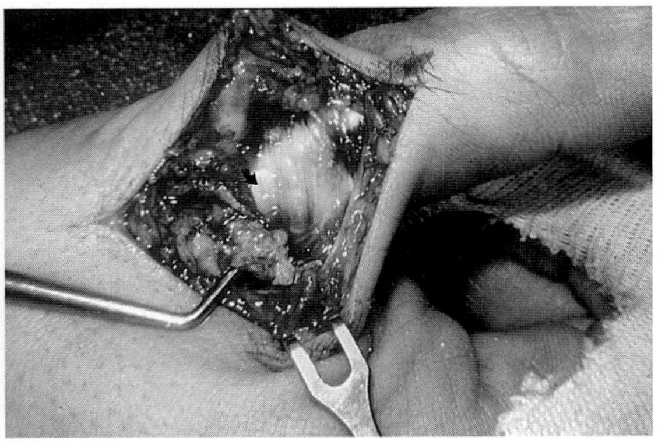

FIGURE 21-6. **A,** Thumb instability after rupture of the ulnar collateral ligament. The marked degree of instability of almost 90° indicated that there was probably a Stener lesion. **B,** This was confirmed at surgery (probe on the avulsed ligament, *arrow* on adductor aponeurosis).

joints of the fingers, which are normally lax in extension and stable in full flexion, the metacarpophalangeal joint of a thumb must be stable in extension and flexion to function effectively.

Management for a partial collateral ligament injury is immobilization of the thumb using a palm-based orthosis or a thumb spica cast (Fig. 21-8). Initially, it may be difficult to differentiate between a first- and second-degree injury, although marked swelling and ecchymoses would be consistent with the more severe sprain. If after the first week, swelling and local tenderness have almost completely resolved, the injury can be considered first degree.

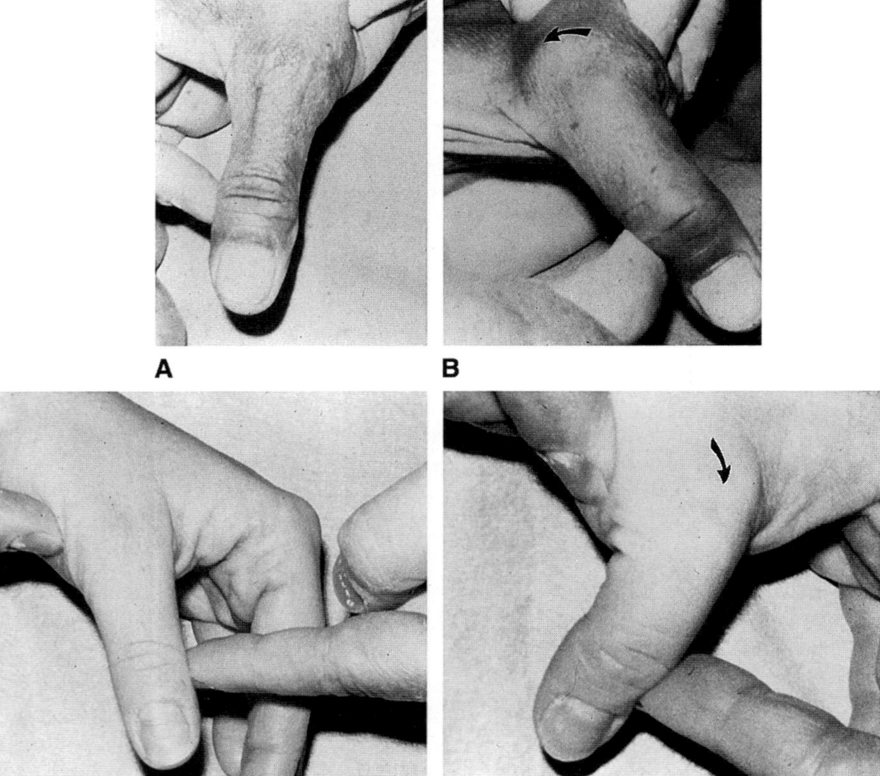

FIGURE 21-7. Stress testing two healthy thumbs in extension and flexion. **A** and **B,** The apparent angulation of the metacarpophalangeal joint when stressed in flexion was actually normal rotation occurring at the trapeziometacarpal joint. **C** and **D,** In this thumb, there was also no abnormal angulation at the metacarpophalangeal joint. The joint rotated when stressed in flexion because of normal laxity of its dorsal capsule.

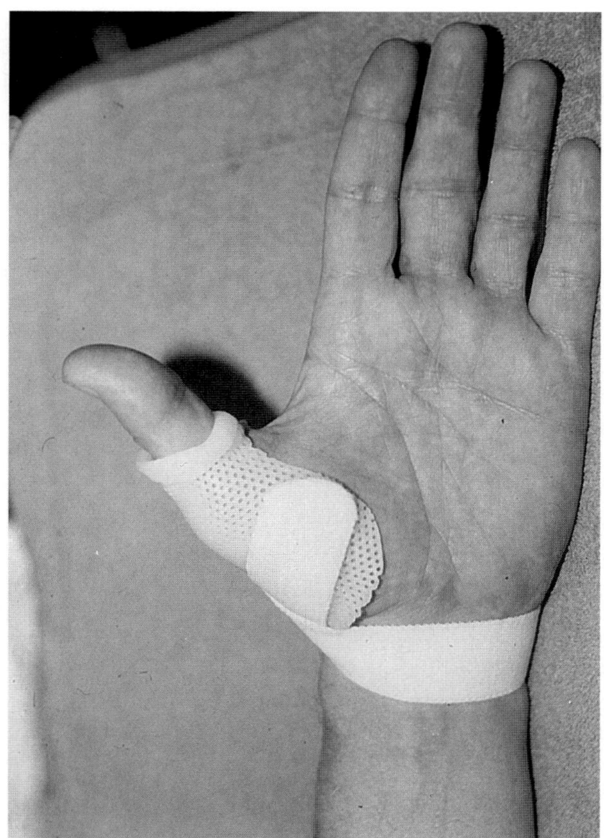

FIGURE 21-8. A palm-based thumb splint provides effective immobilization of a thumb metacarpophalangeal joint. When worn under a glove (i.e., skiing), the velcro strap can be removed.

The splint or cast can then be discontinued, and active range of motion exercises started. Return to full sport activities can be expected within days, although adhesive taping of the thumb or immobilizing it with a small splint for an additional week or two is recommended. If, however, tenderness persists and if there is slight laxity when stressing the joint, the injury should be considered second degree and thumb immobilization continued for 3 to 4 weeks.

A third-degree or complete ligament rupture requires surgery. If surgery is carried out within 3 weeks of the injury, the likelihood of achieving a pain-free, stable thumb can almost be assured. After surgery, the thumb is immobilized for 4 to 5 weeks. The splint is then removed several times each day for active range of motion exercises and discontinued after another week. Resistive exercises to improve muscle strength are important. For the intrinsic muscles, abducting the thumb against the resistance of a rubberband wrapped around it and the palm will strengthen the abductors, and adducting the thumb against the resistance of a sponge in the first web space will strengthen the adductors.

Dorsal dislocations of the metacarpophalangeal joint are more common than volar dislocations and result from hyperextension injuries that tear the volar plate.[51] The metacarpal head protrudes through the intrinsic muscles that pass on both sides of it and insert on the radial and ulnar sesamoids and the sides of the base of the proximal phalanx. A lateral radiograph will show the dislocation, and the position of the sesamoids will aid in determining the site of the tear in the volar plate. If the sesamoids remain close to the dislocated phalanx, which is the usual situation, the plate has torn proximally and is interposed between the phalanx and dorsal surface of the metacarpal head. A closed reduction should be attempted, generally under regional block anesthesia. Pressure is applied to the base of the phalanx in a distal direction to push it over the metacarpal head. Relaxing the intrinsic muscles and flexor pollicis longus by flexing and adducting the metacarpal is often helpful. Applying severe force to the phalanx must be avoided, particularly in the skeletally immature patient, because it could result in damage to the epiphyseal plate. Some dorsal dislocations are irreducible and require surgery. After reduction, either by closed manipulation or surgery, a dorsal extension block splint is used for several weeks.

Interphalangeal Joint. Dislocations of the interphalangeal joint are almost always dorsal and are often compound because the soft tissue envelope around the distal phalanx is firmly anchored by dense, strong skin ligaments. Lateral dislocations are less common than at the distal interphalangeal joints of fingers because the transverse diameter of the condyles of the proximal phalanx in a thumb is wider than the transverse diameter of the condyles of the middle phalanx in a finger. Careful wound lavage and debridement are important, and parenteral antibiotics should be administered. Occasionally, surgery is necessary when the dislocation is irreducible because of entrapment of the distal phalanx by the volar plate or flexor pollicis longus tendon. Stability after reduction, either closed or open, is excellent, and a dorsal extension block splint is used for several weeks.

Fingers

Carpometacarpal Joint. Sprains of the carpometacarpal joint(s) are frequently dismissed by athletes as "bone bruises," and treatment is rarely sought until the problem is chronic. Even acute third-degree sprains, which are often associated with an avulsion fracture from the base of the metacarpal(s) or the contiguous surface of the carpal bone, are sometimes ignored. Clinically, these injuries are accompanied by local swelling and tenderness, and there is often a bony prominence resulting from dorsal displacement of the metacarpal base. Stability is determined by completely flexing the metacarpophalangeal joint, which locks the metacarpal head, and then grasping the proximal phalanx, pushing the finger upward and pulling it downward. This maneuver will demonstrate that the second and third carpometacarpal joints are normally rigid, whereas the fourth and fifth carpometacarpal joints have some laxity (about 15° for the fourth and about 30° for the fifth). The laxity of the fourth and fifth carpometacarpal joints is important for maintaining the normal curvature of the distal metacarpal arch when making a fist.

Visualizing a subluxation of any of the carpometacarpal joints requires oblique radiographs to profile the injured joint. Almost all subluxations and dislocations are dorsal, and if recognized early they can easily be reduced by manipulation. However, they have a propensity to displace, particularly the carpometacarpal joints of the index and middle fingers because of contraction of the powerful extensor carpi radialis longus and brevis tendons.[52] Generally, plaster immobilization is inadequate for these injuries, and percutaneous Kirschner wire fixation of the joint is advisable. Care is taken when inserting the wires to avoid injuring the dorsal sensory branches of the radial and ulnar nerves and the extensor tendons. The radiocarpal joint should not be transfixed, and if possible the midcarpal joint also should be left free. A volar wrist splint is applied, which is removed several times daily for active range of motion exercises. The Kirschner wires, which are generally left out of the skin, are removed after 8 weeks. Despite prolonged immobilization, later subluxations can occur, and follow-up observations are required for at least 6 to 9 months.

Most carpometacarpal sprains are not seen until the condition is chronic and the athlete has a significant disability. This chronic condition is common in amateur and professional boxers, particularly when the instability affects the carpometacarpal joints of the index and/or middle fingers—joints that are normally rigid and comprise the solid base for the longitudinal arch of the hand. As the condition worsens, the athlete experiences increasing pain and swelling that persist for progressively longer periods of time after each successive bout. When the athlete realizes that he is unable to continue with the sport, surgery is warranted. Arthrodesis is the most effective procedure, even for the normally mobile fourth and fifth carpometacarpal joints, provided they are fused in sufficient flexion to maintain the normal curvature of the transverse metacarpal arch.

Metacarpophalangeal Joint. Direct trauma to the knuckle usually causes a contusion to the soft tissues, including the extensor tendon. Sometimes the sagittal fibers are injured, although sudden torsion on the finger is more likely the mechanism of injury than direct trauma. The extensor tendon displaces, usually in an ulnar direction because the radial sagittal fibers are more commonly injured than the ulnar sagittal fibers. If direct trauma is severe, such as a hard blow to the knuckle or repetitive blows during a single episode as may occur in boxing or karate, the dorsal joint capsule can also rupture.[46] Generally, these injuries are not diagnosed until there is a chronic problem. Clinically, the most significant finding is a palpable defect in the joint capsule, which would not be present if the injury was confined to the tendon or its dorsal hood mechanism. Surgery is usually necessary, and the capsule can always be repaired, regardless of the chronicity of the injury, because of the way it tears. Invariably, the tear is in a longitudinal direction, and although the two edges of the capsule may have retracted, they can be brought together for repair.

Unlike the thumb, collateral ligament injuries of the finger metacarpophalangeal joints are rare for several reasons. Each joint is protected by its recessed position in the palm, is supported by an adjacent finger(s), and in extension can easily deviate when a laterally directed force is applied to it. However, when that same force is applied to the joint when flexed, it is likely to cause ligamentous damage because in that position the ligaments are normally taut and do not permit lateral deviation. After a collateral ligament injury, the patient will complain of pain in the general area of the knuckle but will rarely localize it to the ligament itself, which is a reason these injuries are often overlooked. Clinically, there will be tenderness over the injured ligament. The radial collateral ligaments of the ring and little fingers are most commonly injured because these two fingers are most prone to be forcefully deviated ulnarly when in flexed positions. Stability is tested by stressing the joint in complete flexion (Fig. 21-9). For a first- or second-degree injury, rest and splinting the joint are effective, but for a third-degree injury surgery is usually necessary, particularly when there is gross instability. In some patients, the finger will deviate ulnarly simply by the effect of gravity (Fig. 21-10). At surgery, the ligament, which tears with equal frequency at its metacarpal and phalangeal attachments, is reinserted into the bone.

Tears of the volar plate result from sudden hyperextension of the metacarpophalangeal joint. The plate tears at its proximal membranous attachment to the neck of the metacarpal and displaces dorsally with the proximal phalanx, to which it remains attached. The metacarpophalangeal joint of the index finger is most frequently dislocated, followed by the metacarpophalangeal joint of the little finger. Usually, dorsal dislocations cannot be reduced by closed manipulation because, in addition to the volar plate that is displaced behind the metacarpal head, there are structures on both sides of the metacarpal head that entrap it. This anatomic entrapment resembles a child's Chinese fingertrap; the more traction placed on the finger, the tighter the structures become, and the more difficult the reduction. It is for this reason that these dislocations have been referred to as "complex dislocations."[19]

When the metacarpophalangeal joint of the index finger is dislocated, the finger is flexed at both interphalangeal

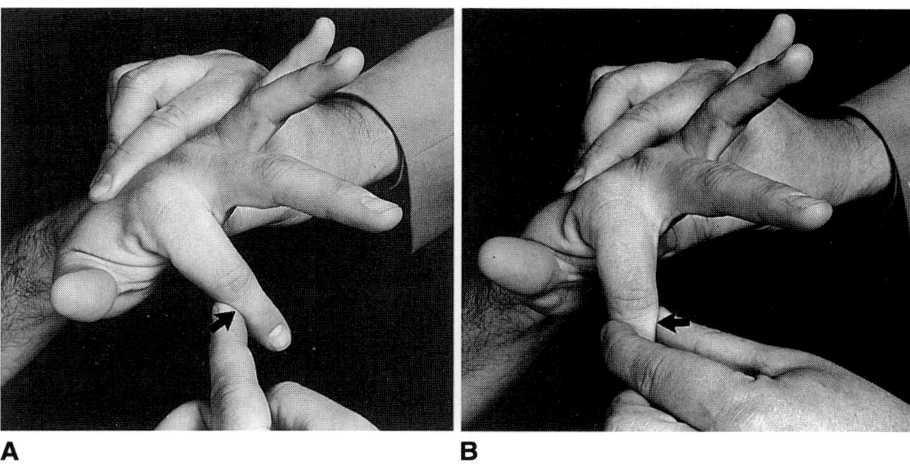

FIGURE 21-9. A and **B,** Unlike the metacarpophalangeal joint of the thumb, evaluating stability of the collateral ligaments of a finger metacarpophalangeal joint requires stressing the joint in full flexion.

joints, hyperextended at its metacarpophalangeal joint, and slightly deviated toward the adjacent fingers. The palmar skin is dimpled or puckered at the proximal palmar crease, which is an important diagnostic clue. Dorsally, a defect can usually be palpated just proximal to the base of the dislocated phalanx. When the joint is subluxated rather than dislocated, there is no lateral deviation of the finger, and the articular surface of the proximal phalanx, which may be hyperextended as much as 90°, still is in contact with the dorsal surface of the metacarpal head.[15] Radiographs of a subluxation or dislocation will show widening of the joint space on the anteroposterior view. The lateral view in a complex dislocation will show the sesamoids to be within the joint because they remain attached to the volar plate, which displaced with the phalanx.[36,61]

The classical surgical approach is volar, and the incision must be carried out with great care because the neurovascular bundle (radial neurovascular bundle for the index finger and ulnar neurovascular bundle for the little finger) is tented over the metacarpal head and can be cut inadvertently. Because of this risk, a dorsal surgical approach is preferred. A longitudinal incision is made in the joint capsule, and the volar plate, which is the structure primarily responsible for preventing reduction, is levered back to its normal position. After surgery, active flexion exercises are begun immediately because there is an inverse relationship between the duration of immobilization and the ultimate mobility of the joint.[29] During the first 2 weeks, a dorsal block splint is worn to protect the joint from hyperextending. If the patient has difficulty regaining active flexion of the metacarpophalangeal joint, a dynamic flexion splint is used. The elastic attached to the cuff over the dorsal aspect of the proximal segment should be of sufficient tension to prevent hyperextension, but it should not prevent full active extension.

Proximal Interphalangeal Joints. Injuries to the proximal interphalangeal joints are among the most common injuries that affect the hand. Many athletes dismiss the injury as a "jammed finger" and neglect to seek treatment. A "jammed finger" is not a medical diagnosis; it neither refers to a specific pathologic condition nor, in most cases, does it accurately describe the mechanism of injury. Fortunately, most are first-degree sprains, but occasionally they are third-degree sprains or even fracture–dislocations of the joint.

Injuries to the dorsal capsule are always associated with damage to the central extensor tendon because both structures are intimately connected. Because the tendon is the more important dorsal stabilizer of the joint, management is directed at restoring its function. The most severe injury is a volar dislocation, which results from a violent flexion force on the joint that tears the capsule and central extensor tendon. Reduction is achieved by closed manipulation, which is confirmed on a lateral radiograph. Although primary repair of the tendon has been recommended for these injuries,[30,56] preferred management is extension splinting as used for an acute boutonnière deformity without a dislocation.

Some volar dislocations are caused by a violent torsional injury on the joint. The middle phalanx rotates volarly, which tears the collateral ligament, and the condyle of the proximal phalanx herniates through the extensor mechanism. The lateral band on that side, alone or with the central slip, which remains attached at its insertion, slips volar to the condyle and entraps it.[33,35,45] Radiographs will not show complete volar displacement of the middle phalanx but rather incongruity of the joint surfaces. Because the joint is twisted, the proximal and middle phalanges will project differently: one will appear lateral, whereas the other will appear oblique (Fig. 21-11). A closed reduction should be attempted with the metacarpophalangeal joint flexed to relax the displaced lateral band. The proximal interphalangeal joint is then derotated and extended, and the lateral band should slip back into its normal position.[8] If this maneuver is not successful, surgery is necessary. Paradoxically, the

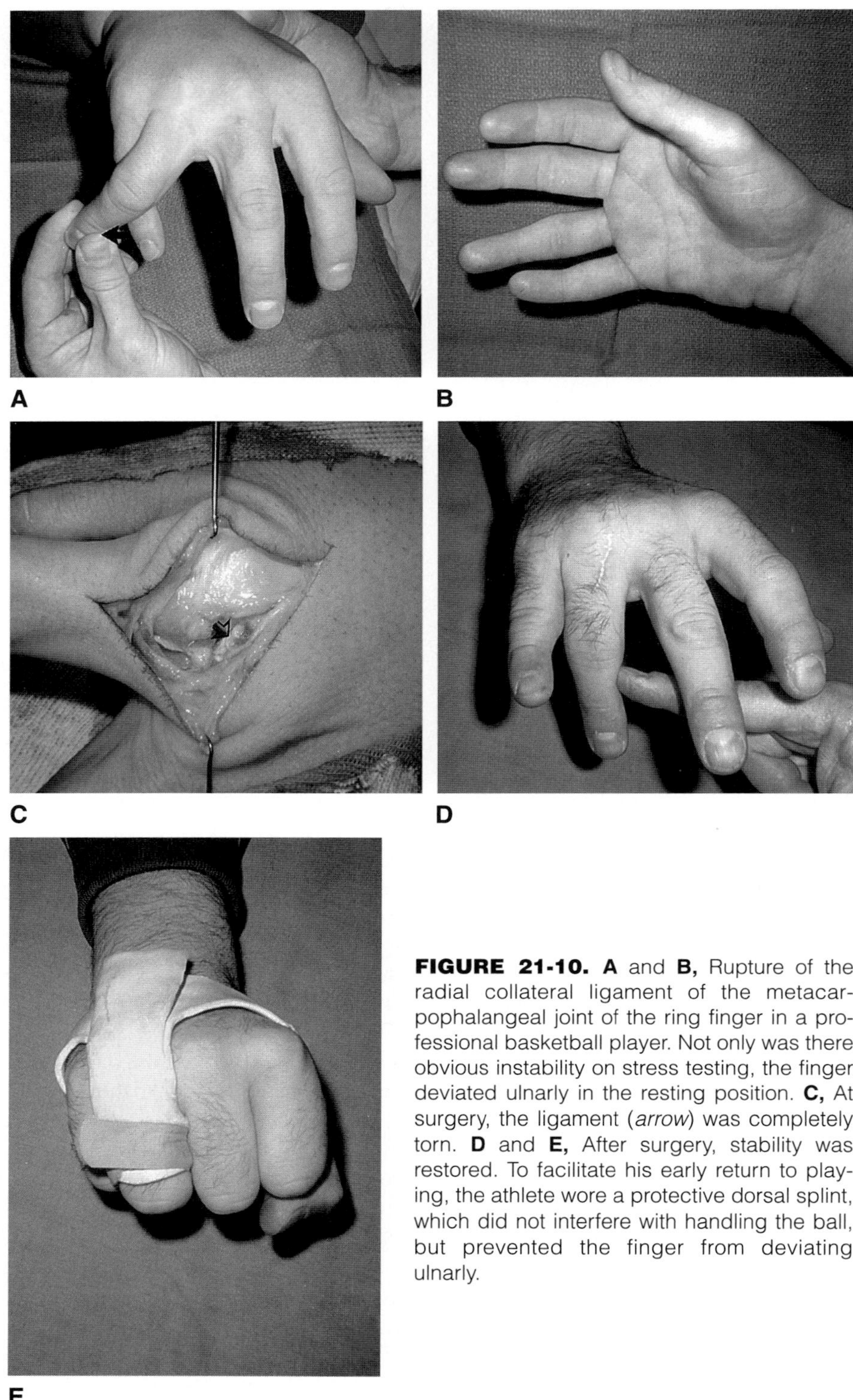

FIGURE 21-10. **A** and **B,** Rupture of the radial collateral ligament of the metacarpophalangeal joint of the ring finger in a professional basketball player. Not only was there obvious instability on stress testing, the finger deviated ulnarly in the resting position. **C,** At surgery, the ligament (*arrow*) was completely torn. **D** and **E,** After surgery, stability was restored. To facilitate his early return to playing, the athlete wore a protective dorsal splint, which did not interfere with handling the ball, but prevented the finger from deviating ulnarly.

prognosis is better for this injury, even if surgery is required, than the volar dislocation that is easily reduced. In the irreducible dislocation, the extensor tendon mechanism is displaced, but not disrupted, and active range of motion exercises can begin within one week of surgery, whereas in the reducible dislocation, the central tendon is torn, which requires more prolonged immobilization and frequently leads to some permanent loss of mobility.

Injuries to the collateral ligaments and volar plate almost always occur together, although their severity may differ. A lateral dislocation that completely tears either the radial or ulnar collateral ligament will also tear the

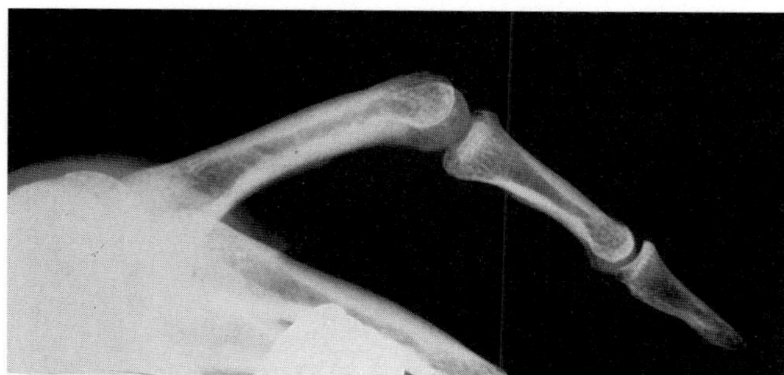

FIGURE 21-11. Lateral radiograph of an irreducible volar subluxation of a proximal interphalangeal joint. The key to the diagnosis is not only the incongruity of the joint surfaces, but also its twisted appearance. The radiograph shows a lateral view of the middle phalanx, but an oblique view of the proximal phalanx.

volar plate. However, a dorsal dislocation that disrupts the volar plate will not necessarily tear either collateral ligament unless the extension force is also directed radially or ulnarly. Injuries to the collateral ligaments and volar plate are exceedingly common. The majority of these injuries never receive medical attention, and fortunately, because most are first-degree sprains, they rarely cause any residual problem. Even second- and third-degree sprains may leave the athlete unscathed, although these injuries, particularly when they involve the volar plate, can result in later joint stiffness and cause a significant disability. Commonly, individuals who sustain proximal interphalangeal joint injuries seek treatment because they are more concerned about the swelling that has persisted for weeks or even months than about any slight loss of mobility. Swelling after most joint injuries in the hand will persist for many months, and it takes generally up to 18 months until it reaches maximum improvement. Even at that time there will often be some permanent enlargement of the joint, and educating patients to this fact will allay their fears.

After a lateral dislocation, the joint hinges either radially or ulnarly, depending on which ligament remains intact. Generally, the joint hinges ulnarly because most third-degree sprains involve the radial collateral ligament. Usually, the dislocation is easily reduced, and often the reduction is carried out immediately after the injury by the athlete who "pulled on the finger." Although the volar plate has also been disrupted, usually at its insertion, and only one collateral ligament remains intact, the joint is relatively stable after reduction.[28,48] Stability results from the normal congruity of the tongue-and-groove configuration of the articular surfaces of the proximal and middle phalanges, and from the compressive effect of the intact flexor and extensor tendon systems. Although many proximal interphalangeal dislocations are never treated and others are simply "buddy taped" to an adjacent finger for 1 to 2 weeks, proper management requires a more careful approach. A radiograph should always be taken to rule out a more serious problem, such as an intraarticular fracture, which will be discussed in a later section. The injured joint is splinted for 2 to 3 weeks in slight flexion. Active range of motion exercises are then begun, and the joint is protected for several more weeks. During this time, buddy taping is effective, and, if possible, the injured finger is taped to the finger on the side of the ligament rupture because it will provide better protection. Surgery for the acute dislocation is necessary only in those very rare cases in which reduction cannot be achieved because of interposition of capsular tissue or if there is unstressed instability.

Failure to provide adequate management for the acute dislocation can result in chronic instability, which is generally seen in athletes who report multiple dislocations, none of which ever received any treatment. Clinically, the joint is enlarged on the side of the injured collateral ligament, usually the radial, and on stress testing, there is more than 20° of instability.[20] In mild cases, buddy taping during sports activities may suffice, but when there is a significant disability, surgery is necessary. If possible, the avulsed ligament is reinserted into the proximal phalanx. If, however, there is no recognizable ligamentous tissue, a new ligament must be reconstructed, and in such cases, a portion of the volar plate can be used[12] or one slip of the flexor superficialis tendon.[22]

The volar plate is the primary static restraint limiting extension at the proximal interphalangeal joint. Experimental studies have shown that when an extension force is applied slowly to the joint, the proximal attachments of the plate gradually attenuate.[4] If that extension force continues, the middle phalanx dislocates dorsally with the volar plate, which then becomes trapped over the head of the proximal phalanx and blocks reduction. Because slow hyperextension is a rare mechanism of injury, irreducible dorsal dislocations are exceedingly uncommon.[16,21] Rather, the usual method of injury is rapid loading, which tears the plate at its distal attachments.

There are two types of distal ruptures, and each may be associated with a bone chip from the base of the middle phalanx.[4,5] In the type I rupture, the damage is confined to the thin central portion of the plate, and its corner attachments remain intact. Although these injuries can be painful and the joint swells, there is no instability. Over-treatment must be avoided, and immobilization of the joint should not exceed one week. Because there is always some bleeding with these injuries, scarring occurs, which can result in a later flexion contracture of the joint. It is, therefore, important to monitor the athlete's condition to ensure that complete joint mobility is restored. A dynamic extension (or flexion) splint is sometimes required if mobility remains restricted after a few weeks. In the type II rupture, which results when the hyperextension force on the joint is more severe, the entire distal attachment of the plate tears, and the lateral capsule also tears between the collateral ligaments and the accessory collateral ligaments. The middle phalanx shifts dorsally hinged on both collateral ligaments. If the split is between the collateral and accessory collateral ligaments, the joint will hyperextend, sometimes as much as 70° to 80°, but the articular surfaces still remain in contact as the middle phalanx articulates with the dorsal aspect of the head of the proximal phalanx. However, when the tears in the lateral capsule are more severe, the middle phalanx will completely dislocate dorsally and produce a bayonet deformity with the proximal phalanx. Closed reduction after these injuries is achieved by simply pushing the base of the middle phalanx over the head of the proximal phalanx. Traction should be avoided because it can entrap soft tissues within the joint and convert a reducible dislocation into an irreducible one.[5] Rarely is there any lateral instability after reduction because the collateral ligaments remain intact. A dorsal block splint is worn for 2 to 3 weeks, which blocks the last 20° to 30° of joint extension, but permits active and passive flexion exercises.

Chronic volar instability is a less common problem than a flexion contracture and is probably related to the normally poor vascularity at the distal attachment of the volar plate. After a volar plate rupture, particularly if it occurred without a bone fragment, there may be no "fracture bleeding" to cause later scarring.[5,38] In addition, if the joint was not immobilized after injury or if there were multiple injuries, any small clots would have been washed away by the synovial fluid. The distal end of the ruptured plate would therefore fail to scar under such circumstances. Instead, its torn end becomes smooth, similar to the end of an unrepaired flexor tendon that is severed within its digital synovial sheath.

In mild cases of volar instability, a small extension block splint can be used to correct the hyperextended joint. Double-connected rings are also effective because they are lightweight and do not interfere with joint flexion. In severe cases, the middle phalanx can get stuck in its hyperextended position, and the patient is unable to flex the finger. For the joint to be flexed, it must first be "unlocked" by passively flexing the middle phalanx. Surgery is often necessary for these problems, and the objective is to construct a constraint that prevents complete joint extension. A variety of surgical procedures have been described, but the most predictable is a tenodesis of the proximal interphalangeal joint using the flexor superficialis tendon.[47]

Distal Interphalangeal Joint. Stability of the distal interphalangeal joints is greater than the proximal interphalangeal joints because of the short lever arm of the distal phalanx and the insertion of the flexor profundus, which is immediately adjacent to the joint. When dislocations occur, they are usually lateral or dorsal and often compound because of the strong connections that anchor the skin to the bone. Wound lavage and antibiotics are necessary and, as with dislocations of the interphalangeal joint of the thumb, some may be irreducible because of entrapment of the volar plate,[41] flexor tendon,[43] or osteochondral fragment.[60] After reduction, joint stability is excellent, and active range of motion exercises are begun within 2 weeks. Chronic instability is a rare problem.

FRACTURES

Thumb

The most significant fractures of the thumb involve the metacarpal, and they account for 25% of all metacarpal fractures.[42] They distinguish themselves from fractures of the other metacarpals by their potential to cause an adduction contraction and their potential deleterious effect on function of the important trapeziometacarpal joint. The latter problem usually occurs as a result of an intraarticular fracture at the base of the bone of which there are two types: the Bennett's fracture and the Rolando fracture.

The Bennett's fracture is an oblique fracture that does not disturb the position of the volar beak of the bone, which is held in place by the intact volar ligament. However, the main portion of the metacarpal often displaces radially and sometimes dorsally because of pull of the abductor pollicis longus tendon. The subluxation component of the fracture is more important than the size of the volar fragment because, if not reduced and articular congruity is not restored, secondary arthritis is likely. Therefore, a careful radiographic examination is necessary to visualize the articular surface, and if conventional radiographs are inadequate, computed tomography is required. If the fracture is nondisplaced or minimally displaced (less than 2 mm), plaster immobilization with a thumb spica cast will suffice. However, when there is greater than 2 mm of articular incongruity, the fracture should be reduced and the joint stabilized. The method of reduction is important. As discussed in the section dealing with ligamentous injuries of the trapeziometacarpal joint, the volar beak of the metacarpal is closest to the contiguous surface of the trapezium when the metacarpal is flexed and pronated. It is in this position that the metacarpal is held as a 0.032-inch Kirschner wire is drilled percutaneously across the joint. Pinning the fracture fragment itself is avoided because pressure of the wire tip against it can cause it to shift in position. If an accurate reduction cannot be achieved by closed means, operative reduction and internal fixation is required using either a Kirschner wire or a small cortical screw, provided the fracture fragment is of ample size.

A Rolando intraarticular fracture is characterized by its T- or Y-shaped configuration. Because these fractures are more comminuted than Bennett's fractures, restoring articular congruity is more difficult to achieve by closed means, and surgery is usually necessary. Occasionally, an intraarticular fracture of the metacarpal base may be so severely comminuted that skeletal traction is the only feasible method of management.[14,62]

Fingers

The first step in evaluating any fracture is a clinical examination, and its importance cannot be overstated. Observing the relationship of the injured finger to the other fingers at rest and during gentle active motions will provide important clues to any abnormal rotation, angulation, or shortening at the fracture site. Not infrequently, the clinical examination is more important than the radiographic examination, and it should always precede it, particularly to assess any rotational deformity of the finger (Fig. 21-12). For each degree of malrotation at the fracture site, as much as 5° of malrotation occurs at the finger tip.[39] A metacarpal fracture that is rotated only 5° can therefore cause 1.5 cm of finger overlap, which is an unacceptable condition that requires correction.

Metacarpal Fractures. Most metacarpal fractures can be successfully managed nonoperatively. Although circular plaster casts are frequently applied to the hand and injured finger in hospital emergency rooms, they are often troublesome to the patient and to the physician

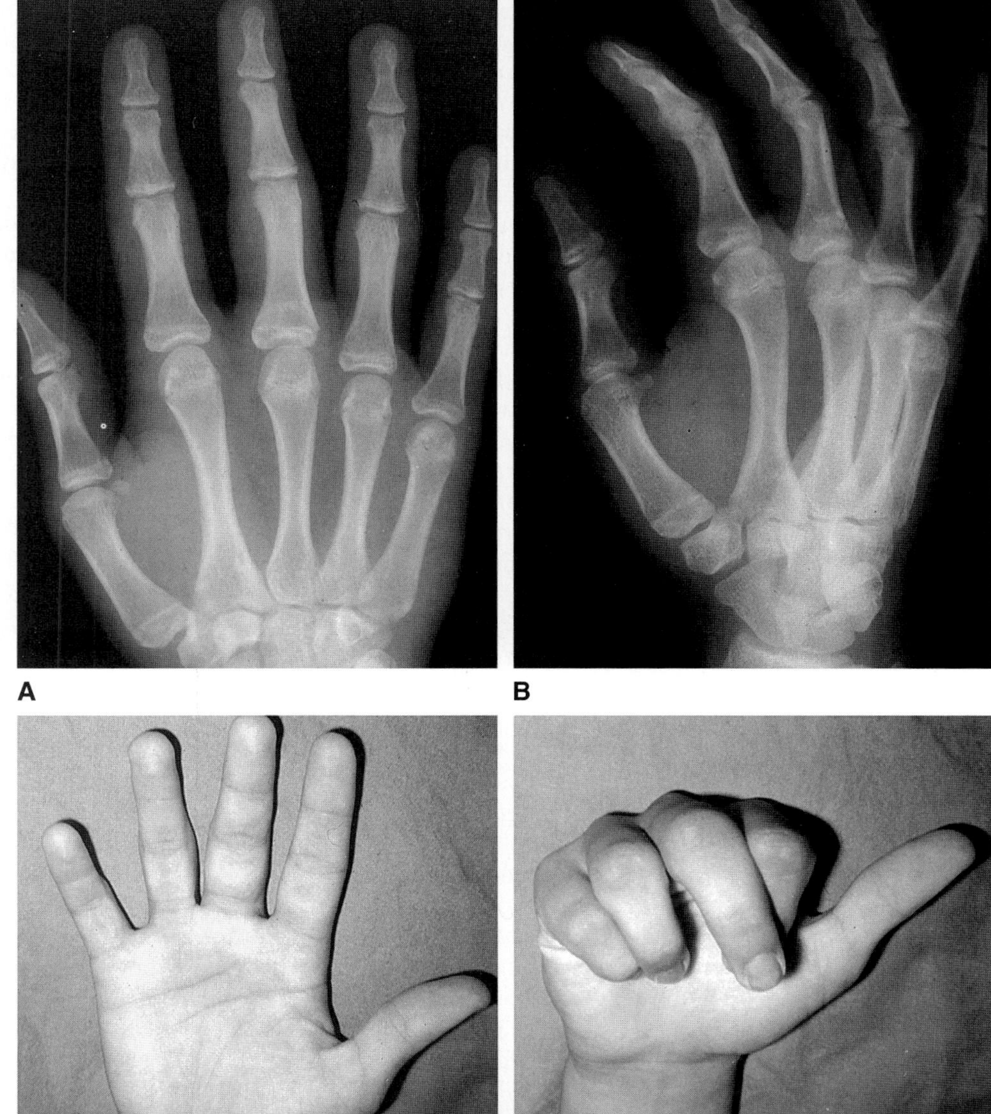

FIGURE 21-12. **A** and **B**, Posterior–anterior and oblique radiographs show what appears to be a nondisplaced fracture through the base of the proximal phalanx of the middle finger. **C** and **D**, Clinically, however, there was obvious malrotation of the finger.

providing follow-up care. It is preferable to immobilize the injured finger with a padded aluminum splint that is sandwiched into a plaster splint that immobilizes the wrist in slight extension. The metacarpophalangeal joint of the finger is immobilized in flexion to keep the collateral ligaments stretched, which reduces the risk of a later extension contracture of the joint. It is important that the splint is bent to conform to the position of the finger and never the reverse. The normal capsular laxity of a metacarpophalangeal joint can permit a malrotated or angulated fracture to appear to be reduced if the finger is taped to a splint that has been bent to conform to the desired position of the finger. The improvement in alignment or rotation of the injured finger is illusory, and as soon as the splint is removed, the deformity will be obvious.

With stable fractures treated nonoperatively, active range of motion exercises can usually be started within 2 to 3 weeks. The splint is removed several times each day for the exercises, which are carried out in warm water, and then reapplied and worn at all other times. With less stable fractures, the period of immobilization is longer before active exercises are begun, but that period should not exceed 3 weeks. If longer immobilization is required, the fracture probably should have been initially treated with some type of internal fixation. Although uninjured fingers are frequently immobilized in the belief that it provides more rigid fixation of the fracture, this practice should be avoided because of its propensity to cause permanent stiffness of those fingers. If a fracture is so unstable that immobilization of an adjacent finger(s) is contemplated, the fracture should be internally fixed. At each follow-up visit, it is important to obtain not only new radiographs to determine if there is any fracture displacement but also to clinically evaluate the finger for any deformity. Generally, fractures that remain stable after 2 to 3 weeks are unlikely to displace. The original aluminum and plaster splint can then be replaced with a more molded splint held in place by several Velcro fasteners. The new splint that is fabricated by the hand therapist facilitates removal and re-application by the patient who is instructed to remove it several times each day for active range of motion exercises. The splint is worn at all other times and is continued until there is radiographic evidence that healing is complete.

Metacarpal fractures are classified as oblique (spiral), which is the most common type, transverse, and comminuted. Transverse fractures are commonly angulated with the apex dorsal. An attempt should be made to correct the angulation by closed reduction following injection of the fracture site with a local anesthetic. If the fracture fragments can be "locked" together, the reduction will usually remain stable. Opinions vary as to the degree of fracture angulation that is acceptable for each metacarpal. Because the fourth and fifth metacarpals are normally mobile, acceptable angulation for the fourth has been reported to be 20° and for the fifth, 35°.[13,55] These figures serve only as reference points, and they should not be applied to every patient. Rather, each fracture must be managed on the basis of the demands placed on the individual athlete's hand. For the individual who participates in racquet sports, an angulated fracture of the fourth or fifth metacarpal with the head of the bone in the palm may interfere with effective grasp. For the amateur or professional boxer any angulation, regardless of the metacarpal that is fractured, is unacceptable and requires correction. The tremendous compressive forces applied to a boxer's hand will likely refracture a metacarpal that is permitted to heal in angulation. The surgical options are crossed Kirschner wires at the fracture site or a plate and screws. Kirschner wires are effective for stabilizing fractures at the neck or metaphyseal area of the bone. The wires are often inserted in a percutaneous fashion on either side of the metacarpal head to avoid damage to the articular cartilage that can lead to pain and stiffness. For fractures through the diaphysis of the bone, crossed Kirschner wires can also be used, but they do not provide as rigid fixation as a plate and screws.[44]

Oblique (spiral) and comminuted fractures are more likely to displace than transverse fractures, and they require close follow-up evaluation, particularly during the first 2 weeks. When there is displacement and shortening of the bone, an operative reduction and internal fixation is necessary. A variety of techniques have been recommended. Kirschner wires are probably used most frequently, but if the configuration of the fragments permits, cortical screws are preferred because they provide more rigid fixation (Fig. 21-13). Generally, it is unnecessary to insert the screws in a lag fashion. In addition to fractures of the shaft of the bone, intraarticular fractures also occur. The priority of treatment for these injuries is to restore articular congruity, and surgery is almost always necessary (Fig. 21-14). These fractures can result in avascular necrosis of the fracture fragment and the patient should be alerted to this possibility.

Regardless of the type of fracture, when internal fixation is rigid, active range of motion exercises are begun within the first postoperative week, often earlier than for fractures treated nonoperatively. As soon as postoperative swelling has subsided, and this is usually about the same time that exercises are begun, the plaster splint that was applied in the operating room is replaced with a more molded splint fabricated by a hand therapist. The splint immobilizes the wrist in slight extension and the MP joint of the finger in about 60° of flexion; the interphalangeal joints do not have to be immobilized. The patient is instructed to remove the splint 3 to 4 times each day for active range of motion exercises, but to wear it at all other times. As with fractures treated nonoperatively, the splint is continued until there is radiographic evidence of bone healing.

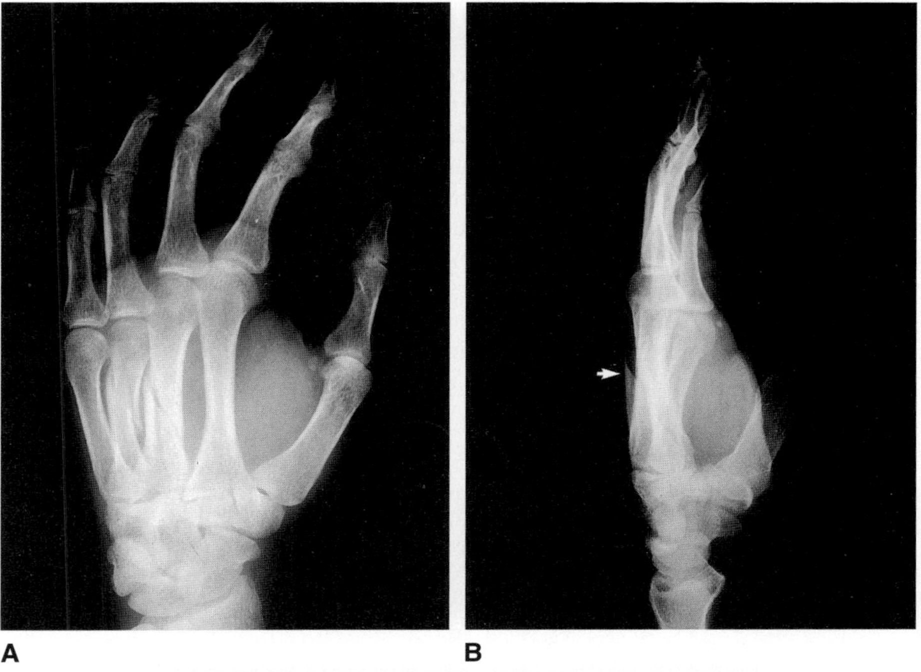

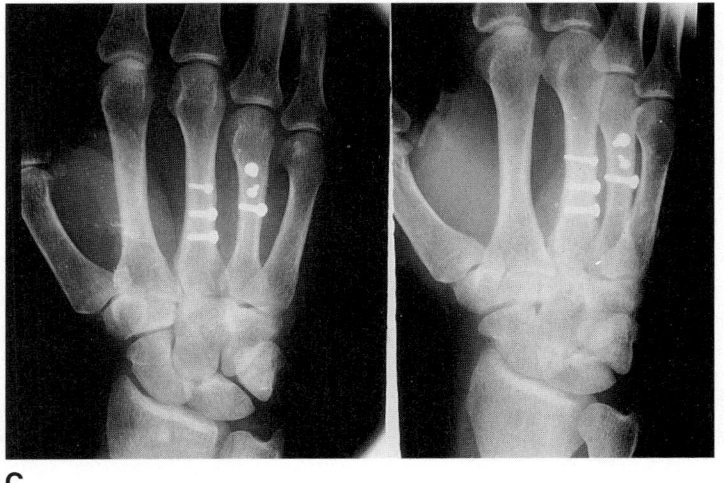

FIGURE 21-13. A and **B,** Oblique and spiral fractures of the third and fourth metacarpals. There was significant displacement evident on the lateral radiograph (*arrow*). **C,** Rigid internal fixation was obtained using 1.5 mm and 2.0 mm cortical screws.

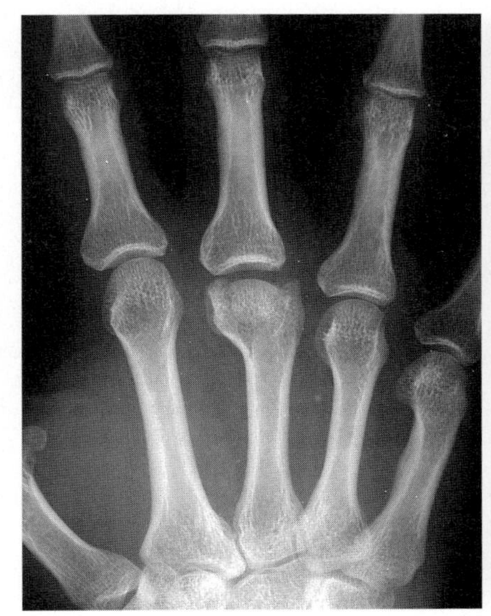

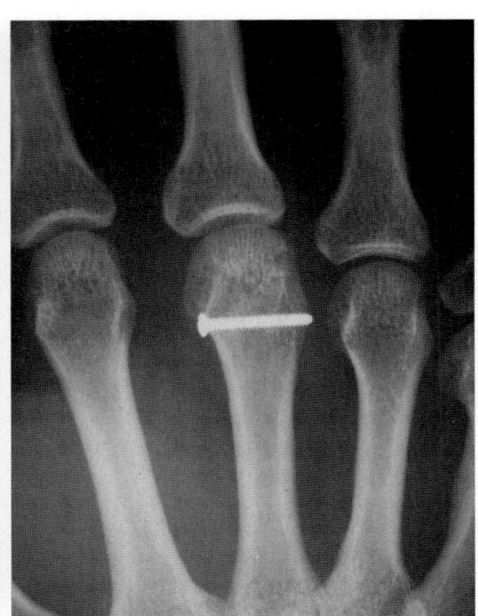

FIGURE 21-14. A, A professional baseball player sustained an intraarticular fracture to the head of his right third metacarpal. His hand was holding a baseball bat when the knuckle was struck by a pitched ball. **B,** At surgery, the depressed fracture fragment was elevated and fixed with a cortical screw inserted on the side of the metacarpal just proximal to the origin of the collateral ligaments.

Phalangeal Fractures. Phalangeal fractures can be classified in a similar fashion as metacarpal fractures, and they require the same meticulous care. Restoring alignment and articular congruity, when the fracture is intraarticular, are the immediate goals of treatment. Many phalangeal fractures require operative reduction and internal fixation. For oblique fractures, cortical screws are preferable to Kirschner wires because they provide more rigid fixation and permit earlier postoperative exercises. Plates and screws are less frequently used than for metacarpal fractures where the soft tissue envelope around the bones is greater. However, they are sometimes indicated for unstable fractures (Fig. 21-15).

The operative approach is important to minimize scarring of the extensor tendon mechanism that can lead to significant postoperative stiffness. For fractures of the proximal and middle phalanx, a mid-axial incision is far more preferable to a dorsal, tendon splitting incision. The side on which the mid-axial incision is made for transverse fractures is determined by what is more comfortable for the surgeon. Generally, this is on the radial sides of the index and middle fingers, and the ulnar

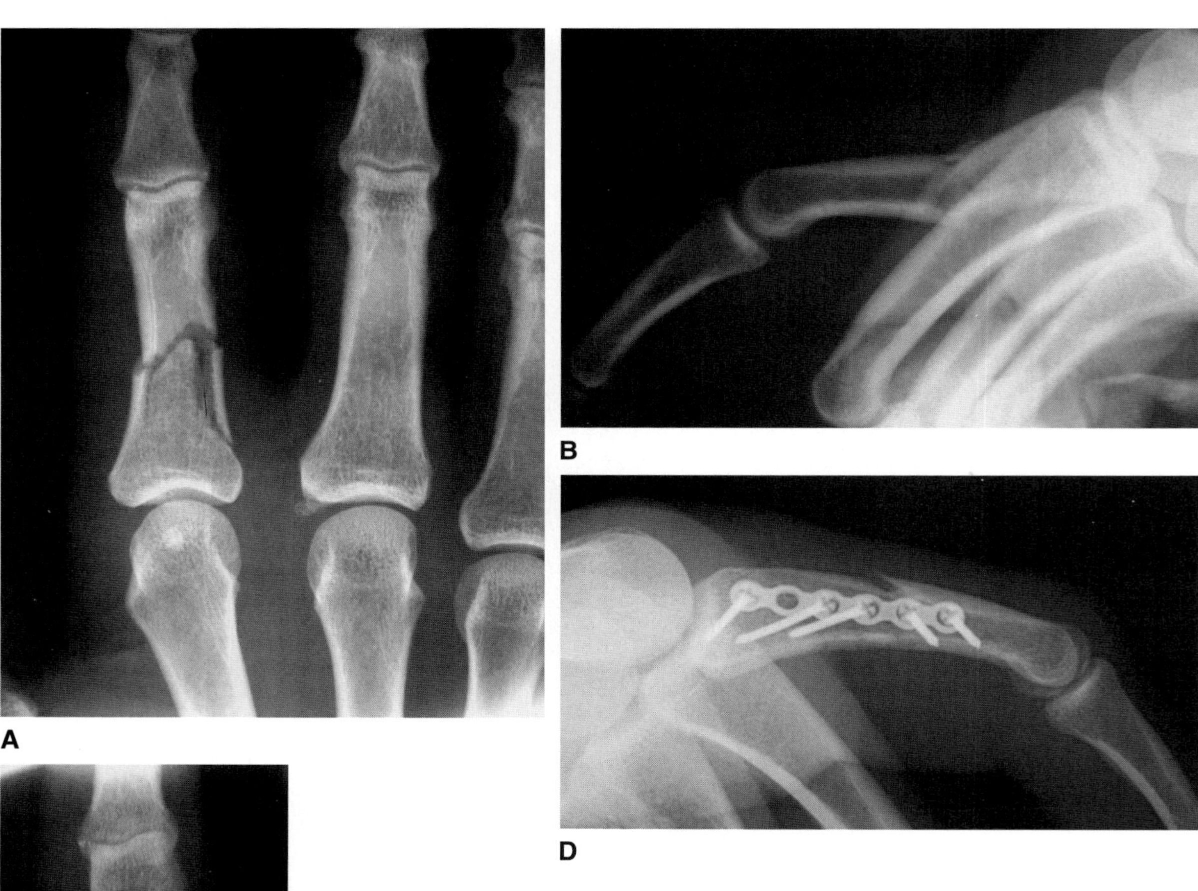

FIGURE 21-15. **A** and **B,** Professional hockey player sustained a comminuted fracture to the proximal phalanx of his right index finger when it was struck by a puck. The initial angulation of the fracture was severe because it tore the volar skin. **C** and **D,** Rigid fixation was provided with a plate and screws. Because the longitudinal fracture fragment was on the ulnar side of the bone, the plate was placed on that side.

sides of the ring and little fingers. For oblique fractures, the incision must be made on the side of the finger to which the distal fracture fragment has displaced in order to identify the fracture site and to shift the distal fragment back into position. The intrinsic lateral band is retracted for fractures in the distal portion of the proximal phalanx and in the middle phalanx. For fractures involving the middle and proximal portions of the proximal phalanx, the lateral band is moved adjacent to the central tendon and then repaired with fine, 6-0 nylon sutures.

Intra-operative fractures involving proximal interphalangeal joints require special attention because of the propensity of these injuries to lead to later arthritis if anatomical alignment is not restored. A condylar fracture of the proximal phalanx is fixed with Kirschner wires or thin cortical screws (Fig. 21-16). At surgery, care must be taken not to detach the collateral ligament from the fracture fragment. Comminuted fractures involving the base of the middle phalanx are challenging injuries that are likely to result in joint stiffness. Patients should always be informed prior to surgery that they will probably not regain normal mobility and that rehabilitation is a lengthy process that takes months and frequently requires the use of dynamic flexion and/or extension splints. A later capsulectomy is sometimes necessary if sufficient mobility cannot be restored with effective therapy. To visualize the fracture site, a volar operative approach is used. The flexor sheath between the A2 and A4 annular pulleys is excised and the flexor tendons retracted. Both collateral ligaments are then sectioned (the volar plate is often avulsed from the base of the

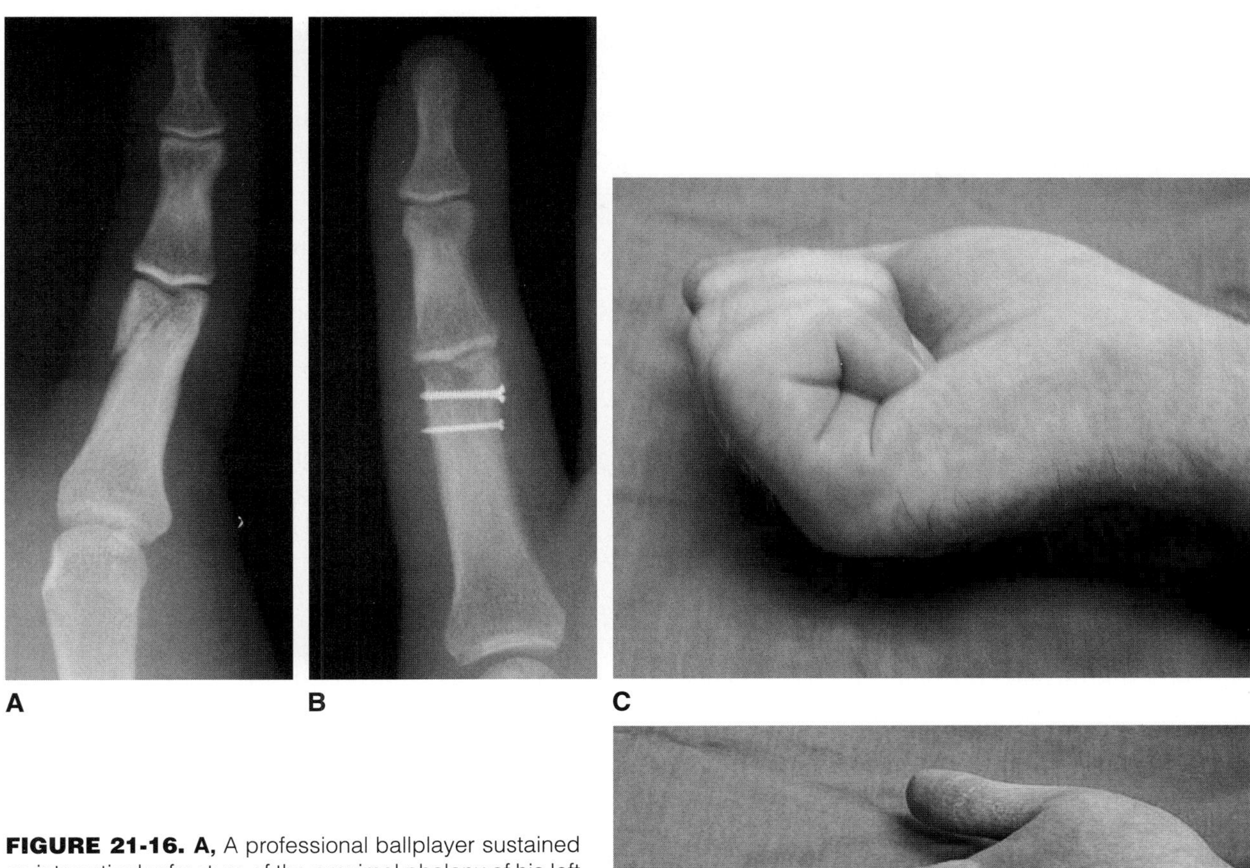

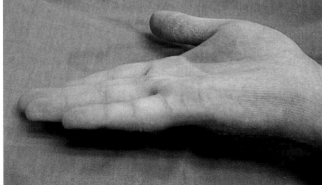

FIGURE 21-16. A, A professional ballplayer sustained an intraarticular fracture of the proximal phalanx of his left little finger when a teammate ran into him. **B,** The displaced condyle was reduced and fixed with 2 cortical screws (1.5 mm and 1.0 mm). **C** and **D,** Because fixation was secure, active range of motion exercises were started after 1 week and the patient regained complete mobility within 8 weeks.

middle phalanx) to permit hyperextension of the joint. When the fracture fragment is depressed, a small bone graft (autograft, allograft, or bone substitute) is inserted behind the fragment to elevate it. A small fragment comprising the volar base of the phalanx is best treated by excision of the fragment and advancing the volar plate into the defect (volar plate arthroplaty). Postoperatively, the initial splint includes the wrist, but the subsequent splint fabricated by a hand therapist is palm based and immobilization is limited to the finger.

CONCLUSION

The majority of hand injuries are minor and heal without the need for any specific medical attention. However, there are many injuries that, if not properly managed, can result in significant and permanent disabilities. Therefore, every injury requires a careful evaluation, the importance of which cannot be overstated. Except for fractures, the physical examination is more important than radiographs.

REFERENCES

1. Abouna JM, Brown H: The treatment of mallet finger: The results of a series of 148 consecutive cases and a review of the literature. Br J Surg 55:652, 1968.
2. Aubriot JH: The metacarpophalangeal joint of the thumb. In Tubiana R (ed): The Hand, vol 1. Philadelphia, WB Saunders, 1981.
3. Bowers WH: Sprains and joint injuries in the hand. Hand Clin 2:93, 1986.
4. Bowers WH: The proximal interphalangeal joint. II. A clinical study of hyperextension. J Hand Surg 6:77, 1981.
5. Bowers WH, Hurst LC: Gamekeeper's thumb: Evaluation by arthrography and stress roentgenography. J Bone Joint Surg 59A:519, 1977.
6. Bynum DK, Gilbert JA: Avulsion of the flexor digitorum profundus: Anatomic and biomechanical considerations. J Hand Surg 13A:222, 1988.
7. Campbell CS: Gamekeeper's thumb. J Bone Joint Surg 37B:148, 1955.
8. Dray GJ, Eaton RG: Dislocations and ligament injuries in the digits. In Green DP (ed): Operative Hand Surgery, 2nd ed. New York, Churchill Livingstone, 1988.
9. Eaton RG: Acute and chronic ligamentous injuries of the fingers and thumb. In Tubiana R (ed): The Hand, vol 2. Philadelphia, WB Saunders, 1985.
10. Eaton RG, Littler JW: Ligament reconstruction for the painful thumb carpometacarpal joint. J Bone Joint Surg 55A:1655, 1973.
11. Engkvist O, Balkfors B, Lindsjo U: Thumb injuries in downhill skiing. Int J Sports Med 3:50, 1982.
12. Faithfull DK: Treatment of chronic instability of the digital joints using a strip of volar plate. Hand 13:36, 1981.
13. Flatt AE: Fractures: Care of Minor Hand Injuries, 3rd ed. St. Louis, CV Mosby, 1972.
14. Gelberman RH, Vance RM, Zakaib GS: Fractures at the base of the thumb. Treatment with oblique traction. J Bone Joint Surg 61A:260, 1979.
15. Green DP, Terry GC: Complex dislocation of the metacarpophalangeal joint: Corrective pathological anatomy. J Bone Joint Surg 55A:1480, 1973.
16. Green S, Posner MA: Irreducible dorsal dislocation of the proximal interphalangeal joint. J Hand Surg 10A:85, 1985.
17. Gunter GS: Traumatic avulsion of the insertion of the flexor digitorum profundus. Aust NZ J Surg 30:1, 1960.
18. Joseph J: Further studies of the metacarpophalangeal and interphalangeal joints of the thumb. J Anat 85:221, 1951.
19. Kaplan EB: Dorsal dislocation of the metacarpophalangeal joint of the index finger. J Bone Joint Surg 39A:1081, 1957.
20. Kiefhaber TR, Stern PJ, Grood ES: Lateral stability of the proximal interphalangeal joint. J Hand Surg 11A:661, 1986.
21. Kjeldal I: Irreducible compound dorsal dislocation of the proximal interphalangeal joint of a finger. J Hand Surg 11B:49, 1986.
22. Lane CS: Reconstruction of the unstable proximal interphalangeal joint: The double superficialis tenodesis. J Hand Surg 3:368, 1978.
23. Langa V, Posner MA: Unusual rupture of a flexor profundus tendon. J Hand Surg 11A:227, 1986.
24. Leddy JP: Flexor tendon: Acute injuries. In Green DP (ed): Operative Hand Surgery, 2nd ed. New York, Churchill Livingston, 1988.
25. Leddy JP, Packer JT: Avulsion of the profundus insertion in athletes. J Hand Surg 2:66, 1977.
26. Louis DS, Buckwater KA: Magnetic resonance imagery of the collateral ligaments of the thumbs. J Hand Surg 14A:739, 1989.
27. Manske PR, Lesker PA: Avulsion of the ring finger flexor digitorum profundus: An experimental study. Hand 10:52, 1978.
28. McCue FC, Honner R, Johnson MC, Geick JH: Athletic injuries of the proximal interphalangeal joint requiring surgical treatment. J Bone Joint Surg 52A:937, 1970.
29. McLaughlin HL: Complex "locked" dislocation of the metacarpophalangeal joints. J Trauma 5:683, 1965.
30. Melone CP: Joint injuries of the fingers and thumb. Emerg Med Clin North Am 3:319, 1985.
31. Miller RJ: Dislocation and fracture dislocations of the metacarpophalangeal joint of the thumb. Hand Clin 4:45, 1988.

32. Moberg E, Stener B: Injuries to the ligaments of the thumb and fingers: Diagnosis, treatment and prognosis. Acta Chir Scand 106:166, 1953.
33. Murakam Y: Irreducible volar dislocation of the proximal interphalangeal joint of the finger. Hand 6:87, 1974.
34. Napier JR: The form and function of the carpometacarpal joint of the thumb. J Anat 89:362, 1955.
35. Neviaser RJ, Wilson JN: Interposition of the extensor tendon resulting in persistent subluxation of the proximal interphalangeal joint of the finger. Clin Orthop 8:118, 1972.
36. Nutter PD: Interposition of sesamoids into metacarpophalangeal dislocations. J Bone Joint Surg 22:730, 1940.
37. O'Brien ET: Fractures of the metacarpals and phalanges. In Green DP (ed): Operative Hand Surgery, 2nd ed. New York, Churchill Livingston, 1988.
38. Ochiai N, et al: Vascular anatomy of flexor tendons. I. Vascular system and blood supply of the profundus tendon in the digital sheath. J Hand Surg 4:321, 1979.
39. Opgrande JD, Westphal SA: Fractures of the hand. Orthop Clin North Am 14:669, 1983.
40. Palmar AK, Linscheid RL: Irreducible dorsal dislocation of the distal interphalangeal joint of the finger. J Hand Surg 2:406, 1977.
41. Palmar AK, Louis DS: Assessing ulnar instability of the metacarpophalangeal joint of the thumb. J Hand Surg 3:542, 1978.
42. Pellegrini UD: Fractures of the base of the thumb. Hand Clin 4:87, 1988.
43. Pohl AL: Irreducible dislocation of a distal interphalangeal joint. Br J Plast Surg 29:227, 1976.
44. Posner MA: Hand injuries. In Nicholas JA, Hershman EB, Posner MA (eds): The Upper Extremity in Sports Medicine, 2nd ed. St. Louis, CV Mosby, 1995.
45. Posner MA: Injuries to the hand and wrist in athletes. Orthop Clin North Am 8:593, 1977.
46. Posner MA, Ambrose L: The boxer's knuckle; dorsal capsule rupture of the metacarpophalangeal joint of a finger. J Hand Surg 14A:229, 1989.
47. Posner MA, Wilenski M: Irreducible volar dislocation of the proximal interphalangeal joint of a finger caused by interposition of an intact central slip: A case report. J Bone Joint Surg 60A:133, 1978.
48. Redler I, Williams JT: Rupture of a collateral ligament of the proximal interphalangeal joint of the finger: Analysis of 18 cases. J Bone Joint Surg 49A:322, 1967.
49. Riordan DC, Kaplan EB: The thumb. In Spinner M (ed): Kaplan's Functional and Surgical Anatomy of the Hand. Philadelphia, JB Lippincott, 1984.
50. Schneider LH: Tendon injuries of the hand. In Nicholas JA, Hershman EB, Posner MA (eds): The Upper Extremity in Sports Medicine. St. Louis, CV Mosby, 1990.
51. Sedel L: Dislocation of the carpometacarpal joints. In Tubiana R (ed): The Hand, vol 2. Philadelphia, WB Saunders, 1985.
52. Sedel L: Dislocation of the metacarpophalangeal joint. In Tubiana R (ed): The Hand, vol 2. Philadelphia, WB Saunders, 1985.
53. Smith JH: Avulsion of a profundus tendon with simultaneous intraarticular fracture of the distal phalanx: Case report. J Hand Surg 6:600, 1981.
54. Smith RJ: Post-traumatic instability of the metacarpophalangeal joint of the thumb. J Bone Joint Surg 59A:14, 1977.
55. Smith RJ, Peimer CA: Injuries to the metacarpal bones and joints. Adv Surg 2:341, 1977.
56. Spinner M, Choi BY: Anterior dislocation of the proximal interphalangeal joint: A care of rupture of the central slip of the extensor mechanism. J Bone Joint Surg 52A:1329, 1970.
57. Stener B: Acute injuries to the metacarpophalangeal joint of the thumb. In Tubiana R (ed): The Hand, vol 2. Philadelphia, WB Saunders, 1985.
58. Stener B: Displacement of the ruptured ulnar collateral ligament of the metacarpophalangeal joint of the thumb: A clinical and anatomical study. J Bone Joint Surg 44B:869, 1962.
59. Stothard J, Caird DM: Experience with arthrography of the first metacarpophalangeal joint. Hand 13:257, 1981.
60. Stripling WD: Displaced intra-articular osteochondral fracture: Cause for irreducible dislocation of the distal interphalangeal joint. J Hand Surg 7:77, 1982.
61. Sweterlitsch PR, Torg JS, Pollack H: Entrapment of a sesamoid on the index metacarpophalangeal joint: Report of two cases. J Bone Joint Surg 51A:995, 1969.
62. Thoren L: A new method of extension treatment in Bennett's fracture. Acta Chir Scand 110:485, 1956.
63. Webbe MA, Schneider LH: Mallet fractures. J Bone Joint Surg 66A:658, 1984.

22 Pelvis, Hip, and Thigh

Steven F. Harwin

INTRODUCTION

Although sports injuries of the pelvis, hip, and thigh may not receive the same attention as those of the knee, ankle, and upper extremities, these areas are equally important to the athlete's performance. These injuries occur at all levels of competition and with all types of activities, including throwing, running, jumping, and changing directions. Older athletes are at increased risk for injuries to the pelvis, hip, and thigh as a result of previous injuries, diminished elasticity, and decreased injury repair mechanisms[51] of a body region that constantly bears a significant amount of stress and strain with activities of daily living.

The region of the pelvis, hip, and thigh includes the largest bone in the body, the femur, and the most powerful and largest muscles, the glutei, the quadriceps, and the hamstrings. They provide a link and support system, connecting the trunk to the lower extremity for weight bearing and locomotion, while providing visceral protection as well. It is obvious that injuries that disable such structures would cause difficulties with sports and activities of daily living. The ability to diagnose and manage injuries of this body region in a timely fashion is of paramount importance to the athlete.

ANATOMY

Understanding the complex anatomy of this region is essential to diagnose and manage injuries affecting the pelvis, hip, and thigh. A complete review of the anatomy is beyond the scope of this chapter; however, an overview of the pertinent anatomy is appropriate.

The bony pelvis (Fig. 22-1) is composed of the two innominate bones, each of which contains three bones: the ilium, the ischium, and the pubis. The three converge at the acetabulum, the pelvic portion of the hip joint. The sacrum and coccyx, which are cradled by the innominate bones, compose the posterior bony pelvis. These articulate posteriorly with the paired innominate bones to form the sacroiliac joint. The innominate bones articulate anteriorly via the pubis and the ischium to form the symphysis pubis. Neither of these joints has any gross motion across it, nor is there muscle action across them. However, the entire pelvis is capable of moving as a unit. These motions include anterior–posterior tilt, lateral tilt, and rotation.

The femur, or thigh bone, has a head and neck region that articulates with the acetabulum to form the hip joint, a complex ball and socket joint. It also has a greater and lesser trochanter to which muscles attach. The average angle between the head and the neck is 125° to 135°.[37] The hip is capable of motion in several planes, but most motion occurs in the sagittal plane (flexion).[63] Activities of daily living require 100° to 120° of flexion, 20° of abduction, and 20° of external rotation.[43] Sporting activities require more motion.[43] The hip is subjected to significant joint forces of up to three times body weight in the early and late stance phase of walking and up to five times body weight with running.[61,63,79] The bony configuration, ligaments, the labrum surrounding the acetabulum, and the muscles surrounding the hip joint all contribute to hip joint stability .

There are several major muscle groups affecting the motion of the pelvis, hip, and thigh. The abdominal group—the external obliques, the internal obliques, the transversus abdominis, and the rectus abdominis—is often overlooked regarding this function. They insert on the iliac wing and flex the trunk if the pelvis is fixed. Conversely, they flex the pelvis when the trunk is fixed. They are segmentally innervated. Also often ignored are the muscles and fascia of the pelvic floor, including the levator ani, coccygeus, and the piriformis.

The three gluteal muscles—the gluteus maximus, medius, and minimus—originate from the posterior and lateral ilium and insert onto the posterior femur and the greater trochanter. The gluteus maximus is the strongest hip joint extensor, which makes it especially important for running and jumping activities. It is innervated by the inferior gluteal nerve. The gluteus medius and minimus are abductors and internal rotators of the hip, as is the tensor fascia femoris. Their innervation is derived from the superior gluteal nerve.

The three adductors—the adductor brevis, longus, and magnus—originate from the pubis and insert onto the medial aspect of the femur. These muscles adduct the hip and thigh. The gracilis and pectineus are often grouped with the adductors because they share a similar origin. However, the pectineus is actually a minor hip flexor, innervated by the femoral nerve, whereas the adductors and the gracilis are innervated by the obturator nerve.

The iliopsoas is the primary muscle responsible for hip flexion. It originates from the transverse processes of the lumbar vertebrae and inserts onto the lesser

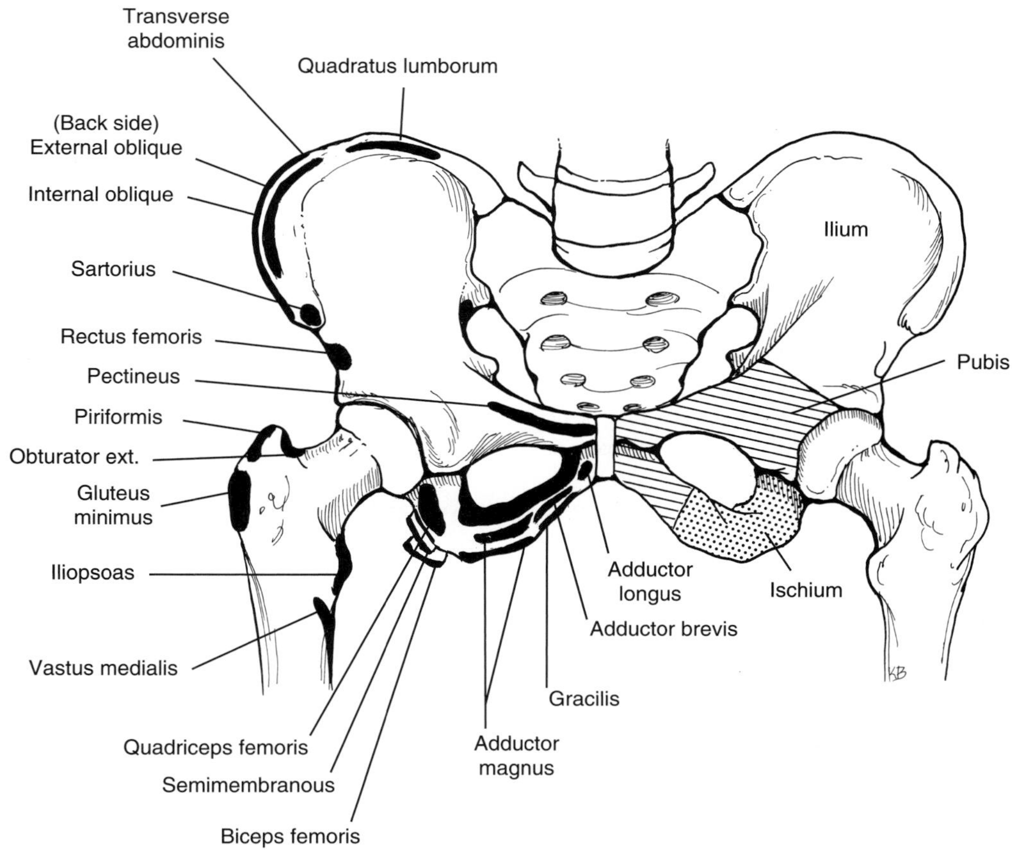

FIGURE 22-1. Diagram of the bony anatomy of the pelvis, hip, and thigh. Also included are selected muscle origins.

trochanter of the femur. It is important for jumping, stair climbing, and uphill running. Depending on position of the hip, it also can serve as an external rotator.

The sartorius muscle is a minor hip flexor and external rotator. Its origin is from the anterior superior iliac spine of the pelvis, and it inserts onto the proximal medial tibia. Therefore, it crosses two joints and is subject to significant stresses; it is innervated by the femoral nerve.

The short external rotators of the hip include the piriformis, the obturator externus and internus, the superior and inferior gemelli, and the quadratus femoris. The gluteus maximus is the primary external rotator of the hip. As a group, the short external rotators originate from the pelvis about the ischium and insert onto and around the posterior greater trochanter of the femur.

For simplicity, it is easier to view the thigh as being composed of two compartments: the anterior (or flexor) and posterior (or extensor) compartments, respectively. The anterior muscles are referred to as the quadriceps femoris, composed of the rectus femoris, vastus medialis, vastus lateralis, and vastus intermedius, which is the deepest. The rectus femoris originates from the anterior inferior iliac spine of the pelvis and the anterior acetabulum inserting via the patella onto the tibial tubercle of the proximal tibia. The other quadriceps muscles originate from the anterior proximal femur and share the same insertion as the rectus femoris. The rectus femoris is a hip flexor and a knee extensor. It crosses the hip and knee joints, and, like the sartorius, it is more prone to injury because of the greater applied stresses. The quadriceps muscle group is innervated by the femoral nerve.

The posterior thigh compartment contains the injury-prone hamstring muscles. These include the semimembranosus, the semitendinosus, and the short and long head of the biceps femoris. The hamstrings originate from the ischial tuberosity and insert onto the proximal tibia and fibular head, thereby also crossing two joints The semimembranosus has a complex insertion that makes up a significant portion of the supporting posterior medial structures of the knee. The semitendinosus shares a common insertion onto the antero-medial tibia with the sartorius and the gracilis comprising the pes anserinus (named thus since it loosely resembles a *goose's foot*).

The hamstrings cross the hip and knee joint and are also susceptible to injury because of this arrangement. Primarily, they are hip extensors and knee flexors.

However, they also affect rotatory motions of the thigh. The biceps femoris is an external rotator, and the semitendinosus affects internal rotation.[28] All of the hamstrings are innervated by the tibial division of the sciatic nerve, except for the short head of the biceps femoris, which is innervated by the peroneal division of the sciatic nerve (Fig. 22-2 and Table 22-1).

The iliotibial band (or tract) is the fascial extension of the tensor fascia femoris and the gluteus maximus. It traverses down the posterior lateral thigh to the lateral intermuscular septum and the vastus lateralis onto the proximal lateral tibia at Gerdy's tubercle.[29] It assists knee flexion and extension, depending on the starting position of the knee. This two-joint muscle–tendon unit is not infrequently injured, causing ilio-tibial band syndrome.

The major ligaments of the pelvis include those of the sacroiliac joint and symphysis pubis. The suprapubic, arcuate pubic, and interpubic ligaments support the symphysis pubis. The dorsal and anterior sacroiliac ligaments and the posterior interosseous ligaments are the primary ligaments supporting the sacroiliac joint. The sacrospinous and sacrotuberous ligaments are accessory supporting ligaments of the complex of the sacroiliac joint. Sacroiliac ligament sprains, often associated with lumbar spine pathology, are not uncommon.

The hip joint has two major ligaments: the iliofemoral ligament anteriorly and the ischiofemoral posteriorly. The pubofemoral is a minor hip joint ligament. These three ligaments compose the hip capsule, which extends from the acetabulum anterior and posterior to the proximal femoral neck. The capsule tightens with internal rotation of the hip. This accounts for the often externally rotated position of the hip after injury, allowing relaxation and greater volume.

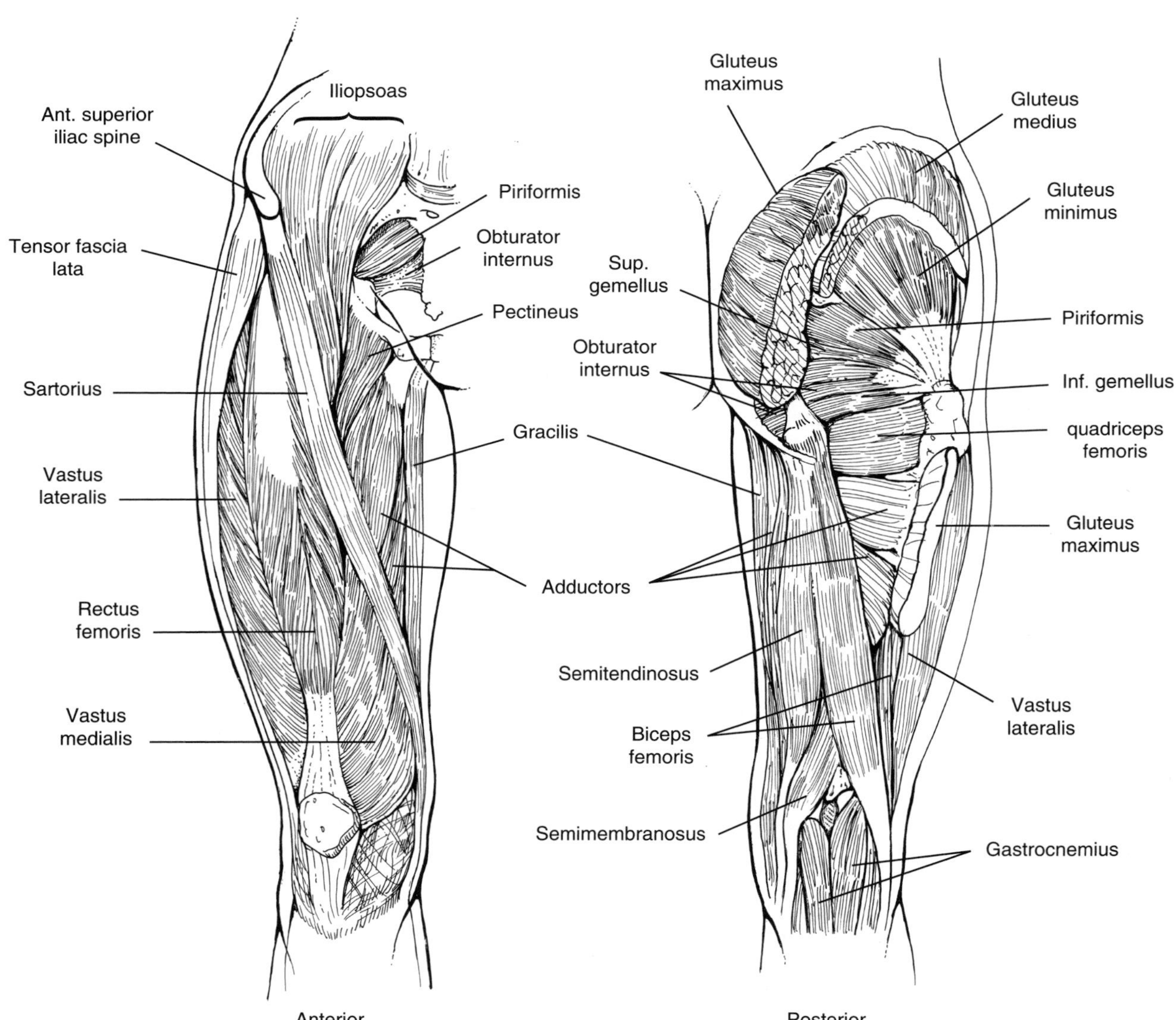

FIGURE 22-2. Diagram of the muscles of the pelvis, hip, and thigh.

Muscle Group Functions

TABLE 22-1

Muscle	Primary	Secondary
Hip flexors	Iliopsoas	Sartorius, quadriceps
Hip extensors		Gluteus maximus
Hamstrings		
Hip abductors and internal rotators	Gluteus medius, gluteus minimus, tensor fascia lata	Gracilis
Hip adductors	Adductor magnus, adductor longus, adductor brevis	Pectineus, posterior gluteus maximus, quadratus femoris, hamstrings
External rotators	Gluteus maximus	Piriformis, biceps femoris, obturator internus and externus, superior and inferior gemelli, quadratus femoris

The intracapsular blood supply to the femoral head and neck are from the retinacular vessels, which are branches of the medial and lateral circumflex femoral arteries. Interruption of this important blood supply can cause osteonecrosis of the hip.

The sensory dermatomes of the hip and thigh are important to know and assess during the physical examination. The inner thigh has a distribution of innervation from L1 to L4. The lateral thigh is innervated from L5, and the posterior thigh from S1 and S2 (Fig. 22-3).[38]

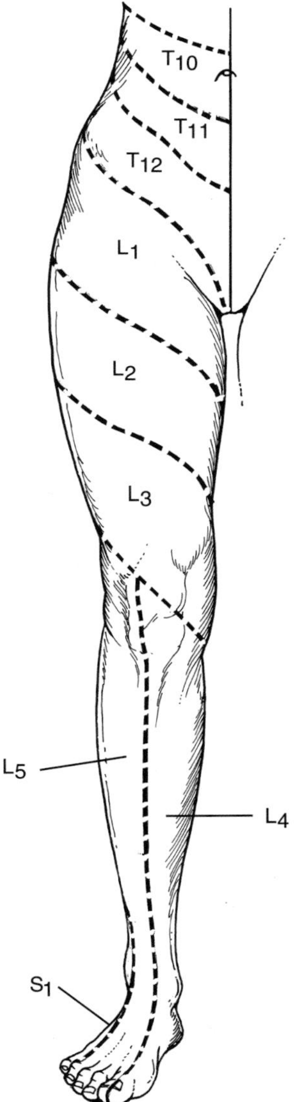

FIGURE 22-3. Sensory dermatome innervation of the pelvis, hip, and thigh (anterior view).

HISTORY AND PHYSICAL EXAMINATION

A time-honored adage of all medical disciplines is certainly applicable to the sports medicine physician: nothing can take the place of a thorough history and physical examination. This assessment must include the hip, knee, pelvis, and spine. The examiner must be aware of remote causes of hip or groin pain such as abdominal pathology, gynecological problems, abnormalities of the genitalia, and pain from remote causes including the kidneys.

The history of injury is vital. We must ascertain when, where, how, and why the injury occurred. The mechanism of injury will help significantly. We must elicit whether or not any sound, snap, click, clunk, or crunch was heard. The character of the pain will also help. Obviously the site of the pain is key, but the type of pain—whether sharp, dull, ache, or cramp—is equally important. We should know whether the pain is present at rest or only with motion. Any numbness, tingling, weakness, or paralysis (even transient) must be noted. Any past injuries, especially similar in nature, and any surgery should be known.

Particularly with the pelvis, hip, and thigh, the physical examination should proceed through several sequential steps, including examination standing, supine, and at times sitting and side lying. Observation and inspection of the athlete is the first step. This includes observation in both stance and during the gait cycle. The standing examination will look for deformities, tilting, swelling, masses, ecchymosis, and gait abnormalities. Limps observed may be antalgic or due to weakness of the abductors or extensors. The patient's posture, alignment, and ability to sit and stand are checked. Any atrophy or muscle asymmetry or wasting is noted. A patient walking with a hand stabilizing the anterior thigh can be suspect for a quadriceps injury or extensor mechanism disruption. It is obviously helpful to ask the patient to point precisely to the source of pain. The spine and low back region is examined, as is the hip.

Palpation should next be performed, eliciting asymmetry, tenderness, and spasm. The range of motion of the joints can then be assessed. The joints above and below the affected area should be examined and ruled out as the source of pathology. The pelvis should be thoroughly examined as well. Palpation of the bony prominences and soft tissue landmarks should be carried out, including the anterior superior iliac spines, ischial tuberosities, pubic symphysis, sciatic nerve, and inguinal region. Swelling and tenderness in the groin region can be indicative of lymphadenopathy, hematoma, hernia, or rarely a tumor.

Range of motion of the hip is assessed supine and prone. Normal hip flexion is 120°. Any contractures should be noted. Extension of the hip, normally about 30°, is best assessed prone. The pelvis is stabilized and abduction is tested, which is usually about 45°. Adduction of the hip approaches 30°. Internal and external rotation is variable, depending on the degree of anteversion of the hips, and usually reaches up to 45°. The more anteversion present, the more internal rotation and less external rotation will be found. People with retroverted hips will have more external and less internal rotation.

The performance of some specific diagnostic physical tests will aid in assessing the joints and muscles. Passive straight leg raising should be examined. If the knee begins to flex when the hip is flexed less than 60°, then the hamstrings are tight, indicating spasm or contracture. The Thomas test, whereby both hips are initially fully flexed, then one hip extended, is performed. A lack of complete extension indicates a flexion contracture of the hip. The Ober test checks for contracture of the tensor fascia lata. The patient lies on the unaffected side with that hip flexed. The upper limb is then abducted and extended. If the limb cannot be lowered to an adducted position, then tightness exists. The Ely test is performed prone and the knee is flexed. If full flexion is not possible or the hip begins to flex, then there is tightness of the anterior muscles.

The Trendelenburg test will reveal weakness of the abductors. If standing on the single affected limb allows dropping of the pelvis on the other side, or tilting of the trunk toward the affected side, weakness is present. The Patrick test (also referred to by the acronym FABER test) brings the hip into flexion, abduction, and external rotation. Pain and limitation of motion is usually indicative of intrinsic hip pathology and may be one of the first signs of osteoarthritis.

A tendency for the hip to externally rotate upon flexion is indicative of a positive Whitman sign, indicating a possible deformity such as is seen with a slipped capital femoral epiphysis.

A neurological exam, including sensory and motor function, should be performed. Circulation and pulses also must be documented.

The next step is a radiographic analysis based on the findings elicited during the history and physical examination. Radiographs are a routine part of the examination because it may be difficult to differentiate a sprain from a more serious injury such as an avulsion fracture, especially in athletes with open growth centers. For pelvic injuries, an anteroposterior radiograph and inlet and outlet views (Fig. 22-4) and oblique or Judet[44] (Fig. 22-5) views in some combination are necessary. A hip series includes anteroposterior and lateral radiographs. Anteroposterior radiographs with internal or external rotation of the hip can also be helpful at times. The femur requires anteroposterior and lateral radiographs of the entire shaft and should include the hip and knee joints. Oblique views may be needed to view lesions such as myositis ossificans or tumors.

Radiographs of the spine would include anteroposterior, lateral, oblique, and cone down views. Depending on findings, a CT scan, MRI scan, and bone scans may be required.

Laboratory studies would be indicated based on the working diagnosis. These might include a CBC, chemistry profile, arthritis profile, and urinalysis.

SOFT-TISSUE INJURIES

Contusions and Sprains

Soft-tissue injuries are common in all sports, and frequently occur in the pelvis, hip, and thigh. Contusions, or bruises, are the most common of these injuries, involving any structure from the skin, superficially, all the way down to the bone and periosteum. Usually, they are of minor severity and are managed symptomatically,[94] although some can cause significant hematoma formation requiring more extensive treatment.[30] Radiographs of the affected area are necessary to exclude the possibility of a fracture or dislocation.

Contusions of the skin run the gamut of a simple ecchymosis to a more significant "raspberry," where the dermis is scraped, scabbed, rough, and tender. These are caused during sliding activities, especially on artificial turf or hard dirt. Management involves cleansing the area and applying topical antimicrobial agents. With activities, the region must be protected from further injury.

Muscle contusions are very common in the anterior and anterolateral thigh. Often these contusions involve

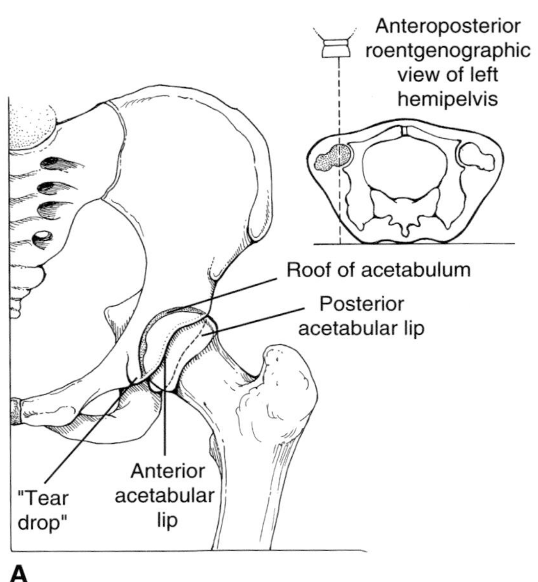

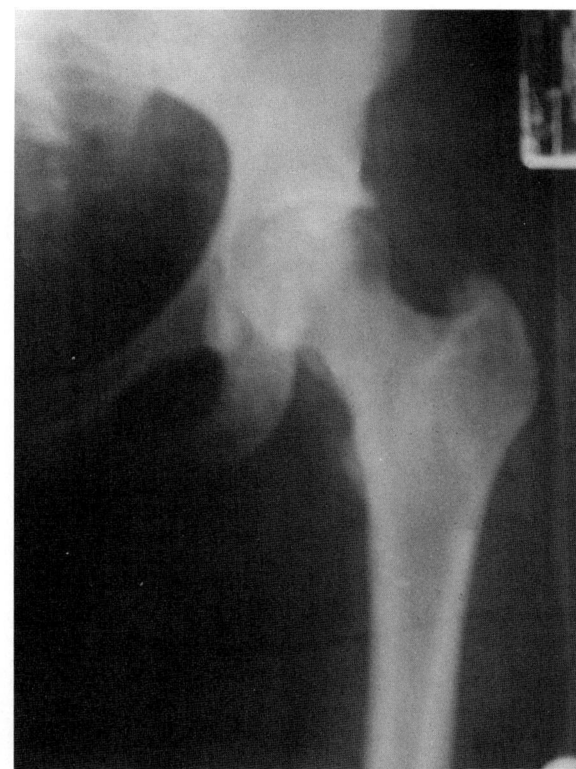

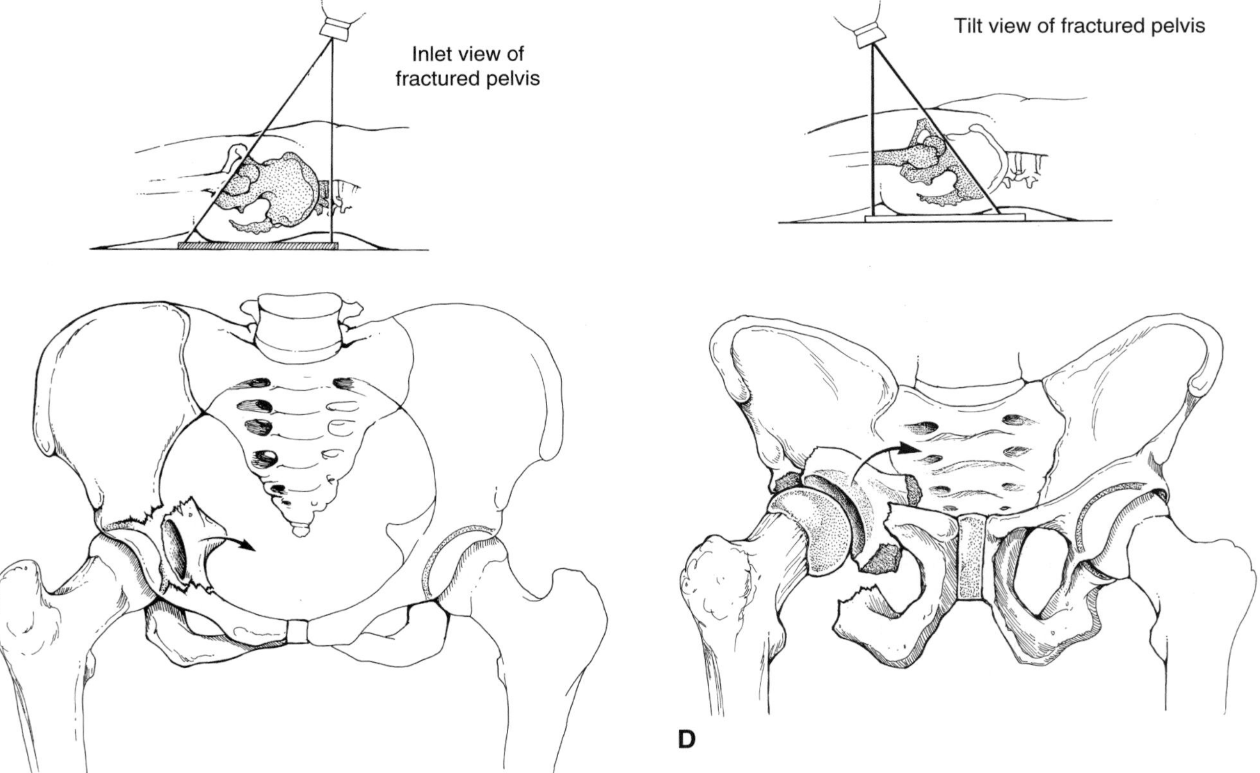

FIGURE 22-4. **A,** Illustration of the technique used for patient positioning to obtain radiographs of the hemipelvis. **B,** An anteroposterior radiograph of a hemipelvis. **C,** Illustration of a pelvic inlet view. The same position of the patient as for an anteroposterior view with the x-ray beam angled 25° caudally. **D,** Illustration of a pelvic outlet view. The x-ray beam is angled 35° cephalad.

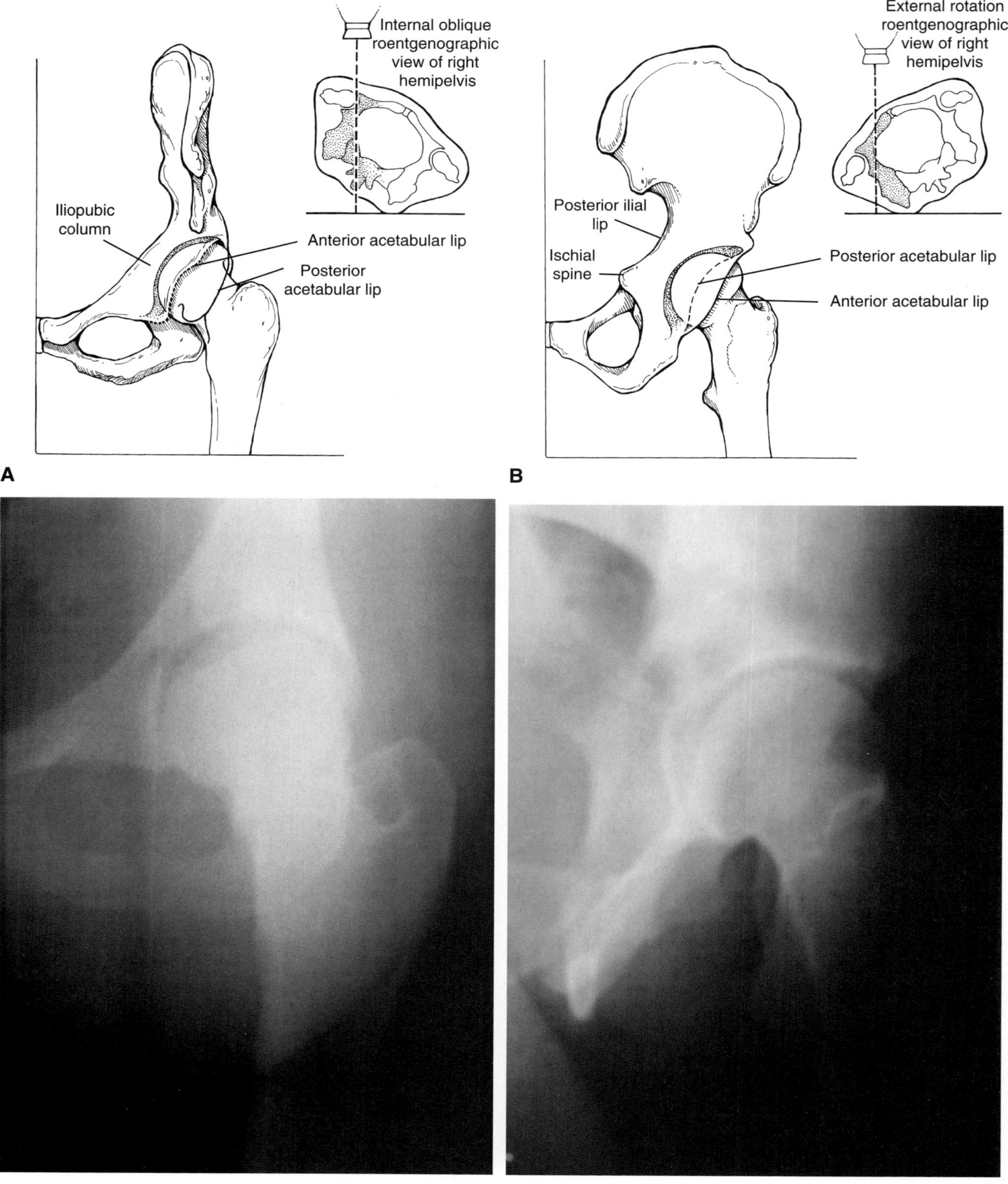

FIGURE 22-5. Oblique (Judet) views of the pelvis to better view the acetabulum. **A,** Anterior oblique view (internal oblique); an anteroposterior pelvic radiograph with the patient rotated 45° away from the injured side, visualizing the iliopubic column and the posterior acetabular lip. **B,** Posterior oblique view (external oblique). The patient is rotated toward the affected side, which visualizes the posterior column and the anterior acetabular lip.**C,** Radiograph illustrating anterior oblique view. **D,** Radiograph illustrating posterior oblique view.

the sartorius and the rectus femoris and are commonly referred to as the "charley horse" injury. They are caused by a significant blunt force being applied directly to the thigh and may lead to hematoma or heterotopic ossification formation.

Bone bruises or contusions are deeper, involve greater force application, and take longer to resolve. The most common locations are the greater trochanter, ischial tuberosity, pubic ramus, and the sacrum. These bony areas are more superficial, with less soft-tissue coverings. Hip pointers are included among these injuries (Fig. 22-6). This term is ambiguous, but it typically involves a blunt-force injury to the iliac crest with subperiosteal hematoma formation.[49] The hip pointer injury includes apophyseal avulsions and fractures and contusions of the iliac crest.[49] With a hip pointer, the athlete experiences difficulty with ambulation and with standing upright secondary to muscle spasm and pain.

In general, the symptoms involved with soft-tissue contusions are localized pain and tenderness acutely, which can become diffuse with time. The patient often will experience decreased range of motion and muscle spasm. Disuse atrophy of the surrounding musculature may ensue if the recovery process is prolonged by symptoms.

Management is similar to that used for all soft-tissue injuries. Initial treatment consists of rest, ice, compression, and elevation. A graduated therapy program then begins and is progressed as the patient tolerates. Later, heat and massage therapies as well as ultrasound and transcutaneous electrical stimulation may be used as adjunctive pain therapeutic modalities.

The first goal of the therapy program is to improve the symptoms. Then, restoring flexibility by stretching the surrounding muscles is instituted. Once the acute symptoms have resolved, restoration of power, strength, and speed are the next goals to be attained. Therapy involves a progression from isometric exercises to isotonic exercises and then on to isokinetic and dynamic resistant exercises. Aerobic reconditioning is essential. The final step of therapy is sports-specific rehabilitation (see box, Physiotherapy Principles). Aspirin and nonsteroidal anti-inflammatory drugs (NSAIDs) must be used cautiously because they may increase the bleeding into the soft tissue[30] and aggravate the initial insult. Physiotherapy modalities and regimens will be discussed in greater detail in another chapter.

Return to sports is guided by the athlete's symptoms and objective evidence of functional normalcy, including coordination, strength, speed, endurance, and painless athletic participation.[30]

More serious diagnoses must be considered when a severe soft-tissue contusion is encountered about the pelvis, hip, and thigh in the athlete, such as a sciatic nerve contusion. Buttock pain with radiation in the sciatic nerve distribution, down the back of the thigh and calf, would be reported. Also, crush injuries and compartment syndrome must be included in the differential diagnosis with severe soft-tissue injuries. Crush injuries and compartment syndrome exhibit a rather tense thigh with the mechanism of injury imparting a significant amount of energy to the region. The examining physician must have a high index of suspicion of thigh compartment syndrome because the symptoms may be subtle with pain and sensory abnormalities and only a mildly swollen thigh. If this diagnosis is suspected, compartment pressures must be measured in the offending compartment. If they are significantly elevated, emergent operative release of all offending fascial compartments must be performed.

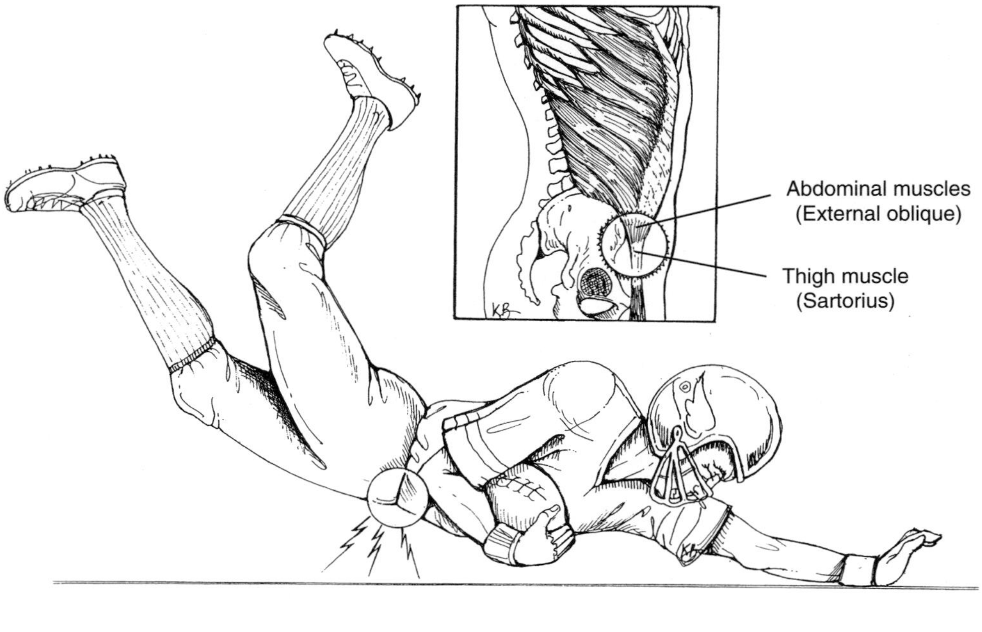

FIGURE 22-6. Illustration of the mechanism of a hip pointer. A direct blow causes a contusion to the iliac crest.

CHECKLIST

Physiotherapy Principles

1. First resolve symptoms*
2. Stretch affected muscles
3. Regain muscle power, strength, and flexibility
4. Regain endurance and aerobic conditioning†
5. Sport-specific training‡

*Rest, ice, NSAIDs, etc.
†When 95% ROM, 75% strength of uninjured leg attained.
‡Sports return when 90% strength of uninjured leg attained.

CHECKLIST

Etiology of Muscle Injuries

- ☐ Poor flexibility
- ☐ Poor coordination
- ☐ Poor warm-up
- ☐ Muscle strength imbalance
- ☐ Muscle weakness
- ☐ Fatigue
- ☐ Electrolyte imbalance
- ☐ Poor technique with sports activity
- ☐ Increased age

The most common long-term complications of soft-tissue contusions are bursitis and the formation of heterotopic ossification, or myositis ossificans. Either one of these conditions can significantly prolong and impede an athlete's rehabilitation and return to sporting activities.

Sprain of the ligaments about the hip is less common than those of the spine and sacroiliac joint, knee, and ankle. Injuries that cause more than tolerated motion may result in sprain of the capsule and ligaments. Exact, precise diagnosis by physical exam is difficult because of the remote location.

In an aging and yet vigorous population, we must be aware that all of these conditions may be superimposed on concomitant entities such as osteoarthritis. The older athlete will take longer to heal and must be counseled.

Muscle Injuries

Muscle injuries are extremely common in sports, and are the most common athletic injuries of the pelvis, hip, and thigh. Contusions were mentioned in the preceding section. Most injuries are minor strains, which are tears or "pulls" at the musculo-tendonous junction.[100] It is important for the examining and treating physician to distinguish between partial and complete tears. The mechanism of injury involves violent contractions with forceful stretching of the involved muscle.[23] This contracting and stretching causes increased energy to be absorbed in the muscle, which exceeds its ultimate tensile strength. This same mechanism causes avulsion fractures in skeletally immature athletes because the tendons are stronger than the cartilage growth plate.

Risk factors for muscle injuries include inadequate flexibility and warm-up, muscle strength imbalances, muscle weakness, electrolyte imbalance, and increased age. Preconditioning and stretching to increase blood flow to the muscles and to increase their ability to absorb energy decreases the incidence of muscle injuries (see box, Etiology of Muscle Injuries).[48,80]

Physical therapy regimens are progressed as was previously discussed with soft-tissue contusions. Surgery is warranted only for complete tears of essential muscle tendon units.

Hamstrings. The hamstring muscles are the most commonly involved muscle injury of the pelvis, hip, and thigh.[49] The injuries often occur at the musculo-tendonous junction with forced flexion of the hip with a fully extended knee, or when the hamstrings are maximally stretched. The symptoms are posterior thigh pain, possibly a "pop" being felt, and difficulty ambulating. Sports activities are inhibited, and a defect may be palpated with the athlete prone with the knee flexed against resistance. The symptoms are exacerbated by knee extension while the hip is flexed. The medial hamstrings—the semimembranosus and semitendinosus—are usually injured during the swing phase of the gait cycle, whereas the lateral hamstrings—the biceps femoris—are injured during the foot take-off phase of the gait cycle.[10] The biceps femoris are the more commonly injured muscles. Hamstring injuries occur primarily in runners because they are antagonists to hip flexion and knee extension, which is an important position of the limb during running. The hamstrings are at increased risk for injury because they cross both the hip and knee joints.

Risk factors for hamstring injuries are poor technique with athletic activities such as warm-up, stretching, and posture. Poor flexibility, endurance, leg length discrepancy, and muscle strength imbalance will increase the susceptibility to hamstring injuries.[52] These and all muscle injuries are clinically classified according to the degree of symptoms and injury. Symptom severity can increase up to 2 weeks after the injury.[41]

A first-degree hamstring injury resolves in a few days with little hemorrhage, no structural damage, and without any objective evidence of functional loss. Second-degree injuries are of moderate severity and represent a partial tear of the muscle with some functional loss. A "pop" is usually heard, and structural damage is present. A painful mass may be palpated posteriorly in the muscle belly. Third-degree injuries are severe, complete tears, usually occurring near the origin or insertion of the muscle. A mass is also palpable in the muscle belly (Table 22-2).[52] Radiographs should be taken to rule out an avulsion fracture of the ischial tuberosity.

Return to sports activities is allowed when the isokinetic strength is within 10% of the uninjured side and

TABLE 22-2 Muscle Injury Classification

Degree	Severity	Structural Damage	Functional Loss	Recovery Time
1st	Mild	None	None to mild	Several days
2nd	Moderate	Partial tear	Mild to moderate	1–3 weeks
3rd	Severe	Complete tear	Moderate to severe	Several weeks

when the other criteria that were previously discussed with soft-tissue injuries are attained.[52]

Quadriceps Femoris. The quadriceps femoris consists of four muscles, of which only the rectus femoris crosses the hip and knee joints. Maximal activity in this muscle group occurs during the heel-off phase of the gait cycle,[17] which coincides with maximal hamstring activity. The quadriceps also function as a decelerator during the support phase of running.[87] The classification of injuries is similar to that for hamstring injuries, except that knee range of motion is also used as a criterion to classify quadriceps injuries. In a first-degree injury, the athlete can flex the knee at least 90°. With a second-degree injury, the knee can flex between 45° and 90°, and a third-degree injury limits flexion to less than 45° (Table 22-3).[41]

The symptoms experienced with quadriceps injuries include pain, spasm, and diminished knee flexion. The limited motion becomes more evident with hip extension if the rectus femoris is primarily involved. The more significantly the motion is restricted, the longer the recovery takes. Hematoma formation is usually evident, but a mass may not be palpable. Radiographic examination is important to rule out a fracture and to assess any heterotopic ossification, especially in chronic injuries.

Complications are relatively common with major anterior thigh muscle injuries. The most common is an extensor lag or weakness and decreased knee flexion. Reruptures and heterotopic ossification formation are more common with complete tears.

Therapy progresses as described in the preceding section. Operative repair usually is necessary for complete tears of the lower-to-middle third of the quadriceps.[41] Return to sport is guided by the principles previously stated. The athlete should have painless motion of the knee within 10° of the uninjured side.[41]

Adductors. The adductors are injured when the thigh is externally rotated and the hip is abducted.[57] This position places maximal stretch on this muscle group. An injury to the adductors at their origin is commonly called the "groin pull."[30] It also has been referred to as "horse rider's strain." This injury is more common in professional and older athletes. The etiology of adductor strains is an imbalance of strength between muscle groups and within the adductor group itself.[57]

Symptoms include pain from the groin to the middle medial thigh, especially in the region of the adductor longus tendon. The pain is worsened with hip abduction.[57] A defect or mass may be palpable over the medial thigh if the tear is complete. These injuries are rarely severe, although power deficits up to 25% have been reported.[58] The differential diagnosis includes an abdominal muscle injury, [89] avulsion fracture of the pubis, or osteitis pubis. A bone scan is useful in the early detection of the latter two entities.

Management proceeds as previously mentioned. Rarely, an operative tenotomy of the adductor longus can be performed for a chronic injury.[74] Return to sport is guided by the same parameters as for quadriceps injuries.

Other Muscles. The external oblique abdominal muscles can be torn at their insertion onto the iliac crests. This injury results from muscle contraction while the trunk is flexed toward the opposite side. The symptoms include tenderness with pain while flexing toward the contralateral side and difficulty straightening the torso. Management is guided by the symptoms and involves restriction from activities, a protective pad, and possibly an abdominal binder.

The iliopsoas can also be injured and strained, especially with muscle contraction when the hip is fixed in extension. The symptoms are deep groin pain or lower

TABLE 22-3 Quadriceps Contusion Classification

Contusion	Knee Motion (°)	Gait	Physical Examination
Mild	>90	Normal	Mildly tender
Moderate	45–90	Antalgic	Tender, large thigh
Severe	<45	Antalgic	Very swollen thigh, painful contraction

abdominal tenderness. Passive external rotation of the hip exacerbates the pain because this position increases the stretch of the iliopsoas.

Rarely, the gluteus medius may be torn or avulsed from the greater trochanter. Partial tears are treated nonoperatively, but complete tears or avulsion of the greater trochanter must be repaired. When the gluteus medius is injured chronically, tendonitis will often ensue. The athlete will experience posterior greater trochanteric pain and tenderness.

The gracilis is often injured with the adductor muscles. Its symptoms and management are the same as for that muscle group.

Myositis Ossificans Traumatica

Myositis ossificans traumatica is heterotopic or ectopic ossification that occurs in a muscle belly or the periosteum after trauma, particularly blunt trauma. It is second only to muscle injuries in frequency of injury in the thigh. The thigh is more commonly involved than the hip (Fig. 22-7).

This is a reactive condition[42] secondary to a soft-tissue injury with hematoma formation. Granulation and scar tissue form secondarily,[93] with calcification developing in the affected area in approximately 3 to 4 weeks.[65] Myositis ossificans is usually located deep near muscle origins, especially about fractures and joints.[2] The exact etiology has not been determined.[99] However, athletes with blood dyscrasias may be predisposed to develop this condition with even minor injuries. Risk factors for development of myositis ossificans include a severe injury, reinjury during the early healing stage, delay in management of muscle injury, a previous history of development of myositis, early vigorous or over-zealous physiotherapy, and surgical treatment before maturation of the lesion (see box, Risk Factors for Myositis Ossificans Traumatica). The overall prognosis is usually excellent.[41,53]

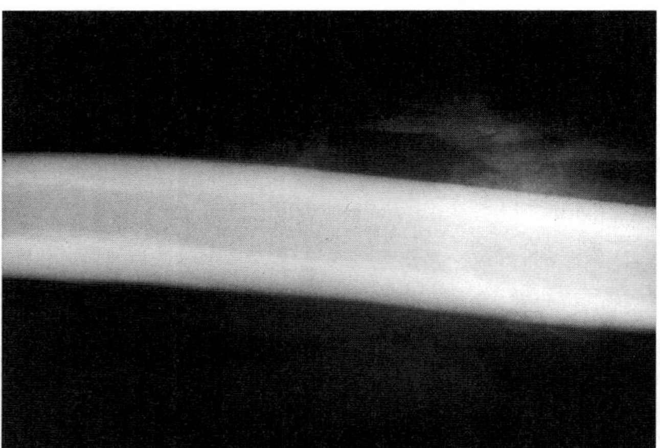

FIGURE 22-7. A lateral radiograph of the mid-shaft of the femur demonstrating myositis ossificans traumatica adjacent to, but not connected to, the femoral cortex.

Myositis ossificans traumatica has been reported to occur in up to 20% of military recruits with thigh contusions.[41] It is less common after thigh muscle strains. The diagnosis should be considered in any athlete with a firm mass at the original sight of injury that develops after 3 to 4 weeks.[1] The athlete will present with a painful and sometimes palpable mass that causes a decreased range of motion.[30] The symptoms also include local swelling, tenderness, and possibly erythema and increased local temperature.

Radiographic examination of the affected area is important to exclude a fracture and to sequentially follow the development and maturation of the myositis. However, the radiographs may not be positive for 2 to 4 weeks.[1,49] The growth of the mass on radiographs stabilizes at 6 months. Ultrasonography has been reported to detect early changes in the soft tissues indicative of the development of myositis ossificans (Fig. 22-8).[47]

Myositis ossificans may be confused with a periosteal osteogenic sarcoma. These two entities are distinguished based on the history, radiographic location of the mass, and the histologic analysis. Myositis ossificans has an antecedent traumatic event, and the athlete is usually younger than 30 years of age. The mass involves the anterior thigh in the majority of patients and stabilizes at 6 months. The alkaline phosphatase is normal, and the radiographs usually will demonstrate a separation between the cortex of the bone and the mass.

With periosteal osteogenic sarcoma, however, the affected individuals are usually older, without an antecedent traumatic event being elicited in the history. The alkaline phosphatase is elevated, and the mass demonstrates continued growth. On radiographic analysis, the mass is contiguous with the cortex of the bone.[65] Furthermore, on histologic examination, the abnormal cells are noted at the periphery of the lesion of the sarcoma, whereas they are centrally located with myositis ossificans. These points of differentiation should help avoid performing a biopsy (Table 22-4).[65]

Management of myositis ossificans is similar to that for other soft-tissue injuries. Bed rest may be necessary if the symptoms are severe. Partial weight bearing with

CHECKLIST

Risk Factors for Myositis Ossificans Traumatica

- ☐ Severe injury
- ☐ Reinjury during early recovery phase
- ☐ Delay in treatment of muscle injury
- ☐ Previous history of myositis ossificans
- ☐ Early vigorous massage and heat with physiotherapy
- ☐ Surgery before lesion maturity

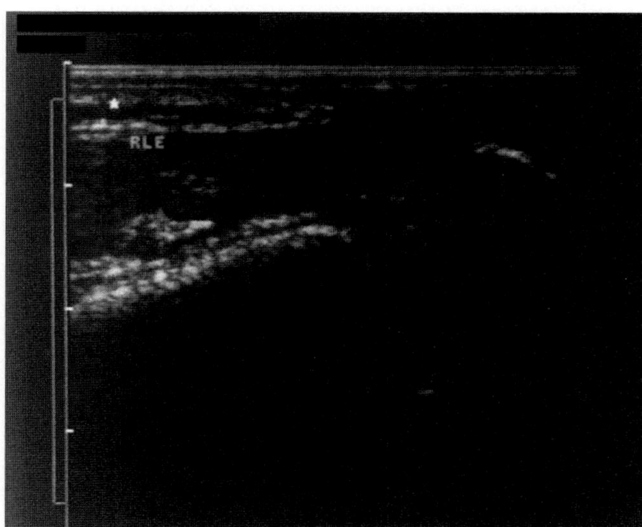

FIGURE 22-8. Ultrasound image demonstrating myositis ossificans.

crutches may be instituted until the pain subsides. NSAIDs should be used cautiously because they can exacerbate the condition by increasing the local bleeding at the injury sight. Massage and manipulation must be avoided because they can increase hematoma formation.[2]

The physiotherapy program begins when the athlete is pain free. Passive range of motion should be avoided for 4 to 6 months.[30] If the functional return is inhibited by the soft-tissue mass, surgery and excision may be necessary. Surgery and excision should not be performed until the mass matures at 9 to 12 months.[66] If surgery is done before the mass is mature, the myositis will recur with greater intensity and quantity. Aspiration and injection of proteolytic enzymes have been used but are better considered experimental modalities at this time.[1,66]

Return to sports is allowed when full strength and agility are obtained, and the athlete can flex the knee 120°.[41] A protective pad over the affected area should be worn.

BURSITIS

The development of a bursitis is very common. Pathology involves an inflammation of the lining, bursa, surrounding bony edges, and joints. The condition is caused by friction from overuse or after trauma from a direct blow to the area that produces an inflammatory response. Classically, the athlete experiences pain that increases with motion and localized tenderness and fullness. Motion is restricted secondary to the pain, and audible "snapping" or crepitation may develop if the condition is chronic.

Bursitis usually develops over the ischial tuberosity, iliopectineal region (Fig. 22-9), and the greater trochanter.[66] Ischial bursitis, commonly called "benchwarmer's bursitis," is painful when seated and must be differentiated from a hamstring injury.[71] Some of the pain is likely secondary to sciatic nerve irritation.

Iliopectineal bursitis causes anterior hip pain and an antalgic gait. The symptoms are lessened with flexion and external rotation of the hip.[21] With trochanteric bursitis, adduction and external rotation of the hip worsens the symptoms. Risk factors for developing trochanteric bursitis include a broad pelvis, which is postulated as the reason for the increased incidence in female athletes. Leg length discrepancy, pronated feet, previous injuries to the area, and abnormal running mechanics such as the feet crossing the midline, are other factors that increase the likelihood of developing this condition.[30]

Management is similar to that for other soft-tissue injuries. NSAIDs play a major role. Aspiration of the bursa and steroid injection may be beneficial if the symptoms persist. With chronicity of the condition, operative excision or release of the offending bursa may be indicated,[68] but only as a final resort.

SNAPPING HIP SYNDROME

Snapping hip syndrome refers to conditions about the hip that cause an audible or palpable "snapping" sound.[82] In addition, the athlete may experience tenderness or

TABLE 22-4 Differential Diagnosis of Myositis Ossificans Traumatica and Osteogenic Sarcoma

	Myositis Ossificans	Osteogenic Sarcoma
Antecedent trauma	+	–
Location of mass	Diaphyseal	Metaphyseal
Status of cortex	Intact	Violated
Histology	Peripheral cells mature	Central cells mature
Symptoms	Pain with activity	Rest and night pain
Size	Decreases with time	Increases with time
Alkaline phosphatase	Normal	Increased

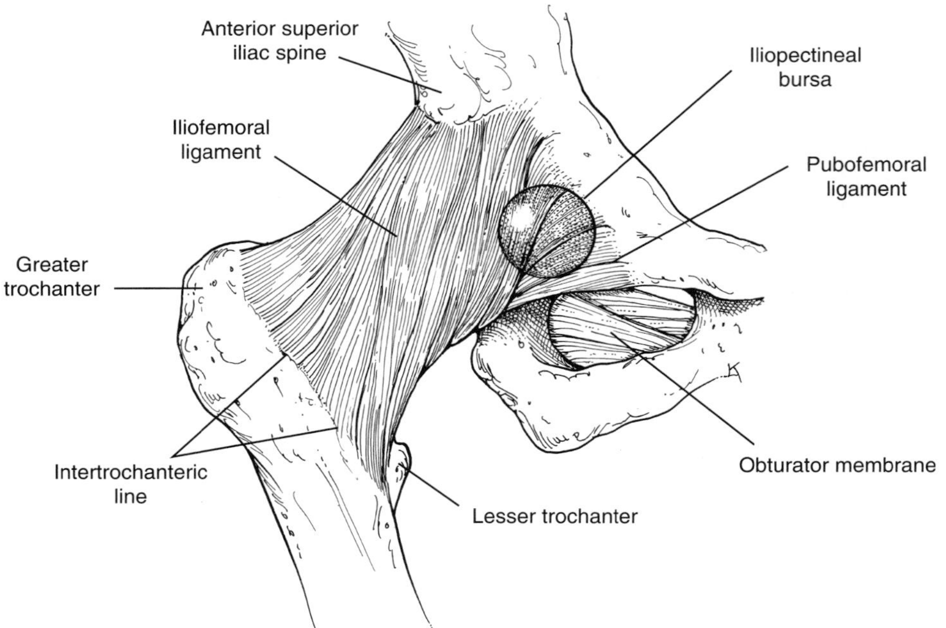

FIGURE 22-9. Illustration of the iliopectineal bursa.

occasional pain, crepitation, and local warmth. This syndrome rarely impairs the athlete's performance.

There are intra-articular and extra-articular etiologies for this syndrome.[101] The most common etiology involves the iliotibial band or tensor fascia lata moving over the greater trochanter.[94] It can also involve the iliopsoas tendon gliding over the iliopectineal eminence in the pelvis or the iliofemoral ligament moving over the femoral head.[94] Posteriorly, the long head of the biceps femoris tendon gliding over the ischial tuberosity can cause this syndrome. Loose bodies, labral tears, synovial chondromatosis, bony exostosis, and subluxation of the hip joint can also produce the snapping hip syndrome.[60,101] Furthermore, women with a wide pelvis, prominent trochanter, and ligament laxity are at increased risk for this condition.

Management involves observation and is symptomatically guided. If signs of inflammation are elicited, NSAIDs should be used. Surgery is rare, but when needed, arthroscopic surgery of the hip can effective, especially for loose bodies and labral tears.

OSTEITIS PUBIS

Osteitis pubis is a self-limited[67] condition caused by inflammation and a reactive periostitis leading to bony changes of the symphysis pubis. Histologic analysis demonstrates a nonspecific inflammatory response with bone resorption and fibrous tissue replacement. The etiologies are a continuum along the spectrum of musculoskeletal injuries and include muscle strains with degenerative changes secondary to overuse, avascular necrosis, an osteochondral defect, fatigue fracture, and avulsion fracture by the gracilis tendon.[97] The condition has also been seen in postpartum women.

The athlete may experience gradual, insidious groin pain, possibly with radiation to the medial thigh and lower abdomen.[30] Tenderness over the pubis may also be elicited. Muscle spasm may be present, particularly in the rectus abdominis and the adductors. Abduction and resisted adduction and pivoting with sports activities increase the pain. Severe symptoms can cause an antalgic or a waddling gait and a clicking sensation. This condition is also known to occur after surgery on the bladder and prostate.[4]

Radiographic findings take approximately 2 to 3 weeks to appear.[97] The findings include symmetrical bone resorption medially, widening of the symphysis, rarefaction or sclerosis of the symphysis, and possibly cystic changes (Fig. 22-10).[33] If cystic changes are present, the physician must also consider hyperparathyroidism, myelomatosis, sarcoidosis, hemochromatosis, rheumatoid arthritis, and osteomyelitis in the differential diagnosis.[33,34] Clinically, the differential diagnosis includes a hernia.

Bone scans demonstrating increased uptake can aid in the early detection of this syndrome.[97] Comparison, weight-bearing views, so-called "flamingo" views, will detect if instability is present. These are taken as two separate radiographs, each one in single leg stance, one with the right leg down and the second with the left leg down. A difference of more than 2 mm in height from a line drawn parallel to the top of the superior pubic ramus on one side of the symphysis pubis to the other is indicative of instability.[7]

Management is symptomatically based. Rest and NSAIDs are the mainstays of treatment. Injection of

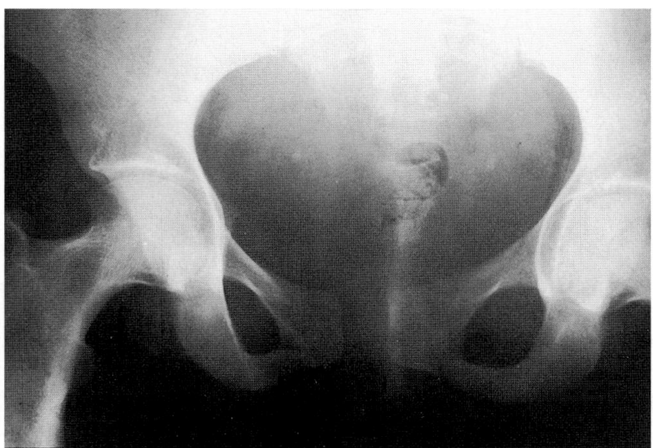

FIGURE 22-10. An anteroposterior radiograph of the pelvis demonstrating widening of the symphysis pubis consistent with osteitis pubis.

steroids may also be used. Rarely, recalcitrant symptoms may necessitate fusion or debridement of the symphysis.[67,97]

ADDUCTOR CANAL SYNDROME

Another condition that may affect the athlete's thigh is the rare adductor canal syndrome, which involves a disruption or compression[3] of the femoral artery at Hunter's canal in the middle third of the anterior thigh. This canal is bordered by the vastus medialis anterolaterally, the sartorius medially, and the adductor longus posterolaterally.[29] The femoral artery and vein and the saphenous nerve pass through this space.

The exact etiology of this syndrome is unclear. It is usually caused by direct trauma leading to thrombosis of the femoral artery. However, an abnormal muscle band from the adductor magnus to the vastus medialis has also been implicated.[91]

Symptoms include leg claudication that worsens with activity and resolves with rest. The physical examination is normal except for absent or diminished pulses. The athlete will have an abnormal response to exercise, with claudication developing, and will have a decreased ankle-brachial index.[91] When the saphenous nerve is affected by the syndrome, the athlete will experience anterior and medial knee pain and possibly dysesthesias.[77] In this case, the symptoms may resolve with injection of a local anesthetic.

The diagnostic work-up includes pulse volume recordings[50] or arteriography[91] to diagnose arterial abnormalities. The Doppler ankle-brachial index can be used as a noninvasive screening test. If results are abnormal, arteriography must be performed. If the superficial femoral artery is determined to be occluded, operative intervention to bypass this lesion is necessary. When recovered, a protective pad for the region should be used during sports participation.

FRACTURES

Pelvis

Pelvic fractures result from very high-energy forces in young patients and from lower-energy injuries in the elderly (Fig. 22-11). Pelvic fractures are rarely incurred by the athlete. The mechanism of injury is either a direct or rotational force application to the pelvis. Collision sports such as football or rugby can cause this injury. Other high-risk sports include hang gliding, auto racing, and snowmobiling. A thorough physical examination is necessary to assess the neurovascular status of the limbs and to exclude any visceral damage to the gastrointestinal or genitourinary tracts; 10% to 30% of pelvic fractures have these associated injuries.[9]

Pelvic fractures are classified as either stable or unstable. One third of all pelvic fractures are unstable.[9] Stable fractures are single-bone fractures that do not involve displacement of the fracture or disruption of the pelvic ring. They are caused by a direct blow to the affected bone. Management is symptomatically guided. A fracture of the iliac wing, sacrum, coccyx, and ischium are examples of stable fractures (Fig. 22-12). With these single-bone fractures, it is essential that the examining physician exclude the possibility of second fracture site in the pelvic ring, indicating potential instability.

Three classic examination maneuvers are performed to assess instability. First, posterior pressure is applied to the iliac crests, and then lateral-to-medial pressure is applied. Finally, downward pressure on the symphysis pubis is performed. Excessive pain or gross motion may indicate an unstable injury pattern.[45] Even in the most experienced hands, pelvic fractures are difficult to assess by physical examination alone.

Unstable pelvis or acetabular fractures less commonly result from sports activities.[94] Unstable fractures include displaced fractures, fractures with dislocations, or joint

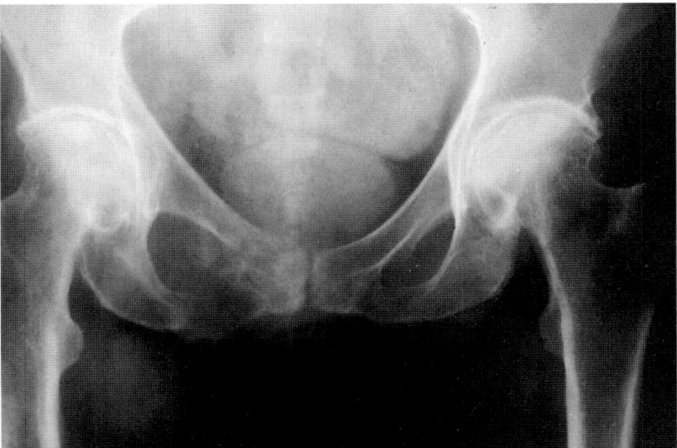

FIGURE 22-11. An anteroposterior radiograph of the pelvis demonstrating superior and inferior pubic rami fractures on the right side.

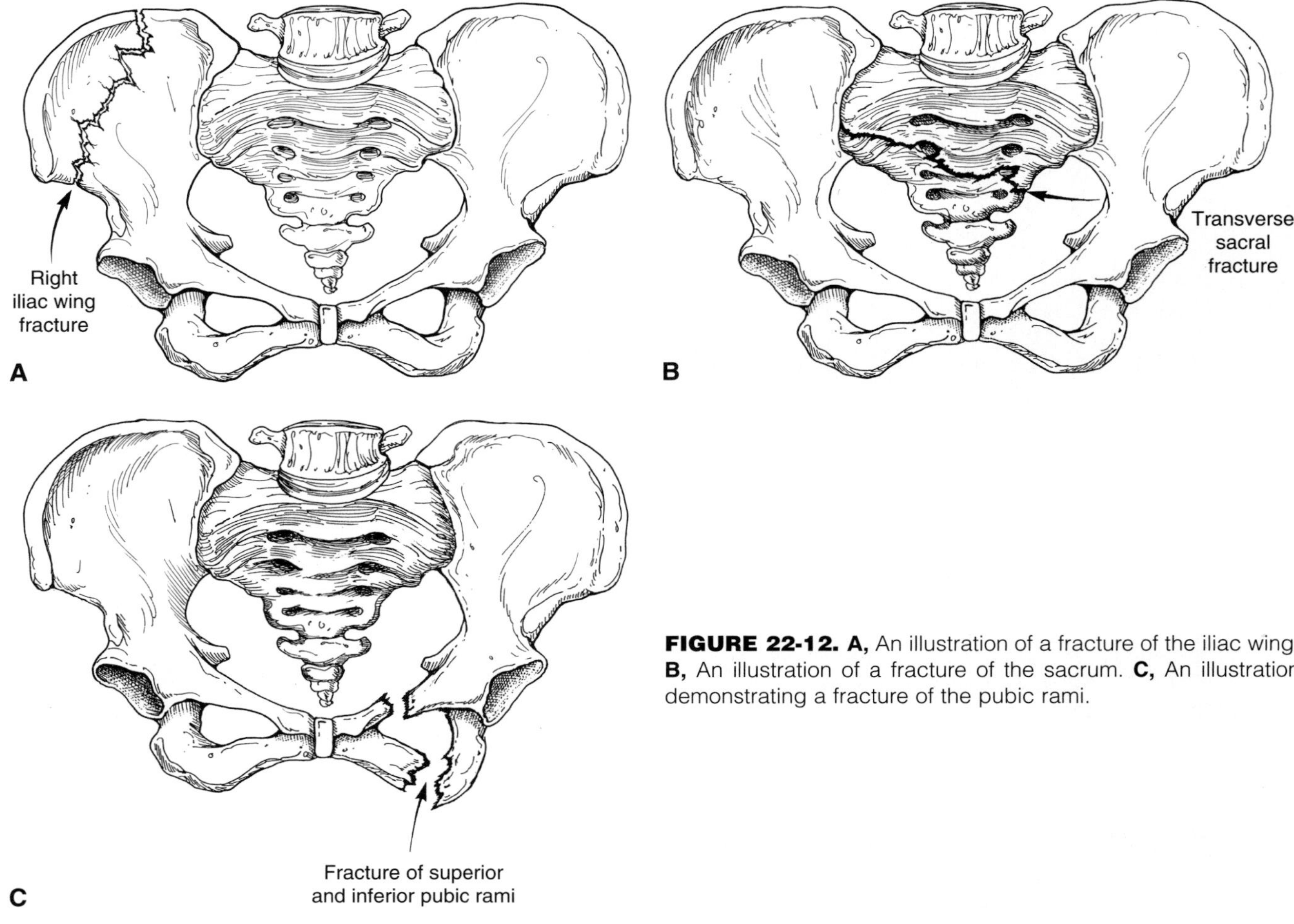

FIGURE 22-12. **A,** An illustration of a fracture of the iliac wing. **B,** An illustration of a fracture of the sacrum. **C,** An illustration demonstrating a fracture of the pubic rami.

separations[95] (Fig. 22-13). Accurate reduction of these fractures and maintenance of the reduction are imperative.

Radiographic analysis must include anteroposterior, lateral, inlet and outlet, and oblique views of the pelvis. Analgesics and appropriate intravenous hydration or blood products are the initial mainstays of treatment. The fracture type guides additional management. Protected weight bearing is begun when tolerated if the fracture is stable or after operative fixation and satisfactory healing of unstable fractures.

Coccyx

Fractures of the coccyx do not commonly result from sports activities. These fractures are sustained when the athlete falls in a seated position or by a direct blow.[30] Symptoms include lower spine and buttock pain that is worse when seated. The pain is localized over the coccyx either externally or internally elicited by a rectal examination. Radiographs should be taken, although they may be difficult to interpret because of the overlying bowel gas patterns. Management is symptomatically guided with NSAIDs or analgesics and donut pads while seated. Warm baths may reduce local muscle spasm. Sports activities are begun when the athlete is pain free. A protective pad should be used over the coccyx. Rarely, a painful ununited fracture may require operative excision.

Hip

Hip fractures also rarely result from athletic participation. The mechanism of injury involves a high-energy trauma applied to the femoral shaft, a rotational force applied to the proximal femur, especially in an older patient, or a direct blow to the greater trochanter. Symptoms include severe groin pain and often deformity. The athlete is unable to bear weight unless the fracture is an impacted subcapital hip fracture or a rare greenstick fracture, occurring in a skeletally immature athlete. With displacement, the leg is held in an externally rotated and shortened position. With nondisplaced fractures, the athlete holds the leg externally rotated because this position is comfortable. Attempts at motion are resisted secondary to pain (Fig. 22-14).

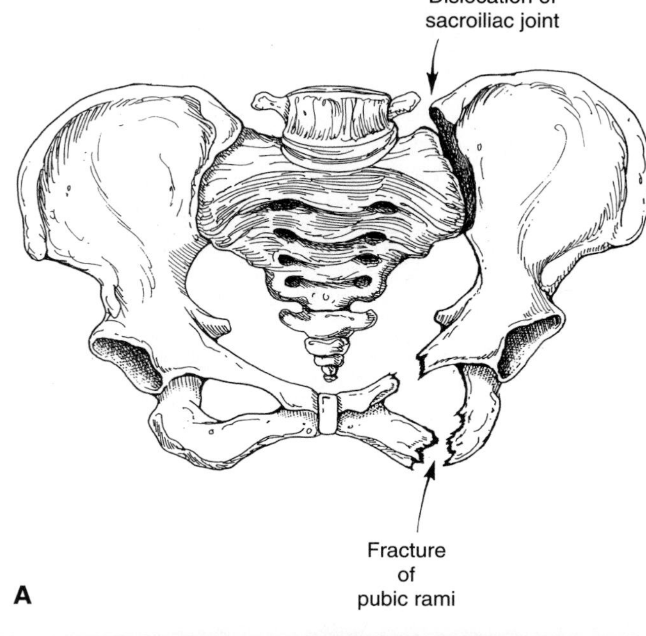

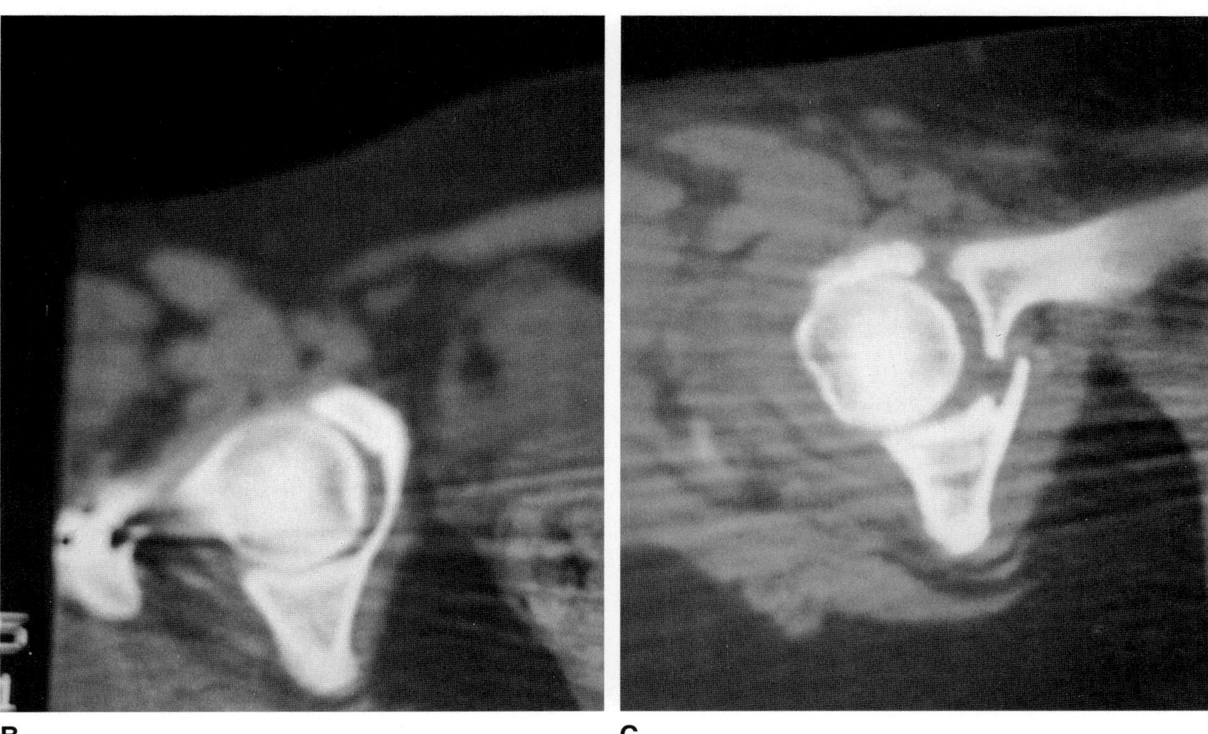

FIGURE 22-13. A, An illustration of an unstable Malgaigne fracture, which involves two vertical fractures on the same side of the pelvis with a dislocation of sacroiliac joint. **B,** A CAT scan demonstrating the normal relationship between the acetabulum and the femoral head. **C,** A CAT scan showing a fracture of the acetabulum with disruption of the normal congruity between the acetabulum and the femoral head with medial wall fracture.

Management is urgent reduction to attain anatomic union because the athlete cannot function well with a significant leg length discrepancy or rotational malalignment. Disruption of the blood supply to the femoral head with ensuing avascular necrosis[21] can be devastating and may occur even with prompt intervention. Skeletally immature athletes may develop premature growth-plate closure, causing a varus deformity as a result of this injury.[14]

The classification of hip injuries in skeletally immature patients is based on location in relation to the growth plate. Commonly, the athlete affected is aged 11 to 13 years.[72] A type I fracture is transepiphyseal; type II is transcervical; type III is cervicotrochanteric; and type IV is an intertrochanteric fracture (Fig. 22-15). Surgery is indicated for type I and II fractures and for a type III fracture if it is displaced. The type IV fracture can be managed either by open reduction and internal fixation

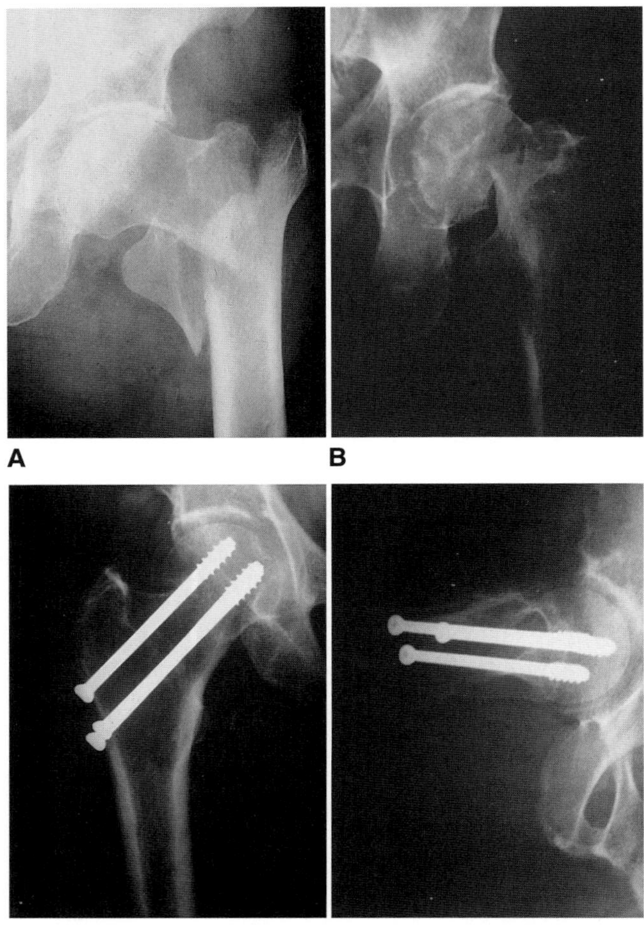

FIGURE 22-14. Radiographic examples of intertrochanteric and femoral neck hip fractures. **A,** Three-part intertrochanteric fracture. **B,** Femoral neck fracture. **C,** Anteroposterior view after open reduction and internal fixation with cannulated lag screws for a nondisplaced femoral neck fracture. **D,** Lateral view.

or with traction and spica casting in the very young skeletally immature athlete.[12,13] The adolescent will need operative fixation.

Potential complications from hip fractures can occur in up to 60% of patients.[85] Avascular necrosis of the femoral head may occur in up to one third of hip fractures. The chance of developing avascular necrosis depends on fracture location and the amount of displacement.[90] The rate with a type I fracture is 100%; with type II fracture the incidence is 15% to 50%; and with a type III fracture the reported incidence is 30% to 40%.[40] Avascular necrosis rarely develops with intertrochanteric fractures. Varus deformity secondary to physeal injury can also occur.

Avulsion

Avulsion fractures more commonly occur in skeletally immature athletes because the tendons are stronger than the cartilaginous growth centers. However, adults can sustain this injury, too. The age range of patients affected is reported to be from 14 to 25 years of age.[96] In the skeletally immature athlete, these fractures occur at secondary growth centers, apophyses, which become separated from the underlying bone. The fractures occur before the secondary ossification centers appear on radiographs. The fractures do not displace widely due to the surrounding thick periosteum. The mechanism of injury involves a very strong muscular contraction against the weaker cartilage apophysis (Fig. 22-16).[58] Radiographic analysis is used to exclude apophysitis, which is an inflammation of the secondary growth centers which causes symptoms similar to avulsion fractures.

Symptoms include localized pain, tenderness, swelling, and sometimes ecchymosis. The functional limitations depend on the specific muscle involved. Radiographs of the affected location must be taken along with comparison views of the uninjured side. Management is symptomatically guided with positioning to relieve the tension of the offending muscle. Protected weight bearing and a graduated therapy program ensue as the symptoms subside. Usually, these fractures can be managed nonoperatively. Some authors recommend operative fixation in competitive athletes to avoid late onset functional disability.[83]

Iliac Crest. Iliac crest avulsion fractures result from a twisting injury while the trunk is abducted. The iliac crest fuses at age 16 years in boys and at age 14 in girls. It fuses beginning on the anterolateral crest and progressing to the posterior crest.[75] Pain to palpation over the iliac crest that worsens with resisted abduction is a characteristic finding with this avulsion fracture. Oblique radiographs and comparison views are needed to diagnose this condition.[27] Management involves partial weight bearing with crutches for 5 to 7 days with analgesics as needed. The symptoms will resolve within 4 to 6 weeks. At that time, the weight-bearing status can be advanced, and sporting activities resumed as symptoms resolve.

Anterior Superior and Anterior Inferior Iliac Spine. The sartorius is the muscle that causes an anterior superior iliac spine avulsion fracture, which is more common in running and jumping sports.[21] Active flexion and passive extension of the hip worsen the symptoms. The avulsed fragment may be palpated in some patients.

The direct head of the rectus femoris causes anterior inferior iliac spine avulsions (Fig. 22-17), which are less common than anterior superior iliac spine avulsions because less stresses are borne here and because this apophysis fuses at an earlier age.[73] Localized pain and weakness with hip flexion are experienced by the athlete. Active hip flexion exacerbates the symptoms. Radiographs of comparison views are needed. An accessory ossicle of the acetabulum, a normal variant, should be excluded. If present, it often will be noted bilaterally. Management is similar to that for other avulsion fractures.

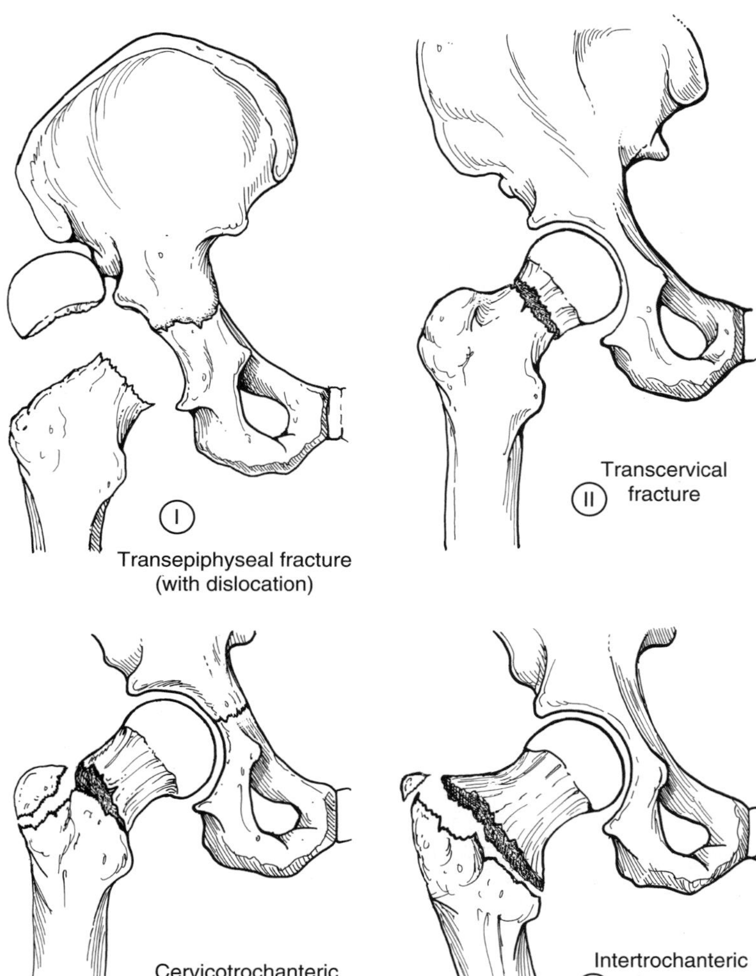

FIGURE 22-15. Pediatric hip fracture classification. **I,** transepiphyseal; **II,** transcervical; **III,** cervicotrochanteric; and **IV,** intertrochanteric.

Ischial Apophysis. Avulsion fractures of the ischial apophysis are also called "hurdler's fractures." The hamstrings are responsible for this avulsion fracture, which occurs at a later age because the ischial apophysis fuses when the athlete is aged 20 to 25 years.[13] This fracture occurs when the hamstrings strongly contract while the pelvis is fixed and flexed and the knee is extended. The patient experiences substantial disability and difficulty with prolonged sitting and pain when the thigh is flexed with the knee extended. A controversy exists regarding conservative management versus excising the fragment. A 68% rate of ununited fractures has been reported.[58] Most orthopedists would consider operative excision only for exuberant, painful callus formation.

Greater and Lesser Trochanter and Acetabular Lip. Avulsion fractures of the greater and lesser trochanter are very rare; accounting for only 1% of all hip injuries.[58] Still more rare is the acetabular lip avulsion fracture (Fig. 22-18).

Avulsions of the lesser trochanter are caused by the pull of the iliopsoas muscle. Eighty-five percent of these fractures occur when the athlete is younger than 20 years of age.[16] The patient will experience anteromedial thigh pain and difficulty elevating the leg with the knee extended. The athlete holds the thigh flexed and adducted. The radiograph must be taken in slight external rotation of the hip to demonstrate the fracture. Management is the same as for other avulsion fractures.

Greater trochanter avulsion fractures are caused by the pull of the abductor muscles (Fig. 22-19). If displacement is significant, then operative repair is considered. Acetabular lip avulsions are caused by the forceful pull of the hip capsule and rarely need surgery.

Stress Fractures

The etiology of stress fractures is not fully elucidated. However, they involve a progressive imbalance between the force absorbed by the bone and the ability of the bone to withstand this force. Thus, they involve an imbalance between the degree of force application and the bone strength.[22] It has been postulated that repeated submaximal stress causes muscle fatigue,[11,31] as the

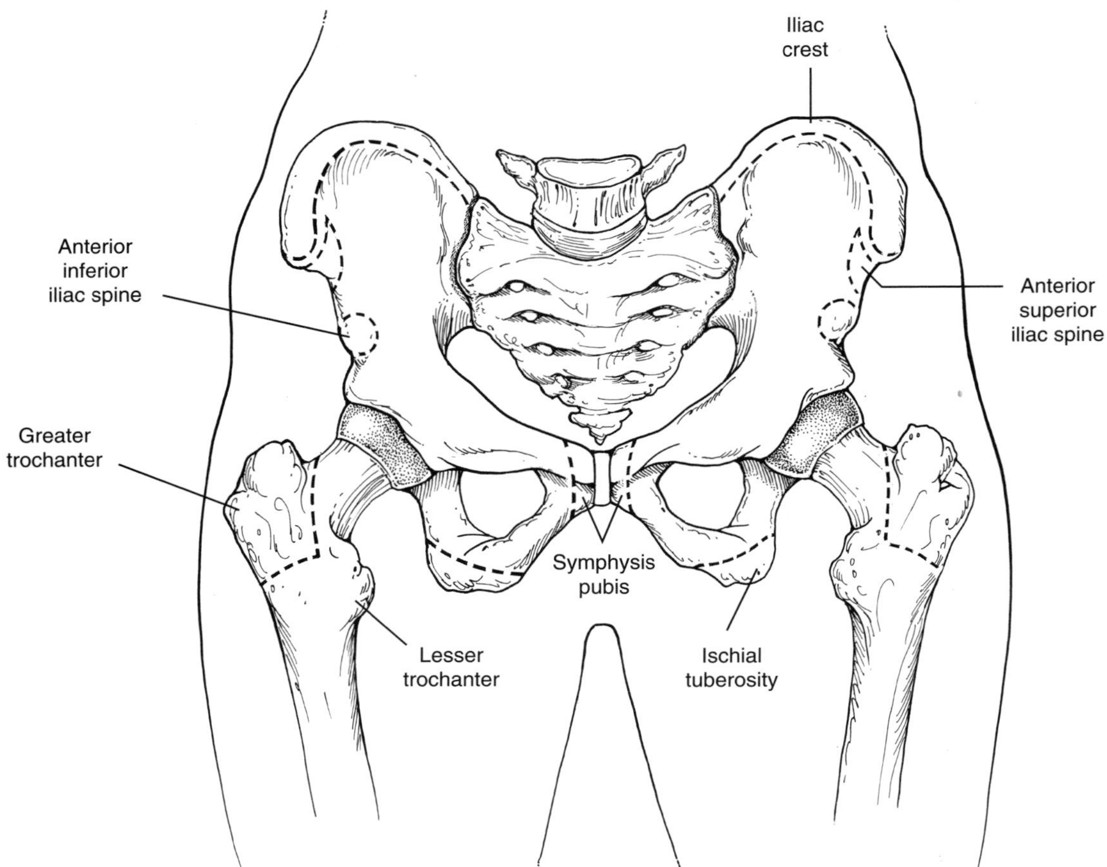

FIGURE 22-16. Diagram of areas of potential avulsion fractures from the pelvic apophyses.

constant back and forth bending of a coat hanger will weaken and eventually break it. This fatigue allows excessive force to be transferred to bone that may be greater than the capacity of the bone to absorb such force. There is a 2% incidence of stress fractures of the proximal thigh in the general population.[54] Stress fractures are diagnosed first by bone scans and later by radiographic changes.[78]

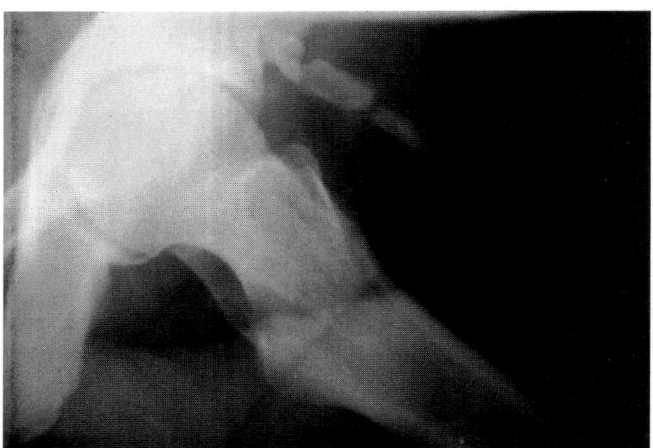

FIGURE 22-17. A skeletally mature individual sustained an avulsion fracture of the anterior inferior iliac spine from the pull of the rectus. Lateral radiograph shows mature calcification of the proximal rectus muscle.

Pelvis. The pubic ramus is the most common bone of this region to be afflicted by stress fractures. Although the incidence of this fracture is low in athletes in general, long-distance runners are more susceptible to this injury. The difference in tensile muscle forces and gait are the main reasons women are more commonly affected than men.[69] The patient experiences inguinal or peroneal pain and an antalgic gait. Weight-bearing capacity may be diminished because of pain. A "standing sign" is indicative of this injury, that is, the inability to stand on the affected limb without support.[62] A bone scan can aid in the early detection of this entity if the clinician has a high index of suspicion (Fig. 22-20).[24,25,64] Radiographic findings are usually positive after several weeks. Activity should be restricted for several months, depending on the radiographic evidence of healing and the symptoms. Supportive taping or strapping may be used adjunctively.

Femoral Neck. Femoral neck stress fractures are more common in military recruits and runners than in other

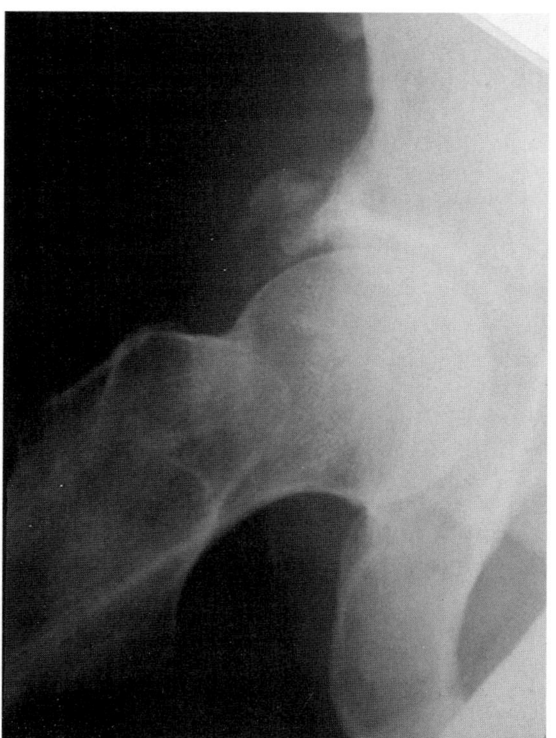

FIGURE 22-18. A skeletally mature individual sustained an avulsion fracture of the anterior acetabular lip from the pull of the hip capsule and the acetabular labrum.

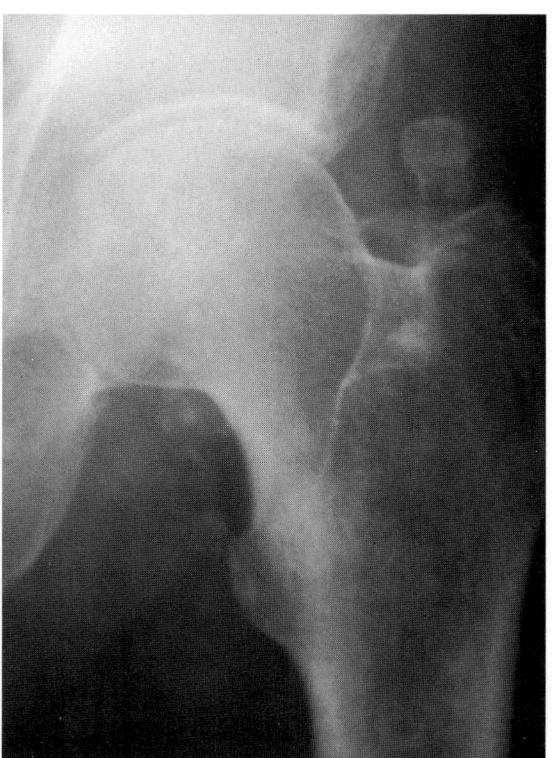

FIGURE 22-19. A radiograph demonstrating an avulsion fracture of the greater trochanter, caused by the pull from the abductor muscles.

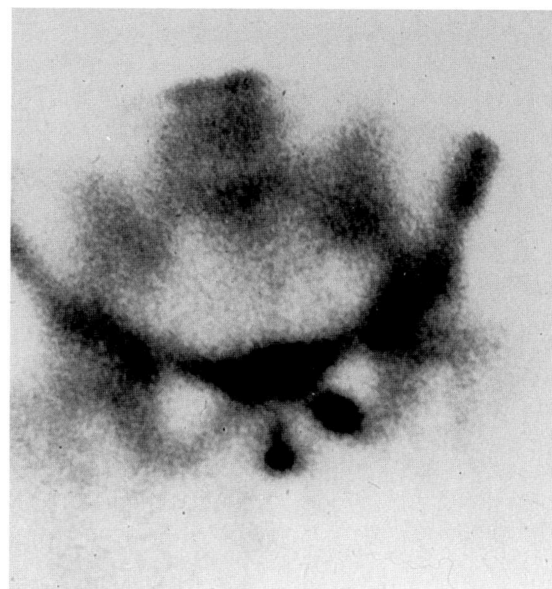

FIGURE 22-20. A technetium-labeled bone scan demonstrating increased uptake in the left inferior pubic ramus consistent with a stress fracture.

athletes (Fig. 22-21).[31,59] The proposed etiology is the loss of shock absorption with muscle fatigue.[6] Training errors, poor footwear, and poor running surfaces may contribute to the development of this condition. Coxa vara will increase athletes' susceptibility to developing femoral neck stress fractures[30] because of the changes in biomechanical stresses incurred at the hip with this condition. There are two main types: a transverse fracture that begins at the superior femoral neck, and a compression type that develops at the inferior femoral neck. The transverse type is potentially unstable and more likely to displace.[21] Compression-type fractures are more common in younger athletes.

Results of bone scans are positive earlier than radiographs. Tomograms and computerized tomographic scans or magnetic resonance imaging may also be useful to help diagnose this condition. These stress fractures have been classified according to Blickenstaff based on the radiographic findings.[6] A type I fracture has callus evident, but no fracture line is visible. These fractures are managed with rest. A type II stress fracture has a fracture line present on radiographs but is not displaced. Management involves either casting or operative fixation. A type III fracture is displaced and necessitates operative fixation. There are more complications with a type III fracture (Table 22-5).

The symptoms include pain in the groin, thigh, or knee that is worsened with weight bearing. An antalgic gait is present, and motion is decreased, particularly

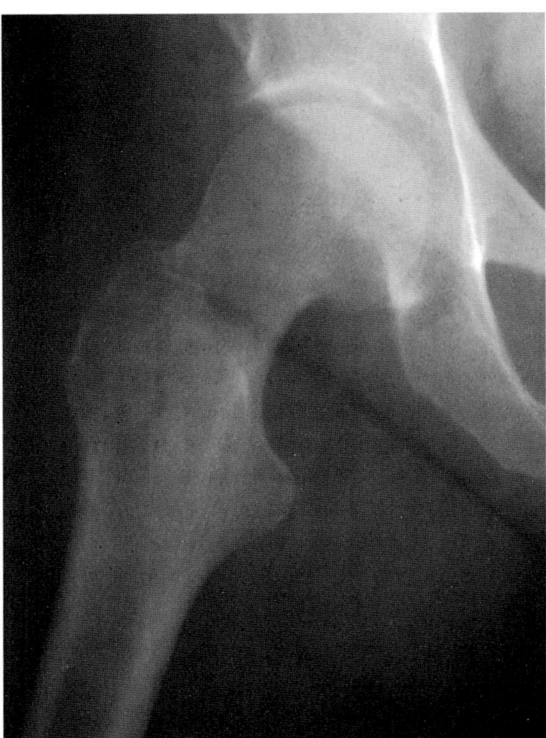

FIGURE 22-21. An anteroposterior radiograph of the hip showing a femoral neck stress fracture at inferior femoral neck.

internal rotation of the hip. If the diagnosis is uncertain, an athlete should have an initial radiograph taken and be empirically treated with rest and not allowed to bear weight on the extremity for 1 week. Radiographs are repeated then and a bone scan is done. If results of both are negative, they are repeated again in 1 week. Again, if they are both negative, a new diagnosis should be entertained. Patients who have a positive bone scan with a negative radiograph should be treated as a "stress reaction" with protected weight bearing (Fig. 22-22).[22]

There is potential for serious complications such as avascular necrosis, nonunion, and varus deformity, especially with displacement. The athlete can resume activities when radiographs demonstrate full healing and when the bone scan does not show increased activity. The indication for surgery includes nondisplaced fractures that do not heal with conservative management or fractures that continue to cause pain even with cessation of activities.[56]

Femoral Shaft. Stress fractures can occur anywhere along the femoral shaft[70]; most commonly they occur at the junction of the proximal and middle third of the femur. Runners are the most susceptible to sustaining this injury, and the incidence is related to training intensity.[20] Osteoporosis[15] and external rotation of the hip beyond 65° increases the risk of developing this stress fracture.[26]

The symptoms include insidious thigh or groin pain that is usually described as aching. Occasionally, the pain may be acute. Swelling and diminished motion are common. Any activity increases the pain, whereas rest relieves the symptoms.

The radiographic findings are delayed.[6,81,98] Bone scans can demonstrate early increased uptake along the femoral shaft.[8] The radiographs should be repeated every 3 months to evaluate the healing process. The physician must be aware of the nutrient artery penetrating the femoral cortex, which can be mistaken for a fracture.

Management includes partial weight bearing for 1 to 4 weeks and cessation of athletic activities.[32,54] Once the athlete is pain free, then full weight bearing is begun. These fractures usually heal in 4 to 8 weeks.[21] During this period a phased rehabilitation program is instituted. Sports activities can be resumed after 8 to 16 weeks.

The diagnosis of femoral periostitis also must be considered; it is an overuse syndrome that affects the mid-thigh at the adductor insertion. It was first reported in female military recruits, particularly those who were noted to over-stride with sports activities.[70] Bone scan will demonstrate linear uptake in the upper half to middle third of the femur. It commonly occurs bilaterally and can occur with femoral shaft stress fractures.[81]

HIP DISLOCATIONS

Hip dislocations rarely result from participation in athletics (Fig. 22-23). The mechanism of injury involves either falling on a flexed knee or a direct force application along the length of the femur, as would occur against the dashboard in a vehicular accident (Fig. 22-24).

TABLE 22-5 Classification of Femoral Neck Stress Fractures

Type	Callus	Fracture Visible on Radiograph	Treatment
I	+	–	Rest
II	+	+, nondisplaced	Cast vs. operative
III	+	+, displaced	Operative

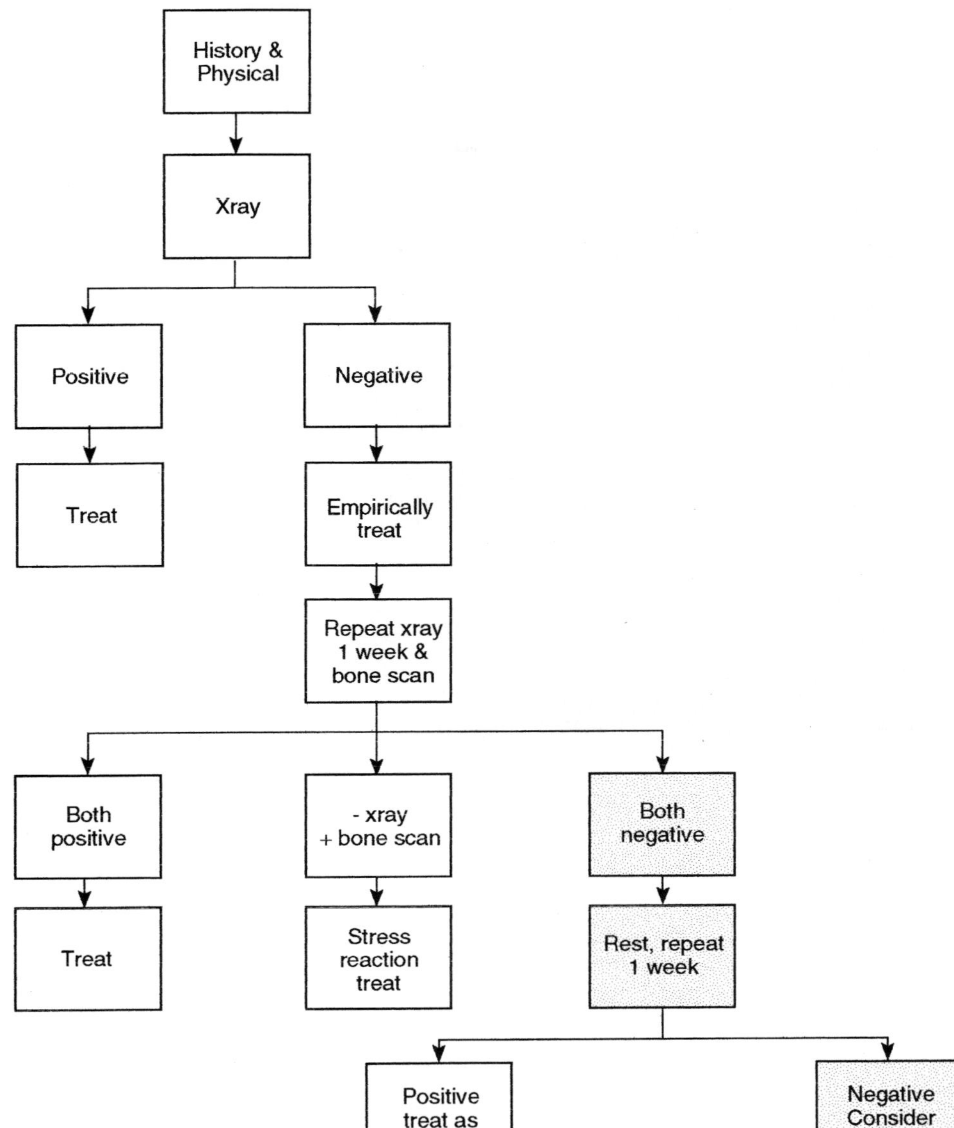

FIGURE 22-22. An algorithm to guide the practitioner in the work-up of stress fractures.

These injuries are surgical emergencies that necessitate immediate reduction of the dislocated joint. It is important to minimize any vascular disruption to the femoral head and injury to the sciatic nerve. If the blood supply is disrupted, avascular necrosis will certainly leave the athlete disabled in activities of daily living and sports. The neurovascular status of the extremity must also be assessed acutely, and the athlete must be immobilized and transported emergently to a hospital.

Symptoms include extreme pain that is worsened with any motion. The athlete is unable to bear weight and is completely immobile. Muscle spasm is present, and motion is restricted secondary to pain. Posterior dislocations are more common than anterior ones.[92] The leg is held in a flexed, adducted, and internally rotated position. Concurrent sciatic nerve injury must be excluded. With anterior dislocations, the leg may be flexed, and usually is abducted, but could be adducted. It is almost always externally rotated. Sometimes the femoral head can be palpated anteriorly.[18] Femoral nerve injuries must be excluded (Fig. 22-25). No attempt to reduce a dislocation should be carried out before an accurate diagnosis is made.

A child is likely to sustain a hip dislocation without an associated fracture of the acetabulum. Adolescents and adults, however, often sustain a fracture of the acetabulum with hip dislocations.

A thorough neurological examination and radiographs of the hip joint, including anteroposterior, lateral, and oblique, Judet[44] images, must be performed before

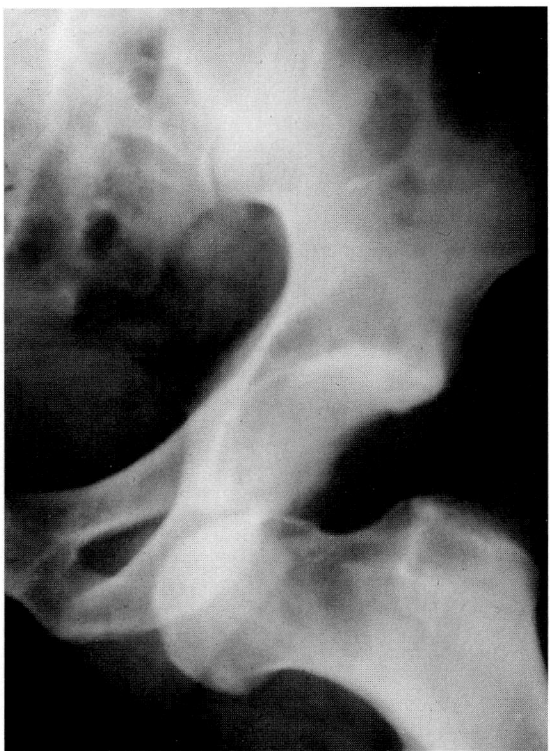

FIGURE 22-23. An anteroposterior view of the left hip demonstrating an inferior dislocation of the hip. A lateral radiograph is necessary to determine if this was an anterior or posterior hip dislocation.

attempting a reduction maneuver on the hip, preferably under anesthesia. Once the hip is relocated, a CAT scan or MRI may be performed to exclude any intra-articular fragments remaining in the joint. Also, the stability of the hip joint and the neurovascular status of the limb must be assessed after the reduction of the joint. If the joint is unstable after the reduction and a fracture is present, operative fixation is required. Concurrent knee ligament injuries can be assessed once the hip is reduced into position.

Avascular necrosis is a potential complication of hip dislocations (Fig. 22-26). The incidence is between 10% and 20%[76] and is directly related to the time delay in reducing the dislocation. The goal is to obtain a reduction as soon as possible and certainly within 24 hours. Avascular necrosis can take up to 2 years to become apparent. There is no correlation between early weight bearing and the development of avascular necrosis.[85]

After a stable reduction, the leg is placed in skin traction until the pain and muscle spasm subsides. Range of motion exercises can be instituted subsequently. Full weight bearing should be delayed for 3 to 4 weeks[85] until the soft tissues have had time to heal. Sports return is allowed when full motion, agility, and strength are regained. Radiographic evaluation should be followed every 3 months for 1 year and then every 6 months for 2 years.[18]

SLIPPED CAPITAL FEMORAL EPIPHYSIS

A slipped capital femoral epiphysis is the most common hip disorder in adolescents.[88] The etiology is not fully elucidated, however, and may involve hormonal factors, genetic factors, or mechanical factors, with concomitant trauma. Patients afflicted are usually aged 10 to 15 years and at the time of the growth spurt. It has been postulated that an increase in growth hormone relative to sex

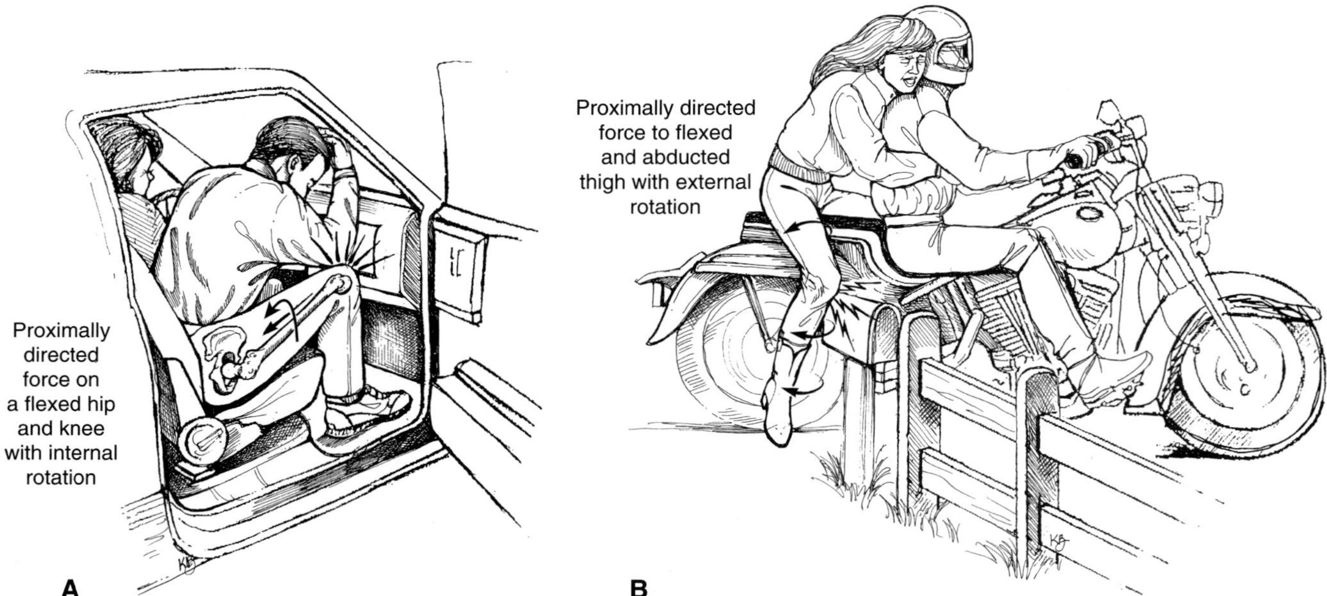

FIGURE 22-24. Illustration of the mechanism of injury of hip dislocations. **A,** Posterior dislocation. **B,** Anterior dislocation.

FIGURE 22-25. Position of the lower extremity with hip dislocations. **A,** With anterior hip dislocations, the leg is held in a flexed, abducted, and externally rotated position. **B,** With posterior dislocations, the leg is shortened, adducted, and internally rotated.

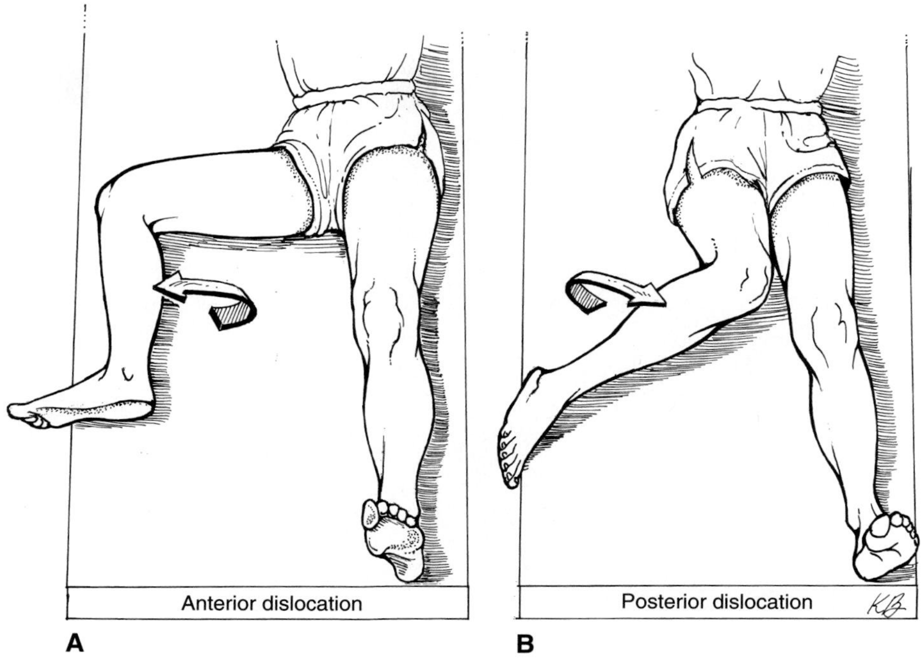

Anterior dislocation

A

Posterior dislocation

B

hormone may be causative because it decreases the shear strength of the physeal plate.[35] More than 50% of affected children are in the ninety-fifth or greater percentile in weight for their age.[46] Boys are more commonly affected than girls.[5] African American males are the group with the highest incidence.[55]

The symptoms include groin, anteromedial thigh, and possibly knee pain. Motion is usually restricted, especially internal rotation of the hip. An antalgic, externally rotated gait is seen. In chronic cases, thigh atrophy and a shortened limb can be observed.

Radiographs, including anteroposterior true and frog lateral views, are used to diagnose this condition. Sometimes this condition is demonstrated on only one radiographic view (Fig. 22-27). The affected side should be compared with the contralateral side. The capital epiphysis is seen to displace posteriorly and downward, whereas the femoral neck displaces upward and anteriorly.

A slipped capital femoral epiphysis is classified as either acute, acute on chronic, or chronic. Further classification requires a lateral radiograph of the hip. A type I involves a slip of less than one-third the width of the femoral epiphysis. Type II involves a 33% to 50% slip, and a type III, severe, slip involves more than 50% of the width of the femoral epiphysis (Table 22-6).[55]

Management is operative fixation of the slipped femoral epiphysis. In the pre-slip phase, with only irregularity and widening of the physis evident on radiographs, in situ operative fixation is recommended.[5] Crutch use and no weight bearing is recommended. Weight bearing is begun at 6 weeks. A displaced epiphysis may require reduction before fixation.

LEGG-CALVÉ-PERTHES DISEASE

Legg-Calvé-Perthes disease is a self-limited, noninflammatory condition that causes avascular necrosis to develop in the hip of patients usually aged 4 to 8 years (Fig. 22-28).[88] This condition must be suspected in any child younger than 12 years with hip pain.[55] The etiology, although uncertain, may involve a vascular insult to the femoral head. Antecedent trauma has been noted in 25% of children with Legg-Calvé-Perthes.[85]

The symptoms of Legg-Calvé-Perthes involve groin, hip, anteromedial, and thigh pain. Knee pain alone has been noted to be present 15% of the time.[55] The patient will also experience muscle spasm, an antalgic gait, and decreased hip motion, especially internal rotation. Chronically, this condition can cause the development of a flexion and adduction contracture of the hip.[88]

Management involves regaining full motion of the hip; specifically, the gluteus medius and maximus and quadriceps must be reconditioned.[55] Anti-inflammatory medications and bed rest may help reduce the pain and increase the motion. Traction may also be necessary. The goal of management is containment of the femoral head within the acetabulum, either by bracing or surgical osteotomy.[88] If the patient wears a brace, he or she is weaned from it, and full activities are allowed when the femoral head demonstrates re-ossification on radiographs.[55]

A poor prognosis with Legg-Calvé-Perthes is associated with the affected child being older than 8 years, the majority of the femoral head being involved, and premature physeal closure.[55]

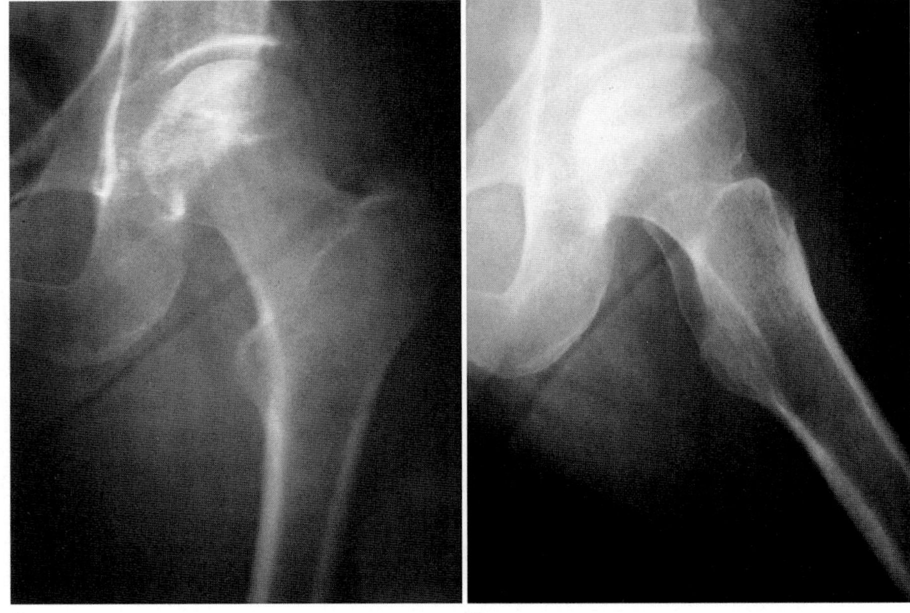

ANT/POS PELV-Tc 99ANT ANT/POS PELV-Tc 99POST

C

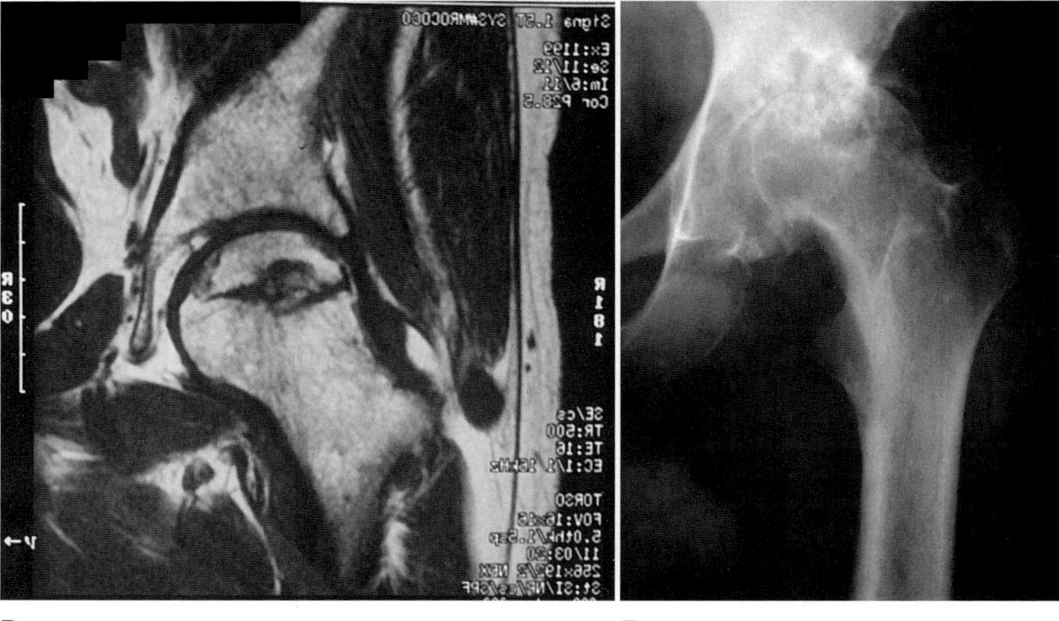

FIGURE 22-26. A, An anteroposterior radiograph of the hip demonstrating avascular necrosis. **B,** The same hip as seen on a lateral radiograph. **C,** A bone scan of the hip demonstrating changes consistent with avascular necrosis. **D,** A magnetic resonance imaging scan showing avascular necrosis. **E,** An anteroposterior radiograph of the hip demonstrating advanced changes secondary to avascular necrosis.

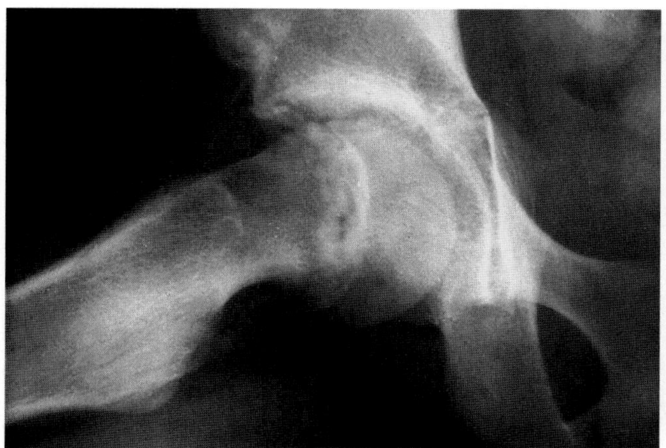

FIGURE 22-27. A frog lateral view of the hip demonstrating a slipped capital femoral epiphysis, which is the best view to visualize minimal slips of the capital epiphysis. Note posterior displacement of the epiphysis.

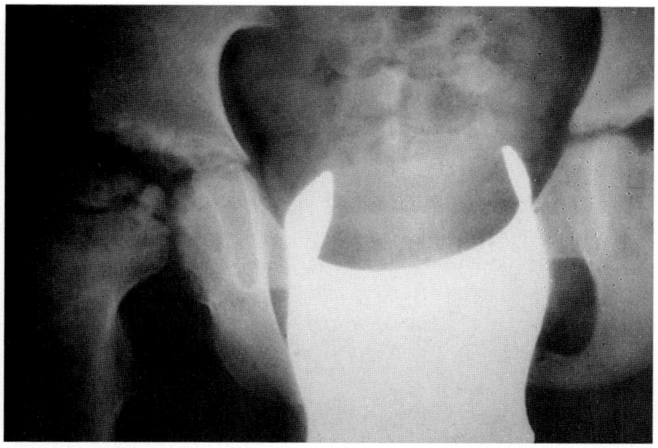

FIGURE 22-28. A radiograph demonstrating the findings of Legg-Calvé-Perthes disease, with lateral extrusion and fragmentation of the epiphysis.

TRANSIENT SYNOVITIS OF THE HIP

Transient synovitis is a self-limited, rapidly resolving inflammation of the hip joint. It is the most common cause of hip pain in children,[55] particularly those younger than 10 years. The etiology may be viral, allergic, or post-traumatic.[55] It is a diagnosis of exclusion, requiring that the physician have a high index of suspicion. Other diagnostic tests must be performed to exclude slipped capital femoral epiphysis, Legg-Calvé-Perthes disease, or arthritis.

The child experiences inguinal, thigh, or knee pain. Motion at the hip is painful, and the child will guard against it. If the child will ambulate, an antalgic gait will be observed. Management involves bed rest, possibly with traction. The child will usually recover in 48 hours.[55] Activities are resumed gradually because early return to activities has been shown to cause recurrences.[36] This condition will precede Legg-Calvé-Perthes disease up to 10% of the time.[88]

ACETABULAR LABRAL TEARS

Acetabular labral tears are an unusual cause of mechanical hip pain. A high index of suspicion is necessary to reach this diagnosis. The athlete will experience a sharp, catching pain in the groin that radiates into the anterior thigh, particularly with rotation of the hip while arising from a seated position.[39] A feeling of "giving way" is sometimes encountered. A palpable and audible click may be elicited with extension and internal rotation of the hip, mimicking snapping hip syndrome.

Arthrography will demonstrate a filling defect.[85] Magnetic resonance imaging and arthroscopy can diagnose this condition. Injection of a local anesthetic can be therapeutic and diagnostic. This condition is treated nonoperatively with physiotherapy and analgesics as needed. Arthroscopic or open operative excision may be necessary for the athlete with recurrent symptoms despite conservative treatment modalities.[19]

TABLE 22-6 Slipped Capital Femoral Epiphysis Classification

Type	Epiphyseal Width Involvement (%)
I	<33
II	33–50
III	>50

MISCELLANEOUS INJURIES

Sacroiliac Joint Pain

There are great stresses borne across the sacroiliac in the young athlete, which are controlled by the supporting ligaments.[85] Pain in this region is caused by sudden twisting motions, improper weightlifting, or a fall on the buttocks. Runners with short legs and poor running mechanics are susceptible to developing sacroiliac joint pain.[85]

Symptoms involve localized pain and tenderness. A positive Lasègue test can be elicited, which is straight leg raising with forced passive dorsiflexion of the foot increasing the pain. Results of a Gaenslen test may also be positive. This test involves the athlete lying on the unaffected side and flexing the hip while the injured hip is extended. An increase in pain in the sacroiliac joint is encountered. The condition is managed symptomatically. Abdominal strengthening and postural exercises are part of the rehabilitation protocol. An abdominal supportive band or lumbosacral corset may help alleviate the pain. NSAIDs, and, rarely, local injections, can be helpful.

Pelvic Floor Myalgia

Pelvic floor myalgia is an unusual condition of increased tension involving the muscles and fascia of the pelvic cavity and causing pain.[84] It includes levator ani syndrome, piriformis syndrome, ano-rectal pain, and coccydynia. The main muscles affected are the levator ani, coccygeus, and piriformis. The coccygeus and levator ani compose the pelvic diaphragm that surrounds the excretory and reproductive sphincters.

The signs and symptoms include back and leg pain, a heavy feeling in the pelvis, possibly pain with bowel movements, constipation, rectal pain, and dyspareunia.[86] A rectal examination will elicit pain. Management is guided by the symptoms, and includes deep heat, mobilization of the sacro-coccygeal joint, stretching, relaxation, and abdominal strengthening.[86]

Neurologic Conditions

Aside from typical referred pain from the spine, some local nerve dysfunction can be disabling for the athlete. Myralgia paresthetica, or irritation of the lateral femoral cutaneous nerve of the thigh, can occur after direct injury or due to entrapment. Treatment is symptomatic, often responding to NSAIDs, physical therapy, and injections. Rarely is surgery necessary.

Ilio-inguinal neuralgia can present with burning pain, tenderness, and sensory dysesthesia. It arises from the L1, L2 root and supplies sensation to the genitalia and medial thigh. The nerve can be injured by direct trauma or entrapment. Confirmation of the diagnosis as well as treatment can be provided by local anesthetic block and steroids. Surgery is rarely needed.

CHECKLIST

Etiology of Hip Pain

Primary pelvis or hip pain
- ☐ Pathology
- ☐ Injury

Referred pain
- ☐ Lumbar sacral spine
- ☐ Pelvic viscera

Inflammatory conditions
- ☐ Ankylosing spondylitis
- ☐ Reiter's syndrome
- ☐ Spondylosis
- ☐ Mono-articular arthritis

Infectious conditions
- ☐ Osteomyelitis
- ☐ Septic arthritis

Neoplasms
- ☐ Primary bone or soft tissue tumors
- ☐ Metastatic lesions

Metabolic bone disorders
- ☐ Paget's disease
- ☐ Endocrine disorders

Hernias

In an otherwise healthy, active athlete, the onset of groin pain can be indicative of a hernia, either inguinal or femoral. Inguinal hernias are more common in males and occur usually above and medial to the pubic tubercle. Femoral hernias are commonly seen in females and appear below and lateral to the tubercle. Each can present with pain and/or swelling, with increased symptoms on any activity that increases the intra-abdominal pressure. These are usually due to a tear or defect in the muscles of the wall of the canal.

The so-called "sports hernia" does not necessarily exhibit a bulge or defect, but rather is due to a weakness or tear of the associated muscles of the abdominal wall. Another clinical entity, "slap shot gut," seen in hockey players, involves a tear of the external oblique aponeurosis with injury to the inguinal nerve.

If the index of suspicion for hernia is high, the athlete should be referred to a surgeon specializing in this entity.

SUMMARY

There are many causes of pelvic, hip, and thigh pain in athletes. In addition to the entities discussed in this chapter, the practitioner must always consider metabolic bone diseases, neoplasms, infections, and inflammatory conditions (see box, Etiology of Hip Pain).[85]

With these entities in mind, guided by a thorough history and physical examination, the sports medicine physician will be well armed to diagnose and begin the treatment of the athletes with injuries to the pelvis, hip, and thigh.

REFERENCES

1. American Academy of Orthopaedic Surgeons (eds): Athletic Training and Sports Medicine. Chicago, American Academy of Orthopaedic Surgeons, 1984.
2. Antao NA: Myositis ossificans of the hip in a professional soccer player. Am J Sports Med 16:82, 1988.
3. Balaji MR, DeWeese JA: Adductor canal outlet syndrome. JAMA 245:167–170, 1981.
4. Beer E: Periostitis and osteitis of the symphysis pubis following suprapubic cystotomies. J Urol 20:233, 1928.
5. Bianco AJ Jr: Treatment of slipping of the capital femoral epiphysis. Clin Orthop 48:103, 1966.

6. Blickenstaff LP, Morris JM: Fatigue fracture of the femoral neck. J Bone Joint Surg 48A:1031–1046, 1966.
7. Bowerman JW: Radiology and Injury in Sport. New York, Appleton-Century-Crofts, 1977.
8. Brunet ME, Hontas RB: The thigh. In DeLee JC, Drez D Jr (eds): Orthopaedic Sports Medicine. Philadelphia, WB Saunders, 1994.
9. Burgess AR, Tile M: Fractures of the pelvis. In Rockwood CA Jr, Green DP, Bucholz RW (eds): Fractures in Adults. Philadelphia, JB Lippincott, 1991.
10. Burkett LN: Investigation into hamstring strains: The case of the hybrid muscle. J Sports Med 3:228–231, 1976.
11. Butler JE, Eggert AW: Fracture of the iliac crest apophysis: An unusual hip pointer. J Sports Med 3:192, 1975.
12. Canale ST, Bourland WL: Fracture of the neck and intertrochanteric region of the femur in children. J Bone Joint Surg 59A:431, 1977.
13. Canale ST, King RE: Pelvic and hip fractures. In Rockwood CA Jr, Wilkins KE, King RE (eds): Fractures in Children. Philadelphia, JB Lippincott, 1991.
14. Colonna PC: Fractures of the neck of the femur in children. Am J Surg 6:793, 1929.
15. Cook SD, et al: Trabecular bone density in menstrual function in women runners. Am J Sports Med 15:503–507, 1987.
16. DeLee JC: Fractures and dislocations of the hip. In Rockwood CA Jr, Green DP, Bucholz RW (eds): Fractures in Adults. Philadelphia, JB Lippincott, 1991.
17. Elliott BC, Blanksby BA: The synchronization of muscle activity and body segment movements during a running cycle. Med Sci Sports Exerc 11:322–327, 1979.
18. Epstein HC: Traumatic dislocations of the hip. Clin Orthop 92:116, 1973.
19. Eriksson E, Arvidsson I, Arvidsson H: Diagnostic and operative arthroscopy of the hip. Orthopaedics 9(2):169–176, 1986.
20. Fitch KD: Stress fractures of the lower limbs in runners. Aust Fam Phys 13:511–515, 1984.
21. Fox JM: Thigh. In Nicholas JA, Hershman, EB (eds): The Lower Extremity and Spine in Sports Medicine. St. Louis, CV Mosby, 1986.
22. Fullerton LR, Snowdy HA: Femoral neck stress fractures. Am J Sports Med 16:365, 1988.
23. Garrett WE, et al: Biomechanical comparison of stimulated and nonstimulated muscle pulled to failure. Am J Sports Med 15:448, 1987.
24. Garrick JG, et al: Early diagnosis of stress fractures and their precursors. J Bone Joint Surg 58A:733, 1976.
25. Geslien GE, et al: Early detection of stress fractures using ^{99}mTc-polyphosphate. Radiology 121:683, 1976.
26. Giladi M, et al: External rotation of the hip: A predictor of risk for stress fractures. Clin Orthop 216:131–134, 1987.
27. Godshall RW, Hansen CA: Incomplete avulsion of a portion of the iliac epiphysis: An injury to young athletes. J Bone Joint Surg 55A:1301, 1973.
28. Grant JCB: The lower limb. In Anderson JE (ed): Grant's Atlas of Anatomy, 8th ed. Baltimore, Williams & Wilkins, 1983.
29. Gray AH: Anatomy of the Human Body. Philadelphia, Lea & Febiger, 1959.
30. Gross ML, Nasser S, Finerman GAM: In DeLee JC, Drez D Jr (eds): Orthopaedic Sports Medicine. Philadelphia, WB Saunders, 1994.
31. Hajek MR, Noble HB: Stress fractures of the femoral neck in runners. Am J Sports Med 10:112, 1982.
32. Hallel T, Amit S, Sega D: Fatigue fractures of the tibial and femoral shaft in soldiers. Clin Orthop 118:35–43, 1976.
33. Hanson PG, Angevine M, Juhl JH: Osteitis pubis in sports activities. Phys Sports Med 6:111, 1978.
34. Harris NH, Murray RO: Lesions of the symphysis in athletes. BMJ 4:211, 1974.
35. Harris WR: The endocrine basis for slipping of the upper femoral epiphysis. J Bone Joint Surg 32B:5, 1950.
36. Hermel MB, Albert SM: Transient synovitis of the hip. Clin Orthop 22:21, 1962.
37. Hollingshead WH: Anatomy for Surgeons, The Back and Limbs, vol 3. Philadelphia, Harper & Row, 1958.
38. Hoppenfeld S: Orthopaedic Neurology. Philadelphia, JB Lippincott, 1977.
39. Ikeda T, et al: Torn acetabular labrum in young patients. Arthroscopic diagnosis and management. J Bone Joint Surg 70B(1):13–16, 1988.
40. Ingram AJ, Bachynski B: Fractures of the hip in children. Treatment and results. J Bone Joint Surg 35A:867, 1953.
41. Jackson DW, Feagin JA: Quadriceps contusions in young athletes: Relation of severity of injury to treatment and prognosis. J Bone Joint Surg 55A:95–105, 1973.
42. Jeffreys TE: Pseudomalignant osseous tumor of soft tissue. J Bone Joint Surg 48B:488, 1966.
43. Johnson RC, Schmidt GL: Hip motion measurements for selected activities of daily living. Clin Orthop 72:205, 1970.
44. Judet R, Judet J, LeTournel E: Fractures of the acetabulum: Classification and surgical approaches for open reduction. J Bone Joint Surg 46A:1615, 1964.

45. Kane WJ: Fractures of the pelvis. In Rockwood CA Jr, Green DP (eds): Fractures in Adults. Philadelphia, JB Lippincott, 1984.
46. Kelsey JL, Acheson DM, Keggi KJ: The body build of patients with slipped capital femoral epiphysis. Am J Dis Child 124:276, 1972.
47. Kirkpatrick JS, Koman LA, Rovere GD: The role of ultrasound in the early diagnosis of myositis ossificans: A case report. Am J Sports Med 15: 179–181, 1987.
48. Komi PV, Burskirk ER: Effect of eccentric and concentric muscle conditioning on tension and electric activity of human muscle. Ergonomics 15: 417–434, 1972.
49. Kulund DN: The Injured Athlete. Philadelphia, JB Lippincott, 1982.
50. Lee BY, LaPointe DG, Madden JL: The adductor canal syndrome: Description of a case with quantification of arterial pulsatile blood flow. Am J Surg 123:617–620, 1972.
51. Levinthal DH: Sports injuries in persons over 30 years of age. Postgrad Med 28:121, 1960.
52. Liemohn W: Factors related to hamstring strains. J Sports Med 18:71–76, 1978.
53. Lipscomb AB, Thomas ED, Johnston RK: Treatment of myositis ossificans traumatica in athletes. Am J Sports Med 4:111–120, 1976.
54. Lombardo SJ, Benson DW: Stress fractures of the femur in runners. Am J Sports Med 10:219–227, 1982.
55. MacEwen GD, Bunnell WP, Ramsey PL: The hip. In Lovell WW, Winter RB (eds): Pediatric Orthopaedics. Philadelphia, JB Lippincott, 1993.
56. McBryde AM Jr: Stress fractures in athletes. J Sports Med 3:212, 1975.
57. Merrifield HH, Cowan RFJ: Groin strain injuries in ice hockey. J Sports Med 1(2):41–42, 1973.
58. Metzmaker JN, Pappas AM: Avulsion fractures of the pelvis. Am J Sports Med 13:349, 1985.
59. Meurmann KOA, Elfving S: Stress fractures in soldiers: A multifocal bone disorder. Radiology 134: 483, 1980.
60. Micheli LJ: Overuse injuries in children's sports: The growth factor. Orthop Clin North Am 14: 337–361, 1983.
61. Morris JM: Biomechanical aspects of the hip joint. Orthop Clin North Am 2:33, 1971.
62. Noakes TD, Smith JA, Lindenberg G: Pelvic stress fractures in long-distance runners. Am J Sports Med 13:120, 1985.
63. Nordin M, Frankel VH: Biomechanics of the hip. In Frankel VH, Burstein AH (eds): Orthopaedic Biomechanics. Philadelphia, Lea & Febiger, 1970.
64. Norfray JF, et al: Early confirmation of stress fractures in joggers. JAMA 243:1647–1649, 1980.
65. Norman A, Dorfman HD: Juxtacortical circumscribed myositis ossificans: Evolution and radiographic features. Radiology 96:301, 1970.
66. O'Donoghue DH: Treatment of Injuries to Athletes, 4th ed. Philadelphia, WB Saunders, 1984.
67. Olerud S, Gerusten S: Chronic pubic symphysiolysis. J Bone Joint Surg 56A:799, 1974.
68. O'Neil DB, Micheli LJ: Overuse injuries in young athletes. Clin Sports Med 7:591, 1988.
69. Pavlov H, et al: Stress fractures of the pubic ramus. J Bone Joint Surg 64A:1020, 1982.
70. Provost RA, Morris JM: Fatigue fracture of the femoral shaft. J Bone Joint Surg 51A:487–498, 1969.
71. Puranen J, Orava S: The hamstring syndrome. Am J Sports Med 16:517, 1988.
72. Ratliff AHC: Fractures of the neck of the femur in children. J Bone Joint Surg 44B:528, 1962.
73. Reed MH: Pelvic fractures in children. J Can Assoc Radiol 27:255, 1976.
74. Renstrom PA, Peterson L: Groin injuries in athletes. Br J Sports Med 14:30–36, 1980.
75. Risser JC: The iliac apophysis: An invaluable sign in the management of scoliosis. Clin Orthop 11:111, 1958.
76. Robertson RC, Peterson HA: Traumatic dislocations of the hip in children: Review of Mayo Clinic series. In Harris WH (ed): The Hip. St. Louis, CV Mosby, 1974.
77. Romanoff ME, et al: Saphenous nerve entrapment at the adductor canal. Am J Sports Med 17:478–481, 1989.
78. Rupani HD, et al: Three-phase radionuclide bone imaging in sports medicine. Radiology 156: 187–196, 1985.
79. Rydell N: Biomechanics of the hip joint. Clin Orthop 92:6, 1973.
80. Safran MR, et al: The role of warm-up in muscular injury and prevention. Am J Sports Med 16:123, 1988.
81. Savoca C: Stress fractures: a classification of the earliest radiographic signs. Radiology 100:519–524, 1971.
82. Scharberg JE, Harper MC, Allen WC: The snapping hip syndrome. Am J Sports Med 12:361, 1984.
83. Schlonsky J, Olix ML: Functional disability following avulsion fracture of the ischial epiphysis. J Bone Joint Surg 54A:641, 1972.
84. Segura JW, Opitz JL, Greene LF: Prostatosis, prostatitis or pelvic floor tension myalgia? J Urol 122(2):168–169, 1979.
85. Sim FH, Scott HG: Injuries of the pelvis and hip in athletes. In Nicholas JA, Hershmann EB (eds): The Lower Extremity and Spine in Sports Medicine. St. Louis, CV Mosby, 1986.
86. Sinaki M, Merritt JL, Stillwell GK: Tension myalgia of the pelvic floor. Mayo Clin Proc 52:717, 1977.

87. Slocum DB, James SL: Biomechanics of running. JAMA 205:721–728, 1968.
88. Tachdjian MO: Pediatric Orthopaedics, vol 1. Philadelphia, WB Saunders, 1972.
89. Taylor DC, et al: Groin pain in athletes due to abdominal musculature abnormalities. Am J Sports Med 13:239–242, 1991.
90. Trueta J, Harrison MHM: The normal vascular anatomy of the femoral head in adult man. J Bone Joint Surg 35B:442, 1953.
91. Verta MJ, Vitello J, Fuller J: Adductor canal compression syndrome. Arch Surg 119:345–346, 1984.
92. Walsh ZT, Micheli LJ: Hip dislocation in a high school football player. Phys Sports Med 17:112, 1989.
93. Walton M, Rothwell AG: Reactions of thigh tissues of sheep to blunt trauma. Clin Orthop 176:273–281, 1983.
94. Waters PM, Millis MB: Hip and pelvic injuries in the young athlete. Clin Sports Med 7:513, 1988.
95. Watson-Jones R: Dislocations and fracture—dislocations of the pelvis. Br J Surg 25:773, 1938.
96. Watts HG: Fractures of the pelvis in children. Orthop Clin North Am 7:615, 1976.
97. Wiley JJ: Traumatic osteitis pubis: the gracilis syndrome. Am J Sports Med 11:360, 1983.
98. Wilson E: Stress fractures. Radiology 92:481–486, 1969.
99. Zaccalini PS, Urist MR: Traumatic periosteal proliferations in rabbits: The enigma of experimental myositis ossificans traumatica. J Trauma 4:344, 1964.
100. Zarins B, Ciullo JV: Acute muscle and tendon injuries in athletes. Clin Sports 2:167–182, 1983.
101. Zoltan DJ, Clancy WG, Keene JS: A new operative approach to snapping hip and refractory trochanteric bursitis in athletes. Am J Sports Med 14:201, 1986.

23 Knee Injuries

David Diduch, Giles R. Scuderi, and W. Norman Scott

The knee is the most frequently injured joint managed in sports medicine.[100] Twenty percent of all football-related injuries involve the knee, including an estimated 42 anterior cruciate ligament tears per 1000 players per year.[37] In addition, skiing accounts for at least one anterior cruciate tear per day at major ski areas.[26] Yet, with advancements in surgical and therapeutic techniques, knee injuries are increasingly treatable toward a return to full participation. The primary care physician frequently must evaluate overuse injuries and acute sprains and strains, both of which can often involve significant intraarticular pathology. Therefore, the treating physician must be completely comfortable with his or her ability to diagnose most common knee injuries, have an understanding of treatment algorithms, and know when it is appropriate to refer the patient to a surgical specialist.

This chapter will help to provide the primary care physician with the diagnostic tools for evaluating the majority of knee injuries, which often result from sports activities. It will also help to provide an understanding of the anatomy as it relates to the biomechanics of the joint and common mechanisms of injury. Finally, the chapter will offer readily available algorithms for appropriate diagnostic work-ups, therapeutic intervention, and indications for referral.

ANATOMY

The knee is composed of three distinct and partially separated joint compartments: the medial and lateral femorotibial joints and the patellofemoral joint. In addition, the proximal tibiofibular joint is included in the knee but is rarely involved in sports-related injuries. Articular cartilage, primarily type II collagen with a high water content, covers each of these joint compartments and provides lubricated gliding surfaces for knee motion. Softening and early wear and tear of this surface is referred to as *chondromalacia*. Frank erosion is technically arthritis. Virtually every adult has at least some degree of wear and tear of these surfaces, but most are minimally symptomatic. Localized traumatic defects of the articular surface are termed *cartilage fractures* or *osteochondral defects* if they involve a "divot" of subchondral bone. A preexisting dysvascular contribution to the etiology of the osteochondral defect confers the term *osteochondritis dissecans*, although the exact etiology most often cannot be determined.

The shapes of the bony articulations provide very little inherent stability to the knee joint, unlike the hip "ball and socket" model. Proper function depends on intact ligamentous structures. Very substantial cruciate ligaments cross in the center of the knee joint. Although they are intraarticular, a surrounding synovial sleeve makes them technically extrasynovial. The anterior cruciate ligament (ACL) is on average 11 mm wide × 38 mm long, originating on the posteromedial part of the lateral femoral condyle (Figs. 23-1 and 23-2).[97] It runs distally in an anteromedial direction to a rather long attachment site on the tibial plateau between the tibial spines (Fig. 23-3). An easy way to remember this orientation is that the direction mimics one's hand in a pocket. The ACL functions as the main stabilizer to resist anterior translation, especially when the knee is in the extended position.[36] The ACL is a secondary stabilizer to excessive varus or valgus stress, to rotation, and to hyperextension.

The posterior cruciate ligament (PCL) is slightly larger at 38 mm × 13 mm and up to 50% stronger than the ACL.[47] It originates from a broad attachment site on the lateral side of the medial femoral condyle and runs distally in a posterior–lateral direction to insert on the back of the tibia approximately 1 cm below the articular surface. Accessory meniscofemoral ligaments often run either anterior (ligament of Humphrey) or posterior (ligament of Wrisberg) to the PCL from the femur to the lateral meniscus rim. Up to 50% of the size of the PCL, at least one of these accessory ligaments is usually (71% of knees) present, but rarely (6% of knees) both are present.[19,47] The PCL is the main stabilizer to posterior translation of the knee, especially in flexion. It serves as a secondary stabilizer to varus or valgus stress.

The collateral ligaments on either side of the knee are the main stabilizers to side-to-side stresses. The medial collateral, or tibial collateral, ligament (MCL) consists of a stronger superficial layer and a deep layer, which attaches to the medial meniscus. The superficial MCL originates from the medial femoral epicondyle and inserts almost 5 cm below the joint line on the medial tibia. Just posterior and confluent with the superficial MCL is the posterior oblique ligament. More of a combination of capsule and supporting retinacular layers, including the insertion of the semimembranosus tendon, than a clearly defined ligament, the posterior oblique ligament is taut in extension and is important in resisting

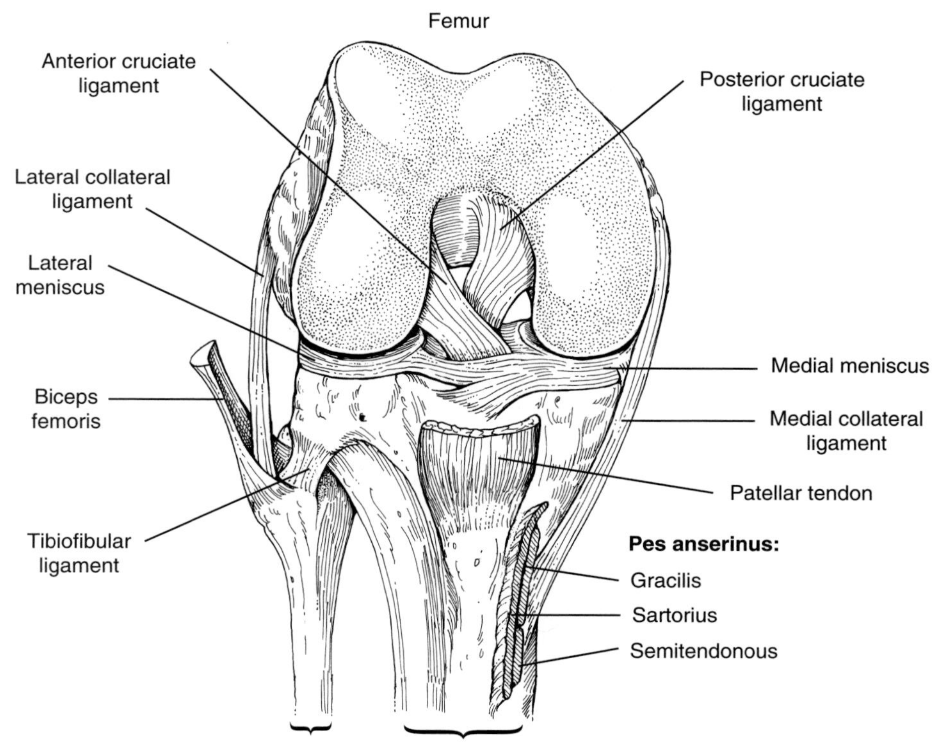

FIGURE 23-1. Anterior view of the knee.

valgus stress and external rotation. Completing the medial structures is the pes anserinus, the common insertion of the sartorius, gracilis, and semitendinosus on the anteromedial tibia.

The lateral collateral, or fibular collateral, ligament (LCL) consists of a single layer and runs from the lateral femoral epicondyle to the fibular head (Fig. 23-4). Superficial to the LCL is the iliotibial band, the fascial continuation of the fascia lata from the lateral hip and thigh, attaching to the anterolateral tibia at Gerdy's tubercle. Because of its muscular origin, the iliotibial band acts as a dynamic stabilizer and, along with the LCL, a static stabilizer, to varus stress. The posterolateral structures are termed the *arcuate complex* and include the LCL, the popliteus muscle and tendon, and the arcuate ligament, which is a thickening of the posterolateral capsule. These structures function to resist varus and internal rotation of the tibia. Deep to all of these

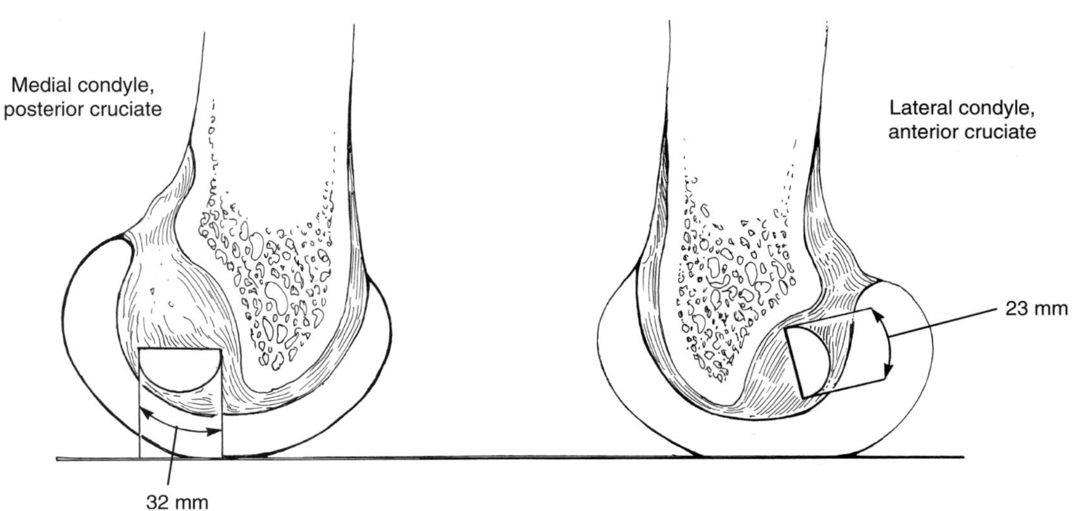

FIGURE 23-2. Origin of the anterior and posterior cruciate ligaments on the femur.

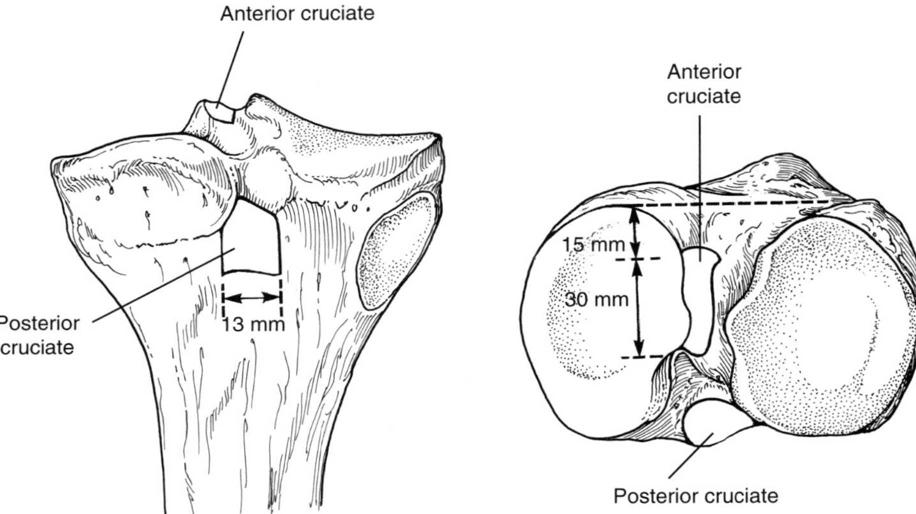

FIGURE 23-3. Attachment sites of the anterior and posterior cruciate ligaments on the tibia.

structures is the knee joint capsule, surrounding the entire joint with an inner layer of synovium. This synovial layer produces the synovial fluid that is essential to joint lubrication and nutrition for articular and meniscal cartilage.

The medial and lateral menisci are wedge-shaped, semicircular structures composed primarily of type I cartilage (fibrocartilage). The collagen fibers are oriented circumferentially, allowing the menisci to absorb 40% to 50% of the compressive forces across the knee joint.[77]

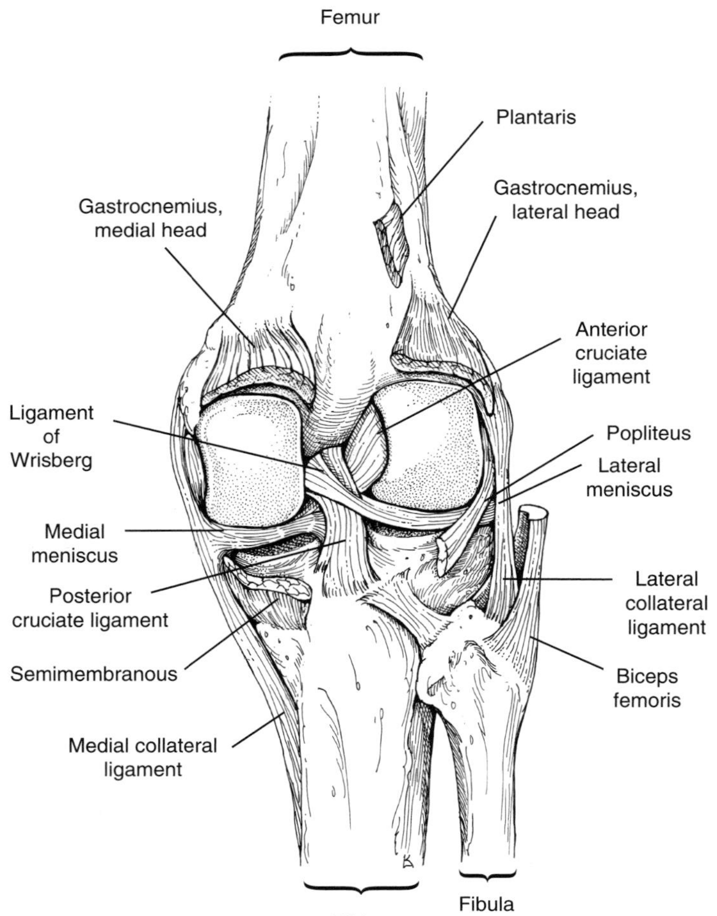

FIGURE 23-4. Posterior view of the knee.

In addition, the menisci act as secondary stabilizers to anteroposterior-directed forces by way of increasing the conformity between the rounded femoral and relatively flat tibial articular surfaces. The vascular supply is restricted to the outer third of the meniscal width, a significant factor in the inability of most meniscal tears to heal.

CLINICAL EVALUATION

History

As with much of medicine, a thorough history regarding knee injuries often makes the diagnosis (Fig. 23-5). For acute injuries, careful attention should be paid to determining the mechanism of injury. Did the knee suffer a twisting injury, often indicating a meniscal or ACL tear? Was this a contact (i.e., clip in football) or noncontact (i.e., change in direction in basketball) injury? What caused the force, from what direction, of what magnitude, and in what position was the patient's leg at the time of injury? Answers to these questions will often suggest a mechanism putting specific structures under stress, such as a valgus force causing injury to the MCL and ACL.

An audible "pop" often signifies an acute tear of the ACL or sometimes a meniscal tear. The extent and onset of swelling is a helpful sign. A knee that swells rapidly over minutes to a couple of hours suggests a hemarthrosis, as seen with a cruciate ligament tear, patella dislocation, or intraarticular bony injury. An effusion that develops over several hours to the next day suggests a meniscal tear. Other important questions include knowledge about previous symptoms, injuries, and treatments to the affected knee and whether the athlete was able to continue sports participation after the acute injury.

Chronic injuries require additional questions regarding the nature of the training regimen, including mileage or duration and intervals, stretching, shoe wear, surfaces, and recent changes in the routine. Onset of symptoms and precipitating activities and whether the athlete had any self-administrated relief are also important.

Physical Examination

Observation and Palpation. An initial evaluation should determine the specific location of pain and any associated crepitus that may be associated with a fracture. A gentle varus and valgus and anteroposterior stress will elicit any gross instability that precludes further examination modalities and necessitates immediate splint stabilization and transfer for orthopedic evaluation. The presence of an intraarticular effusion can be determined by a fullness in the suprapatellar pouch, a fullness surrounding the patella obliterating the usual depressed contour on slight

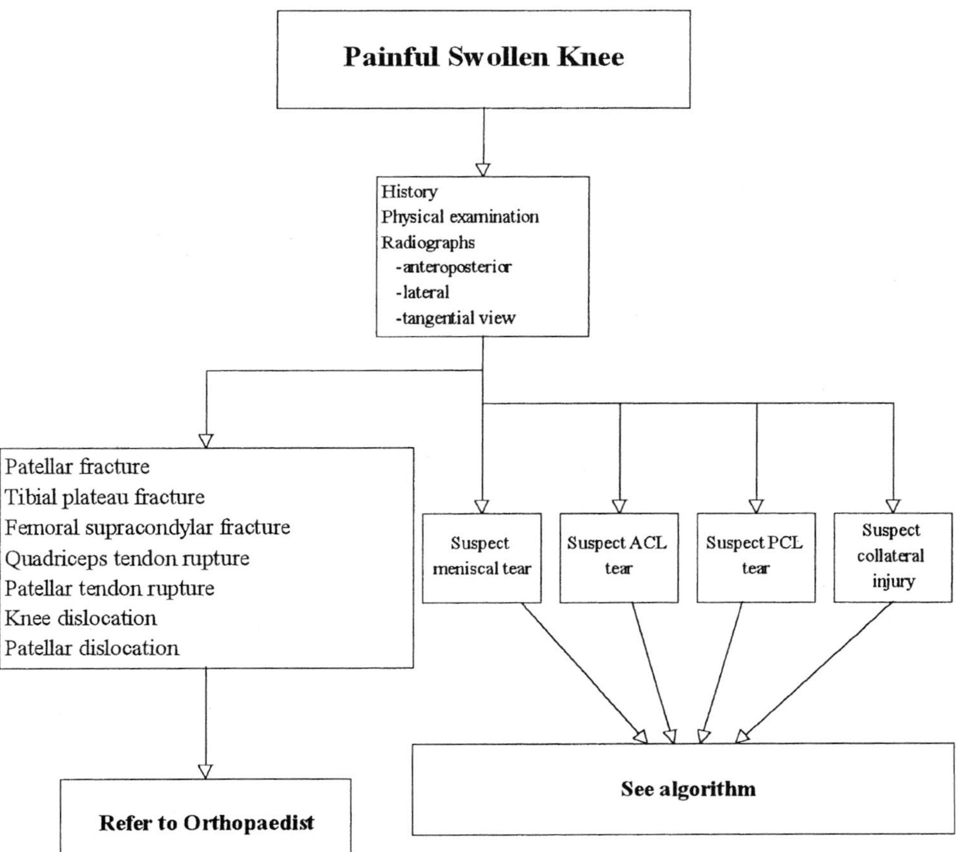

FIGURE 23-5. Algorithm for the acutely swollen knee. (Adapted from the AAOS National Orthopedic Leadership Conference 1995.)

flexion, and possibly the presence of a fluid wave from side to side. A large effusion will result in a ballotable patella that "floats" above its articulating femoral trochlea, making contact only when a posteriorly directed force is applied to bounce the patella up and down (Fig. 23-6). Effusions can be rated as grade I (slight), grade II (mild lift-off of patella), grade III (ballottable patella), or grade IV (tense). In contrast to an intraarticular effusion, extraarticular soft-tissue swelling is more localized and superficial, usually overriding a bony prominence as with prepatellar bursitis. Chronic intraarticular synovitis, as is seen with arthritic knees, has a boggy texture that cannot be "milked" to other knee compartments.

Patella and Extensor Mechanism Evaluation. In the absence of an acute fracture, all patients must be able to actively extend the knee to demonstrate an intact extensor mechanism. One useful method is to have the patient raise the extended leg off the table. Patients need to be coaxed through pain. Inability to extend the knee indicates rupture of the quadriceps tendon or patella tendon, or fracture of the patella and requires immediate referral to an orthopedic surgeon for reconstruction. Often a palpable, painful defect can be determined at the site of disruption. Assuming an intact extensor mechanism, one can determine the active range of motion, from a normal 5° of hyperextension to a maximum of 135° of flexion (Fig. 23-7). Attention can also be directed toward any

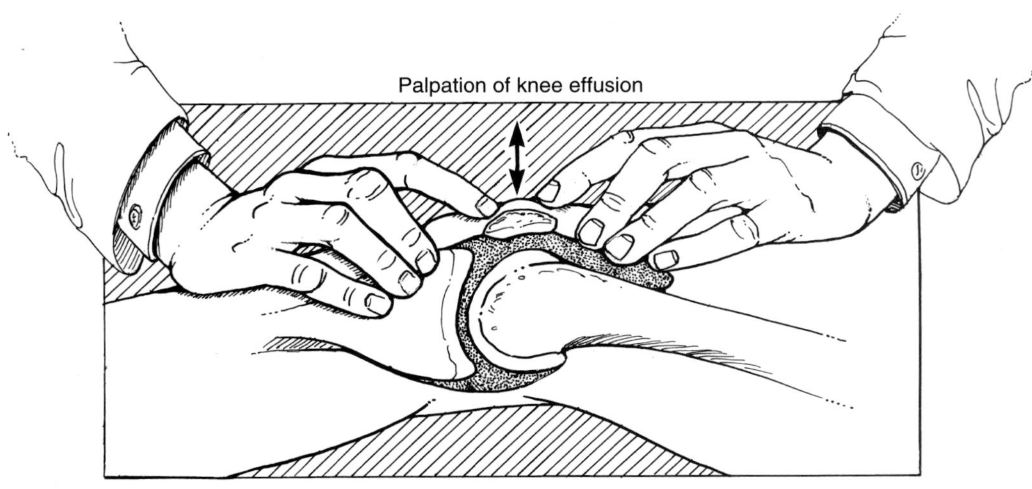

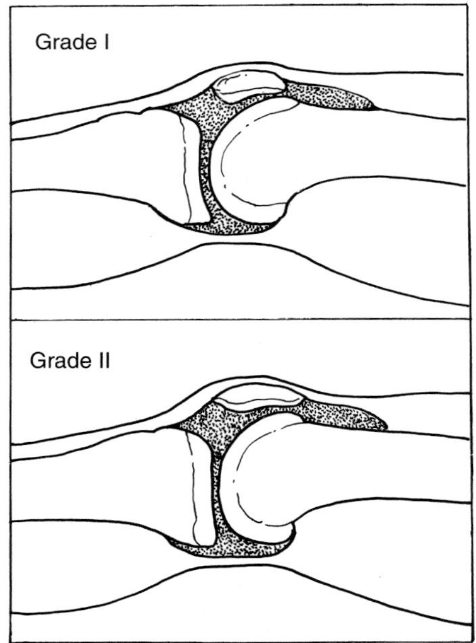

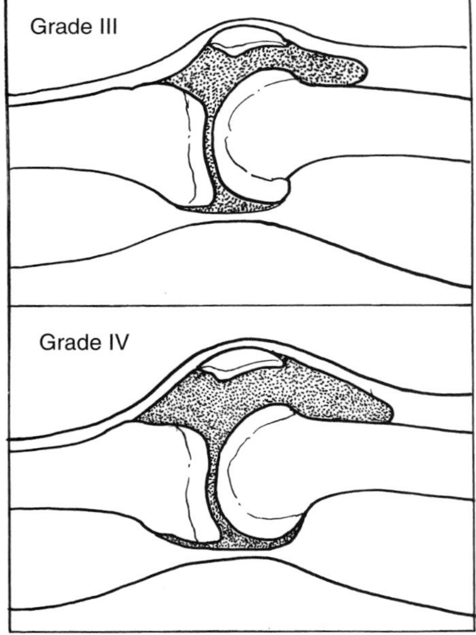

FIGURE 23-6. Knee effusions, graded from I to IV.

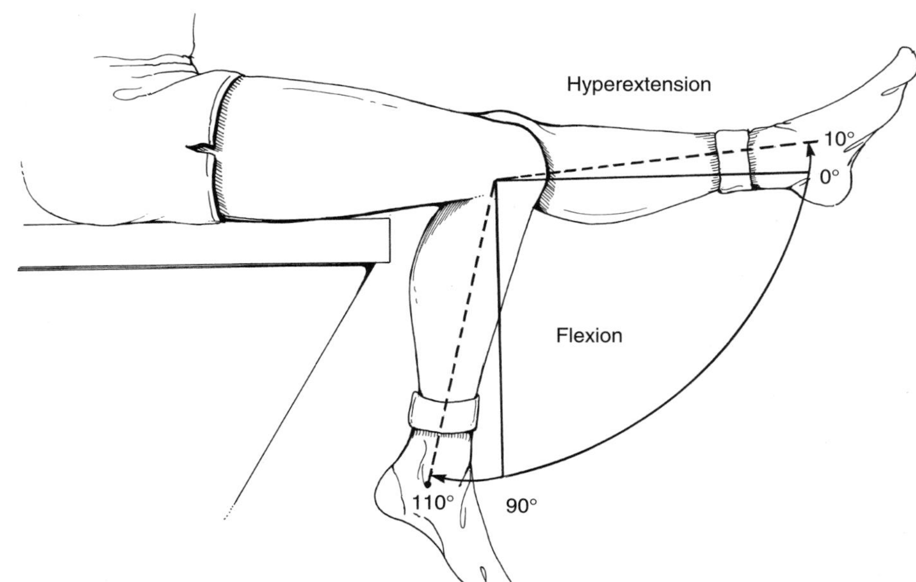

FIGURE 23-7. Normal knee range of motion is from 5° to 10° of hyperextension to 135° of flexion.

degree of quadriceps atrophy, easily measured circumferentially at a common reference point (i.e., 10 cm) above the patella in extension.

Patella tracking in the femoral sulcus groove can be assessed by observation and palpation through a range of motion. Gentle medial-to-lateral pressure against the medial side of the patella during the passive arc of motion represents the "apprehension test" for patella subluxation. A positive test result elicits discomfort and a sensation of impending dislocation laterally. A recent patella dislocation will demonstrate medial retinacular tenderness and an effusion. A knee with a large Q angle is considered anatomically predisposed to patella tracking problems because the quadriceps muscle vector pulls in a more lateral direction. The Q angle is measured in extension as the intersection of lines drawn from the anterior–superior iliac spine to the center of the patella and a second line from the center of the patella to the tibial tubercle (Fig. 23-8). Normal Q angles in men are 8° to 10° and in women are from 10° to 20°.[3] Anterior knee pain can be effectively localized to the patellofemoral articulation by provocative palpation of the undersurface of the patella. In extension with the quadriceps relaxed, the patella can be gently subluxed medially and laterally, affording an opportunity to palpate the articular side with the thumb (Fig. 23-9). Tenderness suggests chondromalacia-type problems. Additionally, the lateral retinaculum adjacent to the patella can be palpated for tight, fibrous bands, which prevent the usual medial displacement on attempted medial subluxation. These bands may cause lateral tilt or tracking of the patella in the femoral sulcus, leading to chondromalacia-type symptoms or patella subluxation and dislocation.

Meniscus Evaluation. Medial or lateral joint line tenderness is very useful to identify meniscal tears. Firm palpation is directed over the meniscal rim with the knee flexed 90° either over the examining table or supine. A knee inflamed from degenerative arthritis or recent injury can give false positive results. Other examination techniques seek to mechanically impinge the torn flap of meniscal tissue between moving articular surfaces, which is essentially the cause of symptomatic knee buckling or giving way that patients report in the history. The Steinmann test is performed with the knee relaxed and flexed 90° off the side of the table. While stabilizing the calf with one hand, the opposite hand grasps the foot and sharply internally and externally rotates the leg (Fig. 23-10). Pain at the joint line suggests a meniscal tear. The McMurray test is performed in the supine position by grasping the heel with one hand while stabilizing the leg with the other hand on the thigh and simultaneously palpating the medial and lateral joint lines. In full flexion, a valgus, external rotation force is applied to the foot, which is then brought into varus, internal rotation. A modification of this test involves moving from full flexion to extension while applying valgus, external rotation and then varus, internal rotation (Fig. 23-11). A positive test result is indicated by joint line pain or a palpable click.[98] The Apley test, a variation of the McMurray test, is performed in the prone position with the knee flexed 90° (Fig. 23-12). While grasping the foot, the tibia is axially loaded to compress the menisci while simultaneously internally and externally rotating the leg. Again, a palpable click or joint line pain represents a positive test result. False positive tests resulting from ligamentous or soft-tissue pain can be differentiated from meniscal pain by repeating the

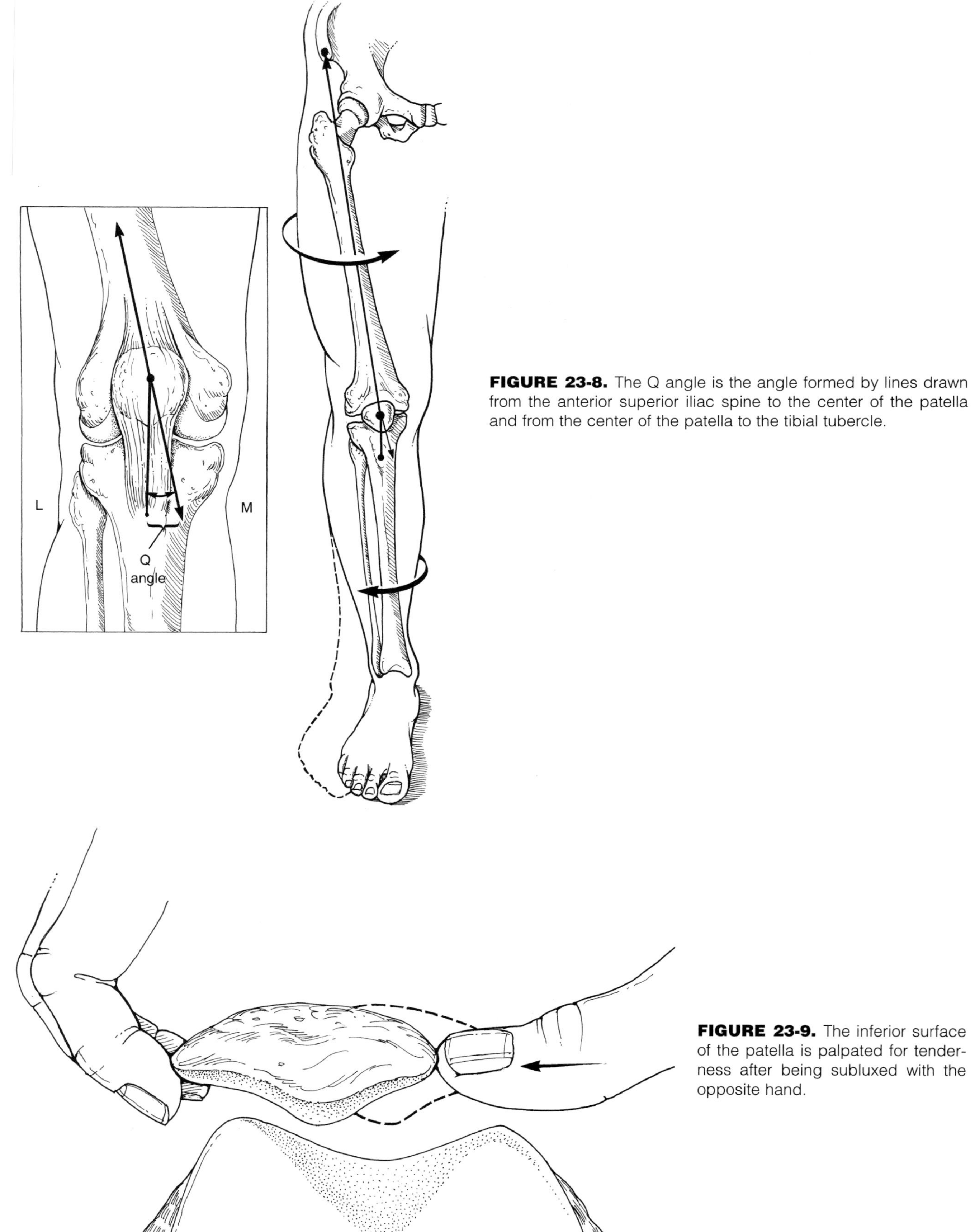

FIGURE 23-8. The Q angle is the angle formed by lines drawn from the anterior superior iliac spine to the center of the patella and from the center of the patella to the tibial tubercle.

FIGURE 23-9. The inferior surface of the patella is palpated for tenderness after being subluxed with the opposite hand.

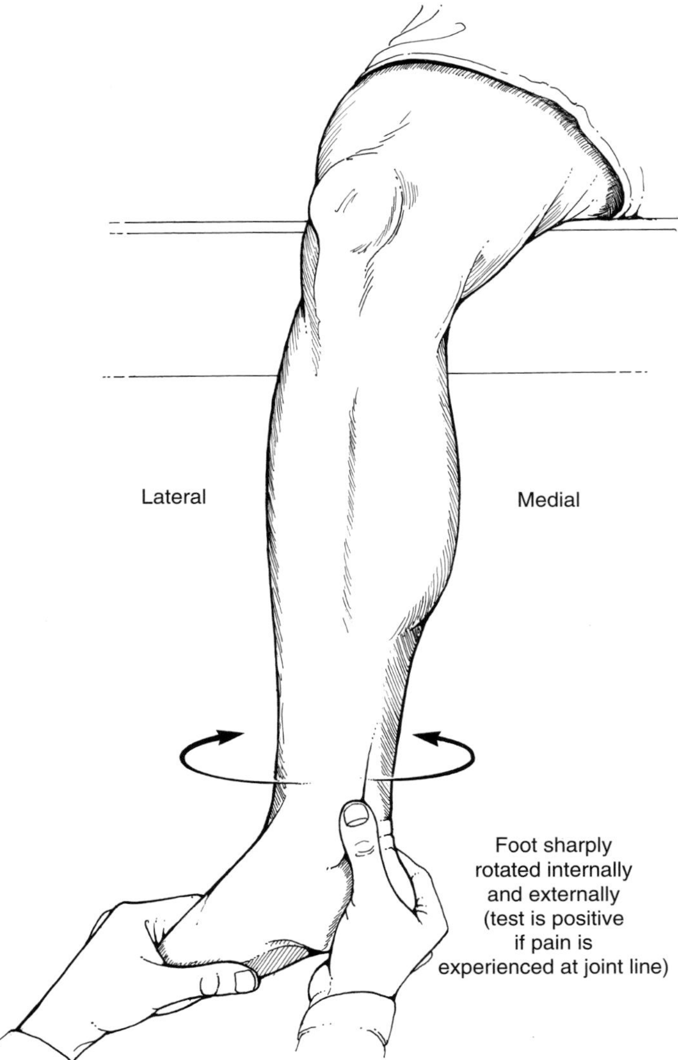
Lateral
Medial
Foot sharply rotated internally and externally (test is positive if pain is experienced at joint line)

FIGURE 23-10. The Steinmann test for meniscal tears. A positive test result is demonstrated by joint line pain with sharp rotation.

test while distracting the leg to unload the meniscus, which should result in the absence of pain or click.

Collateral Ligament Evaluation. The collateral ligaments on either side of the knee are evaluated by stress examinations. The valgus stress test assesses the MCL and supporting structures (Fig. 23-13). With the knee in 30° of flexion, a gentle valgus stress is applied to the knee by grasping the ankle with one hand and applying stabilizing pressure to the lateral thigh with the opposite hand. It is important to perform the test in slight flexion to relax the posterior capsule and effectively isolate stress to the MCL. In full extension, the tight posterior capsule will give a false negative test result. The test can be repeated in full extension to demonstrate additional laxity of the posterior oblique ligament and posteromedial capsule and possibly tears of the ACL or PCL. Specifically, instability to valgus stress at 30° of knee flexion indicates isolated MCL injury; instability at 0° implies MCL and posteromedial capsule injury; and laxity at −10° of hyperextension suggests MCL, posteromedial capsule, and posterior oblique ligament injury and possibly PCL or ACL tears.

The varus stress test is performed in similar fashion, in 30° of flexion to isolate the LCL, and in full extension and hyperextension to assess secondary stabilizers (Fig. 23-14). Instability to varus stress at 30° of flexion suggests isolated LCL injury; instability at 0° suggests LCL and lateral capsular injury; and instability at −10° (hyperextension) implies LCL, lateral capsule, and arcuate complex injury and possibly a PCL tear.

With varus and valgus stress tests, a positive result is graded as follows: grade 1 is up to 5 mm of opening, grade 2 is 6 to 10 mm of opening, or grade 3, which is 11 to 15 mm of opening. It is important with these and all stress examinations to perform the test on the healthy, contralateral leg to differentiate any component of physiologic laxity. If the examiner has difficulty controlling a

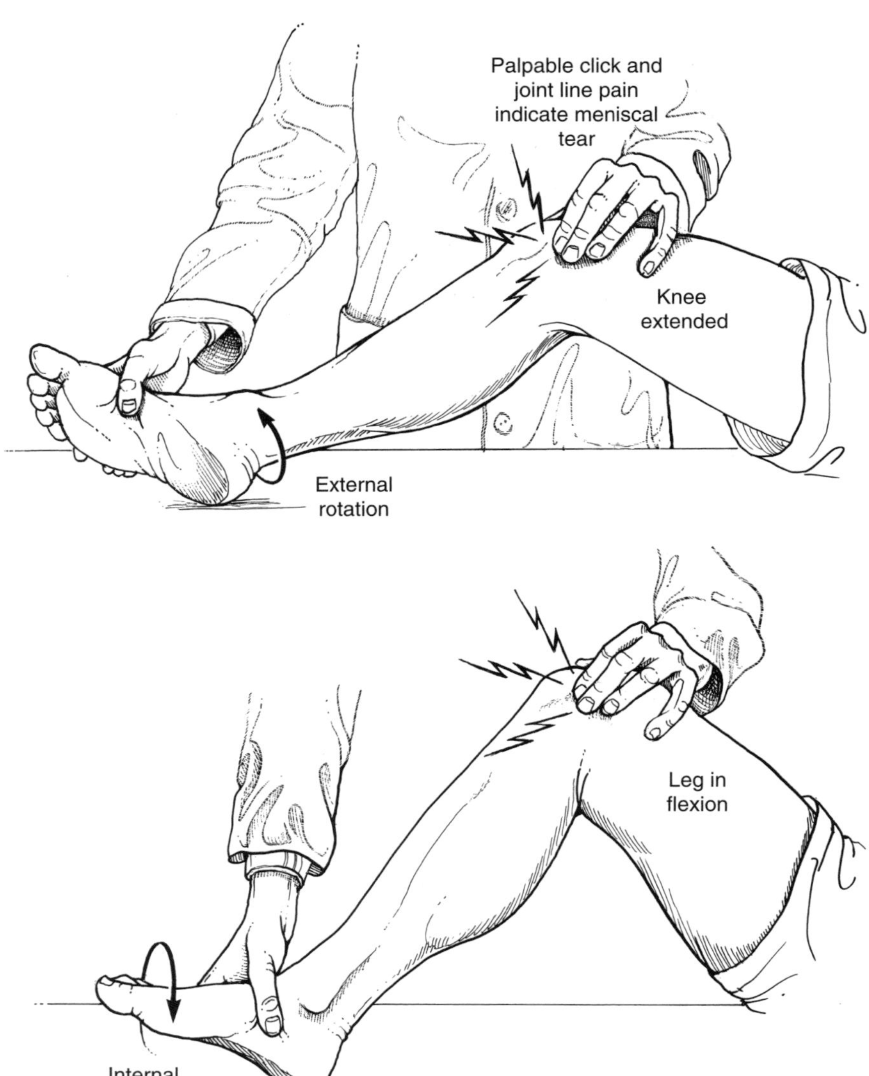

FIGURE 23-11. The McMurray test. The leg in flexion is moved from valgus, external rotation to varus, internal rotation. Alternatively, the knee can be extended during the maneuver. A meniscal tear is suspected with a palpable click or joint line pain.

very large leg, optional variations of the varus or valgus stress test involve cradling the lower leg under the examiner's arm, while applying stress just below the knee with the hands (Fig. 23-15). Alternatively, the leg can be swung partially off the side of the table with the thigh supported and stabilized with one hand while the other hand applies stress at the ankle.

Anterior Cruciate Ligament Evaluation. Numerous tests have been described for ACL instability. The most sensitive and the easiest to perform in the presence of a painful, acutely swollen knee is the Lachman test.[86] With the knee in 20° to 30° of flexion, the leg is grasped with one hand and stabilized at the distal thigh with the other hand. Muscle relaxation is critical to accurate test results. An anteriorly directed force is applied to the proximal tibia to stress the ACL (Fig. 23-16). Anterior displacement compared with the normal contralateral leg is graded as 1+ (0 to 5 mm), 2+ (6 to 10 mm), or 3+ (11 to 15 mm). Additionally, one can comment on whether the endpoint is firm or soft. For problems with a large leg, one may perform the same test with the patient prone.

The anterior drawer test also assesses the integrity of the ACL by an anteriorly directed force on the leg (Fig. 23-17). The patient is supine with the knees flexed to 90°, and the examiner sits on the patient's feet to stabilize the leg. Both hands grasp behind the proximal calf, palpating the hamstring tendons to ensure relaxation, and an anteriorly directed force is applied. Anterior translation is again assessed as 1 to 3+ with a firm or soft endpoint. The test can be repeated with the foot fixed in an internally or externally rotated position to test the integrity of the posterolateral or posteromedial capsules, respectively.

Several additional tests have been described to evaluate the rotational component of ACL instability, termed

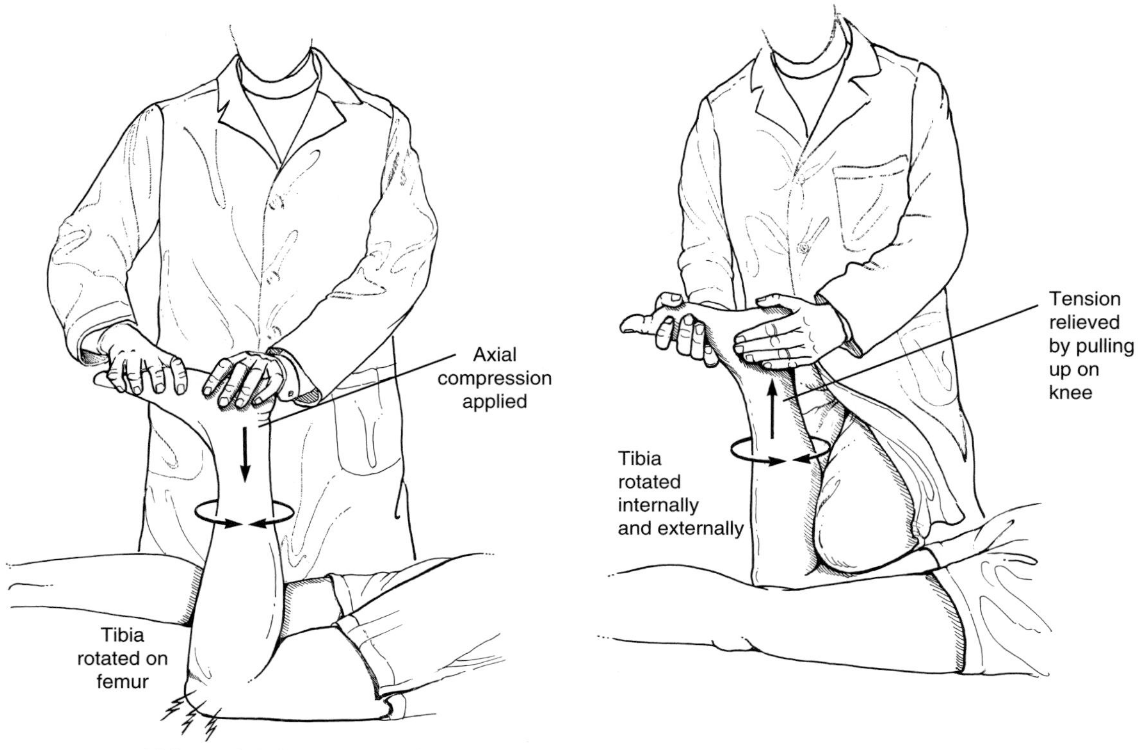

FIGURE 23-12. The Apley test. The knee is axially loaded with the patient prone while subjected to internal and external rotation. Pain or palpable click suggest a meniscal tear. Distraction of the knee should relieve the symptoms.

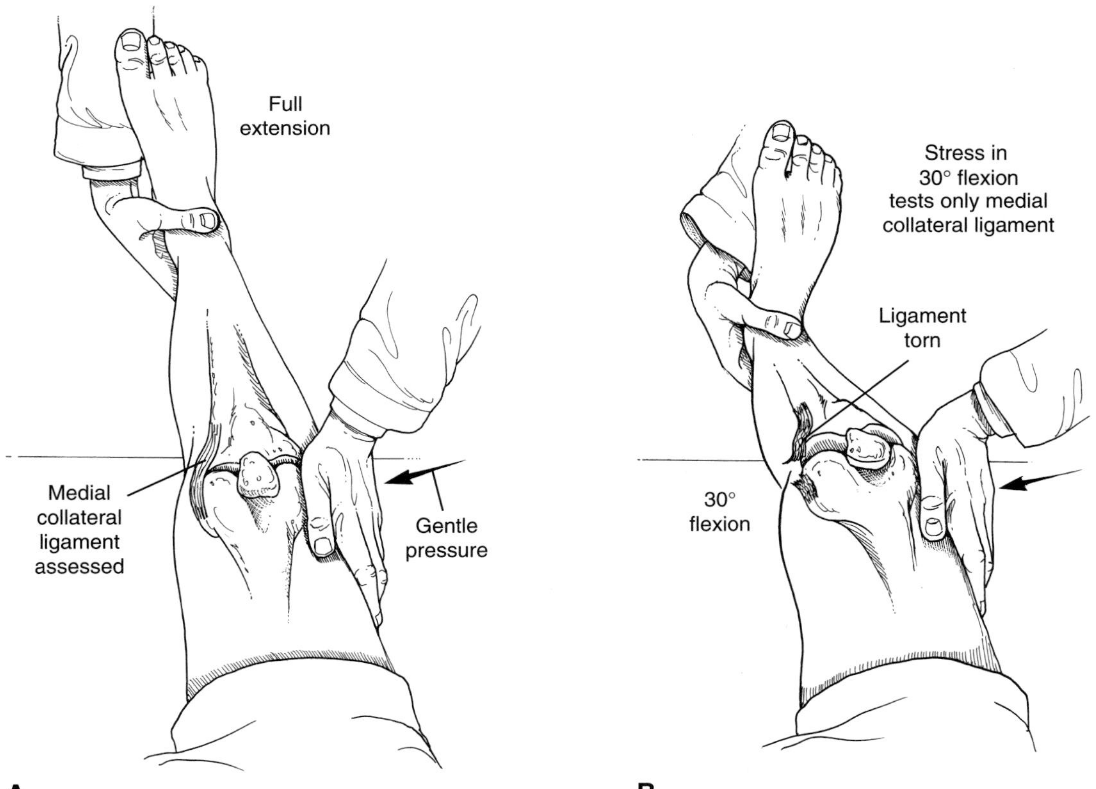

FIGURE 23-13. The valgus stress test is performed at full extension to assess secondary restraints **(A)** and at 30° of flexion to assess the medial collateral ligament **(B)**.

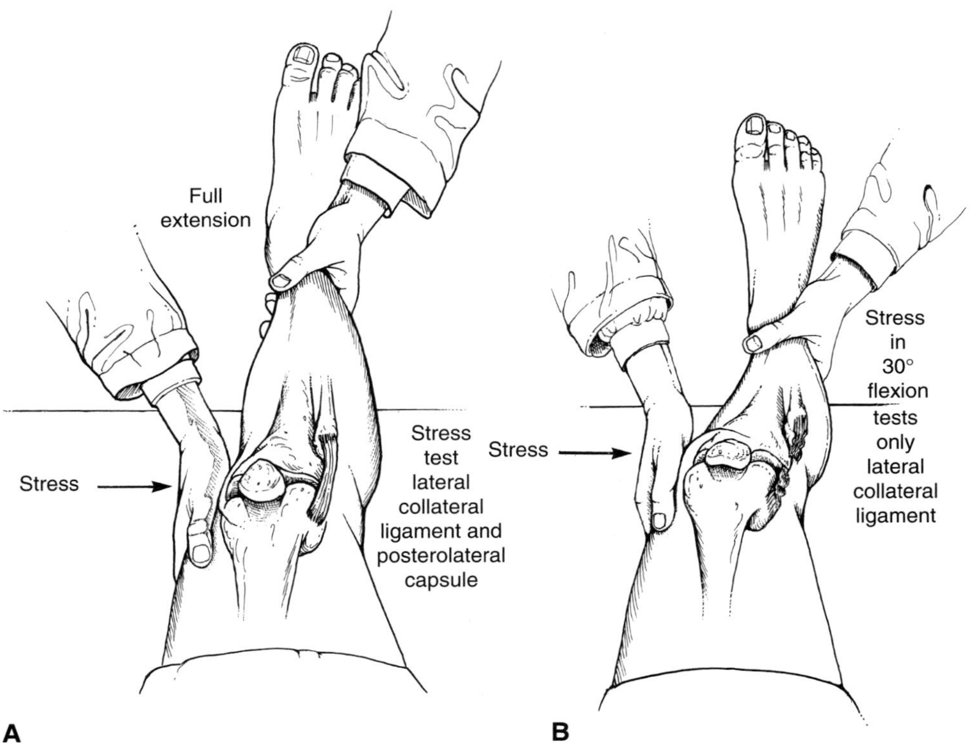

FIGURE 23-14. The varus stress test is performed at full extension to assess secondary restraints **(A)** and at 30° of flexion to assess the lateral collateral ligament **(B)**.

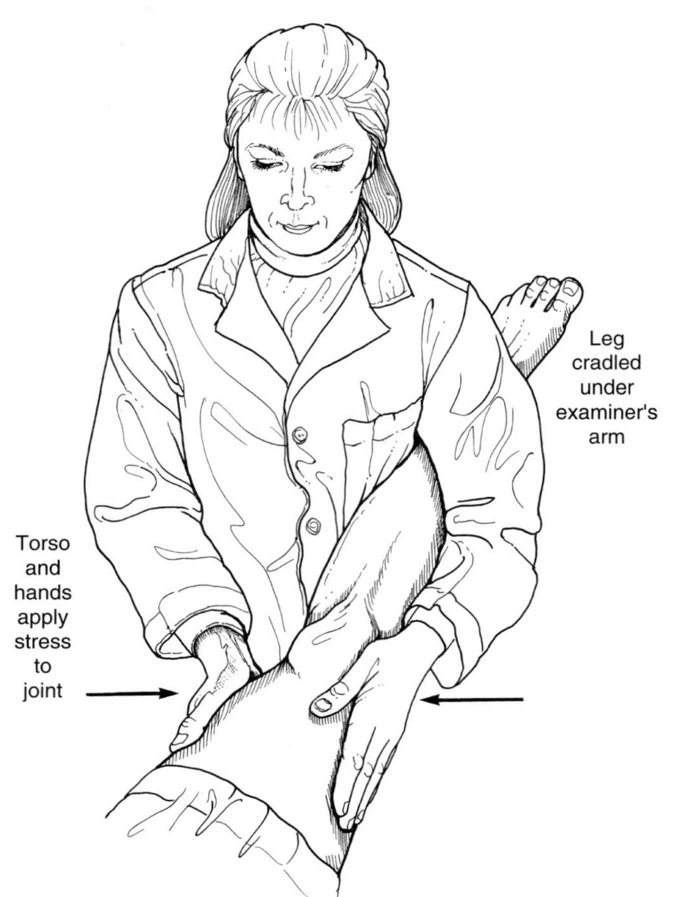

FIGURE 23-15. An alternative method of performing varus and valgus stress testing is with the leg cradled under the examiner's arm while the torso and hands apply the stress.

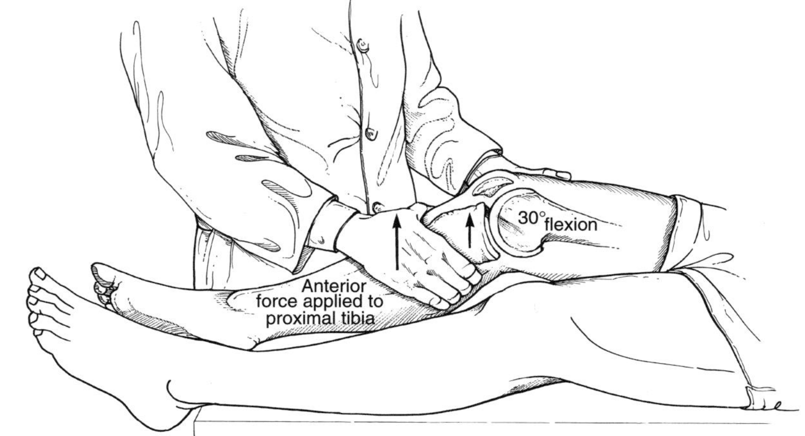

FIGURE 23-16. The Lachman test is performed at 30° of flexion with an anteriorly directed force applied to the proximal tibia while the opposite hand stabilizes the thigh.

anterolateral rotatory instability. This rotatory instability better reflects the functional giving way episode experienced by patients than the straight anterior instability tested by the anterior drawer and Lachman tests. The most commonly used of these tests is the pivot shift test of MacIntosh.[31] With the patient supine, the examiner grasps the ankle with one hand while placing the opposite hand laterally at the knee behind the fibular head, directing pressure anteriorly (Fig. 23-18). With the knee extended, the leg is internally rotated, and a valgus force applied. In this position, the tibia is subluxed anteriorly in an ACL-deficient knee. As the knee is flexed, the iliotibial band tightens and reduces the tibia posteriorly to its normal position with a palpable clunk if the test result is positive. This reduction clunk can be graded 1 (glide), 2 (shift), or 3 (shift and clunk or momentary locking). The Losee test is similar to the pivot shift test except the leg begins in an externally rotated, flexed position and is moved into extension. In this case, the examiner looks for a jump into an anteriorly subluxed position. The flexion–rotation drawer test is a combination of the Lachman and pivot shift tests (Fig. 23-19). Both hands are placed behind the calf to sublux the tibia anteriorly in extension while the leg is stabilized by cradling the ankle under the arm. Flexing the knee to 45° results in a palpable clunk as the tibia reduces posteriorly.

Posterior Cruciate Ligament Evaluation. Tests for PCL disruption in general are less sensitive than those developed for ACL tears. The posterior sag sign is noted by flexing both knees to 90° and observing the contour from the side (Fig. 23-20). A PCL-deficient knee will sag posteriorly, resulting in a less prominent tibial tubercle compared with the opposite knee. The examiner can perform the posterior drawer test by applying posteriorly directed pressure to the tibial tubercle to further demonstrate the degree of laxity. The posterior translation is graded as 1 to 3+ as previously described with documentation of endpoint resistance. One potential difficulty in evaluating the PCL is determining the neutral starting position of the tibia in relation to the femoral condyles, which can be determined by the quadriceps active test. The patient is asked to contract the quadriceps with the

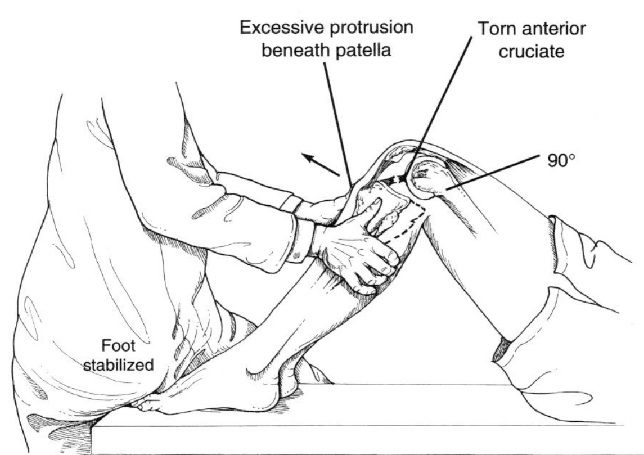

FIGURE 23-17. The anterior drawer test is performed at 90° of flexion with an anteriorly directed force applied to the proximal tibia.

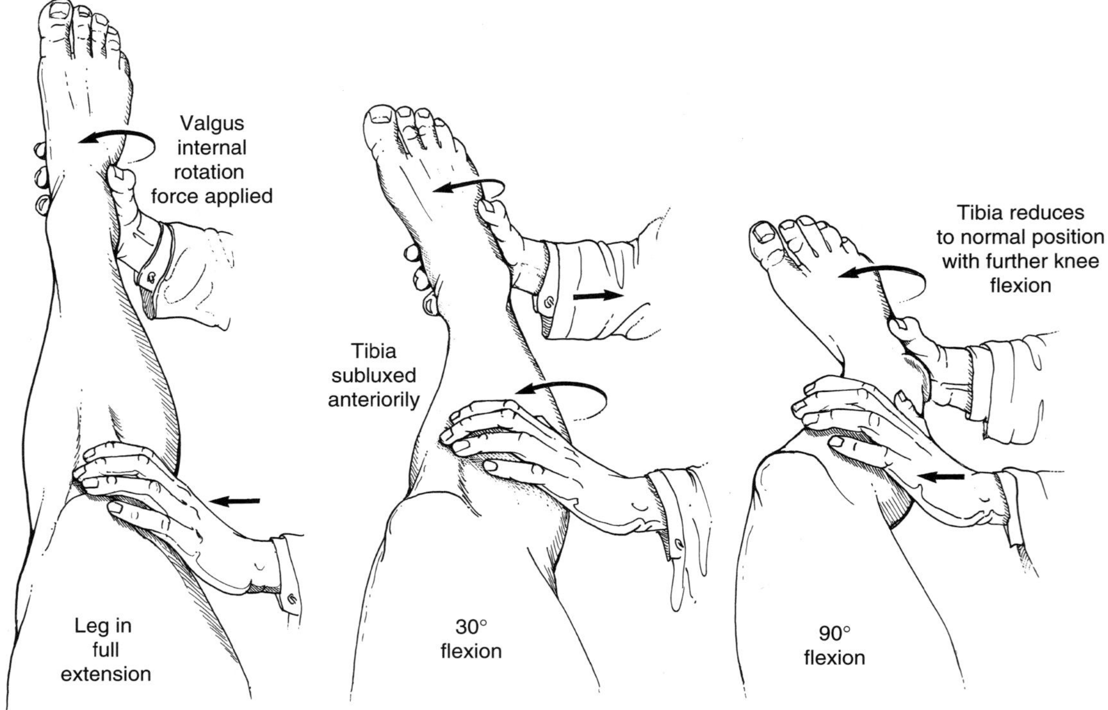

FIGURE 23-18. The pivot shift test begins in extension with a valgus, internal rotation force applied to the leg. In this position, the tibia is subluxed anteriorly. As the knee is flexed, the tibia subluxes posteriorly to its normal position, and a clunk is seen and felt by the examiner.

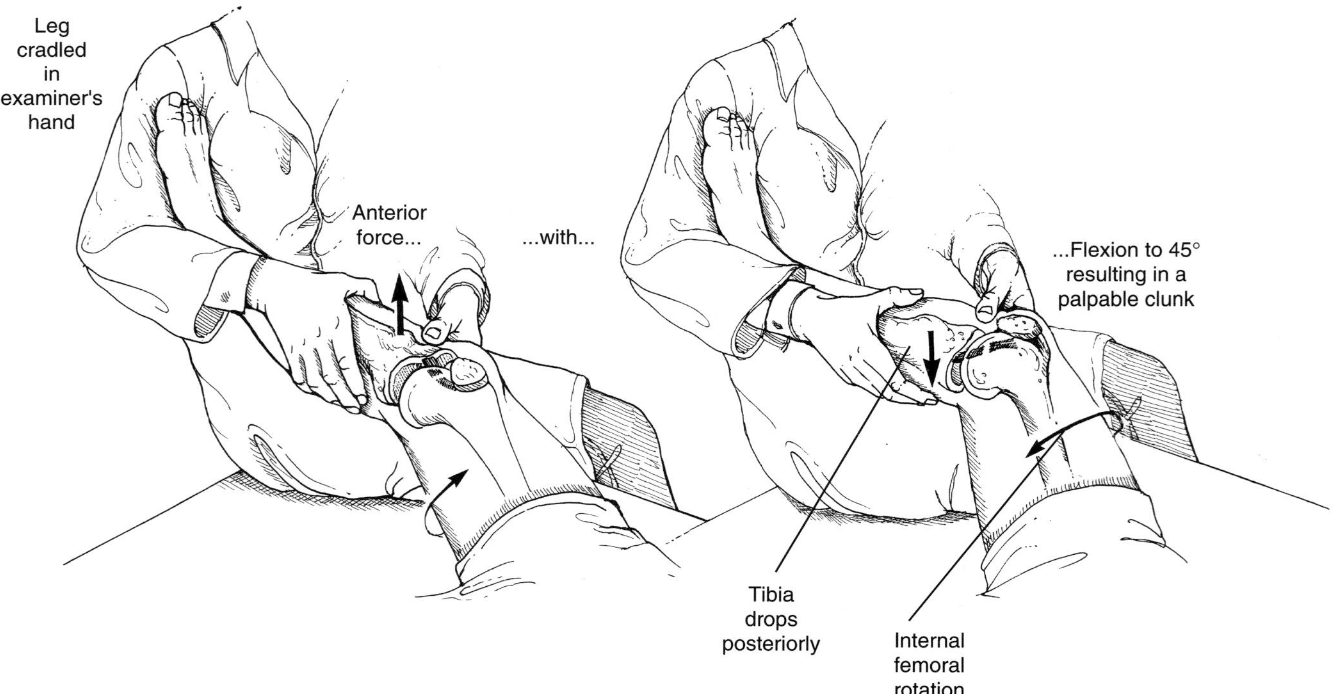

FIGURE 23-19. The flexion–rotation drawer test is performed by cradling the leg in the examiner's hands with an anteriorly directed force to sublux the tibia anteriorly. Flexion to 45° results in a palpable clunk as the tibia reduces posteriorly.

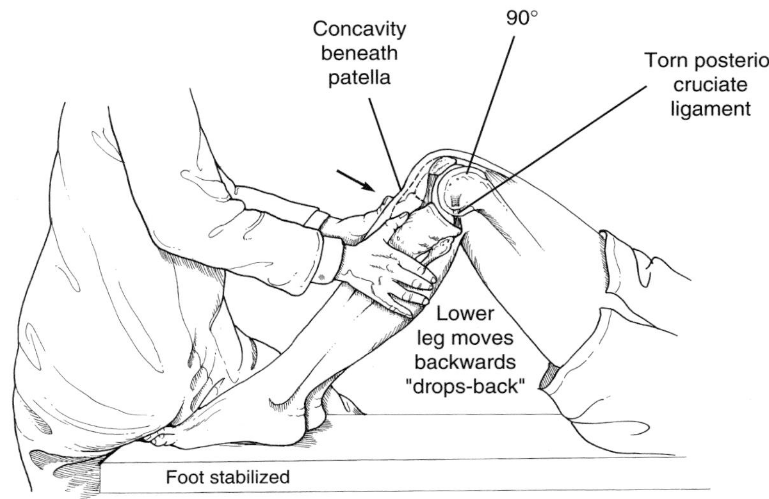

FIGURE 23-20. Posterior cruciate ligament deficiency results in a posterior sag in the resting position, which can be appreciated at 90° of flexion by comparing the contour of the anterior knee with the opposite side. Further posteriorly directed force produces the posterior drawer test to assess the extent of laxity.

knee in 90° of flexion while the examiner stabilizes the foot (Fig. 23-21). A posteriorly subluxed tibia caused by PCL laxity will reduce to a neutral position on quadriceps contraction. This reference point can then be used to perform a posterior Lachman test in 30° of flexion (Fig. 23-22). Another useful reference for quantification is to compare the anterior border of the tibia with that of the femoral condyles. Normally, the tibia is 5 mm anterior to the femoral condyles. If the tibia is flush with the condyles on the posterior drawer or Lachman test, this corresponds to 5 to 10 mm of posterior displacement (2+). An endpoint anterior to the condyles is less than 5 mm (1+), and an endpoint posterior to the condyles is more than 10 mm (3+). Comparison with the contralateral, uninvolved knee is critical.

IMAGING STUDIES

At the initial evaluation of an injured knee, the standard radiographic evaluation should include a standing anteroposterior view, a lateral view, a tunnel view, and a merchant view. The standing anteroposterior view is useful because it allows evaluation of the loaded knee joint and permits measurement of knee alignment. The tunnel view in 30° of flexion demonstrates the intercondylar notch, and delineates the posterior femoral condyles, which may have an osteochondral defect (Fig. 23-23). If a fracture is suspected, additional oblique views can be obtained. Stress views in varus and valgus can be helpful in diagnosing occult physeal fractures in the skeletally immature patient, but they have little role in routine evaluation of ligamentous injuries in the adult.

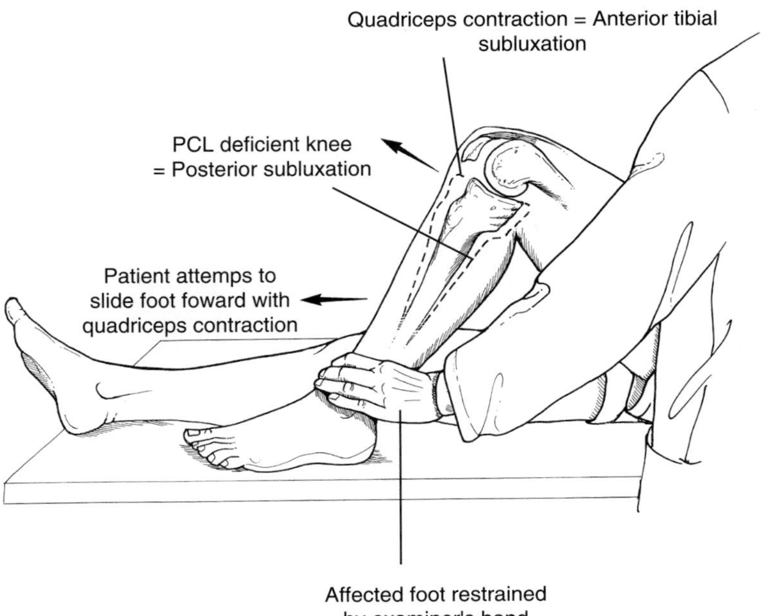

FIGURE 23-21. The quadriceps active test is performed with the knee flexed 90° and the examiner stabilizing the foot on the table. In the posterior cruciate ligament–deficient knee, the tibia is at a posteriorly subluxed starting point. Active contraction of the quadriceps causes a forward translation of the tibia to a neutral position.

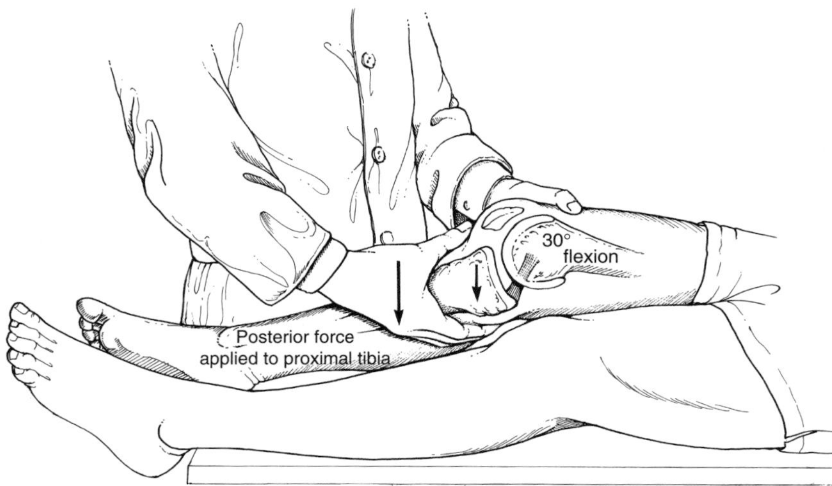

FIGURE 23-22. The posterior Lachman test is performed with the knee flexed 30°. A posteriorly directed force is applied to the tibia and translation and endpoint assessed.

The sunrise or Merchant view is obtained with the patient supine and the knee flexed 45°, with the x-ray beam 30° from horizontal and directed distally toward the cassette (Fig. 23-24). This view demonstrates the alignment of the patellofemoral joint and is used to determine subluxation or tilt of the patella. Other axial views of the patella have been popularized, including the Laurin and Hughston views. Bipartite patella, a normal anatomic variant, can be visualized on the merchant view or on the anteroposterior projection (Fig. 23-25). These well-corticated bony fragments usually are bilateral and occur at the superolateral pole. They are the result of accessory, ununited ossification centers.[66,78]

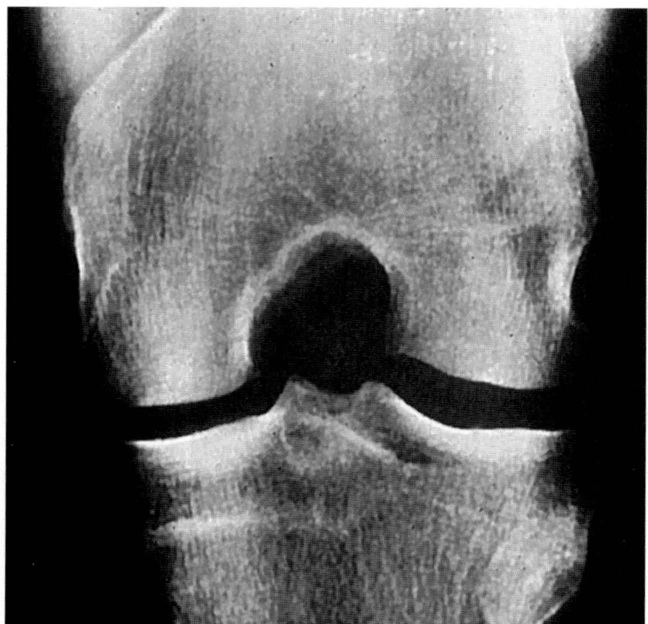

FIGURE 23-23. Standing anteroposterior tunnel or notch view of the knee.

Before the advent of magnetic resonance imaging (MRI), arthrograms were helpful in diagnosing meniscal or cruciate ligament pathology with an accuracy of 60% to 87%.[40] Currently, MRI has become the diagnostic procedure of choice for assessment of intraarticular knee pathology. Accuracy for diagnosing intraarticular pathology ranges from 88% to 97%[12,28] and offers the advantage of providing additional information about the collateral ligaments and bone. Normal meniscal and ligamentous tissue is relatively dark and homogeneous on T1- and T2-weighted images because of the low water and fat content (Fig. 23-26). Findings on MRI compatable with a meniscal tear include change in the usual dark meniscal signal to lighter signal, consistent with interposed joint fluid. Early intrasubstance degeneration is radiographically a grade 1 signal, whereas an intrasubstance tear extending up to but not through the meniscal surface represents a grade 2 signal. Complete tears through the meniscal surface are termed grade 3 signals (Fig. 23-27). Meniscal degeneration, as opposed to a complete tear, often requires arthroscopic confirmation. Cruciate ligament tears are identified by disruption in the normal dark ligament signal with bright joint fluid (Fig. 23-28). Failure to adequately visualize the ACL may be technique-related, resulting from the oblique course of the ligament, or may represent a tear. Therefore, it is important to look in the anteroposterior and lateral projections for the ACL and PCL images. Bone bruises are seen in conjunction with an acute ACL tear 56% to 85% of the time.[33,54] These are usually seen on the distal aspect of the lateral femoral condyle and the posterior lateral tibia (Fig. 23-29).

MENISCAL INJURIES

Meniscal tears usually result from a twisting mechanism in either a contact or noncontact activity. The shear force of the twisting event mechanically catches the meniscus

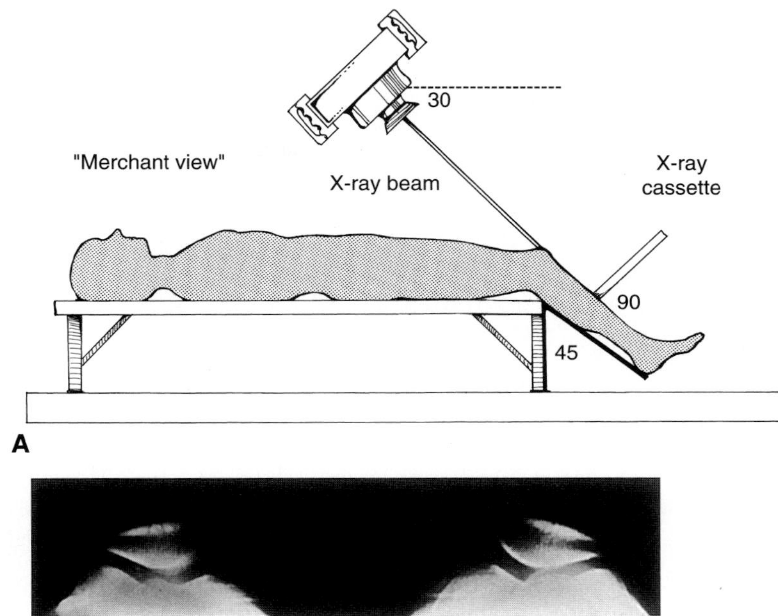

FIGURE 23-24. A, Technique for obtaining the Merchant view of the patella. **B,** Representative normal radiographic Merchant view.

between the femoral condyle and tibial articular surface, creating the tear. Because the medial meniscus is less mobile than the lateral meniscus, it has a greater chance of becoming entrapped between the condyles, resulting in a higher incidence of medial meniscal tears. Although most meniscal injuries result from an acute traumatic event, the patient may relate a relatively minor precipitating event, such as squatting down or getting up from a chair, which correlates with a meniscus with preexisting, intrasubstance degenerative changes. This can appear as grade 1 or 2 signals on MRI scans, indicating damage within the meniscus not extending to the surface of the meniscus. Acute tears in a previously normal meniscus may be associated with collateral or cruciate ligament injuries. Because symptoms from associated ligamentous injuries usually overshadow meniscal symptoms, meniscal tears should always be entertained with a high index of suspicion.

The patient with an acute meniscal tear usually relates moderate pain that gradually subsides, allowing the individual to ambulate with a slight limp and possibly even to continue play in some cases. A joint effusion usually occurs over the ensuing 24 hours and may be slight to moderate. With large, displaced, bucket-handle–type tears, the torn fragment will get trapped between the femoral condyle and tibial plateau, preventing full knee extension. Bucket-handle–type tears are more common on the medial side compared with the lateral side and result in the classic locked knee, which necessitates early referral to an orthopedist for arthroscopy to restore motion.

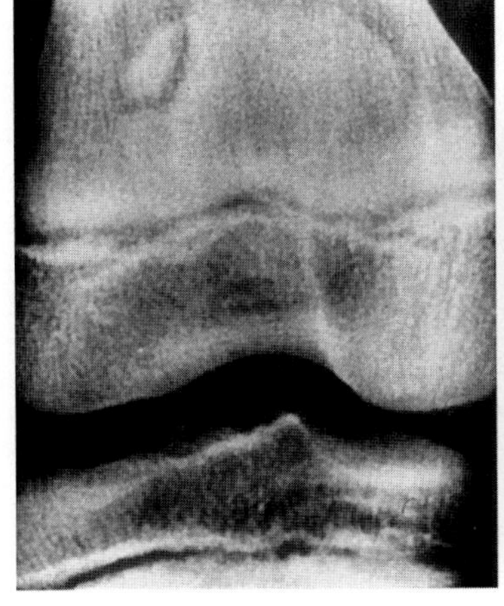

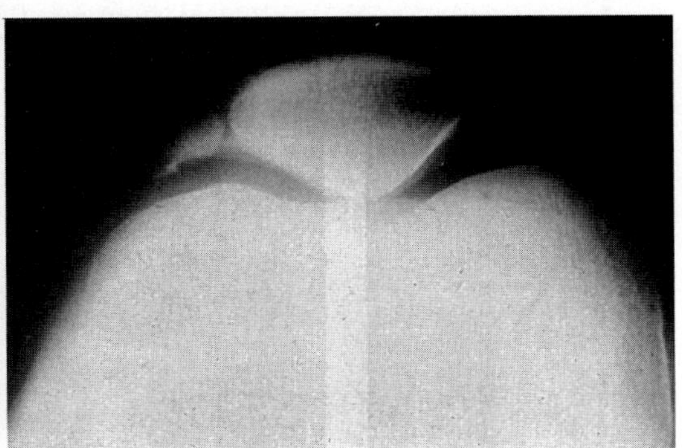

FIGURE 23-25. Bipartite patella is demonstrated on anteroposterior **(A)** and Merchant **(B)** views of the knee. A well-corticated, separate fragment forms the superolateral pole of the patella.

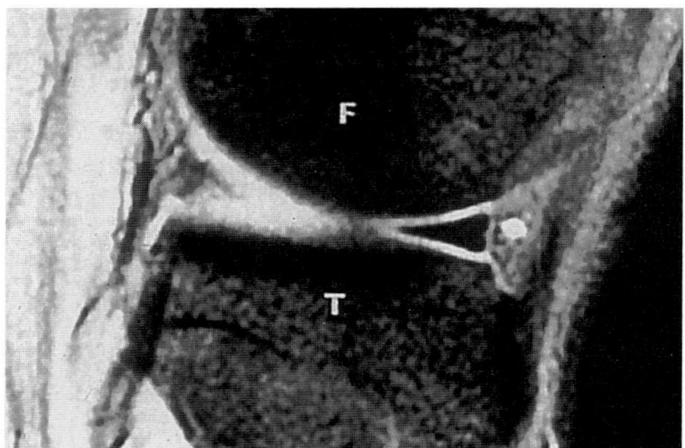

FIGURE 23-26. Magnetic resonance imaging of normal meniscus is illustrated on T2-weighted view.

Most patients with meniscal tears will have full motion and present days to weeks after the initiating event with a history of painful locking, catching, or giving way, especially with twisting movements, which reflects the torn meniscal fragment being mechanically caught between the condyles. It is this mechanical impingement that causes abrasion and arthritic changes of the articular surfaces. Therefore, arthroscopic debridement or repair of the tear is usually recommended, even if symptoms at present may be minimal.

The physical examination reflects tenderness to palpation along the joint line overlying the tear. Provocative maneuvers to recreate impingement of the torn fragment are helpful in confirming the diagnosis. These include the Steinmann test, McMurray test, or Apley test. Localization of a palpable click and associated pain is helpful but not specific. Loose bodies and impinging synovial soft tissue should be entertained in the difficult

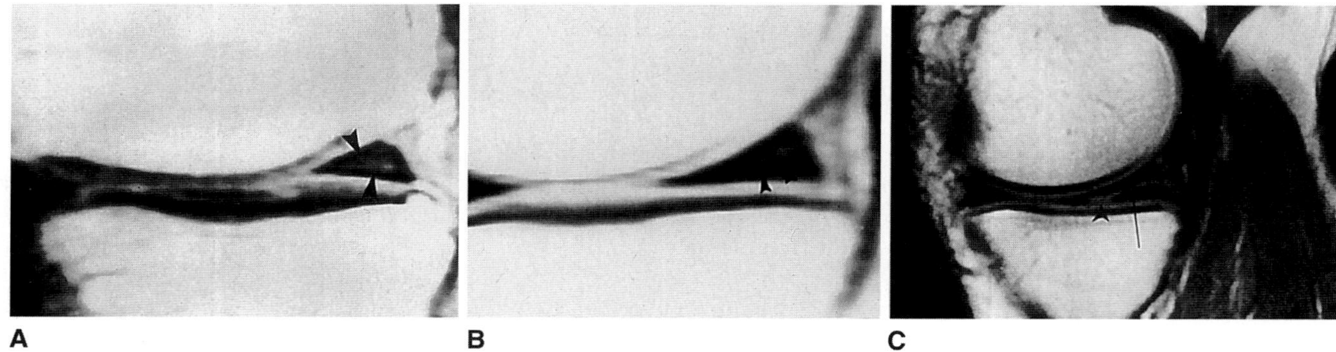

FIGURE 23-27. Magnetic resonance imaging of meniscal tears. **A,** Grade I degeneration is seen as a small area of signal change within the substance of the meniscus. **B,** Grade II degeneration represents signal change that extends up to but not through the meniscal surface. **C,** Grade III tears are complete, extending through the meniscal surface.

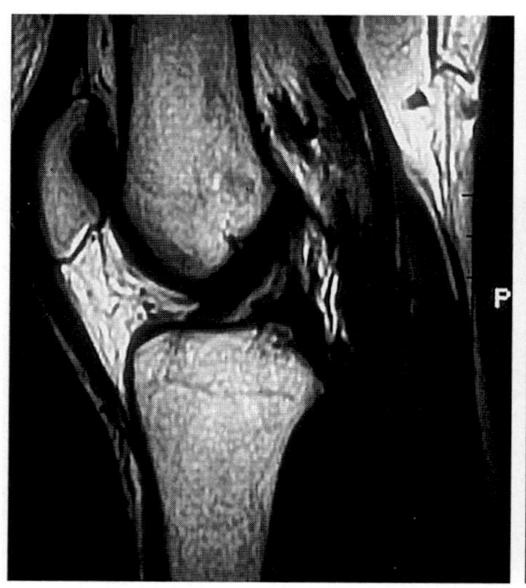

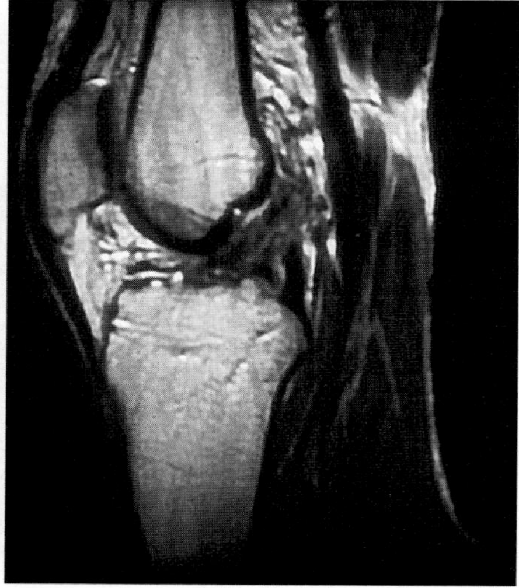

FIGURE 23-28. Magnetic resonance imaging of a healthy anterior cruciate ligament **(A),** and a completely torn anterior cruciate ligament **(B)**.

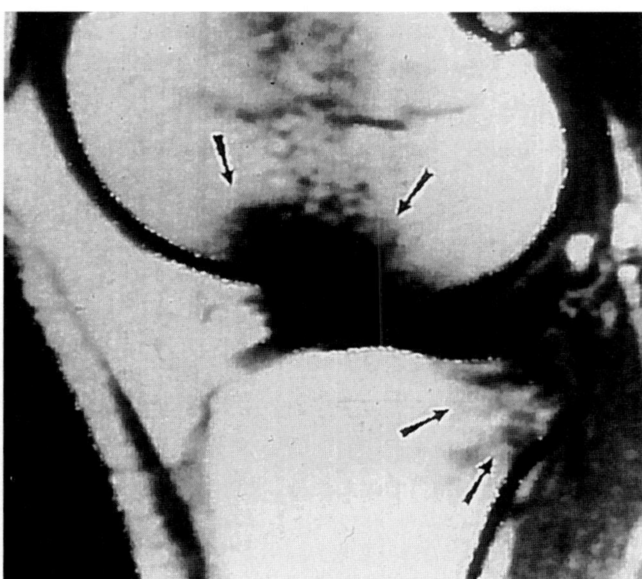

FIGURE 23-29. Magnetic resonance imaging of the knee demonstrating the contrasting dark signal characteristic of a bone bruise in the lateral femoral condyle adjacent to the articular surface and extending proximally into the cancellous bone. Corresponding lesion can be seen in the posterolateral tibia.

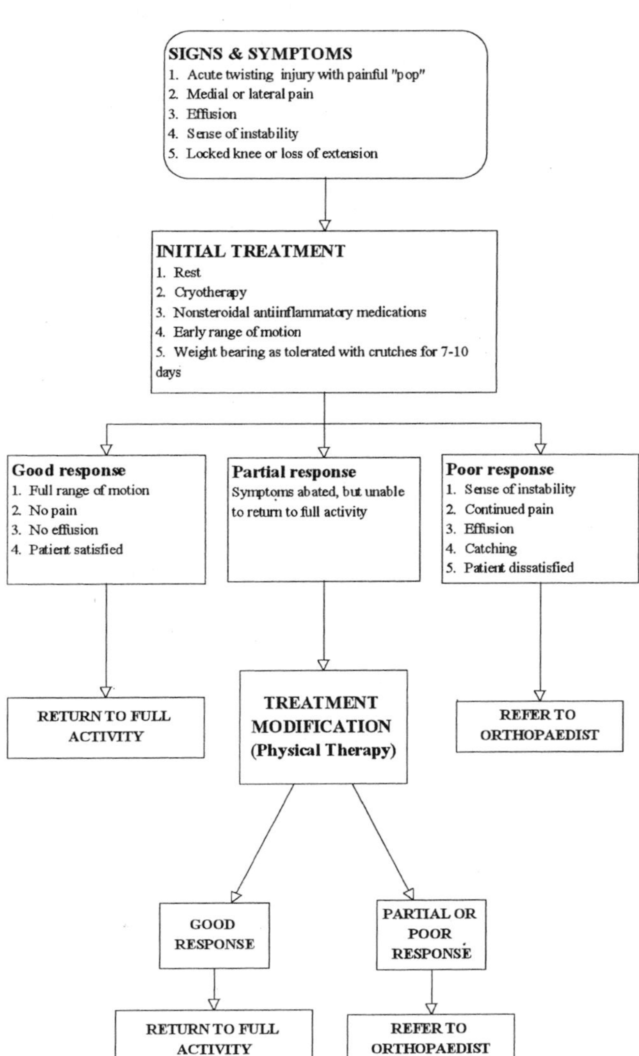

Meniscal Injury
SIGNS & SYMPTOMS
1. Acute twisting injury with painful "pop"
2. Medial or lateral pain
3. Effusion
4. Sense of instability
5. Locked knee or loss of extension
INITIAL TREATMENT
1. Rest
2. Cryotherapy
3. Nonsteroidal antiinflammatory medications
4. Early range of motion
5. Weight bearing as tolerated with crutches for 7-10 days
Good response
1. Full range of motion
2. No pain
3. No effusion
4. Patient satisfied
Partial response
Symptoms abated, but unable to return to full activity
Poor response
1. Sense of instability
2. Continued pain
3. Effusion
4. Catching
5. Patient dissatisfied
RETURN TO FULL ACTIVITY
TREATMENT MODIFICATION (Physical Therapy)
REFER TO ORTHOPAEDIST
GOOD RESPONSE
PARTIAL OR POOR RESPONSE
RETURN TO FULL ACTIVITY
REFER TO ORTHOPAEDIST

FIGURE 23-30. Suspected meniscal tear algorithm. (Adapted from the AAOS National Orthopedic Leadership Conference 1995.)

diagnosis because they can give false positive results. As previously stated, MRI evaluation is more than 90% accurate in diagnosing meniscal pathology (see Fig. 23-27). One should, however, interpret the MRI findings in the context of the history and examination because an MRI often identifies grade 1 or 2 changes in asymptomatic individuals who do not require intervention.[48,69] Clinically asymptomatic discoid menisci represent a congenital anomaly that may not require intervention in the absence of a tear.

A treatment algorithm for suspected meniscal pathology is presented in Figure 23-30. Initial history and physical examination is usually accompanied by plain radiographs to exclude bony pathology, such as osteochondritis dissecans or a loose osteochondral fragment. If the examination suggests associated ligamentous instability, early referral to an orthopedist is appropriate. Otherwise, initial treatment with ice, a brief period of rest, and a short course of nonsteroidal anti-inflammatory drugs (NSAIDs) is indicated. Failure to respond to nonoperative therapy or repeated episodes of catching or giving way suggests a meniscal tear, which should be referred to an orthopedic surgeon. These types of meniscal lesions are successfully managed with arthroscopic surgery. Most tears require debridement to a stable rim. Tears in the peripheral one third or red zone potentially have an adequate blood supply to attempt meniscal repair. Degenerative type patterns, radial tears, horizontal cleavage tears, or tears more than 4 cm in length generally do not heal and are usually addressed by a partial menisectomy. Performing a meniscal repair in conjunction with a cruciate reconstruction has been shown to enhance healing, possibly because of the beneficial healing properties of the bloody, postoperative effusion and subsequent clot. Meniscal repairs in the face of an unstable knee usually fail and are not recommended. The underlying theme in addressing meniscal pathology at arthroscopy is to retain as much of the meniscus as possible to help prevent future arthritic changes.

After arthroscopic surgery, patients should aggressively rehabilitate the knee to restore motion and strength. Most patients are able to restore quadriceps strength with a cycling program and progressive, resistive exercises with light weights.[11] Other patients who lack individual motivation may benefit from a supervised physical therapy program. Return to sports depends on restoration of full range of motion and equal strength, usually obtained in 3 to 6 weeks. Office work can be resumed immediately as pain permits.

LIGAMENTOUS INJURIES

Collateral Ligament Injuries

Collateral ligament injuries often result from a direct injury. A medially directed force against the lateral side of the knee, as occurs from a clip or tackle in football, creates a valgus-deforming force that injures the medial structures. If no rotational component is involved, an isolated MCL injury may occur. Additional rotational force is more likely to result in an associated meniscal tear and ACL injury. Likewise, a laterally directed force against the medial side of the knee can result in injury to the LCL and supporting lateral structures. Injury to the LCL is less common than injury to the medial side. Noncontact injuries can also result from deceleration or pivot mechanisms. The addition of rotational forces to the noncontact mechanism results in an increased incidence of ACL injuries.

Varus and valgus stress testing is performed at 30° of flexion, full extension or 0°, and hyperextension. Laxity only in flexion suggests isolated collateral ligament injury, whereas laxity at full extension suggests additional injury to the posteromedial or posterolateral capsule. Laxity in hyperextension may imply injury to the posterior oblique ligament medially or the arcuate ligamentous complex laterally and possibly injury to the PCL or ACL, depending on the magnitude of force. Laxity to varus or valgus stress should be compared with the opposite, noninvolved knee. In less severe injuries, laxity may not be present, but the patient will report pain on stress of the involved collateral ligament.

Patients usually localize pain well to either side of the knee, although, if an associated cruciate ligament injury is present, these intraarticular symptoms will dominate the examination. With significantly lax knees, the patient may complain of giving way and a sense of instability. Swelling, if present, may be localized to one side of the knee. Tenderness along the course of the collateral ligament or at the femoral origin or tibial insertion is a helpful finding.

Plain radiographs are helpful to rule out osseous abnormalities, including avulsion fractures or growth plate injuries that often mimic collateral injuries in skeletally immature patients. Chronic MCL injuries can demonstrate calcification along the course of the ligament (Pellegrini-Stieda sign). Stress films can be helpful if a physeal fracture is suspected. Otherwise, MRI is best to delineate collateral ligament injuries and any associated pathology. The normal low signal ligament is interrupted by the high signal of edema and hemorrhage (Fig. 23-31).

Collateral ligament injuries, like all ligament sprains, are graded as first degree if microscopic disruption of collagen fibers is present without gross elongation or any clinically detectable laxity.[76] Pain on stress testing and local tenderness and swelling are the dominant findings. Management consists of ice and rest as needed, with early range of motion exercises (Fig. 23-32). Bracing is generally not needed unless used purely for increased patient comfort during the first several days. An off-the-shelf knee immobilizer is adequate. It is important to encourage motion to prevent the rapid onset of stiffness that can occur with a brace. A neoprene knee sleeve that permits full motion gives patients a feeling of support and is preferred. Return to sports is usually within 6 to 8 weeks of injury.

A second-degree sprain represents macroscopic, partial tearing of the ligament with clinically detectable elongation of 0.5 to 1 cm on stress testing. Pain with

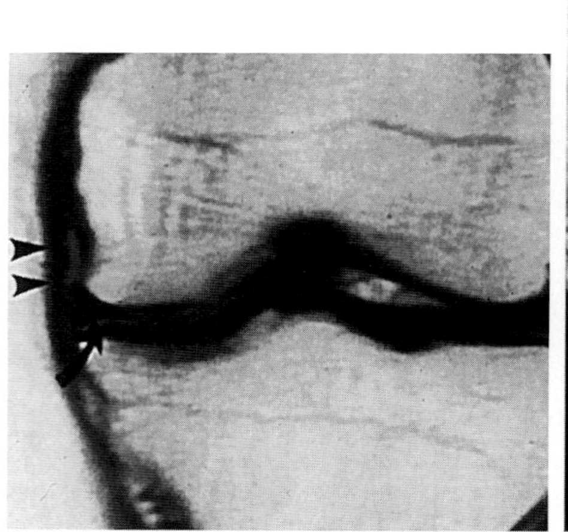
A

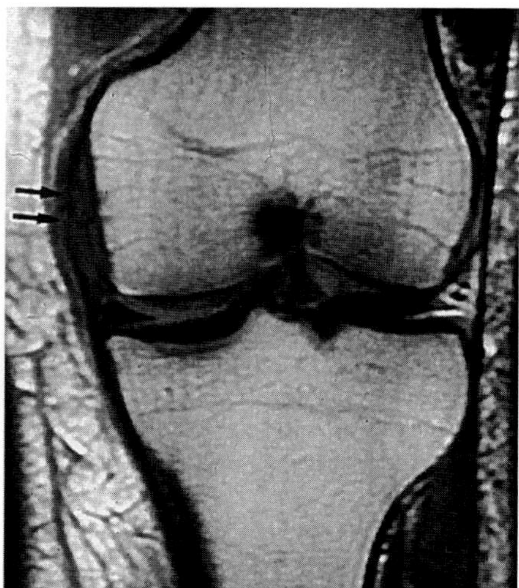
B

FIGURE 23-31. Magnetic resonance imaging of intact **(A)** and torn **(B)** medial collateral ligament (arrows).

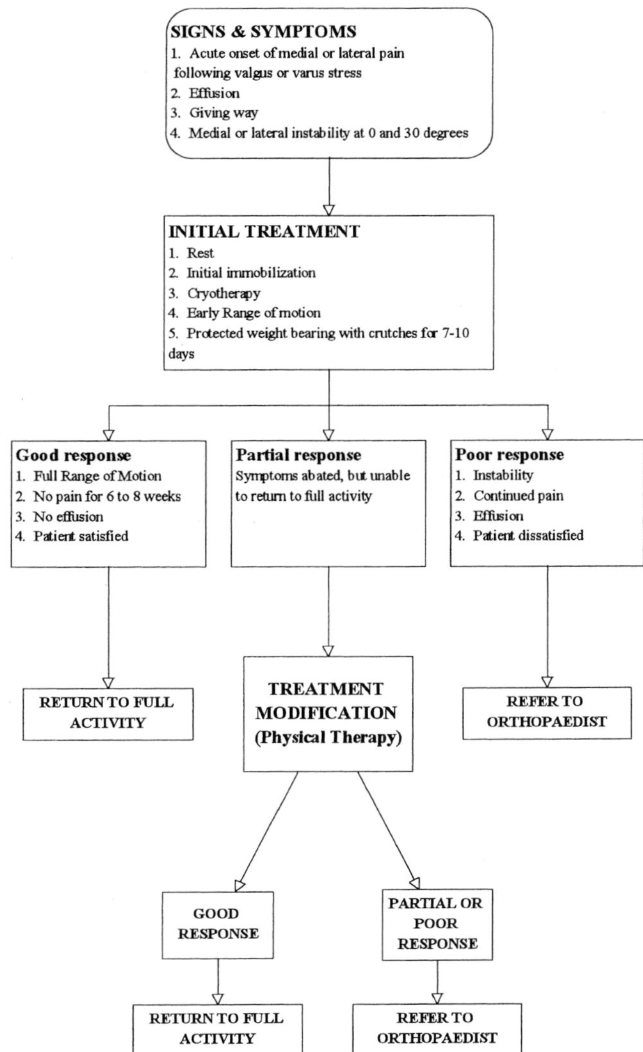

FIGURE 23-32. Treatment algorithm for collateral ligament injuries. (Adapted from the AAOS National Orthopedic Leadership Conference 1995.)

stress testing, local tenderness, and swelling are more pronounced. Grade II collateral injuries can also be managed symptomatically with brace immobilization only temporarily (less than 5 days) as needed for patient comfort. Thereafter, a hinged knee brace permitting motion is recommended only if the patient has significant pain. Cane or crutch support for the first week may facilitate ambulation. Cryotherapy and a short course of NSAIDs may be helpful as the patient works to achieve a full range of motion. Once motion has been obtained, isometric, isotonic, and eventually isokinetic progressive resistive exercises are performed for quadriceps strengthening under physical therapist supervision. Once equal strength is achieved and pain is absent to stress test or palpation, the athlete may return to competitive sports, usually 6 to 8 weeks after injury. Vague, nagging pain can sometimes persist for 3 to 6 months.

A third-degree collateral ligament sprain is a complete disruption with more than 1 cm of joint line opening on stress examination. Pain on stress testing may be disproportionately low because no fibers are actually being stressed in a completely torn ligament. Tenderness along the ligament is significant, and a large effusion is also present, resulting from the associated capsular disruption. A high level of suspicion should be maintained for concomitant ACL injury.

Management is an initial period of immobilization followed by early motion protected by a hinged knee brace. Physical therapy for motion and strengthening is recommended. Full return to activities generally occurs 2 to 3 months after injury, when the patient achieves 90% strength of the opposite side and can perform an agility program similar to that required in the athlete's sport. Patient comfort and athletic performance are better indicators of readiness to return to sport than a specified time period.[38] A small amount of residual laxity is common and does not appear to be a functional problem. Patients may wear the hinged knee brace up to 6 months during return to activites, and pain with activities even with the brace frequently persists for that length of time.

Previous recommendations for operative management of grade III collateral ligament tears are less popular, and nonoperative management appears to provide comparable results in terms of stability without surgical morbidity and with an earlier return to sports participation.[39] Current recommendations for combined injuries of the ACL and MCL are to manage the MCL injury nonoperatively.[79] A delay of 4 to 8 weeks allows the initial inflammatory phase of healing to subside and full motion to be restored. This delays allows adequate and predictable healing of the MCL with less risk of stiffness after ACL reconstruction than if both ligaments were reconstructed. All grade II and grade III collateral ligament tears should be referred to an orthopedist because there is a very high incidence of associated knee pathology with collateral ligament injuries.

Anterior Cruciate Ligament Injuries

ACL tears are becoming increasingly common, with an incidence of 250,000 cases per year in the United States.[42] Women experience up to a sevenfold increase in ACL tears compared with men in competitive sports.[97] This increase perhaps results from anatomic variations of a tighter intercondylar notch, which theoretically could shear the ligament.[70] Women also tend to be more ligamentously lax, which may put the knee at increased risk for injury. As surgical techniques improve and become more predictable, the management of ACL injuries has shifted toward early surgical reconstruction.

Understanding of the natural history of the ACL-deficient knee has also influenced decision making.

The ACL is often torn during running sports when the foot is planted and the knee twists when changing directions. Alternatively, the ACL can be torn by contact to the lateral knee with a valgus, external rotation force; by hyperextension; or rarely by varus, internal rotation force. Classically, the athlete feels a "pop" in the knee, is unable to continue to participate, feels the knee is unsteady, and complains of significant pain. The swelling, secondary to an intraarticular effusion, usually occurs quickly over a few hours. Aspiration is generally reserved for large, tense effusions to provide pain relief. The finding of a hemarthrosis is very helpful, but somewhat nonspecific, and could be found for an osteochondral fracture, a patellar dislocation, a peripheral meniscal tear, or an intraarticular fracture.

The examination of an acute ACL tear is most productive immediately after the injury on the field or court before the onset of swelling. Otherwise, the subsequent pain and swelling obscure a clear examination and make diagnosis more difficult. Examination techniques include a Lachman test at 30° and, if the patient's pain and range of motion permit, an anterior drawer test at 90° to assess anterior translation of the tibia with respect to the femur. A pivot shift maneuver (or one of its variations) is diagnostic if present. The findings are compared with the contralateral normal knee, because laxity may represent a normal, physiologic variant. Careful attention should also be directed to any possible associated collateral ligament injuries or meniscal tears. Meniscal tears in association with an acute ACL and MCL injury occur more often on the lateral side than on the medial side (Fig. 23-33). Additionally, grade II MCL injuries result in a higher incidence of meniscal tears (71%) than seen with grade III MCL injuries (51%),[79] which may result from a distractive mechanism of injury associated with grade III MCL tears as opposed to a compressive mechanism for grade II MCL tears.

Although standard radiographs are of limited value in diagnosing a torn ACL, they provide useful information and should be performed routinely. It would not be unusual to note an avulsion of the tibial spine, a Segond fracture, or an intraarticular fracture.[73] MRI is the imaging modality of choice to supplement the physical examination and to provide supportive information about related structures (Fig. 23-34). Because partial tears of the ACL are very difficult to assess on clinical examination and by MRI, arthroscopic visualization remains the gold standard for diagnosis.

Although no study has shown conclusively that ACL tears directly lead to arthritis, a number of studies confirm that ACL-deficient knees progress to further meniscal and articular surface injuries. Finsterbush et al.[27] showed a 33% incidence of additional intraarticular injuries over 28 months after an isolated ACL tear. Irvine and Glasgow[41] showed an 86% incidence of meniscal tears at an average of 3 years after injury. Other studies have shown that the variable that best correlates

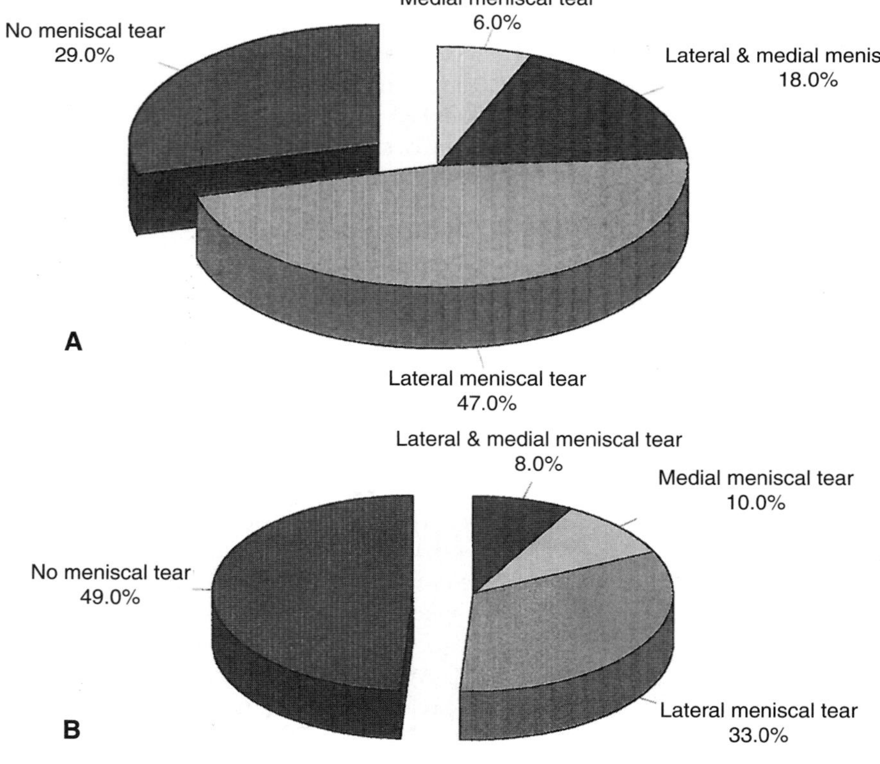

FIGURE 23-33. A, Distribution of meniscal tears in patients with an acute tear of anterior cruciate ligament and an associated grade II sprain of the medial collateral ligament. **B,** Distribution of meniscal tears in patients with an acute injury of the anterior cruciate ligament and an associated grade III sprain of the medial collateral ligament. (From Shelbourne KD, Patel DK: Management of combined injuries of the anterior cruciate ligament and medial collateral ligament. J Bone Joint Surg 77A:800, 1995.)

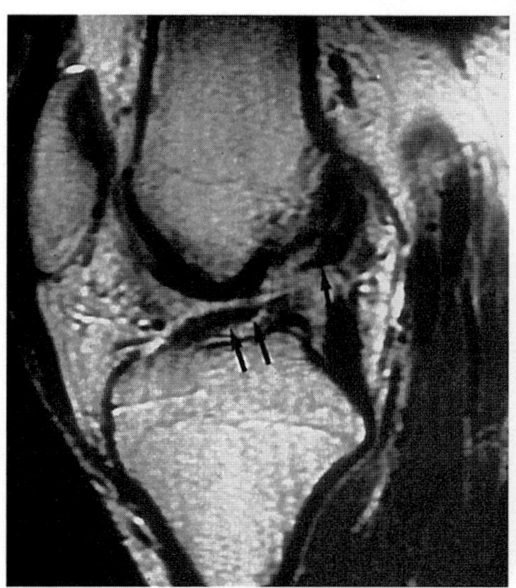
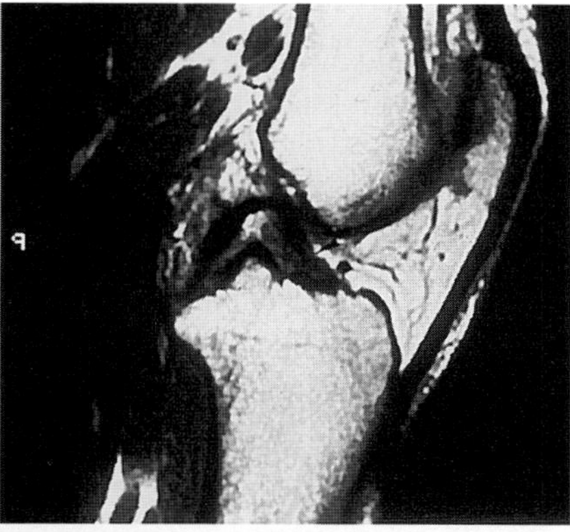
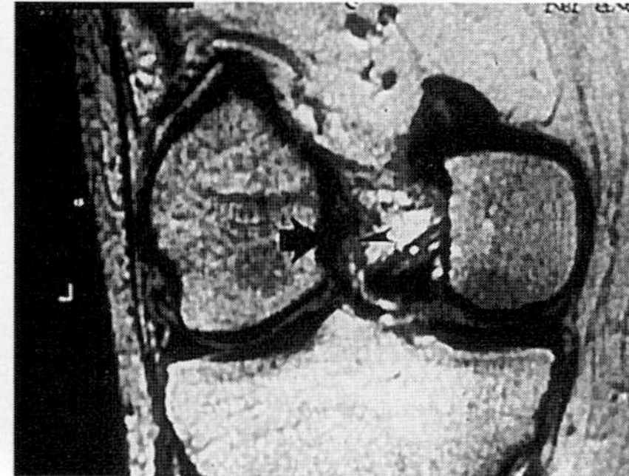

FIGURE 23-34. A, Magnetic resonance imaging of complete anterior cruciate ligament tear demonstrates bright edema signal within the ligament fibers and poor visualization of fiber continuity. **B,** Partial tear on magnetic resonance imaging is seen as interposed edema with fiber continuity.

with arthritic changes and pain in an ACL-injured knee is meniscal injury.[58,94] Therefore, reconstructing the ACL to help preserve the menisci theoretically should help prevent arthritic changes. Unfortunately, no prospective, randomized, blinded study has successfully proven that reconstruction of the torn ACL will prevent arthritis. However, there is general agreement in the orthopedic community that young persons should have ACL reconstructions to minimize future knee injury and to maintain the level of activities. "Young" is a relative term and level of activity may be more important as a person ages. In general, the physician can advise an athlete that if he or she is willing to discontinue sports that involve running, jumping, or pivoting activities, he or she may be content without a reconstruction. Episodes of giving way with activities of daily living would be a strong indication for reconstruction, regardless of a person's athletic activities. Giving way episodes with whatever sports activities a person chooses is another indication to reconstruct the ACL to prevent further knee injury. If a person wants to remain more active than walking-, biking-, and swimming-type activities, a reconstruction is warranted, even if that person is somewhat older (i.e., aged 40 to 50 years). An excellent natural history and outcome study by Daniel[22] showed that the best predictors of a late reconstruction for an ACL tear were preinjury hours more than 200 per year of sports requiring cutting, jumping, pivoting, and a significant degree of laxity compared with the opposite knee by KT-1000 arthrometer measurement. A KT-1000 measurement on the manual maximum test that is 3 mm different than the opposite, uninvolved side is considered abnormal.[20] A side-to-side difference more than 7 mm puts the athlete at a high risk for needing late reconstruction because of repeated giving way episodes. This information is summarized in Table 23-1.[21,22] Level I sports include basketball, football, and soccer and involve jumping, pivoting, and hard cutting. Level II sports include baseball, racket sports, and skiing and involve less jumping or hard cutting.

Current reconstruction techniques use the arthroscopic approach. These endoscopic techniques implant a ligament substitute in the normal femoral and tibial attachment sites of the ACL. The graft choices for ligament substitution include the central one-third bone–patella tendon–bone autograft or allograft, autograft

TABLE 23-1 Surgical Risk Factors

Maximum Difference (mm) Side-to-Side Level I or II Sports	Sports Hours per year		
	<50 hr	50–199 hr	>200 hr
<5	Low	Low	Moderate
5–7	Low	Moderate	High
>7	Moderate	High	High

hamstring tendons, allograft Achilles tendon, or artificial ligament substitutes. Allograft tendons are most useful for revision situations or in older individuals whose patella tendon may be relatively weak because of age-related degenerative changes. If an allograft is chosen, the patient needs to be counseled regarding disease transmission. Artificial ligament substitutes have shown failure rates in excess of 50% and are not recommended.[43,97] Today's gold standard is the central third bone–patella tendon–bone autograft. With this endoscopic technique, aside from the arthroscopic portals, the only incision necessary is an approximately 6-cm anterior incision used to harvest the bone–patella tendon–bone graft (Fig. 23-35). Arthroscopically positioned guides enable the surgeon to prepare the femoral and tibial tunnels, which are necessary to pass and secure the graft. In this manner, the graft is positioned in the knee along the course of the native ACL (Fig. 23-36).[43] Various options for rigid graft fixation allow immediate motion and weight bearing for rapid rehabilitation.[50] After an initial period of exercises to restore motion, therapy focuses on strengthening and eventually proprioceptive, agility, and sports-specific activities. In general, rehabilitation programs have become increasingly aggressive, with most

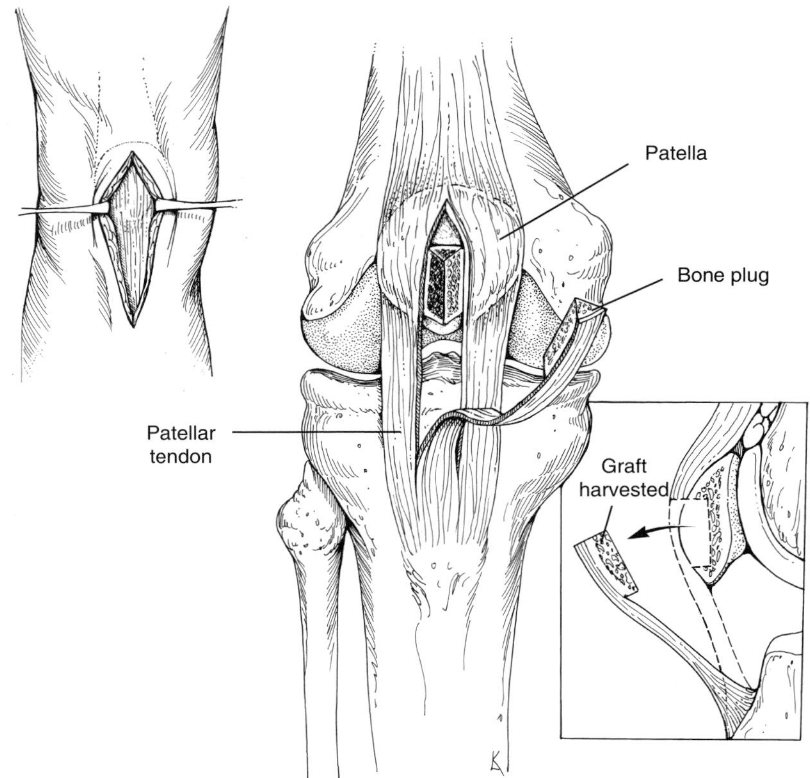

A

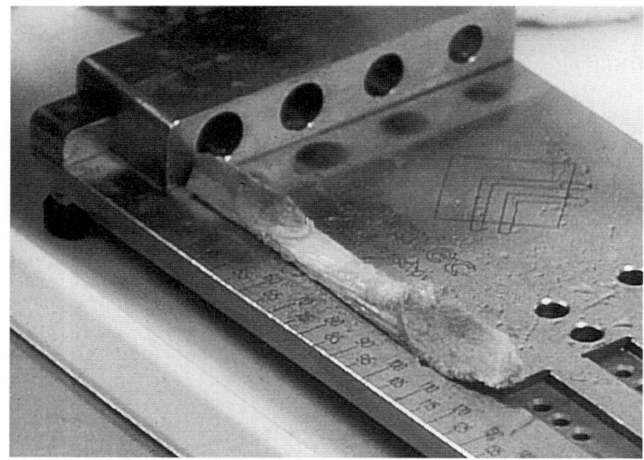
B

FIGURE 23-35. Patella tendon autograft for anterior cruciate ligament reconstruction. **A,** The middle third of the patella tendon is harvested with attached bone plugs from the patella and tibial ends. **B,** Photograph of the patella tendon autograft.

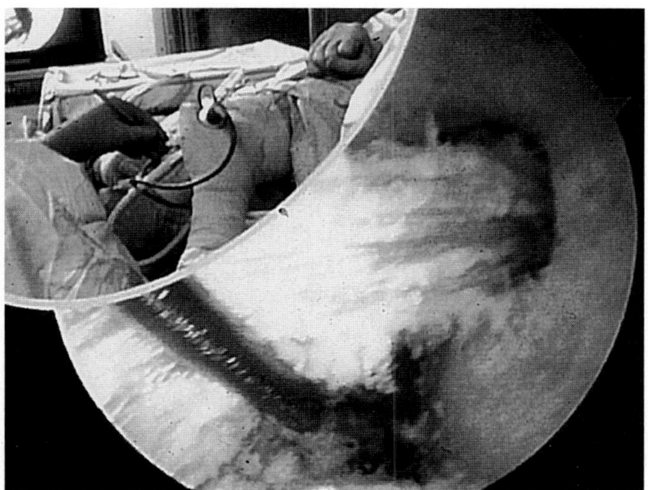

FIGURE 23-36. The bone–patella tendon–bone autograft is passed through tunnels drilled with arthroscopic guides to reproduce the orientation of the native anterior cruciate ligament. Fixation of the bone plugs is achieved with interference fit screws within the tunnel or screw and suture combinations.

athletes now returning to sports by 6 to 8 months after surgery.

Nonoperative management of an ACL tear involves physical therapy for restoration of motion and strengthening. Quadriceps muscle conditioning should ideally be a life-long endeavor. Most athletes can return to sports without surgery by 6 weeks, assuming they have achieved 90% of the strength of the uninvolved knee. The use of a brace provides largely subjective benefit and is controversial, but most athletes seem to prefer their use. The proposed mechanisms by which a brace works include mechanical constraint of joint motion, although this has been documented only at low loads and has not been shown to be effective at the high loads involved with sports. Also, a brace provides a proprioceptive feedback mechanism, serving as a "reminder" to the athlete to avoid positions that may result in a giving way episode.[49,50] If an athlete suffers giving way episodes with sports, one can assume that this places the knee at significant risk for further meniscal and articular cartilage injury, and one should recommend reconstruction.

Any meniscal tear initially present may be repairable, and every attempt should be made to preserve the meniscus. Healing rates are improved from roughly 50% to 93% when performed in conjunction with an ACL reconstruction.[14] This increased rate of healing results from restoration of the normal knee biomechanics, the beneficial healing effects of a postoperative hemarthrosis, including the associated fibrin clot and growth factors, and the lack of degeneration in the meniscus before acute injury.[7,15] Healing rates of meniscal repair in the ACL-deficient knee in the absence of cruciate reconstruction fall off to approximately 30%.[93]

An important component in the nonoperative management of the ACL-deficient knee is counseling the athlete for activity modification. Avoiding activities involving jumping, twisting, pivoting, or cutting is generally necessary for nonoperative management to succeed. If an athlete is not willing to make these modifications, reconstruction should be recommended. This approach to ACL tear management is summarized in the algorithm in Figure 23-37.

Partial tears of the ACL occur in 10% to 28% of all ligament injuries and can be confusing for prognosis and management considerations.[59,92] The amount of ligament torn cannot be accurately assessed by MRI, and arthroscopic visualization and probing can also be misleading and subjective. Progression of a partial tear to a functionally complete ligament tear occurs 38% to 56% of

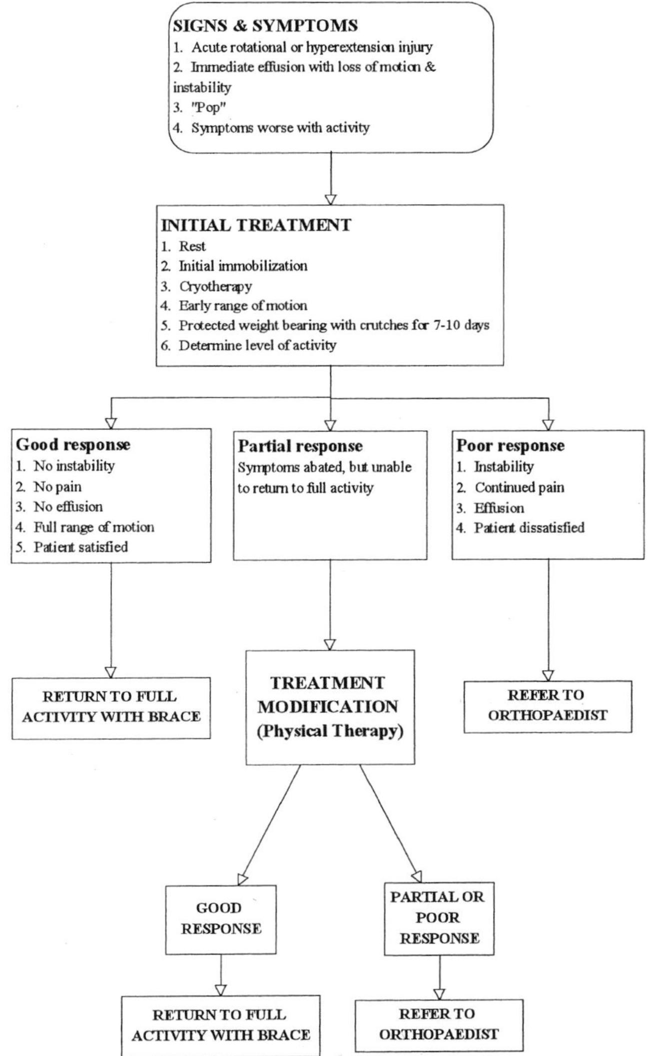

FIGURE 23-37. Anterior cruciate ligament tear treatment algorithm.

the time, with ligaments 25% torn rarely progressing, 50% torn progressing 50% of the time, and 75% torn progressing 86% of the time.[51,60] Current recommendations involve the same lifestyle modifications used for decision making for a complete tear and any history or examination evidence of recurrent instability. If an athlete reports no giving way episodes during activities, has a stable examination, and has less than 50% of the ligament torn at arthroscopy, nonoperative treatment is chosen. However, if the patient has laxity on examination or by history, reconstruction is warranted because the partial tear is functionally a complete tear.[43]

Posterior Cruciate Ligament (PCL) Injuries

PCL injuries occur less often than ACL tears, with an incidence of 3% to 20% of all knee ligament injuries.[18,19] Often these injuries go undetected, as demonstrated by a 2% incidence in asymptomatic collegiate football players.[65] With the advent of MRI, an increasing number of these injuries are being recognized earlier.

The mechanism of injury usually involves a posteriorly directed force against the proximal tibia while the knee is flexed. A fall directly on the knee with the foot plantar flexed causes such posterior displacement. Another common etiology is striking the dashboard against the knee in a motor vehicle accident. PCL injuries have been documented to occur in 44% of major trauma patients with acute hemarthroses.[24] Hyperflexion, possibly with internal rotation, can also cause an isolated PCL tear.[84] Other mechanisms usually involve injury to other ligamentous structures, including extreme varus or valgus injury with combined collateral ligament tears and hyperextension with associated ACL tear.[19,44] One should be suspicious of a knee dislocation if multiple ligaments are injured or if the mechanism involves hyperextension. Any suspicion of a knee dislocation demands immediate orthopedic and vascular evaluation.

The posterior drawer test performed at 90° of flexion is the most helpful test in the physical examination to determine the status of the PCL.[77,90] Normally, the anterior surface of the tibial condyles rests approximately 10 mm anterior to the anterior surface of the femoral condyles, providing a useful reference for displacement with a posterior force. Displacement up to 5 mm is a grade I injury, with the tibial condyles remaining anterior to the femoral condyles. When the tibia and femur are flush, this implies posterior translation of 5 to 10 mm, consistent with a grade II injury. Displacement of the anterior surface of the tibia further posteriorly (more than 10 mm) than the anterior surface of the femoral condyles implies a grade III injury.[90] A posterior sag sign and a positive quadriceps active test are other useful tests for confirming the diagnosis. The posterior Lachman test is somewhat more difficult to use because the proper starting point can be difficult to determine, sometimes giving the false impression of anterior laxity if the posteriorly subluxed starting point is not appreciated. Assessment of the quality of the endpoint to stress and looking for a posterior sag can help avoid this confusion, as can comparison with the healthy knee. Additionally, the KT-2000 arthrometer is very useful to quantitate the degree of posterior laxity and for management decision making similar to the ACL-deficient knee (Fig. 23-38).

An important determination in selecting management options involves the assessment of associated injuries, including the posterolateral corner. Comparing external rotation, posterior translation, and varus laxity with the contralateral knee is useful in assessing injury to the posterolateral corner. Increased external rotation, varus angulation, and posterior translation at 30° and 90° suggests injury to the PCL and the posterolateral corner. However, when the increased rotation, laxity, and translation at 30° decreases at 90° of flexion, the examiner should suspect an isolated injury to the posterolateral corner.[32] Alternatively, injury to the posterolateral corner can be diagnosed by increased passive external rotation of the tibia relative to the femur with the patient prone on the examining table.[19]

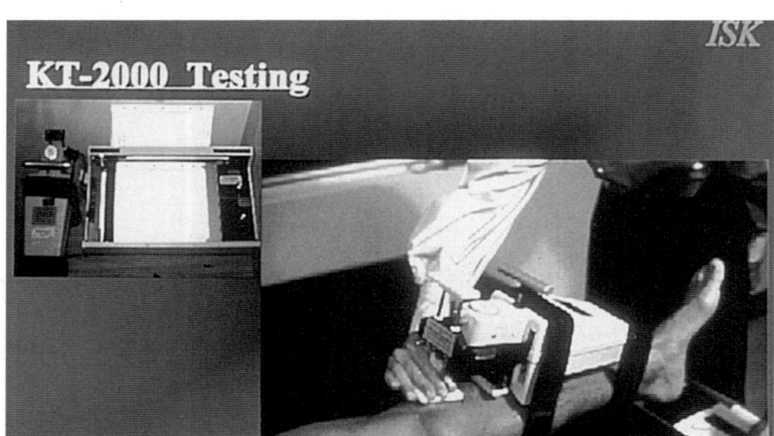

FIGURE 23-38. KT-2000 arthrometer.

Plain radiographs are helpful to look for bony avulsions, which occur in greater frequency in PCL injuries than in ACL injuries. In the chronic PCL-deficient knee, radiographs should be obtained in the standing, weight-bearing mode if possible to assess any degenerative changes that will affect management choices. An additional anteroposterior weight-bearing view with the knee in 45° of flexion often better demonstrates degenerative changes (Fig. 23-39). These degenerative, unstable knees often are in varus alignment and best evaluated on long-length standing films. MRI is the most reliable imaging study to confirm injury to the PCL (Fig. 23-40). The accuracy rate for visualizing a PCL injury is the best of all intraarticular structures and has been shown to be 98% to 100%.[28,35] Because of the posterior orientation of the PCL and its inferior attachment site on the tibial plateau, arthroscopy can yield false negative results without additional posteromedial portal visualization.[25]

Knowledgeable management recommendations for PCL injuries depend on an understanding of the natural history of this injury. Parolie and Bergfeld[65] emphasized quadriceps rehabilitation until strength was equal to the opposite side. With nonoperative treatment, these authors noted that 84% of their athletes had returned to sports and were able to continue to participate for an average of 6.2 years, although only 68% performed at their previous levels.[65] The influence of combined ligamentous injuries has been previously reported, as these patients had significantly worse functional results than those with isolated PCL injuries.[85] Other authors have demonstrated progressive degenerative changes with chronic pain. Clancy[16,17] has confirmed the progression of arthritic changes in the PCL-deficient knee, as substantiated by radiographic evaluation, nuclear imaging, and arthroscopy. Degenerative changes were also confirmed by Keller,[45] who noted a 65% incidence of arthritic changes and a 90% incidence of pain at 6 years. Based on these observations, the nonoperative management of PCL injuries is currently undergoing scrutiny; however, no good prospective study documents that reconstruction prevents arthritic changes.

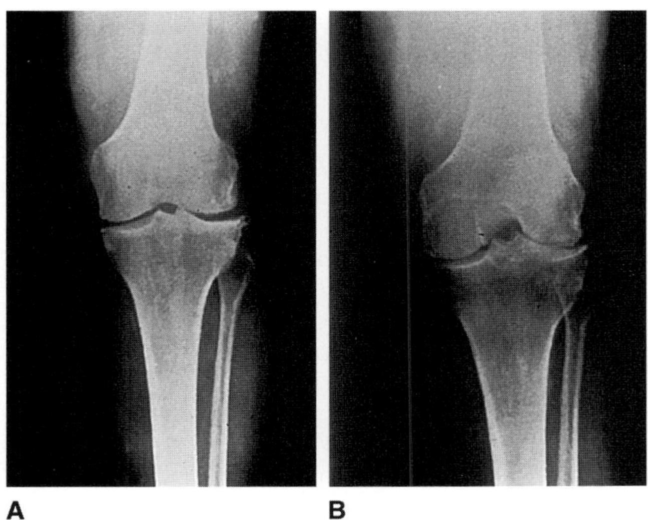

A **B**

FIGURE 23-39. Standing anteroposterior radiograph of the knee **(A)** shows moderate joint space narrowing that is much more evident on the standing, flexed posteroanterior view **(B)**.

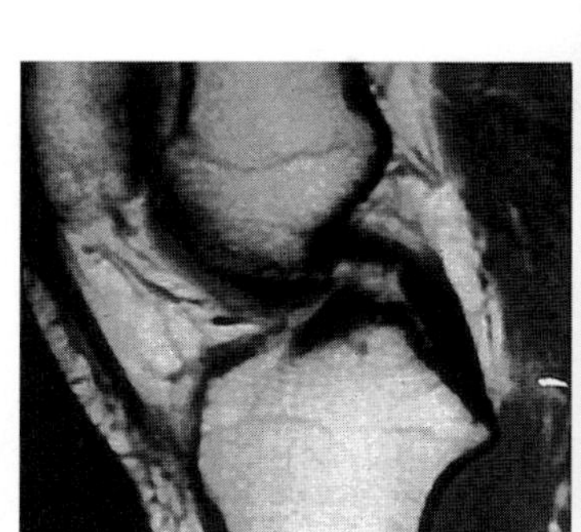

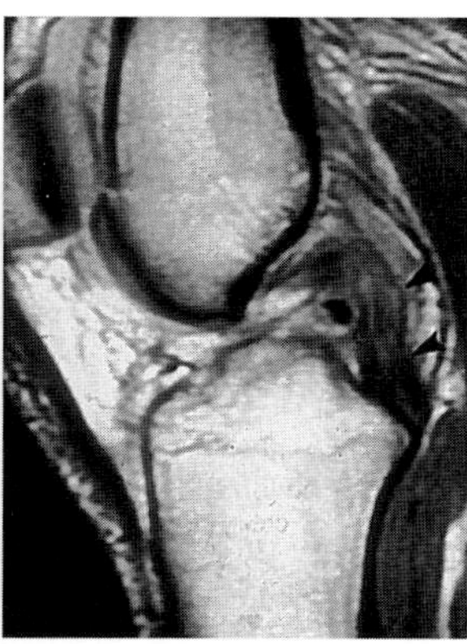

A **B**

FIGURE 23-40. Magnetic resonance imaging of healthy **(A)** and torn **(B)** posterior cruciate ligament. The ligament signal is interrupted by edema with nonhomogeneous fiber appearance.

Current consensus is to manage acute, isolated PCL tears with less than 10 mm of posterior translation on posterior drawer nonoperatively,[25,77,90] which involves quadriceps rehabilitation using closed kinetic-chain exercises, such as squats and leg presses. Open kinetic-chain extension exercises (e.g., seated knee extensions with weights) are to be avoided because of increased pressure on the patellofemoral joint, a common source of pain in the PCL-deficient knee resulting from increased posterior tibial translation.[90] The athlete may return to sports after achieving at least 90% of equal strength, usually within 3 to 4 weeks. Any associated meniscal or chondral injury warrants arthroscopic management if symptomatic. Acute PCL injuries combined with other ligament injuries or if associated with more than 10 mm of posterior translation should be considered for surgical reconstruction. Reconstruction of associated posterolateral, collateral, and ACL injuries is generally recommended. This approach to PCL injuries is summarized in the algorithm from Veltri and Warren (Fig. 23-41).[90]

Chronic PCL tears focus on the presence or absence of associated posterolateral instability and whether posterior translation is more than 10 mm. An initial trial of quadriceps rehabilitation is attempted to improve symptoms, but if unsuccessful, a reconstruction of the PCL is warranted. This assumes that significant radiographic degenerative changes and varus malalignment are not present, in which case a valgus high tibial osteotomy may be indicated. Management of the chronic PCL-deficient knee is summarized in an algorithm in Figure 23-42.[90]

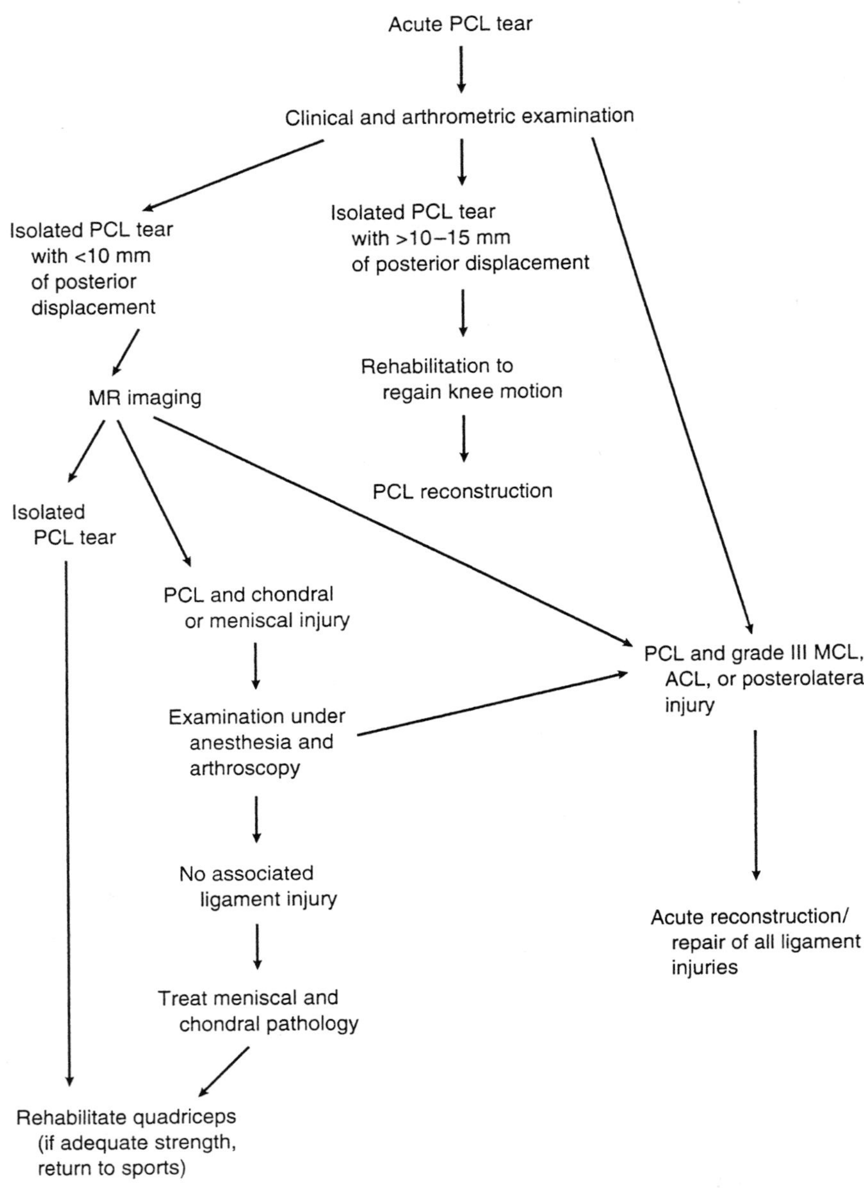

FIGURE 23-41. Acute posterior cruciate ligament tear algorithm. (From Veltri DM, Warren RF: Posterior cruciate ligament injuries. J Am Acad Orthop Surg 1:73, 1993.)

PCL reconstruction is technically more demanding than ACL surgery, primarily because of the posterior location of the PCL and proximity to neurovascular structures. The principles are similar, with arthroscopic-assisted placement of tunnels in the tibia and femur to pass a graft in the position of the native PCL. Because of the longer overall length needed for the graft and common patellofemoral complaints with a chronically posteriorly subluxed knee, many surgeons are using alternatives to the central third–patella tendon autograft. Popular choices include Achilles tendon or patella tendon allograft or, less commonly, hamstring tendons. The Achilles tendon allograft is the most popular because of its additional intrinsic strength and ease in passing through the bone tunnels. Results have generally been good, with Clancy[16] reporting all 10 acute tears and 11 of 13 chronic tears reconstructed with good or excellent results at 2 years. Fanelli[25] has reported similar results.

An avulsion of the PCL occurs more commonly than the ACL, and can be managed nonoperatively by cast immobilization with good results only if the fragment is truly nondisplaced. Displaced fragments reduced and fixed surgically generally yield excellent results (Fig. 23-43), and anatomic reapproximation is the procedure of choice.[1,9,23,52,64,67,87,89] Small fragments not amenable to screw fixation can be treated nonoperatively if there is less than 10 mm of posterior laxity. However, more than 10 mm of laxity warrants reconstruction. This management algorithm is found in Figure 23-44.[90]

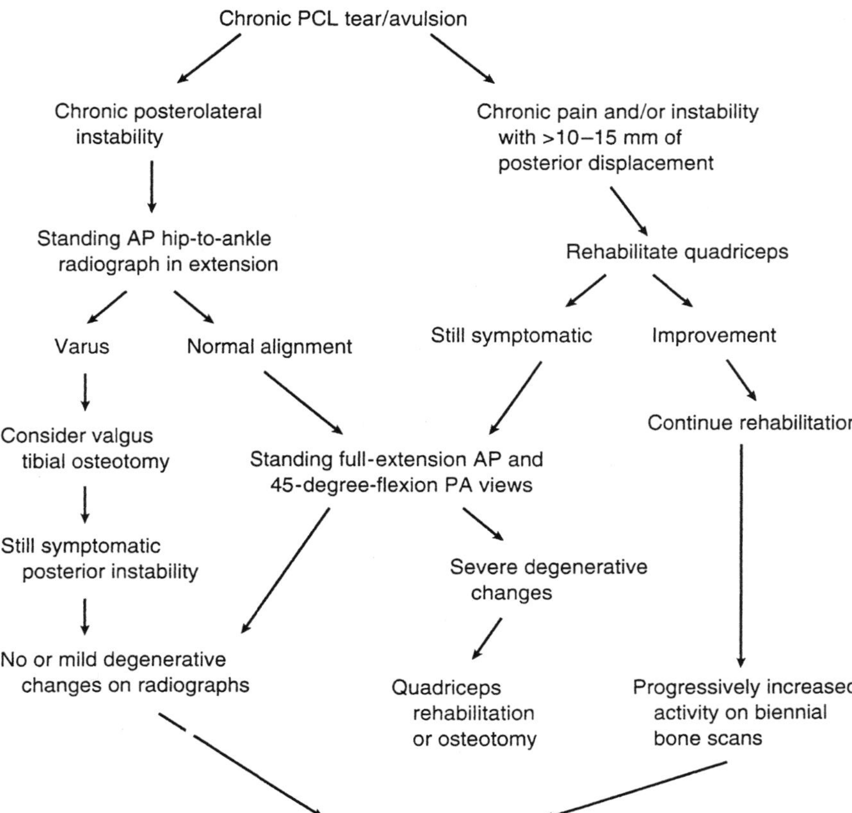

FIGURE 23-42. Chronic posterior cruciate ligament tear algorithm. (From Veltri DM, Warren RF: Posterior cruciate ligament injuries. J Am Acad Orthop Surg 1:74, 1993.)

KNEE DISLOCATIONS

Knee dislocations are relatively infrequent events that result from significant trauma to the knee, usually as a result of motor vehicle accidents or falls, but can also occur in contact sports, such as hyperextension in a football tackle. Dislocation results in major ligamentous injury, usually tearing ACL and PCL, collateral ligaments, and capsular structures.[96] Perhaps more importantly, arterial injury occurs in knee dislocations with a frequency of 29% to 40%.[34,81,88] Intimal arterial injury may be present even in the face of initially intact pedal pulses.[55,80] Therefore, arteriograms or Doppler examinations are essentially mandatory in the acute knee dislocation. Additionally, neurologic injuries occur in 9% to 49% of knee dislocations with recovery rates ranging from 13% to 80%.[6] Because of the significant risk of neurovascular and extensive ligamentous injury, immediate referral to an orthopedist with access to vascular surgery evaluation is mandatory. Arterial repair is necessary within the first 6 to 8 hours to minimize the risk of amputation. Risk of compartment syndrome necessitating fasciotomy also increases with prolonged limb ischemia (Fig. 23-45).

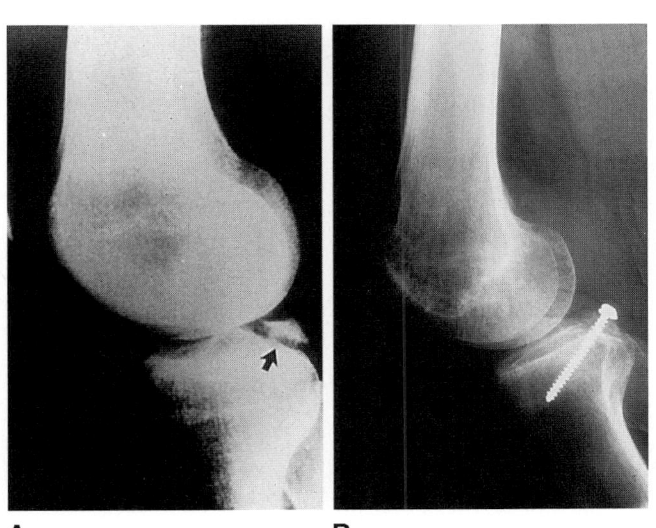

FIGURE 23-43. A, Posterior cruciate ligament avulsion fracture from the tibial insertion. **B,** After open reduction and internal fixation.

Management consists of immediate closed reduction on the playing field or at the scene of the accident, followed by splinting. Often the reduction has occurred spontaneously before physician evaluation, and one must be suspicious for dislocation if the examination demonstrates multiple ligamentous injuries or popliteal fossa tenderness and ecchymosis. Open reduction is often

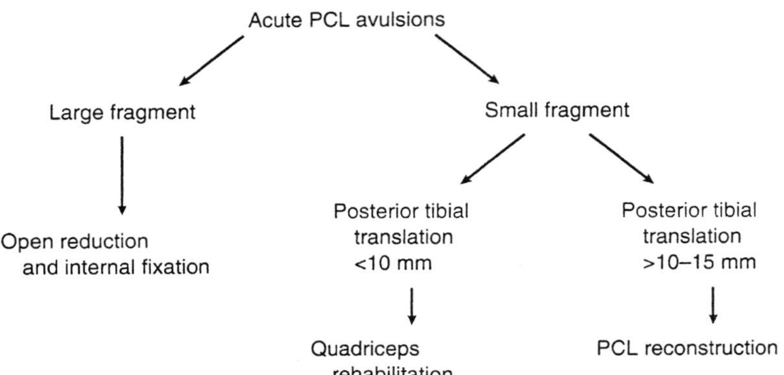

FIGURE 23-44. Posterior cruciate ligament avulsion algorithm. (From Veltri DM, Warren RF: Posterior cruciate ligament injuries. J Am Acad Orthop Surg 1:71, 1993.)

necessary for posterolateral dislocations because of interposition of the joint capsule preventing closed reduction.[46,68] Surgical reconstruction of ligamentous injuries should be performed in cases requiring open reduction or open vascular repair. Ligament reconstruction should be delayed if limb ischemia or a tenuous vascular repair precludes early intervention. Current orthopedic opinion favors early reconstruction of all ligamentous injuries, with primary repair of bony avulsions if possible, or using autograft or allograft techniques.[82,95]

PATELLOFEMORAL JOINT

Patella Subluxation and Dislocation

Anterior knee pain can be a frustrating complaint for the physician and the patient. The exact etiology is often elusive, and nonoperative management may take an extensive period of time before symptoms improve. Surgical intervention can also be frustrating because of the lack of predictability for achieving good results. Sources of pain include malalignment, chondromalacia patella, osteoarthritis, osteochondral fractures, synovial plicae, bursitis, tendonitis, patella subluxation or dislocation, and others. Merchant's classification of patellofemoral disorders demonstrates an extensive list of possible etiologies (Table 23-2).[56] A thorough understanding of the anatomy as it relates to the biomechanics of the patellofemoral joint can help the physician considerably when confronted with this common complaint.

The extensor mechanism includes the quadriceps musculature, the quadriceps and patellar tendons, the patella, and the femoral sulcus. The Q angle (see Fig. 23-8), measured by the angle made from the anterior–superior iliac spine to the patella and from the patella to the tibial tubercle, reflects the vector of the extensor mechanism. An abnormal Q angle more than 10° in men and more than 20° in women should be put in context with the rest of the history and physical examination. The underlying assumption is that an abnormally high Q angle with a more laterally directed quadriceps pull places excessive pressure on the lateral patellofemoral joint and predisposes to subluxation and possibly dislocation. Additionally, an imbalance in the medial and lateral quadriceps muscle forces may accentuate lateral patellar tracking, which may be further affected by a tight lateral retinaculum. Anatomic variations in the shape or contour of the femoral sulcus and patella are also influential in disorders of the extensor

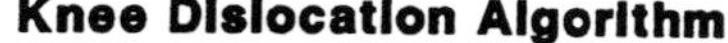

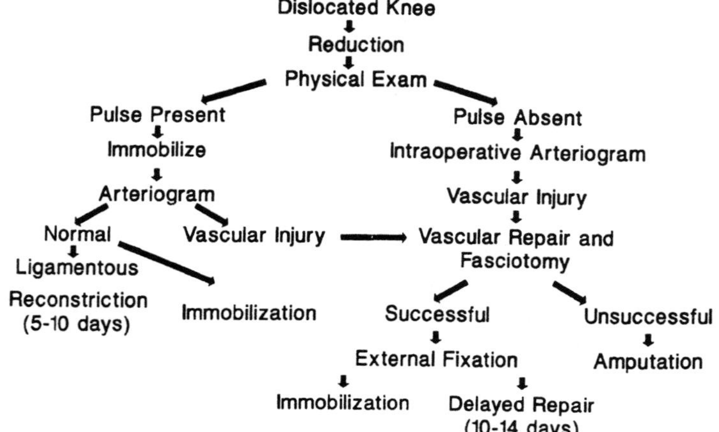

FIGURE 23-45. Management algorithm for knee dislocations. (From Montgomery M, et al: Orthopedic management of knee dislocations. Am J Knee Surg 8(3): 97–103, 1995.)

TABLE 23-2 Merchant Classification of Patellofemoral Disorders

- Trauma (conditions caused by trauma in the otherwise healthy knee)
  - Acute trauma
    - Contusion (924.11)
    - Fracture
      - Patella (822)
      - Femoral trochlea (821.2)
      - Proximal tibial epiphysis (tubercle) (823.0)
    - Dislocation (rare in the healthy knee) (836.3)
    - Rupture
      - Quadriceps tendon (843.8)
      - Patellar tendon (844.8)
  - Repetitive trauma (overuse syndromes)
    - Patellar tendinitis ("jumper's knee") (726.64)
    - Quadriceps tendinitis (726.69)
    - Peripatellar tendinitis (e.g., anterior knee pain of the adolescent caused by hamstring contracture) (726.699)
    - Prepatellar bursitis ("housemaid's knee") (726.65)
    - Apophysitis
      - Osgood-Schlatter disease (732.43)
      - Sinding-Larsen-Johanssen's disease (732.42)
  - Late effects of trauma (905)
    - Post-traumatic chondromalacia patellae
    - Post-traumatic patellofemoral arthritis
    - Anterior fat pad syndrome (post-traumatic fibrosis)
    - Reflex sympathetic dystrophy of the patella
    - Patellar osseous dystrophy
    - Acquired patella infera (718.366)
    - Acquired quadriceps fibrosis
    - Patellofemoral dysplasia
  - Lateral patellar compression syndrome (LPCS) (718.365)
    - Secondary chondromalacia patellae (717.7)
    - Secondary patellofemoral arthritis (715.289)
  - Chronic subluxation of the patella (CSP) (718.364)
    - Secondary chondromalacia patellae (717.7)
    - Secondary patellofemoral arthritis (715.289)
  - Chronic dislocation of the patella (718.362)
    - Developmental
    - Acquired
    - Idiopathic chondromalacia patellae (717.7)
    - Osteochondritis dissecans
  - Patella (732.704)
  - Femoral trochlea (732.703)

Continued

TABLE 23-2—Cont'd Merchant Classification of Patellofemoral Disorders

- Synovial plicae (727.8916) (anatomic variants made symptomatic by acute or repetitive trauma)
  - Pathologic medial patellar plica ("shelf") (727.89161)
  - Pathologic suprapatellar plica (727.89165)
  - Pathologic lateral patellar plica (727.89165)
- Iatrogenic disorders
  - Iatrogenic medial patellar compression syndrome
  - Iatrogenic chronic medial subluxation of the patella
  - Iatrogenic patella infera (718.366)

Orthopaedic ICD-9-CM Expanded Diagnostic Codes in parentheses.

From Merchant AC: Clinical classification of patellofemoral disorders. Sports Med Arthroscopy Rev 2:26–27, 1994.

mechanism. Patella height has also been shown to be a contributing factor.[2,72,74]

One of the most severe injuries to the extensor mechanism is a patellar dislocation. The athlete with a patellar dislocation describes a dramatic event, resulting in a knee with a bizarre appearance because of the laterally displaced patella and significant pain. The patella dislocates laterally as a result of a sudden quadriceps contraction with the knee in partial flexion, often with a twisting component, causing the patella to displace over the lateral femoral condyle. Many times, the patella will spontaneously reduce as the patient straightens the leg, producing a palpable and audible clunk. Other times, the patella remains dislocated and requires closed reduction by medical personnel. The reduction involves slowly, but forcefully extending the knee, often with associated analgesia. A large, painful, bloody effusion quickly develops secondary to disruption of the medial retinaculum. The patient is reluctant to flex the knee but must be coaxed to perform a straight leg raise against resistance to document an intact extensor mechanism. Tenderness is greatest over the medial retinaculum.

Once reduced, plain radiographs, including a Merchant or sunrise view of the patella, should be obtained to look for any osteochondral fracture and possible loose body from the undersurface of the patella (Fig. 23-46). The Merchant view is obtained with the knee in 45° of flexion with the x-ray beam directed caudally at an angle 30° from the plane of the femur (see Fig. 23-24). Also, the articular congruence of the patellofemoral articulation can be measured by drawing lines between the lowest point on the femoral sulcus and the highest points on the medial (AC) and lateral (AB) femoral condyles (Fig. 23-47). This sulcus angle is bisected to provide a reference for the patella position (AO). The lowest point on the femoral sulcus is then connected to the lowest point on the articular surface of

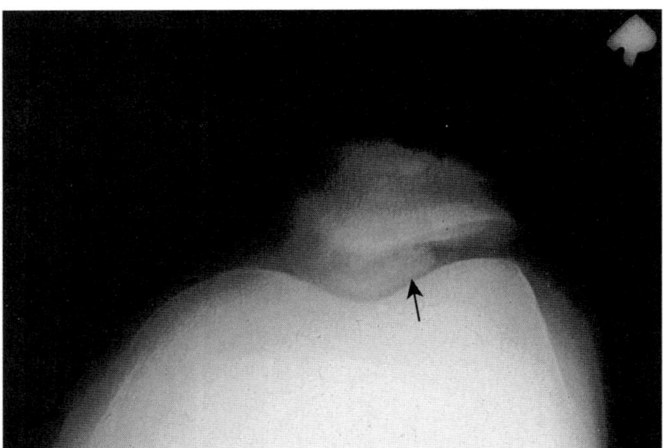

FIGURE 23-46. Osteochondral fracture from the articular surface of the patella (arrow).

the patella (AD) to create the congruence angle. An angle medial to the bisector reference line (AO) is considered to be negative, and an angle lateral to the bisector reference line (AO) is positive. The patella apex or central ridge should lie at or medial to the bisector of the sulcus angle, the normal congruence angle being −6°. If the ridge is displaced laterally with a congruence angle more than 4°, the patella is considered subluxed.[30,66]

This Merchant view also demonstrates lateral tilt, with a disproportionately widened medial patellofemoral joint space as compared with the lateral. Variability in bony morphology makes this assessment of tilt less reproducible. Chronic complaints of patella instability can be further evaluated if necessary with computed tomography scans at 15°, 30°, and 45° of knee flexion to demonstrate abnormal tracking sometimes not evident on standard Merchant views. Assessment of patella height can be performed on the lateral radiograph using the Insall-Salvatti ratio (Fig. 23-48). The ratio of the length of the patella tendon divided by the length of the patella is 1.02 ± 0.13. Variation more than 20% is considered abnormal and evidence of patella baja or alta.[2] Another method of determining patella height has been described by Caton and Linclau.[72]

An athlete with a reduced patella dislocation should be immobilized in extension and referred to an orthopedist. Cryotherapy is recommended for the initial period of swelling and weight bearing can be to tolerance. Evidence of an osteochondral fracture or loose body warrants arthroscopic surgery for fixation or removal, depending on the size and degree of comminution of the fragment. If the medial retinaculum is torn, it can be surgically repaired with imbrication at the same time. If the athlete reports a chronic history of repeated dislocations or if the patella is displaced laterally or tilted on the Merchant view, then a medial proximal realignment with a lateral retinacular release are indicated.[74] In the absence of a fracture in an acute dislocation, MRI can help delineate the extent of pathology. Negative MRI evaluation without patella malalignment on Merchant view can be managed with simple immobilization in extension in a

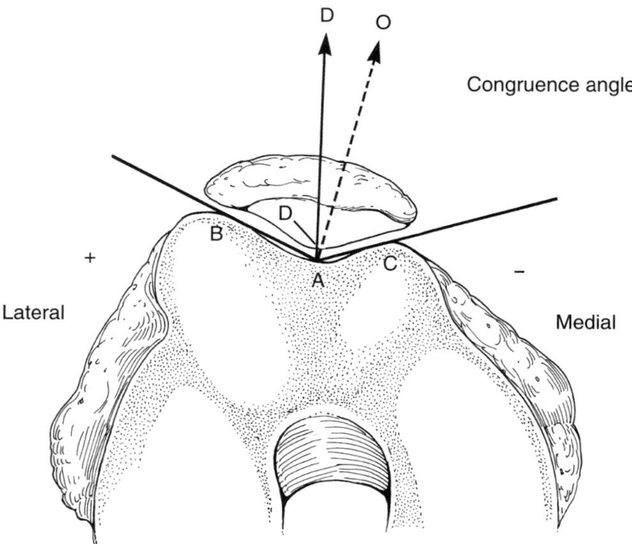

FIGURE 23-47. The congruence angle of the patellofemoral joint as seen on the Merchant view.

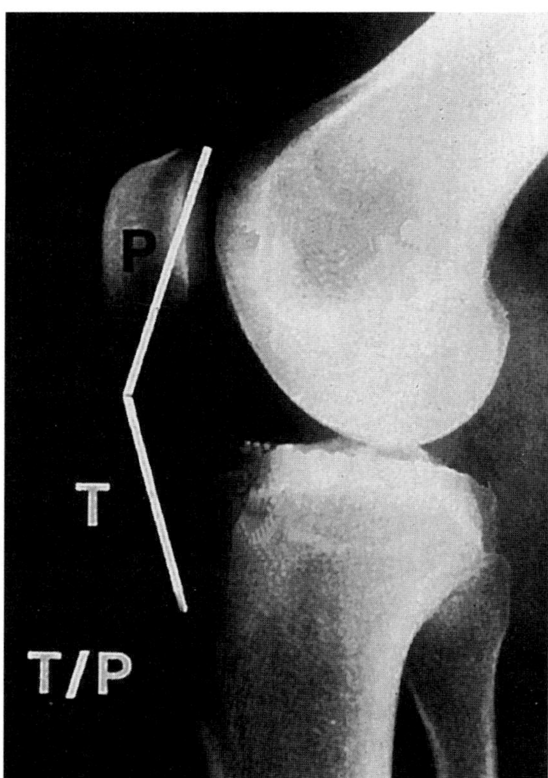

FIGURE 23-48. The Insall-Salvatti ratio of patella height is obtained from the lateral radiograph. The length of the patella tendon as measured on its deep or posterior surface (*T*) is divided by the length of the patella (*P*). The ratio of T/P is 1.02 ± 0.13.

knee immobilizer for 1 to 2 weeks until swelling and pain subside. Physical therapy to restore motion and, most important, for medial quadriceps strengthening should be instituted. This approach to the acute patella dislocation is summarized in the algorithm in Figure 23-49.[29]

Recurrent episodes of patella subluxation can be elicited during patient history as a sensation of the patella slipping laterally with associated giving way of the knee. Pain is usually temporary and swelling mild if present. Physical examination may reveal a tight lateral retinaculum on attempted medial mobilization of the patella or on attempted lifting of the tilted patella to horizontal (Fig. 23-50). Passively ranging the knee with laterally directed pressure against the medial border of the patella—the patella apprehension test—may reproduce a sensation of impending dislocation and pain. Plain radiographs, including a Merchant view, rule out osteochondral injury and look for tilt or radiographic subluxation, which may be separate or combined, as shown in Figure 23-51.

Management of patella subluxation should initially be nonoperative with quadriceps strengthening exercises, especially the vastus medialis. Usually, it is beneficial for the athlete to begin these exercises under the supervision of a physical therapist or an athletic trainer. The athlete should be prevented from flexion beyond 90° because it creates excessive contact pressures on the patellofemoral articulation. A patella-stabilizing brace may be of some benefit. Recently, McConnell taping has become popular in centralizing the patella.[53,99] This technique has variable success because of the difficulty with patient compliance. If the athlete fails an extensive course of therapy, with documented evidence of quadriceps strengthening, he or she may be a candidate for a lateral retinacular release and possibly a proximal patellar realignment.[75] One must be certain, however, that the patient truly participated in a supervised physical therapy program without improvement before choosing operative intervention.

Patellofemoral Syndrome and Chondromalacia

Malalignment and acute or repetitive trauma can lead to degenerative changes on the articular surface of the patella and of the femoral sulcus. Softening and early erosive changes are referred to as chondromalacia. Chondromalacia has been graded by clinical and microscopic appearance

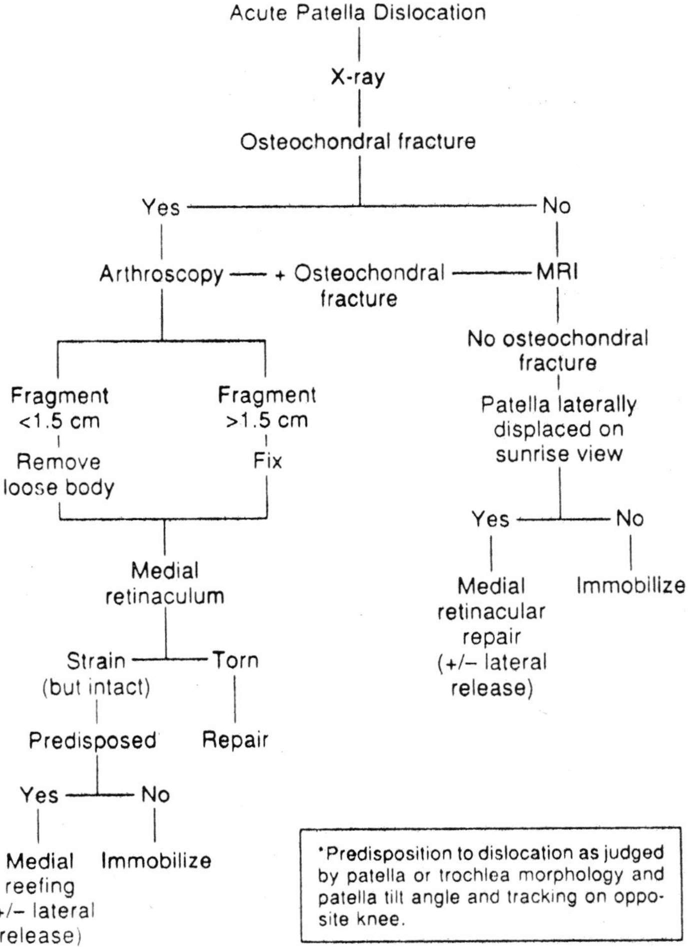

FIGURE 23-49. Acute patella dislocation algorithm. (From Fox JM, Del Pizzo W [eds]: The Patellofemoral Joint. New York, McGraw-Hill, 1993.)

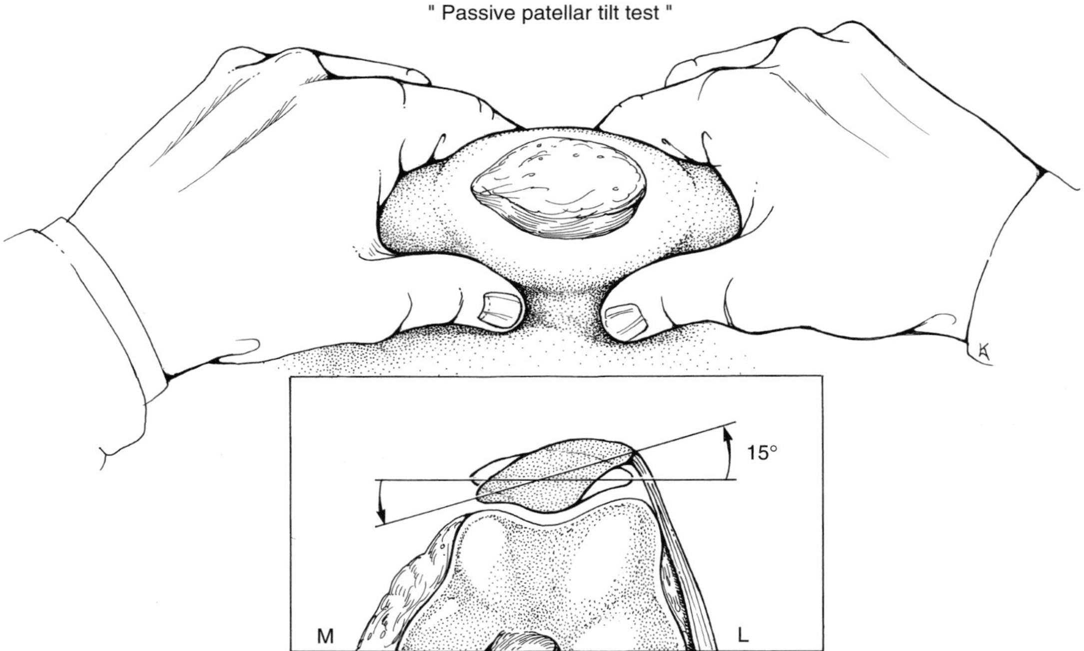

FIGURE 23-50. Passive patella tilt test. In full extension, one should be able to lift the lateral border of the patella beyond horizontal. Inability to do so may indicate a tight lateral retinaculum.

by Outerbridge.[63] Grade I chondromalacia is edema, softening, and possibly some blister lesions. Grade II chondromalacia has chondral fissures extending down to subchondral bone, and grade III has chondral fibrillation and further thinning or wear. Further erosion to eburnated bone is grade IV chondromalacia or osteoarthritis.[91] Often the exact etiology is difficult to establish, but a careful history may elicit overuse activities, especially high-impact activities or activities that necessitate repetitive knee flexion. These activities include running, step machines, squats, or weights beyond 90° of flexion. Maintaining the knee for long periods in a bent position, such as seated in a theatre or on a plane, aggravates symptoms because the extensor mechanism is under tension, compressing the patella against the femur.

The athlete will localize pain diffusely to the anterior knee on history, often describing an aching that increases with activity. Crepitus or cracking noises may be felt or heard during a range of motion, also nonspecific findings. Tenderness on the undersurface of the patella can be elicited by manually subluxing the patella to either side and palpating the surface with the opposite hand, which is a more specific finding. Careful attention should be made to determine any anatomic predisposition to instability or malalignment, including determining any history of dislocation or subluxation or trauma. A tight lateral retinaculum can be identified on attempted medial subluxation and tilt to neutral. If there is no evidence of subluxation or dislocation on history or examination but tenderness on the undersurface of the patella exists with normal alignment, the athlete has lateral patellar compression syndrome (Fig. 23-52). This is a radiographic diagnosis (abnormal patellar tilt without subluxation) and a clinical diagnosis (tight lateral retinaculum, normal mobility, normal Q angle).[57]

Initial management should be nonoperative to include activity modification. Impact activities are to be restricted to recreational status (done on occasion for "fun" but not on a regular basis for conditioning), which would include running, step machines, or aerobics. An aggressive conditioning program for quadriceps strengthening should be performed in nonimpact fashion and include such activities as an exercise bicycle, cross-country ski machine, or swimming for aerobic conditioning. Ice is used for pain and swelling control after work-outs and as needed. Short courses of NSAIDs are used on occasion. If after 6 to 12 weeks of documented rehabilitation and activity modification no benefit is seen, arthroscopic debridement and possibly lateral release may be indicated. The majority of patients do not require surgery for this diagnosis and improve if adequate effort is invested in nonoperative therapy.

Extensor Mechanism Disruptions

Ruptures of the patella or quadriceps tendons are more common in middle-aged or older patients than in young athletes. The patient will note sudden, dramatic pain often in association with an audible "pop." The individual is unable to walk without assistance or a brace. A large,

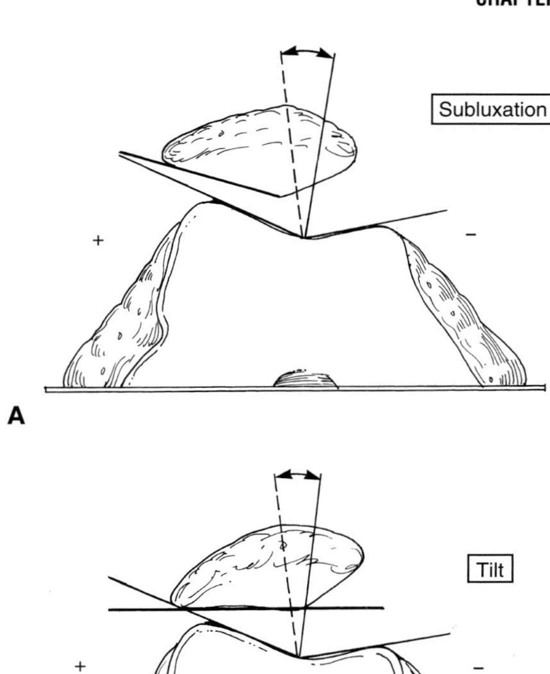

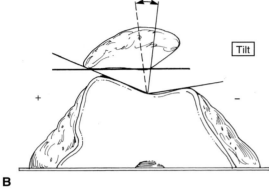

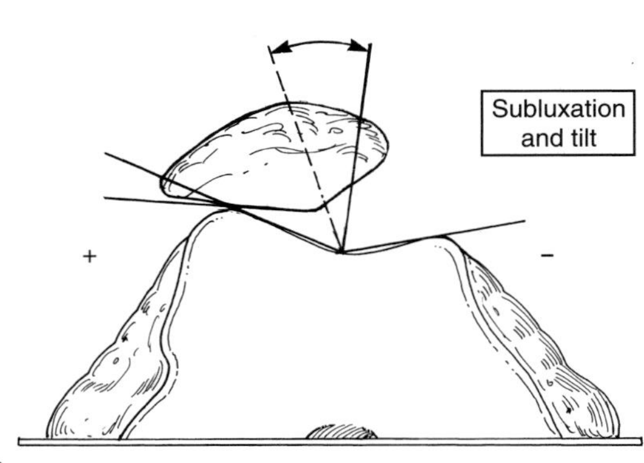

FIGURE 23-51. Patella tracking abnormalities include subluxation **(A),** lateral tilt **(B),** or both **(C).**

bloody effusion is almost immediate. Radiographs confirm the effusion and usually demonstrate a high-riding patella—patella alta—for patella tendon rupture, or possibly a low-lying patella—patella baja—for a quadriceps tendon rupture (Fig. 23-53). On examination, the patient is unable to actively extend the knee against gravity or any resistance. Other injuries can be misinterpreted as an extensor mechanism disruption if the patient cannot be coaxed through the pain to perform a straight leg raise off of the table. If the swelling is not too severe, one can appreciate a palpable, tender defect in either the quadriceps or patella tendon, which is accentuated by

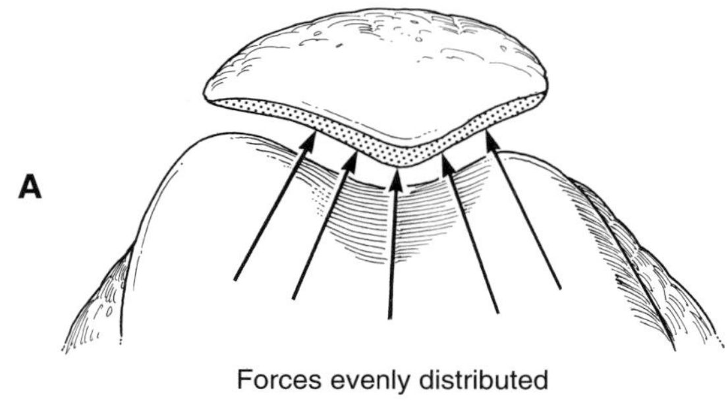

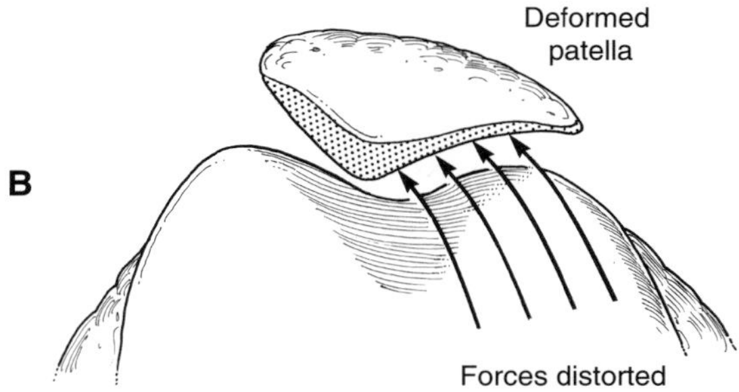

FIGURE 23-52. A, Normal equal distribution of contact forces across the patellofemoral joint. **B,** In lateral patella compression syndrome, the forces are unevenly distributed toward the lateral facet, resulting in deformation and thinning of the articular cartilage.

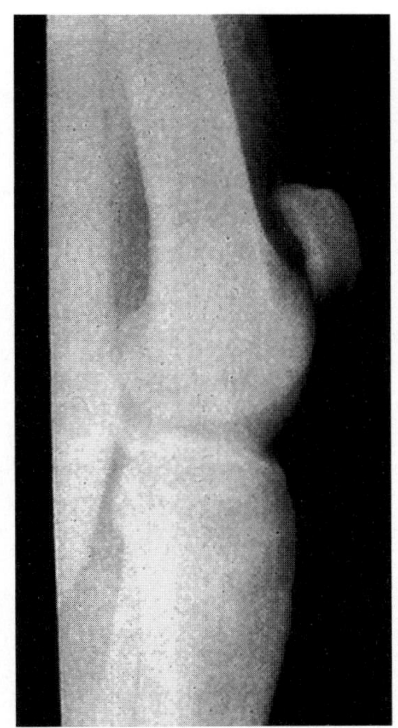

FIGURE 23-53. Extensor mechanism disruption results in an acute hemarthrosis, and for patella tendon rupture results in a high-riding patella.

attempts at lifting the leg. Ruptures most often occur in close proximity to the attachment to the patella on either side.[8]

Management of extensor mechanism disruptions is surgical anatomic repair, possibly with augmentation.[71] For this reason, the athlete should be placed in a knee immobilizer in extension with a gentle compressive wrap and ice to help control swelling. Consultation with an orthopedic surgeon should be obtained as soon as possible. Delays in reconstruction more than a few days make repair significantly more difficult because of progressive retraction of tendon ends.

TENDONITIS AND BURSITIS

Patella Tendonitis (Jumper's Knee)

Patella tendonitis is a diagnosis consistent with overuse or repetitive trauma to the extensor mechanism of the knee, which commonly results from jumping or running sports such as basketball and volleyball. Athletes will present with anterior knee pain and intermittent swelling. On examination, tenderness localizes to the patellar tendon, primarily at its origin on the inferior pole of the patella. Tenderness is most easily appreciated with the knee in extension.[57] Radiographic evaluation is helpful in visualizing any bony abnormality, such as elongation or fragmentation of the inferior pole of the patella, periosteal reactive bone, or calcification within the patella tendon.[8] MRI is reserved for recalcitrant cases and is helpful in diagnosing tendon degeneration (Fig. 23-54).

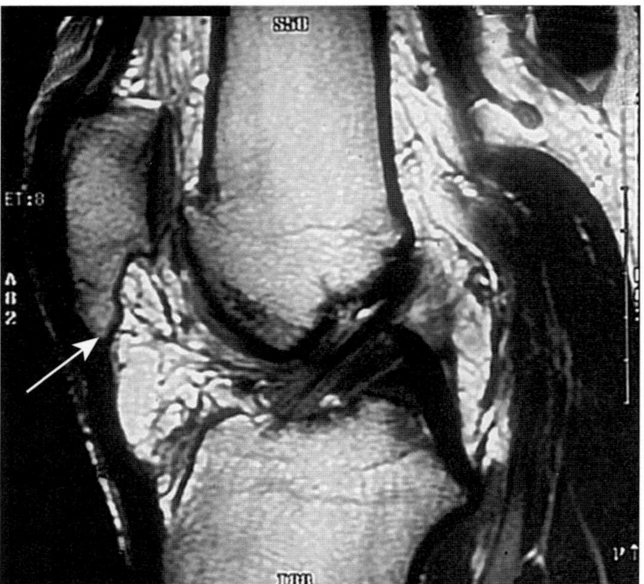

FIGURE 23-54. Chronic patella tendonitis may demonstrate elongation of the patella inferior pole or calcification within the tendon *(arrow).*

Nonoperative management is directed toward a period of rest to allow symptoms to subside, followed by activity modification that limits high-impact sports. Stretching of the quadriceps and hamstrings is helpful, as is a strengthening program. Isokinetic and plyometric exercises aggravate symptoms and should be avoided.[57] Short arc quadriceps strengthening exercises are performed within the painless range of motion. Ice and short courses of NSAIDs are helpful adjuncts. Local steroid injections are to be avoided because they have been shown to cause tendon degeneration and potential rupture. Nonoperative treatment is successful in roughly 90% of patients.[83] A patellar tendon strap can be of subjective benefit as the athlete returns to sports. Rarely is operative intervention to remove a portion of degenerative tendon or the lower pole of the patella necessary.

Iliotibial Band Syndrome

Iliotibial band friction syndrome is a descriptive diagnosis for another overuse syndrome involving repetitive friction between the iliotibial band and the lateral femoral condyle. Runners and cyclists most commonly experience these symptoms. Tenderness and pain are localized to the iliotibial band overlying the lateral femoral epicondyle. This area is palpated during knee range of motion. Tenderness is maximal at 30° of flexion.[57] Pain can also be elicited by having the patient lie on the contralateral side while attempting to abduct the leg in extension. Resisting abduction exacerbates pain over the lateral femoral epicondyle and can be enhanced by palpation.

Nonoperative management includes rest and modification of the training routine. Runners are instructed to shorten their distance and stride length as needed to stop symptoms. Ice and occasional short courses of NSAIDs can be helpful. Stretching exercises are recommended with a gradual return to sports-specific training. Rarely, steroid injections are useful for recalcitrant cases. For those unusual cases that fail to respond to a supervised nonoperative program, operative intervention is considered to partially release a small portion of the posterior iliotibial band.

Bursitis

The bursae are synovial-lined cavities normally containing a thin film of fluid that overlie bony prominences around the knee (Fig. 23-55*A*). Bursae reduce friction during knee motion. Repetitive trauma from overuse or, more commonly, chronic irritation results in local inflammation and fluid collection within the bursa. The prepatellar bursa is the most commonly affected and is termed "housemaid's knee" (Fig. 23-55*B*). Inflammation can occur from repetitive kneeling or a direct blow.

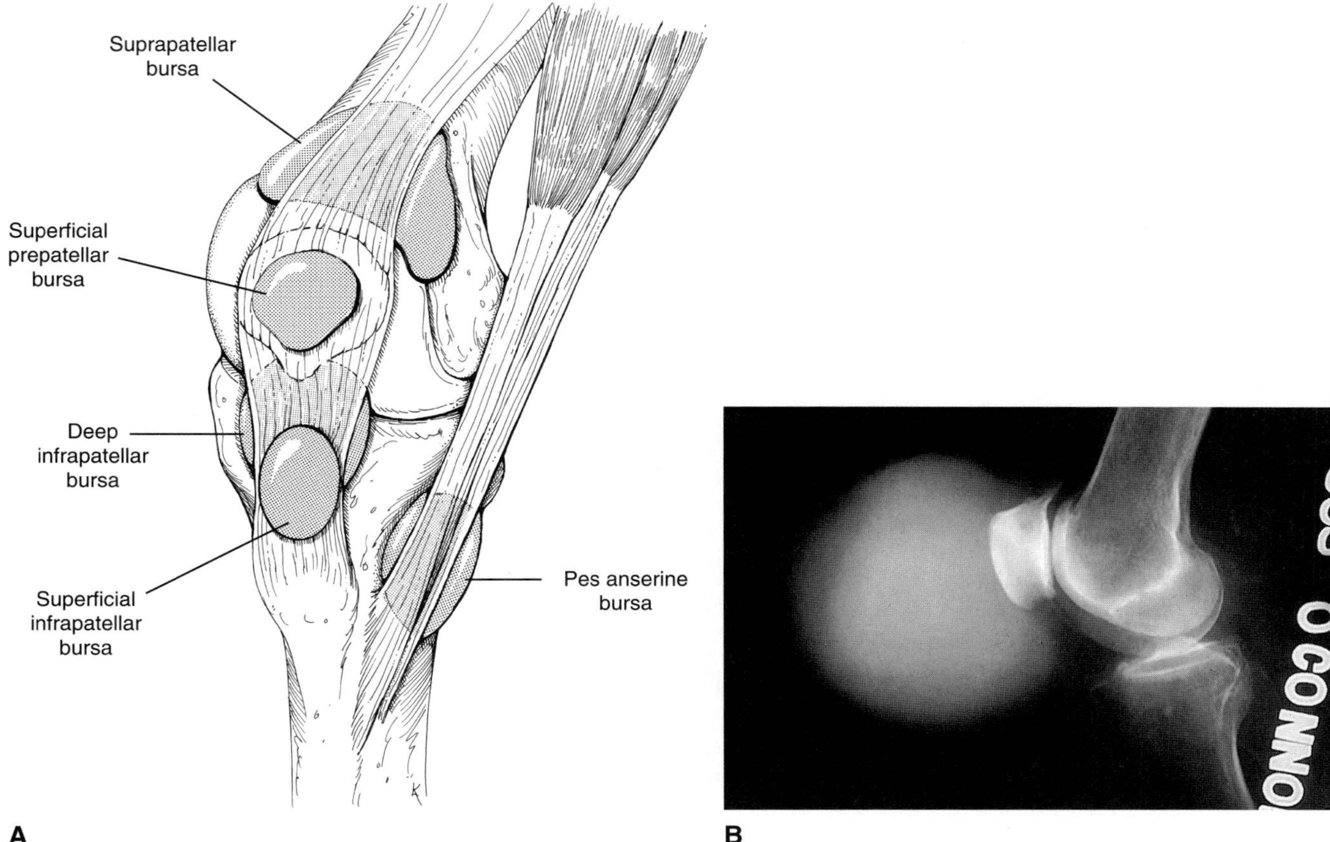

FIGURE 23-55. **A,** Bursae around the knee. **B,** Markedly swollen prepatellar bursa.

Penetrating trauma to the prepatellar region can result in a septic bursitis caused by innoculation with skin flora.

Inferior to the patella are the superficial and deep infrapatellar bursae. Chronic kneeling or acute trauma can cause inflammation of these bursae. Bursitis here is often difficult to distinguish from patellar tendonitis or intraarticular pathology. Under the common insertion of the sartorius, semitendonosis, and gracilis tendons, termed the *pes anserinus,* is the pes anserinus bursa. Overuse activities such as running can produce inflammation here, but this is perhaps overdiagnosed as a misinterpretation of meniscal or other intraarticular pathology. An additional bursa rests under the semimembranosis tendon attachment on the proximal tibia, but it is not often inflamed.

Patients present with swelling, pain, and tenderness well localized to the inflamed bursa. The history of chronic irritating activities is usually obtained. Swelling can be dramatic, but it is always confined to the general area of the inflamed bursa. For prepatellar bursitis, the bony contours of the patella are obscured, unlike an intraarticular effusion. Weight bearing or gentle range of motion does not significantly increase pain, although the patient will note tightness and secondary pain as flexion is increased, which helps distinguish bursitis from septic intraarticular arthritis, which is markedly painful to any range of motion or weight bearing.

Management is directed at stopping the irritating activity—such as kneeling. Ice and short courses of NSAIDs are used. A gentle compressive wrap can help reduce swelling. Occasionally, a period of immobilization in a knee immobilizer brace is necessary. Aspiration can be performed diagnostically and therapeutically.[77] Drainage relieves distention and, as a result, pain. Septic bursitis is managed with aspiration and antibiotics. Advanced or resistant cases can be improved more rapidly with local incision and drainage in the outpatient setting. Chronic, recurrent cases rarely require surgical excision of the chronically thickened bursa.

Synovial Plica

Plicae are normal synovial septums that can sometimes become inflamed and symptomatic. The suprapatellar plica traverses the suprapatellar pouch. The infrapatellar plica, or ligamentum mucosum, loosely connects the fat pad to the superior part of the intercondylar notch. The medial patellar plica and the less common lateral patellar plica run obliquely from the respective sides of the suprapatellar pouch to the anterior fat pad (Fig. 23-56).

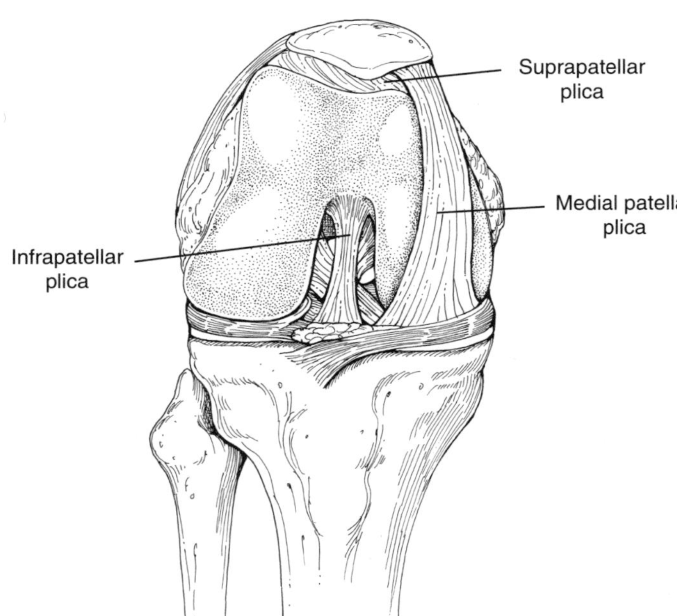

FIGURE 23-56. Synovial plicae of the knee.

The incidence of plica as an anatomic structure in the population ranges 20% to 60%.[77]

Athletes complain of vague anterior knee pain often associated with overuse activities such as running or biking. Symptoms may occur only after a period of exercise as the synovium becomes progressively irritated. Patients may complain of clicking or catching, sometimes occurring at a specific point during flexion as the inflamed plica snaps over the femoral condyle. Sometimes this snapping plica can be palpated and usually is tender. The medial patellar plica is most commonly involved as it becomes inflamed by rubbing over the medial femoral condyle. The mere existance of a plica is not diagnostic because it is a normal structure. In the absence of irritation, other causes should be ruled out.

Management is initially nonoperative and directed toward rest and cessation of the irritating activity. Ice and a short course of NSAIDs can be helpful. Arthroscopy confirms the diagnosis in recalcitrant cases by visualizing a thickened and inflamed synovial band rubbing over the adjacent femoral condyle, sometimes with a matching abraded bony lesion. Arthroscopic resection of the plica is easily performed and effective in 70% to 92% of patients.[77]

Osgood-Schlatter Apophysitis

The proximal tibial growth plate slopes distally in the anterior portion to lie beneath the attachment of the patella tendon on the tibial tubercle. Excessive activity can create a traction apophysitis at the tendon insertion. Osgood-Schlatter apophysitis occurs in active, growing adolescents, usually boys. Athletes present with activity-related pain, swelling, and tenderness localized to the tibial tubercle. Findings are bilateral in 20% to 30% of cases.[57] Radiographs in chronic cases show thickening of the patella tendon, soft-tissue swelling, and sometimes fragmentation of the tibial tubercle (Fig. 23-57).

Rest and activity modification are recommended until symptoms subside. Nonoperative management is almost always successful. Advanced apophysitis essentially represents a stress fracture, and significant symptoms not responding to rest should be reason to immobilize the knee. Symptoms are also limited to the duration of skeletal growth. Occasionally, chronic symptoms caused by painful ossicles in the tendon respond to excision, although surgery

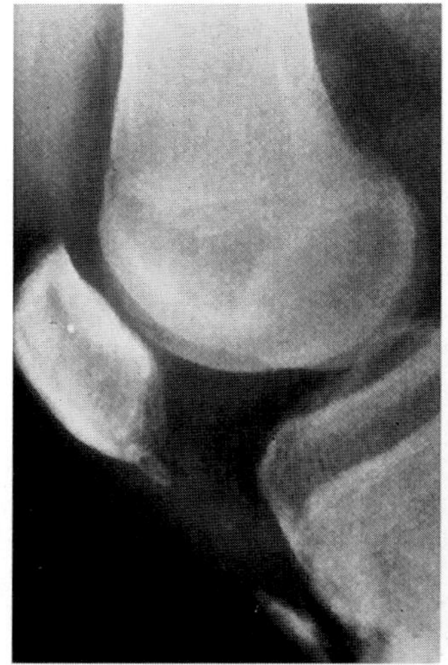
A

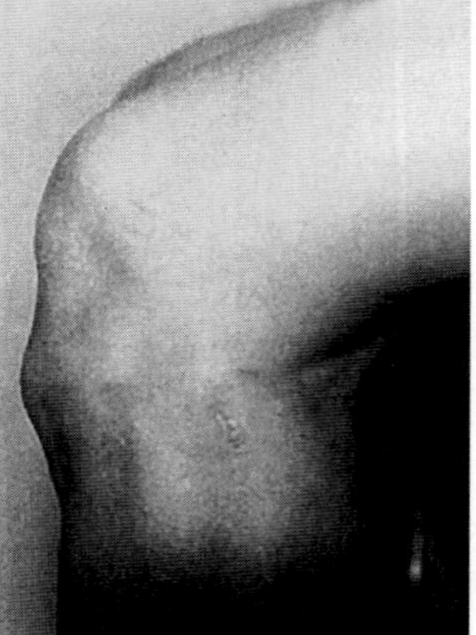
B

FIGURE 23-57. A, Radiograph of Osgood-Schlatter disease demonstrating thickening of patella tendon, fragmentation of the tibial tubercle, and soft tissue swelling. **B,** Clinical picture of bony prominence anteriorly at the tibial tubercle.

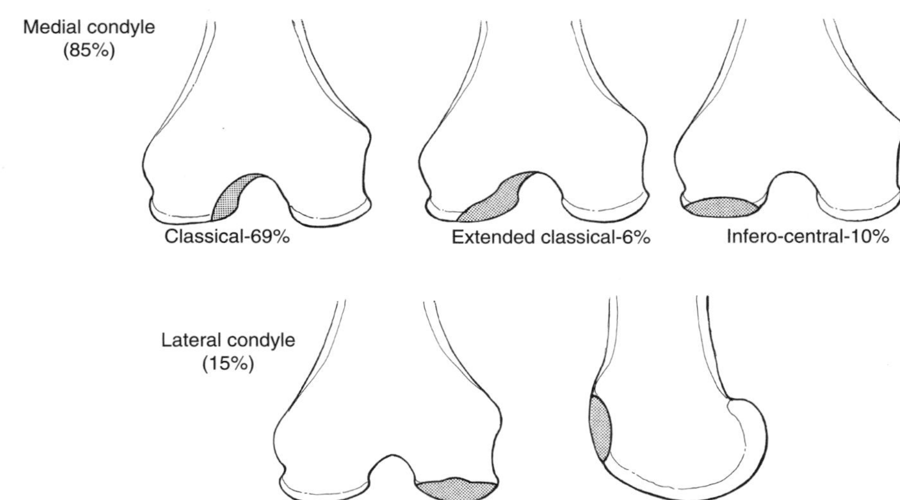

FIGURE 23-58. Locations of osteochondritis dissecans on the distal femur.

is rarely necessary. In even more rare instances, continued activity or acute trauma can result in an avulsion fracture of the tibial tubercle, which requires surgical repair.

Osteochondritis Dissecans

Osteochondritis dissecans is separation of a fragment of subchondral bone with its overlying articular cartilage, leaving a "divot" in the remaining bone. The etiology is likely traumatic, especially in young patients, but is not clear. The most common location is the lateral aspect of the medial femoral condyle, and less often it occurs in the central portion of the lateral femoral condyle (Fig. 23-58).[4,5] An anteroposterior tunnel or notch view can help visualize the lesion (Fig. 23-59). Osteochondritis dissecans occurs during the second to fourth decades, most often in adolescents.[4,77] The osteochondral fragment can be classified by appearance at arthroscopy as intact (grade I), early separation (grade II), partial detachment (grade III), or loose fragment (grade IV).[13]

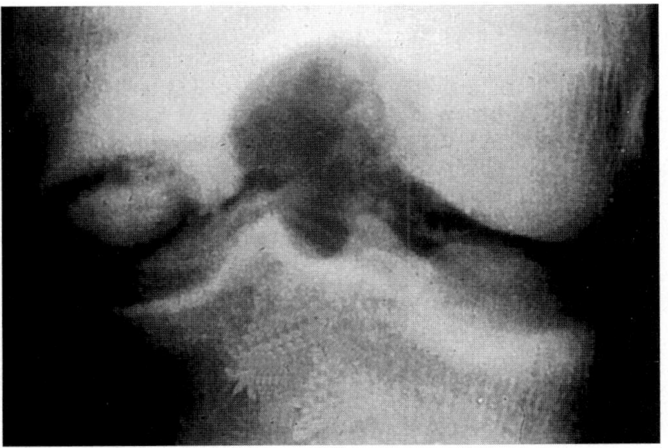

FIGURE 23-59. Anteroposterior tunnel or notch view demonstrating osteochondritis dissecans of the medial femoral condyle.

Patients usually complain of vague, poorly localized knee pain that increases with weight bearing or activity. Plain radiographs to include the notch or tunnel view are usually sufficient, but MRI can add information about the subchondral extent of the lesion. However, the only precise way to assess stability of the fragment is by arthroscopic probing. Large or loose lesions present with a knee effusion, tenderness, and mechanical symptoms of locking, catching, or giving way.

Patients with osteochondritis dissecans should be examined by an orthopedic surgeon. Prognosis is strongly related to size and displacement of the lesion and age of the patient. Young patients (boys younger than 14 years and girls younger than 12 years) generally do well, and the fragment is less likely to displace and require fixation.[57] Smaller fragments and loose bodies causing mechanical symptoms are removed arthroscopically. Large fragments, especially those larger than 25% of the joint surface area, should be fixed in place.[5,13] Metal pins or screws are being replaced in favor of biodegradable pins as the fixation method of choice. Cartilage autograft transplantation is considered experimental and has recently been reported.[10] Arthroscopic drilling of the crater in unrepairable cases promotes proliferation of fibrocartilage in young patients and may give partial relief of symptoms, but it tends to deteriorate with time.

Proximal Tibiofibular Joint Dislocations

The proximal tibiofibular joint is a synovial joint surrounded by a thickened capsule, allowing little significant motion between the tibia and fibular head. Proximal

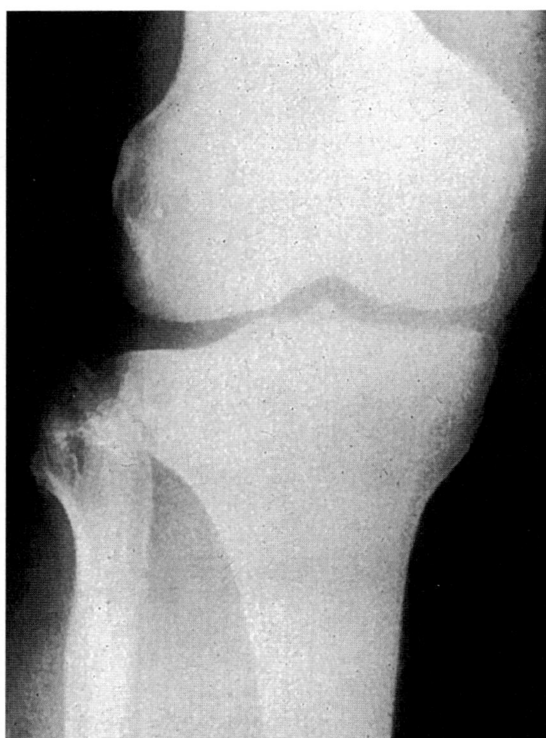

FIGURE 23-60. Proximal tibiofibular joint dislocation.

tibiofibular joint dislocations are rare injuries that can occur as an isolated injury or in conjunction with other injuries in major trauma to the knee. When an isolated injury, the dislocation most often occurs with the knee in flexion and subjected to a twisting mechanism. The LCL attaches to the fibular head and acts to stabilize the proximal tibiofibular joint when the collateral ligament is tight in knee extension. On flexion, the collateral ligament is relatively relaxed, allowing the dislocation to occur given sufficient twisting force.

Ogden[61,62] classified proximal tibiofibular dislocations into three types based on direction of fibular displacement. Anterolateral dislocation is the most common, followed by posteromedial, and superior. Subluxation of the joint can also occur in ligamentously lax individuals, including those with connective tissue disorders, such as Ehlers-Danlos syndrome. The diagnosis is frequently missed when it occurs in conjunction with other major knee trauma. Comparison radiographic views of the opposite knee are helpful when the diagnosis is in doubt. Plain films are generally sufficient (Fig. 23-60). Patients complain of pain and tenderness localized to the proximal fibula that is increased with movement of the fibular head. Flexing the knee helps to relax the collateral ligament to allow stressing the joint.

Management involves closed reduction of the dislocation by applying manual pressure over the fibular head in a direction that will achieve reduction. Flexion of the knee is beneficial to relax the collateral ligament, and muscle relaxation is often necessary. An audible snap is often heard on reduction. Non–weight bearing with crutches for 2 weeks is followed by eventual return to full activities, usually by 6 weeks. Rarely, closed reduction is not possible or cannot be maintained. In these cases, surgical management may include internal fixation with Kirschner wires or resection of the proximal fibular head. Arthrodesis can lead to later ankle discomfort and is not generally recommended. Peroneal nerve palsies can occur in roughly 5% of patients, especially in cases of posterior fibular dislocation. Resection of the fibular head can be helpful in patients with peroneal nerve symptoms.[95]

REFERENCES

1. Abbott LC, Saunders JB, Bosh FC, Anderson CE: Injuries to the ligaments of the knee joint. J Bone Joint Surg 16A:503, 1944.
2. Aglietti P, Buzzi R, Insall JN: Disorders of the patellofemoral joint. In Insall JI (ed): Surgery of the Knee, 2nd ed. New York, Churchill-Livingston, 1993.
3. Aglietti P, Insall JN, Cerulli G: Patella pain and incongruence. Clin Orthop 176:217, 1983.
4. Aichroth PM: Osteochondritis dissecans of the knee. J Bone Joint Surg 53B:440, 1971.
5. Aichroth PM: Osteochondritis dissecans. In Insall JN ed: Surgery of the Knee, 2nd ed. New York, Churchill-Livingston, 1993.
6. Alicea J, Scuderi GS: Knee dislocations. In Tria F (ed): Ligaments of the Knee. New York, Churchill-Livingston, 1995, pp 261–274.
7. Belzer JP, Cannon WD Jr: Meniscus tears: Treatment in the stable and unstable knee. J AAOS 1:41, 1993.
8. Bono J, Haas S, Scuderi GR: Traumatic maladies of the extensor mechanism. In Scuderi GR (ed): The Patella. New York, Springer Verlag, 1995.
9. Brenn JJ: Avulsion injuries of the posterior cruciate ligament. Clin Orthop 18:157, 1960.
10. Brittberg M, Lindahl A, Nilsson A, et al: Treatment of deep cartilage defects in the knee with autologous chondrocyte transplantation. N Engl J Med 331:889, 1994.
11. Bullock D, Scuderi GR: Getting your patient back in action after a meniscal tear. J Musc Med 11(5):68, 1994.
12. Burk DL, Mitchell DG, Rifkin MD, et al: Recent advances in the MRI of the knee. Radiol Clin North Am 28(1):379, 1990.
13. Burks RT, Butorac RB: Injuries and diseases of articular surfaces of the knee. In Scott WN (ed): The Knee. St. Louis, Mosby, 1994.
14. Cannon WD Jr, Vittori JM: The incidence of healing in arthroscopic meniscal repairs in ACL reconstructed knees versus stable knees. Am J Sports Med 20:176, 1992.

15. Cannon WD Jr, Vittori JM: Meniscal repair. In Aichroth PM, Cannon WD Jr (eds): Knee Surgery: Current Practice. New York, Raven Press, 1992.
16. Clancy WG, Shelbourne KD, Zoellner GB, et al: Treatment of knee joint instability secondary to rupture of the posterior cruciate ligament. J Bone Joint Surg 65A:310, 1983.
17. Clancy WG: Repair and reconstruction of the posterior cruciate ligament. In Chapman MW (ed): Operative Orthopedics 3:1651, 1988.
18. Clendenin MB, DeLee JC, Hechman JD: Interstitial tears of the posterior cruciate ligament of the knee. Orthopedics 3:764, 1980.
19. Cooper DE, Warren RF, Warner JP: The posterior cruciate ligament and posterolateral structures of the knee: Anatomy, function, and patterns of injury. American Academy of Orthopedic Surgeons, Instructional Course Lectures, 40:249, 1991.
20. Daniel DM: Principles of knee ligament surgery. In Daniel DM, Akeson WH, O'Connor J (eds): Knee Ligaments: Structure, Function, Injury, and Repair. New York, Raven Press, 1990.
21. Daniel DM, Fithian DC: Current concepts: Indications for anterior cruciate ligament surgery. Arthroscopy 10(4):434, 1994.
22. Daniel DM, Stone ML, Dobson BE, et al: Fate of the ACL-injured patient. Am J Sports Med 22:632, 1994.
23. Drucker MM, Wynne GF: Avulsion of the posterior cruciate ligament from its femoral attachment. J Trauma 15:616, 1975.
24. Fanelli GC: Posterior cruciate ligament injuries in trauma patients. Arthroscopy 9(3):291, 1993.
25. Fanelli GC, Giannotti BF, Edson CJ: The posterior cruciate ligament, arthroscopic evaluation and treatment. Arthroscopy 10(6):673, 1994.
26. Feagin JA, Lambert KL, Cunningham RR, et al: Consideration of the anterior cruciate ligament injury in skiing. Clin Orthop 216:13, 1987.
27. Finsterbush A, Frankl U, Matan Y, Mann G: Secondary damage to the knee after isolated injury of the anterior cruciate ligament. Am J Sports Med 18: 47, 1990.
28. Fischer SP, Fox JM, DelPizzo W, et al: Accuracy of diagnosis from MRI of the knee. J Bone Joint Surg 73A:2, 1991.
29. Fox JM, DelPizzo W (eds): The Patellofemoral Joint. New York, McGraw-Hill, 1991.
30. Fulkerson JP: Patellofemoral pain disorders: Evaluation and management. J AAOS 2:124, 1994.
31. Galway RD, Beaupre A, MacIntosh DL: Pivot shift: A clinical sign of symptomatic anterior cruciate insufficiency. J Bone Joint Surg 54B:763, 1972.
32. Gollehon DL, Torzilli PA, Warren RF: The role of the posterolateral and cruciate ligaments in the stability of the human knee. J Bone Joint Surg 69A: 233, 1987.
33. Graf BK, Cook DA, DeSmet AA, Keene JS: Bone bruises on MRI evaluation of ACL injuries. Am J Sports Med 21:220, 1993.
34. Green NE, Allen BL: Vascular injuries associated with dislocation of the knee. J Bone Joint Surg 59A:236, 1977.
35. Gross ML, Grover JS, Bassett LW, Seeger LL, Finerman GA: Magnetic resonance imaging of the posterior cruciate ligament. Am J Sports Med 20:732, 1992.
36. Guan Y, Butler DL, Dormer SG, et al: Contribution of ACL subunits during anterior drawer in the human knee. Trans Orthop 16:589, 1991.
37. Hewson GF, Mendini RA, Wang JB: Prophylactic knee bracing in college football. Am J Sports Med 14:262, 1986.
38. Indelicato PA: Isolated MCL injuries in the knee. J AAOS 3:9, 1995.
39. Indelicato PA: Non-operative treatment of complete tears of the medial collateral ligament of the knee. J Bone Joint Surg 65A:323, 1983.
40. Ireland J, Trickey EL, Stoker DJ: Arthroscopy and arthrography of the knee. J Bone Joint Surg 62B:3, 1980.
41. Irvine GB, Glasgow MMS: The natural history of the meniscus in anterior cruciate insufficiency. J Bone Joint Surg 74B:403, 1992.
42. Johnson D, Warner JJP: Diagnosis for ACL surgery. Clin Sports Med 12:671, 1993.
43. Johnson RJ, Beynnon BD, Nichols CE, Renstrom PA: Current concepts review: The treatment of injuries of the ACL. J Bone Joint Surg 74A:140, 1992.
44. Kannus P, Bergfeld J, Jarvinen M, et al: Injuries to the posterior cruciate ligament of the knee. Sports Med 12:110, 1991.
45. Keller PM, Shelbourne KD, McCarroll JR, Rettig AC: Non-operatively treated isolated posterior cruciate ligament injuries. Am J Sports Med 12:132, 1993.
46. Kennedy JC: Complete dislocation of the knee joint. J Bone Joint Surg 45A:889, 1963.
47. Kennedy JC, Hawkins RJ, Willis RB, Danylchuck KD: Tension studies of human knee ligaments. J Bone Joint Surg 58A:350, 1976.
48. Kornick J, Trefelner E, McCarthy S, et al: Meniscal abnormalities in the asymptomatic population at magnetic resonance imaging. Radiology 177:463, 1990.
49. Lance EP, Paulos LE: Knee bracing. J Am Acad Orthop Surg 2:281, 1994.
50. Larson RL, Taillon M: Anterior cruciate ligament insufficiency: principles of treatment. J AAOS 2:26, 1994.
51. Lehnert M, Eisenschenk A, Zellner A: Results of conservative treatment of partial tears of the ACL. Int Orthop 17:219, 1993.

52. Lee HG: Avulsion fractures of the tibial attachments of the cruciate ligaments. J Bone Joint Surg 19:460, 1937.
53. Maurer SS, Carlin G, Butters R, Scuderi GR: Rehabilitation of the patellofemoral joint. In Scuderi GR (ed): The Patella. New York, Springer Verlag, 1995.
54. McCauley TR, Moses M, Kier R, et al: Magnetic resonance diagnosis of tears of the anterior cruciate ligament of the knee. Am J Radiol 162:115, 1994.
55. McCoy GF, Hannon DG, Barr RJ, Templeton J: Vascular injury associated with low velocity dislocation of the knee joint. J Bone Joint Surg 69B:285, 1987.
56. Merchant AC: Clinical classification of patellofemoral disorders. Sports Med Arthroscopy 2:26–27, 1994.
57. Miller MD, Cooper DE, Warner JJP: The Knee. Review of Sports Medicine and Arthroscopy. Philadelphia, WB Saunders, 1995.
58. Noyes FR, Mooar P, Matthews DS, Butler DL: The symptomatic anterior cruciate deficient knee. J Bone Joint Surg 65A:154, 1983.
59. Noyes FR, Mooar P, Moorman III CT: Partial tear of the ACL: Progression to complete ligament deficiency. J Bone Joint Surg 71B:825, 1989.
60. Noyes FR, Mooar LA, Moorman III CT, McGinniss GH: Partial tears of the anterior cruciate ligament. J Bone Joint Surg 71B:825, 1989.
61. Ogden JA: Subluxation and dislocation of the proximal tibio-fibular joint. J Bone Joint Surg 56A:145, 1974.
62. Ogden JA: Subluxation of the proximal fibula. Radiology 105:547, 1972.
63. Outerbridge RE: The etiology of chondromalacia patella. J Bone Joint Surg 43B:752, 1961.
64. Palmer I: On the injuries to the ligaments of the knee joint. Acta Chir Scand Suppl 81:3, 1938.
65. Parolie JM, Bergfeld JA: Long-term results of nonoperative treatment of isolated posterior cruciate ligament injuries in the athlete. Am J Sports Med 14:35, 1986.
66. Pavlov H: Radiographic examination. In Insall JN (ed): Surgery of the Knee, 2nd ed. New York, Churchill Livingston, 1993.
67. Pringle JH: Avulsion of the spine of the tibia. Ann Surg 46:169, 1907.
68. Quinlan AG, Sharrard WJW: Posterolateral dislocation of the knee with capsular interposition. J Bone Joint Surg 40B:660, 1958.
69. Raunest J, Hotzinger H, Burrig KF: MRI and arthroscopy in the detection of meniscal degenerations: Correlation of arthroscopy and MRI with histology findings. Arthroscopy 10:634, 1994.
70. Scuderi GR: The femoral intercondylar roof angle: Radiographic and MRI measurement. Am J Knee Surg 6:10, 1993.
71. Scuderi GR: Patellar and quadriceps tendon disruptions. In Scott WN (ed): The Knee. St. Louis, Mosby, 1994.
72. Scuderi GR: Radiographic assessment of patella length, thickness and height. Med Sci Sports Exerc 24(Suppl 5):147, 1992.
73. Scuderi GR: The segond fracture. Am J Knee Surg 4(1):32, 1991.
74. Scuderi GR: The surgical management of patellar instability. In Scuderi GR (ed): The Patella. New York, Springer Verlag, 1995.
75. Scuderi GR: Surgical treatment for patellar instability. Orthop Clin North Am 23:619, 1992.
76. Scuderi GR, Scott WN: Classification of ligament injuries. In Insall JN (ed): Surgery of the Knee. New York, Churchill Livingston, 1993.
77. Scuderi GR, Scott WN, Insall JN: Knee injuries. In Rockwood CA, Green DP (eds): Fractures in Adults, 4th ed. Philadelphia, JB Lippincott, 1996, pp 2001–2126.
78. Scuderi GR, Scuderi DM: Patellar fragmentation. Am J Knee Surg 7:125, 1994.
79. Shelbourne KD, Patel DV: Management of combined injuries of the anterior cruciate and medial collateral ligaments. J Bone Joint Surg 77A:800, 1995.
80. Shelbourne KD, Porter DA, Clingman JA, et al: Low velocity knee dislocations. Orthop Rev 20:995, 1991.
81. Shields L, Mitral M, Cave EF: Complete dislocation of the knee: Experience at the Massachusetts General Hospital. J Trauma 9:192, 1969.
82. Sisto DJ, Warren RF: Complete knee dislocation. Clin Orthop 198:94, 1985.
83. Stanish WD, Curwin S, Rubinovich RM: Tendonitis: The analysis and treatment for running. Clin Sports Med 4:21, 1985.
84. Stanish WO, Rubinovich M, Armason T, Lapenskie G: Posterior cruciate ligament tears in wrestlers. Can J Appl Sports Sci 4:173, 1986.
85. Torg JS, Barton TM, Pavlov H, et al: Natural history of the PCL deficient knee. Clin Orthop 246:208, 1989.
86. Torg JS, Conrad W, Kalen V: Clinical diagnosis of ACL instability in the athlete. Am J Sports Med 4:84, 1976.
87. Toriso T: Avulsion fracture of the tibial attachment of the posterior cruciate ligament. Clin Orthop 143:107, 1979.
88. Treiman GS, Yellin AE, Weaver FA, et al: Examination of the patient with a knee dislocation: The case for selective arteriography. Arch Surg 127:1056, 1992.
89. Trickey EL: Rupture of the posterior cruciate ligament of the knee. J Bone Joint Surg 50B:334, 1968.
90. Veltri DM, Warren RF: Isolated and combined posterior cruciate ligament injuries. J Am Acad Orthop Surg 1:67, 1993.

91. Vigorita VJ, Morgan D: Pathology of the patella. In Scuderi GR (ed): The Patella, 2nd ed. New York, Springer Verlag, 1995.
92. Warner JJP, Warren RF, Cooper DE: Management of acute anterior cruciate ligament injuries. AAOS Inst Course Lect XL:201, 1991.
93. Warren RF: Menisectomy and repair in the ACL deficient patient. Clin Orthop 252:55, 1990.
94. Warren RF, Friederich NF, Muller W, et al: Degenerative arthritis of the knee following anterior cruciate ligament injury. Orthop Trans 13(3):546, 1989.
95. Windsor RE: Knee dislocations. In Insall JN (ed): Surgery of the Knee, 2nd ed. New York, Churchill Livingstone, 1993.
96. Windsor RE: Soft tissue disorders. In Insall JN (ed): Surgery of the Knee, 2nd ed. New York, Churchill Livingstone, 1993.
97. Woztzs EM: The ACL Deficient Knee, Rosemont, IL, AAOS Monograph Series, 1994.
98. Yormak JH, Scuderi GR: Physical examination of the knee. In Tria F (ed): Ligaments of the Knee. New York, Churchill Livingstone, 1995.
99. Zappala F, Taffel C, Scuderi GR: Rehabilitation of the patellofemoral joint. Orthop Clin North Am 23:555, 1992.
100. Zarins B, Adams M: Knee injuries in sports. N Engl J Med 318:950, 1988.

24 The Leg

Edward C. Brown III and Michael A. Kelly

The leg is a common site of acute and chronic sports-related injuries. Many of these clinical entities are either overuse disorders or the result of training errors. Patients with these problems are often first seen in the primary care or sports medicine specialty setting. It is relevant, therefore, for any clinician who evaluates athletes to be familiar with the more common problems.

Common clinical conditions in the leg causing symptoms in athletes include acute compartment syndrome, chronic exertional compartment syndrome, medial tibial stress syndrome (shin splints), stress fractures, and musculotendinous disruptions. The differential diagnosis also includes tendinitis, popliteal artery entrapment syndrome, arterial occlusion, effort-induced venous thrombosis, peripheral nerve entrapment syndromes, and radiculopathies.[31,128]

Although some of these conditions require surgery, knowledge of proper training techniques is essential to both prevent and rehabilitate many of these injuries. The basics of injury prevention include maintenance of a consistent baseline conditioning program, gradual increases in activity, and appropriate shoe wear. In addition, an adequate warm-up period and stretching prior to activity is important, especially in the aging population.

COMPARTMENT SYNDROME

Compartment syndrome is a condition of increased pressure within a closed osseofascial space that causes reduced blood flow and tissue perfusion in that space and leads to ischemic pain and potentially irreversible damage to the soft-tissue contents of the closed space.[64,102] The late sequelae of an undiagnosed or untreated compartment syndrome may include myonecrosis and scarring, decreased nerve and extremity function, and permanent deformity. Clinical recognition of compartment syndrome is attributed to Richard von Volkmann based on his 1881 description of post-traumatic irreversible forearm contractures, which he believed to be of ischemic origin.[133] The leg is the most common site for compartment syndrome in the body and this condition is more common in the anterior and deep posterior compartments where there are less compliant fascial boundaries (Fig. 24-1).[96]

Compartment syndrome can be classified as acute or chronic, and each has different etiologies and presentations. Acute compartment syndrome (ACS) is a well-known clinical entity that requires immediate fasciotomy to avoid irreversible tissue damage. It is characterized by progressive severe pain that does not resolve with rest and is exacerbated by passive stretch of the muscles. Acute compartment syndrome is typically induced by trauma and occurs most commonly after tibial fracture or muscle injury.[3] Other causes of ACS include reperfusion or post-ischemic swelling, arterial injury, limb compression, constrictive dressings or casts, burns, gunshot wounds, and snakebites.[138]

Chronic exertional compartment syndrome (CECS) is an exertional phenomenon involving intermittent compartment pressure elevation with exercise. CECS is often recurrent in nature and occurs with exercise-induced increases in muscle volume in an otherwise healthy compartment. It is typically seen in athletes such as long-distance runners and military recruits whose exercise level elevates the intramuscular pressure to a point that the tissues in the affected compartment become tight and painful, thereby preventing further activity.[31] The pain resolves quickly after rest, and there are usually no permanent sequelae in the affected tissue.

Anatomy

The leg is divided into four fascial compartments: the anterior, lateral, superficial posterior, and deep posterior compartments. These anatomic spaces are bounded by dense fascia and osseous borders. Pertinent anatomy of each compartment includes the major neurovascular structures within each compartment (see Fig. 24-1). Davey et al.[24] described a fifth separate compartment containing the posterior tibialis muscle. Each of the four major compartments contains a sensory nerve that may be affected by elevated compartment pressures. The deep peroneal nerve lies in the anterior compartment; the superficial peroneal nerve lies in the lateral compartment; the posterior tibial nerve lies in the deep posterior compartment; and the sural nerve lies in the superficial posterior compartment. Understanding the anatomy and contents of each compartment is critical for proper diagnosis and treatment of affected compartments. Evaluation for compartment syndrome includes localizing symptoms to the involved muscles and an assessment of the distal sensory component of the involved nerve.

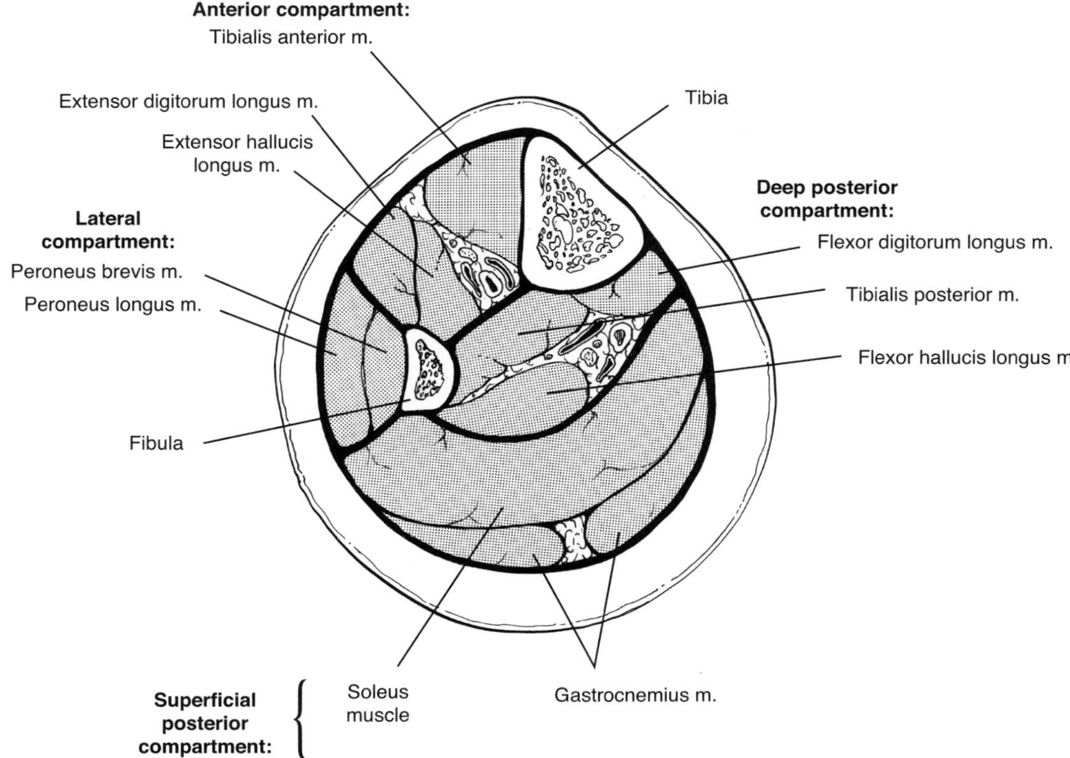

FIGURE 24-1. Four compartments of the leg: transverse section through the middle section of the leg. (Redrawn from Mubarek SJ, Ownes CA: Double incision fasciotomy of the leg for decompression in compartment syndromes. J Bone Joint Surg 59A:184, 1977.)

ACUTE COMPARTMENT SYNDROME

Clinical Evaluation

Acute compartment syndrome is nonreversible by definition because compartment pressure remains elevated above physiologic limits. The diagnosis of acute compartment syndrome may be subtle and clinical suspicion is critical. The diagnosis, while clinical, may be supported by measurements of compartment pressure.

In the athlete, acute compartment syndrome is most commonly seen with tibial fracture and muscle rupture.[3] Rarely, an acute compartment syndrome has been reported with extreme exertional overuse, ankle fractures or sprains, crush injuries, and with medical illnesses including influenza B virus and sickle cell trait.[1,10,22,48,80,92] The patient presents with a history of injury, progressive severe and unrelenting pain in the involved compartment, diffuse firmness with exquisite tenderness running the length of the involved compartment, and exacerbation of pain with passive stretch of the involved muscle group. Often, the pain described is out of proportion to the injury and is not relieved with rest, immobilization, ice, elevation, or narcotics. Pain with passive stretch is a hallmark of ischemia. One clinical study found that elevation of compartment pressure to 30 to 40 mm Hg caused significant patient discomfort and pain with passive stretching.[111]

Historically, compartment syndrome was associated with "the five P's": pain, pallor, paresthesias, paralysis, and pulselessness. However, these may be misleading.[94] The "true P's" of compartment syndrome include pain out of proportion, pain with passive stretch, a pink extremity, palpable pulses, and in later phases, paresthesias and paresis (slight or partial paralysis). Early, the most reproducible finding is severe pain. Other early signs, such as pain on passive stretch and dysesthesias in the involved compartment's neural component are variable, yet may herald an impending compartment syndrome. Paresthesias and paralysis are late clinical findings and may suggest impending compartment necrosis. The arterial examination is most often normal, eliminating any large vessel occlusive process. Abnormal pulses or pallor in the presence of ischemia suggest an arterial inflow injury or disruption.

Pathophysiology

The common feature of compartment syndrome is elevated pressure within the osseofascial compartment that causes ischemia and tissue necrosis.[138] When viewed as a closed space, pressure within the compartment can be elevated by two separate processes; either by increasing the internal volume, such as acute hemorrhage or muscle hypertrophy, or by extrinsic compression, such as a constrictive cast. Clinical and laboratory studies have established basics of the pathophysiology. Each osseofascial compartment has its own unique pressure–volume relationship. Because bone and fascia are relatively inelastic, small increases in intracompartmental volume may lead to large increases of intracompartmental pressure.

It is critical to understand that the development of a compartment syndrome depends on multiple factors. These factors include tissue compartment pressure, duration of elevated pressure, systemic blood pressure, especially diastolic pressure, muscle status, and comorbidities.[138]

The development of a compartment syndrome depends on the magnitude of pressure elevation and the duration of increased pressure. A compartment syndrome can occur rapidly with significant pressure elevations or have a gradual onset with prolonged moderate elevations of pressure. Interference with muscle perfusion and nerve conduction becomes progressively severe with the duration of applied pressure.[104] In the earliest phases, ischemia is associated with pain, but in the later stages, ischemia causes tissue necrosis. Broad pressure–time thresholds for permanent injury are difficult to define, because each musculoskeletal tissue has its own sensitivity. In addition, the antecedent condition of the tissue and comorbid factors, such as muscle trauma and hypotension, also affect subsequent tissue damage from ischemia.

In experimental injuries that produced complete ischemia, skeletal muscle remained electrically responsive for up to 3 hours and survived for as long as 4 hours without irreversible damage. Total ischemia of 8 hours' duration produced complete irreversible changes whereas variable results occurred after 6 hours of total ischemia. Similarly, peripheral nerves conducted impulses for 1 hour after the onset of total ischemia and could survive for 4 hours with only neuropraxic damage.[137] Animal studies have shown that loss of nerve conduction occurs within 2 hours after the onset on ischemia.[13] After 8 hours of total ischemia, axonotmesis was usual and irreversible changes in the nerve commonly occurred.[137]

Tissue viability depends on capillary perfusion. In normotensive humans, normal resting compartment pressures range from 0 to 14 mm Hg and capillary blood pressure ranges between 20 and 30 mm Hg.[85,138] Elevation of interstitial fluid pressure above 30 mm Hg in a normotensive individual subsequently results in progressive decrease in capillary perfusion.[137] This threshold marks the beginning of capillary hypoperfusion and may not reflect the threshold for overt compartment necrosis. Tissue pressure levels greater than 30 to 40 mm Hg are associated with microvascular disturbances that can lead to muscle and nerve ischemia.[83] Muscle necrosis may ensue when tissue pressure elevates to 40 to 50 mm Hg.[135,136] However, other investigators found that high intramuscular pressure may be tolerated without permanent adverse sequelae. Matsen et al.[64] suggested that the critical pressure threshold in patients was greater than 45 mm Hg. Canine studies have demonstrated that peroneal nerve conduction begins to change after 8 hours of pressure elevation to 30 mm Hg in the anterior compartments of the leg.[103,104] If higher pressures are applied, these conduction velocity changes are seen sooner. The appearance of paresthesia in the distribution of the deep peroneal nerve has been documented with pressure greater than 30 mm Hg.[134]

Alternately, the degree of relative pressure difference between compartment pressure and perfusion pressure may be essential. Experimentally measured terminal arterial pressure is equal to diastolic pressure, prompting some to use diastolic pressure as the critical measurement.[139] Microvascular ischemia has been demonstrated to occur in healthy skeletal muscle when tissue pressure is elevated to within 10 mm Hg of diastolic blood pressure.[42,45,61,135,136,137] The presence of muscle injury or trauma adversely affects muscle's ability to tolerate ischemia. As opposed to healthy muscle, tissue perfusion has been demonstrated to be significantly reduced in injured tissue, causing ischemia and ischemic changes when tissue pressure is elevated to within 20 mm Hg of diastolic blood pressure.[138]

More recently, a series of physiological experiments by Heppenstall et al.[45–47] suggested that fasciotomy should be considered whenever compartment pressure is within 40 mm Hg of mean arterial pressure. For a normotensive patient with blood pressure of 120/80 mm Hg, the mean arterial pressure is 103 mm Hg, suggesting a threshold tissue pressure of 63 mm Hg prior to fasciotomy. For a hypotensive patient with blood pressure of 90/60 mm Hg, the mean arterial pressure is 80 mm Hg, suggesting a threshold tissue pressure of 40 mm Hg. This principle reflects prior experimental and human studies that have shown individuals with higher diastolic blood pressures are able to withstand higher tissue pressure without ischemic damage compared to those with lower diastolic blood pressures.[138]

Treatment

Surgical consultation should be obtained to assist in the evaluation and management of these patients. Following evaluation of a patient for acute compartment syndrome, one of three treatment options will be appropriate: observation and supportive measures, compartment pressure measurement, or surgical fasciotomy.

In some cases, the clinical picture is so clear that the diagnosis may be made on clinical grounds alone. In these extremely clear cases, it is reasonable to proceed directly to surgical decompression by fasciotomy. It is more common that the clinical picture is suspicious for compartment syndrome. The clinical estimation of intracompartmental pressure is unreliable. Objective measurement of intracompartmental pressure is very helpful for documentation and essential for clinical decision making.

There continues to be some controversy in establishing a maximum tolerable compartment pressure. This reflects the large degree of individual variation and tolerance to elevated pressure. It should be kept in mind that progressive elevation of compartment pressure may be a more reliable sign of an evolving compartment syndrome than any absolute level of increased pressure. Two basic definitions of critical pressure have emerged from the laboratory and clinical studies: an absolute value and a relative value.[134] As described in the pathophysiology section, laboratory and clinical studies suggest the presence of compartment syndrome with ischemia and potential tissue necrosis when intracompartmental pressure exceeds an absolute value of 30 mm Hg (CP > 30 mm Hg) or a derived value within 20 mm Hg of diastolic blood pressure (CP > DBP – 20 mm Hg).

Today, handheld pressure monitors with an interchangeable side-port needle attached to a syringe plunger mechanism are widely available. The handheld monitors have gained clinical acceptance over previously described techniques with needles or wick catheters because of their accuracy and ease of use. The advantages of these devices are that they are totally self-contained, extremely portable, and very simple to use (Fig. 24-2). These units have been shown to be superior to prior needle techniques and comparable to the more cumbersome wick catheter techniques.[57,82,106] Uliasz et al.[129] found Whitesides' simple needle technique was less consistent and indicated higher pressures by 15 to 20 mm Hg than those obtained with a wick catheter or side-port needles.

When a fracture is present, needle location relative to the fracture is important. In one study, compartment pressures were measured at varying distances from the fracture. The highest pressures in the anterior and deep posterior compartments were found adjacent to the fracture and dropped significantly when measured farther than 5 cm from the fracture.[43]

In some cases of borderline ACS, other variables may be controlled that could reverse ischemia and pressure cycle. Such variables include elevation of systemic blood pressure in the hypotensive patient and facilitation of edema reduction with a venous foot pump. Other nonoperative measures that may have merit include elevation of the limb to the level of the heart, application of ice to cool the extremity, and possibly supplemental oxygen.

When performing fasciotomies for acute compartment syndrome, long skin incisions are mandatory. Cohen et al.[21] studied eight patients with compartment syndrome who underwent surgical decompression while compartment pressures were monitored. Initial decompression was through a skin incision 8 cm in length. The pressure remained above 30 mm Hg in 9 compartments of the eight patients and it dropped below 30 mm Hg only after the length of the skin incision was increased to 16 cm.

When the decompression is performed 6 to 8 hours after the onset of elevated pressure, debridement of necrotic tissue may be necessary to prevent infection. In this instance, the wounds after decompression are left open and managed with sterile dressings and a large, nonrestrictive dressing should be applied. A simple posterior leg splint may provide support and comfort for the leg. Constrictive external dressings or a cast should be avoided. Following surgical decompression, the leg is elevated until swelling subsides. After 3 to 7 days of elevation, the swelling typically subsides substantially to allow delayed primary closure, although split thickness skin grafting may be required.

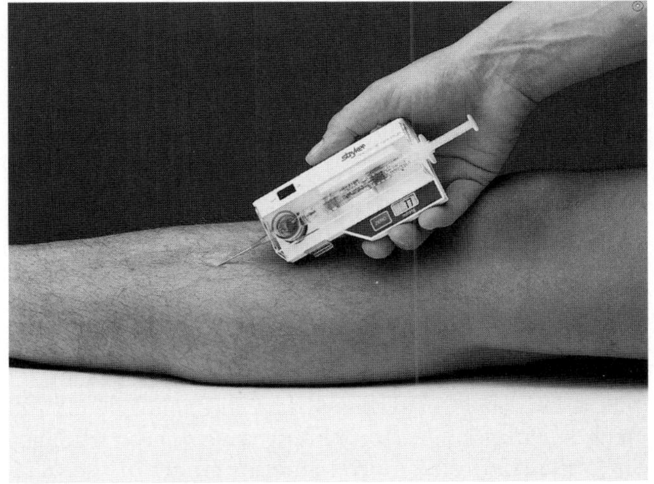

FIGURE 24-2. Stryker STIC pressure monitor device. (Reprinted by permission of Stryker Corporation.)

CHRONIC EXERTIONAL COMPARTMENT SYNDROME

Clinical Evaluation

Chronic exertional compartment syndrome is a reversible event. The typical presentation is a runner who presents with leg pain brought on by exercise and relieved with rest. Initially, the patient notices pain that begins as a dull ache during exertion. If the patient continues to train, the pain increases to the point that the activity must be stopped. As the process progresses, symptoms may linger for an increasing period of time, even into the next day. Another characteristic of CECS is that the onset and degree of pain is often predictable and reproducible, occurring at a similar time during the exercise activity. Patients experience fullness or cramping in the affected compartment during exercise. They may also experience transient numbness and tingling, or weakness in the motor and sensory distribution of involved compartments due to nerve compression secondary to swelling. The development of a foot slap during exercise, for example, suggests involvement of the anterior compartment. Approximately 80% of cases involve either the anterior or deep posterior compartments.[24,93] Bilateral involvement has been reported in up to 82% of patients.[26]

The physical examination of the leg at rest is typically normal. Muscle atrophy and decreased circumference measurements may be present of the condition is unilateral. Examination after exercise may reveal tenderness and fullness of the involved muscle group and there may be an associated decreased sensation or tingling in the distal leg. The presence of a fascial defect may be found at the junction of the middle and distal thirds of the leg and a Tinel's sign occasionally may be present at this site.

Pathophysiology

The exact pathophysiology of CECS is not completely known. During strenuous exercise, muscle fibers can swell up to 20 times their resting size, leading to a 20% increase in muscle volume and weight.[33] Patients with CECS have increased intramuscular pressure at rest and higher than normal intramuscular pressure with exercise compared to normal individuals.[128] During exercise, Mubarek et al.[81] reported intracompartmental pressures to increase to 70 mm Hg in healthy patients and to over 100 mm Hg in patients with CECS. Patients with CECS also possess higher rates of fascial herniation than asymptomatic individuals. Of patients with CECS involving the legs, 39% to 46% have fascial defects over the anterolateral leg compared to asymptomatic individuals who have a <5% incidence.[33,123] These fascial hernias or defects are usually 1 to 2 cm^2 in size and occur near the intermuscular septum between the anterolateral compartments, often at the exit of the superficial peroneal nerve. The superficial peroneal nerve can be compressed by either the edge of the fascial defect or the muscle bulging through the defect. While fascial hernias are a contributing factor, fascial hernias are not present in all patients with CECS. It is likely that a combination of anatomic limitations contributes to the presence and severity of CECS.[96]

Treatment

The diagnosis of chronic exertional compartment pressure relies on objective measurement of compartment pressures, which are measured at rest and after provocative activity. The generally accepted guidelines for the diagnosis of chronic exertional compartment syndrome were established by Pedowitz et al.[93] and include any of the following: (1) a preexercise pressure more than 15 mm Hg, (2) a 1-minute postexercise pressure more than 30 mm Hg, and (3) a prolonged return of pressure to baseline levels with a postexercise pressure more than or equal to 20 mm Hg. Reliable pressure measurement within the deep posterior compartment is often challenging and Wiley et al.[140] proposed using ultrasound as a guide for catheter placement in the deep posterior compartment. Several noninvasive imaging modalities have been evaluated recently, including infrared spectroscopy, MRI scans, and SPECT scans, which may have a greater role in the future.[78,127,131]

Fasciotomy is the mainstay of treatment and is successful in relieving symptoms and allowing a full return to activities.[105,122] Nonoperative treatment is of little benefit for a patient who is unable to modify activities or desires a full return to athletic activity. The results of compartment releases indicate that most patients surgically treated for CECS in the leg experience a high level of pain relief and are satisfied with the results of surgery. Rates of improvement from 81% to 100% have been reported, with greater success rates for patients with anterolateral CECS as compared to deep posterior CECS.[26,33,50,101,105,110,122] Success of deep posterior compartment releases ranges from 50% to 65%.[50,101,105] CECS in the deep posterior compartment is multifactorial and a fasciotomy may not fully alleviate the pain.[50,101,105] Failure to fully release the tibialis posterior muscle (reported by some to be in its own osseofascial compartment), inappropriate diagnosis, and dense postoperative scar formation are believed to be causes of surgical failure when performing a deep posterior compartment fasciotomy.[101,105,110]

Postoperatively, athletes are allowed to bear weight as tolerated and are encouraged to return to aerobic activity using the leg as soon as possible. Most athletes will have returned to full activity within 3 to 12 weeks.[110,128] One recent study suggested that release of the anterior compartment fascia alone may be sufficient and may lead to a quicker recovery and return to sports than the traditional fascial releases of both the anterior and lateral compartments. Patients who underwent anterior compartment release alone returned to sports at an average of 8.1 weeks, but patients who underwent release of both the anterior and lateral compartments returned to sports at an average of 11.4 weeks.[109]

The incidence of perioperative complications ranges from 4.5% to 13% and includes hemorrhage, wound infection, nerve entrapment, artery injury, hematoma, seroma, lymphocele, peripheral cutaneous nerve injury, and deep venous thrombosis.[26,33,101,105,140] The recurrence of symptoms has been reported in 7% to 17% of patients after surgical release.[101,105,110]

MEDIAL TIBIAL STRESS SYNDROME

The term *shin splint syndrome* describes multiple clinical entities without clearly defining location or etiology. Since the shin refers to the anterior aspect of the tibia, the term shin splints has fallen out of favor. Medial tibial stress syndrome (MTSS) is a more appropriate term for this condition. The location of the activity-related pain is along the middle to distal aspect of the posteromedial tibia. Originally, MTSS was used as a nonspecific term referring to overuse syndromes of the leg. Tibial periostitis has been proposed as the more specific diagnosis to explain this clinical entity based on the pathophysiology. This led the AMA to more clearly define the syndrome and suggest the diagnosis be limited to musculotendinous inflammation, excluding stress fractures and ischemic disorders.[2]

Clinical Presentation

Medial tibial stress syndrome is common in distance runners and athletes involved in ballistic sports such as basketball or gymnastics. As with all overuse injuries, significant changes in activity, footwear, terrain, surface, mileage, or intensity of workouts can predispose to the development of medial tibial stress syndrome. This syndrome accounted for 13% of injuries in a runners' clinic and affected 4% of new military recruits.[4,51]

Patients with medial tibial stress syndrome present with gradually progressive and recurrent pain along the posteromedial border of the tibia at the junction of the middle and distal thirds. Initially, the pain is present at the beginning of a workout and may resolve or disappear while exercising, only to return during the cool-down phase. Rest alleviates the symptoms in the early phases of the syndrome. As the syndrome progresses, the pain may change from a dull ache to a more severe pattern and fail to resolve throughout the course of the activity. The process may progress to limit athletic activity and activities of daily living. Bilaterality may occur in 50% of cases.[25]

The physical examination is remarkable for diffuse tenderness along the posteromedial edge of the middle and distal thirds of the tibia. The tenderness is not well localized but extends over approximately one third of the length of the posteromedial tibia. This finding is important in distinguishing stress fractures, characterized by localized point tenderness. Minimal swelling may be present, but no specific mass is seen. The pain may be recreated with resistance to active plantar and dorsiflexion of the foot. The neurovascular examination of the extremity should be normal. In the unclear or vague clinical situation, compartment pressure measurements during activity may be performed to evaluate for the presence of chronic exertional compartment syndrome.

Plain films of the leg are usually normal. Occasionally, radiographs reveal findings including mild cortical hypertrophy of the posteriomedial cortex, a subperiosteal lucency and scalloping of the medial tibia, or a periosteal reaction. Serial radiographs may be helpful.

A bone scan can be the definitive study in the evaluation and diagnosis of medial tibial stress syndrome, particularly in the differentiation from stress fracture of the tibia.[60] The typical findings of three-phase radionuclide imaging involves increased uptake on the soft-tissue (phase III) images that can extend longitudinally from one-third to three-fourths the length of the tibia, which correlates with periostitis of the soleus muscle origins.[55] Radionuclide images (phase I) and blood pool (phase II) images are normal. In tibial stress fractures, uptake is usually well localized, intense, round and fusiform about the tibia, and can be positive on any or all three phases on the bone scan. Radionuclide activity rarely extends beyond 20% of the length of the tibia with stress fractures.[108] Complete scintigraphic evaluation should include medial and lateral views to localize the site of periostitis in medial tibial stress syndrome.

Magnetic resonance imaging can also be beneficial in diagnosing medial tibial stress syndrome. Magnetic resonance imaging findings of medial tibial periosteal edema and bone marrow edema have been reported in professional athletes with the clinical features of medial tibial stress syndrome (Fig. 24-3).[119]

Pathogenesis

The exact pathophysiology of MTSS has not been determined. The soleus and its dense fascia and the flexor digitorum longus muscle originate along the posteromedial border of the middle and distal thirds of the tibia. The tibial posterior muscle has a more proximal and lateral attachment to the tibia. The forces transmitted through these muscles with chronic overuse result in a

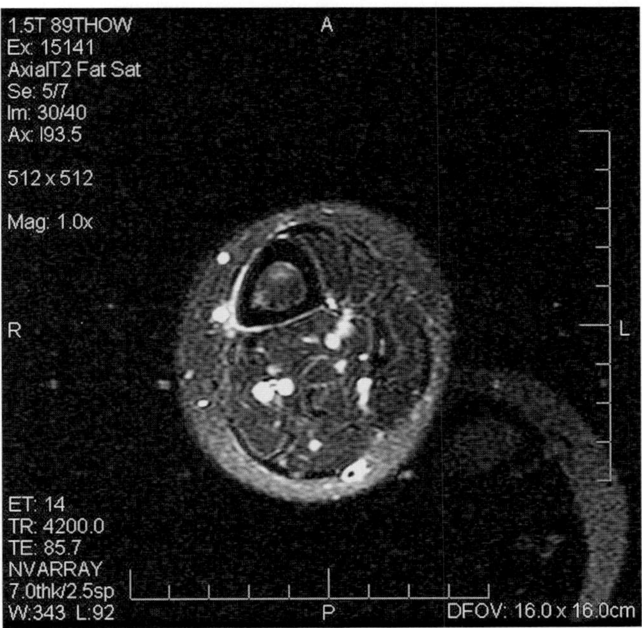

FIGURE 24-3. Axial T-2 magnetic resonance imaging study reveals periosteal edema and fluid findings consistent with medial tibial stress syndrome.

periosteal reaction from microtearing of Sharpey's fibers at the interdigitation of muscle and bone. The reactive inflammation causes a periostitis along this interface. Biopsies of periosteum at the site of tenderness have revealed conflicting results, with the presence of inflammation in one study[81] and its absence in another.[25] The acute phase may represent a periostitis whereas the chronic phase is referred to as a periostalgia, in which the periosteum is potentially disengaged from the cortex by either subperiosteal hemorrhage or avulsion.

Based on two cadaver studies, the soleus appears to be the most likely anatomic structure that contributes to MTSS. Michael et al.[68] found the site of increased tenderness and the site of increased activity on bone scans corresponded to the medial origin of the soleus in cadaveric dissections. The soleus muscle was found to have aponeurotic coverings both anteriorly and posteriorly that enveloped the muscle. The aponeurotic coverings fuse to form a strong fascial layer, referred to as the "soleus bridge," that attaches directly to the posteromedial border of the tibia for three-fourths of its length. Similarly, Beck and Osternig[9] dissected 50 cadaver legs to identify the structures that attach to the tibia at the site of MTSS symptoms. They found the soleus, the flexor digitorum longus, and the deep crural fascia attached most frequently at the site of pain in MTSS. In no specimen was the tibialis posterior muscle, first speculated to be the cause, attached in the vicinity of the clinical symptoms.

Intrinsic biomechanical properties in feet may predispose to the development of MTSS. These include excessive foot pronation, hindfoot and forefoot varus alignment, and heel cord tightness. Several authors have noted an association between excessive pronation of the foot with the development of MTSS.[66,117,132] With normal running and foot pronation, there is lengthening or eccentric contraction of the soleus. Excessive foot pronation leads to increased tension on the soleus and flexor digitorum longus fascial attachments to the tibia. Foot posture has also been shown to play a role in the occurrence of MTSS. Sommer and Vallentyne[117] found both hindfoot and forefoot varus alignment occurred more often in subjects with a history of MTSS than in controls. Finally, a tight heel cord has been observed in association with medial tibial stress syndrome.[132]

Treatment

Rest is the mainstay of treatment for MTSS. Abstaining from the offending activity from a few days to several weeks allows the inflammation at the musculofascial origins to subside. No management combinations have been shown to work better than rest alone. Andrisch et al.[4] prospectively treated 97 subjects with MTSS with five different treatment regimens. No treatment combination hastened recovery faster than rest alone. Although unproven in clinical trials, several treatments are reasonable adjuvants and may be beneficial. These include ice locally, heel cord stretching, anti-inflammatory medications, and orthotic support for excessive pronation. Rest need not be absolute, but rather individualized depending on the intensity, mileage, and terrain of the athlete's workout.

Recurrence of symptoms in MTSS is not uncommon and usually occurs within the first few weeks after return to activities. Training errors are usually responsible. A gradual resumption of running over a 4- to 6-week period is recommended.

Surgical treatment is reserved for patients in whom a prolonged course of conservative therapy has failed. Often these subjects have failed two or three well-supervised trials of rest and have been forced to abandon all physical activity. It is critical in these patients to exclude stress fractures and exertional compartment syndrome. Successful relief of pain has been reported by several authors after fasciotomy of the periosteum along the entire posteromedial aspect of the tibia at the site producing pain.[25,49,81]

STRESS FRACTURES OF THE TIBIA AND FIBULA

Stress fractures are overuse injuries of bone to the point of biomechanical failure and are also called fatigue fractures.[79] Originally described as "march fractures" in the metatarsals of German soldiers in the nineteenth century, stress fractures were not reported in athletes until 1939.[15,99] Tibial stress fractures may account for up to 73% of all stress fractures.[39,130] In athletes, the tibia is by far the most common site of involvement.[28,35,38,41,62,63] In one review of 320 athletes with stress fractures, the incidence of tibial stress fractures was nearly 50%, almost twice the incidence of the next most common stress fracture of the tarsal bones.[63] The reported incidence of tibial stress fracture in the general athletic population is less than 1%.[89] In runners, however, the incidence ranges from 4%[89] to more than 15%.[62] Women runners have been found to have up to 12 times more risk for stress fracture than men.[8,89] These stress fractures in runners frequently follow an increase in mileage or intensity of running. Bilateral stress fractures have been noted in 16.6% of cases.[63] The risk factor for men is not as clear as it is for women, however, general risk factors include increasing age, poor fitness, and non-black race.[72] Risk factors for women include a history of menstrual disturbance, narrow tibial width, lower bone density, lower lean leg mass, and a lower fat diet.[8,36,58] Hyperpronation and tibia vara also predispose the athlete to stress fractures.[62,124]

Stress fractures can occur in all regions of the tibia and may be multiple.[3,16,75,84,87] Tibial stress fractures have been reported in the proximal, central, and distal thirds of the tibia, and no one level is clearly more common than another.[58,59,73,74,88,89,91,107,124] However, tibial stress fractures are exceedingly more common on the compression side of the tibia (posteromedially) than the tension side of the tibia (anterolaterally).[23,114] Compression-type stress fractures tend to develop slowly, allowing ample time for bone remodeling and cortical hypertrophy. Tension-type stress fractures, particularly those occurring in the central third of the anterior cortex, are worrisome injuries as they are more likely to display poor healing and require surgical intervention.[11,40,59,90,91,98] The tension-type stress fracture is more commonly seen in athletes who engage in repetitive jumping activities such as gymnastics, basketball, and ballet.[59,98] These frequently problematic tibial stress fractures have the potential to progress to complete fractures.[40,98] Due to its radiographic appearance, these fractures are sometimes referred to as the "dreaded black line."

Stress fractures of the fibula represent the fifth most common site overall for athletes, with a reported incidence of 6.6%.[63] These fractures have findings similar to tibial stress fractures in the history, examination, and imaging evaluation. Fibular stress fractures are usually seen in long-distance runners and typically occur 3 to 7 cm above the lateral malleolus.[29] The usual site is just proximal to the inferior tibiofibular ligamens at the junction of the cortical and cancellous bone.[56] Devas and Sweetnam[29] postulated that the rhythmic contraction of the long toe flexors causes micromotion of the fibula as an underlying etiology for the stress fracture. Fibular stress fractures have also been reported in association with tibiofibular synostosis.[52] Proximal fibular stress fractures are rare.

Pathophysiology

Stress fractures in athletes result from excessive repetitive loads on the bone that cause an imbalance between bone resorption and bone formation. The exact mechanism responsible for initiating stress fractures remains unclear. Bone remodeling is initiated with a process of osteoclastic resorption followed by osteoblastic new bone formation. Normally, stress-induced remodeling leads to cortical hypertrophy and increased mineralization outpacing resorption. An abrupt increase in the duration, intensity, or frequency of physical activity without adequate periods of rest may lead to a relative escalation of osteoclastic activity.[54] Persistent, repetitive stress on weakened bone leads to overload and occurrence of a fracture. Speculation has also focused on the contribution of muscle in the occurrence of a stress fracture. One theory holds that excessive forces are transmitted to bone when the surrounding muscles become fatigued.[56,67] Alternatively, muscles may contribute to stress fractures by concentrating forces across a localized area of bone, thereby resulting in mechanical insults above the stress-bearing capacity of the bone.[121] In addition to local mechanical influences, systemic factors such as nutritional deficiencies, sleep deprivation, collagen abnormalities, and metabolic bone disorders may also contribute to the development of stress fractures.[12]

Clinical Evaluation

Typical of overuse syndromes, the athlete with a stress fracture presents with leg pain. The onset of pain is insidious over a period of days to weeks. Symptoms are aggravated by activity and relieved with rest. There may be a history of a change in training habits, including mileage, training surface, or inadequate shoe wear. In the early stages, pain occurs at the end of activity and is relieved with rest. As the process progresses, pain may be present with any impact activity including walking. Unlike medial tibial stress syndrome, a short period of rest does not relieve the symptoms. Early diagnosis is essential for avoiding complications and returning the athlete to play as soon as possible. Physical examination is remarkable for localized point tenderness along the tibia or fibula. There may also be a dense soft-tissue mass or local warmth associated with the callus. Hopping on the affected leg may elicit pain.

Results of radiographs may be normal in the first 2 to 3 weeks. Later radiographic changes may include periosteal new bone formation, subperiosteal resorption, endosteal thickening, cortical hypertrophy, or a radiolucent line (Figs. 24-4 and 24-5). However, these findings

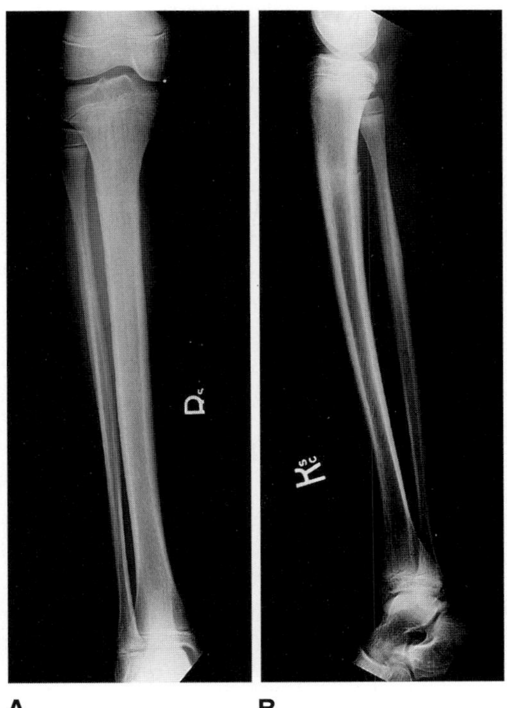

FIGURE 24-4. Anterioposterior (**A**) and lateral (**B**) radiographs demonstrating early presentation of stress fracture in proximal third of tibia. Subtle changes are noted.

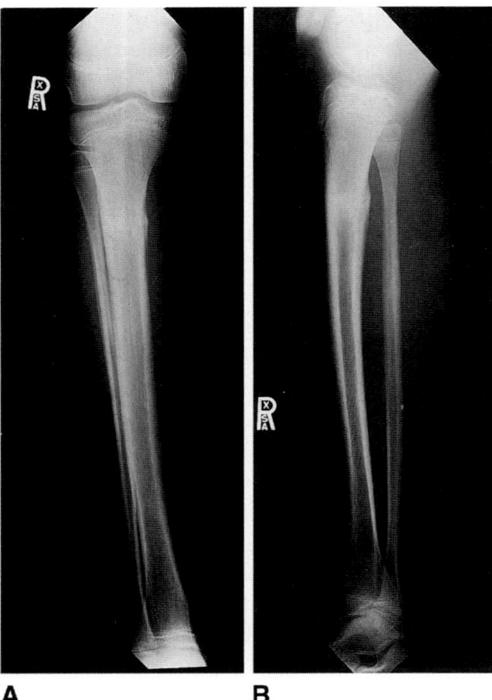

FIGURE 24-5. Anterioposterior (**A**) and lateral (**B**) radiographs of same tibial stress fracture four weeks after presentation. Fracture callus and periosteal new bone are present at fracture site.

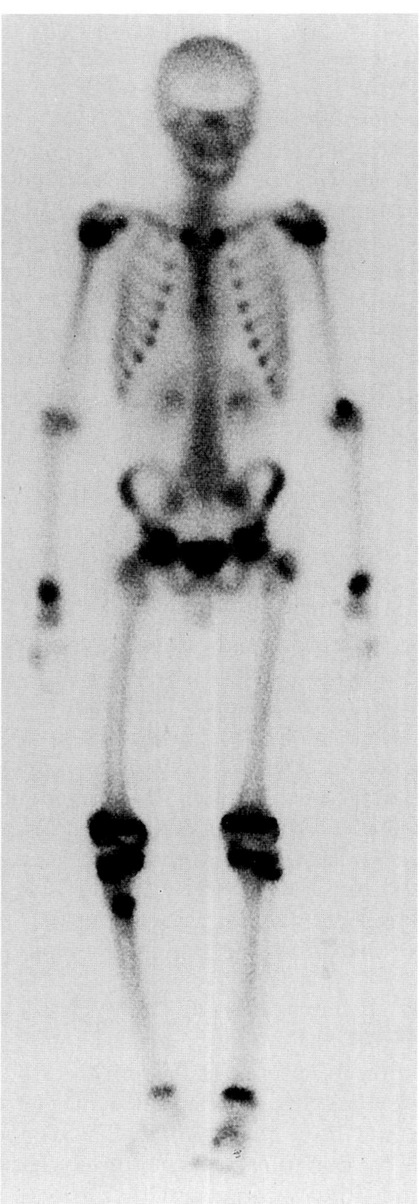

FIGURE 24-6. Bone scan depicting focal changes in proximal third (*right*) tibia consistent with tibial stress fracture.

are variable and can be subtle. Initially, only 50% of patients with stress fractures will have positive radiographic findings.[86,95] Tibial stress fractures are usually transverse, although longitudinal stress fractures of the tibia have been reported.[19,77,130] The initial radiographs for an anterior tibial cortex or tension-type stress fracture also are often normal. Subsequent radiographs, however, may reveal a characteristic Y-shaped or wedge-shaped defect in the anterior cortex with the open end directed anteriorly.[98] The appearance of this pattern is often referred to as the "dreaded black line."

The most sensitive indicator of a stress fracture is the three-phase technetium bone scan, which may be positive in 2 to 7 days after presentation. A negative bone scan virtually excludes the diagnosis of stress fracture. The three-phase bone scan is essentially 100% sensitive for stress fractures during the time of symptoms.[70,86,87,107,108,144] The bone scan reveals a well-localized area of intensely increased radionuclide activity (Fig. 24-6). Stress fractures may be positive in any or all phases of the bone scan. Positive findings on the delayed images may reflect stress remodeling or healing. When symptoms peak with increased hyperemia, bone turnover, and repair, results of the bone scan may be positive in all three phases.[59,108] The intensity of activity on delayed images typically decreases over 3 to 12 months, but it is important to recognize that minor abnormalities may persist for 12 to 18 months, even with resolution of symptoms and an athlete's return to activities.[84] A bone scan for an anterior tibial cortex stress fracture may demonstrate minimal activity indicating nonunion of the stress fracture.[11] Bone scans, unfortunately, have a low specificity, and multifocal synchronous areas of increased uptake are common in the lower extremity. Several reports have documented up to 50% of patients with a positive bone scan correlating to a specific site of pain will have increased uptake in other areas from accelerated bone remodeling.[62,69,84,87] The clinical significance of these findings is controversial. Some lesions may progress to a stress fracture, but other lesions resolve despite continuous training.[18] A brief period of rest is appropriate for these lesions. Finally, a bone scan is an excellent imaging technique for differentiating a stress fracture from medial tibial stress syndrome. In contrast to stress fractures, MTSS is identified by linear increased uptake along the posteromedial aspect of the middle and distal tibia that is present on delayed or phase III images only.

Magnetic resonance imaging (MRI) has emerged as an increasingly important imaging technique in the evaluation of stress fractures. Numerous recent studies have demonstrated the efficacy of MRI imaging in the evaluation of stress injuries to bone.[6,30,119,141] MRI allows depiction of abnormalities weeks before the development of radiographic abnormalities and has comparable sensitivity and superior specificity compared with radionuclide techniques for the detection of osseous abnormalities.[27,97] MRI is noninvasive, has no ionizing radiation, and is more rapidly performed than bone scintigraphy. MRI is effective in diagnosing the spectrum of soft-tissue and osseous injuries, including bone stress reactions, medial tibial stress syndrome (see Fig. 24-3), and stress fractures (Fig. 24-7). In most cases of tibial stress fractures, the fracture extends through a single cortex, with abnormal signal in the marrow cavity and in the adjacent soft tissue.[130] The most common pattern of a fatigue-type fracture is a fracture line that is low signal on all pulse sequences, surrounded by a larger, ill-defined zone of edema (see Fig. 24-7).

Treatment

Most tibial and fibular stress fractures can by treated by cessation of activity and a period of rest. The inciting impact activity must be stopped and a period of impact-free time to allow adequate repair and remodeling is required. Rates of delayed union or nonunion up to 10% may occur if these activities are not sufficiently curtailed.[89] Ideally, stress fractures are best managed through prevention. Training techniques should be reviewed because training errors are a common cause of stress fractures. There is usually complete resolution of compression-type tibial stress fractures after 6 to 8 weeks of relative rest. The return to full training activities may take 3 months.

An effective treatment regimen for the more common posteromedial compression-type tibial stress fracture is a two-phase protocol.[20] Phase one includes cessation of running and local pain control with local physiotherapy, ice massage, and possibly a short course of nonsteroidal anti-inflammatory medication. Weight bearing for daily activities is permitted. During this first phase, alternative aerobic, strengthening, and flexibility activities are prescribed such as cycling, swimming, and water running. The second phase begins when the athlete has been pain-free for at least two weeks with any impact activity. Activities are gradually progressed. If symptoms persist or recur, the impact activities are tapered or stopped. The recurrence rates of stress fractures approach 10% at either the original or a metachronous site.[37,71,89] The average time to return to full activity with this protocol may be 3 months for a compression-type tibial stress fracture and 1 to 2 months for a fibular stress fracture.

Traditional treatment excluded casts or braces, but supplemental use of a pneumatic brace may allow athletes with tibial stress fractures to return to activity

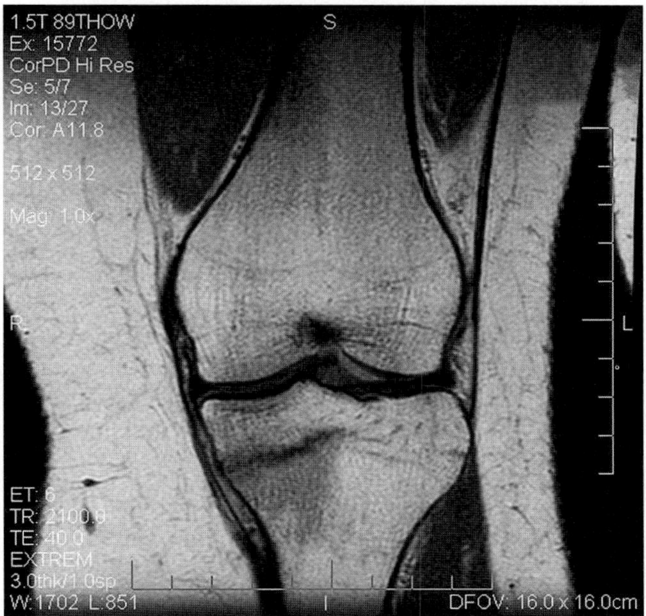

A

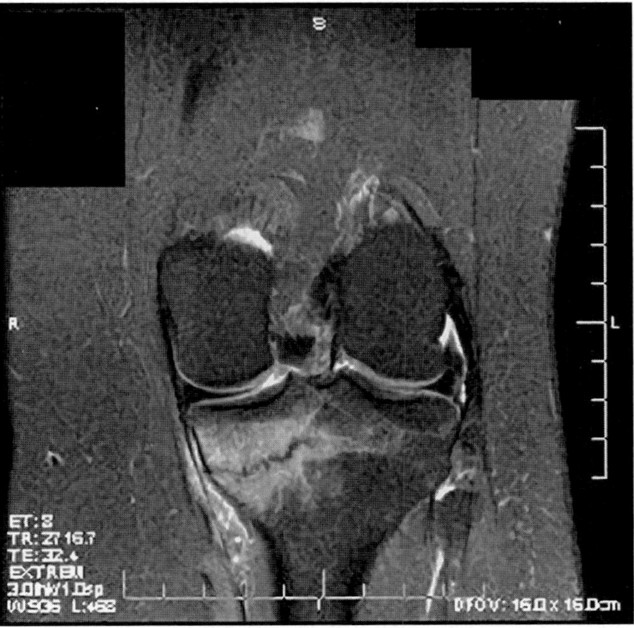

B

FIGURE 24-7. Coronal (**A**) T-1, Coronal (**B**) T-2, and Sagittal. *Continued*

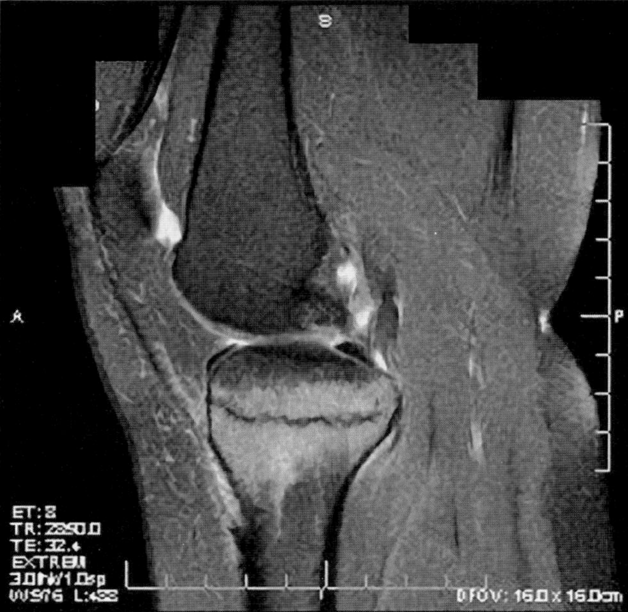

C

FIGURE 24-7, cont'd. (**C**) T-2 magnetic resonance imaging studies reveal proximal tibial stress fracture at previous physeal line in skeletally mature patient.

sooner than traditional treatment alone. In a randomized, prospective study comparing treatment modalities, Swenson et al.[126] found that patients in the pneumatic brace group returned to full, unrestricted activity at 21 days. This return to activity was significantly sooner than the average of 77 days for the group treated with rest alone.

The tension-type anterior tibial stress fracture seen in repetitive jumping athletes requires special attention. This stress fracture is prone to delayed healing, nonunion, and fracture completion and displacement because of poor biomechanics and limited blood supply.[14,40,98] This notorious overuse injury is traditionally treated with prolonged immobilization.[59,98] A short leg non-weight-bearing cast is used initially and may be converted to a walking cast or cast brace if the radiographs and examination demonstrate healing. However, these stress fractures have been reported to fail to heal with simple immobilization.[40] Numerous treatment regimens have been proposed to achieve healing in these recalcitrant fractures. The addition of pulsed external electromagnetic stimulation may facilitate healing but can take up to six months, and reports vary on its effectiveness.[98] Surgical alternatives may be considered when closed treatments are deemed to have failed. Prompt healing has been reported after excision and bone grafting of the lesion.[40] Intramedullary tibial nailing has been shown to produce good to excellent results after failed immobilization.[17] The role of early surgical intervention is not yet defined in athletes, but prophylactic intramedullary internal fixation has successfully treated a professional athlete.[7] Surgery is also effective for recalcitrant fibular stress fractures associated with tibio-fibular synostosis.[52]

MEDIAL GASTROCNEMIUS MUSCLE TEARS

Acute tears of the medial head of the gastrocnemius muscle typically occur in middle-aged individuals during recreational athletics and have been referred to as tennis leg.[32] The tear usually occurs at a time of maximal force during running, jumping, or change of direction. Patients describe a sudden acute pain in the calf and often the sensation of having been struck in the calf. Pain, swelling, and ecchymosis usually progressively increase during the subsequent 24 to 48 hours. This injury was commonly misinterpreted in the past as a rupture of the plantaris tendon. This view was dispelled by a comprehensive review, among other studies, that found no supporting surgical or autopsy evidence of an isolated rupture of the plantaris tendon.[44,53,112] It is now widely accepted that this injury involves the medial head of the gastrocnemius.

Anatomy and Pathophysiology

The gastrocnemius muscle is comprised of a lateral and medial head. Both originate from the femoral condyles and posterior capsule with the muscle mass tapering distally into a broad aponeurosis before blending with the deeper soleus muscle to form the Achilles tendon, which inserts onto the posterior tuberosity of the calcaneus. The medial head of the gastrocnemius muscle possesses some unique and important differences from the lateral head that may predispose it to rupture.[125] The medial head has a larger muscle mass, originates more superiorly on the femur, and has a more oblique fiber orientation than the vertically directed lateral head. Additionally, the gastrocnemius muscle fibers are fast-twitch fibers compared with the soleus, which is primarily slow-twitch.[116] The gastrocnemius muscle has been described as a "short action" muscle, making it vulnerable to overstretch and rupture.[32] It crosses two joints, the knee and the ankle, which makes it prone to injury.[5] Rupture of the medial head occurs with a high-force eccentric muscle contraction, which often occurs during the mechanism of combined extension of the knee and forced ankle dorsiflexion as may occur during tennis, jogging, or landing from a jump.[3,76,113,125] Rupture usually occurs at the musculotendinous junction.[65,76,118,125] Decreased elasticity, dysvascular changes, and atrophy seen with aging or disease reduce the threshold force, causing musculotendinous rupture.[142,143]

Clinical Evaluation

The patient usually gives a history of sudden pain in the calf while running, cutting, accelerating, or stopping.

Often, there is a feeling of having been hit in the calf or the sensation of a "pop." Swelling and pain in the calf usually progressively worsen during the next 24 hours. Ecchymosis of the entire leg can be significant and is usually maximal after a few days. These signs vary with severity of injury. On physical examination, there is usually localized tenderness at the musculotendinous junction and a palpable defect may develop over time. The foot rests most comfortably in an equinus position. The patient should demonstrate evidence of an intact Achilles mechanism with active plantarflexion of the ankle and passive plantarflexion of the ankle on compression of the calf (Thompson test). Guarding to standing toe raises and pain with active or passive ankle dorsiflexion may be present. The neurovascular examination is typically normal. The diagnosis usually can be made on clinical evaluation. Although plain radiographs are typically normal, magnetic resonance imaging can conclusively demonstrate tears of the medial head of the gastrocnemius with surrounding hematoma (Fig. 24-8).

Differential diagnosis includes acute compartment syndrome, acute deep venous thromboembolism, and popliteal cyst rupture. Often, the clinical history will prove helpful in establishing the diagnosis. However, the clinician should be aware that these conditions may coexist simultaneously.[100,115] Acute compartment syndrome may occur after rupture of the medial head of the gastrocnemius, but is rare.[5,120] Deep venous thromboembolism may result as a complication of rupture of the medial head of the gastrocnemius muscle.[115] Doppler ultrasound should be used to evaluate suspected deep venous thromboembolism. The use of anticoagulants in the setting of medial gastrocnemius muscle rupture may cause complications from increased bleeding from the torn muscle and lead to a potential compartment syndrome.[120] Popliteal cyst rupture is usually seen in patients with inflammatory arthritis. The diagnosis may be difficult, and magnetic resonance imaging is helpful in establishing the diagnosis.

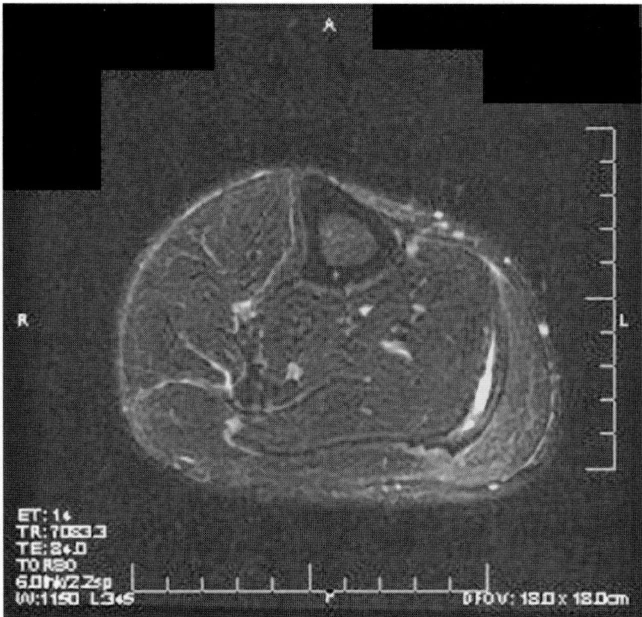

A

B

FIGURE 24-8. Sequential Axial (**A**) and (**B**) T-2 magnetic resonance imaging axial study reveals traumatic hemorrhage at site of rupture of the medial gastrocnemius musculotendinous junction.

Treatment

Treatment of tears of the medial head of the gastrocnemius is nonoperative and is directed toward symptomatic relief. Many nonoperative protocols have yielded good results.[34,53,76] Early management consists of ice and elevation to minimize pain and swelling. Ankle motion is initiated as tolerated. A short course of nonsteroidal anti-inflammatory medication is prescribed. Crutches are useful if weight bearing is painful and a heel lift in the shoe may be used for a short period of time.[32] An aggressive rehabilitation program is initiated within 48 to 72 hours when the bleeding has stopped. Such a program resulted in full rehabilitation of 85% of patients by 2 weeks in a study of 720 patients.[76] Stretching and strengthening after injury continues to be the mainstay of treatment for muscle injuries. Passive stretching of the calf using a towel or elastic band is performed with the knee extended and progresses to standing stretch exercises of the calf as tolerated. Similarly, strengthening progresses as the pain subsides from isometric ankle dorsiflexion and plantarflexion to resistance exercises. These can be performed as active resistance exercises with an elastic band and toe raises against progressive resistance or weight. For a complete muscle tear, full return to athletic participation can typically be expected in 3 to 12 weeks.

REFERENCES

1. Admundsen DE: The spectrum of heat related injury with compartment syndrome. Milit Med 154(9):450–453, 1989.
2. American Medical Association, Subcommittee of Classification of Sports Injuries: Standard Nomenclature of Athletic Injuries. Chicago, American Medical Association, 1966, pp 122–126.
3. Andrisch JT: The Leg in Orthopaedic Sports Medicine, vol 2. St. Louis, Mosby, 1993.
4. Andrisch JT, Bergfeld JA, Walheim J: A prospective study of the management of shin splints. J Bone Joint Surg Am 56:1697–1700, 1974.
5. Anouchi Y, Parker R, Seitz W: Posterior compartment syndrome of the calf resulting from misdiagnosis of a rupture of the medial head of the gastrocnemius. J Trauma 27(6):678–680, 1987.
6. Arendt EA, Griffiths HJ: The use of MR imaging in the assessment and clinical management of stress reactions of bone in high-performance athletes. Clin Sports Med 16:291–306, 1997.
7. Barrick EF, Jackson CB: Prophylactic intramedullary fixation of the tibia for stress fracture in a professional athlete. J Orthop Trauma 6(2):241–244, 1992.
8. Barrow GW, Saha S: Menstrual irregularity and stress fractures in collegiate female distance runners. Am J Sports Med 16(3):209–216, 1988.
9. Beck BR, Osternig LR: Medial tibial stress syndrome. The location of muscles in the leg in relation to symptoms. J Bone Joint Surg Am 76A:1057–1061, 1994.
10. Blaiser D, Barry RJ, Weaver T: Force march-induced peroneal compartment syndrome. Clin Orthop 284: 189–192, 1992.
11. Blank S: Transverse tibial stress fractures: A special problem. Am J Sports Med 15:597–602, 1987.
12. Boden BP, Speer KP: Femoral stress fractures. Clin Sports Med 16:307–317, 1997.
13. Bradley EL III: The anterior tibial compartment syndrome. Surg Gynecol Obstet 136:289–297, 1973.
14. Brahms MA, Fumich RJ, Ippolito VD: A typical stress fracture of the tibia in a professional athlete. Am J Sports Med 8:131–132, 1980.
15. Briethaupt MD: Zur pathologie des menschlischen Fusses. Med Zeitung 24:169, 1855.
16. Burrows HJ: Fatigue fracture of the middle third of the tibia in ballet dancers. J Bone Joint Surg 38:83–94, 1956.
17. Chang PS, Harris RM: Intramedullary nailing for chronic tibial stress fractures. A review of five cases. Am J Sports Med 24:688–692, 1996.
18. Chisin R, Milgrom C, Giladi M, et al: Clinical significance of nonfocal scintigraphic findings in suspected tibial stress fractures. Clin Orthop 220:200–205, 1987.
19. Clayer M, Krishnan J, Lee WK, et al: Longitudinal stress fractures of the tibia. Clin Radiol 46(6): 401–404, 1992.
20. Clement DB: Tibial stress syndrome in athletes. Am J Sports Med 2:81–85, 1974.
21. Cohen MS, Garfin SR, Hargens AR, Mubarek SJ: Acute compartment syndrome. Effect of dermotomy on fascial decompression of the leg. J Bone Joint Surg Br 73(2):287–290, 1991.
22. Cook T, Brown D, Roe J: Hypokalemia, hypophosphatemia and compartment syndrome of the leg after downhill skiing on moguls. J Emerg Med 11(6): 709–715, 1993.
23. Daffner RH, Martinez S, Gehweiler JA: Stress fractures of the proximal tibia in runners. Radiology 142:53–65, 1982.
24. Davey J, Rorabeck CH, Fowler P: The tibialis posterior muscle compartment: An unrecognized cause of exertional compartment syndrome. Am J Sports Med 12(5):391–397, 1984.
25. Detmer DE: Chronic shin splints. Classification and management of medial tibial stress syndrome. Sports Med 3:436–446, 1986.
26. Detmer DE, Sharp K, Sufit RL, Girdley FM: Chronic compartment syndrome: Diagnosis, management and outcomes. Am J Sports Med 13:162, 1985.
27. Deutsch AL, Coel MN, Mink JH: Imaging of stress injuries to bone: Radiology, scintigraphy, and MR imaging. Clin Sports Med 16:275–290, 1997.
28. Devas MB: Stress fractures in athletes. Proc R Soc Med 62:933–937, 1969.
29. Devas MB, Sweetnam R: Stress fractures of the fibula. A review of fifty cases in athletes. J Bone Joint Surg Br 38B:818–829, 1956.
30. Fredericson M, Bergman G, Hoffman KL, et al: Tibial stress reaction in runners: Correlation of clinical symptoms and scintigraphy with a new magnetic resonance imaging grading system. Am J Sports Med 23:472–481, 1995.
31. Friapont MJ, Adamson GJ: Chronic exertional compartment syndrome. J Am Assoc Orthop Surg 11(4): 268–274, 2003.
32. Froisom A: Tennis leg. JAMA 209:415–416, 1969.
33. Fronek J, Mubarek SJ, Hargens AR, et al: Management of chronic exertional anterior compartment syndrome of the lower extremity. Clin Orthop 207: 253–262, 1986.
34. Gecha S, Torg E: Knee injuries in tennis. Clin Sports Med 7(2):435–452, 1988.

35. Giladi M, Ahronson Z, Stein M, et al: Unusual distribution and onset of stress fractures in soldiers. Clin Orthop 192:142–146, 1985.
36. Giladi M, Milgrom C, Simkim A, et al: Stress fractures and tibial bone width. J Bone Joint Surg 69B:326–329, 1987.
37. Giladi M, Ziv Y, Aharonson Z, Nli E, Danon Y: Comparison between radiography, bone scan and ultrasound in the diagnosis of stress fractures. Milit Med 149:459–461, 1984.
38. Gilbert RS, Johnson HA: Stress fractures in military recruits: A review of twelve years experience. Milit Med 131: 716–722, 1966.
39 Greaney RB, Gerber FH, Laughlin RL: Distribution and natural history of stress fractures in U.S. Marine recruits. Radiology 146:338–346, 1983.
40. Green NE, Rogers RA, Lipscomb AB: Nonunions of stress fractures of the tibia. Am J Sports Med 13(3):171–176, 1985.
41. Hallel T, Amis S, Segal D: Fatigue fractures of tibia and femoral shafts in soldiers. Clin Orthop 118: 35–43, 1976.
42. Heckman MM, Whitesides TE Jr, Grewe SR, et al: Histologic determination of the ischemic threshold of muscle in the canine compartment syndrome model. J Orthop Trauma 7:199–210, 1993.
43. Heckman MM, Whitesides TE Jr, Grewe SR, et al: Compartment pressure in association with closed tibial fractures: The relationship between tissue pressure compartment and the distance from the site of fracture. J Bone Joint Surg Am 76:1285–1292, 1994.
44. Helms CA, Fritz RC, Garvin GJ: Plantaris muscle injury: Evaluation with MR imaging. Radiology 195(1):201–203, 1995.
45. Heppenstall RB, Sapega AA, Izant T, et al: Compartment syndrome: A quantitative study of high-energy phosphorus compounds using 31P-magnetic resonance spectroscopy. J Trauma 29:1113–1119, 1989.
46. Heppenstall RB, Sapega AA, Scott R, et al: The compartment syndrome: An experimental and clinical study of muscular energy metabolism using phosphorus magnetic resonance spectroscopy. Clin Orthop 226:138–155, 1988.
47. Heppenstall RB, Scott R, Sapega A, et al: A comparative study of the tolerance of skeletal muscle to ischemia: Tourniquet application compared with acute compartment syndrome. J Bone Joint Surg Am 68: 820–828, 1986.
48. Hieb LD, Alexander AH: Bilateral anterior and lateral compartment syndromes in a patient with sickle-cell trait. A case report and a review of the literature. Clin Orthop 228:190–193, 1988.
49. Holen KJ, Engebretsen L, Gronvoldt, et al: Surgical treatment of medial tibial stress syndrome (shin splints) by fasciotomy of the superficial posterior compartment of the leg. Scan J Med Sci Sports 5:40–43, 1995.
50. Howard JL, Mohtadi NG, Wiley JP: Evaluation of outcomes in patients following surgical treatment of chronic exertional compartment syndrome in the leg. Clin J Sports Med 10:176–184, 2000.
51. James SL, Bates BT, Osterling LR: Injuries to runners. Am J Sports Med 6(2):40–50, 1978.
52. Kottmeier SA, Hanks GA, Kalenak A: Fibular stress fracture associated with distal tibiofibular synostosis in an athlete. Clin Orthop 281:195–198, 1992.
53. Leach R: Leg and foot injuries in racquet sports. Clin Sports Med 7(2):359–370, 1988.
54. Li G, Zhang S, Chen G, et al: Radiologic and histologic analysis of stress fractures in rabbit tibias. Am J Sports Med 13:285–294, 1985.
55. Lieberman CM, Hemingway DL: Scintigraphy of shin splints. Clin Nucl Med 5:31, 1980.
56. McBryde AM: Stress fractures in athletes. J Sports Med 3:212–217, 1976.
57. McDermott AGP, Marble AE, Yabsley RH, et al: Monitoring dynamic anterior compartment pressures during exercise. A new technique using the STIC catheter. Am J Sports Med 10:83–89, 1982.
58. Margulies J, Simkim A, Leighter I, et al: Effect of intense physical activity on the bone mineral content in the lower limbs of young adults. J Bone Joint Surg 68A(7):1090–1093, 1986.
59. Martire JR: The role of nuclear medicine bone scans in evaluating pain in athletic injuries. Clin Sports Med 6(4):713–737, 1987.
60. Martire JR: Differentiating stress fractures from periostitis: The finer points of bone scans. Phys Sports Med 22(10):71–81, 1994.
61. Matava MJ, Whitesides TE Jr, Seiler JG III, et al: Determination of the compartment pressure threshold of muscle ischemia in a canine model. J Trauma 37:50–58, 1994.
62. Matheson GO, Clement DB, McKenzie, et al: Scintigraphic uptake of 99m Tc at nonpainful sites in athletes with stress fractures: the concept of bone strain. Sports Med 4:65–75, 1987.
63. Matheson GO, Clement DB, McKenzie, et al: Stress fractures in athletes: A study of 320 cases. Am J Sports Med 15(1):46–58, 1987.
64. Matsen FA, Winquist RA, Krugmire RB: Diagnosis and management of compartment syndromes. J Bone Joint Surg Am 62A:286–291, 1980.
65. Menz MJ, Lucas GL: Magnetic resonance imaging of the gastrocnemius muscle. J Bone Joint Surg 73:1260–1262, 1991.
66. Messier SP, Pittala KA: Etiologic factors associated with selected running injuries. Med Sci Sports Exerc 20:501–505, 1988.

67. Meyer SA, Saltzman CL, Albright JP: Stress fractures of the foot and leg. Clin Sports Med 12:395–413, 1993.
68. Michael RH, Holder LE: The soleus syndrome. A cause of medial tibial stress (shin splints). Am J Sports Med 13:87–94, 1985.
69. Milgrom C, Chisin R, Giladi M, et al: Multiple stress fractures. Clin Orthop 192:174–179, 1985.
70. Milgrom C, Chisin R, Giladi M, et al: Negative bone scans in impending tibial stress fractures. Am J Sports Med 12(4):488–491, 1984.
71. Milgrom C, Giladi M, Chisin R, Dizian R: The long term follow-up of soldiers with stress fractures. Am J Sports Med 13(6):398–400, 1985.
72. Milgrom C, Giladi M Simkim A, et al: An analysis of the biomechanical mechanism of tibial stress fractures among Israeli infantry recruits. Clin Orthop 231:216–221, 1988.
73. Milgrom C, Giladi M, Stein M, et al: Stress fractures in military recruits. J Bone Joint Surg 67B:732–735, 1985.
74. Milgrom C, Giladi M, Stein M, et al: Medial tibial pain. Clin Orthop 213:167–171, 1986.
75. Miller EH, Schneider HJ, Bronson JL, et al: A new consideration in athletic injuries: The classical ballet dancer. Clin Orthop 111:181–191, 1975.
76. Miller WA: Rupture of the musculotendinous juncture of the medial head of the gastrocnemius muscle. Am J Sports Med 5:191–193, 1977.
77. Miniaci A, McLaren AC, Haddad RG: Longitudinal stress fractures of the tibia. Can Assoc Radiol J 39(3):221–223, 1988.
78. Mohler LR, Styf JR, Pedowitz RA, et al: Intramuscular deoxygenation during exercise in patients who have chronic anterior compartment syndrome of the leg. J Bone Joint Surg Am 79:844–849, 1997.
79. Morris JM, Blickenstaff LD: Fatigue Fractures: A Clinical Study. Springfield, IL, 1967.
80. Moyer RA, Boden BP, Marchetto PA, Kleinhart F, Kelly JD: Acute compartment syndrome of the lower extremity secondary to noncontact injury. Foot Ankle 14(9):534–537, 1993.
81. Mubarek SJ, Gould RN, Lee YF, et al: The medial tibial stress syndrome. A cause of shin splints. Am J Sports Med 10(4):201–205, 1982.
82. Mubarek SJ, Hargens AR, Owen CA, et al: The Wick catheter technique for measurement of intramuscular pressure. A new research and clinical tool. J Bone Joint Surg Am 58A:1016–1020, 1976.
83. Mubarek SJ, Owens CA, Hargens AR et al: Acute compartment syndrome: Diagnosis and treatment with the aid of the Wick catheter. J Bone Joint Surg Am 60A:1091–1095, 1978.
84. Nielsen MB, Hansen K, Hlmer P, Dyrbe M: Tibial periosteal reactions in soldiers. Acta Orthop Scanda 62(6):531–534, 1991.
85. Nkele C, Aindow J, Grant L: Study of the pressure of the normal anterior tibial compartment in different age groups using the slit-catheter method. J Bone Joint Surg 70A:98, 1988.
86. Norfray J, Schlacter L, Kernahan W, et al: Early confirmation of stress fractures in joggers. JAMA 243(16):1647–1649, 1980.
87. Nussbaum AR, Treves ST, Mischeli L: Bone stress lesions in ballet dancers: scintigraphic assessment. Am J Roentgenol 150(4):851–855, 1988.
88. Orava S: Stress fractures. Br J Sports Med 14: 40–44, 1980.
89. Orava S, Hulkko A: Stress fractures in athletes. Int J Sports Med 8:221–226, 1987.
90. Orava S, Hulkko A: Stress fractures of the mid-tibial shaft. Acta Orthop Scand 55:35–37, 1984.
91. Orava S, Puranen J, Ala-hetola L: Stress fractures caused by physical exercise. Acta Orthop Scand 49:19–27, 1978.
92. Paletta CE, Lynch R, Knutsen AP: Rhabdomyolysis and lower extremity compartment syndrome due to influenza B virus. Ann Plast Surg 30:272–273, 1993.
93. Pedowitz R, Hargens A, Mubarek S, Gershuni D: Modified criteria for the objective diagnosis of chronic compartment syndrome of the leg. Am J Sports Med 18(1):35–40, 1990.
94. Pelligrini VD, Evarts CM: Complications in Rockwood and Green's Fractures in Adults. Philadelphia, JB Lippincott, 1991.
95. Prather JL, Nusynowitz ML, Snowdy HA, et al: Scintigraphic findings in stress fractures. J Bone Joint Surg 59:869–874, 1977.
96. Reneman RR: The anterior and lateral compartment syndrome of the leg due to intensive use of muscles. Clin Orthop 113:69–80, 1975.
97. Resnick D. The Diagnosis of Bone and Joint Disorders, 3rd ed. Philadelphia, WB Saunders, 1995.
98. Rettig AC, Shelbourn KD, McCarroll JR, et al: The natural history and treatment of delayed union stress fractures of the anterior cortex of the tibia. Am J Sports Med 16:250–255, 1988.
99. Roberts SM, Vogt EC: Pseudofracture of the tibia. J Bone Joint Surg 21(4):891–901, 1939.
100. Robinson N: Spontaneous rupture of the gastrocnemius muscle presenting as acute thrombophlebitis. Am Surg 38(7):385–388, 1972.
101. Rorabeck CH, Bourne RB, Fowler PJ: The surgical treatment of exertional compartment syndrome in athletes. J Bone Joint Surg Am 65:1245–1251, 1983.
102. Rorabeck CH, Bourne R, Fowler P, et al: The role of tissue pressure measurement in diagnosing chromic anterior compartment syndrome. Am J Sports Med 16:143–146, 1988
103. Rorabeck CH, Castle GSP, Hardie R, Logan J: Compartmental pressure measurements: An

experimental investigation using the slit catheter. J Trauma 21:446–449, 1991.
104. Rorabeck CH, Clarke KM: The pathophysiology of the anterior tibial compartment syndrome. J Trauma 18:299, 1978.
105. Rorabeck CH, Fowler PJ, Nott L: The results of fasciotomy in the management of chronic exertional compartment syndrome. Am J Sports Med 16: 224–227, 1988.
106. Rorabeck CH, Hardie PC, Logan J: Compartmental pressure measurement. An experimental investigation using the slit catheter. J Trauma 21:446–449, 1981.
107. Roub L, Gumerman L, Hanley E, et al: Bone stress: A radionuclide imaging perspective. Radiology 132:431–438, 1979.
108. Rupani MD, Molder LE, Espinola DA: The three-phase of radionuclide bone-imaging in sports medicine. Radiology 156:187–196, 1985.
109. Schepsis AA, Gill SS, Foster TA: Fasciotomy for exertional anterior compartment syndrome: Is lateral compartment release necessary? Am J Sports Med 27(4):430–435, 1999.
110. Schepsis AA, Martini D, Corbett M: Surgical management of exertional compartment syndrome of the lower leg: Long-term follow-up. Am J Sports Med 21:811–817, 1993.
111. Seiler JG III, Womack S, De L'Aune WR, et al: Intracompartmental pressure measurements in the normal forearm. J Orthop Trauma 7:414–416, 1993.
112. Severance H, Bassett F: Rupture of the plantaris—Does it exist? J Bone Joint Surg 64(9):1387–1388, 1982.
113. Shields CL, Redix L, Brewster CE: Acute tears of the gastrocnemius. Foot Ankle 5:186–190, 1985.
114. Singer M, Maudsley RH: Fatigue fractures in the lower tibia. J Bone Joint Surg 36B:647–649, 1954.
115. Slawski DP: Deep venous thrombosis complicating rupture of the medial head of the gastrocnemius muscle. J Orthop Trauma 8(3):263–264, 1994.
116. Smith MJ: Muscle fiber types. Orthop Clin North Am 14:403–411, 1983.
117. Sommer HM, Vallentyne SW: Effect of foot posture on the incidence of medial tibial stress syndrome. Med Sci Sports Exerc 27:800–804, 1995.
118. Speer KP, Lohnes J, Garrett WE: Radiographic imaging of muscle strain injury. Am J Sports Med 21(1):89–95, 1993.
119. Spitz DJ, Newberg AH: Imaging of stress fractures in the athlete. Radiol Clin North Am 40:313–331, 2002.
120. Staehley D, Jones W: Acute compartment syndrome following tear of the medial head of the gastrocnemius muscle. Am J Sports Med 14(1): 96–99, 1986.
121. Stanitsk CL, McMaster JH, Scranton PE: On the nature of stress fractures. Am J Sports Med 6: 391–396, 1978.
122. Styf JR, Korner LM: Chronic anterior compartment syndrome of the leg: Results of treatment by fasciotomy. J Bone Joint Surg Am 68:1338–1347, 1986.
123. Styf JR, Korner LM: Microcapillary infusion technique for measurement of intramuscular pressure during exercise. Clin Orthop 207:253–262, 1986.
124. Sullivan D, Warren RF, Pavlov H, Kelman G: Stress fractures in 51 runners. Clin Orthop 187:188–192, 1984.
125. Sutro C, Sutro W: The medial head of the gastrocnemius: A review of the basis for partial rupture and for intermittent claudication. Bull Hosp Joint Dis Orthop Inst 45(2):150–157, 1985.
126. Swenson AJ, DeHaven KE, Sebastianelli WJ, et al: The effect of a pneumatic leg brace on return to play in athletes with tibial stress fractures. Am J Sports Med 25(3):322–328, 1997.
127. Takebayashi S, Takazawa H, Sasaki R, et al: Chronic exertional compartment syndrome in lower legs: Localization of follow-up with thallium-201 SPECT imaging. J Nucl Med 38:972–976, 1997.
128. Toulipolous S, Herschman EB: Lower leg pain. Diagnosis and treatment of compartment syndromes and other pain syndromes of the leg. Sports Med 27(3):193–204, 1999.
129. Uliasz A, Ishida JT, Fleming KJ, Yamamoto LG: Comparing the methods of measuring compartment pressures in acute compartment syndrome. Am Emerg Med 21(2):143–145, 2003.
130. Umans H, Kaye J: Longitudinal stress fractures of the tibia: Diagnosis by magnetic resonance imaging. Skeletal Radiol 25:319–324, 1996.
131. Verleisdonk EJ, van Gils A, van der Werken C: The diagnostic value of MRI scans for the diagnosis of chronic exertional compartment syndrome of the lower leg. Skeletal Radiol 30:321–325, 2001.
132. Viitasalo JT, Kvist M: Some biomechanical aspects of the foot and ankle in athletes with and without shin splints. Am J Sports Med 11:125–130, 1983.
133. Volkman R: Die ischaemischen muskellamungen und kontrakturen. Zentabl Chir 8:801, 1881.
134. Watson JT: Knee and Leg: Bone Trauma, OKU-6:533–558. Rosemont, IL, AAOS, 1999.
135. Whitesides TE Jr, Haney TC, Harada H: Tissue perfusion measurements as a determinant for the need of fasciotomy. Clin Orthop 113:43, 1975.
136. Whitesides TE Jr, Harada H, Morimoto K: The response of skeletal muscle to temporary ischemia: An experimental study. J Bone Joint Surg 53A:1027, 1971.

137. Whitesides TE Jr, Harada H, Morimoto K: Compartment syndromes and the role of fasciotomy, its parameters, and techniques. Instr Course Lect 26:179–196, 1977.
138. Whitesides TE Jr, Heckman MM: Acute compartment syndrome: Update on diagnosis and treatment. J Am Assoc Orthop Surg 4(4):209–218, 1996.
139. Wiederhelm CA, Weston BV: Microvascular, lymphatic and tissue pressures in the unanesthetized mammal. Am J Physiol 225:992–996, 1973.
140. Wiley JP, Short WB, Wiseman DA, Miller SD: Ultrasound catheter placement for deep posterior compartment pressure measurements in chronic compartment syndrome. Am J Sports Med 18:74–79, 1990.
141. Yao L, Johnson C, et al: Stress injuries of bone: An analysis of MR imaging staging criteria. Acad Radiol 5:34–40, 1998.
142. Zarins B, Ciullo JV: Acute muscle and tendon injuries in athletes. Clin Sports Med 2:167–182, 1983.
143. Zarins B, Ciullo JV: Biomechanics of the musculotendinous unity: Relation to athletic performance and injuries. Clin Sports Med 2:71–86, 1983.
144. Zwas S, Elkanovitch R, Frank G: Interpretation and classification of bone scintigraphic findings in stress fractures. J Nucl Med 28(4):452–457, 1987.

25 The Foot and Ankle

Christopher E. Hubbard

EVALUATION

Evaluation of the foot and ankle begins with a carefully recorded history, thorough but focused physical examination, and ordering and interpretation of pertinent radiographic studies. Both acute and chronic sports problems require a detailed history of factors that led to or contributed to the injury. In the acute injury, it is helpful to attempt to determine the mechanism of injury, the position of the foot and ankle at the time of impact or twist, and whether it was a low- or high-impact event (i.e., ankle inversion during a tennis match or crash while skiing). Did the foot or ankle become swollen right away, and if so, on what part of the lower leg? Was the patient able to bear weight on the leg right away? Did the patient go to the emergency room? All these answers can help determine the severity of injury. In the chronic injury, it is helpful to learn what activities contribute to the symptoms. Does the patient have pain with walking, or after running a few miles? Is it an annoyance or disability? Does it prevent the patient from participating in certain activities? Do certain shoes or sneakers make a difference? Does the patient feel this is a pain problem versus a weakness or instability problem? Pain can be described in many ways: sharp and intense, burning, or dull and achy. Different types of pain suggest different pathology.

Past medical, surgical, and family history are important to review. Inflammatory and infectious disease can mimic or contribute to various tendon and joint symptoms. Prior and current athletic history indicates certain overuse syndromes, and might reveal similar problems in the past. Certain medical conditions might preclude the use of nonsteroidal anti-inflammatories.

Physical examination should start in an orderly and consistent manner. The physician should become familiar with a certain methodology and try to duplicate the exam with each new patient. Both lower extremities of the patient should be visualized, and the examiner should be positioned in a comfortable manner when assessing the patient. In the acute setting, inspection for areas of edema and ecchymosis can help in localizing the injured body part. Abrasions, blisters, or lacerations may indicate a serious underlying injury. Deformity can indicate a joint dislocation or severe fracture. If the patient is able to bear weight, then knee, ankle, and foot alignment should be assessed. Observation of valgus or varus alignment of the hindfoot is pertinent for certain ankle and foot disorders.

Palpation is important to localize the injured area. This part of the exam should still be in an orderly fashion, but start at the presumed uninvolved areas and then finish at the anticipated area of injury to maximize patient cooperation. In the ankle, focal points should include the lateral ankle ligaments, medial deltoid ligament, peroneal, Achilles, posterior and anterior tibial tendons, and the lateral and medial ankle malleoli. Any tenderness, thickening, or incontinuity should be noted. The lateral ankle ligaments include the anterior talofibular and calcaneofibular ligaments. The anterior inferior tibiofibular ligament is part of the distal ankle syndesmosis and is palpated just proximal to the anterolateral joint line of the ankle. The medial deltoid ligament is palpated just inferior to the medial malleolus. The peroneal tendons course just inferior to the distal fibula, and any crepitus or subluxation should be noted. The Achilles tendon can be tender proximally or distally, thickened due to a tendinosis, or in complete discontinuity after a rupture. The posterior tibial tendon runs just inferior to the medial malleolus along the ankle, and when injured, is most often tender at the tip of the medial malleolus. The anterior tibial tendon courses along the anteromedial ankle, inserts at the medial cuneiform of the foot, and should be palpated for tenderness and continuity. Tenderness along the lateral or medial malleolus of the ankle can be suggestive of fracture.

Focal points of palpation in the foot include the heel, base of the fifth metatarsal, anterior process of the calcaneus, dorsal navicular, third intermetatarsal webspace, second metatarsalphalangeal joint, and plantar to the metatarsal heads. Tenderness at the plantar-medial heel is suggestive of plantar fasciitis. Common fractures occur along the fifth metatarsal, anterior process of the calcaneus, and less commonly at the navicular. A synovitis of the metatarsalphalangeal joints usually occurs at the second metatarsal, and metatarsalgia is most common under the second or third metatarsal heads. Other areas to palpate include the sesamoids, located plantar to the first metatarsal head, and the metatarsal necks or shafts, locations of potential stress fractures.

Neurovascular testing includes palpating the dorsal pedis artery, located between the base of the first and second metatarsals, and the posterior tibial artery, palpated posterior and inferior to the medial malleolus. Sensory testing includes the superficial peroneal, deep peroneal, saphenous, posterior tibial, and sural nerves. The superficial peroneal nerve courses along the anterolateral ankle and supplies sensation to the dorsum of the foot. The deep peroneal nerve supplies the skin in the first webspace of the toes. The saphenous nerve supplies sensation to parts of the medial foot. The posterior tibial nerve supplies sensation to the plantar foot, and the sural nerve to the lateral aspect of the foot.

Range of motion should be evaluated at the ankle, subtalar, transverse tarsal, and first metatarsalphalangeal joints. Ranges can vary according to different individuals but are listed as:

- Ankle: 15° dorsiflexion/45° plantarflexion
- Subtalar: 20–50° combined eversion/inversion
- 1st MTP: 50–70° dorsiflexion/10–25° plantarflexion

Strength testing includes dorsiflexion, plantarflexion, inversion, and eversion of the ankle and foot. Muscle testing can be graded on a scale of 0/5 to 5/5 for normal strength.

The dorsiflexors of the ankle and foot include the anterior tibial tendon (AT), extensor hallucis longus (EHL), extensor digitorum longus (EDL), extensor hallucis brevis (EHB), and extensor digitorum brevis (EDB). The AT is the major dorsiflexor of the ankle and can be tested by asking the patient to bring the foot into a dorsiflexed and slightly inverted position against resistance. The EHL and EHB can be evaluated against resistance to extension at the metatarsalphalangeal and interphalangeal joints of the first toe, respectively. The EDL and EDB are evaluated by active extension of the lesser toes and against resistance.

The plantarflexors of the ankle and foot are the Achilles tendon, flexor digitorum longus (FDL), and flexor hallucis longus (FHL). The Achilles tendon is tested by forced plantarflexion of the ankle. The FDL and the FHL are evaluated by forced plantarflexion of the lesser and greater toes, respectively.

The posterior tibial tendon (PTT) is the primary invertor of the ankle. It is isolated by starting in a position of plantarflexion and eversion and instructing the patient to invert the foot. The PTT is also tested by the ability to perform a single-stance heel rise.

The peroneal longus and brevis (PL and PB) are the major evertors of the ankle. These are tested by again starting the foot in a plantarflexed position, and instructing the patient to evert the foot against resistance (Fig. 25-1). The PL also plantarflexes the first ray and can be tested by instructing the patient to force the first ray down against resistance.

Dynamic testing of the ankle includes evaluating for peroneal subluxation or dislocation. This is accomplished by placing the examiner's fingers on the peroneals, just posterior to the tip of fibula, and instructing the patient to dorsiflex and evert the ankle (Fig. 25-2). If the tendons subluxate or dislocate, the examiner will feel the tendons slip anterior over the fibula.

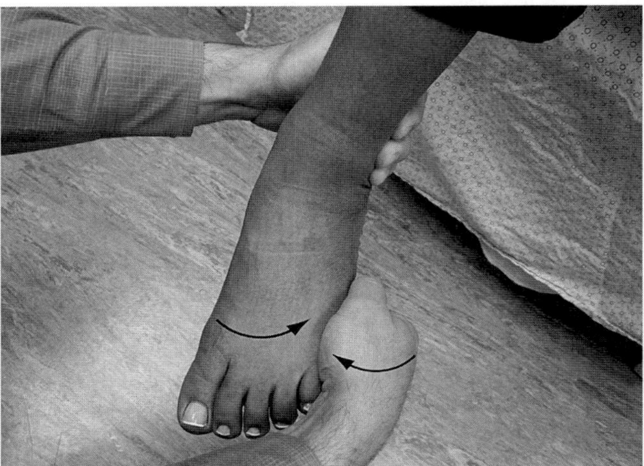

FIGURE 25-1. Testing for peroneal tendon strength. The patient everts against resistance in a position of plantarflexion.

The anterior drawer test evaluates instability of the ankle (Fig. 25-3). The examiner stabilizes the distal tibia with one hand and then, with the other hand gripping the posterior hindfoot, applies an anterior directed force to the foot. Instability is graded as +1, +2, and +3 based on the anterior motion.

Metatarsalphalangeal synovitis or instability is determined by the vertical stress test, or Lachman test. In this maneuver, the distal metatarsal is stabilized with one hand, and a dorsal directed force is applied with the other hand to the affected toe (Fig. 25-4). Pain is suggestive of an inflamed and possibly unstable joint.

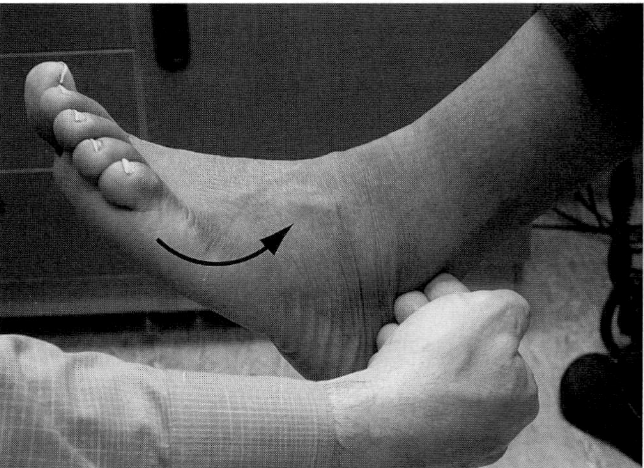

FIGURE 25-2. Testing for subluxation of the peroneal tendons. The examiner places two fingers posterior along the distal fibula and the patient dorsiflexes and everts. Any anterior subluxation is noted.

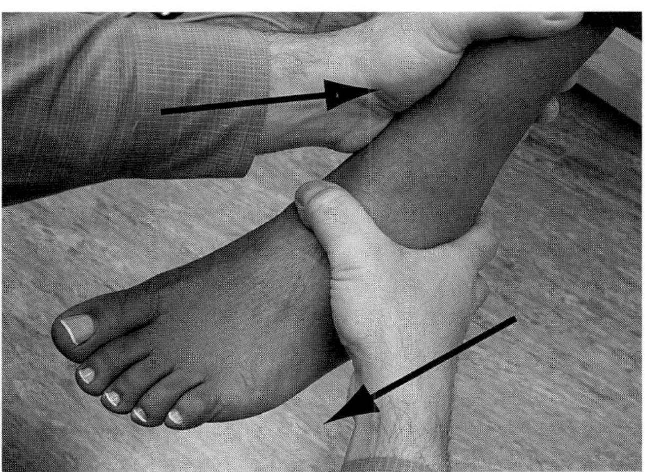

FIGURE 25-3. The anterior drawer test. One hand of the examiner stabilizes the distal tibia, and the other grasps the posterior heel and applies an anterior force.

Finally, gait should be evaluated in the patient without an acute injury. This requires visualizing the lower leg, including the knee, for any rotational, or antalgic patterns.

ANKLE DISORDERS

Sprains

Ankle sprains are one of the most common ankle injuries the primary care provider will see. These injuries account for 7% to 10% of all emergency room visits.[13] A sprain represents an injury to the constraining ligaments and capsule of the ankle joint caused by a twisting or rotational motion of the talus in the ankle mortise. This injury can range from a stretching to a complete disruption of these ligaments. Most sprains represent an inversion injury, leading to injury of the lateral ankle ligament complex.

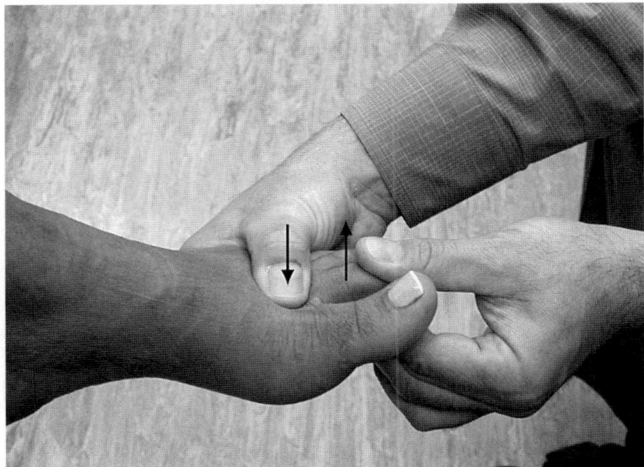

FIGURE 25-4. The vertical stress test for metatarsalphalangeal synovitis/inflammation. The distal metatarsal is stabilized with one hand, while the other hand grasps the toe and applies a vertical stress. A positive test results in pain or laxity of the joint.

The stability of the ankle joint results from the static stabilizers, the bony geometry and ligaments, and the dynamic stabilizers, the muscles and tendons that cross the ankle joint. The bony geometry is composed of the truncated shaped talus surrounded by the medial and lateral malleoli, which are the distal projections of the distal tibia and fibula, respectively. The ligaments of the lateral ligament complex include the anterior talofibular (ATF), calcaneofibular (CF), and the posterior talofibular ligament (PTF). The ATF is a thickening of the anterior capsule of the ankle joint, which originates from the anterior distal fibula and attaches to the neck of the talus. The CF originates from the distal tip of the fibula and attaches to the lateral calcaneus. The PTF courses from the distal fibula and attaches to the posterior process of the talus. The ATF and the CF ligaments are the most important to anterior and lateral stresses of the ankle joint.

Other crucial ligaments to ankle stability include the medial deltoid ligament, composed of superficial and deep layers, which courses from the medial malleolus to the navicular and talus, and is a restraint to eversion stress on the ankle. The anterior inferior tibiofibular ligament comprises part of the distal syndesmosis, and can be injured in an external rotational force.

Lateral sprains of the ankle can be defined as a grade I, II, or III injury depending on their severity. Although this is not always a precise classification in terms of exact injury to the ligaments, it can serve as a guideline to treatment. Grade I represents a partial disruption of ligament fibers, usually involving one (ATF) ligament. Grade II is a more severe sprain, often a disruption of the ATF ligament and partial disruption of the CF ligament. Grade III sprains represent a complete disruption to the ATF and CF ligaments.

Patient history is important in initial evaluation. Does the patient know the position of the foot during the injury? Was the patient able to walk right away? Did the ankle become swollen right away, and if so, on what part first? Is there a history of previous sprains?

On exam, areas of edema and ecchymosis should be noted. Differential diagnosis includes peroneal tendon subluxation, lateral malleolus fracture, anterior process of the calcaneus fracture, proximal fifth metatarsal fracture, and Achilles injury. Tenderness along the lateral ligaments will be present after an inversion sprain. Any bony tenderness along the lateral malleolus, proximal fibula (suggestive of fracture with distal ankle syndesmosis disruption), or foot should necessitate radiographs of the appropriate area. The anterior drawer test should be performed, but can be painful during the initial evaluation.

Initial treatment of ankle sprains is nonsurgical unless there is other severe pathology, and consists of rest, ice, elevation, limited immobilization, and rehabilitation. Generally, grade I ankle sprains are stable and can be treated with ice, nonsteroidal anti-inflammatories, and weight bearing when comfortable, with ankle stirrup brace if needed. Pain and discomfort is the gauge to return to normal activity, and a supportive brace may be helpful on resumption of sports. Peroneal strengthening exercises can be taught using a Theraband as resistance (Fig. 25-5). Grade II and III ankle sprains are more severe and should be referred to an orthopedic surgeon for treatment. A removable walking boot and crutches are initially beneficial, and reduction of swelling through icing, elevation, and compression stocking is the short-term goal. Icing consists of 20-minute sessions three to four times during the initial 72 hours. Gentle range of motion exercises are started to maintain flexibility. After the edema has started to subside, weight bearing as tolerated in the walker boot is allowed, and the start of peroneal and proprioceptive exercises under the supervision of a physical therapist is begun. Rehabilitation continues until ankle stability increases and more sports specific conditioning starts. The ability to single stance hop on the affected side without pain signifies return to sports. Bracing or taping can be used in the transition to full activity.

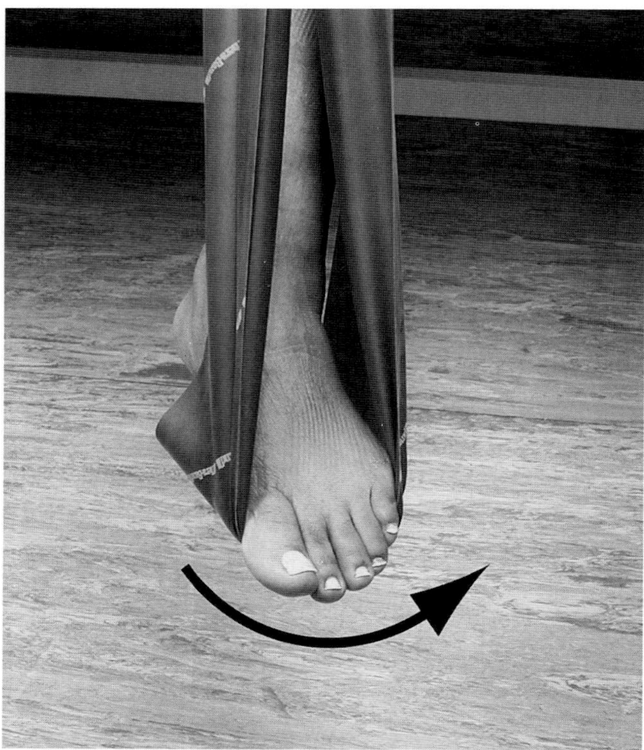

FIGURE 25-5. Peroneal strengthening exercises. A Theraband is used as resistance to eversion. The patient is instructed to start in a position of plantarflexion, and roll out in eversion against the band. Start with 20 repetitions, 3 sets at a time, 2 times a day and increase repetitions and sets as tolerated.

Syndesmotic Injuries

The "high" ankle sprain is an injury to the distal syndesmosis of the ankle. This complex includes anterior and posterior inferior tibiofibular ligaments, the interosseous ligament, and the interosseous membrane that connects the tibia to the fibula along the length of the lower leg. These structures provide stability to the ankle mortise and allow rotational and translational motions at the ankle joint.

An injury to the syndesmosis is typically an external rotation of the ankle with resulting dorsiflexion and eversion of the foot. Examination should consist of palpation of the AITF ligament and external stressing to the foot to reproduce the pain. The Cotton test involves compressing the mid-tibia and fibula, thereby stressing the syndesmosis, and is positive if pain is felt at the ankle. Palpation of the proximal fibula is important for detection of a Maisonneuve fracture, which is a fracture often associated with a distal syndesmotic injury. Radiographs of the ankle, and tibia/fibula if proximal tenderness is present, can detect more serious injury such as a deltoid ligament disruption, syndesmotic widening, or fibula fracture, all of which might require surgical intervention. A stable sprain of the syndesmosis can be treated similar to a grade II or III lateral sprain, but typically requires a longer recovery process. Any widening of the distal syndesmosis requires surgical fixation with a transsyndesmotic screw.

Chronic Ankle Instability

Estimates are that chronic ankle instability occurs in up to 42% of patients with acute ankle sprains.[5] Instability can be functional or mechanical. In functional instability, the patient subjectively feels that the ankle gives way, but on exam the ankle has a physiologic normal range of motion. Mechanical instability refers to anterolateral ankle motion beyond the physiologic normal and can be objectively evaluated by the examiner. Athletes might state that the ankle gives way with little inciting trauma, such as uneven pavement. Specific tests on exam include the anterior drawer and talar tilt, and comparing both to the contralateral side. The talar tilt test involves stabilizing the distal tibia with one hand, and applying an inversion force to the hindfoot with the other hand (Fig. 25-6). Both of these tests can be done under x-ray or fluoroscopy for a more objective measurement. Physical therapy, including peroneal tendon strengthening and proprioceptive training, and taping or bracing for athletic activities, are the mainstays of conservative treatment. Surgical reconstruction can be considered for the patient with mechanical instability who has failed conservative treatment.

Anterolateral Soft Tissue Ankle Impingement

Up to 40% of patients after sprains report chronic pain.[5] Ferkel has a described pathway in which an inversion

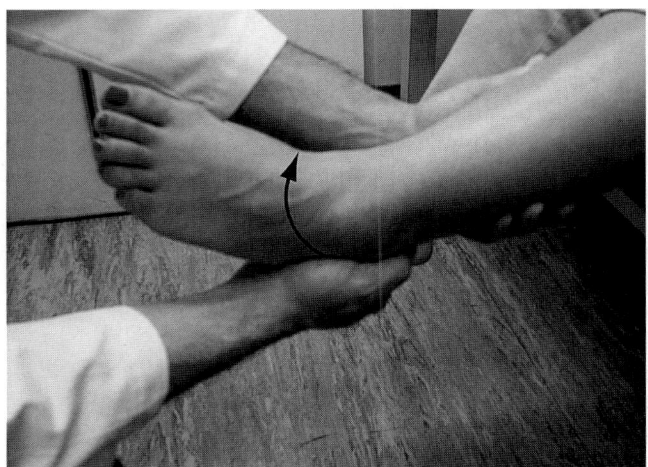

FIGURE 25-6. The talar tilt test. The examiner stabilizes the distal tibia with one hand, and inverts the hindfoot with the other. The contralateral side is used for comparison for any differences in laxity.

sprain leads to a torn ATF or CFL, incomplete healing, repetitive motion, inflamed ligament ends, synovitis and scar tissue, hypertrophic soft tissue, impingement, and, finally, chronic lateral ankle pain.[8] Patients report a vague pain along the lateral ankle joint, worse with athletic activity and absent at rest. Generally, there are no complaints of instability or giving way. On exam, patients have pain over the anterolateral ankle joint, a stable ankle, and a standing heel squat will often reproduce the pain in the anterolateral ankle joint. Physical therapy, judicial use of a corticosteroid injection, and heel lift can be helpful. Surgical arthroscopy with debridement of scar and inflamed tissue can be performed in recalcitrant cases.

Peroneal Tendon Disorders

The peroneus brevis and longus are the primary evertors of the ankle. At the level of the ankle joint, they pass in a fibro-osseous tunnel formed by a concave groove of the fibula anteriorly, the superior peroneal retinaculum posterolaterally, and the calcaneofibular ligament medially. The brevis inserts onto the base of the fifth metatarsal, and the longus courses inferior to the cuboid and inserts onto the base of the first metatarsal, where it also functions as a plantarflexor of the first ray. The longus can contain an os peroneum just proximal to the cuboid tunnel and is ossified in 20% of cases. Injuries to the tendons can include tendinitis, longitudinal tears, subluxation/dislocation, and occasionally rupture. Tendinitis and tears can result from overuse or repeated inversion sprains. Tenderness just inferior to the tip of the lateral malleolus is suggestive of peroneal injury. Rest, ice, anti-inflammatories, and an air stirrup are the initial treatment.

Subluxation or dislocation of the peroneal tendons typically results from a force resulting in dorsiflexion and eversion of the ankle. Reproducing this motion can produce the anterior translation of the peroneus brevis or longus on the distal fibula (Fig. 25-7). Initial treatment is casting or walker boot, but subacute or chronic presentation may require surgical repair of the superior peroneal retinaculum and possibly a fibula groove deepening procedure.

Rupture is less common and usually involves the peroneus longus just proximal to the os peroneum. In the acute setting, patients might hear a pop; this injury can also occur as an overuse syndrome, and symptoms will then occur more insidiously. On exam, tenderness is noted on the peroneus longus at the lateral wall of the calcaneus. Radiographs might demonstrate an os peroneum that is proximally retracted. Treatment involves repair or a tenodesis of the peroneus longus to the peroneus brevis.

Achilles Tendon Disorders

The Achilles tendon is formed by the coalescence of the medial and lateral heads of the gastrocnemius, and the soleus muscles. The Achilles tendon is 10 to 15 cm in length, is the strongest tendon in the body, and is the major plantarflexor of the foot at the ankle joint. The tendon is surrounded by a paratenon, although no true synovial sheath exists. Disorders to the Achilles tendon can be classified as noninsertional and insertional. Noninsertional disorders include the area 2 to 6 cm above the insertion of the tendon to the calcaneus. Insertional problems occur at the posterior heel at the level of the retrocalcaneal bursae and tendon insertion site.

Puddu described noninsertional tendon pathology as paratendinitis, paratendinitis with tendinosis, and tendinosis.[9] Paratendinitis is characterized as an inflammation

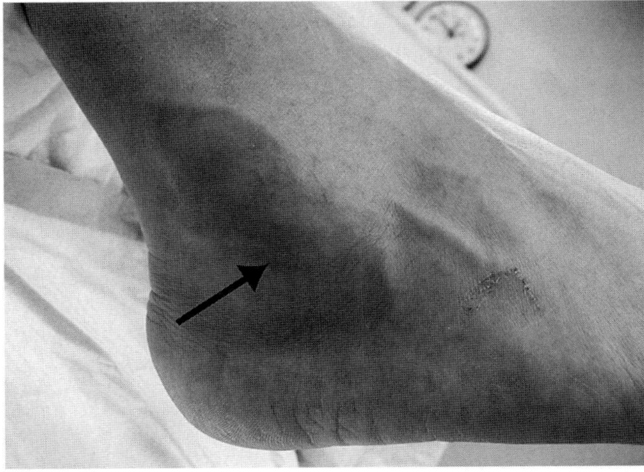

FIGURE 25-7. Dislocation of the peroneal tendons. Note the anterior postion of the tendons along the distal fibula.

of the paratenon. Paratendinitis with tendinosis refers to paratenon inflammation as well as intratendinous degeneration of the Achilles. Tendinosis is a noninflammatory degeneration of fibers of the tendon.

Noninsertional problems typically are seen in the active athlete, such as in runners or those who participate in sports that require cutting, twisting, or jumping. Overpronation of the foot and a tight heelcord have been implicated as factors. Clinically, in acute or subacute paratendinitis, the patient will have diffuse tenderness to palpation along the tendon, a feeling of fullness along the tendon, and at times crepitus. Paratendinitis with tendinosis might present with a more focal tenderness, and tendinosis will present with a discrete nodule or thickening of the tendon, with possible decreased plantarflexion strength. Initial treatment is shoewear modification, including heel lift, rest, ice, and activity modification. At times, immobilization in a walker boot can control the initial inflammatory phase. Stretching and physical therapy are used when the inflammatory component has decreased. Orthotic management to correct overpronation in the appropriate patient also is helpful. Surgical treatment depends on tendon involvement, and can include paratendon and/or tendon debridement, or tendon transfer and augmentation in more severe cases.

The insertional disorders can involve the tendon, the retrocalcaneal bursa, and a Haglund calcaneal deformity. The retrocalcaneal bursae lies just anterior to the Achilles tendon insertion site and posterior to the posterior process of the calcaneus, which when enlarged and prominent, is referred to as a Haglund deformity. The tendon can be involved with a tendinosis with or without calcification, the bursae can be inflamed, and the Haglund deformity can exacerbate both problems. Typically, the patient is older, less athletic, and more sedentary than the patient with noninsertional problems. Initial treatment in these disorders is similar to the noninsertional problems, and consists of heel lift or immobilization, followed by a stretching program. Recovery is slow, and in recalcitrant cases surgical debridement of the tendon, excision of the Haglund deformity, and possible flexor hallucis longus tendon transfer can be successful.

Achilles tendon ruptures occur most commonly in patients between 30 and 40 years old, and the male-female ratio ranges from 5:1 to 10:1 in most studies. Most common in jumping and cutting sports such as basketball and tennis, the mechanism is thought to be pushing off the foot with an extended knee. Patients sometimes describe a feeling as if they were kicked from behind. These injuries are not always very painful, and patients at times can walk with only a minimal limp, and thus this injury can be overlooked. On exam, a gap in the tendon can often be palpated 2 to 6 cm from insertion, and patients are unable to single heel rise. The Thompson test is described as positive for a tear if, upon squeezing the calf with the patient supine and leg pointed upward, there is no plantarflexion of the foot against gravity (Fig. 25-8). Treatment options continue to be somewhat controversial. Generally, recommended treatment in the active, athletic patient is surgical repair.[11] Different techniques can be utilized, but the recent trend is to limit postoperative casting and progress with therapy as early as 2 weeks after surgery using a range of motion walker boot. Nonsurgical casting or functional bracing is an option, although higher rates of rerupture and decreased plantarflexion power are seen, and are recommended for the sedentary, less active, or medically unstable patient.

Posterior Tibial Tendon Disorders

The posterior tibial tendon courses along the medial ankle and inserts onto the medial navicular and plantar aspect of the medial cuneiform. During normal gait, its function is to invert the foot, lock the hindfoot and

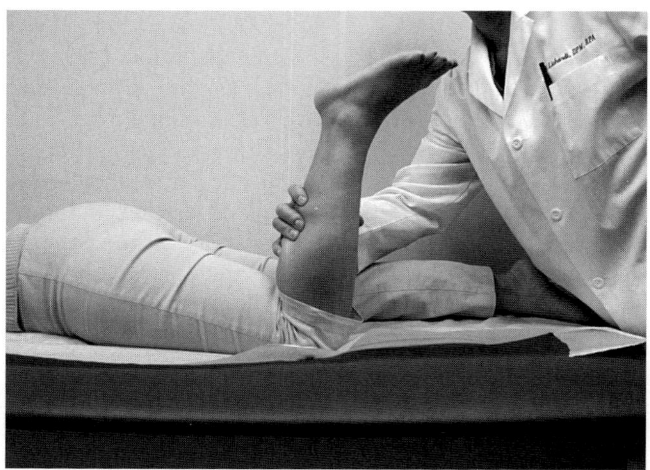

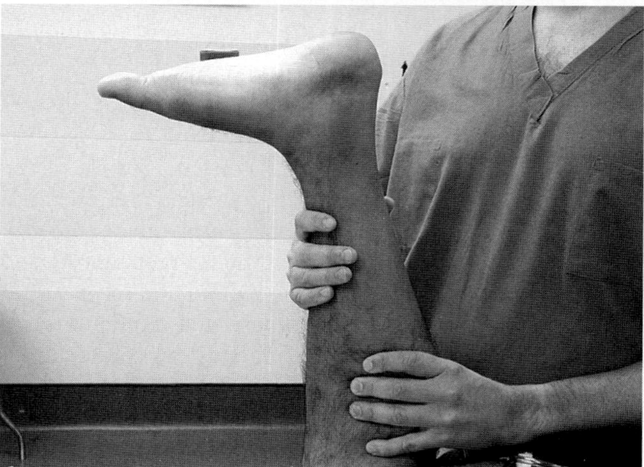

FIGURE 25-8. The Thompson test. With the patient prone, the examiner squeezes the calf. If the Achilles tendon is intact, this should result in plantarflexion of the foot. If the tendon is torn, the foot cannot be plantarflexed, and the test is considered positive.

transverse tarsal joints, and allow the Achilles tendon to plantarflex the foot. Injuries to this tendon in the athlete include tendinitis, tendinosis, and intrasubstance tear with elongation and dysfunction of the tendon. Most commonly seen in the runner, tendinitis is an overuse injury. Patients will describe pain along the inner ankle with activity, and on exam, tenderness is usually localized to the tendon just posterior to the medial malleolus. Single heel rise on the affected side may be painful, and with only a tendinitis, there should be no apparent arch collapse. Treatment includes activity modification, ice, and an anti-inflammatory. An ankle air stirrup or walker boot can be helpful, and in the patient with bilateral pes planus or overpronated feet, an orthoses with a medial arch and/or post can be beneficial in the long term. If there is a tendinosis or longitudinal split in the tendon, a decreased arch is often unilaterally present on exam, and patients will have a decreased strength on single heel rise. The "too many toes" sign refers to viewing the patient's feet from behind; more toes are seen on the involved side due to the collapse of the medial arch and increased forefoot abduction (Fig. 25-9). This is more problematic to treat, and surgical options include tendon transfer of the flexor digitorum longus and medial slide calcaneal osteotomy to correct the increased heel valgus.

Osteochondral Lesions of the Talus

Osteochondral lesions of the talus (OLT) refer to injury to the cartilage and subchondral bone of the dome of the talus, and are generally traumatic in nature. Their incidence has been reported as 6.5% of ankle sprains, and can be a reason for continued pain and dysfunction following a previous ankle sprain.[2] No single mechanism can explain each case, but it is thought that they represent an impaction injury to the cartilage and bone during initial injury. Patients will present with pain, joint effusion, and limitation of athletic activity, and often can recount a specific lateral ankle injury. Exam can be nonspecific, with pain elicited with certain ankle movements, depending in the location of the lesion. Radiographs are negative in most cases, and an MRI is the recommended radiographic exam.

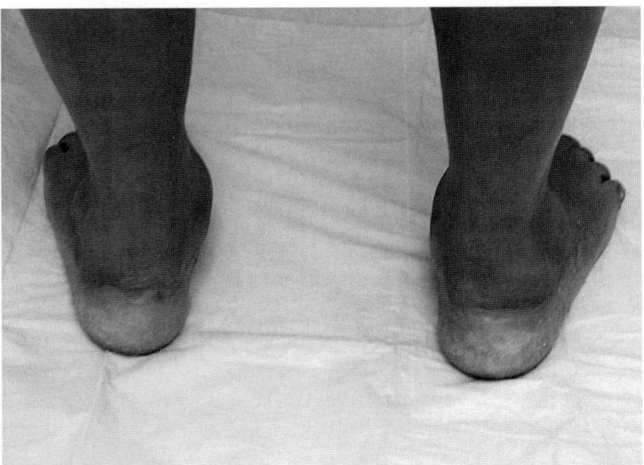

FIGURE 25-9. The "too many toes" sign. By viewing the patient from behind, one can notice more toes visible on one side. This corresponds to an increased pes planus, or flatfoot due to posterior tibial tendon dysfunction.

These lesions are graded based on their size, instability, and displacement. In the skeletally immature patient, cast immobilization with non–weight bearing is recommended for the nondisplaced lesion. In the older patient, depending on instability and displacement, ankle arthroscopy and drilling of the subchondral bone at the base of the lesion is indicated in the symptomatic patient. Larger lesions, and those failing arthroscopic drilling, are candidates for osteochondral transplantation, or autologous chondrocyte transplantation.

DISORDERS OF THE FOOT

Heel Pain

One of the most common athletic foot complaints is heel pain. The most common etiology is due to plantar fascia inflammation, although stress fracture, heel spur, nerve entrapment, and plantar fascia tear have been described as potential sources of heel pain. The plantar fascia originates from the medial tuberosity of the plantar calcaneus, divides into bands that insert onto fibrous tissues along the plantar aspect of the toes. The term *windlass mechanism* refers to the elevation of the longitudinal arch as the toes are extended during walking or running, thus tightening the plantar fascia. Repetitive strain on the plantar fascia is thought to lead to inflammation and microtearing of the fibers that originate along the plantar calcaneus. Athletes will typically describe pain along the heel with the first few steps in the morning, standing after sitting for extended periods, but also with prolonged weight-bearing activity. Symptoms usually have an insidious onset. On exam, plantarmedial calcaneal tenderness is typical.

Initial treatment consists of stretching the heel cord and plantar fascia (Fig. 25-10), viscoelastic heel cups, and a dorsiflexion nightsplint. The purpose of the nightsplint is to keep the plantar fascia in a stretched out position overnight, compared to the typical plantarflexed non–weight bearing position. Recovery can be gradual. A corticosteroid injection is usually just a temporizing measure and can potentially cause rupture of the fascia. Immobilization can be helpful if the above mentioned modalities fail. Lithotripsy has recently been reported to have some benefit in limited studies and, when available, is another treatment option.[1] Surgical intervention with an open or endoscopic release of the medial one-third of the plantar fascia origin is an option in those patients who fail 6 to 12 months of conservative treatment.

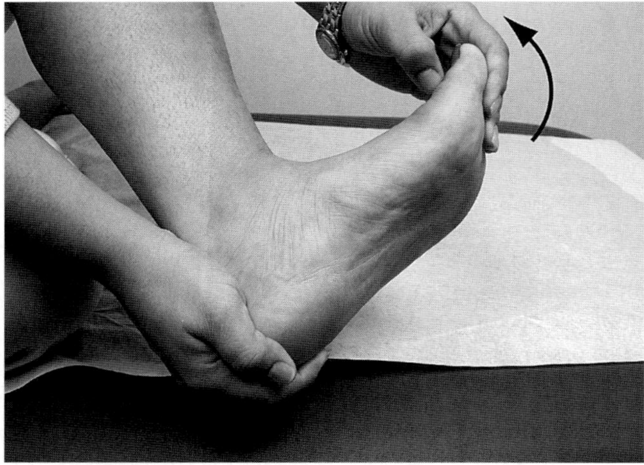

FIGURE 25-10. Plantar fascia stretching. The patient dorsiflexes the toes and ankle, and holds the stretch for 15 seconds. Repeat 5 stretches, 4 to 5 times per day.

Differential diagnosis includes stress fracture of the calcaneus. These patients will have tenderness along the medial and lateral calcaneus, and more proximal to the typical heel pain. Radiographs will occasionally reveal a dense fracture line, but if they are negative and suspicion is high, an MRI will be conclusive. Treatment is a walker boot until the patient is free of symptoms. Entrapment of the first branch of the lateral plantar nerve can be a source of heel pain and can be superimposed on a plantar inflammation. Initial treatment is similar, but surgical treatment includes a release of the nerve in addition to the plantar fascia.

Hallux Rigidus

Hallux rigidus refers to a degenerative joint condition of the first metatarsalphalangeal joint, resulting in pain and decreased motion. This can result in diminished push-off power for the athlete, and the repetitive jamming and impingement of the joint during activity can lead to further degenerative changes. The athlete will describe a sharp or dull pain at the joint, usually dorsal, and discomfort at rest in more severe cases. Typically, on exam there are palpable dorsal and lateral osteophytes, restricted joint range of motion, and synovitis. Dorsiflexion of less than 30° is generally symptomatic for the athlete. Radiographic examination reveals dorsal osteophytes of the metatarsal head and base of the proximal phalanx, and joint space narrowing.

Severity is graded as I, II, and III. Grade I presents as a moderate decreased motion, dorsal osteophytes, but mild to no joint space narrowing. Grade II (Fig. 25-11) involves more severe loss of joint motion, dorsal osteophytes, and moderate degenerative joint change. Grade III is a near complete loss of joint motion, with extensive joint deterioration. Conservative approaches include taping, shoewear modification, and possibly functional orthoses. The goal is to support the joint and limit stresses to motion. A steel or rigid support in the orthoses or athletic shoe can accomplish this goal. Surgical treatments include a cheilectomy, which is a dorsal one-third metatarsal head resection, combined with a closing wedge proximal phalangeal osteotomy for grade I and II. For the more severe grade III, a fusion or capsular arthroplasty can decrease pain, but can limit function.

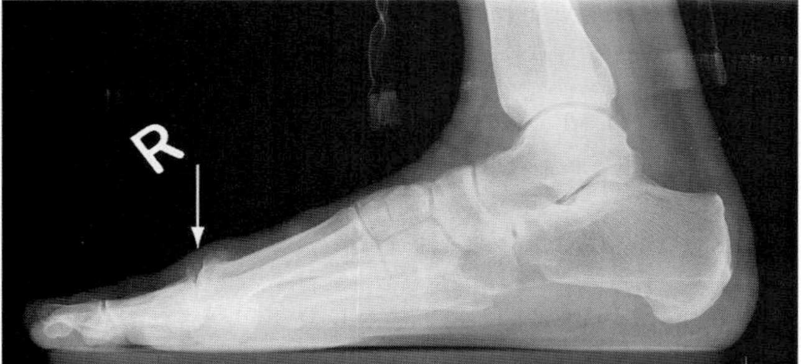

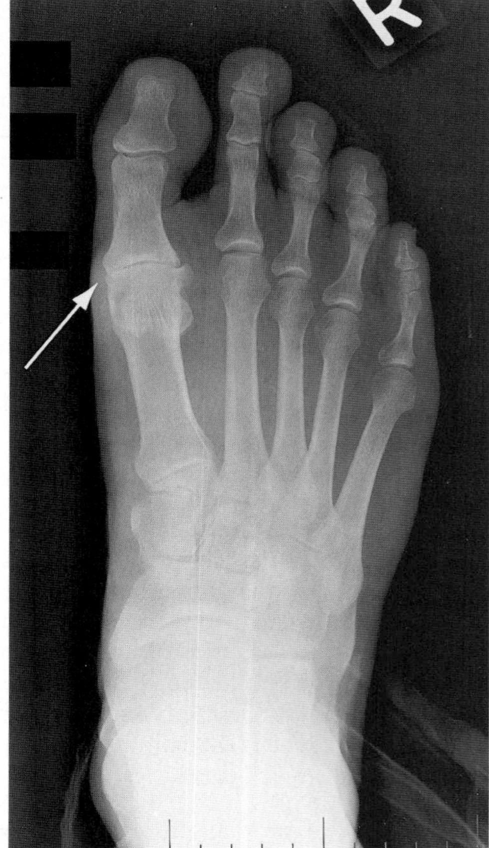

FIGURE 25-11. Hallux rigidus grade II. Note the dorsal osteophytes of the metatarsal head and joint space narrowing.

Turf Toe

Turf toe refers to a hyperextension injury to the first metatarsalphalangeal joint and represents a strain or tear to the capsule and ligament restraints. The stability of the joint results from the collateral ligaments, a thickening of the plantar capsule called the plantar plate, and the flexor hallucis brevis, which contains the medial and lateral sesamoids and attaches to the base of the proximal phalanx. Spectrum of injury includes a sprain or disruption of the plantar plate, collateral ligament injury, sesamoid fracture, complete dislocation of the joint, and chondral damage to the metatarsal head. Upon presentation, the patient should be questioned for toe position at injury. Patients will generally be swollen and ecchymotic at the first toe. Valgus and varus stress testing should be performed for collateral ligament damage, and dorsal and plantar capsule tenderness noted. Radiographs are taken for suspected sesamoid fracture. Treatment in mild sprains requires rest, ice, and taping to restrict dorsiflexion. More severe injuries require immobilization or, for sesamoid disruption, possible surgical repair. A rigid forefoot insole is helpful in return to sports.

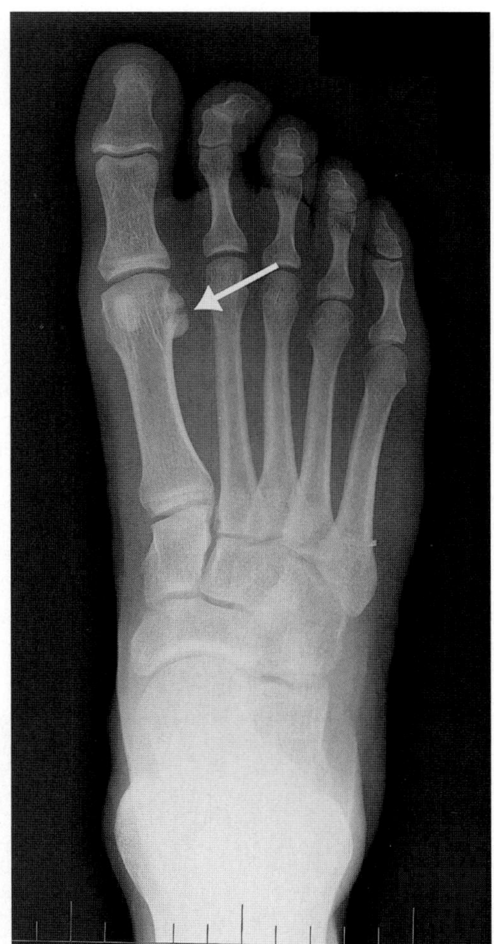

FIGURE 25-12. Acute lateral sesamoid fracture,. Note the diastasis and sharp cortical margins.

Sesamoid Disorders

The medial and lateral sesamoids are located in the flexor hallucis brevis, their dorsal surface is covered with cartilage, and they articulate with the plantar surface of the metatarsal head. The sesamoids are connected to each other by the intersesamoidal ligament and are centered under the metatarsal head by the crista, a small osteochondral ridge. They connect to the base of the proximal phalanx through the FHB and the plantar plate. In 10% to 30% of the population, one sesamoid is bipartite, having never achieved bony fusion, and this is usually the medial sesamoid.[4] Sesamoid dysfunction can include inflammation, stress fracture, and acute fracture of a sesamoid or bipartite sesamoid. Clinically, patients will experience pain under the ball of the first toe and will have swelling in the acute presentation. A patient with an acute fracture (Fig. 25-12) will find it quite difficult to bear weight, but an inflammation or stress fracture might have a more insidious onset and be painful only with athletic activity. Tenderness is usually elicited along the plantar surface of the involved sesamoid. Radiographs can reveal an acute fracture, with or without diastasis, but can be difficult at times to distinguish between a bipartite sesamoid. MRI or CT scan can further clarify the full extent of injury.

Sesamoiditis, an inflammatory condition, can be caused by inflamed bursae, and treatment initially is rest, orthoses with first metatarsal head relief (Fig. 25-13), or a walker boot. An acute fracture with minimal displacement can be treated with cast immobilization, and then orthoses. A stress fracture or bipartite diastasis is treated with a walker boot. Surgical treatment with partial or total sesamoidectomy is generally reserved for stress or bipartite fractures unresponsive to boot or orthotic management. A differential diagnosis in sesamoid disorders is entrapment of the plantarmedial digital nerve. In this condition, tenderness is more medial than plantar, and shoewear modification or orthotic relief can be helpful.

Tarsal Coalition

A *tarsal coalition* refers to an abnormal fibrous or bony connection between the calcaneus and the navicular, or the talocalcaneal joint. Patients will complain of pain along the subtalar joint and will often sustain multiple ankle sprains due to restricted hindfoot motion. The onset of symptoms usually is between the ages of 11 and 20, but can present later in life after a severe ankle sprain. As the subtalar motion becomes more limited, patients will place increased stresses on adjacent joints in the foot, and will experience more pain with activity.

On exam, the patient will have decreased motion at the hindfoot, and will often have a flattening of the arch and increased valgus of the hindfoot. Radiographs can detect a coalition. An oblique view of the foot can

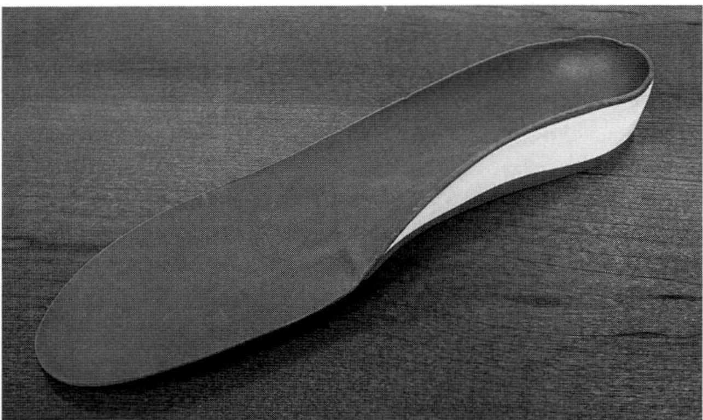

FIGURE 25-13. A custom orthoses. Note the depression in the orthoses at the first metatarsal head for unloading the sesamoids.

demonstrate a calcaneonavicular coalition (Fig. 25-14), and a calcaneal axial view can reveal a talocalcaneal coalition. Beware of multiple coalitions. CT scan can provide confirmation. Treatment begins with cast immobilization. Those patients who fail to respond to conservative treatment are candidates for excision of the coalition. More extensive coalitions might require subtalar or triple arthrodesis.

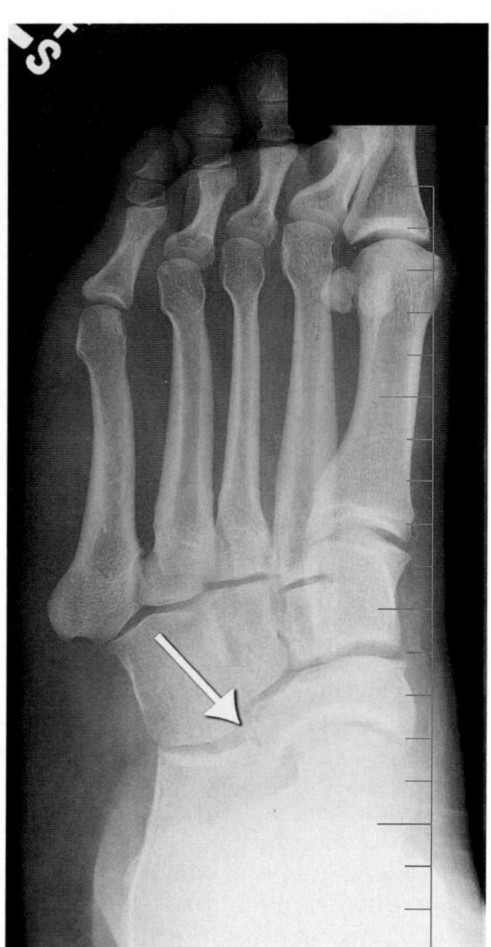

FIGURE 25-14. Fibrous calcaneonavicular coalition. Note the close and uneven appearance of the space between the calcaneus and navicular.

Second Metatarsalphalangeal Synovitis/Instability

Pain and swelling at the second toe is a common problem seen in the athlete, especially the runner. At times mistaken for a neuroma or stress fracture, this condition is commonly caused by an inflammation that can lead to deterioration of the capsule and ligaments, resulting in an instability of the joint. The second metatarsal is often the longest of the five metatarsals, and this is thought to be a factor in why the second metatarsalphalangeal joint is most commonly affected. Chronic synovitis due to overuse and attritional changes of the plantar plate of the joint can lead to a joint instability. The cycle continues with the instability leading to increased inflammation.

Athletes will complain of swelling and pain along the base of the second toe. They might notice the second toe drifting up or to the side, and discomfort is related to activity. The vertical stress test, in which the toe is stressed in a dorsal direction after stabilizing the metatarsal, is positive for this condition. Laxity of the joint also can be appreciated with this maneuver.

Initial treatment includes taping the toe, a metatarsal pad or bar, an anti-inflammatory, and activity modification. A single corticosteroid injection can be helpful, but potentially can worsen the instability. Surgical options include synovectomy with possible flexor to extensor toe tendon transfer to stabilize and reduce the joint. Part of the differential diagnosis is Freiberg disease, which is a osteochondroses, or avascular necrosis of the metatarsal head.

Metatarsalgia

Pain under the plantar metatarsal heads is referred to as *metatarsalgia*. Most commonly seen in runners, metatarsalgia often is present under the second or third metatarsal head. Multiple etiologies exist, including a tight heelcord or anterior ankle impingement, which both can lead to decreased ankle dorsiflexion and increased stresses under the ball of the foot. This can lead to clawing of the toes due to overrecruitment of the toe extensors, and exacerbate the metatarsalgia. Initial treatment includes a heel cord stretching program and metatarsal pad or bar. This usually is successful, but surgical options can be utilized depending on the etiology. A gastrocnemius recession can correct heel cord tightness, an anterior ankle bony debridement can increase ankle dorsiflexion, and a plantar condylectomy or metatarsal osteotomy can decrease forces under the metatarsal head.

Morton's Neuroma

Morton's neuroma refers to an impingement of the common interdigital nerve as it passes under the transverse intermetatarsal ligament at the metatarsal heads. As the toes dorsiflex at the last stage of stance in the gait cycle, the nerve is compressed between the plantar aspect of the foot and the edge of the intermetatarsal ligament. Constrictive shoewear, such as women's fashionable shoes, can exacerabate this impingement. The nerve develops perineural fibrosis, leading to an increased soft tissue thickness, and then increased propensity to be pinched.[12] The third webspace is the most common location for a neuroma, but the reason for this is not completely understood. Patients' symptoms are worse in shoes, and athletes will often feel relief on removing their shoes and rubbing the plantar foot. Patients can also describe a numbness or tingling into the adjacent toes. On exam, tenderness in the webspace along with a Mulders click (the neuroma being pressed between the metatarsal heads) is characteristic for this problem. Treatment begins with a metatarsal pad and/or corticosteroid injection. Recalcitrant cases require surgical excision.

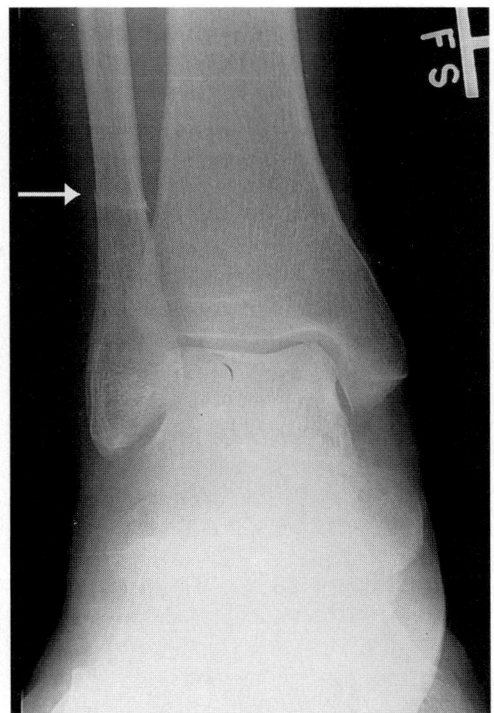

FIGURE 25-15. Stress fracture of the distal fibula.

FRACTURES AND DISLOCATIONS OF THE FOOT AND ANKLE

Stress Fractures

Stress fractures are thought to represent 5% of all sports injuries, with about 50% occurring in the foot and ankle.[6,7] A fatigue fracture refers to normal bone loaded with excessive loads that overwhelm the body's repair processes. An insuffiency fracture refers to weakened bone due to medical condition (i.e., renal disease, osteoporosis, or Paget's disease).

In the athlete, the stress fracture generally is a fatigue fracture. Causes include training errors, improper shoewear, poor biomechanics, changing or uneven surfaces, and anatomic factors. The athlete will complain of activity-related pain with an insidious onset. Swelling can be minimal. The patient's history often is not significant for a specific injury. Recent training habits and any changes in shoewear or orthoses should be determined. On exam, tenderness is usually localized to the involved bone. Radiographs of the affected area are ordered, but can be negative initially. MRI can be diagnostic and is ordered depending on the clinical suspicion and whether it will alter the treatment plan.

Common stress fractures in the ankle include the distal fibula (Fig. 25-15) and medial malleolus. In the foot, common areas are the metatarsals (Fig. 25-16), calcaneus (Fig. 25-17), navicular, and the sesamoids. Most stress fractures are treated with activity modification and immobilization in a walker boot. The navicular and fifth metatarsal stress fracture often requires casting and non–weight bearing, and surgical fixation if there is nonunion.

Ankle Fractures

Acute ankle fractures occur as a result of a severe twisting or rotational force applied to the foot. Fractures to the lateral, medial, and posterior malleolus can occur separately or in combination. The deltoid and syndesmotic

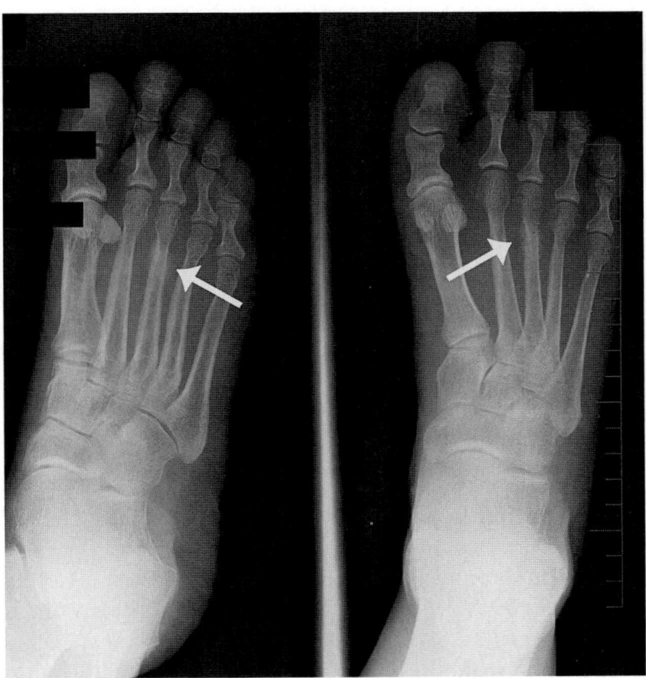

FIGURE 25-16. Stress fracture of the third metatarsal.

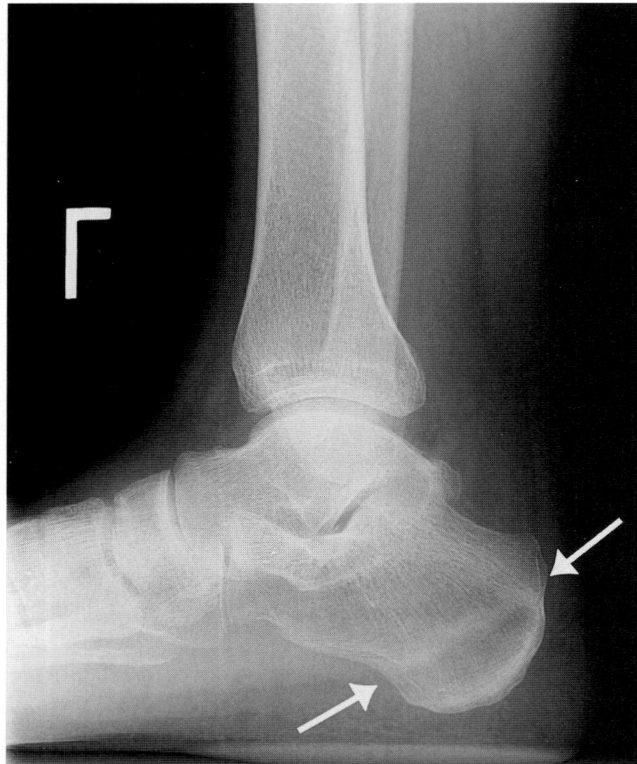

FIGURE 25-17. Stress fracture of the calcaneus.

ligaments also can be disrupted. A dislocated ankle is an emergency and should be reduced as quickly as possible to lessen the severity of injury to the soft tissues. Initial treatment is splinting, elevation, and ice. Depending on the instability and displacement, surgical reduction and fixation can be required.

Subtalar Dislocation

Sometimes referred to as "basketball foot," subtalar dislocations are infrequent. Most are medial dislocations, and in the basketball player, occur when the player's foot forcefully inverts in a plantarflexed postion. Some reduce spontaneously, but they may require open reduction in the operating room. Stiffness at the subtalar joint is a common consequence and can lead to degenerative changes.

Proximal Fifth Metatarsal Fractures

Fractures of the proximal fifth metatarsal are among the most common fractures of the foot. They can be classified according to their location: tuberosity, metaphyseal (Jones fractures), and diaphyseal. Tuberosity fractures are by far the most common type and are a result of an inversion twist of the foot. It is thought that the peroneus brevis insertion or lateral band of the plantar fascia is responsible for the fracture pattern.[10] Usually nondisplaced or minimally displaced, these can be treated symptomatically in either a stiff shoe or walker boot. Significant displacement, or an intraarticular step-off, might indicate surgical reduction and fixation.

The Jones fracture, named after Sir Robert Jones who described his own injury, occurs at the metaphyseal–diaphyseal junction of the base of the fifth metatarsal, and in the athlete, offers alternative treatments. Nonsurgical treatment entails casting and non–weight bearing, and in a significant majority of patients will heal.[3] Surgical treament with intramedual screw fixation allows early weight bearing, return to sports as early as 6 to 7 weeks, and results in a higher union rate (Fig. 25-18). Proximal diaphyseal fractures usually are chronic or acute-on-chronic stress fractures, and typically require fixation with or without bone grafting.

Other Metatarsal Fractures

Most other metatarsal fractures can be managed with a cast shoe or walking boot. Closed or open reduction is indicated for displaced fractures, with alignment in the sagittal plane thought to be most important.

Lisfranc Sprain/Fracture–Dislocation

The Lisfranc midfoot complex, named after the surgeon to Napoleon Bonaparte, refers to the tarsometatarsal joints, and forms the transverse arch of the midfoot. The key to the bony stability of the arch is the second metatarsal, which is recessed compared to the adjacent first and third tarsometatarsal articulations, and due to the trapezoidal shape of these bones, resists displacement. Further stability is a result of dorsal and plantar tarsometatarsal ligaments, and intermetarsal ligaments at the bases of the metatarsals. However, there is no intermetatarsal ligament between the first and second metatarsals, and the second metatarsal is attached to the medial cuneiform through the strong, oblique Lisfranc ligament. Injuries to this complex include a sprain of the Lisfranc ligament or fracture and dislocation of the midfoot complex.

These injuries are sometimes difficult to diagnose initially, and a high index of suspicion should be present for any midfoot injury, because the consequences of improper treatment are severe. The mechanism of injury is a plantarflexion force of the foot, causing the weaker dorsal ligaments to tear and allowing the metatarsals to subluxate dorsally. A combined abduction stress will lead to a strain or rupture of the Lisfranc ligament. Patients will complain of pain in the midfoot with weight bearing, which will vary depending on the severity of the injury.

On exam, there often is dorsal foot swelling, and with tear or rupture of the Lisfranc ligament there can be plantar ecchymosis. Tenderness at the involved tarsometatarsal joints is present, and abduction stressing

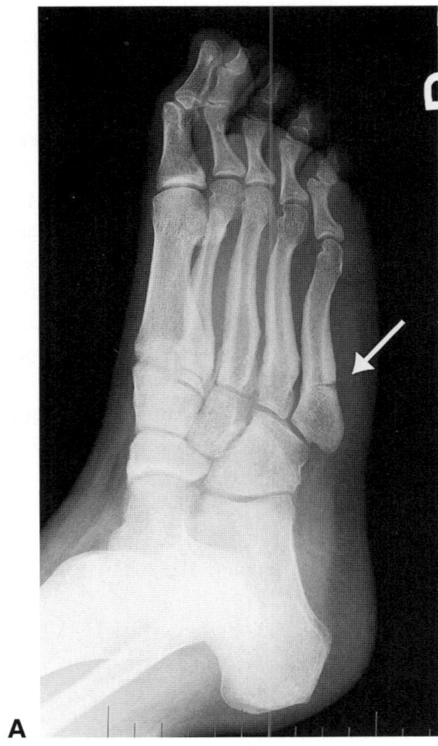

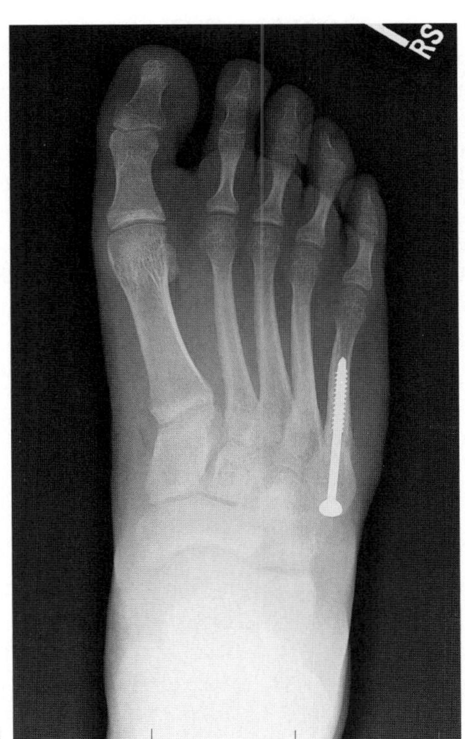

FIGURE 25-18. Jones fracture of the base of the fifth metatarsal. **A,** Preoperative radiograph. **B,** Postoperative radiograph after intramedullary fixation.

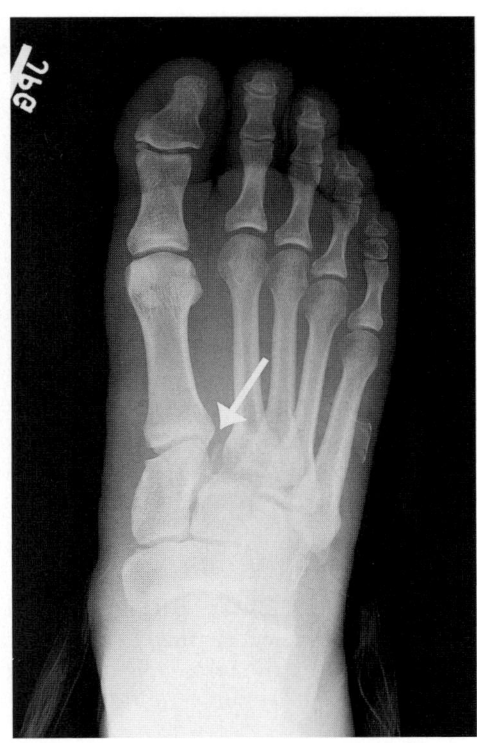

FIGURE 25-19. Lisfranc fracture–dislocation. Note the widening at the space between the bases of the first and second metatarsal, and small fracture fragment.

and compression of the midfoot are painful. Radiographs should be weight bearing, and on the AP view, the medial base of the second metatarsal should line up with the medial border of the middle cuneiform (Fig. 25-19). Any diastasis or step-off indicates injury, and a CT scan or MRI will reveal the severity. A sprain without displacement can be treated with limited weight bearing, a walker boot, rehabilitation, and gradual return to sports. Displacement, instability, and/or fracture requires surgical reduction and fixation.

Anterior Process of the Calcaneus Fractures

Part of the differential diagnosis in ankle and foot inversion injuries is a fracture of the anterior process of the calcaneus, because these fractures can be overlooked. This injury represents an avulsion fracture of the anterior process of the calcaneus at the attachment of the bifurcate ligament. The mechanism of injury is a plantarflexion and inversion of the foot. Patients will describe lateral ankle or foot pain, but will state that it does not feel like the typical sprain. Palpation will reveal tenderness at the anterior process (Fig. 25-20). Radiographs sometimes are inconclusive, but the oblique view of the foot demonstrates this area most clearly. Small, minimally displaced fragments can be treated in a cast or walker boot with progressive weight bearing, but larger, displaced fragments require fixation to minimize future

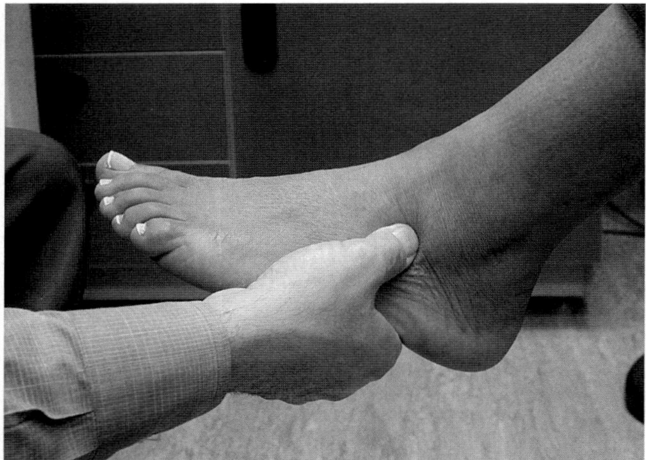

FIGURE 25-20. Palpation of the anterior process of the calcaneus.

degenerative changes at the calcaneocuboid joint. Symptomatic fractures not recognized until months after injury can be treated with steroid injection or surgical excision.

Toe Fractures

Fractures of the toes are the most common injury of the bones in the foot. Most are due to a direct blow, either by stubbing the toe or by a dropped object. Often they can be treated with a stiff-soled shoe, ice, and buddy taping to the adjacent toe. Displaced or intraarticular fractures may require closed reduction with a digital block or open reduction with pinning. Dislocations are less common, but usually can be treated in a similar manner.

REFERENCES

1. Alvarez R: Preliminary results on the safety and efficacy of the OssaTron for treatment of plantar fasciitis. Foot Ankle Int 23:197–203, 2002.
2. Bosien WR, Staples OS, Russell SW: Residual disability following acute ankle sprains. J Bone Joint Surg 37A:1237–1243, 1955.
3. Clapper MF, O'Brien TJ, Lyons PM: Fractures of the fifth metatarsal: Analysis of a fracture registry. Clin Ortho 315:238–241, 1995.
4. Dobas DC, Silvers MD: The frequency of the partite sesamoids of the first metatarsophalangeal joint. J Am Pediatric Assoc 67:880–882, 1977.
5. Gerber JP, Williams GN, Scoville CR, et al: Persistent disability associated with ankle sprains: A prospective examination of an athletic population. Foot Ankle Int 19:653–660, 1998.
6. McBryde AM Jr: Stress fractures. In Baxter DE (ed): The Foot and Ankle in Sport. 1995, pp 81–93.
7. Pecina M, Bojanic I, Dubravcil S: Stress fractures in figure skaters. Am J Sports Med 8:277, 1990.
8. Pfeffer GB: Chronic Ankle Pain in the Athlete. Rosemont, IL, American Academy of Orthopaedic Surgeons, 2000.
9. Puddu G, Ippolito E, Postacchini F: A classification of Achilles tendon disease. Am J Sports Med 4:145, 1976.
10. Richli WR, Rosenthal DJ: Avulsion fractures of the fifth metatarsal: Experimental study of pathomechanics. AFR 143:889–891, 1984.
11. Romanelli DA, Almekinders LC, Mandelbaum BR: Achilles rupture in the athlete: Current science and treatment. Sports Med Arthrosc Rev 8:377–386, 2000.
12. Shereff MJ, Grande DA: Electron microscopic analysis of the interdigital neuroma. Clin Orthop 271:296–299, 1991.
13. Stephens MM, Sammarco GJ: The stabilizing role of the lateral complex around the ankle and subtalar joints. Foot Ankle 13:130–136, 1992.

IV

The Female Athlete

26 Metabolic Conditions in the Female Athlete

Robyn J. Hakanson and
Sara M. Wiskow

Young girls and women are now participating in sports at a higher rate than ever. As a result, physicians are seeing not only musculoskeletal sports injuries in this group, but also a variety of problems related directly or indirectly to the uniquely female hormonal environment. The triad of disordered eating, amenorrhea, and osteoporosis, known as the female athlete triad, is commonly seen in female athletes of all levels. The factors contributing to this syndrome are many, and management of its sequelae requires a multidisciplinary approach. Diagnosis, prevention, and management of the problems seen in the female athlete require not only a high index of suspicion for diagnosis, but also cooperation of all involved members of the sports medicine team.

MENSTRUAL DYSFUNCTION

Menstrual abnormalities, from a few skipped periods to a complete absence of menses, are extremely common in both athletic and nonathletic adolescents and young women. The true incidence of irregular menses is unknown, but has been reported at 1% to 66% among athletes, compared with 2% to 5% of the general population. By definition, primary amenorrhea is the absence of menstruation by age 16 in a girl with secondary sex characteristics. Secondary amenorrhea is the absence of three or more consecutive menstrual cycles in a woman who has had at least one episode of menstrual bleeding. Oligomenorrhea is fewer than eight menses per year.[26] Pregnancy is the most common cause of amenorrhea. Less commonly, structural or hormonal abnormalities can also cause amenorrhea.

The normal menstrual cycle represents a complex interplay of hormones. The 28-day cycle is divided into the follicular phase (FP) in which the follicle matures (days 1–9), the ovulatory period during which ovulation occurs (days 10–14), and the luteal phase (LP) in which the endometrium prepares for the implantation of a fertilized ovum (days 15–28). In the absence of implantation of a fertilized egg, the endometrium is sloughed, and menstruation occurs. This cycle is regulated by luteinizing hormone (LH) and follicle-stimulating hormone (FSH) from the pituitary gland, which is itself controlled by the regular pulsed secretion of gonadotropin-releasing hormone (Fig. 26-1). Any disruption in this balance can lead to hypothalamic pituitary axis (HPA) dysfunction and oligomenorrhea or amenorrhea[60] (Fig. 26-2).

Hypoestrogenism and Menstrual Dysfunction

Normal menstrual function is determined by a complex relationship between nutrition, exercise intensity and volume, body mass index, and psychological stressors. Individual tolerance for changes in these factors is variable. Pathological eating behavior and negative energy balance are common among women in sports that require the maintenance of very low body weight for enhanced performance or aesthetic appearance. Gymnastics and ballet dancing are examples of these activities. In other words, the athlete is likely to take in too few calories to sustain her level of activity, resulting in an “energy drain.” These girls and women quickly become amenorrheic. Warren and Perlroth reported that the reproductive and metabolic hormonal profiles of amenorrheic women engaged in these types of sports closely parallel those of nonathletic amenorrheic women with eating disorders such as anorexia nervosa, indicating that nutritional restriction is directly related to the menstrual dysfunction seen in these athletes.[59]

When periods are suppressed in response to increased athletic activity and/or dietary changes, many athletes find it to be a convenience and may not be concerned. In fact, the short-term absence of menses in and of itself is not the problem; rather, it is the lack of estrogen associated with HPA suppression that can lead to subsequent osteopenia or osteoporosis. The long-term consequences of reduced levels of estrogen and progesterone may include an increased risk of reduced bone mineral density (BMD) and stress fractures. HPA suppression can compromise both bone mineral accrual during adolescence and young adulthood and the maintenance of bone mineral density later in life.[42]

Delayed menarche, the result of low gonadotropin secretion, is seen frequently in young female athletes. One result of delayed menarche may be scoliosis, which has been reported in young ballet dancers. In addition to scoliosis, the ballet dancers in this study had a 61% incidence of fractures.[58] Hypogonadism associated with delayed menarche seems to favor long-bone growth, substantiated by the decreased upper to lower body ratio and increased arm span noted in ballet dancers in particular.[59] Alternatively, perhaps the physical characteristics associated with late maturation are more suitable for successful

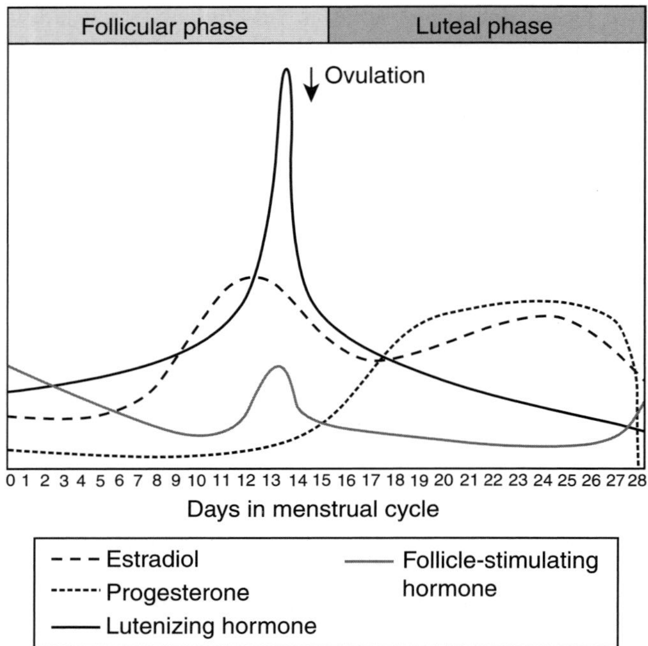

FIGURE 26-1. Hormonal fluctuations in a normal 28-day menstrual cycle.

athletic performance, and the prevalence of delayed menarche and associated physical characteristics among certain female athletes may simply reflect a "natural selection" of sorts based on normal genetic variability.

Hyperandrogenism and Menstrual Dysfunction

Sports that emphasize strength and size over leanness, (e.g., swimming or rowing) are not associated with low body weight and restricted nutrition. However, menstrual cycle dysfunction may occur in these athletes as well. Hyperandrogenism along with elevated LH and LH/FSH ratios is seen in these athletes. This is in direct contrast to the hypoestrogensism observed in athletes engaged in sports requiring thinness, such as gymnastics, long-distance running, or ballet.[16,59] Elevations in androgen concentrations may impair follicular development, which may lead to anovulation and amenorrhea. It certainly is possible, however, that elevated androgens are occurring as a result of normal genetic variability and may simply make the athlete more suited to those sports because of the physical advantages. Hyperandrogenism as a cause for amenorrhea has not been as well studied as

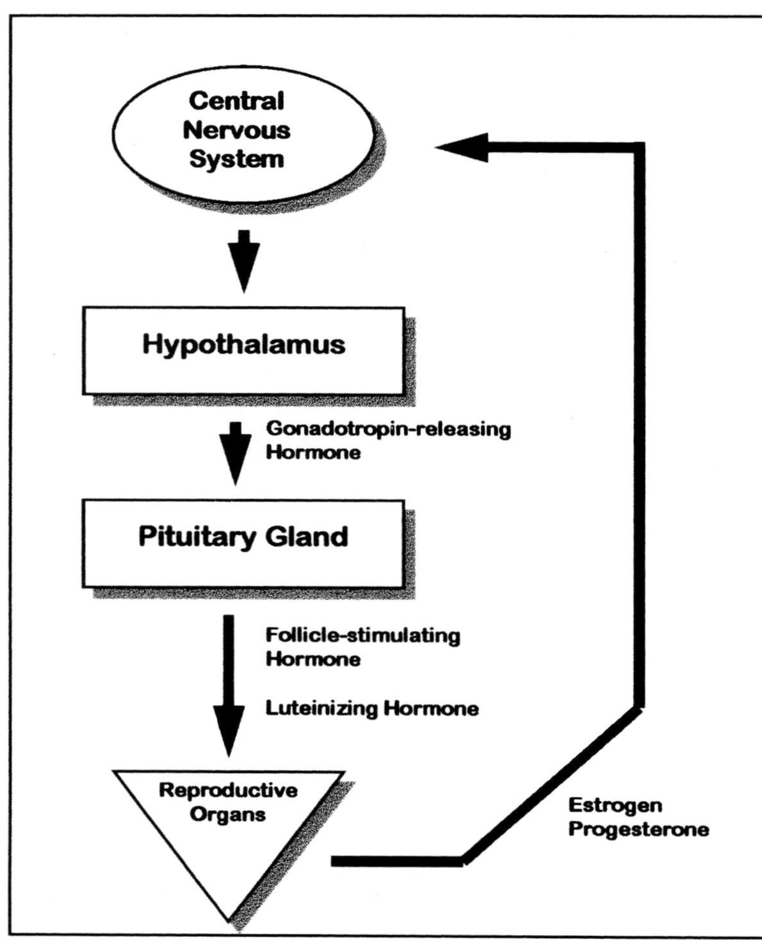

FIGURE 26-2. Hypothalamic pituitary axis.

hypoestrogenism, thus future research is necessary to determine cause and effect.

Although exercise-related menstrual irregularity is not a contraindication to participation in sports, it should trigger an evaluation of the athlete's training schedule and diet, as well as referrals to specialists for a thorough gynecologic, metabolic, and endocrine evaluation if appropriate.

Evaluation of Amenorrhea in the Athlete

Although the primary care physician, often a team physician, should be the coordinator of all aspects of the diagnosis and treatment when dealing with a female athlete, referrals to gynecologists, nutritionists, and other specialists may be appropriate. A complete menstrual history as well as a nutritional history is mandatory. A diagnosis of amenorrhea in the female athlete requires a thorough work-up. A thorough physical examination should include a pelvic exam if the athlete is sexually active. Laboratory tests should also be obtained (Table 26-1).

The laboratory work-up of amenorrhea should include a pregnancy test as well as a complete blood count and chemistry panel to evaluate nutritional status. The hormonal studies that should be obtained are follicle-stimulating hormone (FSH), prolactin, and thyroid-stimulating hormone (TSH). In addition, in the presence of hirsutism, acne, or polycystic ovarian syndrome, free testosterone, dehydroepiandrosterone sulfate (DHEA-S), and luteinizing hormone (LH) have also been suggested. A progesterone challenge test in which a short course of progesterone is given to elicit withdrawal bleeding may also be helpful to assess estrogen status. The presence of withdrawal bleeding indicates that estrogen stores are not likely to be seriously low.[32]

If stress fractures are known or suspected, other radiologic studies such as x-rays, MRI, or bone scans may be indicated. The question of whether a Dual Energy X-ray Absorptiometry (DEXA) scan is indicated is controversial. There are currently no recommendations for the use of DEXA in young women. However, it may be helpful to have a baseline scan if one suspects that osteopenia or osteoporosis is present. It may also be helpful to monitor treatment effects.[32]

THE FEMALE ATHLETE TRIAD (FAT)

The syndrome of amenorrhea, osteoporosis, and disordered eating has become known as the female athlete triad[45] (Fig. 26-3). This common entity will frequently present with noticeable weight loss or with the presence of a stress fracture. In this instance the orthopedic sports medicine physician may be the first point of physician contact for these athletes, and thus it is important for the orthopedic surgeon to ask some simple screening questions about the patients' menstrual and dietary history, and to provide appropriate referral if necessary. A low index of suspicion is mandatory. Once amenorrhea has been identified in an athlete, a preliminary screening for FAT is indicated.

Disordered Eating

Most amenorrheic athletes do not suffer from an eating disorder. However, there is research to suggest that athletic participation in sports, particularly those that emphasize leanness, increases the risk for disordered

TABLE 26-1 Laboratory Evaluation of Athletic Amenorrhea

Diagnosis	βHCG	TSH	Prolactin	LH	FSH	Estradiol	Withdrawal Bleed
Pregnancy	Positive						
Hypothalamic Pituitary Axis Suppression	Negative	Normal	Normal	Low	Low	Low	Weak or absent
Hyperandrogenic Anovulary Syndrome (Polycystic Ovarian Syndrome)	Negative	Normal	Normal	>2:1 LH/FSH ratio	Normal to High	Positive	
Premature Ovarian Failure	Negative	Normal	Normal	Normal	High	Low	Absent

βHCG = beta human chorionic gonadotropin
TSH = thyroid-stimulating hormone
LH = luteinizing hormone
FSH = follicle-stimulating hormone

Harmon KG: Evaluating and treating exercise-related menstrual irregularities. Phys Sportsmed 30(3), 2002. Reprinted with permission.

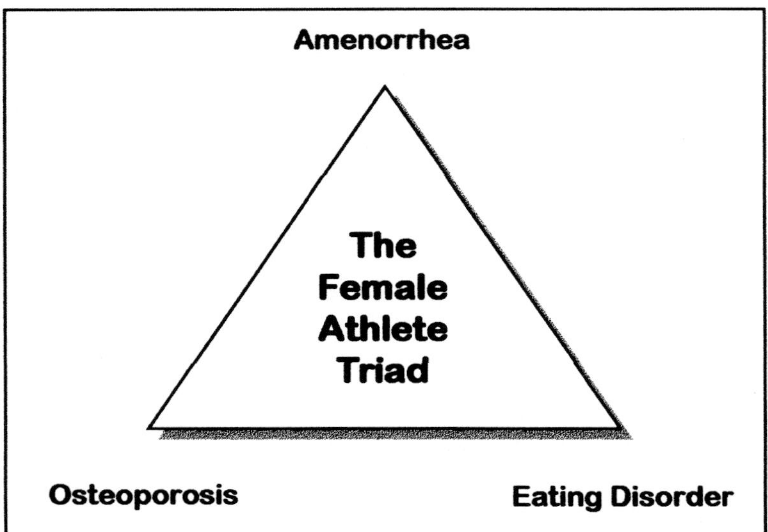

FIGURE 26-3. The female athlete triad.

eating.[5,12] In a study by Barrow and Saha that investigated the prevalence of stress fractures in competitive collegiate female long-distance runners, an alarming trend in disordered eating was noted among the amenorrheic runners. Eating disorders were reported in 47% of the amenorrheic group, 20% of the group experiencing one to five menses/year, 10% of the 6 to 9 menses/year group, and only 7% of the eumenorrheic athletes.[5] Thus, eating disorders are prevalent in this population, and may go unnoticed until a problem occurs.

Anorexia nervosa and bulimia nervosa are the two most prevalent eating disorders, both of which are recognized in the *Diagnostic and Statistical Manual of Mental Disorders*.[2] Anorexia typically involves restricting dietary intake, dramatic loss of weight (at least 15% below ideal body weight), wearing baggy clothes, dramatic mood swings, or extremely controlled exercise regimes. Long-term effects of anorexia include metabolic dysfunction, hormone imbalances, menstrual irregularity, muscle wasting, cardiac pathology, and in severe cases, death. Bulimia nervosa involves eating, sometimes an inordinate amount of calories in a single sitting, then using some method to purge the food from the body. Bulimics are typically not underweight, and because they may be at their ideal weight, or even slightly above that weight, the visible signs and symptoms may go unnoticed longer. Laxatives, diuretics, vomiting, severe dieting, or excessive exercise are ways that bulimics counteract their binge eating. Long-term consequences of bulimia include esophageal ulcers, tooth enamel and gum erosion, gum disease, tooth decay, menstrual irregularity, and throat and mouth cancers.

The psychological aspects to eating disorders are deep-rooted and often passed down from one generation to the next based on sisters', mothers', coaches', or teammates' experiences, eating habits, and body perceptions. The stress to compete at elite levels can motivate an athlete to strive to be leaner in order to be faster, have more endurance, and, most important, maintain her ideal body image.

A communication network is extremely important in the treatment of an eating disorder. Optimally, this network should include roommates, teammates, parents, coaches, certified athletic trainers (ATC), dieticians, physicians, and possibly psychologists or counselors. The presence of a possible eating disorder is frequently identified by an athlete's roommates or teammates. These people spend the most time with the athlete and can identify or verify warning signs of disordered eating. This can become a complicated matter when the athlete is trying the keep her disordered eating a secret from coaches, parents, and trainers. Most athletes know that their competition status can be revoked if the situation is severe enough, and that fact alone is often enough to keep them from revealing the condition to those in authority positions. Parents, too, may notice changes in their child's appearance and/or mood, or seclusion from activities, and may also notice erratic eating rituals, bathroom visits after meals, and may find discarded diuretic or laxative boxes.

Eating disorders are a serious issue, and communication between friends, parents, coaches, and trainers is important to ensure that the athlete gets proper care and doesn't feel alienated or motivated to withhold information or refuse treatment. Frequently the athletic trainer is responsible for referral to a physician. Subsequently, dieticians and counselors may become involved. Regardless of where the referral network begins, the relationship between athlete, parent, coach, athletic trainer, and physician is critical to ensure successful treatment for the eating disordered athlete.

Bone Mineral Density

It is well established that bone mineral density is directly correlated with duration and severity of menstrual dysfunction.[17,57] The longer an athlete is amenorrheic or oligomenorrheic, theoretically, the more bone loss occurs. Increases in BMD have been observed after treatment with oral contraceptives to regulate the menstrual cycle.[52] However, there are also studies to support no change or even bone loss with contraceptive use.[50] Despite the return of normal menses, athletes may never attain the BMD seen in their eumenorrheic peers.[31]

Stress Fractures

The earliest manifestation of the female athlete triad may be a stress fracture secondary to a decrease in bone mineral density. Stress fractures can occur in both male and female athletes, and multiple studies have reported on the prevalence of these.[7,8,10,39] A stress fracture is the result of an imbalance between bone resorption and remodeling. The abnormal hormonal milieu often seen in female athletes provides such an abnormal environment that a healthy balance is disrupted. Studies done in military populations support the fact that females sustain more stress fractures than their male counterparts.[30,51] A retrospective review by Matheson found that the tibia was the most common site for a stress fracture in both men and women (49.1%), followed by the tarsal bones, metatarsals, femur, fibula, sesamoids, and spine.[39] However, literature suggests that women have more femoral and metatarsal stress fractures in addition to pelvic and rib fractures.[7]

A review by Arendt outlines the etiologic theories behind the increased incidence in female stress fractures. These include muscle control and neuromotor differences, anthropomorphic factors, training differences, and overall bone health.[3] Nutritional and hormonal factors combine to affect bone density and subsequent risk of stress fracture. A prospective study by Bennell et al. found that among female track and field athletes, significant risk factors for stress fractures were identifiable. Interestingly, no such risk factors were identifiable in the male athletes. These predictive factors were lower bone density, history of menstrual abnormalities, less lean mass in the lower limb, and a diet lower in fat.[8]

Pubic Ramus. Pubic ramus fractures can occur in both men and women. Presentation is with groin pain and tenderness. These fractures are commonly noted in two situations: cross-over running style in which there is excessive adduction across the line of gait progression, or overstriding, which is excessive flexion during gait. Overstriding is often seen in women, particularly when they train with men, who tend to be taller on average. Commonly the female runner is shorter and has a shorter stride length. Thus, the "overstride" is a way to keep pace with a taller running partner. The resultant chronic pull on the adductors leads to early adductor tendinitis or pubic ramus stress fractures. Treatment is rest and activity modification while healing occurs. Correction of the abnormal gait pattern is important to prevent a recurrence.[56,46]

Ribs. Rib fractures are seen in female rowers and golfers, but also have been reported in female gymnasts, tennis players, and swimmers. These tend to occur posterolaterally where bending stresses from the periscapular muscles are greatest. Posterolateral chest pain is the common presenting complaint, and pain may be exacerbated by coughing and deep breathing. Treatment should include refraining from the offending activity for 4 to 8 weeks, and a gradual return to sports with an emphasis on periscapular stabilization and strengthening.[27]

Femur. Stress fractures of the femur can occur in the neck, shaft, or supracondylar region. These are commonly seen in weight-bearing endurance athletes such as long-distance runners and ballet dancers. Fractures in the supracondylar region are few and have not been adequately classified. Femoral shaft fractures present insidiously with thigh pain and respond to rest and protected weight bearing for up to 4 weeks.[10]

Femoral neck stress fractures are more common and present with insidious groin pain. Diagnosis can be confirmed with a bone scan or MRI. Those that are nondisplaced can be treated with protected weight bearing and frequent radiographic follow-up. However, fractures that occur on the "tension" side of the femoral neck warrant internal fixation to avoid fracture displacement and the risk of avascular necrosis.[19]

Treatment: Oral Contraceptives

Treatment for exercise-related menstrual irregularity and decreased bone mineral density consists of reducing training volume, increasing body weight, and improving nutritional status. The goal is, of course, to resume normal menses. These options, however, may be unacceptable to many athletes because of fears of decreased athletic performance, and noncompliance in this group is high.[26] Hormone replacement therapy (HRT) in the form of postmenopausal hormone replacement regimens or oral contraceptives can be used by most women who have no contraindications. It is recommended that a 0.035 mg oral contraceptive pill should be used for initial hormonal therapy in athletes.[20] Oral contraceptives are usually more convenient and acceptable to premenopausal women than postmenopausal HRT, and many athletes want the contraceptive benefits. Other benefits include a possible decrease in the risk of iron deficiency anemia by decreasing the volume of monthly menstrual blood loss, and allowing manipulation of the menstrual cycle for travel, training, and competition commitments.[6] However, there remains concern about the general side effects of oral contraceptives. These include rare but serious side effects such as cardiovascular complications, hypertension, or thromboembolic disease. Less serious but far more common are complications such as headaches, breast tenderness, nausea, and weight gain.

Weight Gain: Myth or Reality? Athletes may be reluctant to take oral contraceptives for fear of gaining weight. Many studies indicate no overall effect on body weight while taking oral contraceptives,[18,53] although there may be some weight gain hypothesized to be the result of either fluid retention or possibly appetite stimulation.[6] Newer oral contraceptive preparations with lower doses of estrogen and progesterone may have fewer side effects than the older, higher dose pills.

However, a study by Casazza et al. showed that oral contraceptive users significantly increased body weight by 2 to 3 kgs, and fat mass by 1 to 2 kgs, though their data was taken from a eumenorrheic sample of recreational athletes, and not elite endurance runners or gymnasts.[13] Female figure skaters, rowers, and gymnasts may find this 2 kg weight gain to be unacceptable, and thus noncompliance with oral contraceptive treatment may ensue. It should be emphasized to the elite athlete, however, that athletes continuing to train at high exercise intensities may not be as likely to have the weight gain typically associated with oral contraceptive use in the general population.

Performance Effects. As for performance decrements from oral contraceptive use, data is still inconclusive. There have been reversible reductions in $\dot{V}O_{2max}$ associated with oral contraceptive use. However, it is unclear whether these $\dot{V}O_{2max}$ reductions actually translate into changes in performance. Casazza et al. found a decrease in peak $\dot{V}O_{2max}$ with oral contraceptive use over a 4- month period, but no changes in diet, exercise patterns, peak heart rate, minute ventilation, or respiratory exchange ratio.[13] But again, the women in the study were not elite athletes but "moderately physically active young women." A double-blind randomized trial of 14 elite athletes taking low-dose triphasic oral contraceptives showed decreases in $\dot{V}O_{2max}$ in both groups from the follicular to the luteal phase. After two months on the oral contraceptive preparation, the treatment group had a further 5% decrease in $\dot{V}O_{2max}$ while the treatment group had a slight increase (1.5%).[6,36] There were no changes reported in the other variables measured, including maximum heart rate, anaerobic endurance, and aerobic endurance at 90% $\dot{V}O_{2max}$. Notelovitz et al. found in a prospective randomized study of oral contraceptive users over a period of 6 months that $\dot{V}O_{2max}$ did decrease significantly during the period of observation. In this study serum cholesterol, triglycerides, and lipoprotein profiles were unchanged.[48] In a prospective randomized study of 10 women and 15 men as control subjects, Bryner et al. found that low-dose oral contraceptives taken over a single cycle did not affect the $\dot{V}O_{2max}$, endurance test or respiratory rate during treadmill running.[11] However, this was a short-term study. Whether these observed decreases in $\dot{V}O_{2max}$ translate to detrimental effects on performance, particularly at the elite level, is not clear.

Subjectively, women report decreases in PMS symptoms with oral contraceptive use. In addition, oral contraceptives may result in an increase in blood volume due to decreased menstrual blood loss. Theoretically both of these may effectively improve athletic performance by increasing cardiac output, stroke volume, and oxygen delivery to muscle tissue. The overall effects of oral contraceptive use on athletic performance, particularly at the elite level, deserve further study.

The rate of perceived exertion (RPE) has been frequently used to assess the motivational level of subjects during strenuous aerobic exercise, some authors reporting significantly higher RPE during submaximal or maximal intensity exercise in the menstrual phase or luteal phase than in the follicular phase.[22] The impairment of physical performances in the late luteal and menstrual phases is generally attributed to the existence of premenstrual and menstrual syndrome symptoms: fatigue, fluid retention (inducing swelling, congestion, and discomfort), weight gain, mood changes (including irritability, depression, motivation loss), and dysmenorrhea. In a study by Giacomoni et al., maximum power during a vertical jump test was significantly decreased in the menstrual phase compared to the follicular phase in women stating they had menstrual symptoms, while no significant differences were observed in women stating no menstrual symptoms.[22]

Risk of Injury. An association between oral contraceptive use and injury risk has been suggested.[6] It is hypothesized that female sex hormones may have a direct effect on the growth and development of soft-tissue structures. Estrogen and progesterone receptors have been identified in the fibroblasts of the human anterior cruciate ligament.[38] Studies have found that fluctuations in serum estrogen levels lead to alterations in ACL fibroblast metabolism, which may result in structural and compositional changes in the ligament.[63] Therefore, ACL injury may be more likely to occur during certain phases of the menstrual cycle as a result of native hormonal concentrations. Wojtys et al. studied 28 female athletes who had sustained noncontact ACL injuries in the 3 months prior to study. The history taken from the athlete included mechanism of injury, menstrual cycle history, and contraceptive use. This study found a statistically significant difference between the stage of the menstrual cycle and the likelihood for ACL injury. Specifically, more ACL injuries occurred in the ovulatory phase of the cycle (days 10–14). In addition, they found significantly fewer injuries during the follicular phase (days 1–9).[61] However, this study relied solely on an athlete's recall of her menstrual cycle. Subsequently the same researchers studied ACL injuries and were able to validate menstrual cycle phase with urine hormone measurements within 24 hours of injury. The link between cycle phase and risk of injury was statistically confirmed, with the ovulatory phase being the most risk-prone phase. This would coincide with the natural estrogen spike necessary to induce ovulation. Also of interest in that study was the finding that oral contraceptive use diminished the significance of the association, although the number of OC users in this study was small (14/69).[62] Other than this finding, however, there is to date no research which has looked specifically at whether contraceptive use affects rate of athletic injury.

NUTRITION

It is well established that calcium is essential for bone health. Current recommendations are that all women should get between 1000 mg and 1500 mg of calcium daily,[44] but most women get far less than that. Although it is generally accepted that low estrogen levels in postmenopausal or premenopausal women with endocrine dysfunction are related to the osteopenia that is observed in these groups, the role of estrogen in bone dynamics is not fully understood. Because estrogen receptors have not been found in bone, it is generally assumed that the effects of estrogen on bone are indirect.[6]

Bisphosphonates and nasal calcitonin-salmon have also been used to treat osteoporosis, particularly in postmenopausal groups, but have not been as effective in increasing BMD as estrogen replacement therapy.[26] The bisphosphonates have assumed a significant role in the treatment of osteoporosis because they bind strongly to calcium and are easy to use. The precise mechanism is not understood, but it is thought that bisphosphonates inhibit the osteoclast-mediated bone resorption.[24] Lindsay et al. found that postmenopausal women with low BMD showed increased bone mass in the hip and spine following treatment with hormone replacement therapy and alendronate. This study demonstrated that alendronate added to hormonal replacement produced increases in BMD that were greater than hormone replacement therapy alone.[37] However, these therapies have been used only in osteoporotic postmenopausal populations, and their potential use in young athletes is currently unstudied.

Nutritional Counseling

Nutrition counseling is important for all athletes, even if there is no evidence for an eating disorder. Many athletes, especially endurance athletes, eat a diet heavy on carbohydrates, and sacrifice protein and fat to maintain low caloric intake. It is well reported that distance runners consume too few calories to meet their energy expenditure.[5,12,33] This is primarily accomplished by avoiding fat intake. An athlete's diet should include carbohydrate consumption at 60%–65% of daily caloric intake, protein at 15%–20%, and fat intake at 20%–25%.[29] These numbers are not concrete and should vary between individual athletes based on body composition, training season, and sport.

It has been shown in animal models that increasing dietary fat intake can increase the number of mitochondria and fat stores in the muscle; it was thought reasonable that this may apply to humans as well. Following this hypothesis, Horvath et al. found that, contrary to current practice by endurance runners, consuming high carbohydrates and little or no fat in their diets may not benefit running performance. They studied trained male and female runners who were prescribed three different diets: low (15%), medium (30%), and high (45%) fat diets over 7-day periods. Following three months of continued endurance training on each diet, follow-up tests were conducted to determine differences in $\dot{V}O_{2max}$ at baseline, monthly, and at three months following the completion of the study. None of the diets changed the body weight or percent body fat of the runners.[28] In addition, there was no change in the maximal grade, 8.2% to 7.9%, or time to exhaustion by the subjects going from the low to medium fat diets. However, total running time was significantly longer on the high than on the medium fat diet (3%), while grade did not significantly increase (8.6% to 8.8%). Increasing dietary fat did not change $\dot{V}O_{2max}$ (expressed per kg), the expiratory gas exchange ratios, maximal heart rates, or net lactate accumulation. The endurance time of the subjects running on a treadmill in the medium fat diet increased 20% in females and 8% in males compared to the low fat diet. There were no significant differences in endurance time between the high and medium fat diet.

HORMONAL EFFECT ON CARDIAC FUNCTION

Estrogen's involvement in the regulation of cardiac structure and function has been demonstrated in animal and human data. Both endogenous and exogenous estrogens have been reported to have acute and chronic effects on cardiovascular structure and function and cardio-protective effects against heart disease. Specifically, changes include increased plasma volume, stroke volume, and cardiac output during the luteal phase in eumenorrheic females and those taking oral contraceptives.[21] Specific receptor sites for estrogen have been located in the heart and the great vessels, through which estrogens may affect a variety of intracellular changes that may contribute to the previously discussed cardiovascular changes. Data from recent studies indicate that the previously thought cardioprotective effects from hormone replacement therapy may not occur, that endogenous estrogens may contribute to heart health, but that exogenous estrogens may in fact increase serum lipids and subsequently increase the risks of cardiovascular events or myocardial infarction.[54]

The studies involving exogenous estrogen consumption are limited because differences in exercise regimens and intensity are difficult to control. In addition to the lack of information concerning oral contraceptive consumption and exercise hemodynamics, there are a limited number of studies that address the age-controlled influence of menopause on changes in exercise hemodynamics, body mass, fat free mass, and bone density that occur as a result of training.[23]

PREGNANCY IN THE FEMALE ATHLETE

At some point during the life of a female athlete pregnancy may occur. Most will want to continue to participate in some form of athletic activity. According to the most recent committee opinion by the American College of Obstetricians and Gynecologists (ACOG),

> Generally, participation in a wide range of recreational activities appears to be safe during pregnancy; however, each sport should be reviewed individually for its potential risk, and activities with a high risk of falling or those with a high risk of abdominal trauma should be avoided during pregnancy.[1]

Essentially, in the absence of contraindications, women generally benefit from safe, carefully monitored exercise during pregnancy (Table 26-2). A history and physical examination by an athlete's obstetric physician prior to continuing exercise routines, and certainly before undertaking any new activities, is essential to ensure the safety of both mother and child.

The musculoskeletal system benefits from exercise during pregnancy. It has been reported that regular physical exercise prior to pregnancy reduces the risk for back pain during pregnancy.[49] In addition, structured physical therapy regimens during pregnancy and beyond can help prevent or alleviate the back and pelvic pain that plagues many women during a pregnancy.[47]

The changes that will affect a pregnant athlete's body are many. In addition to the obvious increases in weight and change in center of balance, the athlete will also undergo a number of cardiovascular and hormonal changes. These adaptations prepare the athlete's body for the stresses of delivery and to provide a nurturing environment for the growing fetus.

Hemodynamically, the pregnant athlete will experience an increase in blood volume, heart rate, and stroke volume. In addition, cardiac output will increase and peripheral vascular resistance will decrease.[14] Heart rate increases by 20% in the second and third trimesters.[43] After the first trimester, there are also cardiovascular changes related to body position. The supine position results in obstruction of venous return by the uterus, and a subsequent decrease in cardiac output. Motionless standing can also decrease cardiac output. Clark et al. found that, compared to the lateral position, there was a mean fall of 9% in cardiac output while supine. In addition, there was an 18% decrease when patients were standing.[15] Thus, it is important for an athlete to avoid any exercises that may involve the supine position or prolonged motionless standing.

The hormones relaxin and progesterone are both known to mediate joint laxity.[4] Pelvic and low back pain have been attributable to relaxin levels during pregnancy.[35] In addition, joint laxity has been documented during pregnancy.[55] In an unusual case report, Blecher and Richmond reported on a woman who developed transient laxity of an ACL graft which was placed 2 months prior to conception.[9] Clearly, there is some hormonal influence on soft tissues. In theory, laxity during pregnancy may predispose an athlete to injury. However, this remains speculative, as the actual incidence of joint injury during pregnancy has not been prospectively studied.

The type of exercise chosen during pregnancy should minimize risk to the fetus as well as injury to the mother. Participation in sports that place the mother at risk of direct contact (e.g., basketball, ice hockey) or falling, (e.g., downhill skiing, horseback riding, and gymnastics) have a high risk for trauma in the pregnant woman. Scuba diving should be avoided due to the risk of decompression sickness to the fetus. ACOG recommendations call for avoiding exertion at altitudes above 6000 feet.[1] In addition, it is important for the exercising mother to monitor body temperature, because hyperthermia has been associated with neural tube defects.[41] However, there is little research on strenuous, competitive exercise during pregnancy.[25] As with the recreational athlete, the competitive athlete requires close physician supervision as she continues to compete or train.

Nutritional requirements increase progressively during pregnancy. Carbohydrates, in particular, are utilized at a greater rate by pregnant women. Many of the changes associated with pregnancy will persist for several weeks postpartum.[1] However, following delivery a woman's prepregnancy exercise routines should be started as soon as physically and medically safe. A return to exercise in the postpartum period has been associated with a decreased incidence in postpartum depression.[34] In addition, exercise combined with dieting is safer for a lactating mother than dieting alone, because lean body mass is better preserved with exercise.[40]

In summary, exercise during pregnancy can provide mental and physiologic benefits for the mother. However, the specific activity or sport chosen should

TABLE 26-2 Contraindications to Exercise during Pregnancy

Absolute Contraindications to Aerobic Exercise During Pregnancy
Hemodynamically significant heart disease
Restrictive lung disease
Incompetent cervix/cerclage
Multiple gestation at risk for premature labor
Persistent second- or third-trimester bleeding
Placenta previa after 26 weeks of gestation
Premature labor during the current pregnancy
Ruptured membranes
Preeclampsia/pregnancy-induced hypertension
Relative Contraindications to Aerobic Exercise During Pregnancy
Severe anemia
Unevaluated maternal cardiac arrhythmia
Chronic bronchitis
Poorly controlled type 1 diabetes
Extreme morbid obesity
Extreme underweight (BMI < 12)
History of extremely sedentary lifestyle
Intrauterine growth restriction in current pregnancy
Poorly controlled hypertension
Orthopedic limitations
Poorly controlled seizure disorder
Poorly controlled hyperthyroidism
Heavy smoker

Reproduced with permission from the American College of Obstetrics and Gynecology: Exercise during pregnancy and the postpartum period. Technical Bulletin 267, 2002.

be carefully assessed for any potential risk to mother or fetus. Any exercise program should be closely monitored by the patient's physician and adjusted as the pregnancy progresses to meet the changing needs of the mother's body.

CONCLUSION

Although the understanding of the unique physiology of the female athlete has improved, there are many questions left unanswered. Hormonal influences, both endogenous and exogenous, can affect cardiovascular, respiratory, and metabolic parameters, but these changes are probably clinically insignificant for the average recreational athlete. However, small changes in these areas may have a dramatic effect on the elite athlete. Further study is necessary to determine just what, if any, effect hormonal influences have on performance. In addition, individual variation in menstrual cycles, physical traits, and genetic predisposition may make it difficult to generalize, even with the results of well-controlled studies.

The sports medicine team must remain vigilant to the warning signs of the female athlete triad. The detrimental effects of decreased bone mineral density are significant and may mean stress fractures in the athlete, causing loss of playing time and potential morbidity. In addition, once menses return through weight gain, improved nutrition, or treatment with exogenous hormones, there is ample evidence to suggest that bone mineral density may not return to pre-amenorrheic levels. As today's young athletes age, one must wonder whether we will begin to see an entire generation of women who suffer from hip and vertebral fractures in middle age.

As physicians, trainers, and therapists we are obligated to learn as much as we can about the female athlete so that we may successfully guide young girls and women through athletic performance and active lifestyles, to maximize performance and ensure lifelong health.

REFERENCES

1. American College of Obstetricians and Gynecologists: Exercise During Pregnancy and the Postpartum Period. American College of Obstetricians and Gynecologists Technical Bulletin. Washington, DC, American College of Obstetricians and Gynecologists, 2002, p 267.
2. American Psychiatric Association: Diagnostic and Statistical Manual of Mental Disorders: DSM-IV, 4th ed. Washington, DC, American Psychiatric Association, 1994.
3. Arendt EA: Stress fractures and the female athlete. Clin Orthop 372:131–138, 2000.
4. Arnold C, Van Bell C, Rogers V, et al: The relationship between serum relaxin and knee joint laxity in female athletes. Orthopedics 25(6):669–673, 2002.
5. Barrow GW, Saha S.: Menstrual irregularity and stress fractures in collegiate female distance runners. Am J Sports Med 16(3):209–216, 1988.
6. Bennell K, White S, Crossley K: The oral contraceptive pill: a revolution for sportswomen? Br J Sports Med 33:231–238, 1999.
7. Bennell KL, Malcom SA, Thomas SA, et al: The incidence and distribution of stress fractures in competitive track and field athletes. Am J Sports Med 24(2):211–217, 1996.
8. Bennell KL, Malcom SA, Thomas SA, et al: Risk factors for stress fractures in track and field athletes: A twelve-month prospective study. Am J Sports Med 24(6):810–818, 1996.
9. Blecher AM, Richmond JC: Transient laxity of an anterior cruciate ligament-reconstructed knee related to pregnancy. Arthroscopy 14(1):77–79, 1998.
10. Boden BP, Osbahr DC, Jimenez C: Low-risk stress fractures. Am J Sports Med 29(1):100–111, 2001.
11. Bryner, RW, Toffle RC, Ullrich IH, et al: Effect of low dose oral contraceptives on exercise performance. Br J Sports Med 30(1):36–40, 1996.
12. Byrne S, McLean N: Elite athletes: Effects of the pressure to be thin. J Sci Med Sport (5)2:80–94, 2002.
13. Casazza GA, Suh S-H, Miller BF, et al: Effects of oral contraceptives on peak exercise capacity. J Appl Physiol 93(5):1698–1702, 2002.
14. Clark SL, Cotton DB, Lee W, et al: Central hemodynamic assessment of normal term pregnancy. Am J Obstet Gynecol 161(6):1439–1442, 1989.
15. Clark SL, Cotton DB, Pivarnik JM, et al: Position change and central hemodynamic profile during normal third-trimester pregnancy and post partum. Am J Obstet Gynecol 164(3):883–887, 1991.
16. Constantini NW, Warren MP: Menstrual dysfunction in swimmers: a distinct entity. J Clin Endocrinol Metab 80(9):2740–2744, 1995.
17. Drinkwater BL, Bruemner B, Chesnut CH III: Menstrual history as a determinant of current bone density in young athletes. JAMA 263(4):545–548, 1990.
18. Dusterberg B, Ellman H, Muller U, et al: A three-year clinical investigation into efficacy, cycle control and tolerability of a new low-dose monophasic oral contraceptive containing gestodene. Gynecol Endocrinol 10(1):33–39, 1996.
19. Egol KA, Koval KJ, Kummer F, et al: Stress fractures of the femoral neck. Clin Orthop 348:72–78, 1998.
20. Frankovich RJ, Lebrun CM: Menstrual cycle, contraception, and performance. Clin Sports Med 19(2): 251–271, 2000.
21. George KP, Birch KM, Jones B, et al: Estrogen variation and resting left ventricular structure and function in young healthy females. Med Sci Sports Exerc 32(2):297–303, 2000.
22. Giacomoni M, Bernard T, Gavarry O, et al: Influence of the menstrual cycle phase and menstrual symptoms on maximal anaerobic performance. Med Sci Sports Exerc 32(2):486–492, 2000.
23. Green JS, Stanforth PR, Gagnon J, et al: Menopause, estrogen, and training effects on exercise hemodynamics: The HERITAGE study. Med Sci Sports Exerc 34(1):74–82, 2002.
24. Greenspan SL, Harris ST, Bone H, et al: Bisphosphonates: Safety and efficacy in the treatment and prevention of osteoporosis. Am Fam Physician 61(9):2731–2736, 2000.
25. Hale RW, Milne L: The elite athlete and exercise in pregnancy. Semin Perinatol 20(4):277–284, 1996.
26. Harmon KG: Evaluating and treating exercise-related menstrual irregularities. Phys Sportsmed 30(3), 2002.
27. Holden DL, Jackson DW: Stress fracture of the ribs in female rowers. Am J Sports Med 13(5):342–348, 1985.
28. Horvath PJ, Eagen CK, Fisher NM, et al: The effects of varying dietary fat on performance and metabolism in trained male and female runners. J Am Coll Nutr 19(1):52–60, 2000.
29. See http://www.usda.gov
30. Jones BH, Bovee MW, Harris JM, et al: Intrinsic risk factors for exercise-related injuries among male and female army trainees. Am J Sports Med 21(5): 705–710, 1993.
31. Jonnavithula S, Warren MP, Fox RP, et al: Bone density is compromised in amenorrheic women despite return of menses: A 2-year study. Obstet Gynecol 81(5 Pt 1):669–674, 1993.
32. Joy, E., Clark, N., Ireland, M.L., et al: Team management of the female athlete triad: Part 1: What to look for, what to ask. Phys Sportsmed 25(3):1–11, 1997.
33. Kaiserauer S, Snyder AC, Sleeper M, et al: Nutritional, physiological, and menstrual status of distance runners. Med Sci Sports Exerc 21(2): 120–125, 1989.

34. Koltyn KF, Schultes SS: Psychological effects of an aerobic exercise session and a rest session following pregnancy. J Sports Med Phys Fitness 37(4): 287–291, 1997.
35. Kristiansson P, Svardsudd K, von Schoultz B: Serum relaxin, symphyseal pain, and back pain during pregnancy. Am J Obstet Gynecol 175(5):1342–1347, 1996.
36. Lebrun CM: Effect of the different phases of the menstrual cycle and oral contraceptives on athletic performance. Sports Med 16(6):400–430, 1993.
37. Lindsay R, Cosman F, Lobo RA, et al: Addition of alendronate to ongoing hormone replacement therapy in the treatment of osteoporosis: A randomized, controlled clinical trial. J Clin Endocrinol Metab 84(9):3076–3081, 1999.
38. Liu SH, Al-Shaikh R, Panossian V, et al: Primary inmmunolocalization of estrogen and progesterone target cells in the human anterior cruciate ligament. J Orthop Res 14:526–533, 1996.
39. Matheson GO, Clement DB, McKenzie DC, et al: Stress fractures in athletes: A study of 320 cases. Am J Sports Med 15(1):46–58, 1987.
40. McCrory MA, Nommsen-Rivers LA, Mole PA, et al: Randomized trial of the short-term effects of dieting compared with dieting plus aerobic exercise on lactation performance. Am J Clin Nutr 69(5):959–967, 1999.
41. Milunsky A, Ulcickas M, Rothman KJ, et al: Maternal heat exposure and neural tube defects. JAMA 268(7):882–885, 1992.
42. Morris FL, Wark JD: An effective, economic way of monitoring menstrual cycle hormones in at risk female athletes. Med Sci Sports Exerc 33(1):9–14, 2001.
43. Morton MJ, Paul MS, Campos GR, et al: Exercise dynamics in late gestation: Effects of physical training. Am J Obstet Gynecol 152(1):91–97, 1985.
44. National Academy of Sciences. Recommended Dietary Allowances, 10th ed. Washington, DC, National Academy Press, 1989.
45. Nattiv A, Agostini R, Drinkwater B, et al: The female athlete triad. The inter-relatedness of disordered eating, amenorrhea, and osteoporosis. Clin Sports Med 13:405–418, 1994.
46. Noakes TD, Smith JA, Lindenberg G, et al: Pelvic stress fractures in long distance runners. Am J Sports Med 13(2):120–123, 1985.
47. Noren L, Ostgaard S, Johansson G, et al: Lumbar back and posterior pelvic pain during pregnancy: A 3-year follow-up. Eur Spine J 11(3):267–271, 2002.
48. Notelovitz M, Zauner C, McKenzie L, et al: The effect of low-dose oral contraceptives on cardiorespiratory function, coagulation, and lipids in exercising young women: A preliminary report. Am J Obstet Gynecol 156(3):591–598,1987.
49. Ostgaard HC, Zetherstrom G, Roos-Hansson E, et al: Reduction of back and posterior pelvic pain in pregnancy. Spine 19(8):894–900, 1994.
50. Prior JC, Kirkland SA, Joseph L, et al: Oral contraceptive use and bone mineral density in premenopausal women: Cross-sectional population-based data from the Canadian Multicentre Osteoporosis Study. CMAJ 165(8):1023–1029, 2001.
51. Protzman RR, Griffis CC: Stress fractures in men and women undergoing military training. J Bone Joint Surg 59-A(6):825, 1977.
52. Recker RR, Davies KM, Hinders SM, et al: Bone gain in young adult women. JAMA 268(17): 2403–2408, 1992.
53. Rosenberg M: Weight change with oral contraceptive use and during the menstrual cycle. Results of daily measurements. Contraception 58:345–349, 1998.
54. Rossouw JE, Anderson GL, Prentice RL, et al: Risks and benefits of estrogen plus progestin in healthy postmenopausal women: Principal results from the Women's Health Initiative randomized controlled trial. JAMA 288(3):321–333, 2002.
55. Schauberger CW, Rooney BL, Goldsmith L, et al: Peripheral joint laxity increases in pregnancy but does not correlate with serum relaxin levels. Am J Obstet Gynecol 174(2):667–671, 1996.
56. Teitz CC: Stress fractures. In Teitz CC: The Female Athlete. Rosemont, IL, American Academy of Orthopaedic Surgeons, 1997, pp 81–85.
57. Voss LA, Fadale PD, Hulstyn MJ: Exercise-induced loss of bone density in athletes. J Am Acad Orthop Surg 6(6):349–357, 1998.
58. Warren MP, Brooks-Gunn J, Hamilton LH, et al: Scoliosis and fractures in young ballet dancers. Relation to delayed menarche and secondary amenorrhea. N Engl J Med 314(21):1348–1353, 1986.
59. Warren MP, Perlroth NE: The effects of intense exercise on the female reproductive system. J Endocrinol 170:3–11, 2001.
60. Wilson JD, Braunwald E, Isselbacher KJ, et al (eds): Harrison's Principles of Internal Medicine, 12th ed. New York, McGraw-Hill, 1991.
61. Wojtys EM, Huston LJ, Lindenfeld TN, et al: Association between the menstrual cycle and anterior cruciate ligament injuries in female athletes. Am J Sports Med 26(5):614–619, 1998.
62. Wojtys EM, Huston LJ, Boynton MD, et al: The effect of the menstrual cycle on anterior cruciate ligament injuries in women as determined by hormone levels. Am J Sports Med 30(2):182–188, 2002.
63. Yu WD, Panossian V, Hatch JD, et al: Combined effects of estrogen and progesterone on the anterior cruciate ligament. Clin Orthop 383:268–281, 2001.

27

Upper Extremity Injuries in the Female Athlete

Frances Cuomo and Kathleen Cook

GENERAL PRINCIPLES OF PHYSIOLOGY AND ANATOMY

Anatomical variations between men and women lead to differences in performance in certain sports and in incidence of injury. Women generally have shorter limbs, narrower shoulders,[3] and smaller forearm-to-arm ratios than their male counterparts.[2] Women also have smaller articular surfaces to dissipate impact force, resulting in less power for throwing and striking. The shorter lever arm in the female accounts for mechanical differences of the upper extremities that are unrelated to muscularity.[24]

Although there is little qualitative difference in the female's muscle tissue, men have greater muscle mass per total body weight, and thus greater overall upper body strength.[15] Women tend to be weaker in the upper extremities than the lower extremities, but females are capable of increasing upper body strength by 15% to 45% with minimal hypertrophy of muscles.[45] Women should take precautions when using health club equipment for muscle conditioning, as many of the machines, particularly those focused on training the upper extremities, may place excessive strain on the unconditioned female. Equipment that places hands in a starting position behind the vertical plane of the ears can encourage anterior shift of the humeral head in the glenoid, a problem exacerbated by joint laxity.[2]

Stress fractures in athletes have traditionally been reported to affect primarily the bones of the lower extremities with repetitive weight-bearing activity. However, a small number of cases have been reported of fatigue injury to the bone in the upper limbs. Sinha and colleagues reviewed the clinical reports of active patients with a stress fracture in a non-weight-bearing location of the upper extremity or ribs and found that sport-specific patterns of injury exist.[39] Athletes involved in upper extremity weight-bearing activities such as gymnastics, diving, and cheerleading were predominantly female. Gymnasts had the highest overall incidence of stress fractures in the upper extremity.[5] All of the fractures experienced by this population occurred distal to the elbow, indicating that the weak link for weight bearing is distal in the kinetic linkage of the upper extremity.[39] In contrast, throwing athletes experienced stress fractures predominantly at the shoulder girdle, indicating that the throwing motion places a greater force on the proximal upper extremity.

The physiological basis for the occurrence of these stress fractures was situations in which the rate of microdamage incurred by the bone in response to exercise accumulated faster than the rate of active repair. Such a situation can arise when a training program is rapidly intensified. Muscle fatigue was also implicated in the occurrence of upper extremity stress fractures when the neuromuscular system was unable to protect bones and joints from high peak loads.[45]

Skeletally immature individuals and young women with the female athlete triad syndrome are also at a greater risk for stress fractures in the upper extremity resulting from excessive, sudden increases in mechanical load. The female athlete triad, a disorder involving the three-part interplay of disordered eating, amenorrhea, and osteoporosis, has been shown to diminish bone mass density (BMD).[25] Hypoestrogenic states seen in amenorrheic athletes are most detrimental to BMD accretions at the time of menarche (11 to 15 years), when the largest proportion of BMD is amassed.[26]

Although gymnasts are typically at a higher risk for developing the female athlete triad due to the sport's emphasis on physical appearance, gymnastics offers a protective effect on the BMD of the upper extremities. High-impact sports increase strain on the skeleton and stimulate increases in BMD.[35] The osteogenic effect of weight-bearing activity has been extensively documented in the lower extremities; however, because the shoulder is not a weight-bearing joint, it is not commonly studied in the upper extremities. In gymnastics, the upper limbs are extensively subjected to weight-bearing and high-impact loading forces up to 18 times body weight. Upper limb dominance accounts for 6% to 9% increases in BMD in normal individuals, and this percentage increases with participation in unilateral activities.[41] In contrast to unilateral activities such as racquet sports, gymnastics provides uniform benefits for both limbs. In 2002, Proctor demonstrated with DEXA scans for bone mineral content (BMC) and BMD that gymnasts had significantly higher BMD levels in both limbs of the upper extremities in comparison to the control. In the control group, the dominant arm had significantly greater BMC. In the gymnast group, the increase in BMD was uniform across both limbs, indicating that BMD increases caused by participation in gymnastics was significantly greater than the osteogenic benefits of daily life.[35]

Studies show that lean body mass correlates to higher BMD, and women tend to develop less lean body mass than males, which contributes to lower relative BMD levels in women.[26,35] Female deficiency in lean body mass development has been hypothesized to have a hormonal basis.[15,19] Hormones also play a role in joint stability; high levels of progesterone produce relaxation of joints and ligaments in women, which contributes to the high incidence of joint laxity observed in adolescent females around the time of menarche. It is hypothesized that tightness in the joints women experience later in life is due to hormone deficiencies.

MUSCULOSKELETAL INJURIES

Studies have shown that sports injuries are generally more sport- than gender-specific[44]; however, Sallis and colleagues found a gender difference in injury incidence for swimming and water polo.[37] Female swimmers had significantly greater incidence of back/neck and shoulder, as well as hip, knee, and foot injuries, and female water polo players reported more shoulder injuries. Across all the sports investigated in the 15-year, retrospective study conducted by Sallis and colleagues that included a total of 3,767 participants, women had a higher incidence of shoulder injuries overall, particularly problems involving instability and frozen shoulder.[37] Lanese et al. found that although women gymnasts were injured at a greater rate than men, males were more likely to incur injuries to the upper extremities.[23] However, this finding was attributed to disparities between men's and women's gymnastic events and apparatus, noting that men gymnasts use predominantly upper body musculature and women use predominantly lower body musculature. The gender-linked hypothesis of incidence injury has not been substantially supported and remains circumstantial.

SHOULDER INSTABILITY

There is no definitive evidence to support the belief that female shoulders are more lax than male shoulders. Existing data suggests that females may have greater generalized laxity than males, but overall joint laxity does not correspond to shoulder laxity.[7] Laxity is not synonymous with instability and the two may occur mutually exclusive of the other in many cases.[7] *Laxity* is defined as the asymptomatic physiological motion of the glenohumeral joint that allows normal range of motion (ROM). Instability involves the abnormal motion of the glenohumeral joint that results in pain, subluxation, or dislocation of the shoulder.[13] Multidirectional instability (MDI) is symptomatic instability in more than one direction that includes inferior instability as a significant component (Fig. 27-1).

Current evidence is inconclusive in supporting the hypothesis that ligamentous laxity is more common in women, and whether generalized laxity corresponds to shoulder laxity.[11,13,28] Marshall et al. examined the gender basis of joint looseness and whether it is a function of a particular joint or characteristic of the entire person.[27] Multiple joint looseness parameters were examined in 124 preadolescent and adolescent males and females. The findings show that laxity is characteristic of the person, and is not gender-specific. Females showed significantly higher generalized laxity than males, but no significant difference was found in the shoulder. Emery and Mullaji found that shoulders in adolescent females were not

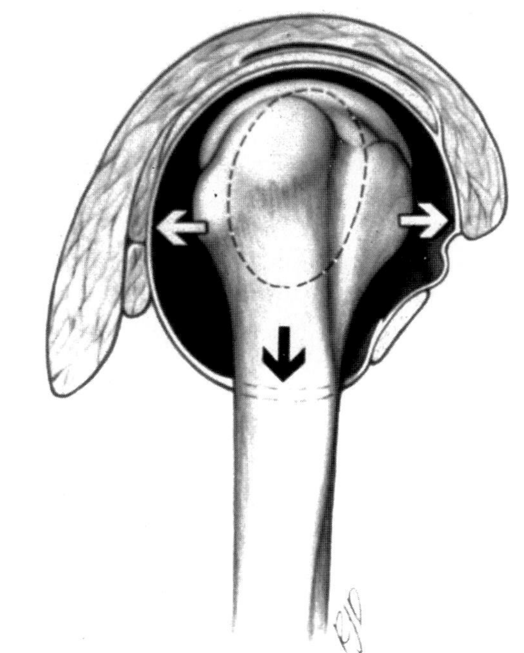

A

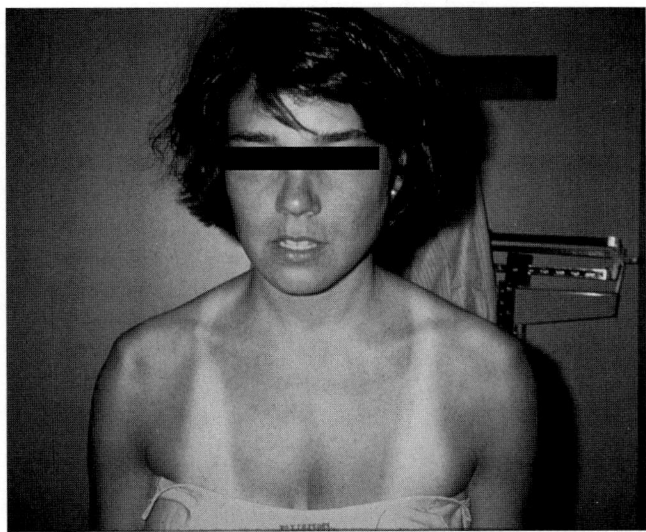

B

FIGURE 27-1. A, Multidirectional instability of the glenohumeral joint caused by capsular redundancy. **B,** Bilateral sulcus signs secondary to inferior capsular stretch.

more lax than shoulders in adolescent males and generalized joint laxity did not correlate with shoulder laxity.[11] In contrast, Grana and Morets found that shoulders of female high school basketball players were more lax than males at any age and that mobility decreased with age across both genders.[14] McFarland et al. found that shoulders in female high school and collegiate athletes were significantly more lax than shoulders in males; however, no raw data was included in the study.[28] Hypermobility syndrome, which is characterized as generalized joint laxity that presents with pain and musculoskeletal complaints, has been shown to be more common in females (Fig. 27-2).[7,21]

Bilateral shoulder instability is indicative of an intrinsic condition such as increased capsuloligamentous laxity and is often seen in patients with multidirectional instability.[38] O'Driscoll and Evans suggest that the occurrence of bilateral instability is more common in females; however, the findings were not statistically significant.[34] The pathophysiology of MDI involves factors other than excessive capsuloligamentous laxity; in many patients the contralateral shoulder is equally lax, yet asymptomatic. The rotator cuff plays an important role in shoulder stability by compressing the humeral head, known as *concavity compression*. The effectivness of concavity compression on maintaining joint stability depends on a number of factors, including the integrity of the labrum and the dynamic forces of the rotator cuff tendons.[38] No conclusive epidemiological study on the gender prevalence of MDI has been conducted; however, Brown et al. found a gender distribution of 45% males and 55% females by combining patient trials of numerous studies.[7] Patients are typically adolescent athletes or adults younger than 30 years of age. Rehabilitation programs for patients with MDI should focus on strengthening the dynamic stabilizers and improving neuromuscular coordination. Operative intervention can be undertaken in patients with persistent instability 6 to 12 months following a rehabilitation trial. Surgical intervention is directed at tightening the inferior capsule and the rotator interval capsule.[7,38] The inferior capsular shift procedure described by Neer and Foster is the standard for correcting capsular redundancy.[32] An arthroscopic stabilization procedure is also performed and the few studies that have examined this approach suggest that the results are comparable to open surgical techniques.[7]

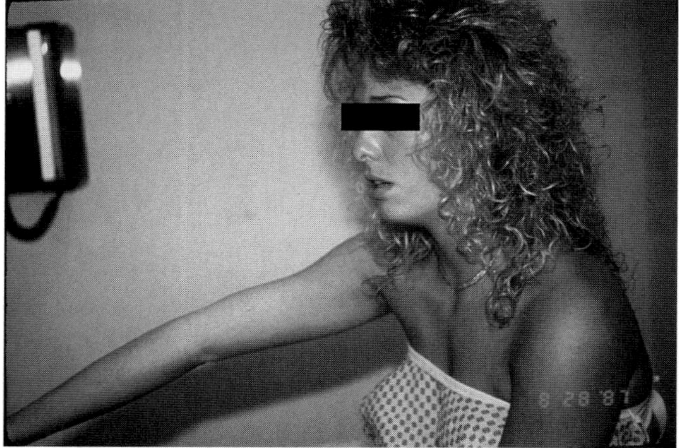

FIGURE 27-2. Hyperextension of the elbow consistent with generalized ligamentous laxity.

Although atraumatic, acquired instability is more common in patients with MDI, unidirectional instability often develops following trauma inflicted by high-energy sports associated with dislocations, such as basketball and gymnastics. Milgram et al. found that post-traumatic shoulder instability is three times more common in women than in men.[30] Repetitive overhead motion in sports such as swimming, volleyball, and tennis causes microtrauma, which can exacerbate preexisting capsular laxity or lead to the primary development of instability over time.

Shoulder instability can lead to the development of an impingement syndrome, because increased laxity allows for the upward and anterior migration of the humeral head in the glenoid, which leads to inflammation beneath the acromion and impinges the rotator cuff tendons.[9] Increased tissue irritation and inflammation inhibits forward flexion and can lead to the development of bursitis and tendinitis, and over time, a tear in the rotator cuff. Frequent extensions of the arm at high speeds contribute to both the development of bursitis and tendinitis; however, the risk increases with age. Tendinitis is more likely to develop in females who begin an aggressive training program with unconditioned muscles.

The kinematics of men's baseball throwing has been well documented, but the biomechanics of windmill softball pitching are less understood. During the overhand pitching motion, forces reaching 80% to 120% of body weight (BW) are produced at the elbow and shoulder. These forces, which occur during specific instances in the pitching motion, have been implicated in rotator cuff tears, subacromial impingement, and labrum tears, particularly SLAP lesions. Studies show that stresses on the shoulder and elbow during underhand pitching are similar to the stresses experienced during overhand throwing.[4] The major difference between the two pitching motions is the timing of the peak values for the resultant forces. The greatest resistance to distractions, which are compressive, superior forces, occurs during the delivery phase for underhand pitching, but occurs during the deceleration phase in overhand pitching. The magnitude of the forces during underhand pitching reaches 80% to 95% of the normalized values for overhand pitching, indicating that underhand pitching produces stress at the shoulder and elbow comparable to overhand pitching. To prevent overuse injuries, women softball pitchers should be instructed in proper pitching mechanics, perform exercises for strengthening the shoulder and rotator cuff musculature, and limit the number of pitches they throw in a given time period (Barrentine).[4]

A high frequency of suprascapular and infraspinatus atrophy has been demonstrated in the shoulder of female volleyball players.[12] Muscle weakness and imbalance of muscle strength between agonists and antagonists is associated with rotator cuff injuries. EMG analysis has shown that the most active stage of the shoulder occurs in the follow-through, during which the subscapularis internally rotates the shoulder while the infraspinatus, suprascapularis, terses minor, and deltoid muscles attempt to decelerate the arm, placing high demands on the eccentric strength of the decelerating muscles. Alfredson et al. found that female volleyball players had significantly higher concentric and eccentric peak torque of the rotator muscles in the shoulder than the nonactive control group.[1] The concentric peak torque of the extensors and eccentric peak torque of the flexors and extensors of the elbow were also greater in the volleyball players. Alfredson et al. concluded that the higher concentric and eccentric strength of the rotator muscles of the shoulder and extensor muscles of the elbow in the volleyball players resulted from muscular adaptation to activity.[1] None of the volleyball players tested had an incidence of shoulder injury. Alfredson et al. attributed this to the finding that none of the volleyball players demonstrated weakness of the external rotators in the dominant arm, indicating a good balance between agonist–antagonist rotator muscles of the shoulder. To prevent overuse injuries, female volleyball players should work to strengthen the internal and external rotator muscles of the shoulder.

Rehabilitation for a patient with instability should emphasize strengthening the rotator cuff and deltoid muscles with below-the-shoulder exercises. In some cases, patients with MDI may develop secondary impingement syndrome, and pain can prevent the patient from completing their rehabilitation program. A subacromial injection of a steroid preparation to take down the swelling of the bursa can provide sufficient relief for the patient to resume the exercise plan.

The standard operative treatment for instability is the anterior-inferior capsular shift procedure to reduce capsular laxity without limiting motion (Fig. 27-3).[6] This method is favored over the Putti-Platt and Magnuson-Stack procedures that shorten the subscapularis, and the Bankart procedure because these procedures have shown a significant loss of external rotation in clinical trials.[40] Such restrictions in ROM are particularly detrimental to athletes involved in overhead sports and can eventually lead to glenohumeral arthritis or joint replacement.[6] Athletes with anterior instability constitute a broad spectrum ranging from unidirectional anterior instability to MDI, with inferior capsular laxity. Inferior capsular shift provided excellent results in 96% of the cases, with patients returning to full athletic activity.[6] However, patients should be carefully selected, avoiding habitual dislocators with accompanying psychiatric disorders. An open surgical approach is preferred over an arthroscopic repair[30] to restore anatomy by correcting capsular laxity or labral avulsion.

FROZEN SHOULDER

Frozen shoulder, also known as adhesive capsulitis, is a painful disorder that results from global limitation of active and passive glenohumeral motion. Primary adhesive capsulitis results from idiopathic, progressive, painful loss of motion in patients whose radiographs are normal and other conditions with similar presentations have been ruled out. Other causes of pain and motion loss include primary glenohumeral arthrosis, rotator cuff pathology, and cervical spine disease. Secondary adhesive capsulitis results from a known extrinsic or intrinsic cause (Fig. 27-4). Primary adhesive capsulitis is relatively rare, with one study citing only a 4.7% incidence of all shoulder referrals.[8] Females are two to four times more likely than men to develop adhesive capsulitis (Fig. 27-5).[20] It is hypothesized that hormonal changes associated with menopause are related to the increased incidence of adhesive capsulitis in the female.[43] However, this theory has not been thoroughly tested and remains speculative. Other risk factors for the development of adhesive capsulitis include cervical disease, hyperthyroidism, ischemic heart disease, chest or breast surgery, autoimmune disorders, and diabetes.[8,31] The incidence of adhesive capsulitis is approximately 2% of all shoulder disorders and is as high as 19% for diabetic patients.[31]

As the name implies, adhesive capsulitis has a perivascular inflammatory component. Neviaser described fibrosis as an additional component of the pathology and suggested that the condition represented a reparative inflammatory process.[33] There is some controversy over whether the underlying pathologic process is a fibrosing condition or an inflammatory condition, but significant evidence suggests that the underlying pathology is synovial inflammation with reactive capsular fibrosis. The extent of fibrosis and inflammation depends on the stage of the disease, but the initial biologic trigger for the transition from inflammation and subsequent fibrosis is unknown (Fig. 27-6).[16]

In contrast, Bunker and Anthony found that inflammation was not significant and not directly associated with the functional or mechanical abnormality. Bunker and Anthony obtained excision specimens of the coracohumeral ligament and, after a histological examination, the main cell populations from the biopsies of the coracohumeral ligament and the rotator interval were found to be fibroblasts and myofibroblasts. Since these cells can be mistaken for inflammatory cells without proper identification with immunocytochemistry, Bunker and Anthony suggest that the condition does not have a significant inflammatory basis and the underlying

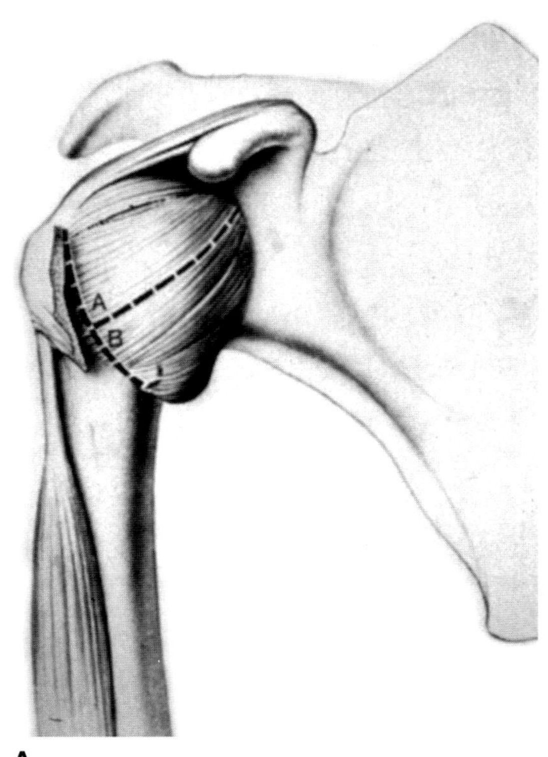

A

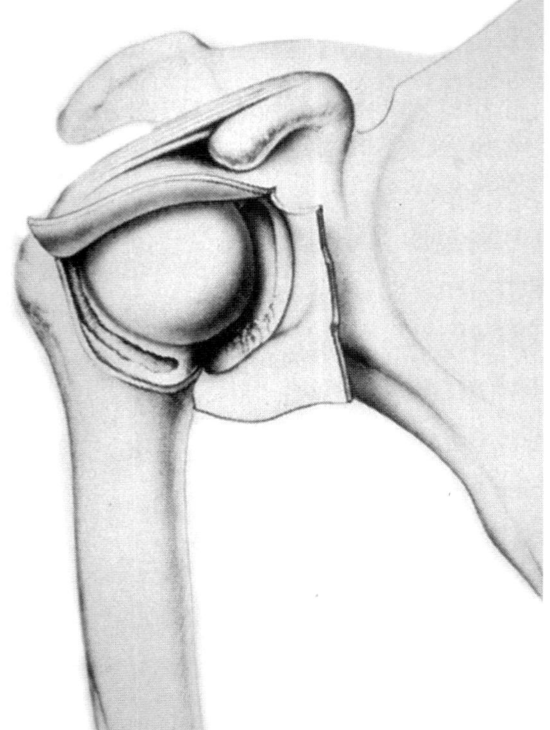

B

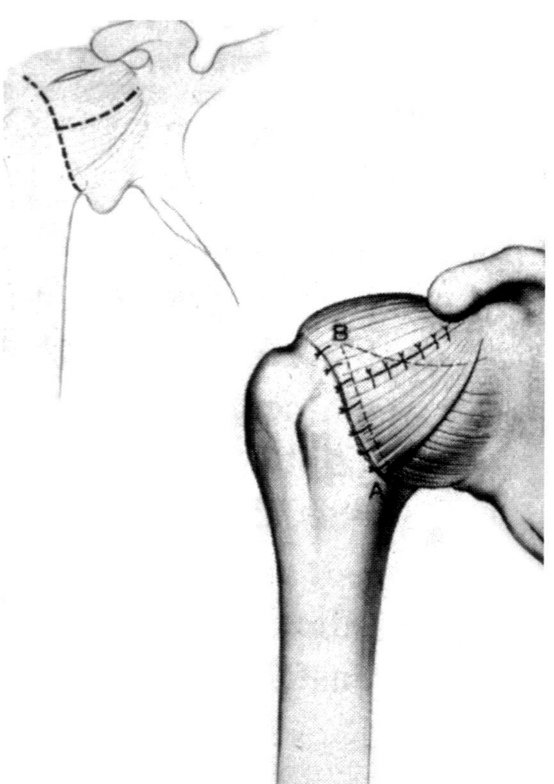

C

FIGURE 27-3. A, Capsular redundancy is demonstrated. **B,** A T-shaped capsulotomy is performed releasing the anterior/inferior capsule. **C,** The inferior flap is shifted superiorly while the superior flap reinforces the anterior repair reducing capsular redundancy on all three sides.

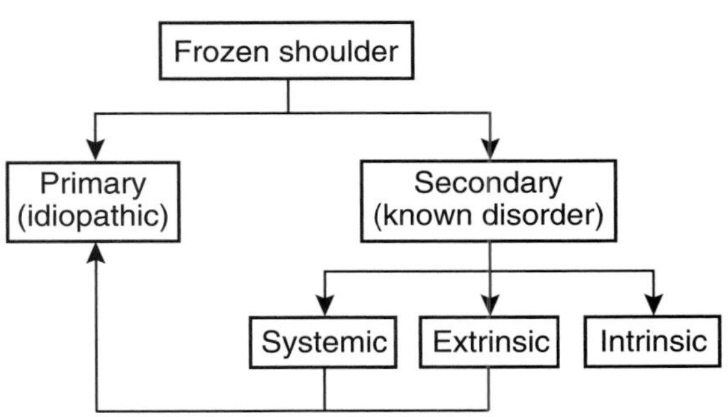

FIGURE 27-4. Frozen shoulder classification as described by Zuckerman and Cuomo. (Zuckerman JD, Cuomo F: Frozen shoulder. In Matsen FA, Fu FH, Hawkins RJ [eds]: The Shoulder: A Balance of Mobility and Stability. Park Ridge, IL, American Academy of Orthopaedic Surgeons, 1993, pp 253–268.)

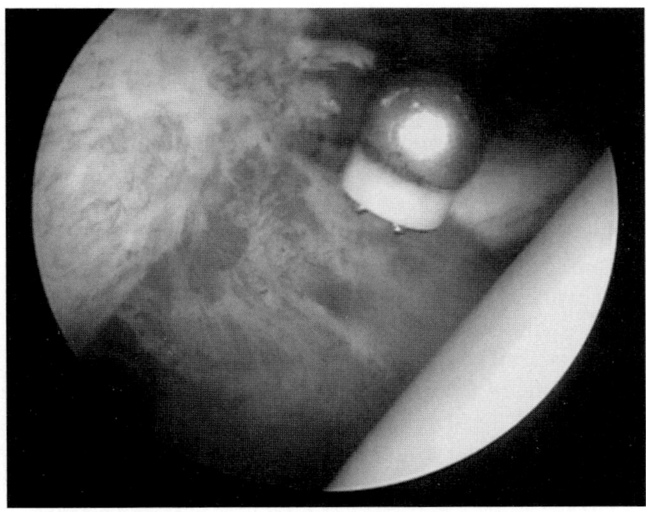

FIGURE 27-6. Synovial inflammation identified during arthroscopy consistent with frozen shoulder syndrome.

pathological process is active fibroblast proliferation coupled with marginal transformation to smooth muscle. However, the progression and stage of the disease in the patients was not specified, and thus it is likely that these patients were in stage 3, and the inflammation component was less prominent. Increased vascularity and collagen production was noted in the lesions. Collagen was produced from the fibroblasts to form thick nodular bands. The biopsy samples were identical to Dupuytren's disease of the hand in microscopic appearance and cell types.[8]

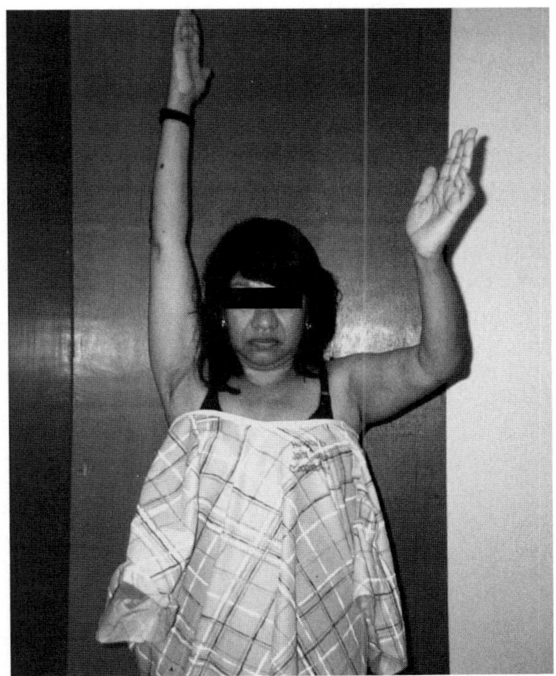

FIGURE 27-5. Profound loss of elevation both actively and passively seen in frozen shoulder syndrome.

Cytokines have recently been identified as playing a role in the inflammation and fibrosis of adhesive capsulitis. Cytokines are known to be involved in the initiation and termination processes in multiple musculoskeletal tissues, and recent studies have shown that their sustained production results in fibrosis.[17] Rodeo et al. identified specific cytokines believed to be involved in the inflammatory and fibrosis spectrum of the disease. The study found an increase in transforming growth factor-β, platelet-derived growth factor, and hepatocyte growth factor in patients with primary and secondary adhesive capsulitis.[36] Matrix metalloproteases may also play a role the development of frozen shoulder. In a study conducted by Hutchinson and colleagues, 6 of 12 patients with inoperable gastric cancer developed adhesive capsulitis or a Dupuytren's-like condition when treated with a synthetic matrix metalloproteinase inhibitor.[18]

Adhesive capsulitis occurs in four stages and involves pathologic changes in the synovium and subsynovium. In stage 1, hypervascular synovitis is apparent with a normal underlying capsule. Fibroblastic hyperplasia and disorganized collagen deposition characterizes stage 2, reflecting a loss of capsular volume and a response to the painful synovitis. No inflammatory infiltrates are found in stage 2. Patients in stage 3 report symptoms lasting 9 to 14 months and show persistent loss of capsular volume and fibrosis of the glenohumeral joint, with minimal synovial hyperplasia. ROM is limited and unchanged with examination following injection of local anesthetic, but the shoulder is typically pain-free. Stage 4, known as the "thawing phase," is characterized by gradual recovery of ROM resulting from capsular remodeling.

Treatment options for adhesive capsulitis vary with the stage of the disease, and range from benign neglect, supervised rehabilitation, nonsteroidal anti-inflammatory medications, intraarticular corticosteroid injections, distention arthrography, and closed manipulation to open surgical release and arthroscopic capsular release.[10,16] Accurate diagnosis of the stage of adhesive capsulitis being treated is critical for achieving optimal results. Intraarticular injections can be extremely helpful in diagnosis and treatment and are recommended for early stages of the disease to distinguish between stage 1 and stage 2. Patients in stage 2 will not have significant improvement of range of motion and only mitigated pain. Patients treated with intraarticular corticosteroids within 3 months of the onset of symptoms demonstrate a rapid recovery within 6 weeks. Patients in stage 2 note a vast improvement in at-rest pain, but results on recovery of range of motion depend on the duration of the symptoms. Patients are evaluated 2 weeks postinjection and a rehabilitation program for increasing scapular stabilization is typically initiated.

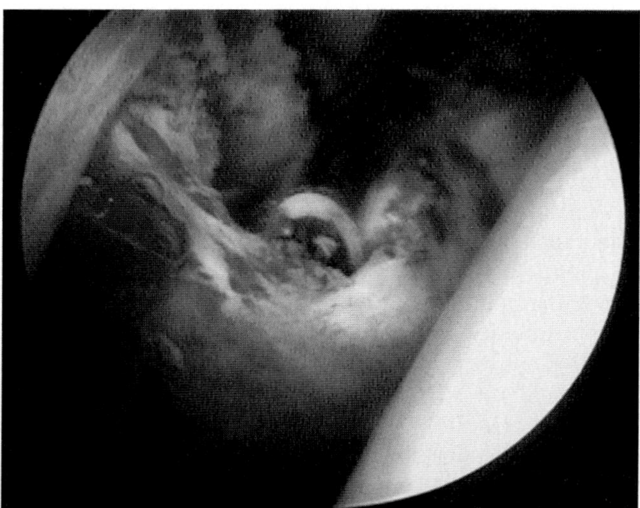

A

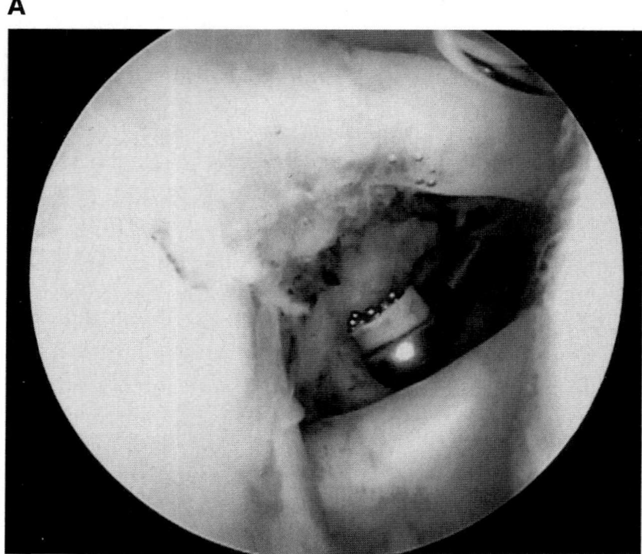

B

FIGURE 27-7. A, Inflamed, thickened rotator interval. **B,** Post-arthroscopic capsular release performed with thermal wand.

In stages 3 and 4, corticosteroid injections are ineffective because the inflammatory phase of the disease has passed. Physical therapy programs prescribed at this phase in the disease are designed to increase range of motion through aggressive stretching. Patient selection is important for considering operative treatment. Closed manipulation is not recommended for patients with osteopenia, recent surgical repair of soft tissue about the shoulder, or in the presence of fractures, neurologic injury, and instability. An arthroscopic inspection is typically completed before a closed manipulation is done. For patients who fail to gain mobility following manipulation, an open soft-tissue release is the traditional alternative, often involving a Z-plasty lengthening of the subscapularis and the anterior aspect of the capsule. Recently, arthroscopic release of capsular contraction has shown advantages over open release, such as reduced postoperative morbidity and precision sectioning of the contracted capsule, with comparable effectiveness (Fig. 27-7).[44,45] The open procedure is preferred for patients who have had a previous operation that has shortened or entrapped extraarticular structures.

Passive range of motion is conducted in the recovery room under anesthesia to maintain the increase in ROM achieved by the surgery. A physical therapy program of aggressive stretching to maximize ROM coupled with modalities for pain and inflammation is commenced immediately postoperatively, and strengthening exercises are gradually incorporated.[17]

REFERENCES

1. Alfredson H, Pietila T, Lorentzon R: Concentric and eccentric shoulder and elbow muscle strength in female volleyball players and non-active females. Scand J Med Sci Sports 8:265–270, 1998.
2. Arendt E: Orthopaedic issues for active and athletic women. In Agostini R (ed): Clinics in Sports Medicine—The Athletic Women. Philadelphia, WB Saunders, 1994.
3. Arnheim D: Modern Principles of Athletic Training, 7th ed. St. Louis, Mosby, 1989, pp 64–111.
4. Barrentine SW, Fleisig GS, Whiteside JA: Biomechanics of windmill softball pitching with implications about injury mechanisms at the shoulder and elbow. J Orthop Sports Phys Ther 28:405–415, 1998.
5. Beunen G, et al: Ulnar variance and skeletal maturity of radius and ulna in female gymnasts. Med Sci Sports Exerc 31:653–657, 1999.
6. Bigliani LU, Kurzweil PR, Schwatzbach CC: Inferior capsular shift procedure for anterior-inferior shoulder instability in athletes. Am J Sports Med 22:578–584, 1994.

7. Brown GA, Tan JL, Kirkley A: The lax shoulder in females: Issues, answers, but many more questions. Clin Orthop 372:110–122, 2000.
8. Bunker RD, Anthony PP: The pathology of frozen shoulder: A Dupuytren-like disease. J Bone Joint Surg 77B:677–683, 1995.
9. Cavallo RJ, Speer KP: Shoulder instability and impingement in throwing athletes. Med Sci Sports Exerc 30:18–25, 1998.
10. Connolly JF: Unfreezing the frozen shoulder. J Musculoskel Med 15(11):47–56, 1998.
11. Emery RJH, Mullaji AB: Glenohumeral joint instability in normal adolescents: Incidence and significance. J Bone Joint Surg 73B:406–408, 1991.
12. Ferretti A, Cerullo G, Russo G: Suprascapular neuropathy in volleyball players. J Bone Joint Surg 69A:260–263, 1987.
13. Flatow EL, Warner JJP: Instability of the shoulder: complex problems and failed repairs: Part I. Relevant biomechanics, multidirectional instability, and severe glenoid loss. Instr Course Lect 47:97–112, 1998.
14. Grana WA, Moretz JA: Ligamentous laxity in secondary school athletes. JAMA 240:1975–1976, 1978.
15. Hale RW: Women and sports: Keeping up with female athletes' needs. Contemp OB/GYN 13:85–95, 1979.
16. Hannafin JA, Chiaia TA: Adhesive capsulitis: A treatment approach. Clin Orthop 372:95–109, 2000.
17. Hannafin JA, Vad VB: Frozen shoulder in women: Evaluation and management. J Musculoskel Med 17:13–28, 2000.
18. Hutchinson JW, Tierney GM, Parsons SL, Davis TR: Dupuytren's disease and frozen shoulder induced by treatment with a matrix metalloproteinase inhibitor. J Bone Joint Surg 80B:907–908, 1998.
19. Ichinose Y, et al: Morphological and functional differences in the elbow extensor muscle between highly trained male and female athletes. Eur J Appl Physiol 78:109–114, 1998.
20. Ireland ML: The special conerns of the female athlete. In Fu F, Stone D (eds): Sports Injuries. Baltimore, Williams & Wilkins, 1994, pp 153–187.
21. Jessee EF, Owen DS, Sagar KB: The benign hypermobile joint syndrome. Arthritis Rheum 23: 1053–1056, 1980.
22. Kadi F, Thornell LE: Concomitant increases in myonuclear and satellite cell content in female trapezius muscle following strength training. Histochem Cell Biol 113:99–103, 2000.
23. Lanese R, et al: Injury and disability in matched men's and women's intercollegiate sports. Am J Pub Health 80(12):1459–1462, 1990.
24. Leone M, Lariviere G, Comtois A: Discriminant analysis of anthropometric and biomotor variables among elite adolescent female athletes in four sports. J Sports Sci 20:443–449, 2002.
25. Loud KJ, Micheli LJ: Common athletic injuries in adolescent girls. Curr Opin Pediatr 13(4):317–322, 2001.
26. Madsen KL, Adams WC, Van Loan MD: Effects of physical activity, body weight and composition, and muscular strength on bone density in young women. Med Sci Sports Exerc 30:114–120, 1998.
27. Marshall JL, Johanson N, Wickiewicz TL: Joint looseness: A function of the person and the joint. Med Sci Sports Exer 12:189–194, 1980.
28. McFarland EG, Campell G, McDowell J: Posterior shoulder laxity in asymptomatic athletes. Am J Sports Med 24:468-471, 1996.
29. McIntyre LF, Caspair RB, Savoie FH III: The arthroscopic treatment of multidirectional shoulder instability: Two-year results of a multiple suture technique. Arthroscopy 13:418–425, 1997.
30. Milgram C, Mann G, Finestone A: A prevalence study of recurrent shoulder dislocations in young adults. J Shoulder Elbow Surg 7:621–624, 1998.
31. Miller MD, Wirth MA, Rockwood CA: Thawing the frozen shoulder, the "patient" patient. Orthopedics 19:849–853, 1996.
32. Neer CS, Foster CR: Inferior capsular shift for involuntary inferior and multidirectional instability of the shoulder. J Bone Joint Surg 62A:897–908, 1980.
33. Neviaser JS: Adhesive capsulitis of the shoulder: Study of pathological findings in periarthritis of the shoulder. J Bone Joint Surg 27:211–222, 1945.
34. O'Driscoll SW, Evans DC: Contralateral shoulder instability following anterior repair: An epidemiological investigation. J Bone Joint Surg 73B: 941–946, 1991.
35. Proctor K, et al: Upper-limb bone mineral density of female collegiate gymnasts versus controls. Med Sci Sports Exerc 34:1830–1835, 2002.
36. Rodeo SA, Hannafin JA, Tom J: Immunolocalization of cytokines and their receptors in adhesive capsulitis of the shoulder. J Orthop Res 15:427–436, 1997.
37. Sallis RE et al: Comparing sports injuries in men and women. Int J Sports Med 22:420–423, 2001.
38. Schenk TJ, Brems JJ: Mulitdirectional instability of the shoulder: Pathophysiology, diagnosis, and management. J Am Acad Orthop Surg 6:65–72, 1998.
39. Sinha A, Kaeding CC, Wadley GM: Upper extremity stress fractures in athletes: Clinical features of 44 cases. Clin J Sports Med 9:199–202, 1999.
40. Symeonides PP: Reconstruction of the Putti-Platt procedure and its mode of action in recurrent traumatic anterior dislocation of the shoulder. Clin Orthop 246:8–15, 1989.

41. Taafe DR, et al: Differential effects of swimming versus weight-bearing activity on bone mineral status of eumenorrheic athletes. J Bone Min Res 10:586–593, 1995.
42. Warner JJP, Allen A, Wong P: Arthroscopic release of postoperative capsular contracture of the shoulder. J Bone Joint Surg Am 79:1151–1158, 1997.
43. Warner JJP, Answorth A, Marks PH: Athroscopic release for chronic, refractory adhesive capsulitis of the shoulder. J Bone Joint Surg Am 78:1808–1816, 1996.
44. Whiteside PA: Men's and women's injuries in comparable sports. Phys Sports Med 8:130–136, 1980.
45. Wilmore JH: Alterations in strength, body composition, and anthropometric measurements consequent to a 10-week weight training program. Med Sci Sports 6:133, 1974.

28 Lower Extremity Injuries in the Female Athlete

Letha Y. Griffin

The lower extremity is a site of frequent injury in the female athlete. In fact, the NCAA's Injury Surveillance System reports 54.2% of all injuries in women participating in all NCAA sports occur to the lower extremity.[99] During the 2001–2002 soccer season, lower extremity injuries accounted for 71.1% of all injuries.[99] As in male athletes, the most common lower extremity injuries in females are sprains, strains, and contusions. However, anatomic, physiologic, and biomechanical differences in males and females account for some variation in injury expression. For example, noncontact ACL injuries, anterior knee pain, stress fractures, and ankle and foot overuse injuries occur more frequently in women than men.

ANTERIOR CRUCIATE LIGAMENT INJURIES

Epidemiology

Although the reported rate of ACL injuries occurring in the general population is 1 in 3,000 individuals, the majority of these injuries occur in young people, from 15 to 25 years of age.[25,41,89] In females, the incidence of those undergoing surgery for this injury appears to drop significantly after age 20 whereas in males it stays elevated until age 40 to 45 (Fig. 28-1).[39] In high-risk sports such as basketball and soccer, the rate of injury in women is greater than that in men.[6,18,33,35,63,65,78,136]

Collegiate female athletes have a one in ten chance of injuring their ACLs during a four-year college career, and high school female athletes have a one in 100 chance of injuring their ACLs during their four-year high school career.[96,99]

Several studies have demonstrated that athletes who sustain an ACL injury are likely to have a parent or sibling who also injured this ligament.[34,51] Once injured, a female athlete under 20 years of age has a one in ten chance of reinjuring the same knee and a slightly greater than one in ten chance of sustaining an ACL injury in the opposite knee.[103]

Significance

Unfortunately, these injuries are frequently associated not only with significant emotional and financial impacts, but they also have been found to have long-lasting health ramifications.[36,82] Although we have made significant advancements in the diagnosis and surgical reconstruction of the injured ACL, we have not been able to reverse the articular cartilage injury that occurs concurrently with the ligament injury. Therefore, despite adequate stabilization of the injured female athlete's knee, there is a significant likelihood of her developing degenerative joint disease within a decade of her injury.[24,103,110]

Prevention

Proposed Strategies. Faced with these outcome statistics, it is not enough to merely diagnose, stabilize, and rehabilitate the injured athlete. Prevention strategies for this injury must be developed if we are going to decrease this injury's long-term consequences (see box, Proposed Prevention Strategies). Early in the 1980s, it was thought that perhaps functional knee bracing was the answer to preventing ACL injuries. However, despite multiple studies, there is no good data demonstrating that a functional knee brace will prevent an ACL injury in an ACL-intact individual.[35,46,108,112,123] Researchers in the Scandinavian countries and others have examined the shoe–surface interface as a potential modifiable risk factor.[68,95,113] These investigators have tried to develop a shoe that has adequate traction to permit optimal sports performance, yet not so much traction that the foot sticks and the body moves around the fixed foot, putting the knee at risk for a ligament injury. Such an ideal surface–shoe interface has not been found, and therefore, there are no prevention programs based on this intriguing idea. Research is ongoing.

Anatomic factors have also been proposed as possible risk factors for ACL injury. In general, females have more femoral anteversion, greater hip varus and knee valgus, a larger Q angle of the knee, more tibial torsion, and greater foot pronation than men (Fig. 28-2).[61,63,65,128] Yet, a direct link between any of these factors with an increased incidence of ACL injury has not been

CHECKLIST

Proposed Prevention Strategies

- Enhanced knee stability through bracing
- Improve shoe–surface interactions
- Manipulate hormonal status
- Alter predisposing anatomic factors
- *Improve biomechanics through neuromuscular conditioning

*Presently, only this latter concept has been the focus for the development of prevention programs.

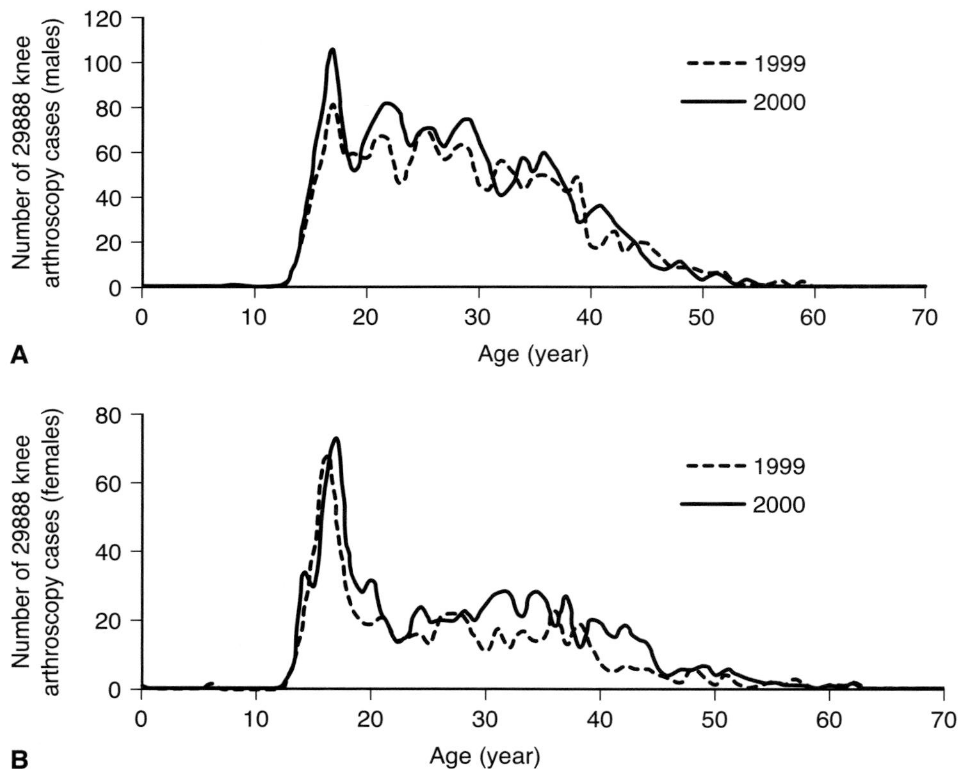

FIGURE 28-1. Statistics gathered by the American Board of Orthopaedic Surgery on surgeries performed by board candidates in orthopaedic surgery during the years 1999–2000. The code 29888 is the procedure code for ACL reconstruction. Graph lists the number of cases per age of patient. **A,** Cases performed in men. **B,** Cases performed in women. (Reprinted with permission from Garrett WE Jr: Non-contact ACL injuries in female athletes: Risk factors and biomechanical considerations, ICLS 78th Annual meeting, American Academy of Orthopaedic Surgeons, February 9, 2003, New Orleans, LA.)

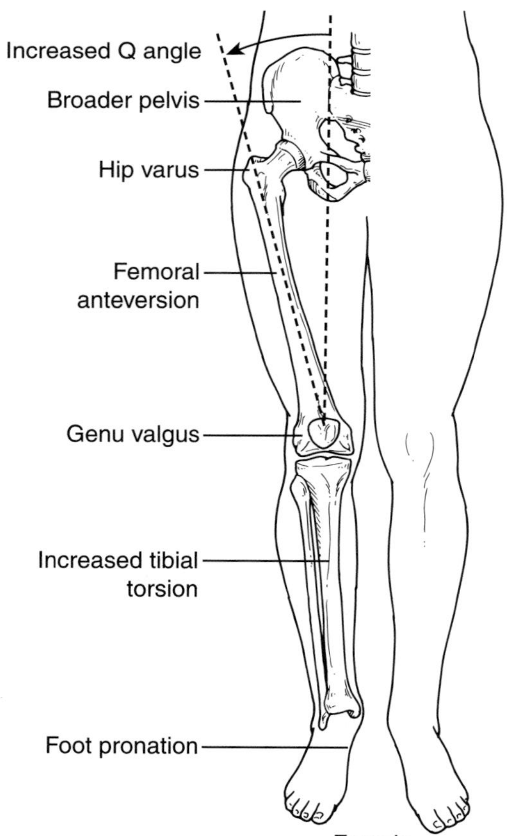

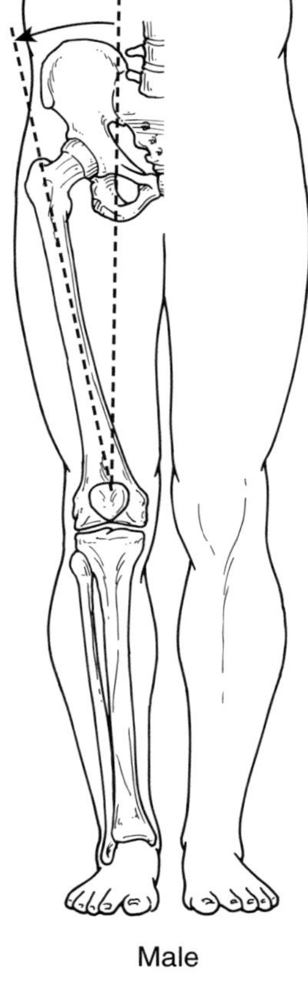

FIGURE 28-2. Anatomic variations in the lower extremity alignment of men and women.

demonstrated. Similarly, although women appeared to have narrower femoral notches and smaller ACLs than men, no definitive association with notch size or size of the ACL with injury has been shown.[4,51,59,71,92,115,118,119,124,127] Generally, women who are smaller anatomically than age-matched males have smaller ACLs, which are housed in smaller notches within smaller femurs.[124] Therefore, although the association of anatomic variables to ACL injuries is intriguing, until one or several factors can be reliably associated with an increase in the rate of ACL injury, prevention strategies based on alteration of anatomic factors are not reasonable.

The association of sex hormones to ACL injury has been intensely studied. Liu et al. reported finding receptor sites for estrogen and progesterone in human ACL cells.[79] Estrogen is known to affect collagen synthesis and fibroblast proliferation.[79,117] Yet, there is no agreement on which of the sex hormones is important in ACL injury.

No clear link between the hormonal fluctuations during the menstrual cycle and the occurrence of ACL injury has been established. Wojtys et al. reported more injuries in the ovulatory phase of the menstrual cycle whereas Myklebust et al. reported a decrease in the injury rate during the midcycle estrogen surge (days 8-14 of the menstrual cycle).[94,112] Several researchers found a greater number of injuries occurring just before or after the onset of menses.[5,90,91,94,117] At present, there is insufficient evidence to suggest that altering hormonal levels or restricting women from sport during any portion of the menstrual cycle is effective in preventing ACL injuries.

Biomechanical risk factors appear to be the key modifiable risk factors in preventing ACL injuries. Seventy to seventy-five percent of all ACL injuries involve no contact with another player.[56,67] At-risk situations for ACL injury are decelerating, cutting or pivoting, changing directions, or landing a jump. Typically when a ligament injury occurs, the athlete has landed, cut, pivoted, or decelerated flat-footed in an upright posture.[47,67,120] Often, there is an unplanned event or perturbation that occurs prior to injury, throwing the athlete "off balance."[67] It is known that a maximum eccentric quadriceps contraction when the foot is planted can create enough force to tear the ACL.[85,86]

Previously, it was felt that if one was strong and flexible, one could prevent an ACL injury from occurring. However, strong, flexible muscles must fire at appropriate times if injuries are to be prevented. This means a conditioned neuromuscular control system is as essential for injury prevention as are strong, flexible muscles.[55,56,75] Pure strength, unchecked by neuromuscular controls, may result in injury. Proprioception plays an integral role in neuromuscular control, providing essential input for "functional joint stability"—that is, joint stability required to perform a functional activity without injury.[76]

Existing Programs. Prevention programs based on altering biomechanical risk factors through neuromuscular training has become popular in the last several years.[17,47,55,84] These programs teach young athletes to practice landing a jump, cutting, pivoting, and stopping in a more flexed position on the balls of the feet with hips and knees bent and the body balanced over the lower extremity. Plyometric jump drills seems to be an effective means to train young athletes to land correctly while helping to develop hamstring strength.[52,54,55,67,74,83,84,131,133] Agility drills improve neuromuscular functional joint stability. Balance drills also enhance proprioception.[17]

In addition, it seems important to develop an awareness of "at-risk" situations and preplan avoidance strategies. Ettlinger et al. found a 62% decrease in serious knee injuries in an awareness-trained group of ski patrollers and instructors from 20 ski areas.[31] These patrollers and instructors analyzed injury videos and developed strategies to avoid the events that can result in an ACL injury while skiing.

In skiing where the risk of ACL injury is 2.2 times greater in women, the majority of injuries occur from what has been termed "the phantom foot mechanism."[91,122] Elements of the phantom foot mechanism include skier off balance to the rear, uphill arm back, hips below the knee, uphill ski unweighted, weight on the inside edge of the downhill ski, and upper body generally facing downhill. If these elements of the phantom foot mechanism begin to fall into place, an appropriate initial response is to keep arms forward, feet together, and hands over skis in an attempt to avoid injury.[1,91,122]

In summary, the five strategies that form the basis for most of the currently available ACL prevention programs are: increased injury awareness, traditional stretching and strengthening exercises, agility drills, plyometric jump drills, and cardiovascular exercises (see box, Five Strategies of Neuromuscular Conditioning for ACL Prevention) These components can be adapted into the pre-season conditioning activities for a sport and can be continued as a part of in-season conditioning routines. More research is needed, but early data suggests that such programs do significantly decrease the incidence of ACL injuries in young female athletes.[17,31,52,54,55,84,131]

Treatment

If an ACL injury does occur in a female athlete, treatment is similar to that of male athletes.[8,22,32,116] Initially, following a thorough evaluation including a comprehensive history and physical examination and indicated diagnostic studies, the athlete begins a rehabilitation program to restore strength, range of motion, and neuromuscular control. Decisions for operative correction (that is, reconstruction of the injured ACL) need to be based on the degree of laxity demonstrated in the female athlete's knee combined with the activity level of the athlete. It is

CHECKLIST

Five Strategies of Neuromuscular Conditioning for ACL Prevention*

- Increase awareness of injury mechanics (may be sports-specific)
- Increase strength and flexibility
- Initiate plyometric drills for the lower extremity
- Enhance proprioception through balance drills
- Maintain cardiovascular conditioning

*Further information on ACL prevention programs can be obtained from the following sources:
Caraffe A. Orthopaedic Clinic, S. Maria Hospital University of Perugia, 1-05106 Terni, Italy
Sportsmetrics Training Program, Cincinnati Sports Medicine Research and Educational Foundation, 311 Straight Street, Cincinnati, OH 45219
The Awareness Program, Vermont Safety Research, PO Box 85, Underhill, VT, 05490
The Prevent Injury Enhance Performance (PEP) Program, Holly Silvers, MPT, 1310 20th Street, Suite 150, Santa Monica, CA, 90404.

not unusual for young female athletes, between the ages of 15 and 35, to have difficulty controlling the increased knee laxity that occurs following ACL injury. Therefore, reconstruction is frequently recommended.[19,57,65]

In the early to mid 1990s, many expressed concern over the potential outcome of ACL reconstructions in women. Investigators feared women would not perform well during rehabilitation, grafts would loosen, and other postoperative complications would be more frequent in women. However, studies have since demonstrated the effectiveness of ACL reconstruction in women athletes using either quadruple hamstring grafts or patella-tendon grafts.[8,21,22,32,57,102,116] No increase in the complication rate was noted.

Initially, quadruple hamstring grafts in women were reported to have increased side-to-side laxity when evaluated objectively with the KT-1000 arthrometer.[9,21,22,32] However, such increases in side-to-side laxity scores were not correlated with inferior results functionally, as indicated by subjective evaluations or objective outcome measures.[3,21,22,32,57,99,116] Moreover, longer-term studies (5 years) demonstrate an equalization of laxity scores between females reconstructed with hamstring grafts and those in whom patella tendon grafts were used.[102]

Few papers have investigated the effect bone density may have on graft fixation in women. Pinczewski and colleagues have theorized that perhaps interference screws, particularly the bioabsorbable interference screws used with hamstring grafts, may predispose to increased laxity because of decreased bone mineral density in the femurs and tibias of injured women undergoing ACL reconstruction.[102,103] However, presently there are very little in the way of supportive data for or against this argument. Further evaluation seems prudent.

Because of the high rate of reinjury in the same extremity or injury to the ACL of the opposite extremity in young female athletes, it is advisable to incorporate prevention strategies into their rehabilitation programs.

ANTERIOR KNEE PAIN

Definition

More prevalent, but not as devastating as an ACL injury, is anterior knee pain in women.[77,104] Garrick has termed anterior knee pain "the most common overuse syndrome that affects athletes."[40] It represents approximately 25% to 30% of all injuries seen in women runners.[77,109] Other names given to this clinical entity that presents with vague symptoms of pain in the front of the knee which increase with bending and squatting activities as well as with stair and hill climbing are patellofemoral stress syndrome (PFSS), patella pain, and patella maltracking abnormality (see box, Interchangeable Terms for the Syndrome of Anterior Knee Pain). An effusion is rarely present in this syndrome and, in fact, this syndrome is associated with very few objective signs. This entity is not synonymous with chondromalacia patella or with subluxation or dislocation of the patella. Goodfellow called this entity the "mythical disease."[44]

Etiology

Its etiology is really unknown.[54] Some feel it is caused by maltracking of the patella, but others feel this entity results from recurrent stress to the patellofemoral joint in the female athlete.[29,62,64,114,121]

Maltracking Theory. At puberty, the pelvis widens and there is an increase in hip varus and knee valgus. At the same time, many young girls involved in running sports develop their vastus lateralis to a greater degree than their vastus medialis. The dominant vastus lateralis combined with one or several of the following—femoral anteversion, foot pronation, anterior pelvic tilt, increased hip varus, or increased knee valgus—results in the patella that sits and tracks laterally in the trochlear groove.[38] Such an altered patellofemoral relationship is felt to be responsible for abnormal patellofemoral forces that can lead to anterior knee pain. Anterior pelvic tilt is felt to be an influencing factor because it is associated with hamstring tightness and tightness of the iliotibial band.[60]

CHECKLIST

Interchangeable Terms for the Syndrome of Anterior Knee Pain

- Anterior knee pain
- Patellofemoral stress syndrome
- Patella pain
- Maltracking patella

Overload Theory. However, Thomee and his colleagues evaluated lower extremity alignment in 40 patients and 20 controls, comparing the alignment of each patient's symptomatic leg to his or her nonsymptomatic leg and to the alignment of the legs in 20 asymptomatic controls.[125] The control population were females of the same age and relative size as those who were symptomatic. The investigators found no predictable relationship between patella maltracking issues and anterior knee pain. Hence, they concluded overload, not maltracking, results in symptomatic anterior knee pain.

The overload theory has been popularized by Scott Dye, MD.[29] This theory is based on each individual having a zone of functional homeostasis or an "envelope of function" (Fig. 28-3). The size of this zone depends on the individual's own uniqueness (such as her anatomy and past injuries). If the athlete keeps her activity (load and duration) within the zone of homeostasis, she functions well. If she increases the amount and intensity of the activity to where it exceeds the zone, symptoms will appear. For example, if a young woman has a laterally tracking patella but walks only on flat-level ground for 15 minutes each day, then she may not develop symptoms of anterior knee pain. However, if this same young woman runs stadium steps for 2 hours a day or does the Stairmaster for 2 hours a day at high intensity, anterior knee pain may occur. This theoretical model for anterior knee pain accepts the idea that this syndrome is probably caused by a combination of factors.

Treatment

Exercise. Treatment of the symptomatic athlete is typically directed at altering patella tracking and at least temporarily decreasing the intensity or type of the offending activity. Exercises designed to strengthen the quadriceps, especially the medial expanse of the quadriceps (vastus medialis and the vastus medialis obliques) to balance the quadriceps' pull of the patella, combined with strengthening of the hip adductors, hip internal rotators, and stretching exercises not only for the quadriceps but also for the hamstring muscle groups, the iliotibial band, and tight lateral retinacular structures frequently improve maltracking.[7,23] The increased strength of the muscle groups around the knee help to stiffen the knee and broaden its envelope of function. Decreasing anterior pelvic tilt through core stability exercises (trunk and abdominal exercises) is also important.

Bracing, Taping, and Orthotics. Bracing and/or taping of the patella to alter patella femoral forces may be effective in some girls.[43,105,106,129] McConnell taping is a taping technique popularized by this physical therapist in 1986.[88] Tape is used to hold the patella in a neutral position in the center of the groove (Fig. 28-4). Braces can encircle the patella, provide a lateral pad, or elevate the patella in the groove. Frequently, braces have straps designed to act as McConnell taping strips do—that is, to dynamically pull or push the patella into the center of the trochlear groove.

Some girls who pronate find adding arch supports to their shoes or using custom shoe orthotics helpful.[30]

One should explain to the female athlete and her parents, in the case of young teenage athletes, that there is not one orthotic, brace, or taping technique that works for everyone just as there is not one exercise routine that works for all athletes. Selecting the proper orthotic, brace, or taping method is most frequently a trial-and-error process.[23,35]

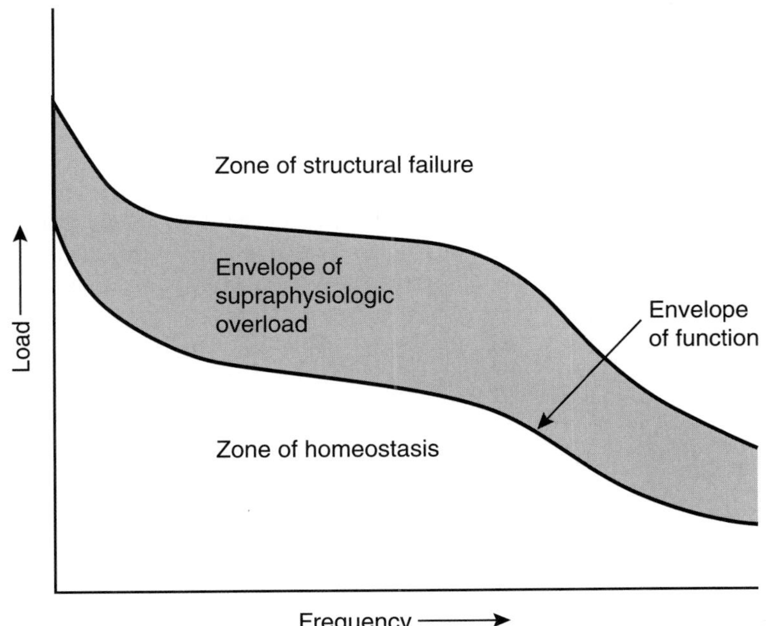

FIGURE 28-3. Dye's concept of the "envelope of function." As load and/or frequency of activity increases, one enters the zone of supraphysiologic overload and ultimately the zone of structural failure. (Adapted from Dye SF: The knee is the biologic transmission with an envelope of function: A theory. Clin Orthop 325:10–18, 1996.)

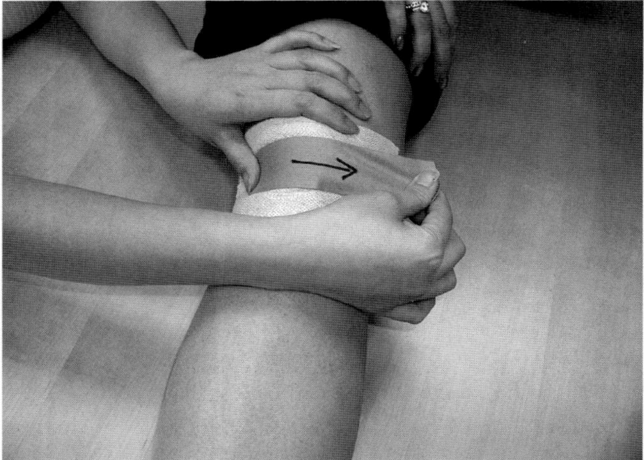

A

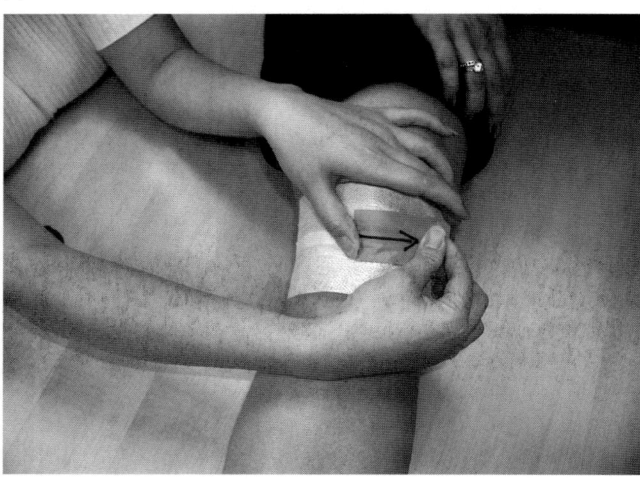

B

FIGURE 28-4. McConnell taping consists of strategically applied strips of adhesive tape designed to "pull" the patella into an anatomic position. To correct lateral tracking of the patella, the patella is taped from its lateral border (**A**). When excessive lateral tilt is encountered, taping is done from the midpoint of the patella (**B**).

Decrease Offending Activities. Decreasing activities that increase patella forces such as wearing high-heeled shoes, sitting with the knee acutely bent (e.g., "Indian-style position"), and running steps or hills for conditioning often aids in decreasing symptoms.[104] Obesity, by increasing the load on the patellofemoral joint, can be a contributing factor and should be addressed.[104]

Set Reasonable Expectations. Most importantly, the physician should help the symptomatic athlete set reasonable expectations. Honestly relate our limited knowledge of the cause of patella pain and the trial-and-error method of treatment (see box, Elements of a Treatment Program for Anterior Knee Pain). Such a discussion typically helps to decrease the patient's anxiety and frustration if symptoms do not immediately improve.

CHECKLIST

Elements of a Treatment Program for Anterior Knee Pain

Instruct in exercise
Apply braces and taping
Fashion shoe orthotics
Decrease offending activity
Address obesity
Set reasonable expectations
Employ surgical options only if repeated attempts of conservative measures fail to relieve symptoms and there exists correctable abnormal anatomy

One should educate the athlete and the athlete's parents (in the case of the young teenage athlete) on the nature of an overuse injury and mechanisms of maltracking and overload in addition to the advantage and the purpose of the various approaches to treatment.

Surgical Options. Multiple surgical procedures have been described to treat patella pain, but, in the opinion of this author, surgery should be reserved for those with true chondromalacia, multiple patella dislocations and/or subluxations, and perhaps those with a markedly tight laterally retinaculum who have failed a prolonged course of nonoperative therapies. When contemplating surgical options for the young female athlete, who despite efforts at nonoperative care continues to complain of severe discomfort (with her complaints frequently echoed by her caring and concerned parents), consider the advice of Dr. Goodfellow who stated, "One would not burr holes in the skull to relieve a headache; therefore do not be lulled into thinking that various surgical procedures will resolve chronic 'anterior' knee pain."[44]

STRESS FRACTURES

Etiology

It may be more the unique hormonal milieu of the female rather than her unique anatomy that results in an increased incidence of stress fractures. A stress fracture occurs in bone when bone is stressed beyond its physiologic capacity to repair itself. That is, stress fractures occur from an imbalance between bone formation and bone loss.[15,72] Stress fractures may be classified as fatigue or insufficiency fractures. The fatigue fracture is one that occurs in normal bone in a healthy person secondary to increased mechanical stress. Less mechanical stress is needed to cause a fracture in bone that has been weakened by osteoporosis, osteomalacia, or other disease states. These fractures are termed *insufficiency fractures*, which implies that the bone is insufficient, not necessarily that this stress is overwhelming.

Incidence in Risk Factors

In military recruits and unconditioned athletes, the risk of stress fractures has been reported to be 10 times higher in women than men.[107] However, it is often difficult to determine a precise incidence rate for stress fractures (i.e., the number of fractures per hours of participation) because the hours of participation, especially in recreational athletes, may be difficult to quantitate.

Similar rates of stress fractures in males and females have been reported for conditioned track athletes.[12] Nattiv et al. reported a difference in stress fracture incidences between males and females, but did not feel that the difference reached statistical significance.[98] Nonetheless, multiple reports have been published on the high rate of stress fractures in athletes where the "lean look" is valued, such as dance, skating, gymnastics, and cross-country.[26,101,111] This same group of athletes also have been found to have a high incidence of disordered eating (up to 62%) and frequently have low estrogenic amenorrhea.[10,13,16,130] This decrease in estrogen can be associated with a decrease in bone mineral density just as the decreased estrogen levels seen following menopause may be associated with an accelerated loss of bone mineral density.[27,28,134] Estrogen decelerates bone absorption, resulting in a slower rate of bone turnover and thus decreases bone loss.[66,69] The association of disordered eating, amenorrhea, and osteoporosis has been termed the *female athlete triad* (see box, Female Athlete Triad).[2,97]

Bone mass is determined by a combination of linear growth, which is completed by approximately age 20, and the consolidation of increased bone mass for the next 10 to 15 years after that date. This means that 80% to 90% of a person's total bone mineral content is typically accrued by the end of adolescence.[70] Young women with low estrogen amenorrhea before bone mass is obtained lose 2% of bone mass per year instead of gaining 2.4% per year.[100] In essence, osteoporosis is a disease that may begin in adolescence even though it may not expressed until late adulthood.[11,126]

In addition to lower body weight and lower body fat, risk factors for stress fractures in women include low dietary calcium, low bone density, delayed menarchy, menstrual irregularities, decreased calf girth, less lower extremity lean mass, and a prior history of stress fractures and increased playing intensity.[12,14,93,98]

CHECKLIST

Female Athlete Triad

- Disordered eating
- Amenorrhea
- Osteoporosis

Techniques Used to Measure Bone Mineral Density (BMD). In girls and women with recurrent stress fractures, particularly in those with abnormal menstrual patterns but also in those with normal menstrual patterns but other risk factors for osteoporosis (positive family history, abnormal menstrual periods during young adulthood, and nicotine or alcohol use), bone mineral density should be measured (Table 28-1). The most common technique to measure bone mineral density is a dual energy x-ray absorptiometry (DEXA or DXA) scan—an x-ray based scanning tool. It is rapid (3 to 7 minutes) and although the most common sites monitored are the spine and hip, the technique can measure density at multiple sites with very little delivered radiation (1–2 m rad).[80] Results are reported as "T-scores" which compare the bone mineral density of the athlete to a reference population of gender-matched, normal 30- to 35-year-olds. The National Osteoporosis Foundation defines osteoporosis as a T-score of less than two standard deviations below normal and osteopenia as a T-score of between one and two standards below normal scores.[69,80] Other, less commonly used measures of bone mineral density include single energy x-ray absorptiometry (SEXA), single photon absorptiometry (SPA), quantitative computed tomography bone scan, and ultrasound. Ultrasound of the calcaneus is a rapid and easy to perform office procedure but does not have the precision of the DEXA scan.[69]

Treatment

In young girls with stress fractures, one must treat not only the injury to bone, but also evaluate and treat the associated causes for this stress reaction. One must examine training schedules, but also make certain to ask about menstrual history and dietary practices, and if aberrations are found, help the young female athlete resolve these critical issues.

Increasing caloric intake and decreasing the intensity of training in young athletes with a delay in menarchy or the presence of secondary amenorrhea has been recommended to try to "trigger" the beginning of normal menstrual cycling. However, data now indicate that even with the return of normal menstrual cycles or with estrogen replacement therapy, normalization of bone mineral density may not occur.[66]

Moreover, it has been theorized that leanness and intense exercise may not be the sole explanation for amenorrhea seen in these athletes.[20] Recently there has been a marked interest in the correlation of leptin levels to nutritional status and levels of bone mineral density.[66] Leptin is synthesized by adipocytes and placenta cells and acts on the hypothalic nuclei to regulate food intake, energy expenditure, growth, and sexual maturation. It is also felt to participate in the regulation of basal metabolic rate and is low in fasting individuals.[3] Amenorrheic females with poor food intake have been found to have

TABLE 28-1 **Techniques for Measuring Bone Mineral Density**

Abbreviation	Name	Comments
DEXA or DX Scan	Dual Energy X-ray Absorptiometry	Very little radiation Can measure trabecular and compact bone Rapid to perform (3-7 min) Excellent precision & accuracy
SEXA	Single Energy X-ray Absorptiometry	Inexpensive Limited to peripheral sites
RA	Radiographic Absorptiometry	Measured density of hands/peripheral sites Relatively low cost Rapid to perform (> 2 min)
SPA	Single Photon Absorptiometry	Measures radius & calcaneus Relatively inexpensive Takes about 15 minutes Relatively low dose radiation
DPA	Dual Photon Absorptiometry	Takes longer than SPA to perform Not commonly used
QCT	Quantitative Computed Tomography	Higher dose radiation than DPA Relatively complex to use
QVS	Quantitative Ultrasound	Lacks precision of DEXA scan Can measure only a few sites Device small and portable No radiation

low leptin levels.[73,134] Warren suggests that leptin turns off reproductive function in response to starvation; therefore, it is related to the amenorrhea seen in athletes who have a compromised nutrition status and altered bone mineral density.[130] At present there is little known regarding the potential direct effects of leptin on bone mineral density.[130] More research is needed.

Warning signs of disordered eating include compulsive exercising above or beyond the requirements of the sport; increasingly restrictive diet; a preoccupation with food, calories, and body weight; dissatisfaction with one's own body; fear of becoming fat even when one's weight is average or below average; frequent bathroom trips after meals for the purposes of purging; binge eating; fasting; eating secretly or avoid eating with others; and wearing baggier or layered clothing.[135] It is important to stress to the young athletes that disordered eating results in significant adverse effects on an athlete's performance, including decreased strength, endurance, speed, and coordination, slower reaction times, a decreased ability to concentrate, electrolyte imbalances and dehydration, and an increased susceptibility to injury and amenorrhea with bone loss and stress fractures.

Recommended Calcium Intake

Recommended calcium intake for athletes with normal menstrual cycles and normal estrogen levels is 1000 mg/day. Calcium intake for athletes with low estrogenic amenorrhea is 1500 mg/day just as it is for postmenopausal women with decreased estrogen levels not on hormonal replacement therapy (HRT) (Table 28-2).

FOOT AND ANKLE OVERUSE INJURIES

Epidemiology

Anterior and posterior soft-tissue ankle impingement, symptomatic bunions, and os trigonum impingement are not infrequent in female gymnasts and dancers. In fact, epidemiologic studies document that approximately 40% of all injuries to dancers are to the lower leg, foot, and ankle.[81] Ankle sprains have also been reported to be more common in women; in fact, women have a 25% greater risk of sustaining a grade I ankle sprain compared with their male counterparts.[58]

Bunions

In 1991, over 200,000 bunionectomies were performed in the United States. No mention was made of the age range or the activity level of those in this group. Hallux valgus is nine times more common in women than men.[37] A great percentage of symptomatic bunions are aggravated by inappropriate footwear. Tight-fitting character shoes or toe shoes in dancers can be problematic, as can skating boots in ice skaters or any ill-fitting sport shoe.

TABLE 28-2 **Recommended Daily Calcium Intake**

Age	mg/Day
Adolescent–young adults	1200–1500
Female Athlete	1500
Euestrogenemia	1000
Hypoestrogenemic Adults	1500
Adults	
Men (25–65 years)	1000
Women (25–50 years)	1500
Post-menopausal women	1500
Post-menopausal women (on HRT)	1000

The athlete should measure the width of her foot and compare this with the width of the shoe to make certain that the shoe is compatible for her. With point shoes, each dancer should try to find the toe box that best suits her foot. Many skating boots are custom-made, and therefore adequate forefoot width can be assured if proper measurements are obtained.

Treatment of symptomatic bunions in an athletic population typically consists of shoe modification, padding, and exercises for the big toe and foot. Rarely is surgery recommended.

Ankle Impingement

Posterior ankle impingement results from forced plantarflexion whereas anterior ankle impingement typically results from over-rotating a tumbling pass in gymnastics or ineffectively decelerating when landing a jump or stopping, resulting in hyperdorsiflexion and impingement of the anterior synovium between the tibia and the talus or impingement of the bony structures themselves. Athletes should be encouraged to use trunk, thigh, and leg muscles to decelerate prior to and upon landing rather than "jamming" their ankles on impact.

The athlete with anterior ankle impingement complains of pain across the front of her ankle at the tibiotalar junction. Swelling may be present in this area. Typically, there is no ankle joint effusion. Palpation of this area is painful. Radiographs may be normal initially, but in cases of chronic anterior ankle impingement, anterior tibial or talar osteophytes can occur.

Attention to strengthening exercises for trunk, thigh, and leg are keys to treating anterior ankle impingement, as is attention to proper landing techniques. Anterior ankle pads can be temporarily taped on the athlete's ankle to remind the athlete not to hyperdorsiflex upon landing. In cases of chronic ankle impingement, even with significant anterior bony osteophytes, rarely is arthroscopic debridement required unless the osteophytes significantly restrict motion. Return to dance or sport following such an arthroscopic procedure may be prolonged (approximately 3 to 4 months).[49]

Soft-tissue posterior ankle impingement may be difficult to differentiate from os trigonum impingement or impingement of the posterior calcaneus against an elongated posterior talar process. All can result from maximum plantarflexion. Pain is typically felt posteriorly behind the lateral malleolus with forced plantarflexion. Diffuse posterior ankle swelling may be present, but a joint effusion is rarely seen. If bony impingement is present, a bone scan will be positive. In such cases, if conservative management consisting of decreasing activity (or in some cases even immobilization), anti-inflammatories, strengthening exercises, and technique modifications fails to relieve symptoms, resection of the symptomatic os trigonum or bone spur may be required.[87]

Posterior medial ankle pain may imply tendinitis of the flexor hallux longer (FHL) alone or in association with bony impingement from an os trigonum.[42,48,50] Conservative measures are initially recommended to treat this entity and only in long-standing recalcitrant cases is tenolysis of the flexor hallucis longer required.[50,87] A posterior medial ankle incision to address both the FHL and a symptomatic os trigonum (if one is associated) is preferred over the traditional posterior lateral incision made for excision of the os trigonum alone. The latter incision has fewer risks because the neurovascular bundle does not have to be mobilized.

Following any surgical procedure, after an initial period of immobilization, aggressive rehabilitation to restore range of motion, strength, neuromuscular control, and balance is required. Return to dance is feasible following such surgery, although months may be required for complete rehabilitation of the dancer.[42,50]

SUMMARY

In general, injuries to female athletes are very similar to those seen in males athletes—that is, injuries are typically more sports-specific than gender-specific. However, there are several injuries, including ACL injuries, patellofemoral stress syndrome, stress fractures, and some overuse injuries of the foot and ankle, that occur more frequently in female athletes than in their male counterparts. This chapter has tried to highlight some of the distinctive features of these injuries in women athletes.

REFERENCES

1. ACL Awareness—A Guide to Knee Friendly Skiing. (Videotape). Underhill Center, VT, Vermont Safety Research, 1993.

2. ACSM: Position stand on the female athlete triad. Med Sci Sports Exerc 29(5):i–ix, 1997.
3. Ahima RS, Prabakaran D, Mantzoros C: Role of leptin in the neuroendocrine response to fasting. Nature 382:250–252, 1996.
4. Anderson AF, Lipscomb AB, Liudahl KJ, Addlestone RB: Analysis of the intercondylar notch by computed tomography. Am J Sports Med 15(6):547–552, 1987.
5. Arendt EA, Bershadsky B, Agel J: Periodicity of non-contact anterior cruciate ligament injuries during the menstrual cycle. J Gend Specif Med 5(2):19–26, 2000.
6. Arendt EA, Dick RW: Knee injury patterns among men and women in collegiate basketball and soccer: NCAA data and review of literature. Am J Sports Med 23(6):694–701, 1995.
7. Arroll B, Ellis-Pegler E, Edwards A, Sutcliff G: Patellofemoral pain syndrome: A critical review of the clinical trials on nonoperative therapy. Am J Sports Med 25(2):207–212, 1997.
8. Barber-Westin SD, Noyes FR, Andrews M: A Rigorous comparison between the sexes of results and complications after anterior cruciate ligament reconstruction. Am J Sports Med 25(4):514–526, 1997.
9. Barrett GR, Noojin FK, Hartzog CW, Nash CR: Reconstruction of the anterior cruciate ligament in females: A comparison of hamstring versus patellar tendon autograft. Arthroscopy 18(1):46–54, 2002.
10. Barrow GW, Saha S. Menstrual irregularity and stress fractures in collegiate female distance runners. Am J Sports Med 16(3):209–216, 1998.
11. Beck BR, Shoemaker MR: Osteoporosis: Understanding key risk factors and therapeutic options. Phys Sports Med 28(2):69–84, 2000.
12. Bennell KL, Brukner PD: Epidemiology and site specificity of stress fractures. Clin Sports Med 16(2): 179–196, 1997.
13. Bennell KL, Malcolm SA, Thomas, SA, et al: Risk factors for stress fractures in female track and field athletes: A retrospective analysis. Clin J Sports Med 5(4):229–235, 1995.
14. Bennell KL, Malcolm SA, Thomas, SA, et al: Risk factors for stress fractures in female track and field athletes. Am J Sports Med 24(6):810–818, 1996.
15. Boden BP, Osbahr DC: High-risk stress fractures: Evaluation and treatment. J Am Acad Orthop Surg 8(6):344–353, 2000.
16. Brownell KD, Steen SN, Wilmore JH: Weight regulation practices in athletes: Analysis of metabolic and health effects. Med Sci Sports Exerc 19(6): 546–556, 1987.
17. Caraffa A, Cerulli G, Projetti M, Aisa G, Rizzo A: Prevention of anterior cruciate ligament injuries in soccer: A prospective controlled study of proprioceptive training. Knee Surg Sports Traumatol Arthrosc 4(1):19–21, 1996.
18. Chandy TA, Granna WA: Secondary school athletic injuries in boys and girls: A three year comparison. Phys Sports Med 13(3):106–111, 1985.
19. Chudik SC, Garrett WE: Addressing ACL injuries in women. Women's Health 4(3):100–107, 2001.
20. Clark N: Athletes with amenorrhea. Phys Sports Med 21(4):45–48, 1993.
21. Colombet P, Allard M, Bousquet V, et al: Anterior cruciate ligament reconstruction using four-strand semintendinosus and gracilis tendon grafts and metal interference screw fixation. Arthroscopy 18(3): 232–237, 2002.
22. Corry IS, Web JM, Clingeleffer AJ, Pinczewski LA: Arthroscopic reconstruction of the anterior cruciate ligament: A comparison of patella tendon autograft and four-strand hamstring tendon autograft. Am J Sports Med 27(4):444–454, 1999.
23. Crossley K, Bennell K, Green S, et al: Physical therapy for patellofemoral pain: A randomized, double blinded placebo-controlled trial. Am J Sports Med 30(6):857–865, 2002.
24. Daniel DM, Stone Ml, Dobson BL, et al: Fate of the ACL-injured patient: A prospective outcome study. Am J Sports Med 22(5):632–644, 1994.
25. Daniel DM, Stone ML, Sachs R, Malcom L: Instrumented measurement of anterior knee laxity in patients with acute anterior cruciate ligament disruption. Am J Sports Med 13(6):401–407, 1985.
26. DeSouza MJ, Maguire MS, Rubin KR, Maresh CM: Effects of menstrual phase and amenorrhea on exercise performance in runners. Med Sci Sports Exerc 22(5):575–580, 1990.
27. Drinkwater BL, Bruemner B, Chesnut CH 3rd: Menstrual history as a determinant of current bone density in young athletes. JAMA 263(4):545–548, 1990.
28. Drinkwater BL, Nilson K, Chestnut CH 3rd , et al: Bone mineral content of amenorrheic and eumenorrheic athletes. N Eng J Med 311(5):277–281, 1984.
29. Dye SF: The knee is the biologic transmission with an envelope of function: A theory. Clin Orthop 325:10–18, 1996.
30. Eng JJ, Pierrynowski MR: Evaluation of soft foot orthotics and the treatment of patellofemoral pain syndrome. Phys Ther 73:62–70, 1993.
31. Ettlinger CF, Johnson RJ, Shealy JE: A method to help reduce the risk of serious knee sprains incurred in alpine skiing. Am J Sports Med 23(5):531–537, 1995.
32. Ferrari JD, Bach BR, Bush-Joseph CA, et al: Anterior cruciate ligament reconstruction in men and women: An outcome analysis comparing gender. Arthroscopy 17(6):588–596, 2001.
33. Ferretti A, Papandrea P, Conteduca F, Mariani P: Knee ligament injuries in volleyball players. Am J Sports Med 20(2):203–207, 1992.

34. Flynn K, Pedersen C, Birmingham T, et al: The familial predisposition toward tearing anterior cruciate ligament: A case control study. AOSSM Specialty Day, February 2003, New Orleans, LA.
35. France EP, Paulos LE: Knee bracing. J Am Acad Orthop Surg 2(5):281–287, 1994.
36. Frank CB, Jackson DW: The science of reconstruction of the anterior cruciate ligament. J Bone Joint Surg 79A:1556–1576, 1997.
37. Frey C: Foot health and shoe wear for women. Clin Orthop 372:32–44, 2000.
38. Fulkerson JP, Arendt EA: Anterior knee pain in females. Clin Orthop 372:69–73, 2000.
39. Garrett WE Jr: Non-contact ACL injuries in female athletes: risk factors and biomechanical considerations, Instructional Course Lecture Series. 78th Annual American Academy of Orthopaedic Surgeons Meeting, February 9, 2003, New Orleans, LA.
40. Garrick JG: Anterior knee pain. Phys Sports Med 17(1):75–84, 1989.
41. Garrick JG, Requa RK: Anterior cruciate ligament injuries in men and women: How common are they? In Griffin LY (eds): Prevention of Non-contact ACL Injuries. Rosemont, IL, American Academy of Orthopaedic Surgeons, 2001, pp 1–9.
42. Garth WP Jr: Flexor hallucis tendonitis in a ballet dancer: A case report. J Bone Joint Surg 63A(9): 1489, 1981.
43. Gilleard W, McConnell J, Parson D: The effect of patella taping on the onset of vastus medialis obiquus and vastus lateralis muscle activity in persons with patellofemoral pain. Phys Ther 78(1): 25–32, 1998.
44. Goodfellow JW: Chondromalcia patella: A mythical disease. Bone Joint Surg 66B:455–456, 1984.
45. Gray J, Taunton JE, McKenzie DC, et al: A survey of injuries to the anterior cruciate ligament of the knee in female basketball players. Int J Sports Med 6(6): 314–316, 1985.
46. Grace T, Skipper B, Newberry J, et al: Prophylatic knee braces and injury to the lower extremity. J Bone Joint Surg 70A(3):422–427, 1988.
47. Griffis ND, Vequist SW, Yearout KN, et al: Injury and prevention of the anterior cruciate ligament. Paper presented at the American Orthopaedic Society for Sports Medicine. 15th Annual Meeting, June 19–22, 1989, Travers City, MI.
48. Hamilton WG: Tendonitis above the ankle joint in classical ballet dancers. Am J Sports Med 5:84–88, 1977.
49. Hamilton WG: Foot and ankle injuries in dancers. Clin Sports Med 7(1):143–173, 1988.
50. Hamilton WG, Geppert MJ, Thompson FM: Pain in the posterior aspect of the ankle in dancers: Differential diagnoses and operative treatment. J Bone Joint Surg 78A:1491–1500, 1996.
51. Harner CD, Paulos LE, Greenwald AE, et al: Detailed analysis of patients with bilateral anterior cruciate ligament injuries. Am J Sports Med 22(1): 37–43, 1994.
52. Heidt RS Jr, Sweeterman LM, Carlonas RL, et al: Avoidance of soccer injuries with pre-season conditioning. Am J Sports Med 28(5):659–662, 2000.
53. Heino-Brechter J, Powers CM: Patellofemoral stress during walking in persons with and without patellofemoral pain. Med Sci Sports Exerc 34(10): 1582–1593, 1996.
54. Hewett TE: Neuromuscular and hormonal factors associated with knee injuries in female athletes: Strategies for intervention. Sports Med 29(5): 313–327, 2000.
55. Hewett TE, Riccobene JV, Lindenfeld TN: The effect of neuromuscular training on the incidence of knee injury in female athletes: A prospective study. Am J Sports Med 27(6):699–706, 1999.
56. Hewett TE, Stroupe AL, Nance TA, Noyes FR: Plyometric training in female athletes: Decreased impact forces and increased hamstring torques. Am J Sports Med 24(6):765–773, 1996.
57. Hofmeister EP, Gillingham BL, Bathgate MB, Mills WJ: Results of anterior cruciate ligament reconstruction in the adolescent female. J Pediatr Orthop 21(3):302–306, 2001.
58. Hosea TM, Carey CC, Harner MF: The gender issue: Epidemiology of ankle injuries in athletes who participate in basketball. Clin Orthop 372:45–49, 2000.
59. Houseworth SW, Mauro VJ, Mellon BA, Kieffer DA: The intercondylar notch in acute tears of the anterior cruciate ligament: A computer graphics study. Am J Sports Med 15(3):221–224, 1987.
60. Hruska R: Pelvic stability influences lower extremity kinematics. Biomechanics 5:23–29, 1998.
61. Huegel M, Meister K, Rolle G, et al: The influence of lower extremity alignment in the female population on the incidence of non-contact ACL tears. Presented at the 23rd Annual Meeting of the American Academy of Orthopaedic Surgeons, June 22–25, 1997, Sun Valley, ID.
62. Hungerford DS, Barry M: Biomechanics of the patellofemoral joint. Clin Orthop 144:9–15, 1979.
63. Huston LJ, Greefield ML, Wojtz EM: Anterior cruciate ligament injuries in the female athlete: Potential risk factors. Clin Orthop 372:50–63, 2000.
64. Hvid I, Andersen LB, Schmidt H: Chondromalacia patellae: The relation to abnormal patellofemoral joint mechanics. Acta Orthop Scand 52(6):661–666, 1981.
65. Ireland ML, Wall C: Abstract: Epidemiology in comparison of knee injuries in elite male and female United States basketball athletes. Med Sci Sports Exerc 22(Suppl):S82, 1990.

66. Kaufman BA, Warren MP, Dominguez JE, et al: Bone density and amenorrhea in ballet dancers are related to a decreased resting metabolic rate and lower leptin levels. J Clin Endocrinol Metab 87(6):2777–2783, 2002.
67. Kirkendall DT, Garrett WE: The anterior cruciate ligament enigma. In Griff LY, Garrick JG (eds): Women's Musculoskeletal Health Update for the New Millennium 372:64–68, 2000.
68. Lambson RB, Barnhill BS, Higgins RW: Football cleat design and its effect on anterior cruciate ligament injuries: A three-year prospective study. Am J Sports Med 24(2):155–159, 1996.
69. Lane JM, Nydick M: Osteoporosis: Current modes of prevention and treatment. J Am Acad Orthop 7(1):19–31, 1999.
70. Lane JM, Russel L, Khan SN: Osteoporosis. Clin Orthop March (372):139–150, 2000.
71. LaPrade RF, Burnett QM: Femoral intercondylar notch stenosis and correlation to anterior cruciate ligament injuries: A perspective study. Am J Sports Med 22(2):198–202, 1994.
72. Lassus J, Tulikoura I, Konttinen YT, et al: Bone stress injuries of the lower extremity: A review. Acta Orthop Scand 73(3):359–368, 2002.
73. Laughlin GA, Yen SS: Hypoleptinemia in women athletes: Absence of a diurnal rhythm with amenorrhea. J Clin Endocrinol Metab 82(1):318–321, 1997.
74. Lephart SM, Ferris CM, Riemann BL, et al: Gender differences in strength and lower extremity kinematics during landing. Clin Orthop 401:162–169, 2002.
75. Lephart SM, Fu H: The role of proprioception and the treatment of sports injuries. Sports Exer Inj 1:96–102, 1995.
76. Lephart SM, Reimann BFH: Introduction to the sensorimotor system. In Lephart SM, Fu FH, (eds): Proprioception and Neuromuscular Control in Joint Stability. Champaign, IL, Human Kinetics, 2000.
77. Lichota DK: Anterior knee pain: symptom or syndrome? Curr Womens Health Rep 3(1):81–86, 2003.
78. Lindenfeld TN, Schmitt DJ, Hendy MP, et al: Incidence of injury in indoor soccer. Am J Sports Med 22(3):364–371, 1994.
79. Liu SH, Al-Shaikh RA, Panossian V, et al: Primary immunolocalization of estrogen and progesterone target cells in the human anterior cruciate ligament. J Orthop Res 14(4):526–533, 1996.
80. Lucas TS, Einhorn TA: Osteoporosis: The role of the orthopaedist. J Am Acad Orthop Surg 1(1): 48–56, 1993.
81. Macintyre J, Joy E: Foot and ankle injuries in dance. Clin Sports Med 19(2):351–368, 2000.
82. Malek MM, DeLuca JY, Kunkle KL, Knable KR: Outpatient ACL surgery: A review of safety, practicality, and economy. Instr Course Lect 45:281–286, 1996.
83. Mandelbaum BR, Silvers HJ, Watanabe DS, et al: ACL prevention strategies in the female athlete and soccer: Implementation of neuromuscular training program to determine its efficacy on the incidence of ACL injury. Presented at the American Orthopaedic Society of Sports Medicine Specialty Day, 2002, Dallas, TX, abstract, p 94.
84. Malinzak RA, Colby SM, Kirkendall DT, et al: A comparison of knee joint motion patterns between men and women in selected athletic tasks. Clin Biomech 16(5):438–445, 2001.
85. Markolf KL, Burchfield DM, Shapiro MM, et al: Combined knee loading states that generate high anterior cruciate ligament forces. J Orthop Res 13(6):930–935, 1995.
86. Markolf KL, Gorek JF, Kabo JM, Shapiro MS: Direct measurements of resultant in forces in the anterior cruciate ligament: An in vitro study performed with a new experimental technique. J Bone Joint Surg. 72A:557–567, 1990.
87. Marotta JJ, Micheli LJ: Os trigonum impingement in dancers. Am J Sports Med 20(5):533–536, 1992.
88. McConnell J: The management of chondromalacia patella: A long-term solution. Aust J Physiother 32: 215–223, 1986.
89. Miyaska KC, Daniel DM, Stone ML, et al: Incidence of knee ligament injuries in the general population. Am J Knee Surg 4:3–8, 1991.
90. Moller-Nielsen J, Hammar M: Women's soccer injuries in relationship to the menstrual cycle and oral contraceptive use. Med Sci Sports Exerc 21(2):126–129, 1989.
91. Moller-Nielsen J, Hammar M: Sports injuries and oral contraceptive use. Is there a relationship? Sports Med 12(3):152–160, 1991.
92. Muneta T, Takakuda K, Yamamoto H: Intercondylar notch width and its relation to the configuration and cross-sectional area of the anterior cruciate ligaments: A cadaveric knee study. Am J Sports Med 25(1):69–72, 1997.
93. Myburgh, KH, Hutchins J, Fataar A, Hough SF, Noakes TD: Low bone density is an etiologic factor for stress fractures in athletes. Ann Intern Med 113(10):754–759, 1990.
94. Myklebust G, Maehlum S, Holm I, Bahr R: A prospective cohort study of anterior cruciate ligament injuries in elite Norwegian team handball. Scand J Med Sci Sports 8(3):149–153, 1998.
95. Myklebust G, Maehlum S, Engerbretsen L, et al: Registration of cruciate ligament injuries in Norwegian top level team handball. A prospective study covering two seasons. Scand J Med Sci Sports 7(5):289–292, 1997.
96. National Federation of High School Press Release: High School Athletics Participation Continues to Rise. Kansas City, MO, 1998.

97. Nattiv A, Agostini R, Drinkwater B, Yeager K: The female athlete triad: The inter-relatedness of disordered eating, amenorrhea and osteoporosis. Clin Sports Med 13(2):405–418, 1994.
98. Nattiv A, Puffer JC, Casper, J, et al: Stress fracture risk factors, incidence, and distribution: A 3-year prospective study in collegiate runners. Med Sci Sports Exerc (Suppl 5):S347, 2000.
99. 2001–2003 NCAA Season–National Injury Surveillance System. National College Athletic Association One NCAA Plaza, 700 West Washington Street, Indianapolis, IN 46204.
100. Otis CL, Lynch L: How to keep your bones healthy. Phys Sports Med 22(1):71–72, 1994.
101. Pecina M, Bojanic I, Dubravcics S: Stress fractures in figure skaters. Am J Sports Med 18(3):277–279, 1990.
102. Pinczewski LA, Deehan DJ, Salmon LJ, Russell VJ, Clingeleffer A: A 5-year comparison of patellar tendon vs four-strand hamstring tendon autograft for arthroscopic reconstruction of the anterior cruciate ligament. Am J Sports Med 30(4):523–536, 2002.
103. Pinczewski LA, Russel BJ, Calmon LJ: Osteoarthritis after ACL reconstruction. A comparison of patella tendon and hamstring tendon grafts for ACL reconstruction over seven years. Presented at the AOSSM Specialty Day, February 8, 2003, New Orleans, LA.
104. Post WR, Welker DM: Patellofemoral problems in women. Women's Health. Orthopaedic Edition 3(4):136–143, 2000.
105. Powers CM, Landel R, Sosnick T, et al: The effects of patellar taping on stride characteristics and joint motion in subjects with patellofemoral pain. J Orthop Sports Phys Ther 26(6):286–291, 1997.
106. Powers CM: Rehabilitation of patellofemoral joint disorders: A critical review. J Orthop Sports Phys Ther 28(5):345–354, 1998.
107. Protzman RR, Griffis CG: Stress fractures in men and women undergoing military training. J Bone Joint Surg 59(A):825, 1977.
108. Randall F, Miller H, Shurr D: The use of prophylactic knee orthoses at Iowa State University. Orthot Prosthet 37:54–57, 1983.
109. Renstrom AF: Mechanisms, diagnosis, and treatment of running injuries. In Heckman JD (ed): Instructional Course Lectures, Vol. 42. Rosemont, IL, AAOS, 1993, pp 225–234.
110. Roos HP, Ornell M, Gardsell P, et al: Soccer after anterior cruciate ligament injury: An incompatible combination? A national survey of incidence and risk factors and 7-year follow up of 310 players. Acta Orthop Scand 66(2):107–112, 1995.
111. Rosen LW, Hongh DO: Pathogenic weight-control behavior of female college gymnasts. Phys Sports Med 16(9):141–144, 1988.
112. Rovere GD, Haupt HA, Yates CS: Prophylactic knee bracing in college football. Am J Sports Med 15(2):111–116, 1987.
113. Scranton PE, Whitesel JP, Powell JW, et al: A review of a selected non-contact anterior cruciate ligament injuries in the national football league. Foot Ankle Int 18(12):772–776, 1997.
114. Shambaugh JP, Klein A, Herbert JH: Structural measures as predictors of injury basketball players. Med Sci Sports Exerc 23(5):522–527, 1991.
115. Shelbourne KD, Davis TJ, Klootwyk TE: The relationship between intercondylar notch width of the femur and the incidence of anterior cruciate ligament tears: A prospective study. Am J Sports Med 26(3):402–408, 1998.
116. Siegel MG, Barber-Westin SD: Arthroscopic-assisted outpatient anterior cruciate ligament reconstruction using the semitendinosus and gracilis tendons. Arthroscopy 14(3):268–277, 1998.
117. Slauterbeck JR, Clevenger C, Lundberg W, Burchfield DM: Estrogen level alters the failure load of the rabbit anterior cruciate ligament. J Orthop Res 17(3):405–408, 1999.
118. Souryal TO, Freeman TR: Intercondylar notch size in anterior cruciate ligament injuries in athletes: A prospective study. Am J Sports Med 21(4):535–539, 1993.
119. Souryal TO, Moore HA, Evans P: Bilaterality in anterior cruciate ligament injuries: Associated intercondylar notch stenosis. Am J Sports Med 16(5):449–454, 1988.
120. Stacoff A, Kalin X, Stussi E: Impact in landing after a volleyball block. In de Groot G, Hollander A. Juijing P, van Ingen Schenau G (eds): Biomechanics XI. Amsterdam, Free University Press, 1988, pp 694–700.
121. Stanitski CL: Knee overuse disorders in the pediatric and adolescent athlete. Instr Course Lect 42:483–495, 1993.
122. Stevenson H, Webster J, Johnson R, Beynnon B: Gender differences in knee injury epidemiology among competitive alpine ski racers. Iowa R Othop J 18:64–66, 1998.
123. Teitz CC, Hermanson BK, Kronmal RA, Diehr PH: Evaluation of the use of braces to prevent injury to the knee in collegiate football players. J Bone Joint Surg 69A:2–9, 1987.
124. Teitz CC, Lind BC, Sacks BM: Symmetry of the femoral notch with index. Am J Sports Med 25(5):687–690, 1997.
125. Thomee R, Renstrom P, Karlsson J, Grimby G: Patellofemoral pain syndrome in young women II. Muscle function in patients and healthy controls. Scand J Med Sci Sports 5(4):245–251, 1995.
126. Tosi LL, Lane JM: Osteoporosis prevention and the orthopaedic surgeon: When fracture care is

not enough. J Bone Joint Surg 80A(11):1567–1569, 1998.

127. Toth AP, Cordasco FA: Anterior cruciate ligament injuries in the female athlete. J Gen Specif Med 4(4):25–34, 2001.
128. Traina SM, Bromberg DF: ACL injury patterns in women. Orthopaedics (20)6:545–549, 1997.
129. Warner S, Knutsson E, Ericksson E: Effective taping the patella on concentric and eccentric torque and EMG of knee extensor and flexor muscles in patients with patellofemoral pain syndrome. Knee Surg Sports Traumatol Arthrosec 1:169–177, 1993.
130. Warren MP, Brooks-Gunn J, Fox RP, et al: Osteopenia in exercise-associated amenorrhea using ballet dances as a model: A longitudinal study. J Clin Endocrinol Metab 87(7):3162–3168, 2002.
131. Wedderkopt N, Kaltoft M, Lundaard B, Rosendahl M, Froberg K. Prevention of injuries in young female players in european team handball. A prospective intervention study. Scand J Med Sci Sports 9(1):41–47, 1999.
132. Wojtys EM, Huston LJ, Lindenfeld TN, Hewett TE, Greenfield MLVH: Association between menstrual cycle and anterior cruciate ligament injuries in female athletes. Am J Sports Med 26(5):614–619, 1998.
133. Wojtys EM, Huston LJ, Taylor PD, Bastran SD: Neuromuscular adaptations in isokinetic, isotomic, and agility training programs. Am J Sports Med 24(2):187–192, 1996.
134. Wolman RL, Clark P, McNally E, Harries M, et al: Menstrual state and exercise as determinants of spinal trabecular bone density in female athletes. Br Med J 301(15):516–518, 1990.
135. Yurko-Griffin L, Harris S: Female athletes. In Sullivan JA, Anderson SJ (eds): Care of the Young Athlete. Rosemont, IL, AAOS, 1999, pp 137–148.
136. Zelisko JA, Noble HB, Porter M: A Comparison of men's and women's professional basketball injuries. Am J Sports Med 10(5):297–299, 1982.

29 Spinal Injuries in the Female Athlete

Lyle J. Micheli and
Michelle McTimoney

Over the 30 years since the inception of Title IX, women have become increasingly interested in sport and physicians have become increasingly interested in the female athlete. Title IX was enacted in 1972 in response to the women's movement of the 1960s. It is a law that prohibits sexual discrimination in federally assisted education programs. Within a few years of Title IX's institution, the Amateur Sports Act of 1978 was passed in an effort to support gender equity (and other antidiscriminatory issues) in sport, a movement that was initiated by Title IX. Although there are still areas in which progress must be made, these laws have facilitated the advancement of women both academically and athletically. Within 25 years of enacting this law, the proportion of females in high school graduating classes increased from 43% to 63% and the proportion of women earning medical degrees increased from 9% to 38%.[62] These advances in the classroom have been paralleled on the playing field. The past 30 years has seen a fourfold increase in women's participation in intercollegiate athletics. As a result, women now comprise 37% of all college athletes, compared with 15% in 1972. In high school, the proportion of females participating in sport is now 1 in 2.5, nearly equal to that of men (1 in 2). This number has significantly increased since 1971 when only 1 in 27 females participated in high school athletics.[72] Young female athletes can now aspire to model the successes of outstanding female individuals such as Mia Hamm, Dr. Dot Richardson, and Hayley Wickenheiser.[62]

The recent increase in athletic achievements of females not only looks great on paper, but also has had a significant impact on the psychosocial development of women. With respect to mental health, young female athletes are less likely to get pregnant (5% versus 11%),[73] less likely to engage in high-risk behavior including smoking marijuana and using other illicit drugs, less likely to experience suicidal ideation, and more likely to have a positive body image.[74] Medically, there is now evidence to suggest that exercise may be more important than calcium to ensure bone health as women age[75] and that sports participation in high school is related to increased bone density in 18- to 31-year-old sedentary women.[59]

As women permeate the world of sport and compete with the same drive and intensity as men, they begin to visit physicians' offices with the same or greater frequency as men.[41,61] Data from the early 1970s indicate that injury rates for female high school athletes were significantly less than for their male counterparts.[9] With the advent of the NCAA Injury Surveillance System, it becomes apparent that women's injury rates are now fast approaching that of men in comparable sports. Men and women have similar injury rates in soccer (20.1 versus 17.2) hockey (19.7 versus 17.2) and basketball (8.6 versus 8.0); however, collegiate-level female soccer players actually sustain a higher proportion of injuries to the head (1.63 versus 1.16) and knee (2.7 versus 2.44).[41] The debate thus ensues: are females at risk for injury because of the sport they play, or because of the anatomy, biomechanics, and physiology of being female? Data published in the 1980s would suggest that many injury rates are sport specific rather than gender specific.[11,65] Much of the NCAA Injury Surveillance data still supports this hypothesis.

There are, however certain injuries for which the risk has been well established to be increased in females. Noncontact ACL injury is an excellent example of this. Women have been shown to be twice as likely as men to sustain a noncontact ACL injury while playing soccer, and almost 5 times as likely while playing basketball.[1] Although several theories have been proposed to explain this phenomenon, there is still no conclusive evidence of a definitively causative factor.

Are women more likely to sustain certain spine injuries at an increased rate because of the differences in anatomy, physiology, and biomechanics? The musculoskeletal and biomechanical differences between men and women are most striking in the lower extremity. It is well known that foot pronation, genu valgum, femoral anteversion, hip varus, and bitrochanteric width are greater in females.[20] The triad of foot pronation, genu valgum, and femoral anteversion, referred to as the "miserable malalignment syndrome," is often implicated in maltracking of the patella and resultant patellar pain as well as other overuse injuries of the lower extremity. Because the spine is the proximal link in the kinetic chain of the lower extremities, it would not be unreasonable to hypothesize that lower extremity alignment may have implications for injury to the spine. Although literature on gender-specific risk factors for spine injury is sparse, Nadler has reported an increase in low back pain in females with acquired lower extremity ligamentous laxity and overuse injuries.[40]

It has been well established that females have a higher risk for developing adolescent idiopathic scoliosis.[7,44,63]

It has been suggested that the spine acts as a "conduit for transferring mechanical power between the upper and lower extremities during rapid and forceful movements."[71,76] In keeping with this, female swimmers have been found to have a higher prevalence of both idiopathic and functional (corrects with recumbency and suspension) scoliosis, with the functional curve being toward the swimmer's dominant side.[3] Similarly, increased curves to the dominant side have been found in javelin throwers and tennis players.[25,27] Delayed puberty and menarche have been identified as risk factors for idiopathic scoliosis in the ballet dancer.[63] The hypoestrogenism associated with delayed menarche also delays the maturation of the osseous centers of the spine, thus predisposing the female to instability and curvature, and the prolonged growth period associated with delayed puberty exposes the spine to deforming forces over a longer period of time.[43,63,76]

An increased lordosis has been demonstrated in skeletally immature female gymnasts in intensive training.[42] Female ballet dancers with increased femoral anteversion are known to develop an increased lumbar lordosis to overcome the limitation in turnout caused by excessive femoral anteversion.

Early studies of general populations suggested that being female was a protective factor with respect to the development of spondylolysis.[46] However, because of the increased risk of developing spondylolysis in certain sports that have high female participation,[13,17,22,29,48,54] spondylolysis is a significant problem for the female athlete.

STRUCTURAL ABNORMALITY OF THE SPINE

Scoliosis

A simple overview of the normal and abnormal alignment of the spine can be useful for the sports physician caring for the female athlete because there is a relatively high incidence of structural spinal deformities in females. The normal spinal alignment in the sagittal plane consists of a lordosis or anterior curvature of the cervical spine, a kyphosis or posterior curvature of the thoracic spine and, again, a lordosis of the lumbar spine. In the coronal dimension, there is normally no lateral deviation. Coronal curvature is defined as scoliosis.

Spinal deformities can be of two types. In the sagittal plane, a spinal deformity is defined as excessive curvature of sites of normal curvature or abnormal location of curvature. For example, thoracic kyphosis of greater than 50° or kyphotic curvature at the thorolumbar junction, which is normally neutral, are sagittal deformities. Similarly, excessive lumbar lordosis, again greater than 50°, is a spinal deformity. This is particularly noteworthy in the young female athlete, because excessive lumbar lordosis is often associated with low back pain.

The second type of spinal deformity, scoliosis, can be present at any level. It is always abnormal. It may have different etiologies. The etiologies of scoliosis include idiopathic, congenital, neurogenic, reactive, and mechanical. Idiopathic scoliosis is the most common etiology encountered in athletes. As its name implies, the exact cause of this deformity is not known. It most commonly has its onset in females in early adolescence. There is often a family history, but not necessarily so. Left untreated, the curvature can become severe, compromising pulmonary function and neurologic function, and contributing to the degeneration of the spine and late onset back pain. Treatment of progressive idiopathic scoliosis includes bracing and exercising; perfusion surgery is necessary for curvatures in excess of 45°.

Congenital scoliosis results from structural abnormalities of the spine such as two vertebrae partially fused together or hemi vertebrae. There often are associated rib fusions or deformities. No treatment may be necessary, but assessment by a pediatric orthopedist is strongly recommended.

Neuromuscular diseases such as polio, muscular dystrophy, or cerebral palsy may have associated spinal deformities. These can include kyphosis, scoliosis, or a combination of the two.

Reactive scoliosis is usually associated with a painful spinal condition such as a herniated disk, infection, or neoplasm.

It must be remembered that idiopathic scoliosis, the most commonly encountered type of scoliosis in the young female athlete, is not painful. Any painful scoliosis must be referred to a spinal specialist, preferably a pediatric orthopedic surgeon.

Risk Factors. The prevalence of idiopathic adolescent scoliosis in the general population is approximately 2% to 3%.[63,64] There is an increased prevalence in female ballet dancers (24%),[63] tennis players (13%),[27] and swimmers (6.9%).[3] Also, 16% of swimmers had a *functional* scoliosis to the dominant side. Unilateral torque forces were felt to account for the increased prevalence of scoliosis in the tennis players and swimmers, whereas in ballet, the dancers were hypothesized to co-inherit scoliosis together with decreased upper-to-lower body ratio and long arm span that represents the ideal body type for classical ballet. A combination of delayed maturity, ligamentous laxity, and asymmetric spinal loading was felt to account for a tenfold increase in the prevalence of scoliosis in one study of rhythmic gymnasts.[58] With respect to gender as a risk factor, the proportion of males and females with small curves is approximately equal; however, as the curve increases in severity, the female to male ratio approaches 4:1.[8]

Presentation. Idiopathic adolescent scoliosis typically presents as a painless spinal deformity often identified by a parent or coach in a pre- or early-pubertal adolescent. There may be a positive family history of scoliosis and a history of participation in one of the previously mentioned sports. It is important to inquire as to the onset of menarche in females to help with decision making for management interventions. If any history of pain or neurologic deficit is elicited, the physician must seriously consider other causes of bony pathology that may induce a reactive scoliosis, such as spondylolysis, Scheuermann's kyphosis, syrinx, herniated disk, and both benign and malignant bony tumors.[45] Interestingly, one study recently revealed that nearly one-quarter of children with idiopathic scoliosis, traditionally felt to be exclusively asymptomatic, complained of back pain at some point.[45]

Physical Examination. It is imperative that the spine be inspected in its entirety with full exposure at all levels, looking for asymmetry of the spine, shoulders, ribs, and pelvis. This should be done with the patient standing in bare feet. There should be no areas of bony tenderness. Range of motion may be limited in lateral flexion and rotation, and an obvious scapular prominence will be noted on forward flexion. Sitting and standing heights can be documented and followed to monitor gain or loss of spine height. A thorough neurological exam is done to assure that there are no deficits that would prompt a more detailed investigation. In idiopathic scoliosis there is no alteration in strength, sensation, or proprioception, and all reflexes are preserved.

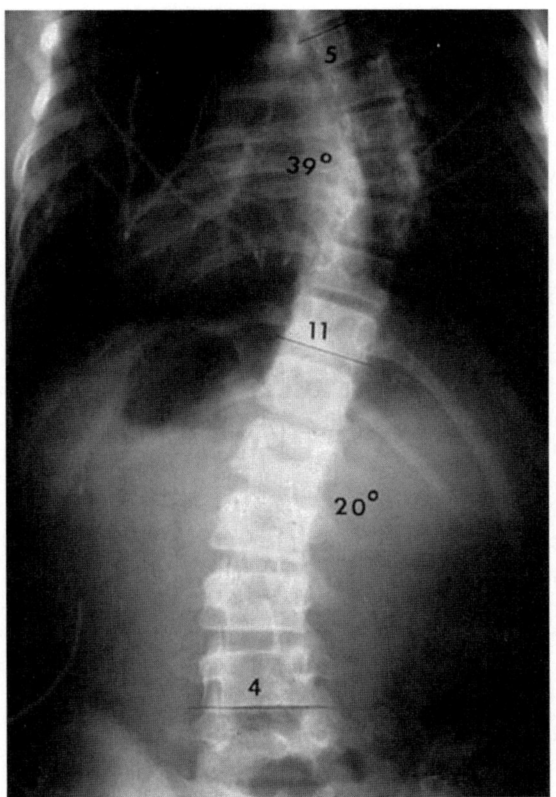

FIGURE 29-1. PA film of scoliosis, displaying technique for measuring the Cobb angle.

Imaging. If there are no complaints of pain, and the neurologic exam is normal (including all reflexes), then only plain films in the PA and lateral views are obtained. Subsequent to the initial assessment, only PA films are needed. The PA film is a standing, long cassette film and should include the lower cervical vertebrae and the pelvis. In idiopathic adolescent scoliosis, there are no bony abnormalities, aside from the obvious curve(s). The curve is measured on the PA by the Cobb technique. A line is drawn parallel to and extending from the superior aspect of the most superior vertebral body involved in the curve. Similarly, a line is drawn parallel to and extending from the inferior border of the most inferior vertebral body involved in the curve. Perpendiculars are drawn to extend from each of these lines and intersect. The Cobb angle is the angle formed by these intersecting lines (Fig. 29-1). This process is performed for each curve identified on the film. Classification of the curve(s) can then be done according to the classification scheme described in the preceding section. The level of skeletal maturity must also be determined by either bone age (x-ray left wrist) or Risser score (progression of iliac apophysis).

Management. Most often, the focus of management is to ensure that the curve does not progress to an extent that would cause significant cosmetic deformity and resultant psychosocial morbidity. Curves rarely progress to an extent that would compromise cardiovascular function or result in mortality. Most patients with scoliosis, at some point in their adult life, will experience a minor degree of back pain.[2] Progression of the curve is most likely in women, those presenting prior to menarche, and those presenting with a Risser score of 0 (skeletal immaturity). It is known that double curves are more likely to progress than single curves and that thoracic curves are more likely to progress than lumbar curves. The angle of curve at presentation also has prognostic significance, with more significant curves having an increased risk of progression.[10]

Treatment options include observation, bracing, and surgery, and decision making is based on the previously discussed risk factors. Usually, children who present with curves of less than 20° can be observed with repeat radiographs every 4 to 6 months, and every 3 to 4 months if the curve is 20° to 25°. Adults who present with curves of less than 20° are unlikely to progress and do not need close follow-up. Physiotherapy may be prescribed if there is an element of back pain associated with the scoliosis, but it will not halt or slow the progression of the curve. If more than 5° of progression is noted over any 6-month interval, or the curve measures more than 25°, referral to an orthopedic surgeon for assessment for bracing is appropriate. If a skeletally immature patient presents with a curve greater than 30°, bracing is considered immediately. If a mature patient presents with a curve of 30° to 40°, the patient should be monitored with yearly radiographs until 2 to 3 years after the end of spine growth and then every 5 years, because recent evidence suggests that curves may continue to progress even once skeletal maturity has been attained.[10]

Bracing options consist of either a cervico-thoraco-lumbo-sacral orthosis (CTLSO) such as the Milwaukee brace or a thoraco-lumbo-sacral orthosis (TLSO) such as the Boston or Charleston brace. Currently, the Boston brace and the Charleston brace are used most frequently. The Boston brace is usually worn 16 to 23 hours/day, and sports participation is possible while wearing the brace. The Charleston brace is worn for 8 hours/day and usually at night. The Boston brace is favored in most studies, which show less curve progression with its use.[15,23] Females have been shown to respond better than males to bracing.[30] It is important for the patients and their families to understand that the objective is to halt further progression of the curve, rather than to return the spine to straight.

In cases in which bracing has failed to slow the progression of the curve, or when the curve has reached 40° to 45° in the immature athlete, surgical management should be considered. The aim is to effectively stabilize the spine and halt the progression of the curve, while fusing as few segments as possible in order to preserve motion and decrease chronic back pain. After fusion, the athlete can still participate in many sports; however, contact sports, gymnastics, and diving should be avoided because they are felt to concentrate significant forces immediately above or below the site of a rigid portion of the spine.[34]

Transitional Vertebrae. Transitional vertebrae occur in 4% to 8% of the population and can be a source of pain in the lumbar spine. This is referred to as Bertolotti's syndrome. To be a true transitional vertebra, at least one transverse process must have fused with or articulate with the ilium or the sacrum (Fig. 29-2). There must also be an intervertebral disk space caudal to the transitional vertebra. If a pseudoarthrosis develops, considerable pain can result. In patients with transitional vertebrae, disk herniation and spinal stenosis are more likely to occur at the level adjacent to the affected vertebra, although the absolute incidence of these conditions is not increased in patients with transitional vertebrae. Elster postulates that this is because of hypermobility at this segment.[14] Transitional vertebrae may be evident on plain films, but occassionally CT or MRI may be necessary for clarification. Rest and NSAIDs are the current treatment of choice for alleviation of the pain associated with the pseudoarthrosis. Rarely is operative intervention necessary.

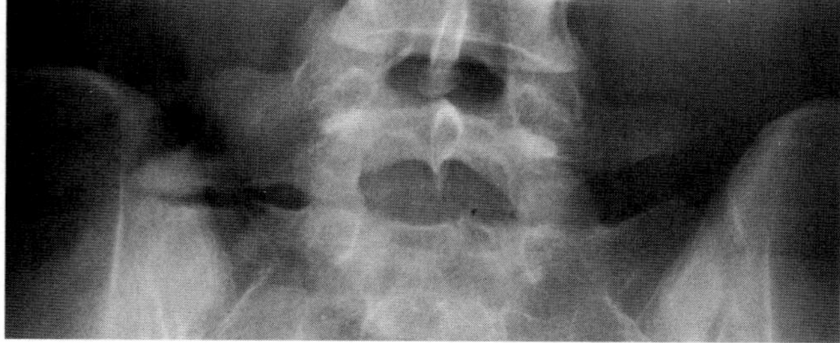

FIGURE 29-2. PA film of transitional vertebra.

OVERUSE INJURIES TO THE THORACIC AND LUMBAR SPINE

Spondylolysis and Spondylolisthesis

Spondylolysis is a defect in the pars interarticularis. It usually occurs in the lower lumbar vertebrae (L5) and can be one of five types.[69] The two types discussed most frequently are dysplastic spondylolysis and isthmic spondylolysis. Dysplastic spondylolysis is the genetic variety of the lesion and occurs in 4% to 6% of the general population.[18,46,77] It is typically asymptomatic and is often coincidentally noted as a radiolucent interruption in the pars on lumbar radiographs. Isthmic spondylolysis is often the variant present in athletes and is secondary to a fatigue fracture of the pars interarticularis. Spondylolysis has been shown to be one of the most common etiologies for low back pain in adolescent athletes. It is significantly less common in adult athletes.[36] Degenerative, traumatic, and pathological spondylolysis comprise the remaining three subclasses of spondylolysis.

Risk Factors. Isthmic spondylolysis has been found to be present in 8% to 83% of athletes, depending on the specific population studied. Type of sport has consistently been identified as a significant risk factor for the development of isthmic spondylolysis. It has been found to occur with increased frequency in divers (83%), cricket fast bowlers (55%), weight lifters (13% to 45%), gymnasts (11% to 38%), wrestlers (33%), high jumpers (24%), and football linemen (24%). Dancing and figure skating have also been shown to have an increased risk of spondylolysis.[13,17,22,29,35,48,54] The common factor among these sports is the element of repetitive hyperextension of the lumbar spine. Heredity is also a significant risk factor for both isthmic and dysplastic spondylolysis, with the highest occurrence being in Alaskan natives.[56,77] Spondylolysis has been shown not to be present at birth or in nonambulatory individuals.[18,47,77] Despite being three times less likely to develop spondylolysis than males, women are at an increased risk of developing the complication of spondylolisthesis (the forward slippage of one vertebral body on the vertebral body below it).[54] Individuals with spondylolysis have been shown to have spina bifida occulta in 22% to 92% of cases, compared with a prevalence of approximately 7% in the general population.[12,18,29,32,55,66,77]

Etiology. The etiology of spondylolysis is still unclear. It appears that a developmental dysplasia of the pars and the erect posture of humans both play a significant role. It is felt that varying amounts of shear stress across the pars will be tolerated, depending on the extent of dysplasia and resultant mechanical weakness of the pars. Athletes participating in high-risk sports will, over time, develop enough force across the pars to result in fracture, even if there is no underlying dysplasia.[66]

Presentation. In athletes, spondylolysis most often presents with the insidious onset of low back pain, although it can present with an acute event. Typically there is an increase in volume and or intensity of training in one of the high-risk/lumbar hyperextension sports. The patient's low back pain is aggravated with lumbar extension. Rarely, signs and symptoms of a radiculopathy may be present secondary to hypertrophy of synovium at the level of the lesion. Most times, however, there are no neurological symptoms. The patient may have found some relief with NSAIDs, rest, or heat.

Physical Examination. On physical exam, there may be no obvious spinal deformity or some degree of lumbar hyperlordosis may be present. There is tenderness to palpation at the affected vertebral level. Range of motion may be limited in both flexion and extension. Flexion is limited by tight hamstrings that are almost universally present. Extension is limited by pain that can be reproduced by having the patient extend the lumbar spine while weight bearing on one or two feet. Single leg lumbar extension will reproduce the pain on the ipsilateral side (Fig. 29-3). A detailed neurologic exam usually reveals no deficits. Examination of flexibility must be compared with the level of flexibility previously present in the athlete to detect the deficit that is often present in the hamstrings. This is especially important with dancers and gymnasts, who normally have extreme hamstring flexibility, thus making it easy to overlook relative hamstring tightness.

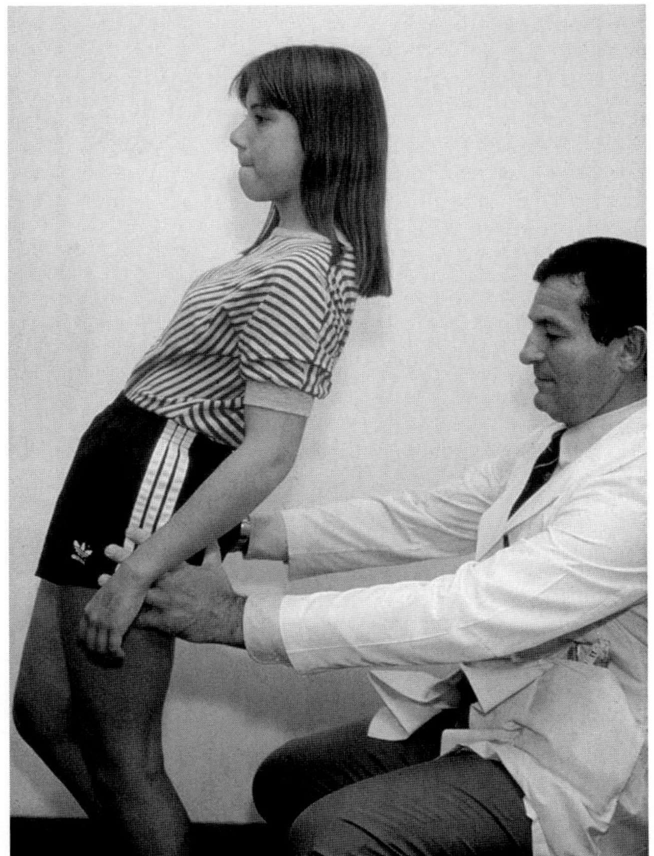

FIGURE 29-3. Physical examination technique for assessing single leg hyperextension. This maneuver will reproduce the patient's pain on the side ipsilateral to the spondylolytic lesion.

Imaging. Plain films are an essential part of the radiographic work-up of spondylolysis. PA, standing lateral, and oblique views are obtained to potentially identify a radiographic lucency of the pars, to look for findings that coexist with spondylolysis, and to rule out other bony abnormalities of the spine. Findings on the PA view that are seen with spondylolysis include lateral deviation of the spinous process and sclerosis of the contralateral pedicle. The classic radiographic finding of spondylolysis is lucency in the neck of the "scotty dog" evident on the oblique views (Fig. 29-4). It should be noted, however, that this sign is present in only 32% of cases of spondylolysis because of the variation in angle of the x-ray beam and plane of the fracture through the pars.[49] The standing lateral view is necessary to evaluate the extent of spondylolisthesis, if it is present. Once plain films have been reviewed, a SPECT (single-photon emission computed tomography) scan is obtained. SPECT is used because it allows the spatial separation of bony structures that overlap on traditional diphosphonate bone scintigraphy, therefore allowing more precise localization of the defect (Fig. 29-5). A negative SPECT scan with negative bone films usually excludes the diagnosis of spondylolysis. If, after a positive SPECT scan, there is still question as to the etiology of the pain, a CT scan may need to be obtained to rule out other bony pathology such as osteoblastoma or osteoid osteoma that may mimic the pain of spondylolysis. CT is used to identify the exact location and character of the lesion and is much more specific than the SPECT scan. CT is also a useful tool in assessing the stage (acute versus chronic) of the lesion and, as a result, its potential for bony healing (Fig. 29-6).[26] MRI is not currently used as part of the radiographic protocol for the work-up of spondylolysis,

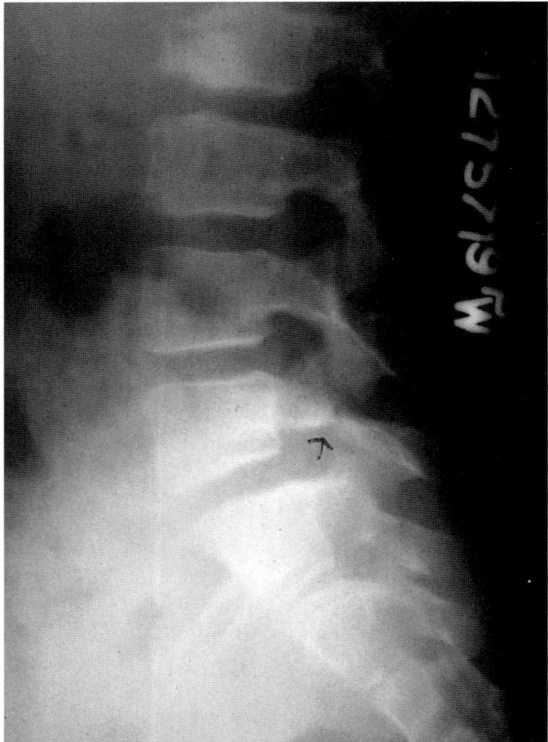

FIGURE 29-4. Oblique film of lumbar spine showing the lucency in the neck of the "scotty dog" associated with spondylolysis.

however recent research seems to be establishing its potential utility in the diagnosis of spondylolysis. As technique develops for visualization of the pars, MRI may prove to be an effective tool in the investigation and management of spondylolysis.

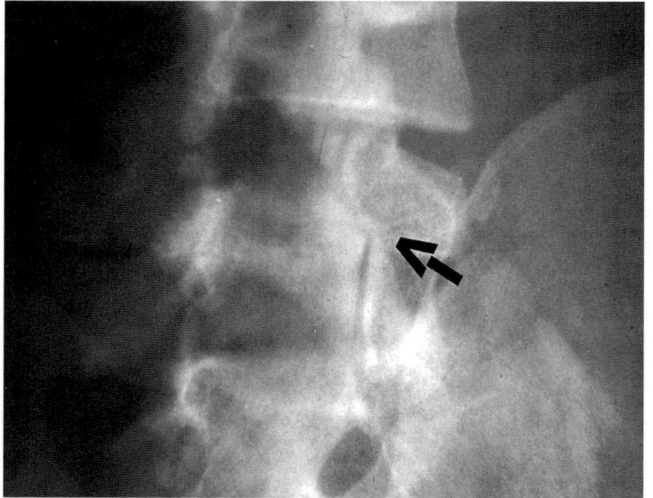

FIGURE 29-5. SPECT scan showing spondylolytic lesion.

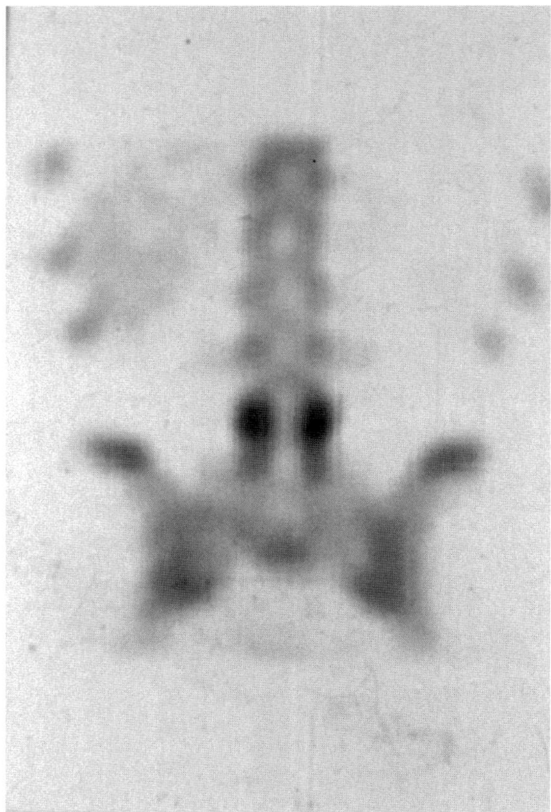

FIGURE 29-6. CT scan showing spondylolytic lesion.

Management. In some circumstances, the pain associated with spondylolysis may be of neurologic origin secondary to inflamed synovium at the fracture site, or concurrent disk disease at a level adjacent to the lesion. In most cases, however, the pain is bony in origin and secondary to movement across the fracture site. The principal goals in the management of spondylolysis are to alleviate this pain and to prevent further slippage in the cases in which bilateral spondylolysis has led to spondylolisthesis. When the spondylolytic lesion is an active stress fracture, bony healing of the lesion is the ultimate goal.

It is felt that fractures of more recent onset are more conducive to complete bony healing than are older lesions. The reason for this is still unclear. It is known that there are distraction forces across the fracture site, and these forces may play a role in delayed healing, as they do at other sites of distraction fracture such as the hip and fifth metatarsal. There is also evidence that with time, a pseudoarthrosis may form across the fracture site, allowing communication of the fracture with the facet joints superior and inferior to it. With the introduction of synovial fluid into this pseudoarthrosis, healing may be impaired.[53] In cases in which bony healing is not possible, a painless fibrous union is the goal.

Spondylolisthesis is a frequent complication of bilateral spondylolysis (Fig. 29-7). In some studies, up to 80%

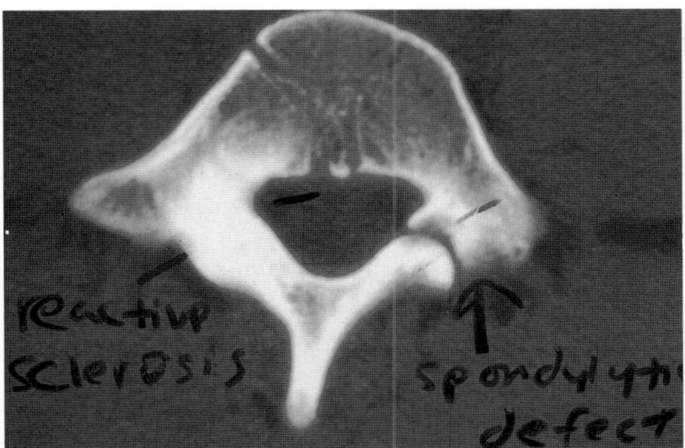

FIGURE 29-7. Lateral film of the lumbar spine demonstrating forward slip of L5 on S1 in spondylolisthesis.

of patients already will have some degree of spondylolisthesis at presentation.[18,50,70] The amount of slip found at presentation is usually 80% to 90% of the total eventual amount of slip.[18,38,51] Progression of the slip occurs in 44% of cases, regardless of athletic involvement.[4,19,38,51] Predicting which patients will develop spondylolisthesis is difficult. Only two risk factors have been consistently shown to be associated with progression of the slip: spondylolisthesis of greater than 20% to 30% at diagnosis and adolescence.[4,18,28,51] The amount of slip is determined by measuring the distance between lines drawn through the posterior border of S1 and L5 (for an L5/S1 slip) as a percentage of the width of S1 (Fig. 29-8). The grading scheme is divided into four intervals: <25% slip is grade 1, 25% to 50% is grade 2, 50% to 75% is grade 3, 75% to 100% is grade 4. A slip greater than 100% is called spondyloptosis. In the cases in which spondylolisthesis is present at diagnosis or develops, bony healing is unlikely to occur, and pain management and prevention of further slip are the goals.

Guidelines for management of spondylolysis and spondylolisthesis remain similar to those published initially by Wiltse[67] and Wiltse and Jackson,[68] although there is considerable variation in the approach to "conservative" therapy. In general, patients with spondylolysis and spondylolisthesis are treated as follows:

1. Asymptomatic child, <25% slip: standing lateral lumbar x-ray every 6 months until age 15, then annually until the end of growth. No activity limitation, but avoid occupations involving heavy labor.
2. Asymptomatic child, 25%–50% slip: same guidelines as (1), but avoid contact sports or hyperextension.
3. Symptomatic child, <50% slip: conservative management (as described in the following paragraphs) including physiotherapy, bracing, and activity modification in addition to the recommendations in (2).
4. More than 50% slip: surgical management is usually indicated and orthopedic consultation is necessary.

Physiotherapy should emphasize hamstring and lumbodorsal fascial stretching and abdominal and antilordotic strengthening.

Bracing is usually instituted with a modified Boston overlapping brace molded in 0° of lumbar lordosis to help unload the posterior elements (Fig. 29-9). This brace is worn 23 hours each day, slowly increasing the time in the brace over the first few weeks. For the first month of treatment, activity is limited to physiotherapy. Following this, sports participation in the brace is permitted, provided there is no pain or lumbar hyperextension. The patient is followed at regular intervals for clinical assessments and imaging for a period of 3 to 6 months (details follow).

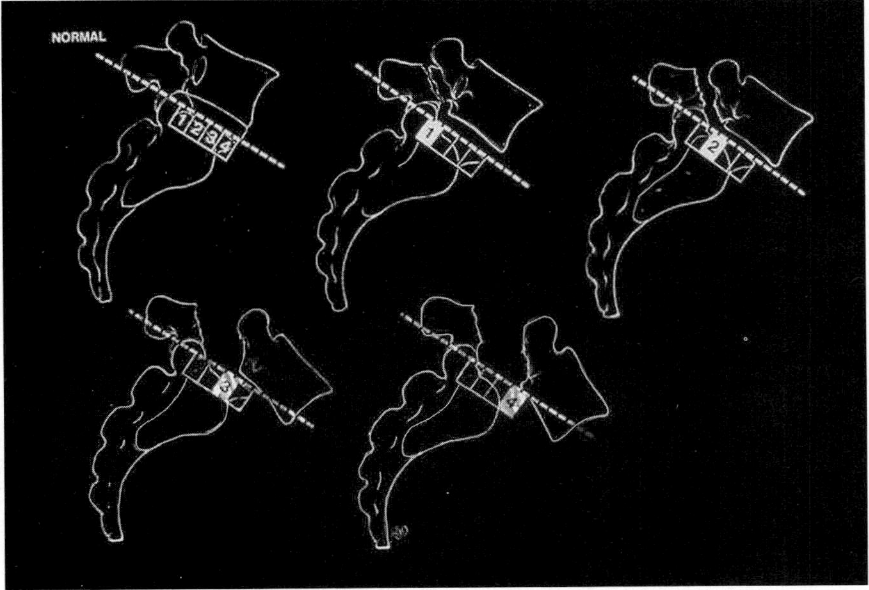

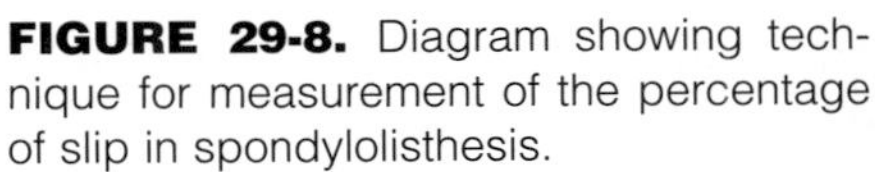

FIGURE 29-8. Diagram showing technique for measurement of the percentage of slip in spondylolisthesis.

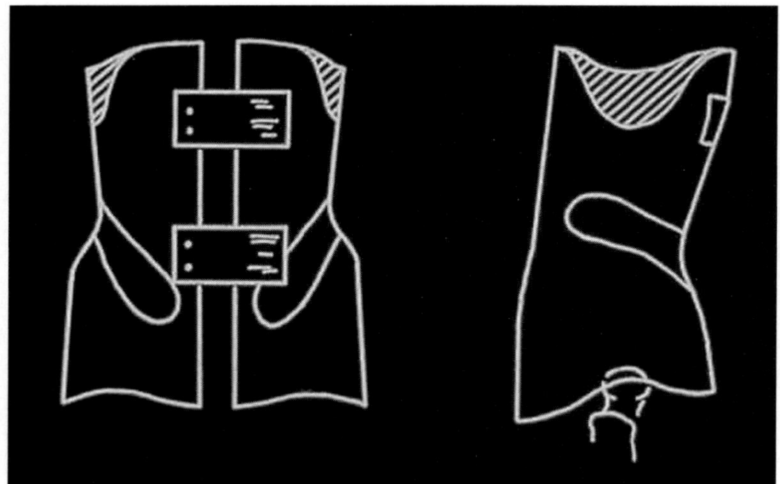

FIGURE 29-9. Boston overlapping brace.

At this point, weaning from the brace is usually possible. Seventy-five percent of patients treated by this protocol have been found to have good or excellent results.[55]

Return to sport is always the paramount question for athletes. Again, following the above protocol, athletes were found to be pain free 4 to 6 weeks after initiation of treatment and able to participate in their sport wearing the brace with a good to excellent outcome in 80% of athletes.[12]

When weaning from the brace is felt to be appropriate, this is commenced first during sleep; if the patient remains asymptomatic, time out of the brace is increased. Sporting activity is the final activity for which brace use will be used.

In patients with persistent pain or delayed healing, there have been a few case reports of successful outcomes with the use of an electromagnetic field bone growth stimulator.[16,33]

The author's current approach to symptomatic patients with spondylolysis and spondylolisthesis of less than 50% is as follows:

1. Initial visit
   Investigations: PA, standing lateral, and oblique plain films and a SPECT bone scan. If diagnosis cannot be confirmed with these investigations, a CT is obtained.
   Interventions: Physiotherapy as described in the preceding paragraphs and a Boston overlapping brace in 0° of lumbar lordosis are prescribed.
2. One-month follow-up visit:
   Investigations: None if patient is improving and asymptomatic.
   Interventions: Trim brace slightly to allow for athletic participation provided sport does not cause pain. Hyperextension activity is contraindicated.
3. Three-month follow-up visit:
   Investigations: CT to follow progress of bony lesion. If bony healing is complete, weaning from the brace may be initiated as described in the following, otherwise continue current management.
4. Six-month follow-up visit:
   Investigations: Standing lateral to assess for slip of spondylolisthesis if bony healing not previously documented; CT to follow progress of bony healing.
   Interventions: Weaning from the brace over a period of 3 to 6 months if healing has been documented. May try pulsed electromagnetic field bone growth stimulation in the cases of painful nonunion; otherwise, surgical intervention may be necessary.
5. One- and two-year visits:
   Standing lateral plain films to assess for spondylolisthesis progression.

If the patient initially presents with a sponylolisthesis of more than 50%, orthopedic consultation is necessary to consider surgical stabilization.

Scheuermann's Disease

Two variants of Scheuermann's kyphosis are known to exist. The classic, or typical, variety is a painless thoracic kyphosis secondary to anterior wedging of 5° or more in each of at least three consecutive vertebrae. It presents as a cosmetic deformity consisting of an inflexible thoracic hyperkyphosis and lumbar hyperlordosis in adults. Atypical Scheuermann's disease is a painful condition localized to the upper lumbar vertebrae. Again, there is anterior wedging of vertebrae, but the criteria allow for variability in the number of affected vertebrae. This condition presents as low back pain in the adolescent athlete.[5] In both of these conditions, there is herniation of disk material into the vertebral bodies.

Risk Factors. Athletes involved in sports that place the spine under increased axial load, especially in forward flexion (gymnastics, diving), have an increased risk for developing atypical Scheuermann's.[21,24] No other risk factors have been identified.

Etiology. The etiology of atypical Scheuermann's is undetermined. There is known to be a protrusion of disk material into the vertebral body resulting in the formation of Schmorl's nodes, the classic finding seen on plain film in Scheuermann's kyphosis.

Presentation. The athlete will complain of low back pain of variable duration that is aggravated by forward flexion. There may be a history of involvement in one of the previously mentioned sports. Although in classic Scheuermann's there is a thoracic hyperkyphosis and a lumbar hyperlordosis, athletes with atypical Scheuermann's may have a "flat back" and an inability to flex through the lumbar spine (Fig. 29-10). Pain may be induced on forward flexion. This motion is accomplished through flexion at the hips rather than the lumbar spine. There are no specific areas of bony tenderness. Hamstring inflexibility is often present and the neurologic examination is normal.

Imaging. Investigations for atypical Scheuermann's include PA and standing lateral radiographs. The lateral film is most helpful and reveals a decreased lumbar lordosis, vertebral endplate abnormalities, Schmorl's nodes, and disk space narrowing (Fig. 29-11).

Management. The goal of management is to reduce pain and increase function. This is done through a combination of relative rest, physiotherapy, and bracing. Rest from the aggravating activities is prescribed. Cross-training in other areas is permitted. A Boston brace with 15° of lumbar lordosis is custom fit for the athlete and worn 23 hours/day. This intervention dramatically reduces pain. Physiotherapy is essential, with an emphasis placed on peripelvic stabilization, lumbodorsal fascial stretching, abdominal strengthening, and hamstring flexibility. After the athlete has been symptom free for one month, weaning from the brace is initiated.

Degenerative Disk Disease

Degenerative disk disease has been shown to account for nearly half of all complaints of low back pain in adult

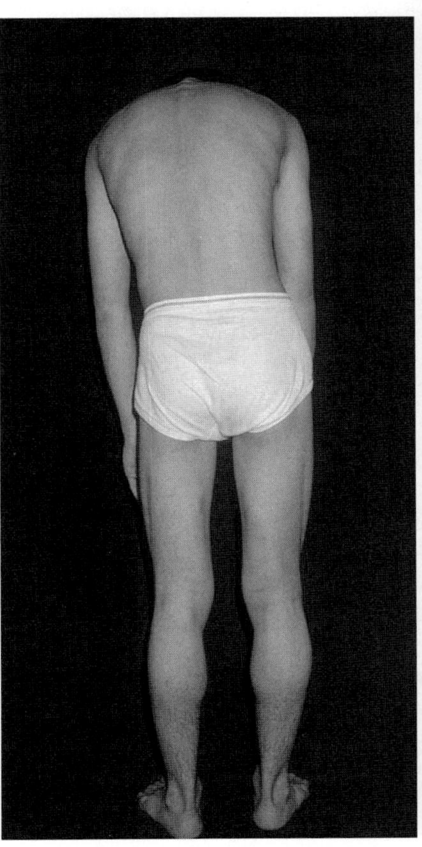

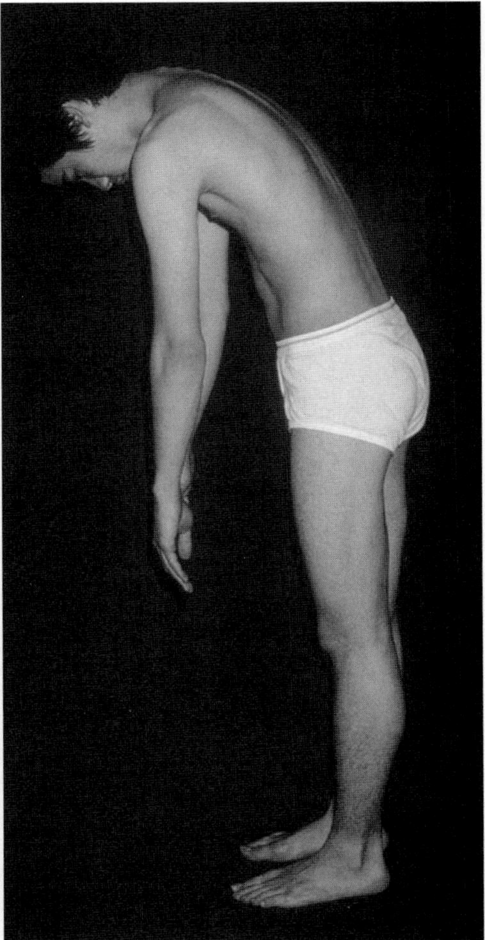

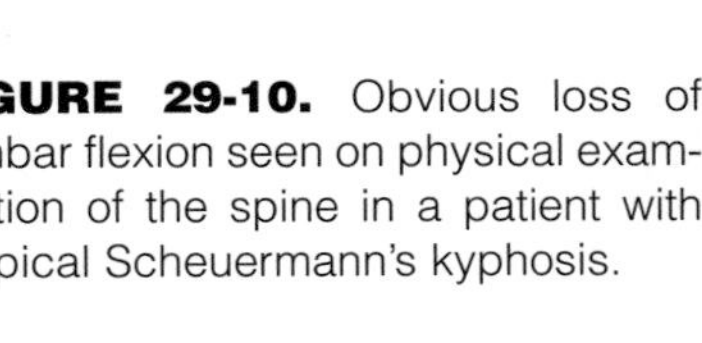

FIGURE 29-10. Obvious loss of lumbar flexion seen on physical examination of the spine in a patient with atypical Scheuermann's kyphosis.

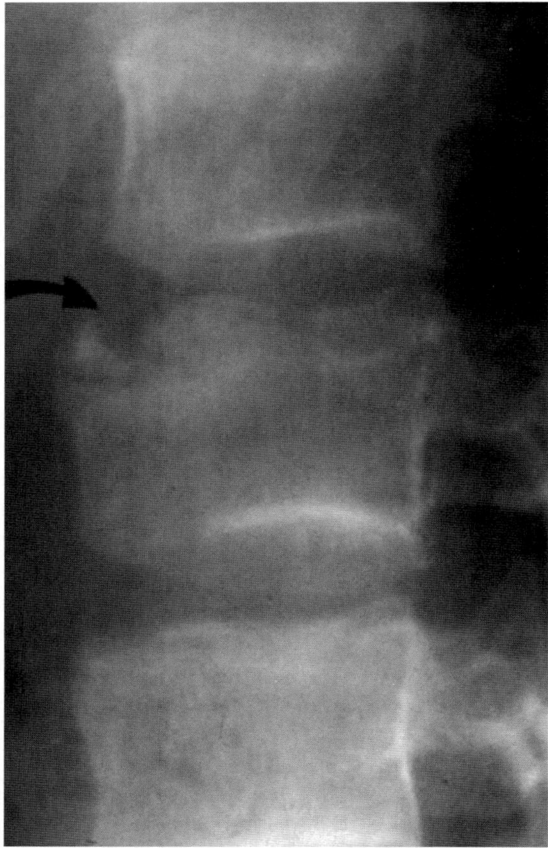

FIGURE 29-11. Lateral plain film of the lumbar spine of a patient with atypical Scheuermann's. Note the Schmorl's nodes and anterior wedging of the vertebrae.

athletes.[72] Pain may arise initially in the annulus; however, as degeneration progresses and forces are transferred to the surrounding osseous and ligamentous structures, facet joint arthrosis can also produce pain.

Risk Factors. Athletes involved in gymnastics have been shown to have an increased risk of disk degeneration.[57,60] Heavy labor and heredity also have been shown to be risk factors for degenerative disk disease. Gender has not been shown to affect risk.

Presentation. Degenerative disk disease presents with intermittent low back pain, which increases with activity and forward flexion. Radicular symptoms or sciatica are more suggestive of an acute herniation. On physical examination, there will be diffuse lumbar tenderness and paravertebral muscle spasm. Both flexion and extension may produce pain, with extension pain indicative of foraminal involvement or central stenosis and facet joint hypertrophy. Examination of flexibility reveals hamstring tightness. No specific neurologic defecits are elicited with isolated disk degeneration.

Imaging. AP and lateral plain radiographs are often normal early in the disease. With further disk degeneration, facet joint hypertrophy and disk space narrowing are evident. MRI is a sensitive tool in detecting changes associated with disk degeneration; however, these changes have also been shown to be present in asymptomatic individuals.[6] Discography is the most effective tool for identifying symptomatic degenerative disk disease. If the degenerative disk is the cause for the patient's back pain, injecting a small amount of saline into the presumed affected disk, under fluoroscopic guidance, will reproduce the patient's pain.

Management. Nonoperative management is usually effective in the control of symptoms associated with degenerative disk disease. Varying degrees of relative rest, bracing, and physiotherapy are prescribed. Avoidance of activities that involve flexion or increased axial load on the spine are essential and often sufficient to significantly decrease pain. A soft lumbar corset may provide some relief, but a rigid thoracolumbar orthosis molded in 15° of lordosis may be necessary. Sports participation within the brace is permitted, provided it does not induce symptoms. Physiotherpy is helpful to regain paraspinal and abdominal strength and lumbodorsal fascia and hamstring flexibility. In recalcitrant cases, orthopedic consultation is necessary for consideration of anterior and/or posterior fusion of the involved segment.

ACUTE INJURY TO THE THORACIC AND LUMBAR SPINE

Acute Herniation of the Nucleus Pulposis

Acute herniation of the nucleus pulposis (HNP) is an important cause of low back pain in the athlete. Although the average age for presentation with HNP is 35,[31] it can occur at any age.

Etiology. It is known that the intervertebral disk is under most pressure when sitting,[39,77] and that rotation and shear forces can produce circumferential and radial tears in the annulus. These tears allow for expulsion of nuclear material through the outer layers of the annulus. This can result in inflammation and chemical neuritis in a richly innervated area, thus causing intense pain and spasm, in addition to any compression of the nerve root itself.

Risk Factors. Research has revealed little in the way of athletic risk factors for HNP, with a recent study implicating only bowling as positively correlated to the occurrence of HNP.[37] Gender has not been found to be a risk factor.

Presentation. The patient with HNP will present with low back pain, often, but not always, following an acute event. In many, but not all, the pain will radiate in a radicular pattern consistent with the level of the injury. The pain is aggravated by sitting (more than standing), flexion, or activities that induce a Valsalva maneuver. It is very important to question the patient about bowel or bladder symptoms, as these may be suggestive of cauda equina syndrome.[52] The physical examination may reveal splinting and scoliosis in reaction to severe lumbar pain. Midline lumbar tenderness is present, with paravertebral muscle spasm. Range of motion of the lumbar spine will be decreased. Motor and sensory testing reveals changes in the distribution of the affected nerve root. Deep tendon reflexes may also be diminished. If the sciatic nerve is involved, straight leg testing will reproduce the back pain and induce pain along the course of the sciatic nerve. Hamstring flexibility is decreased. The presence of a perineal sensory deficit in association with bowel or bladder symptomatology is highly suggestive of cauda equina syndrome. This is a surgical emergency and necessitates immediate consultation with a spine surgeon to avoid irreversible bowel and bladder dysfunction.[52]

Imaging. PA and lateral spine films are negative, with the exception of disk space narrowing in some cases. MRI and CT will reveal disk herniation (Fig. 29-12).

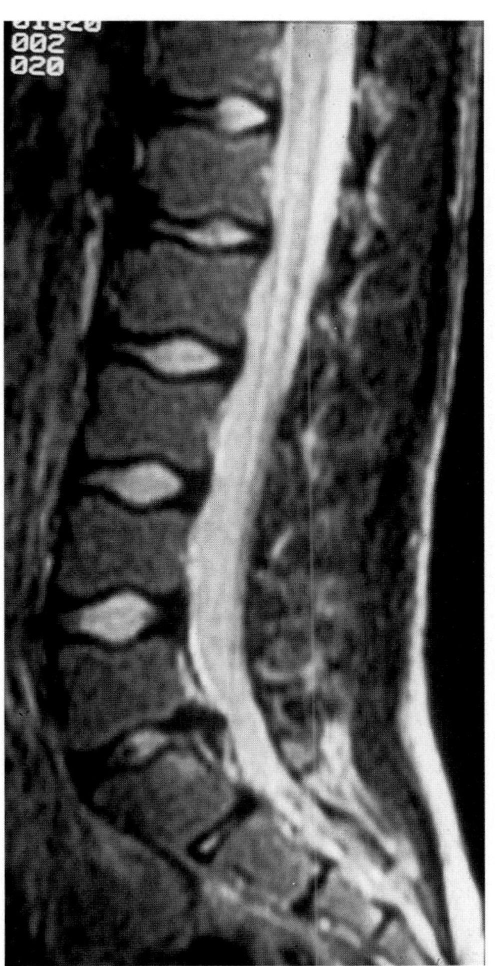

FIGURE 29-12. MRI of the lumbar spine showing herniation of intervertebral disc material.

Management. As in many spine conditions, a combination of relative rest, physiotherapy, and bracing is helpful. A prolonged period of bedrest is no longer prescribed, and actually may lead to worsening back and hamstring flexibility. A few days of bedrest may be appropriate initially to control pain; otherwise, the patient may perform activities as tolerated with the exception of prolonged sitting, jumping, straining, and weight lifting. The patient is encouraged to keep the spine in a neutral position as much as possible. Physiotherapy is useful for increasing abdominal and paraspinous strength and hamstring flexibility. Some patients may benefit from the use of a soft corset, and others may require a rigid thoracolumbar orthosis in 15° of flexion to provide support in a position of comfort and decrease the force across the disk. NSAIDs may be a useful adjunct in decreasing both pain and inflammation associated with herniation of nuclear material. Occasionally a short course of narcotics and/or muscle relaxants may be necessary to decrease pain and muscle spasm. With these measures, most patients will obtain relief within the first few weeks of treatment. If symptoms persist beyond 6 weeks, epidural steroid injections may be necessary. Few patients will fail conservative management and will need to be assessed for surgical intervention.

Other

Sprains, strains, and fractures can also occur in the thoracolumbar region and are discussed elsewhere in this text.

NONTRAUMATIC SOURCES OF PAIN

The differential diagnosis of back pain in the athlete must always include etiologies of infectious (diskitis, osteomyelitis) and neoplastic (osteoblastoma, osteoid osteoma) origins. Nonmusculoskeletal sources of pain must also be considered. In the female athlete, gynecologic pathology may cause pain referred to the low back, and renal, GI, and vascular origins should not be overlooked. A thorough history and review of systems should be obtained to raise or lower the clinician's index of suspicion for these etiologies.

REFERENCES

1. Arendt E, Dick R: Gender specific knee injury patterns in basketball and soccer. Presented at the American Orthopedic Society for Sports Medicine, Sun Valley, ID, 1993.
2. Ascani E, Bartolozzi P, Logroscino CA, et al: Natural history of untreated idiopathic scoliosis after skeletal maturity. Spine 11(8):784–789, 1986.
3. Becker TJ: Scoliosis in swimmers. Clin Sports Med 5:149–158, 1986.

4. Blackburne JS, Velikas EP: Spondylolisthesis in children and adolescents. J Bone Joint Surg 59-B(4): 490–494, 1977.
5. Blumenthal SL, Roach J, Herring JA: Lumbar Scheuermann's. A clinical series and classification. Spine 12(9):929–932, 1987.
6. Boden SD, David SO, Dina TS, et al: Abnormal magnetic resonance scans of the lumbar spine in asymptomatic subjects: A prospective investigation. J Bone Joint Surg 72A:403–408, 1990.
7. Brooks HL. Scoliosis: A prospective epidemiological study. J Bone Joint Surg 57A:968–972, 1975.
8. Brooks HL, Azen SP, Gerberg E, et al: Scoliosis: A prospective epidemiologic study. J Bone Joint Surg Am 57:968–972, 1975.
9. Calvert R: Athletic injuries and deaths in secondary schools and colleges, 1975–76 (National Center for Education and Statistics, Department of Health, Education and Welfare). Washington, DC, US Government Printing Office, 1978.
10. Canale: Campbell's Operative Orthopaedics, 10th ed. St. Louis, Mosby, 2003.
11. Clarke K, Buckley W: Women's injuries in collegiate sports. Am J Sports Med 8:187–191, 1980.
12. d'Hemecourt PA, Zurakowski D, Kriemler S, Micheli LJ: Spondylolysis: Returning the athlete to sports participation with brace treatment. Orthopedics 25(6):653–657, 2002.
13. Elliott BC: Back injuries and the fast bowler in cricket. J Sport Sci 18:983–991, 2000.
14. Elster AD: Bertolotti's syndrome revisited: Transitional vertebrae of the lumbar spine. Spine 14(12):1373–1377, 1989.
15. Emans JB, Kaelin A, Bancel P, et al: The Boston bracing system for idiopathic scoliosis: Follow-up results in 295 patients. Spine 11:792–801, 1986.
16. Fellander-Tsai L, Micheli LJ: Treatment of spondylolysis with external electrical stimulation and bracing in adolescent athletes: A report of two cases. Clin J Sport Med 8(3):232–234, 1998.
17. Ferguson RJ, McMaster JH, Stanitski CL: Low back pain in the college football lineman. Sports Med 2(2):63–69, 1974.
18. Fredrickson BE, Baker D, McHolick WJ, et al: The natural history of spondylolysis and spondylolisthesis. J Bone Joint Surg 66A(5):699–707, 1984.
19. Frennered AK, Danielson BI, Nachemson AL: Natural history of symptomatic isthmic low-grade spondylolisthesis in children and adolescents: A seven-year follow up study. J Pediatr Orthop 11: 209–213, 1991.
20. Frey C: Foot health and shoewear for women. Clin Orthop 372:32–44, 2000.
21. Gerbino PG, Micheli LJ: Back injuries in the young athlete. Clin Sports Med 14(3):571–590, 1995.
22. Germanaud J, Bardet M: Is the female sex a risk factor for acute low back pain? (letter) Revue du Rhumatisme 60(11):850–851, 1993.
23. Green NE: Part-time bracing of adolescent idiopathic scoliosis. J Bone Joint Surg 68A:738–742, 1986.
24. Greene TL, Hensinger RN, Hunter LY: Back pain and vertebral changes simulating Scheuermann's disease. J Pediatr Orthop 5(1):1–7, 1985.
25. Gussbacher A, Rompe G: Die dynamische und statische beanspruchen der Wirbelsaule und ihre moglichen auswirkungen bei verschiedenen sportarnen. Schweiz Z Sportmed 31:119–124, 1983.
26. Harvey CJ, Richenberg JL, Saifuddin A, Wolman RL: Pictoral review: The radiological investigation of lumbar spondylolysis. Clin Radiol 53:723–728, 1998.
27. Hellstrom M, Jacobsson B, Sward L, Peterson L: Radiological abnormalities of the thoraco lumbar spine in athletes. Acta Radiol 31:127–132, 1990.
28. Ikata T, Miyake R Katoh S, et al: Pathogenesis of sports related spondylolisthesis in adolescents. Am J Sports Med 24(1):94–98, 1996.
29. Jackson DW, Wiltse LL, Cirincione RJ: Spondylolysis in the female gymnast. Clin Orthop 117:68–73, 1976.
30. Katz DE, Richards BS, Browne RH, Herring JA: A comparison between the Boston brace and the Charleston bending brace in adolescent idiopathic scoliosis. Spine 22:1302–1312, 1997.
31. Kelsey JL: AN epidemiological study of acute herniated lumbar intervertebral disc. Rheumatol Rehab 14:144–159, 1975.
32. Laurent LE, Einola S: Spondylolisthesis in children and adolescents. Acta Orthop Scand 31:45–64, 1961.
33. Maharam LG, Sharkey I: Electrical stimulation of acute spondylolysis. Med Sci Sports Exerc 24(Suppl): 538, 1992.
34. Micheli LJ: Sports following spinal surgery in the young athlete. Clin Orthop 198:152–157, 1985.
35. Micheli LJ, Micheli ER: Back injuries in dancers. In Shell CG (ed): The Olympic Scientific Congress Proceedings: The Dancer as Athlete. Champaign, IL, Human Kinetics, 1986, pp 91–94.
36. Micheli LJ, Wood R: Back pain in young athletes. Arch Pediatr Adolesc Med 149:15–18, 1995.
37. Mundt DJ, Kelsey JL, Gordan AL, et al: Northeast Collaborative Group on Low Back Pain. An epidemiologic study of sports and weight lifting as possible risk factors for herniated lumbar and cervical discs. Am J Sports Med 21(6):854–860, 1993.
38. Muschik M, Hahnel H, Robinson PN, et al: Competitive sports and the progression of spondylolisthesis. J Pediatr Orthop 16:364–369, 1996.
39. Nachemson A, Morris JM: In vivo measurements of intradiscal pressure. J Bone Joint Surg 46: 1077–1084, 1964.

40. Nadler SF, Wu KD, Galski T: Low back pain in college athletes. A prospective study correlating lower extremity overuse or acquired ligamentous laxity with low back pain. Spine 23(7):828–833, 1998.
41. National Collegiate Athletic Association (NCAA) Injury surveillance system. Accessed April 1, 2003. http://www.ncaa.org/membership/ed_outreach/health-safety/iss/index.html.
42. Ohlen G, Wedmark T, Sprangfort E: Spinal sagital configuration and mobility related to low back pain in the female gymnast. Spine 14:847–850, 1989.
43. Omey ML, Micheli LJ, Gerbino PG: Idiopathic scoliosis and spondylolysis in the female athlete. Clin Orthop 372:74–84, 2000.
44. Payne WK: Does scoliosis have a psychological impact and does gender make a difference? Spine 22:1380–1384, 1997.
45. Ramirez M, Jonsston CE, Browne RH: The prevalence of back pain in children who have idiopathic scoliosis. J Bone Joint Surg 79A:364–368, 1997.
46. Roche MB, Rowe GG: The incidence of separate neural arch and coincident bone variations. Anat Rec 109:233–252, 1951.
47. Rosenberg NJ, Bargar WL, Friedman B: The incidence of spondylolysis and spondylolisthesis in nonambulatory patients. Spine 6(1):35–38, 1981.
48. Rossi F: Spondylolysis, spondylolisthesis and sports. J Sports Med 18(4):317–340, 1978.
49. Saifuddin A, White J, Tucker S, Taylor BA: Orientation of lumbar pars defects. J Bone Joint Surg 80-B(2):208–211, 1998.
50. Saraste H: Long term clinical and radiological follow-up of spondylolysis and spondylolisthesis. J Pediatr Orthop 7:631–638, 1987.
51. Seitsalo S, Osterman K, Hyvarinen H, et al: Progression of spondylolisthesis in children and adolescents. Spine 16(4):417–421, 1991.
52. Shapiro S: Cauda equina syndrome secondary to lumbar disc herniation. Neurosurgery 32:743–746, 1993.
53. Shipley JA, Beukes CA: The nature of the spondylolytic defect. J Bone Joint Surg 80(B):662–664, 1998.
54. Soler T, Calderon C: The prevalence of spondylolysis in the Spanish elite athlete. Am J Sports Med 28(1):57–62, 2000.
55. Steiner ME, Micheli LJ: Treatment of symptomatic spondylolysis and spondylolisthesis with the modified Boston brace. Spine 10(10):937–943, 1985.
56. Stewart TD: The age incidence of neural arch defects in Alaskan natives considered from the standpoint of etiology. J Bone Joint Surg 35A:937–950, 1953.
57. Sward L, Hellstrom M, Jacobsson B, et al: Disc degeneration and associated abnosrmalities of the spine in elite gymnasts: A magenetic resonance imaging study. Spine 16:437–443, 1991.
58. Tanchev PI, Dzherov AD, Parushev AD, et al: Scoliosis in rhythmic gymnasts. Spine 25(11): 1367–1372, 2000.
59. Teegarden D, Proulx WR, Kern M, Sedlock D, et al: Previous physical activity relates to bone mineral measures in young women. Med Sci Sports Exerc 28:105–113, 1996.
60. Tertti M, Paajanen H, Kujala UM, et al: Disc degeneration in young gymnasts, a magnetic imaging study. Am J Sports Med 18:206–208, 1990.
61. Tosi L: Women and the orthopaedic surgeon. Clin Orthop 372:17–31, 2000.
62. US Department of Education: Title IX: 25 Years of Progress, 1997. Accessed April 1, 2003. http://www.ed.gov/pubs/titleIX/index.html.
63. Warren MP, Brooks-Gunn J, Hamilton LH, et al: Scoliosis and fractures in young ballet dancers. Relation delayed menarche and secondary amenorrhea. N Eng J Med 314:1348–1353, 1986.
64. Weinstein SL: Idiopathic scoliosis: Natural history. Spine 11(8):780–783, 1986.
65. Whiteside P: Men's and women's injuries in comparable sports. Phys Sportsmed 8:130–140, 1980.
66. Wiltse LL: The etiology of spondylolisthesis. J Bone Joint Surg 44A(3):539–560, 1962.
67. Wiltse LL: Spondylolisthesis in children. Clin Orthop 21:156–163, 1961.
68. Wiltse LL, Jackson DW: Treatment of spondylolisthesis and spondylolysis in children. Clin Orthop 117:92–100, 1976.
69. Wiltse LL, Newman PH, Macnab I: Classification of spondylolysis and spondylolisthesis. Clin Orthop 117:23–29, 1976.
70. Wiltse LL, Widell EH, Jackson DW: Fatigue fracture: The basic lesion in isthmic spondylolysis. J Bone Joint Surg 57–A(1):17–22, 1975.
71. Wojtys EM: The association between athletic training time and the sagittal curvature of the immature spine. Am J Sports Med 28:490–498, 2000.
72. The Women's Sports Foundation. Accessed April 1, 2003. http://www.womenssportsfoundation.org/cgibin/iowa/index.html.
73. The Women's Sports Foundation. Sport and teen pregnancy, 1998. Accessed April 1, 2003. http://www.womenssportsfoundation.org/binary-data/WSF_ARTICLE/ pdf_file/883.pdf.
74. The Women's Sports Foundation. Health risks and the teen athlete, 2000. Accessed April 1, 2003. http://www.womenssportsfoundation.org/binary-data/WSF_ARTICLE/pdf_file/771.pdf.
75. The Women's Sports Foundation. Women's sports & fitness facts & statistics, 2000. Accessed May 21, 2003. www.womenssportsfoundation.org/binary-data/WSF_ARTICLE/pdf_file/123.pdf.
76. Wood K: Spinal Deformity in the adolescent athlete. Clin Sport Med 21(1):77–92, 2002.
77. Wynne-Davies R, Scott JHS: Inheritance of spondylolisthesis. J Bone Joint Surg 61B(3):301–305, 1979.

V

The Pediatric Athlete

30 The Lower Extremity

Peter G. Gerbino II and
Lyle J. Micheli

Primary care of the pediatric athlete can be a challenging endeavor. The pediatric population sustains many of the same injuries as adults and, in addition, is at risk for other types of injuries. Because of the physeal growth centers and the physiology of growth itself, many more and potentially serious injuries may occur in this population. The physes not only add diagnostic possibilities, they also make treatment more difficult because they must be protected. Conversely, children generally heal more quickly and more completely, which permits early, focused intervention and achieves better results.

Understanding the types of injury that can occur is the first step in effective management. We must then apply our knowledge of pertinent risk factors to arrive at a specific diagnosis. Treatment, rehabilitation, and prevention are effective only if the proper diagnosis has been made. In this chapter we will examine all these variables as they pertain to the lower extremity. Types of injuries, risk factors, diagnosis, treatment, rehabilitation, and prevention will be explored. In addition, three problems that can be particularly frustrating—acute knee effusion, patellofemoral pain, and shin splints—receive special attention. Management algorithms have been provided for these problems.

TYPES OF INJURY

Trauma

In the lower extremity, the athlete can sustain acute macrotrauma or repetitive microtrauma. Trauma can result in fractures, dislocations, muscle–tendon tears, ligament tears, and contusions. Fractures and dislocations can be fairly straightforward to manage, but certain of these—patella subluxation, for example—can be more challenging to correct. In acute trauma, the greatest pitfall is failure to diagnose. We must remain vigilant in our treatment of subtle physeal injuries and internal derangements that frequently are misdiagnosed as contusions, sprains, or strains.

Overuse

All mechanical structures will eventually fail if loaded cyclically for a long enough period of time. The mechanical structures in the young athlete include bone, cartilage, muscles, tendons, and the specialized ligaments, cartilages, and bone of joints. Cyclic loading overuse leads to different problems in each of these structures. In many respects, thinking broadly about the tissue involved and its overuse risk factors will lead to more efficacious management than will affixing a syndrome name to the problem.

Bone. Cyclic loading of diaphyseal long bones will lead to stress or fatigue fracture. Bone follows well-understood mechanical properties of anisotropic materials for crack propagation.[8] Before the fracture occurs, however, the bone undergoing such loads will respond metabolically. In response to Wolff's Law, the stressed bone thickens and strengthens.[24] When the ability of the bone to remodel is outpaced by the loading stresses, microfracture and inflammation occur.[8] Inflammation metabolites eventually cause pain, which is the only warning sign of an impending stress fracture. Ignoring or misdiagnosing this pain can result in a much longer recovery period than if addressed early. A young ballerina ignored pain under her left hallux for several weeks before she was suddenly no longer able to bear weight. Radiographs and bone scan confirmed a medial sesamoid stress fracture and also showed increased uptake in both femurs, both tibiae, and both ankles (Fig. 30-1). Only the sesamoid had been painful.

Joints. Joints are special places where bone, articular cartilage, meniscal cartilage, ligaments, and joint fluid interact. Overuse in a joint can result in joint inflammation, effusion, pain, and eventually degeneration. Pain in a joint can originate at torn or irritated synovium, capsule, retinaculum, or ligament. Mechanical deformation from a torn labrum or meniscus, osteochondral fragment, or excess fluid can indirectly produce pain. Finally, metabolic products from articular cartilage breakdown or synovitis may directly cause pain.[6]

Growth Cartilage. In addition to articular cartilage, there is physeal and apophyseal growth cartilage in the young athlete. Both of these growth cartilages are subject to overuse injury. Cyclic loading can lead to traction apophysitis, apophyseal disruption, or physeal fracture.

Muscle and Tendons. Supervised maximal use of muscles leads to hypertrophy and increased fiber size.[2]

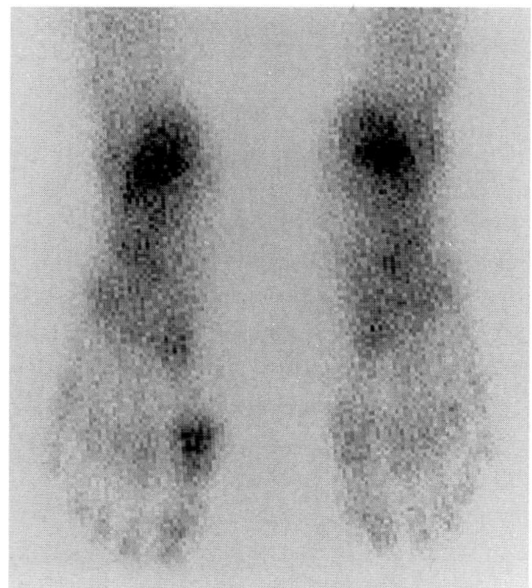

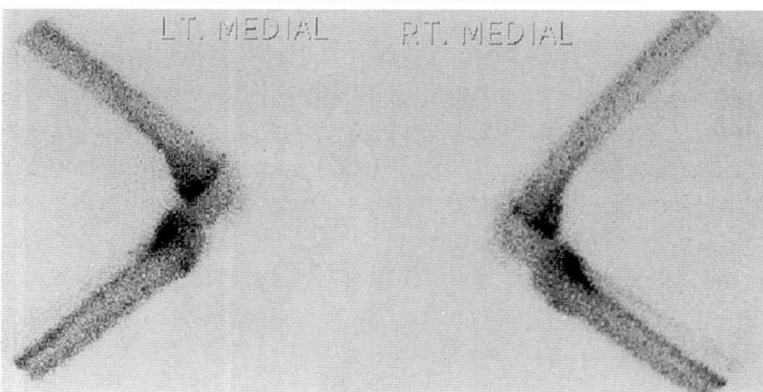

FIGURE 30-1. Bone scan of an 18-year-old ballerina with painful stress fracture of the left medial sesamoid. The additional areas of increased uptake in both ankles, femurs, and tibiae were asymptomatic but mildly tender to palpation. In the presence of pain, each of these other areas would have also been diagnosed as a stress fracture rather than a bone stress reaction.

Unsupervised weight training can lead to muscle tears and scarring.[15] Scarring can cause shortening and exacerbate the tightness that accompanies axial skeleton growth.

Tendons rarely become directly inflamed in children. More common is apophyseal injury or bursitis from excess friction. When muscles and tendons are overused, all risk factors for that injury must be identified and corrected.

RISK FACTORS

Epidemiologic studies of children's overuse injuries have identified several intrinsic and extrinsic risk factors (Table 30-1).[17,42]

Intrinsic Risk Factors

Growth Process. In children, growth and growth spurts are major risk factors for overuse injury of the lower extremity. As the axial skeleton grows, the soft tissues are passively stretched. In a growth spurt, this can cause pathological tightness and several types of overuse injury.

TABLE 30-1 Risk Factors Associated with Overuse Injuries in the Young Athlete

Intrinsic	Extrinsic
Growth process	Training or technique error
Growth tissues	Improper coaching
Anatomic malalignment	Improper footwear or gear
Muscle–tendon imbalance	Playing surface
Psychological factors	Nutrition
Associated disease state	Cultural deconditioning
Gender	

Growth Tissues. The presence of growth tissues is a separate growth-related risk factor. Softer growing bones are at risk for compression injury such as osteochondritis dissecans. Physeal cartilage is weaker than bone and at risk for acute fracture, stress fracture, and apophyseal injury.

Anatomic Malalignment. In the lower extremity, anatomic malalignment can result in several types of injury. Common malalignments such as pes planus or patella alta may never lead to pathology. At other times, these same conditions can lead to relative overuse. For example, a young runner may be able to increase his or her mileage 10% per week normally. If the child has flat feet with decreased shock absorption, 10% per week may be overuse and result in patellofemoral pain or medial tibial pain. A list of anatomic malalignments and some of their possible sequelae is provided in Table 30-2.

Muscle–Tendon Imbalance. Overdevelopment of one muscle group without development of its antagonists can result in overuse injury. An extremely common occurrence in young basketball players is patellofemoral pain and overuse exacerbated by tight, weak hamstrings. Stretching the hamstrings may be all that is needed to end the knee pain. Unfortunately, the recent trend to more single-sport athleticism[49] and the lack of cross-training results in more muscle–tendon imbalance problems.

Psychologic Factors. The mind–body interaction always has a role in illness. In trauma or overuse injury, this interplay may seem less important, but not always. Reflex sympathetic dystrophy (RSD), especially around the knee, was virtually unknown in teenage athletes until several investigators began reporting this phenomenon,

TABLE 30-2 Common Anatomic Malalignments and Possible Resulting Sequelae from Overuse

Malalignment	Injuries	Prevention
Increased femoral anteversion	Hip pain, knee pain, snapping hip	Stretching, activity modification
Leg length inequality	Unilateral shin splints, patellofemoral stress, back pain	Heel lift
Internal tibial torsion	Knee pain	Orthotics
Patellar maltracking	Patellofemoral stress, subluxation	Selective VMO strengthening
Patella alta	Patellofemoral stress, subluxation	Bracing, VMO strengthening
Pes planus	Knee pain	Orthotics

especially in young women.[17,46,54] As in adult RSD, early aggressive treatment with physical therapy and gabapentin or amitriptyline leads to better results. Surgical intervention may exacerbate the problem.

Associated Disease State. Genetic or developmental anomalies and diseases can alter risk for overuse injury. Osteochondritis dissecans, Legg-Calvé-Perthes disease, and slipped capital femoral epiphysis are examples of tissue injury resulting from activity that normally would not be overuse. Although it may be many years before these conditions are completely understood, it is helpful to think of them in terms of at-risk patients with suboptimal tissues.

Gender. It is now conclusive that females are at greater risk for anterior cruciate ligament (ACL) tears than are males. Specifically within the sports of volleyball, soccer, and basketball, women are four to ten times more likely to sustain an ACL tear than are men.[3,27] Attempts to determine whether size of ACL, size of notch, hormones, menstrual cycle, muscle strength, conditioning, and jumping patterns are implicated are inconclusive. The current consensus is that landing patterns and muscle dynamics are most likely responsible.[30]

Extrinsic Risk Factors

Training or Technique Error. Training error is usually too much too soon of mileage, weight lifting, and so forth. It can also be poor technique, such as running on only one side of the road, effectively duplicating leg length discrepancy. Increasing training 10% per week seems to be optimal for avoiding overuse injuries in an otherwise healthy child.[41]

Improper Footwear or Gear. The wrong running shoes can lead to foot, knee, hip, or back pain. Manufacturers work to improve impact absorption quality of shoes while decreasing their weight.[9] Similarly, the wrong gear for a given athlete can precipitate an overuse injury. For example, large, adult-size soccer balls led to many lower extremity injuries in children, and we now have balls of several sizes and weights for different aged children.

Playing Surface. The hardness of the playing surface is causally related to early season shin splints and patellofemoral syndrome.[33] Traction qualities also factor into injury risk calculation. A comparison of natural grass to Astroturf showed significantly higher knee injury rates on the Astroturf.[48]

Nutrition. Intensive research to find performance-enhancing nutrition is underway by manufacturers. More important, however, is the lack of certain nutrients that some children have or the radical dietary practices of other children. All children, but especially females, may be calcium, vitamin D, and iron deficient.[66] Wrestlers may severely restrict fluid intake to make weight and have been shown to develop morphological changes as a result.[60] Drug and substance abuse can be placed in this category as well. Use of diuretics or anabolic steroids may directly and indirectly increase risk for overuse injury.[64]

Cultural Deconditioning. Twenty years ago, children engaged in free-play (usually outdoors) when they were not at school. Now that time is increasingly occupied with sedentary watching of television and playing with computers and video games.[50] Pediatric obesity has become an epidemic.[25,35] These factors create "weekend warriors" of children with all the overuse injuries formerly seen only in their parents.

SPECIFIC LOWER EXTREMITY INJURIES

Hip and Pelvis

Acute trauma about the hip and pelvis in the young athlete is common. Most injuries are contusions and minor muscle strains, but more serious injuries can occur. The most common of these is apophysis avulsion. This can easily be confused with a muscle strain but tends to resolve more slowly. Specific avulsions include sartorius pull-off at the anterosuperior iliac spine or rectus femoris avulsion at the anteroinferior iliac spine. The iliopsoas tendon may avulse the lesser trochanter, and the abdominal obliques may avulse their insertion on the ilium. All will occur as a result of a sudden force and are tender to palpation at the apophysis. Radiographs will show a widened apophyseal clear space and possibly soft-tissue swelling. Iliopsoas avulsion may result in extensive swelling and ecchymosis of the medial thigh.

Treatment is rest, application of ice, and gentle stretching of the involved muscles until resolution of symptoms in 4 to 6 weeks. Because some of the avulsions displaced more than a few millimeters can become chronically painful, operative repair is now being done more often. Rehabilitation involves continued stretching of the involved muscles and, most important, stretching of the antagonist muscles. Prevention requires adequate warm-up and stretching and identifying at-risk athletes. These are children in a growth spurt with generalized lower extremity tightness.

Hip and pelvis fractures and dislocations occasionally occur. These require stabilization and transport to a trauma center for emergent care by the orthopedic traumatologist.

Overuse injuries about the hip and pelvis are also common. Any of the sites of traumatic apophyseal avulsions may present as a chronic apophysitis. Diagnosis is similar to that of the avulsion, except that the radiographs may be normal. If necessary, a bone scan may be done and comparison made to the contralateral apophysis for relative increased uptake on the injured side. Treatment, rehabilitation, and prevention are similar to that for avulsions.

Tendinitis and bursitis occur about the hip. A snapping hip may be caused by the iliopsoas tendon, rectus femoris, or fascia lata. Trochanteric bursitis and snapping fascia lata may be the result of tight adductors and relative overuse of the abductors and hip extensors. Stretching the abductors and fascia lata, strengthening the core peripelvic muscles, and taking anti-inflammatories are frequently effective, but corticosteroid injection of the trochanteric bursa may be necessary. Refractory cases require surgical release.

Snapping psoas and rectus femoris tendons typically occur with hip flexion and external rotation maneuvers. The risk factors seem to be tight posterior capsule and lax anterior hip capsule combined with weak abdominal muscles and a lordotic spine. Primary treatment is rest and stretching of the psoas, quadriceps, hamstrings, and posterior hip capsule. Posture is corrected and abdominal muscles strengthened. Corticosteroid injection of the tendon sheath may be successful, but tendon recession or release may be necessary.

Stress fracture of the femoral neck occurs in young runners. Inguinal pain that persists warrants further investigation. Bone scan may be necessary to confirm the diagnosis. Treatment consists of decreasing activities until symptoms resolve and slowly returning to activities. If the stress fracture is on the superior side of the femoral neck, a screw is placed to prevent fracture.

Slipped capital femoral epiphysis occurs most commonly in preadolescent boys that tend to be overweight and during a growth spurt. Evidence exists that this physeal stress fracture occurs as a result of several factors, including genetic predisposition, hormonal influence, and orientation of the physis itself.[37] A large acute slip will be apparent on plain radiographs. Plain films will be negative in a preslip. Figure 30-2 shows a mild slip. Bone scan may show increased uptake compared with the contralateral physis. MRI may show fluid changes about the physis.[61] Treatment depends on the extent of the problem. Because of the consequences of a displaced physeal fracture, aggressive treatment is warranted. The child should be placed on crutches, and if the diagnosis is confirmed, hospitalization and transphyseal fixation is required. The contralateral hip should be thoroughly investigated because there is a 15% to 30% incidence of bilaterality.[37]

Legg-Calvé-Perthes disease results in avascular necrosis of portions of the femoral head. Figure 30-3 shows the radiographs of the progression of head necrosis. If diagnosed early and treated with decreased weight

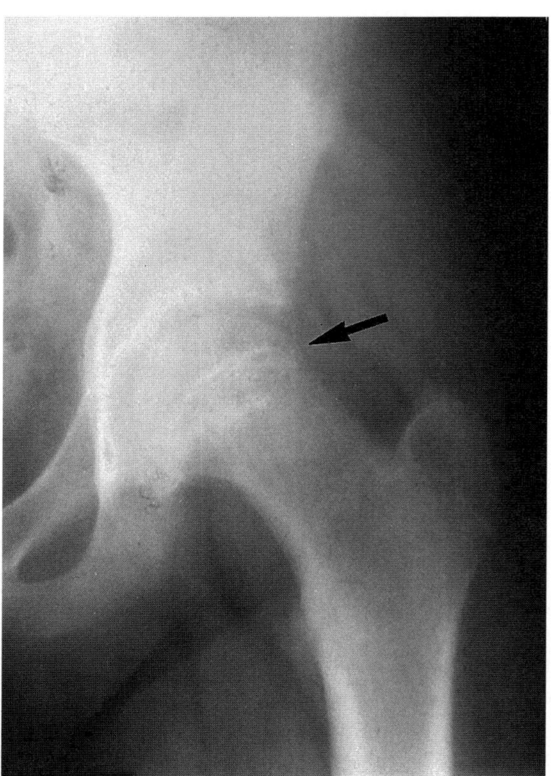

FIGURE 30-2. Radiograph of hip with slipped capital femoral epiphysis. The range of injury is from pre-slip (physeal injury without epiphyseal movement) to mild (1/3 head diameter slip), moderate (1/3 to 1/2 diameter slip), to severe (greater than 1/2 diameter slip). This would be graded as mild.

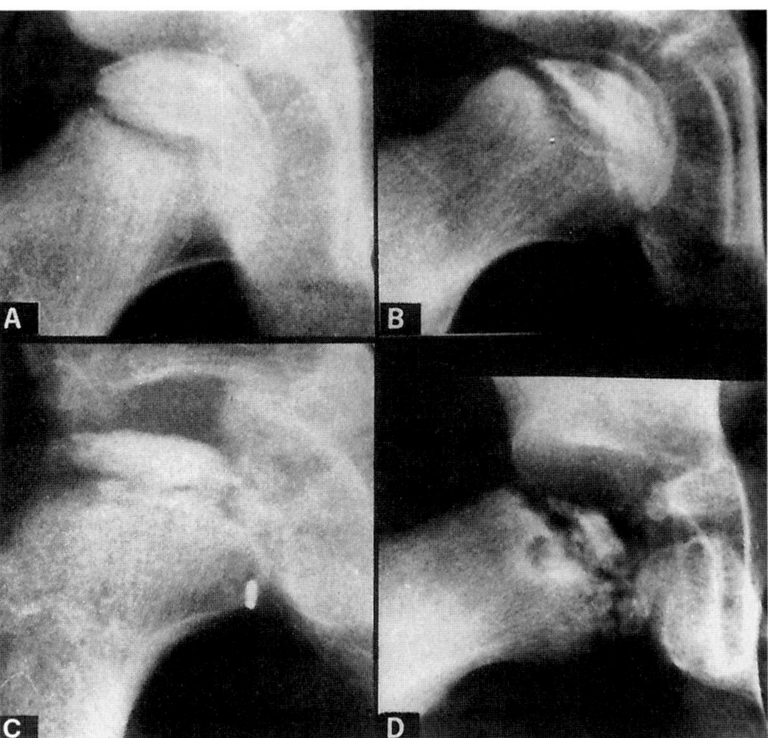

FIGURE 30-3. Radiographs of the progression of necrosis in Legg-Calvé-Perthes disease. The final stage (**D**) is fragmentation of the epiphysis with incongruity of the joint.

bearing, the head will reconstitute without serious sequelae.[47] Risk factors include low birth weight, male sex, and certain socioeconomic backgrounds.[38] Athletic participation is not necessary for the condition to occur. In a predisposed individual, however, athletic activity may amplify the problem.

Thigh and Femur

Acute trauma to the thigh will result in contusion, muscle tears, or femur fracture. Contusions are treated with rest, ice, compression, and elevation (RICE), and one must ensure that myositis ossificans does not develop. There is some evidence that oral nonsteroidal anti-inflammatories (NSAIDs) may help decrease myositis ossificans formation if given after 2 to 3 days of icing.[65]

Muscle strains (tears) occur with both concentric and eccentric muscle loading. Both the electrophysiological status of the muscle (e.g., amount of preexercise stretching) and the rate of muscle fiber loading appear to be causally related to these injuries. After RICE treatment, gentle stretching to maintain flexibility during healing is required. Full recovery can be expected in 4 to 6 weeks.

Overuse injury in the thigh is limited to occasional femur stress fractures. These can occur in runners, ballerinas, and other young athletes who place repetitive demands upon their lower extremities. Modifying the inciting activity will result in resolution of symptoms in a matter of weeks. Stretching the hamstrings and quadriceps may prevent recurrence. Water therapy has been extremely helpful in keeping these athletes in condition while allowing the stress fracture to heal.[34] It is essential to avoid dismissing inguinal or thigh pain as "growing pains."

Knee

The knee sustains more injuries than any other joint. It is useful to think of the knee in terms of its three articulating regions: the patellofemoral joint, the medial compartment, and the lateral compartment. Severe trauma can produce fracture of the femur, patella, or tibia, and may even cause dislocation of the tibia from the femur, a condition requiring thorough assessment of arterial patency after reduction. These topics are beyond the scope of this chapter, and the reader is directed to any of the standard orthopedic fracture texts for additional information. All require urgent (or in the case of dislocation, emergent) orthopedic consultation.

Trauma may also result in patella dislocation, ligament injuries, meniscal tears, and osteochondral fracture. Acute knee trauma in a young athlete is a frequent occurrence, and primary care clinicians caring for these athletes should be comfortable in its management. A diagnosis of "knee sprain" in a young athlete does not address the specific injury and may delay or circumvent appropriate care.

History. In the vast majority of knee injuries, the history alone will lead to the correct diagnosis. An athlete with a twisting injury to the knee resulting in a "pop" with rapid swelling and inability to continue playing has most likely torn the anterior cruciate ligament (ACL). We know that there is a high incidence of meniscal tear associated with ACL tear, so thorough meniscal examination is imperative.[4] This same type of injury without a distinctive "pop" or with more gradual swelling may be the result of a partial ACL tear or simply a meniscal tear.

Nonpainful giving way commonly indicates ACL laxity. Painful giving way may indicate patella subluxation. Locking of the knee, defined as inability to fully extend the joint, is caused by mechanical obstruction. Effusion may limit the final 10° of extension because of discomfort, but a torn meniscus flap, osteochondral fragment, or ACL stump may lock the knee at 30° or 40° of flexion. An acutely locked knee requires urgent referral to the sports medicine orthopedist. This type of internal derangement can only be managed operatively. Forcing the knee into extension (such as would occur by use of a knee immobilizer) can extend a meniscal tear or produce articular cartilage damage. A posterior splint with the knee in a comfortable position is far safer.

A pure varus or valgus stress may result in lateral or medial collateral ligament tear. These injuries may be isolated or occur with meniscus, cruciate, or osteochondral injury. A direct trauma to the knee followed by a "pop" and then another "pop" should be suspect for patellar dislocation and reduction. Before beginning the physical exam, the history should have led the examiner to search for patellofemoral, cruciate ligament, meniscal, and/or collateral ligament pathology.

Physical Examination. Much can be gained by simple inspection of the injured knee. The contralateral knee is almost always available for comparison. A large effusion will not be overlooked, but a small effusion might. A subtle fullness on either side of the injured-side patellar tendon might be the only finding. If the patient holds the knee in a position of flexion, this may indicate effusion or a locked knee.

Examination of the knee with post-traumatic effusion in a young athlete is directed by the history. If ACL tear is suspected, the ACL patency is examined last, because guarding may prevent further examination. Similarly, if patellofemoral injury is suspected by history, this is examined last to minimize pain. Whatever order of examination is chosen, the patellofemoral mechanism, medial structures, lateral structures, and cruciates need to be individually assessed.

An acute, post-traumatic effusion is always presumed to be hemarthrosis. Hemarthrosis may be caused by ligament tear, peripheral meniscus tear, patellar retinaculum tear, or fracture. Of these, only collateral ligament tears are usually treated nonoperatively. All other sources of acute hemarthrosis require consideration of surgical intervention and should be referred to a sports medicine orthopedist within 48 hours. Some confusion exists regarding the differentiation between effusion and edema. Effusion is always symmetric, versus edema, which is more superficial and focal. Edema may be caused by contusion, collateral ligament tears, bursitis, local infection, or other focal conditions. Traumatic effusion is caused by internal derangement. Range of motion, varus and valgus laxity at 30° of flexion, and Lachman or 30° anterior drawer tests should be performed. Joint line tenderness may be the only indicator of meniscal tear. McMurray test[39] will be positive for large tears but may be negative for smaller ones. Internal and external tibial rotation with the knee in full flexion stresses the posterior meniscal horns and can aid with meniscal tear diagnosis. The pivot shift[20] assesses the ACL and posterolateral capsule. Tests for the PCL include the sag,[10] reverse drawer,[10] and quad active test.[12] All these tests are the same in children as in adults and are performed similarly. If the effusion prevents one or more tests, aspiration with or without lidocaine injection can be performed, or one can wait 2 weeks and reevaluate.

Required radiographs are the same as for an adult. Anteroposterior, lateral, tunnel, and skyline views demonstrate all compartments and bony structures. A tibial eminence avulsion is an ACL tear equivalent and will be seen best on the tunnel view.[40] A lateral capsular sign (Segond fracture) frequently indicates that an ACL tear is also present.[28]

A knee may be locked because of a displaced osteochondral fracture fragment making range of motion testing contraindicated, so care must be taken when ordering radiographs for a locked knee. The technologist may try to force the knee into full extension to obtain a standard AP. Instructions should be given to the technician specifying what positions are possible with the particular knee.

Figure 30-4 provides an algorithm for assessment of post-traumatic effusion. Note that MRI is not mandatory and is used to solve diagnostic dilemmas. A primary care provider who has diagnosed an acute traumatic effusion has ample evidence of internal derangement by the effusion alone to obtain orthopedic consultation. MRI has become easier to obtain and less expensive and the information obtained is extensive. Prior to surgery, many surgeons will obtain an MRI to confirm the diagnosis.

Physical examination of the patellofemoral mechanism requires assessing each portion of the mechanism (Fig. 30-5). As in the adult, the quadriceps tendon, patella, medial and lateral retinaculae, and patellar tendon should be palpated. In the child, the tibial tubercle apophysis and distal pole of the patella should also be assessed. Dynamic tracking of the patella is evaluated. Hemarthrosis with a medial retinacular defect and pain indicates patella subluxation or dislocation. An acutely enlarged, painful tibial tubercle may indicate avulsion fracture.

Treatment. Locked knee, for whatever reason, is referred to the sports medicine orthopedist for prompt

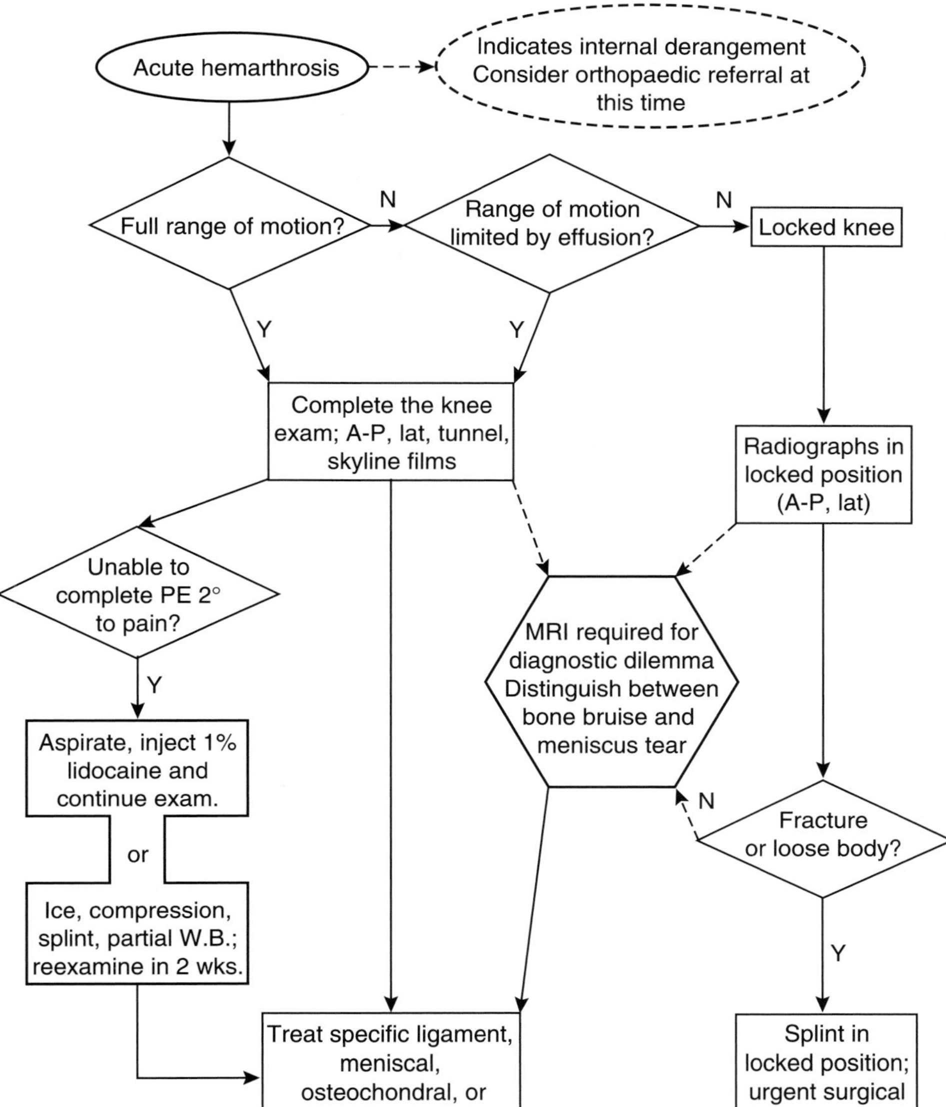

FIGURE 30-4. Algorithm for management of a traumatic effusion of the knee. Traumatic effusion is always presumed to be hemarthrosis, indicating internal derangement and requiring surgical consideration.

operative treatment. Non–weight bearing in a posterior splint with the knee in its locked position is appropriate. An NSAID may prolong bleeding and swelling and so is not a good option for initial pain relief.

An acute effusion also warrants orthopedic evaluation. As the effusion resolves over several weeks, the quadriceps muscles atrophy, altering the patellofemoral mechanics and making rehabilitation more difficult. Meniscal tears almost always require arthroscopic treatment. A reparable meniscus may become irreparable if the child further damages the torn portion during the delay. ACL tears may or may not require reconstruction, but they always require thorough evaluation and rehabilitation. A free osteochondral fragment must be replaced or removed promptly to avoid further chondral injury.

Patella dislocation, tibial tubercle avulsion, and tibial eminence avulsions may or may not require surgical intervention. Treatment recommendations are constantly evolving and depend on several variables.[21,26,31,40] All require orthopedic evaluation.

Rehabilitation after traumatic knee injury is quite specific, depending on the injury. This field is also constantly evolving, and in the past 15 years we have seen ACL reconstruction rehabilitation change dramatically. It was once felt that 6 weeks of immobilization in flexion and 1 year of physical therapy was required to achieve optimal results.[51] Now most surgeons utilize immediate postoperative continuous passive motion and full activities within 6 months.[52]

Prevention is yet another area in which exciting progress has been made. Several studies have now clearly

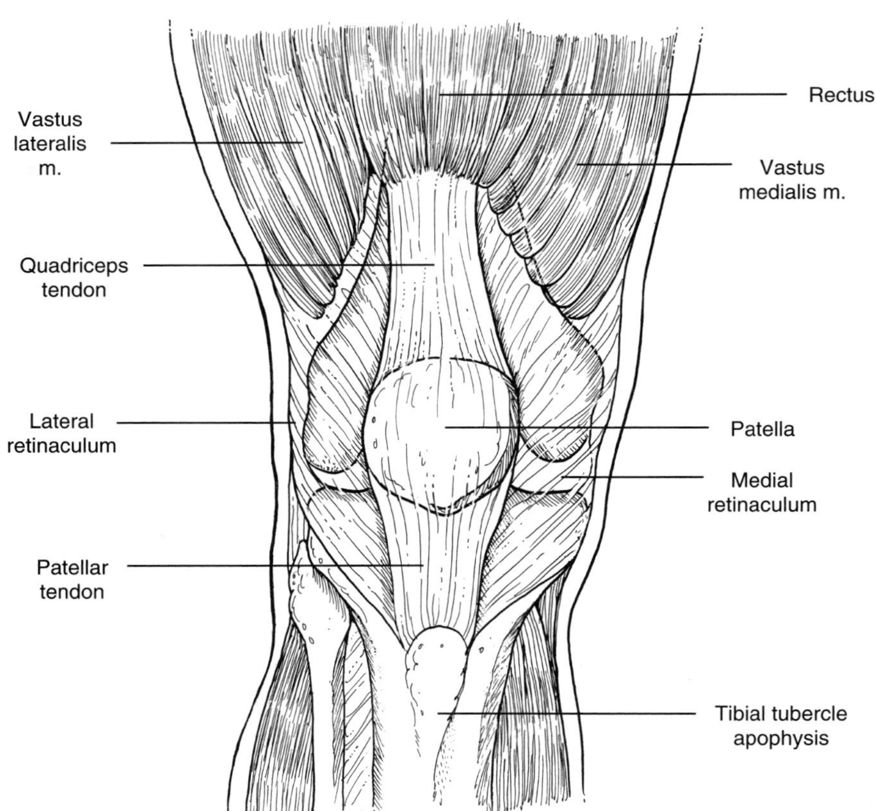

FIGURE 30-5. Anatomy of the extensor mechanism. Each component of the system is evaluated for its contribution to patellofemoral pain or dysfunction.

demonstrated that prophylactic knee bracing does not affect ACL injury rates.[7] This has resulted in considerable cost saving to youth sports teams. Recent and ongoing research into the variables that may predispose certain athletes to ACL tears is generating hypotheses that may aid in preventing some of these injuries.[30,57,58]

Overuse Knee Injuries

Overuse injuries about the knee in the young athlete usually result in extensor mechanism problems. The single other entity which may be regarded as an overuse injury in this age group is osteochondritis dissecans.

Osteochondritis Dissecans. Osteochondritis dissecans (OCD) is an osteochondral lesion of unknown etiology that may or may not result in knee pain. It is most commonly found on the medial femoral condyle weight bearing surface but may also be found on the lateral femoral condyle. The essential lesion is probably recurrent microtrauma to the subchondral bone. Eventually, the bone becomes damaged and blood flow is altered. The vascular insult to a portion of the condyle leads to avascular necrosis, possible fracture along the line of necrosis, and possible separation of the fragment.[22] Early in the process there is no pain or point tenderness, and radiographs of the knee or knees may only show a mottled appearance of the condyle. Continued running and jumping can lead to the avascular lesion that may or may not separate from the femur (Fig. 30-6). MRI shows more detail (Fig. 30-7).

Treatment depends on the stage of disease. If there is not a discrete lesion on imaging studies, simple rest will relieve symptoms and eventually result in normal condyle architecture. Achieving relative rest in this population may be difficult and require casting in extension simply to slow down the child. Focal lesions may require immobilization in extension or arthroscopic drilling if stable. Displaced or loose fragments require internal fixation with pins or screws. All efforts should be made to restore normal condylar architecture, and even long-standing free fragments can be successfully replaced in the young athlete, although they may have to be reshaped to fit the original defect.

Extensor Mechanism. Overuse injuries to the extensor mechanism can occur anywhere from the quadriceps to the tibial tubercle. Two force vectors are responsible for virtually all extensor mechanism problems. The first is the anteroposterior (AP) joint force. This force is proportional to the forces generated by the quadriceps muscles. These forces can be concentric, as in a jump, or eccentric, as in deceleration following a jump when landing. Tight hamstrings and/or quadriceps, such as

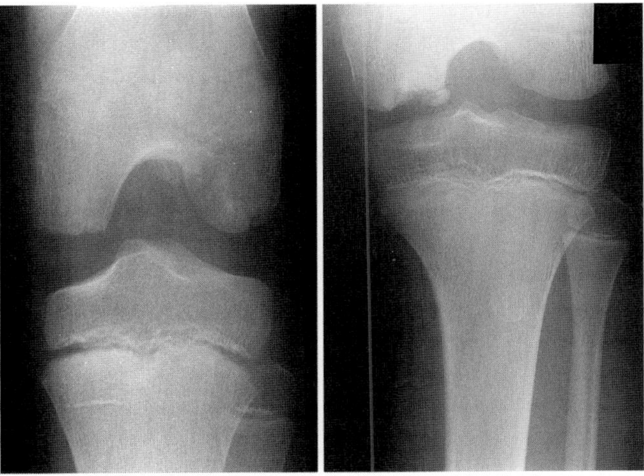

FIGURE 30-6. A, Radiograph of a patient with grade I osteochondritis dissecans (OCD) of the medial femoral condyle and grade II OCD of the lateral condyle. The appearance of the medial condyle can be associated with an asymptomatic as well as exquisitely tender knee. The process is felt to be localized osteomalacia from stress-induced hypervascularity. When the process becomes painful, subchondral microfractures are felt to have occurred. The lateral condyle with grade II OCD shows the avascular region. No displacement of the fragment is present. **B**, Grade III OCD with displacement of the osteochondral fragment.

typically occur during the growth spurts, exacerbate the problem. The cyclic loading of running, jumping, and other vigorous knee extension can lead to partial tendon avulsion at the distal pole of the patella (Sinding-Larsen-Johansson syndrome) (Fig. 30-8) or at the tibial tubercle (Osgood-Schlatter syndrome) (Fig. 30-9).

More difficult to diagnose and treat is peripatellar pain from AP force overload. The source of pain in this condition has remained elusive but is felt to be the medial and lateral patellar retinaculi and possibly the patellar subchondral bone itself.[13,18,19] The history will reveal pain with stair-climbing, after prolonged sitting, or after sports activities. Instead of point tenderness at the tendon or its insertion, there is diffuse tenderness along one or both sides of the patella and increased symptoms with the patella apprehension test[16] or with AP loading of the patella.

A second force vector that frequently leads to patellofemoral pain is excessive lateral pull of the quadriceps as opposed to medial pull. The more severe cases of lateral tracking will lead to recurrent subluxation or dislocation of the patella. The history may be similar to AP overload, but physical exam will demonstrate more lateral retinacular tenderness and will usually demonstrate lateral tracking and decreased patella mobility. If there is also medial retinaculum tenderness, care should be taken to check for a painful medial plica palpable as a tender medial band on flexion–extension. Excessive lateral tracking may pull a previously normal plica into

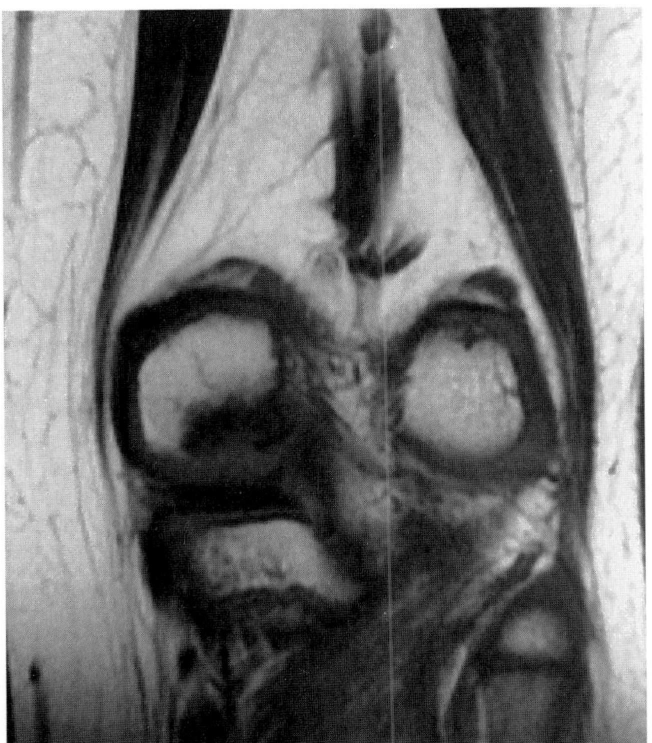

FIGURE 30-7. Magnetic resonance image of the grade III OCD in Figure 30-6B showing extensive edema or hypervascularity in the bone surrounding the areas of the defect.

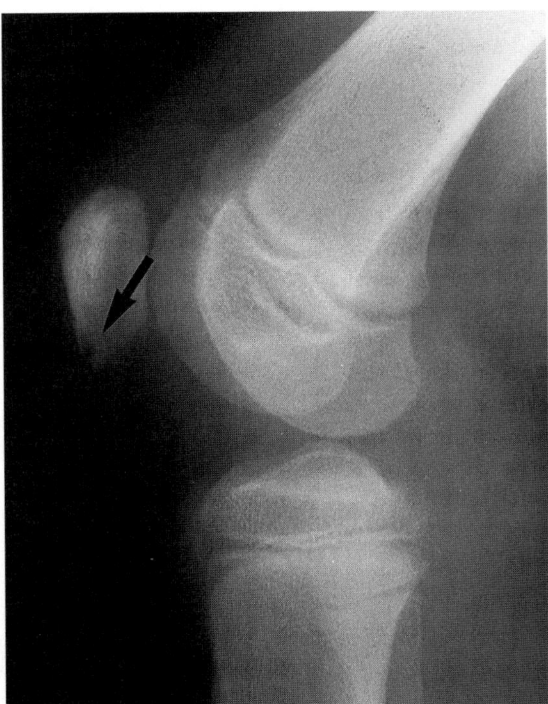

FIGURE 30-8. Sinding-Larsen-Johansson apophysitis of the distal pole of the patella.

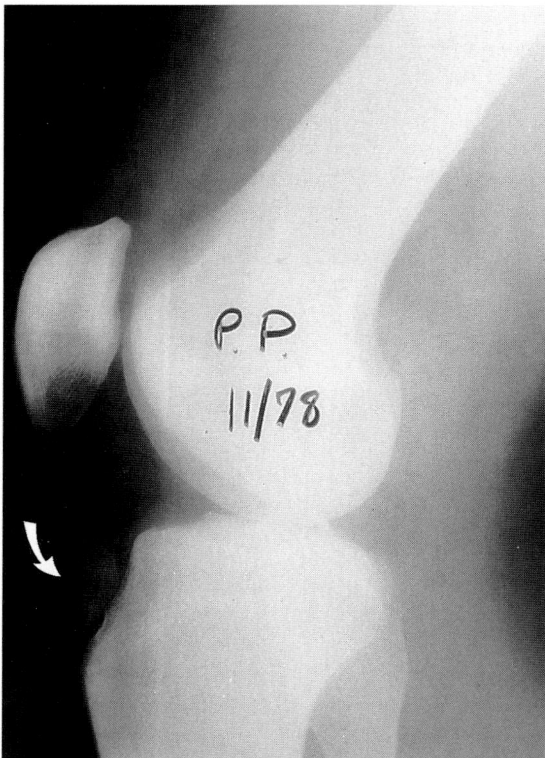

FIGURE 30-9. Osgood-Schlatter's apophysitis of tibial tubercle. Note apophyseal widening and tubercle enlargement.

CHECKLIST

Risk Factors Associated with Extensor Mechanism Pain from Anteroposterior and Lateral Force Overload

Normal alignment with excessive joint reaction forces

- ☐ Extrinsic
  - Training error
  - Hard playing surface
  - Poor footwear
- ☐ Intrinsic
  - Anatomic malalignment (patella alta or infera)
  - Muscle–tendon imbalance (tight hamstrings and/or quadriceps)

Laterally tracking patella

- ☐ Extrinsic
  - Training error ("whip kick" associated with breast stroke)
- ☐ Intrinsic
  - Muscle–tendon imbalance (overdeveloped lateral quads or underdeveloped vastus medialis obliquus)
  - Anatomic malalignment (internal tibial torsion, genu valgum, increased Q-angle, pes planus)

the medial femoral condyle, causing thickening and eventually fibrosis and inflammation.

A large quadriceps or Q-angle and varus–valgus anomalies of the knee may influence patellofemoral stresses, but the significance of these measures is controversial.[16] Evidence of excessive lateral compression may be demonstrated on the skyline view radiograph, but these films are difficult to standardize in a nonresearch setting and, at best, give a static view of a dynamic problem.[14] The box lists risk factors associated with both types of patellofemoral stress overload.

Of special interest is patella alta, a growth spurt–related phenomenon in which the patellar tendon portion of the extensor mechanism elongates more than the quadriceps tendon portion. This leaves the patella higher in the femoral sulcus with increased distal pole compressive forces and greater risk for lateral subluxation in extension. Patella alta is a condition that can exacerbate both AP and lateral patellofemoral stress overload.

Treatment of patellofemoral stress syndrome is based on the specific etiology. With normal tracking and AP overload, emphasis is on hamstring stretching, quad stretching, and decreased running, jumping, and stair-climbing. Symptoms should resolve over several weeks. For lateral tracking, AP forces are decreased and emphasis is on selective vastus medialis obliquus strengthening to dynamically pull the patella medially.[45] Braces that centralize the patella are sometimes helpful.[53] Bands that alter the fulcrum of the patellofemoral mechanism may help.[36]

Despite adequate physical therapy and bracing, it is not always possible to relieve symptoms in a laterally tracking patella. Arthroscopic lateral retinacular release may be necessary to achieve balanced, centralized tracking.[43] For more severe tracking problems or recurrent subluxation or dislocations, lateral release is combined with medial reefing and possible tibial tubercle repositioning.[11] In any of these procedures, the goal is to visualize corrected, centralized tracking during the operation. If true chondromalacia of the retropatellar surface has already developed, it may not be possible to restore the knee to a totally pain-free status.

Other extensor mechanism problems include isolated medial plica syndrome, usually caused by a direct medial blow,[32] and lateral tracking patella. Sinding-Larsen-Johansson syndrome and Osgood-Schlatter's apophysitis are treated precisely the same as normal tracking patellar overload with hamstring and quadriceps stretching, local application of ice acutely and then heat subsequently, and relative rest of the mechanism to restore the pain-free state. As in osteochondritis dissecans, it is occasionally necessary to immobilize overactive youngsters in a cylinder cast to achieve relative rest.

A blow to the medial knee or recurrent patella subluxation may produce inflammation and tenderness in a previously normal medial plica. Examination may elicit a tender focal band of tissue snapping over the medial femoral condyle during knee flexion–extension. If this does not resolve with patella bracing, quad strengthening, oral anti-inflammatories, and arthroscopic debridement is necessary. Occasionally corticosteroid injection into the thickened plica tissue may be effective. An algorithm for evaluation and treatment of patellofemoral pain is presented in Figure 30-10. Repeat examinations may be necessary to fully understand the particular risk factors and etiology.

Other Knee Overuse Problems. When the quadriceps are tight relative to the hamstrings and there is selective adductor or abductor overuse, pes anserinus or iliotibial band bursitis may occur. In pes bursitis, the pes attachment

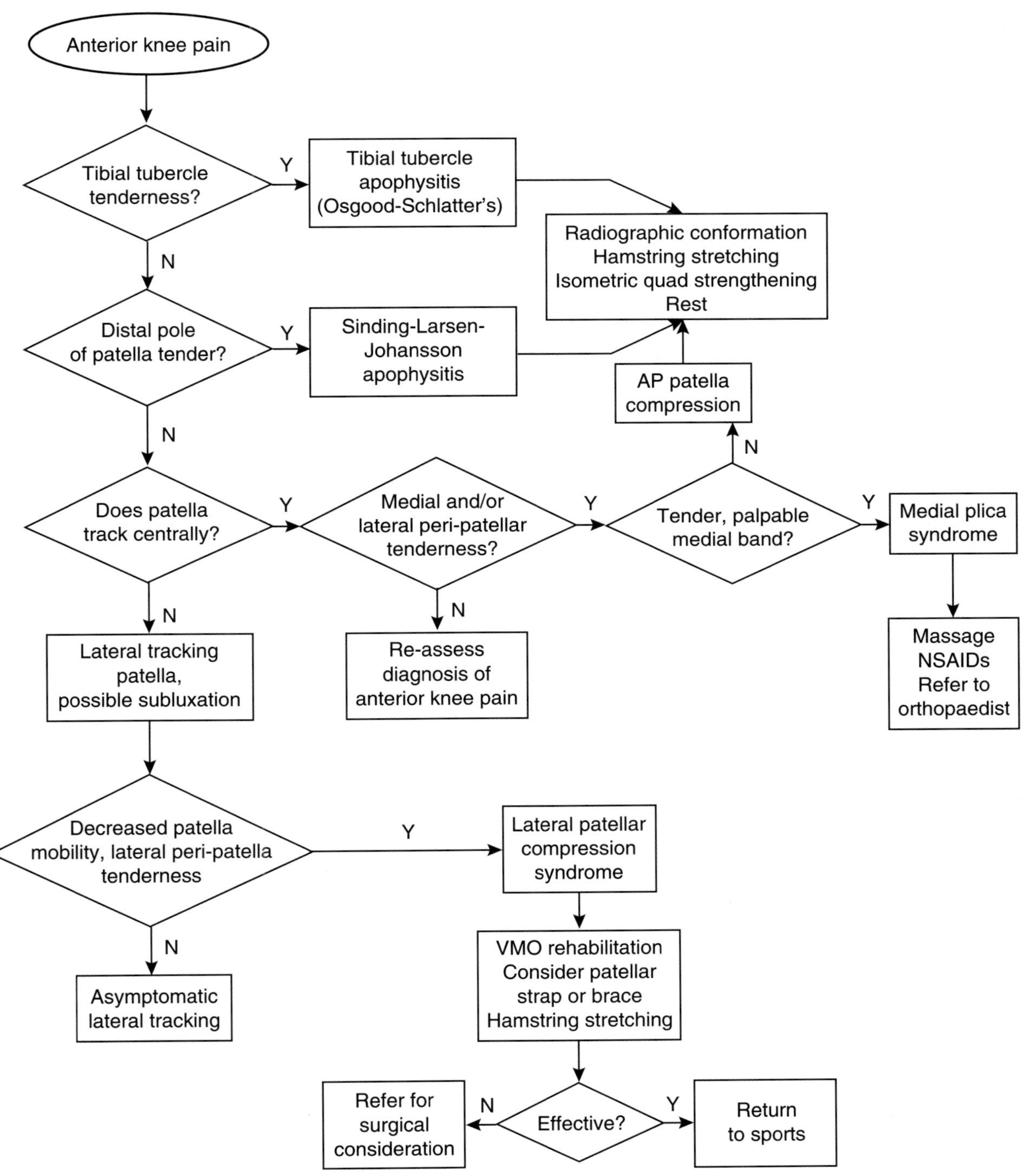

FIGURE 30-10. Algorithm for evaluation and management of knee extensor mechanism pain. Focused treatment based on specific etiology will prevent recurrence.

on the anterior medial tibia is tender to palpation, and there may be palpable fluctuance of the underlying bursa. Similarly, the iliotibial band may be tender laterally, and pain may be exacerbated by adduction stretching of the lateral thigh soft tissues.

Treatment for either condition consists of oral anti-inflammatories, postexercise ice massage, and gentle passive stretching of the affected structures and the antagonist structures. Any relative muscle strength or tightness imbalance should be corrected. Other identified risk factors need to be eliminated or modified. If symptoms persist, the bursa can be injected with a corticosteroid.

Lower Leg

Acute trauma to the leg usually results in contusion but occasionally will cause fracture. Contusions are treated with rest, ice, compression, and elevation for the first 48 to 72 hours. NSAIDs may decrease the incidence of myositis ossificans, but starting them immediately may prolong bleeding and increase swelling.

Tibial fractures in children rarely require surgical management. Physeal injury must be considered, and if a nondisplaced Salter-Harris Type I physeal fracture is suspected (point tenderness at the physis and a normal x-ray), it is better to treat it aggressively with casting until the pain resolves. The low-energy type of tibial fractures that young athletes sustain are readily treated with casting and subsequent rehabilitation. All fractures should be referred to the orthopedist. Any acute trauma can result in excessive swelling to the point where venous outflow is blocked. This condition is tibial compartment syndrome and must be arrested immediately before tissue necrosis occurs. Any post-traumatic extremity that is swollen and elicits pain to passive motion of, for example, a toe, should be emergently referred for compartment syndrome evaluation of the classic five Ps: pain, pallor, paresthesias, pulselessness, and paralysis. Only pain is present before permanent damage has occurred.

Overuse injuries of the leg have been collectively referred to as "shin splints" and are actually one of three types of injury. Lower leg pain may be caused by periostitis, stress fracture, or diffuse compartment swelling. Distinguishing among these conditions is an important skill and requires precise history, physical examination, and imaging studies.

A young athlete with leg pain brought on by exercise should be questioned about the nature of the pain. The pain of exertional compartment syndrome is debilitating pain that intensifies as the workout progresses. The pain usually dissipates over several minutes after cessation of activity. Stress fractures and periostitis tend to cause pain continuously during the activity. Symptoms may intensify over a period of days to weeks, but not usually within an exercise period. Discriminating between stress fracture and periostitis is more difficult, especially because periostitis frequently precedes a stress fracture. Fibular point tenderness is usually a stress fracture or impending stress fracture. Tibia pain may be focal or diffuse and may occur medially or laterally. Focal pain is more likely to be stress fracture, diffuse pain periostitis. Indirect, three-point bending forces applied to the tibia may increase stress fracture pain but should not increase periostitis symptoms. Young runners classically develop a stress fracture of the distal fibula just proximal to the ankle syndesmosis after increasing their mileage.[62] Lateral tibial periostitis arises from tibialis anterior overuse, and medial periostitis from tibialis posterior and soleus overuse.[59]

Resisted ankle dorsiflexion exacerbates lateral tibial periostitis, and resisted pronation and eversion exacerbates medial tibial periostitis. A tight Achilles tendon and strong gastroc-soleus muscles frequently accompany lateral tibial periostitis. Imaging studies for tibial periostitis and stress fractures begin with plain radiographs. Early on, these will be normal, but after 3 or more weeks, diffuse (periostitis) or focal (stress fracture) periosteal reaction may be present. It may be necessary to obtain imaging confirmation of either diagnosis. Some children (or their parents) will be noncompliant without hard evidence, and treatment will vary depending on the precise etiology. A bone scan will show focal uptake for stress fracture, whereas in periostitis there is diffuse activity (Fig. 30-11). MRI has shown fluid changes associated with both conditions in different patterns.[59] If the sensitivity and specificity of MRI are eventually found to be comparable to bone scan, this may become the diagnostic tool of choice.

Relative rest is employed for the treatment of periostitis and stress fractures. Stress fractures will usually heal following 4 to 6 weeks of painless ambulation. Casting is

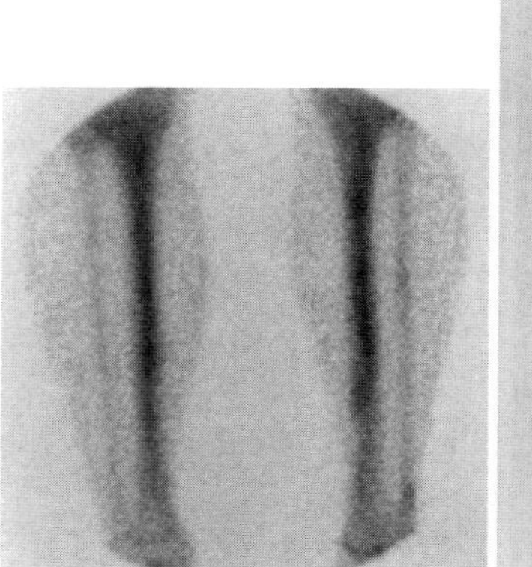

A

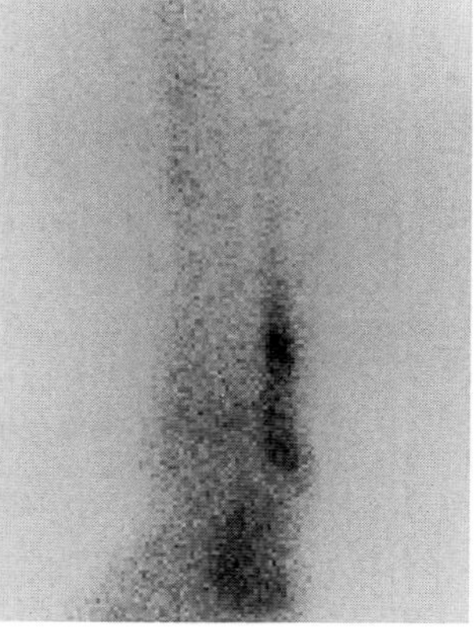

B

FIGURE 30-11. A, Periostitis of both tibiae in a runner. Isotope uptake is all among anterior tibiae, as is tenderness. **B**, Fibular stress fracture showing focal uptake by Tc99m bone scan. Indirect force on fibula elicits pain.

not necessary unless an overt fracture occurs or the child cannot be rested any other way. A tibial coaption brace can decrease pain and potentially speeds healing. Once again, NSAIDs may not be optimal pain relievers for stress fractures because their antiprostaglandin effects theoretically slow bone healing. Once pain and point tenderness have resolved, the child can progress as tolerated to his or her activities. Training error is the most common risk factor for stress fracture, and applying the "10% increase per week" limit on training should prevent recurrence.

In addition to relative rest, periostitis requires identification of risk factors and specific physical therapy. Lateral tibial periostitis is exacerbated by running hills or stairs, by a tight Achilles tendon, or by other situations requiring overuse of the tibialis anterior for ankle dorsiflexion. Likewise, poor running shoes, concrete surfaces, and activities demanding more shock absorption from pronation will overstress the tibialis posterior. These risk factors can be the major cause of medial tibial periostitis. Stretching the gastroc-soleus complex, avoiding repetitive dorsiflexion, and ice massage after activity will aid healing of lateral symptoms. Orthotics help with medial periostitis. Surgery is rarely indicated for these conditions.

If exertional compartment syndrome is suspected, an exercise stress test is done by having the patient exercise until symptoms occur. The anterior, lateral, posterior, deep posterior, and posterior tibial compartments are palpated for tenderness. Objective tests require taking compartment pressure measurements at rest and at 1 and 2 minutes after exercise. A compartment pressure 30 to 40 mm Hg above resting pressure at 1 minute after exercise is abnormal.[1]

A condition that presents similarly to exertional compartment syndrome is muscle hernia through a fascial defect in the leg. A fascial defect may be palpable, and compartment pressures may be elevated after exercise.

Both exertional compartment syndrome and fascial hernia are treated the same. Conservative attempts can be made at deep myofascial massage and slow increase of running distance to avoid the painful threshold. If these treatments fail, and they frequently do, the fascia must be released. In contrast with post-traumatic compartment syndrome, the skin does not have to be widely incised and left open. Only the affected compartments need to be released, and early return to activities is necessary to avoid "bridging" scar formation along the line of release. Operative release is rarely necessary in children and is done only after a positive compartment stress test.

Most fascia hernias are felt to result from high compartment pressures, so closure of the defect will exacerbate the problem. Occasionally, a traumatic fascial defect can be repaired without resulting in exertional compartment syndrome, but this is risky. Full release as in exertional compartment syndrome is typically required. An algorithm for diagnosis and management of shin splints is presented in Figure 30-12.

Foot and Ankle

Trauma to the juvenile athlete about the foot and ankle can cause fracture, dislocation, physeal injury, or ligament sprains. The common inversion ankle injury that causes anterior talofibular ligament tears in the adult commonly results in a nondisplaced Salter-Harris Type I physeal fracture of the distal fibula in the immature athlete. Radiographs are normal. Physical examination elicits tenderness at the distal fibula and possibly also to the lateral ligaments. Experimental work is being done with MRI to identify these injuries,[56] but at present the diagnosis remains a clinical one. In an inversion ankle sprain of any magnitude, the distal fibula itself should not be tender. If it is, physeal fracture must be presumed and treated with 3 weeks of casting with partial weight bearing. If at 3 weeks the tenderness is gone, physical therapy may be begun to restore motion, peroneal strength, and ankle proprioception. If symptoms persist, further casting is required. Follow-up radiographs may be necessary at 3 to 6 month intervals to watch for premature physeal closure.

Routine ankle sprains are treated as adult injuries with the RICE routine initially, followed as quickly as possible (within days) with weight bearing as tolerated. A stirrup Aircast (Summit, New Jersey) splint is helpful in restoring crutch-free ambulation within 1 to 2 weeks. Physical therapy is also begun immediately, and full competition is permitted once symmetrical proprioception and balance have returned. Prophylactic taping does have a place in competition and during the recuperation period.[23]

One possible complication of ankle sprain is chondral or osteochondral injury of the talar dome. This usually occurs on the anterolateral corner or centromedial ridge of the dome. The youngster may complain of ankle sprain that never resolves or may not ever recall a sprain. Physical examination will elicit point tenderness on the talar dome anterolaterally with the foot in plantarflexion, or there may be anterior or posterior tenderness medially on the dome. Radiographs will be normal or show a small osteochondral injury to either corner (Fig. 30-13). MRI will show much more extensive damage to the talus (Fig. 30-14). Treatment is by arthroscopic debridement and drilling. Occasionally, a fragment will be large enough to repair, but this is unusual. A medial injury frequently requires a small posterior arthrotomy to excise the symptomatic chondral flap. Despite this treatment, permanent ankle pain can result.

An ankle sprain that is slow to heal may also be what trainers call a "high" ankle sprain. This is a tear of the anterior tibiofibular syndesmosis ligament and can take 8 to 12 weeks or longer to resolve. Tenderness is found at the area of syndesmosis just proximal to the ankle joint,

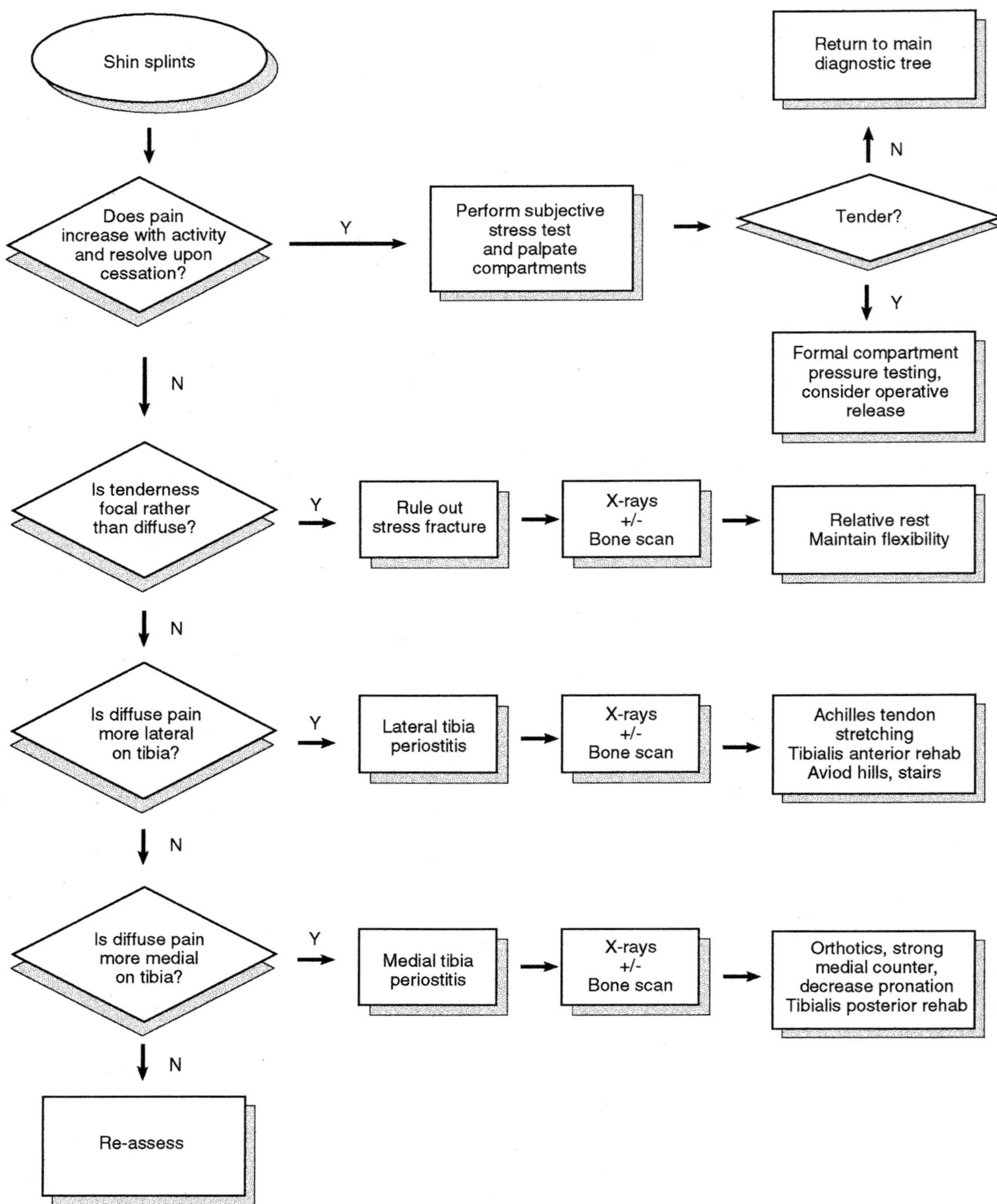

FIGURE 30-12. Algorithm for evaluation and management of shin splints.

and mediolateral compression of the leg above the ankle will be painful. If widening of the syndesmosis is seen on the mortise view of the ankle, AP and lateral views of the entire leg must be obtained to rule out a proximal fibular fracture (Maisonneuve fracture) (Fig. 30-15). Complete syndesmosis disruptions require operative repair with transmalleolar screw fixation. Partial tears require up to 12 weeks of immobilization and protected weight training.

Management of fractures about the ankle requires detailed knowledge of the bony and soft-tissue anatomy. A fracture may appear relatively innocuous on radiographs but may have interposed periosteum preventing proper healing. Medial malleolus and juvenile Tillaux fractures are such examples.[5] Both usually require open reduction and internal fixation.

In the foot, eversion trauma may cause fracture of the navicular apophysis leading to painful accessory navicular.

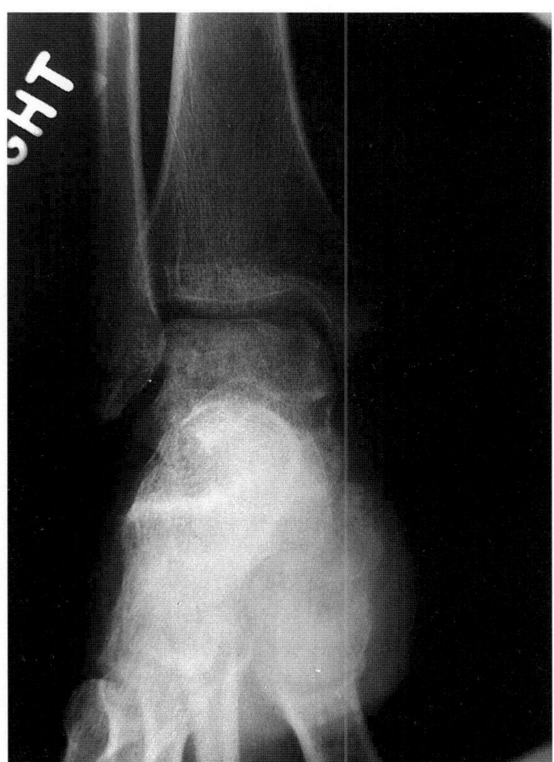

FIGURE 30-13. Osteochondral injury to the medial talar dome in an adult. Note the disuse osteopenia that resulted from prolonged immobilization.

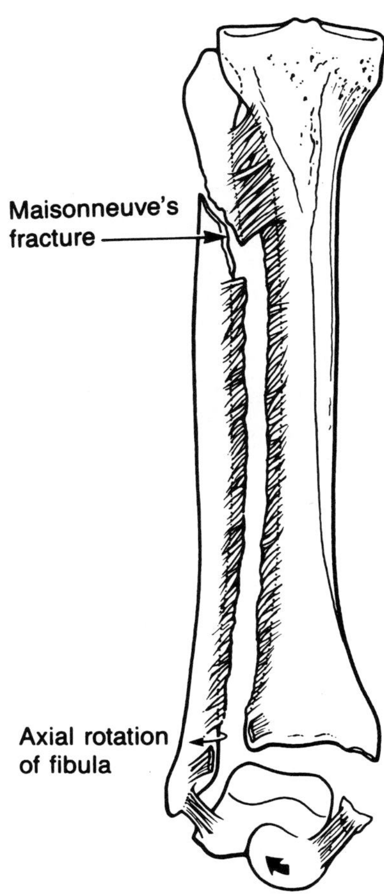

FIGURE 30-15. Drawing of the leg depicting the classic Maisonneuve proximal fibula fracture and its mechanism of injury.

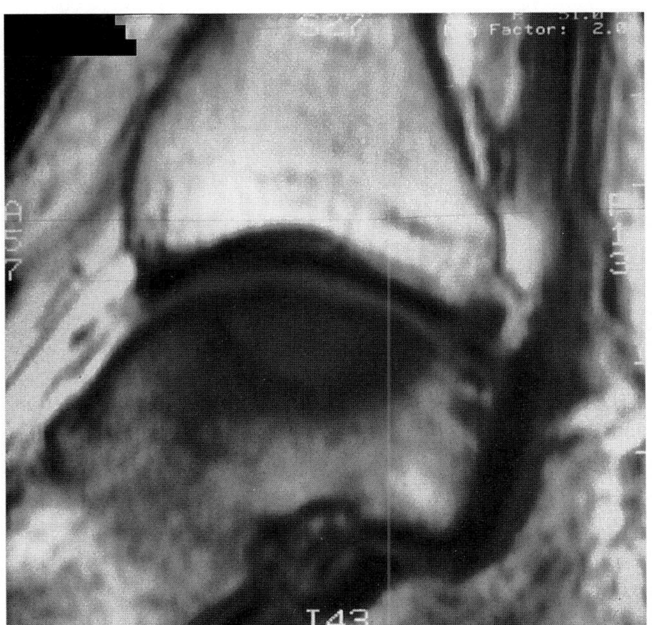

FIGURE 30-14. MRI of a talar dome osteochondritis dissecans lesion.

These may heal and become nontender or can require excision.

Overuse injuries in the ankle and foot include stress fracture, apophysitis, avascular necrosis, plantar fasciitis, and painful accessory ossicle. Stress fractures of almost every bone of the foot have been reported, but most frequently include the sesamoids, metatarsals, and calcaneus. Diagnosis and treatment are similar to other lower extremity stress fractures. Prevention entails identifying and eliminating risk factors.

As in the knee, muscle–tendon overuse in the child produces apophysitis rather than tendinitis. Most common is Achilles tendon apophysitis at the calcaneal insertion, or Sever's disease. This is felt to be a stress injury to the physis caused by overpull of a tight, strong triceps surae. Avoiding running and jumping will resolve pain and, over time, radiographs will show resolution of the increased opacification of apophysis.

Pain, point tenderness, and opacification of the tarsal navicular bone are the hallmarks of Köhler's bone disease. Radiographs show opacification and collapse of the navicular bone (Fig. 30-16) and MRI shows changes

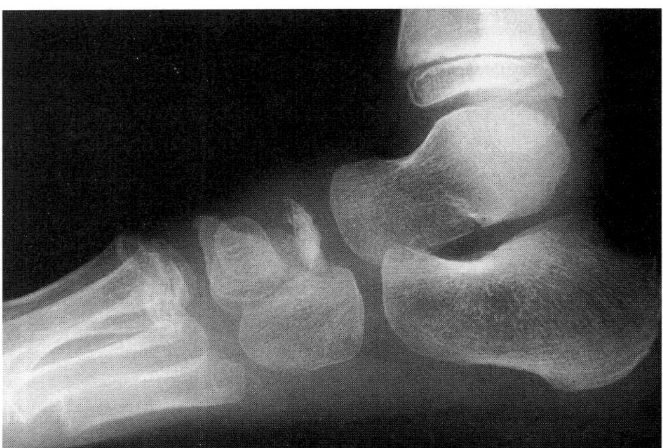

FIGURE 30-16. Köhler's avascular necrosis of the tarsal navicular bone.

consistent with avascular necrosis (AVN). The condition is felt to occur from overuse in predisposed individuals. Even when there is collapse of the navicular, virtually all resolve over 8 months with rest of the foot. Casting for 12 weeks may speed healing.[29]

A similar osteochondrosis is Freiberg's infarction, or AVN of the metatarsal head (usually the second metatarsal). Localized pain is the usual complaint, and radiographs typically show opacification and irregularity of the head consistent with AVN (Fig. 30-17). As in Köhler's bone disease, repetitive microtrauma in a predisposed youngster is felt to be causative.[55] Treatment consists of metatarsal padding or orthotics with relative rest. Three to 4 weeks of casting may be required to relieve symptoms. Collapse of a metatarsal head may not resolve spontaneously and harmlessly. In this regard, Freiberg's infarction behaves more like Legg-Calvé-Perthes disease of the hip rather than Köhler's disease. Chronic pain and degenerative arthritis may follow Freiberg's infarction, requiring surgical intervention.

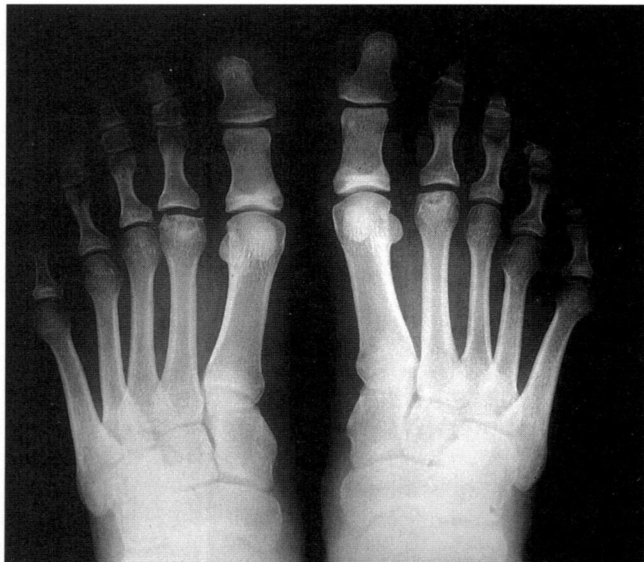

FIGURE 30-17. Freiberg's infarction of the second metatarsal head.

Bony anatomic variations can also lead to overuse problems. In the adolescent foot, these include adolescent bunion, tarsal coalition, and os trigonum. Bunion may be symptomatic in any adolescent, but the demands of competition may exacerbate pain. Initially, treatment consists of footwear modifications and padding, possibly including orthotics. Surgery is reserved for those with persistent symptoms, and many procedures exist for varying amounts of deformity.[63]

Tarsal coalition encompasses bony or fibrous unions of the calcaneus to the talus or cuboid or of the talus to the navicular. Other coalitions are reported but are less common.[44] In the child, presenting symptoms may be rearfoot pain associated with increased activity. Physical examination will show limited or absent subtalar motion and tenderness in the medial or lateral hindfoot. Pes planus is a common associated finding. Routine radiographs are almost always read as negative, but a Harris axial view can demonstrate a talocalcaneal coalition (Fig. 30-18). Computed tomography in the sagittal and coronal planes will best demonstrate the bony relationships (Fig. 30-19).[67]

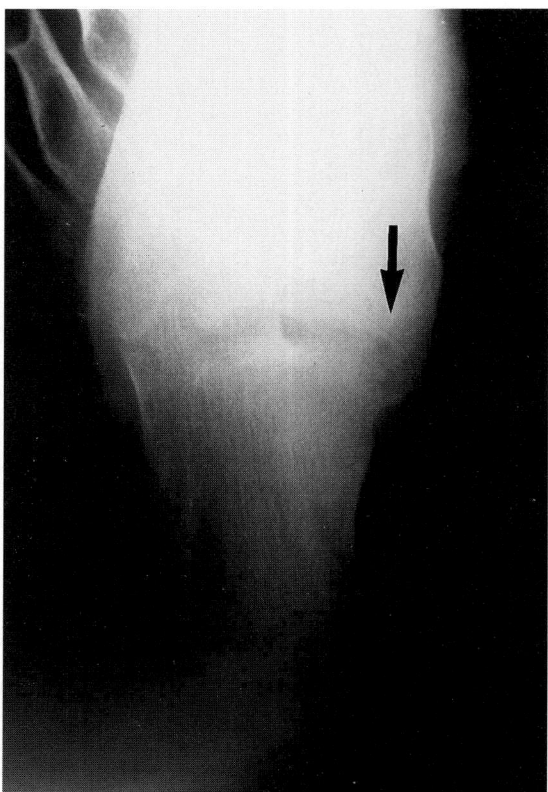

FIGURE 30-18. Harris axial view of the heel showing talocalcaneal coalition *(arrow).*

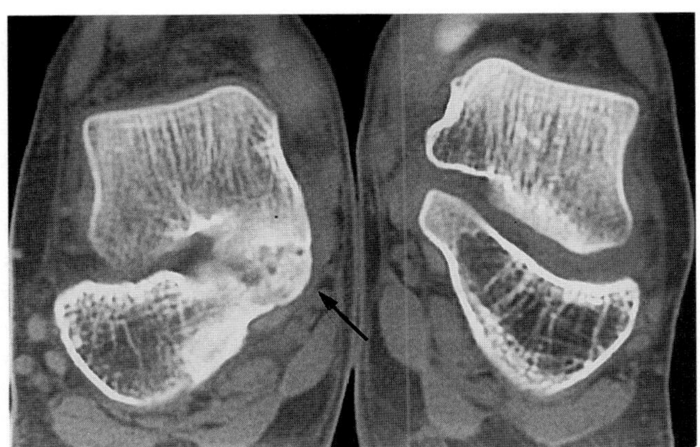

FIGURE 30-19. Computerized tomogram shows talocalcaneal coalition with better detail *(arrow)*. Contralateral foot has normal talocalcaneal joint.

Rest and orthotics may resolve symptoms, but permanent correction requires resection of the bony or fibrous bridge. Long-term results of resection are generally good to excellent with much improved motion.[44]

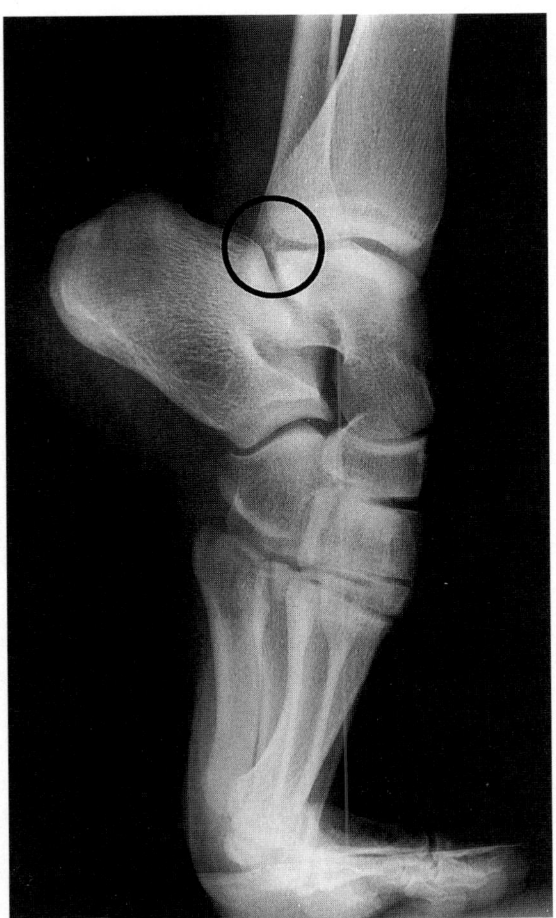

FIGURE 30-20. Radiograph of ankle in demi-pointe. Small os trigonum is seen at center of circle and was responsible for painful impingement in maximal plantarflexion.

Flat feet are common and not usually symptomatic. Because pronation accounts for some shock absorption during running, lack of effective pronation can be a risk factor for overuse injury. Altering the training schedule, obtaining running shoes with a strong medial counter, and utilizing orthotics to regain some of the shock absorption of controlled pronation can be helpful.

Os trigonum tarsi is a normal variant but becomes symptomatic in ballerinas who must achieve and maintain pointe. In this position, the accessory ossicle impinges the posterior ankle capsule (Fig. 30-20) and, if symptomatic, requires excision.

SUMMARY

Lower extremity injuries in children and adolescents include most of those found in adults and also include the apophysitises, osteochondritises, and physeal injuries. The young athlete has unique risk factors associated with both growth and the different mechanical properties of bone, cartilage, and collagen as compared with the adult. Adequate diagnosis and treatment requires detailed knowledge of these properties and risk factors. Despite the knowledge that youngsters heal readily and generally do not suffer long-term sequelae from imprecise diagnosis, this situation is changing. Single-sport athletes and high-demand sports are resulting in more and more debilitating injuries. Identifying risk factors and preventing recurrence is essential to providing quality care.

REFERENCES

1. Abramowitz AJ, Schepsis AA: Chronic exertional compartment syndrome of the lower leg. Orthop Review 23(3):219–225, 1994.
2. Andersen P, Henriksson J: Training induced changes in the subgroups of human type II skeletal muscle fibres. Acta Physiol Scand 99(1):123–125, 1977.
3. Arendt E, Dick R: Knee injury patterns among men and women in collegiate basketball and soccer. NCAA data and review of literature. Am J Sports Med 23(6):694–701, 1995.
4. Balkfors B: The course of knee-ligament injuries. Acta Orthop Scand 198(Suppl):1–99, 1982.
5. Beaty JH, Linton RC: Medial malleolar fracture in a child. A case report. J Bone Joint Surg 70A(8): 1254–1255, 1988.
6. Bollet AJ: Analgesic and anti-inflammatory drugs in therapy of osteoarthritis. Semin Arthritis Rheum 11(1 Suppl):130, 1981.
7. Brewster CE, et al: Rehabilitation of the knee. In Nicholas JA, Hershman EB (eds): The Lower Extremity and Spine in Sports Medicine, 2nd ed. St. Louis, Mosby–Year Book, 1995.

8. Carter DR, Hayes WC: Compact bone fatigue damage: A microscopic examination. Clin Orthop 127:265–274, 1977.
9. Cavanagh PR: The Running Shoe Book. Mountain View, CA, Anderson World, 1980.
10. Clancy WG Jr, et al: Treatment of knee joint instability secondary to rupture of the posterior cruciate ligament: Report of a new procedure. J Bone Joint Surg 65A(3):310–322, 1983.
11. Cox JS: Evaluation of the Roux-Elmslie-Trillat procedure for knee extensor realignment. Am J Sports Med 19(5):303–310, 1982.
12. Daniel DM, et al: Use of the quadriceps active test to diagnose posterior cruciate-ligament disruption and measure posterior laxity of the knee. J Bone Joint Surg 70A(3):386–391, 1988.
13. Darracott J, Vernon-Roberts B: The bony changes in "chondromalacia patellae." Rheumatol Phys Med 11(4):175–179, 1971.
14. Delgado-Martins H: A study of the position of the patella using computerized tomography. J Bone Joint Surg 61B(4):443–444, 1979.
15. Ebbeling CB, Clarkson PM: Exercise-induced muscle damage and adaptation. Sports Med 7(4): 207–234, 1989.
16. Fairbank JC, et al: Mechanical factors in the incidence of knee pain in adolescents and young adults. J Bone Joint Surg 66B(5):685–693, 1984.
17. Forster RS, Fu FH: Reflex sympathetic dystrophy in children. A case report and review of literature. Orthopedics 8(4):475–477, 1985.
18. Fulkerson JP, et al: Histologic evidence of retinacular nerve injury associated with patellofemoral malalignment. Clin Orthop 197:196–205, 1985.
19. Fulkerson JP. Diagnosis and treatment of patients with patellofemoral pain. Am J Sports Med 30(3): 447–456, 2002.
20. Galway RD, Beaupre A, MacIntosh DL: Pivot shift: A clinical sign of symptomatic anterior cruciate ligament insufficiency. J Bone Joint Surg 54B(4):763, 1972.
21. Garcia A, Neer CS: Isolated fractures of the intercondylar eminence of the tibia. Am J Surg 95: 593–598, 1958.
22. Garrett JC: Osteochondritis dissecans. Clin Sports Med 10(3):569–593, 1991.
23. Garrick JG, Requa RK: Role of external support in prevention of ankle sprains. Med Sci Sports Exerc 5(3):200–203, 1973.
24. Goodship AE, Lanyon LE, McFie H: Functional adaptation of bone to increased stress. An experimental study. J Bone Joint Surg 61A(4):539–546, 1979.
25. Gortmaker SL, et al: Increasing pediatric obesity in the United States. Am J Dis Child 141(5):535–540, 1987.
26. Gronkvist H, Hirsch G, Johansson CL: Fracture of the anterior tibial spine in children. J Pediatr Orthop 4(4):465–468, 1984.
27. Henry JC, Kaeding C: Neuromuscular differences between male and female athletes. Curr Womens Health Rep 1(3):241–244, 2001.
28. Hess T, et al: Lateral tibial avulsion fractures and disruptions to the anterior cruciate ligament. A clinical study of their incidence and correlation. Clin Orthop 303:193–197, 1994.
29. Ippolito E, Ricciardi-Pollini PT, Falez F: Köhler's disease of the tarsal navicular: Long-term follow-up of 12 cases. J Pediatr Orthop 4(4):416–417, 1984.
30. Ireland ML. The female ACL: Why is it more prone to injury? Orthop Clin North Am 33(4):637–651, 2002.
31. Janarv P, et al: Long-term follow-up of anterior tibial spine fractures in children. J Pediatr Orthop 15(1):63–68, 1995.
32. Johnson DP, Eastwood DM, Witherow PJ: Symptomatic synovial plicae of the knee. J Bone Joint Surg 75A(10):1485–1496, 1993.
33. Jones DC, James SL: Overuse injuries of the lower extremity: Shin splints, iliotibial band friction syndrome, and exertional compartment syndromes. Clin Sports Med 6(2):273–290, 1987.
34. Kelsey DD, Tyson E: A new method of training for the lower extremity using unloading. J Orthop Sports Phys Ther 19(4):218–223, 1994.
35. Kimm SY, Obarzanek E: Childhood obesity: A new pandemic of the new millennium. Pediatrics 110(5): 1003–1007, 2002.
36. Levine J, Splain S: Use of the infrapatella strap in the treatment of patellofemoral pain. Clin Orthop 139:179–181, 1979.
37. Loder RT, Aronson DD, Greenfield ML: The epidemiology of bilateral slipped capital femoral epiphysis. A study of children in Michigan. J Bone Joint Surg 75A(8):1141–1147, 1993.
38. Loder RT, Schwartz EM, Hensinger RN: Behavioral characteristics of children with Legg-Calvé-Perthes disease. J Pediatr Orthop 13(5):598–601, 1993.
39. McMurray TP: The semilunar cartilages. Br J Med 29:407, 1942.
40. Meyers MH, McKeever FM: Fracture of the intercondylar eminence of the tibia. J Bone Joint Surg 52A(8):1677–1684, 1970.
41. Micheli LJ: The child and adolescent. In Harris M, et al (eds): Oxford Textbook of Sports Medicine. New York, Oxford University Press, 1994.
42. Micheli LJ: The incidence of injuries in children's sports: A medical perspective. In Brown E, Branta CF (eds): Competitive Sports for Children and Youth: An Overview of Research and Issues. Champaign, IL, Human Kinetics, 1988.

43. Micheli LJ, Stanitski CL: Lateral patellar retinacular release. Am J Sports Med 9(5):330–336, 1981.
44. O'Neill DB, Micheli LJ: Tarsal coalition: A follow-up of adolescent athletes. Am J Sports Med 17(4): 544–549, 1989.
45. Outerbridge RE, Dunlop JA: The problem of chondromalacia patellae. Clin Orthop 110:177–196, 1975.
46. Pillemer FG, Micheli LJ: Psychological considerations in youth sports. Clin Sports Med 7(3):679–689, 1988.
47. Poussa M, et al: Prognosis after conservative and operative treatment in Perthes disease. Clin Orthop 297:82–86, 1993.
48. Powell JW, Schootman M: A multivariate risk analysis of selected playing surfaces in the National Football League: 1980–1989. An epidemiologic study of knee injuries. Am J Sports Med 20(6): 686–694, 1992.
49. Requa RK: The scope of the problem: The impact of sports-related injuries. In National Institutes of Health Publication #93-3444: Conference on Sports Injuries in Youth: Surveillance Strategies. Proceedings. April 8-9, 1991, Bethesda, Maryland.
50. Salminen JJ, et al: Leisure time physical activity in the young. Correlation with low-back pain, spinal mobility and trunk muscle strength in 15-year-old school children. Int J Sports Med 14(7):406–410, 1993.
51. Shelbourne KD, et al: Arthrofibrosis in acute anterior cruciate ligament reconstruction. The effect of timing of reconstruction and rehabilitation. Am J Sports Med 19(4):332, 1991.
52. Shelbourne KD, Wilckens JH: Current concepts in anterior cruciate ligament rehabilitation. Orthop Review 19(11):957–964, 1990.
53. Shellock FG, et al: Effect of a patellar realignment brace on patellofemoral relationships: Evaluation with kinematic MR imaging. J Magnetic Resonance Imaging 4(4):590–594, 1994.
54. Silber TJ, Majd M: Reflex sympathetic dystrophy syndrome in children and adolescents. Report of 18 cases and review of the literature. Am J Dis Child 142(12):1325–1330, 1988.
55. Smille IS: Freiberg's infraction (Köhler's second disease). J Bone Joint Surg 39B:580, 1957.
56. Smith BG, et al: Early MR imaging of lower-extremity physeal fracture-separations: A preliminary report. J Pediatr Orthop 14(4):526–533, 1994.
57. Souryal TO, Freeman TR: Intercondylar notch size and anterior cruciate ligament injuries in athletes. A prospective study, Am J Sports Med 21(4):535–539, 1993.
58. Souryal TO, Moore HA, Evans JP: Bilaterality in anterior cruciate ligament injuries: Associated intercondylar notch stenosis. Am J Sports Med 16(5):449–454, 1988.
59. Spaeth HJ, et al: Magnetic resonance imaging detection of early experimental periostitis. Comparison of magnetic resonance imaging, computed tomography, and plain radiography with histopathologic correlation. Investigative Radiol 26(4):304–308, 1991.
60. Steen SN, Brownell KD: Patterns of weight loss and regain in wrestlers: Has the tradition changed? Med Sci Sports Exerc 22(6):762–768, 1990.
61. Stover B, et al: Early changes in the hip joint following epiphysiolysis of the femoral head. Results of an MRT study. Radiologe 34(1):46–51, 1994.
62. Sullivan D, et al: Stress fractures in 51 runners. Clin Orthop 187:188–192, 1984.
63. Trott A: Hallux valgus in the adolescent. AAOS Instructional Course Lect 21:262, 1975.
64. Wagner JC: Enhancement of athletic performance with drugs. An overview. Sports Med 12(4):250–265, 1991.
65. Wahlstrom O, et al: Heterotopic bone formation prevented by diclofenac. Prospective study of 100 hip arthroplasties. Acta Orthop Scand 62(5): 419–421, 1991.
66. Warren MP: Excessive dieting and exercise: The dangers for young athletes. J Musculoskel Med 4:31–40, 1987.
67. Wechsler RJ, et al: Tarsal coalition: Depiction and characterization with CT and MR imaging. Radiology 193(2):447–452, 1994.

31 The Upper Extremity

Laura Forese and Joshua Hyman

INTRODUCTION

Children and adolescents are engaging in sports in greater numbers than ever before and, unfortunately, along with the positive benefits of athletic endeavor, they are also experiencing sports injuries in greater numbers. The upper extremity is the site of many problems for the young athlete. Certain sports predispose the immature upper extremity to injury, but virtually all sports (as well as free play) expose the young athlete to the dangers of falls that can lead to fractures. The sports-related upper extremity disorders can be broken down into two major categories: overuse injuries or fractures and dislocations.

For the purposes of general classification, the pediatric upper extremity will be divided into five anatomic areas: hand, wrist, elbow, shoulder, and clavicle, and each will be addressed for both overuse injuries and typical fractures and dislocations. Because this is not a comprehensive text on trauma, only selected fractures and dislocations will be discussed.

GENERAL PRINCIPLES

It is trite but true that children and adolescents are not simply small versions of adults. The importance of the growing musculoskeletal system cannot be overemphasized. Growth plate injuries are common and may have important sequelae. Ligamentous injuries, in contrast, are much less common because of the relative strength of soft tissues compared to immature bone.

Children may have real difficulty localizing pain or other symptoms. Children and adolescents may also underestimate the importance of reporting pain, especially if they believe that this may keep them out of sports and other play activities. Careful attention must be paid to the physical examination of the child with a sports injury. Comparison must always be made with the uninvolved side.

Radiographs can be confusing in the immature skeleton; therefore it is critical that comparison views of the contralateral extremity be used. CT scans and MRIs may be necessary to image the osteocartilaginous structures. An arthrogram may provide vital information in properly diagnosing and treating an elbow injury.

Overuse injuries arise because of repetitive microtrauma to the growing skeleton.[16] Overuse can produce stress fractures, tendonitis, and bursitis. Rest is often the treatment of choice. Children and adolescents are often at the mercy of adults who establish and supervise training regimens and athletic events. It is critical that appropriate technique be used and that strict guidelines about rest are observed, even before an injury occurs.[13,22]

HAND

General Examination

Athletic injuries of the hand and wrist are quite common, accounting for up to 9% of all sports injuries.[18] The physical examination must assess for tenderness of the involved part, swelling, tendon integrity, range of motion, joint stability, finger alignment, sensation, and vascular status. Radiographs, although often necessary, do not take the place of a careful examination because there are many soft tissue injuries that occur. Anteroposterior, lateral, and oblique radiographs provide sufficient information for most hand injuries. In general, pediatric injuries are treated conservatively with good results.[15]

Fractures and Dislocations

FDP Avulsion. Avulsion of the flexor digitorum profundus tendon off of the distal phalanx is often called a “jersey finger,” because a player catches the fingertip in another player’s jersey while trying to tackle the other player. Bony injury is rare in this problem, and it can often go undetected because the only deficit is inability to actively flex at the distal interphalangeal (DIP) joint.[17] The most common digit involved is the ring finger. Prompt surgical repair is indicated to reattach the tendon as soon as possible. Delay in diagnosis may lead to compromised results. Injuries seen late may be treated with “benign neglect,” DIP fusion, or free tendon grafting (Fig. 31-1).[11]

Mallet Finger. In distinction to the flexor digitorum profundus avulsion is the mallet finger, which results from an injury around the insertion of the extensor tendon. Depending on the forces involved and the age of the athlete, this injury can produce a fracture, an avulsion of the tendon, or a tendon disruption.[3] On examination, the DIP joint will demonstrate full passive extension, but lack active extension. AP and lateral radiographs must be obtained to evaluate the presence and degree of bony

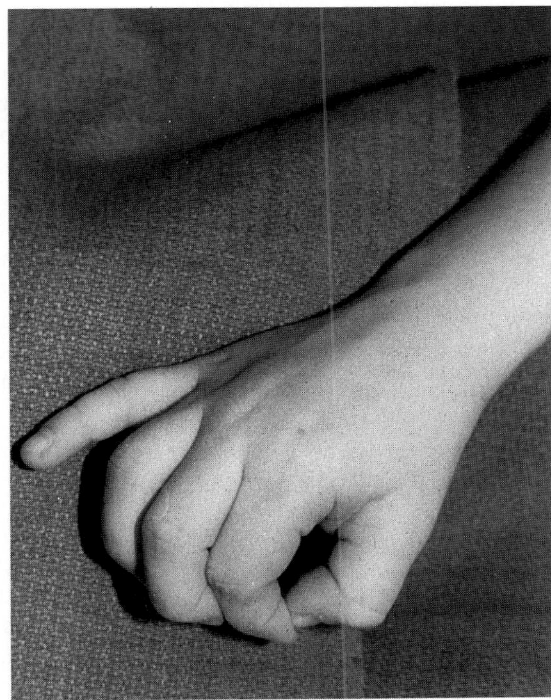

FIGURE 31-1. This child avulsed the FDP of the fifth finger while playing on the sports field.

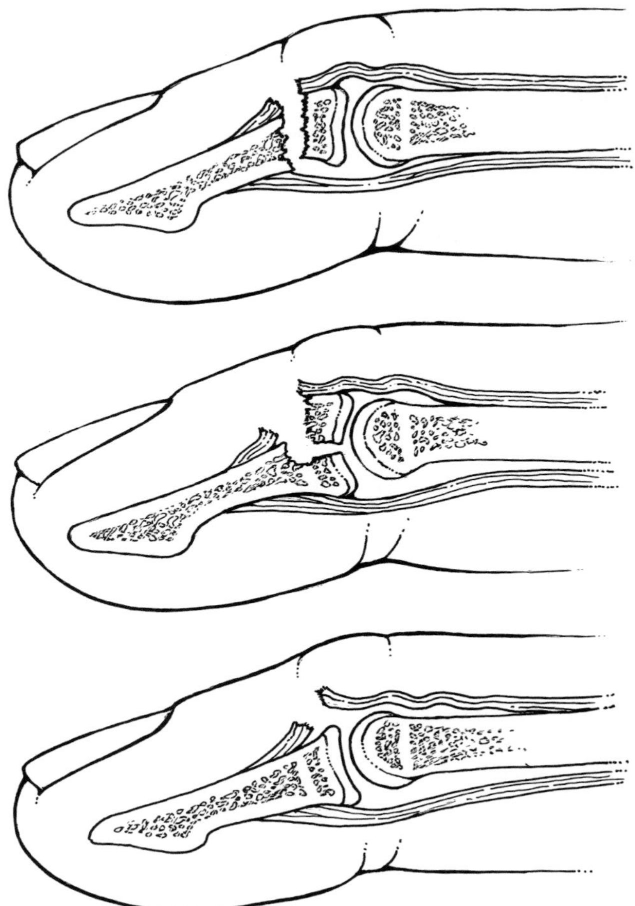

FIGURE 31-2. Three types of mallet finger.

involvement and joint subluxation. Most mallet finger deformities can be treated with splinting the DIP joint in neutral extension for 8 weeks followed by gentle progressive exercises until motion has reached 35–40° of flexion and full extension. Surgery is rarely indicated except for those injuries associated with open tendon lacerations, physeal fractures with avulsions of the nail from the matrix, and intraarticular fractures with volar subluxation of the distal fragment (Fig. 31-2).[5]

Jammed Finger. A jammed finger is the result of a significant force on the extended finger, which causes pain and swelling at the proximal interphalangeal joint. There is no bony or ligamentous injury and the joint is stable. After other problems are ruled out, the jammed finger is protected with rest and a slow return to range of motion and full activity. The joint may remain persistently sore for many months, and the swollen appearance around this joint may never fully resolve.

Metacarpal and Phalangeal Fractures and Dislocations. A full discussion of all the different types of metacarpal and phalangeal fractures and dislocations is far beyond the scope of this text; however, there are some important general principles for the primary care provider. At least two radiographs at right angles to each other are critically important because of the problems with malunion. A fracture that appears adequately reduced on an anteroposterior view and on an oblique view may be significantly displaced on the lateral view. A rotatory deformity of just a small amount can cause real problems of overlapping of the fingers with the hand closed. As with most fractures in children, closed methods are usually sufficient; however, open reductions are sometimes indicated, and an early diagnosis and treatment plan is far superior to a late one (Fig. 31-3).

Dislocations are often easily reduced by a well-meaning person or by the child or adolescent himself on the playing field. However, the dislocation still requires a careful physical examination, including testing of range of motion and stability of the ligamentous complex. Radiographs are also necessary to rule out any associated bony injury. Some dislocations are not reducible by closed methods, and thus persistent reduction attempts are not appropriate.

Overuse Injuries

There are no specific overuse injuries of the hand in children and adolescents.

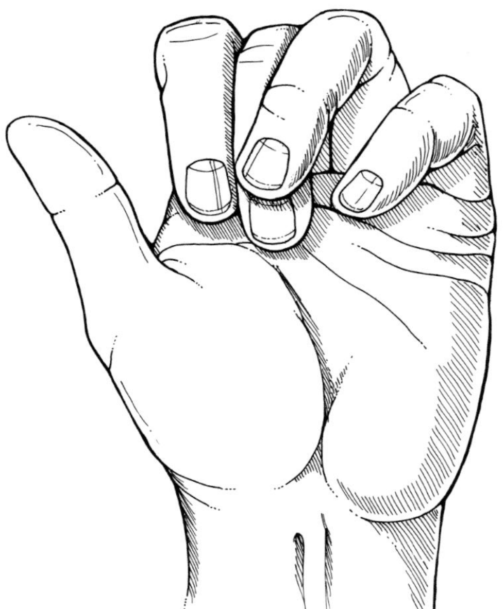

FIGURE 31-3. Malrotated fingers as a result of malunion of a phalanx fracture.

WRIST

General Examination

It can be difficult to sort out the site of injury in the wrist because of the close anatomic relationship of the structures. Again, a careful examination of the contralateral wrist is necessary. The centers of ossification of the carpal bones and the distal radius and ulna do not all have the same timing of ossification, so radiographs can be misleading. Comparison views are highly recommended.

Fractures and Dislocations

Scaphoid Fractures. The scaphoid is by far the most commonly injured of the carpal bones in children and adolescents. This injury usually results from a fall on the outstretched hand. Initial examination does not demonstrate any deformity; however, the anatomic snuffbox, the area between the extensor pollicis longus and brevis, may be tender. Unfortunately, this injury often goes unnoticed even when radiographs are taken because initial radiographs are often negative. If an injury is suspected, but radiographs are normal, immobilization in a thumb spica cast is indicated. Although most pediatric scaphoid fractures heal with immobilization, some will go onto nonunion, particularly if untreated. Displaced fractures and nonunions often require surgical intervention.[8]

Radius and Ulna Fractures. It is usually not difficult to diagnose a fracture of the radius and/or ulna. The mechanism of injury is also from a fall on the outstretched hand, and the child is usually exquisitely tender at the site of the fracture. A complete fracture of either or both bones typically has an obvious deformity. There are few indications for surgical intervention in radius and ulna fractures in children. Most of them can be treated quite successfully with closed reduction and casting or splinting. Although distal radius growth plate fractures are common, they rarely lead to any significant problem with subsequent growth arrest.

Of note is the torus (or buckle) fracture, which is a cortical compression without significant displacement. Torus fractures can go completely unnoticed and are often only mildly painful. Often the diagnosis is delayed because of the lack of symptoms. These fractures do not require reduction and are often treated with simple splinting for comfort.

Overuse Injuries

Overuse injuries of the wrist are common in young athletes. Tendonitis and tenosynovitis occur frequently in athletes who perform repetitive motions with their wrists. Tenosynovitis of the first dorsal compartment of the hand, or de Quervain's disease, occurs in activities that require hyperabduction of the thumb, such as golf and racquet sports. Tendonitis of the flexor carpi ulnaris occurs in athletes who participate in racquet sports and rowing. These patients will exhibit pain over the dorsal aspect wrist that is exacerbated by wrist extension against resistance. In general, anti-inflammatory medications, rest, and short-term immobilization are helpful in treating these conditions.

A repetitive stress response that has been seen in gymnasts is overuse syndrome in the distal radius.[21] The patients complain of pain, particularly with weight bearing on the hand and placement of the wrist in dorsiflexion. Radiographs may be slow to show the findings that are typical of stress changes to the open growth plates: cystic changes and widening of the growth plate.[20] The suggestion has been made that those who are treated prior to radiographic changes will recover faster. The treatment has been rest and, typically, the patients recover completely. There is no evidence of sequelae in those who rest (Fig. 31-4).

ELBOW

General Examination

Much of the elbow anatomy is palpable, and an examination should include careful inspection and palpation in an attempt to pinpoint the exact area of pain (Fig. 31-5). Full range of motion is from 0° of flexion to over 130° of flexion. People with laxity actually have hyperextension of the elbow beyond 0° of flexion. This full range of motion is not actually necessary for most activities, and an athlete can easily hide a somewhat limited range of motion. The ulnar nerve is in close proximity to the bony structures and must be carefully assessed.

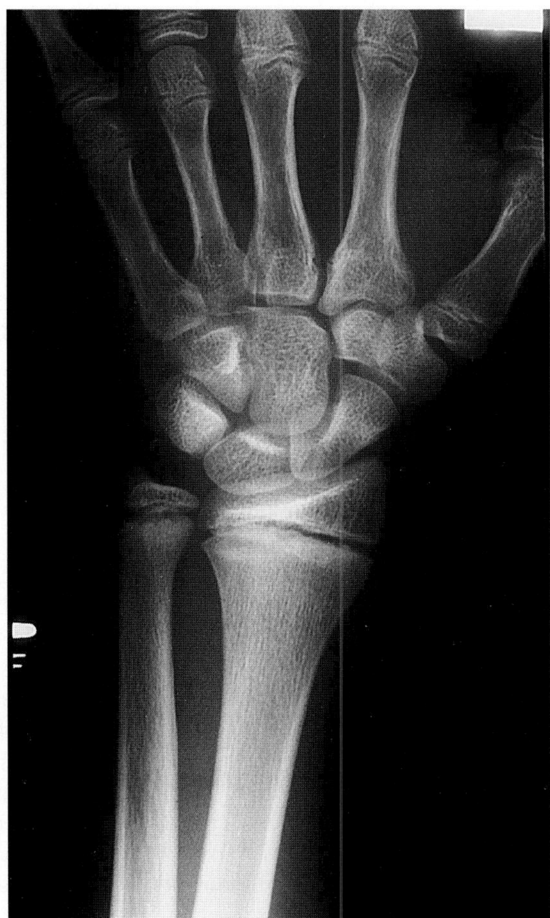

FIGURE 31-4. This child, a competitive gymnast, had chronic wrist pain and tenderness over the growth plate that responded to rest and modified activity.

The immature elbow is a particularly vulnerable joint in throwing sports and in gymnastics. In baseball, there may be throws that are particularly damaging to the elbow, and in gymnastics the elbow is a weight-bearing joint.[4] Common in these sports is the presence of chronic pain.

Fractures and Dislocations

Dislocation of the elbow is particularly rare in children.[6] Unfortunately, fractures about the elbow are common. The mechanism of injury can vary with the specific type of elbow fracture, but most are from falls onto the arm or the outstretched hand. Because much of the immature elbow is unossified, radiographs can be deceptive or at least difficult to interpret. Unlike the principles of treatment for many other upper extremity fractures discussed here, fractures around the elbow in children and adolescents often require open or closed surgical reduction with percutaneous pinning to prevent displacement. This is due to the significant forces around the elbow that tend to displace fractures, which could result in functional and cosmetic problems in the future (Fig. 31-6).

Overuse Injuries

During the acceleration phase of throwing, compression forces act on the lateral side of the elbow and tensile forces act on the medial side. Medial tension can lead to strain of the flexor muscles, medial epicondylitis, and medial epicondyle fractures. Lateral compression forces may cause radial head hypertrophy, capitellar fractures, and osteochondritis dissecans.[10] Historically, this constellation of injuries has been called “Little Leaguer’s elbow.”[2] This term, however, does not accurately describe the specific injury to the child’s elbow and for this reason should be avoided. Rather, each condition should be thought of as a separate injury that may occur in conjunction with others.

Osteochondritis dissecans is a term used to describe vascular compromise of the capitellum that is related to repetitive compressive forces. It typically occurs in children 10 to 14 years of age. Panner’s disease is a similar condition occurring in younger children. Patients will frequently complain of pain along the lateral elbow, loss of motion, and symptoms of locking. Radiographs may demonstrate fragmentation of the capitellum. Treatment is guided by the age of the patient, degree of fragmentation of the capitellum, and the presence of loose bodies.

In general, Panner’s disease is a self-limited condition that does not create loose bodies or lead to long-term problems. Patients with Panner’s disease should be encouraged to avoid activities that cause axial stress and valgus loading of the elbow, such as throwing and gymnastics. With rest, symptoms will resolve, and eventually full, symmetrical ossification of the capitellum will be seen on radiographs.

Patients with osteochondritis dissecans have a more guarded prognosis. In general, the younger the patient presents, the better the outcome. As patients approach skeletal maturity, the potential for spontaneous healing diminishes. The presence of loose bodies and symptomatic locking are indications for elbow surgical removal of loose bodies. Typically this is performed arthroscopically. Occasionally, large loose fragments may be reduced and fixed in place with wires, screws, or bioabsorbable implants. The long-term prognosis for the older adolescent athlete with osteochondritis is guarded. If the surface of the capitellum is irregular at the completion of growth, pain, stiffness, and arthrosis will likely occur.

Medial Epicondylitis. The classic injury is a repetitive valgus stress reaction of the medial epicondylar apophysis. This stress produces age-dependent injury patterns, such as apophysitis in childhood and epicondylar avulsion fractures in the more mature athlete. Older adolescents and young adults are less prone to bony injury and more

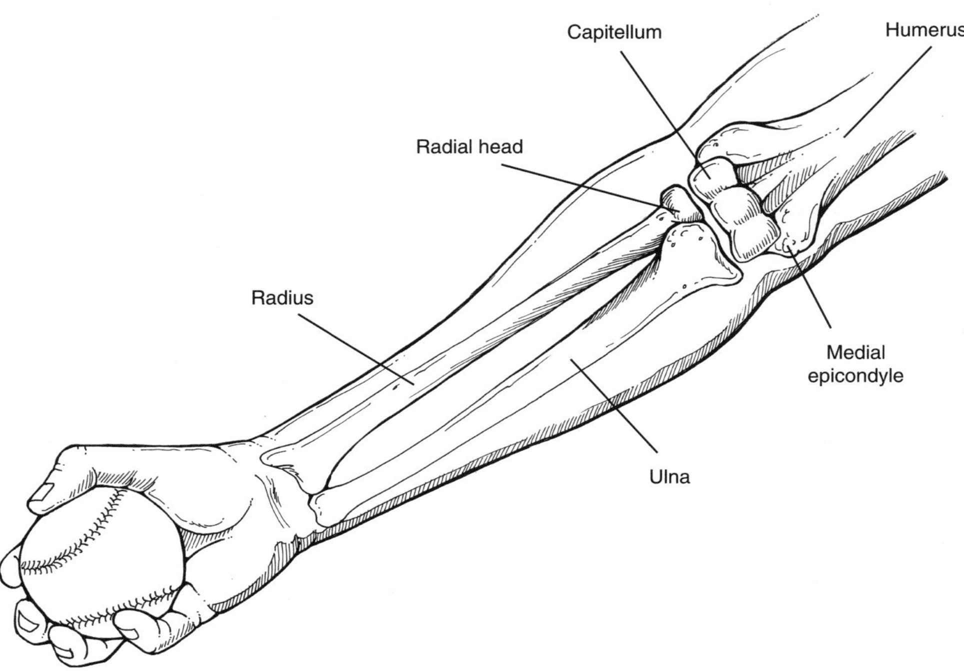

FIGURE 31-5. Anatomy of the elbow.

likely to sustain muscle injury on the medial side of the elbow. Typically, there is pain and swelling along the medial elbow, flexion contracture, and tenderness at the medial epicondyle. Pain is exacerbated with throwing and when valgus stress is applied with 20° of elbow flexion.

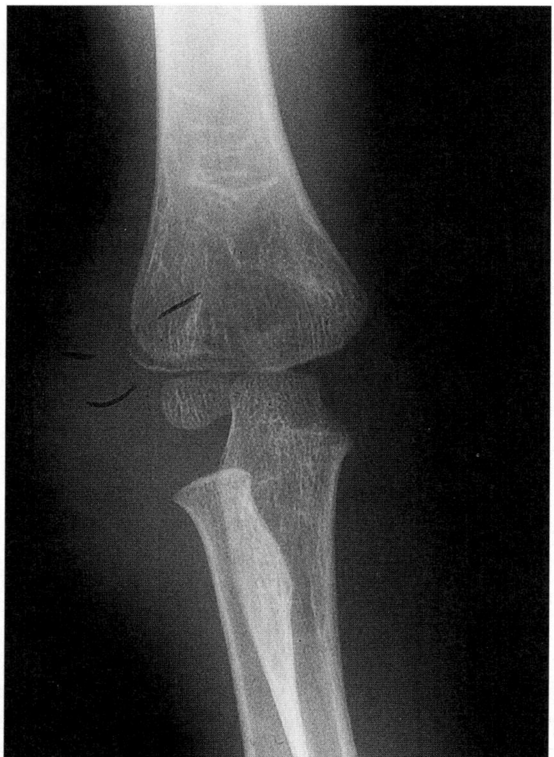

FIGURE 31-6. A lateral condyle fracture that required pinning to prevent malunion or nonunion.

Radiographs usually are normal, however they may show fragmentation of the medial epicondyle. Contralateral views may be helpful.

Treatment comprises rest and anti-inflammatory medication until the elbow is asymptomatic, followed by stretching and gradual strengthening to regain full range of motion and forearm strength. Throwing should resume only after pain has subsided. Prevention is even more effective than treatment, and it is for this reason that there should be some restrictions on the number of innings pitched in a given week. Controversy exists as to the contribution of throwing sidearm and pitching curveballs. Nonetheless, proper pitching mechanics must be taught to young aspiring pitchers.[12]

SHOULDER

General Examination

A systematic shoulder examination is critical to properly evaluate shoulder injuries to prevent missing important clinical findings. Both shoulders must be exposed from the neck to the hands. The examination should begin with thorough observation of the alignment of the limb, paying special attention to any deformities that might herald a fracture or dislocation. Inspect the skin for redness, swelling, and bruising. Note any muscle atrophy. Comparison with the contralateral limb is very useful. Next, the bony landmarks of the shoulder should be palpated for evidence of point tenderness. The specific areas that should be examined are the sternoclavicular joint, the entire clavicle, the acromioclavicular joint, the acromion, and the scapular spine. Range of motion must be assessed and compared with the opposite side.

Specifically, one must evaluate forward elevation, abduction, and external and internal rotation in both 0° and 90° of abduction. Strength testing must be performed. Finally, ligamentous stability should be evaluated. Glenohumeral stability can be assessed with the patient supine and the shoulder abducted 90° and the elbow flexed. The humeral head is centered within the glenoid fossa by axial loading, and then gentle manipulation is performed in all directions, noting any excessive movement or pain relative to the opposite side. The anterior apprehension test is performed with the shoulder abducted 90° and then gently externally rotating the shoulder to 90°. A patient with anterior shoulder instability will note discomfort or "apprehension" with this maneuver. Finally, bear in mind that cervical spine disorders may cause pain referred to the shoulder. Therefore the neck should be evaluated in any patient with shoulder pain.

Fractures and Dislocations

Clavicle. Midshaft clavicle fractures are among the most common injuries for children and adolescents. The typical cause is a fall on the outstretched hand. Examination reveals swelling, deformity, and tenderness at the fracture site. The clavicle has tremendous potential to remodel and therefore is virtually always treated closed, often with just a sling or a figure of eight bandage that attempts to stabilize the fracture and provide some comfort. Judicious use of nonsteroidal anti-inflammatory drugs provides adequate pain relief. Immobilization and activity restriction for 3 to 6 weeks is sufficient to treat most clavicle fractures. These fractures lay down abundant callus and thus a bump is often visible and palpable long after healing has taken place (Fig. 31-7). An exception to closed treatment is the case in which the bone ends have become fixed in muscle and are not reducible closed. Another rare exception is a fracture that is causing pressure on the brachial plexus, which may also have to be treated by open reduction and perhaps internal fixation.

Sternoclavicular injuries are much less common than fractures of the midshaft or the distal portion of the clavicle. A significant force is usually required to cause injury that will present with pain at the junction of the sternum and clavicle. Dislocations of this joint in the immature skeleton are virtually unheard of since the growth plate does not close until the late teens or early twenties. Instead, an epiphyseal fracture occurs. Radiographic confirmation is notoriously difficult to obtain with plain radiographs, so other imaging such as a CT scan or MRI may be necessary. Treatment, other than rest, is rarely necessary unless there is some compression of the great vessels.

At the distal end of the clavicle, fractures also occur, especially through the distal growth plate or metaphysis. The mechanism of injury is typically a fall directly on the point of the shoulder. This is the equivalent of an acromioclavicular separation in an adult. In the mid- to late teens, acromioclavicular separation can occur and this should be treated as adult injury. The treatment for most distal clavicle injuries is rest, typically a sling, for those injuries that are non- to minimally displaced. Even those with moderate displacement are often treated with observation because of the remodeling potential of the clavicle. Fractures with major or fixed displacement and those causing neurovascular symptoms may require more extensive, operative treatment.

Humerus. Fractures of the proximal humerus are classified as either physeal or diaphyseal fractures. All injuries to the shoulder should be evaluated with AP, lateral and axillary lateral views. In the adolescent athlete, Salter-Harris II fractures are fairly common because the proximal humeral physis is one of the last to close. Because the proximal humeral physis account for 80% of the growth of the entire bone, displaced fractures in the skeletally immature athlete have an incredible ability to remodel. For this reason, most of these fractures can be treated nonoperatively with a sling for 4 to 6 weeks.[14] Fractures with greater than 50% displacement or angulation greater than 45° should be referred to a specialist for further evaluation (Fig. 31-8).

Dislocation of the glenohumeral joint occurs in adolescents in much the same way that it occurs in adults. The shoulder has the least stability of all the major joints

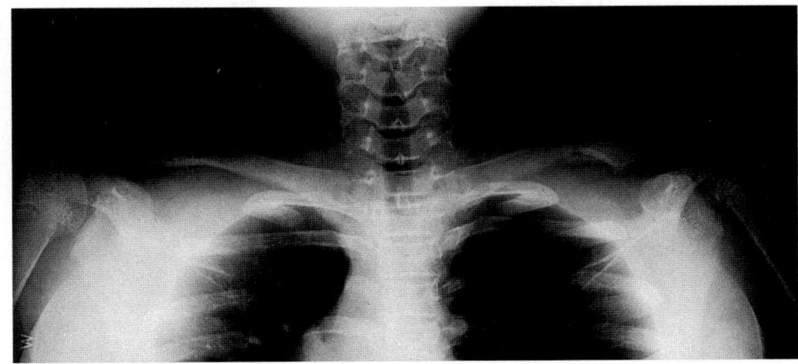

FIGURE 31-7. A typical left, midshaft clavicle fracture with early healing.

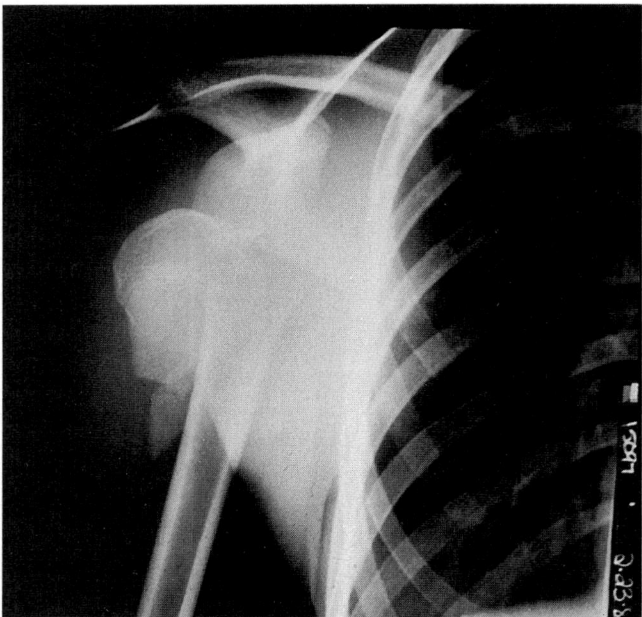

FIGURE 31-8. A fracture sustained on the football field that did require a manipulative reduction.

because it has soft tissue rather than bony stability. This injury is not common in children, who tend to sustain fractures rather than dislocations, but as children age into adolescence and then into young adulthood, the shoulder becomes more vulnerable. Anterior dislocation is far more common than posterior dislocation.

Treatment is by closed reduction, which should not be attempted without radiographs to rule out any associated bony pathology. The first dislocation is usually treated by immobilization in a sling after the reduction and rest for several weeks, followed by a rehabilitation program that strengthens the shoulder musculature. Some athletes have no further problems after a single dislocation. Unfortunately, many young athletes go on to recurrent dislocations, which can be a major problem.[9] Although recurrent dislocations are often easily reduced, even by the athlete on the playing field, the instability in the joint can be very uncomfortable and may make the athlete extremely apprehensive. Surgery may be the only option to allow these athletes to return to competition.

Overuse Injuries

Little Leaguer's Shoulder. Little Leaguer's shoulder is a classic overuse injury in which the immature skeleton responds to constant low levels of stress from pitching with changes at the growth plate.[23] Although this syndrome is called Little League shoulder because of the high incidence in pitchers in organized activity, a similar syndrome has also been described in tennis players.[7] The mechanism of injury appears to be the repetitive overhead rotational motion. Afflicted children and adolescents have pain and some mild loss of range of motion, which seems to respond rapidly to cessation of pitching and rest.[1] Potential injury to the site of future growth is what causes concern in this syndrome, but there do not appear to be cases of actual growth problems (Fig. 31-9).

Impingement Syndrome. Impingement occurs when the supraspinatus tendon (part of the rotator cuff) is progressively irritated by rubbing on the undersurface of the acromion. This is brought about by forward elevation activities, precisely those that are used in certain swimming and tennis strokes and overhead throwing.

While the impingement is in the initial stages of pain with forward elevation, rest is once again the treatment of choice. Modification of training practices may be critical to getting the athlete back to competition.[19] Full range of motion must also be regained. Acromioplasty, the surgical removal of some offending bone from the undersurface of the acromion, is sometimes necessary if conservative care does not resolve the problem.

CONCLUSION

Fractures and related trauma of the upper extremity in children and adolescents are commonplace occurrences. We expect those falls and are often aware of the potential sequelae. The overuse injuries to the upper extremity are less common and receive much less attention in print and in the training of health care professionals.

Children and adolescents who participate in sports, particularly organized sports, are directed by parents and coaches to perform certain training and practice activities. It is incumbent upon those adults to pay careful attention to time spent on certain stressful activities

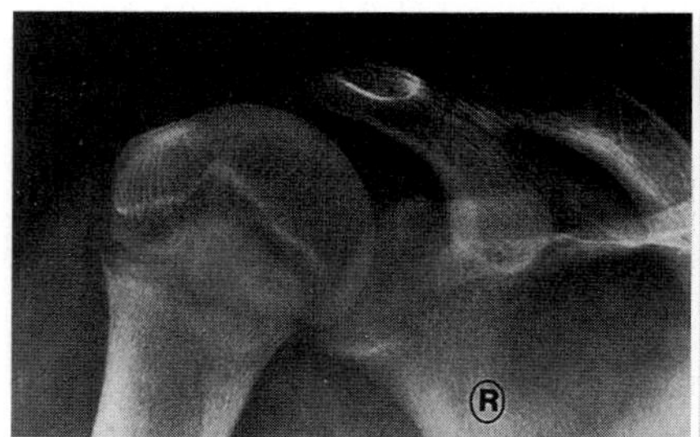

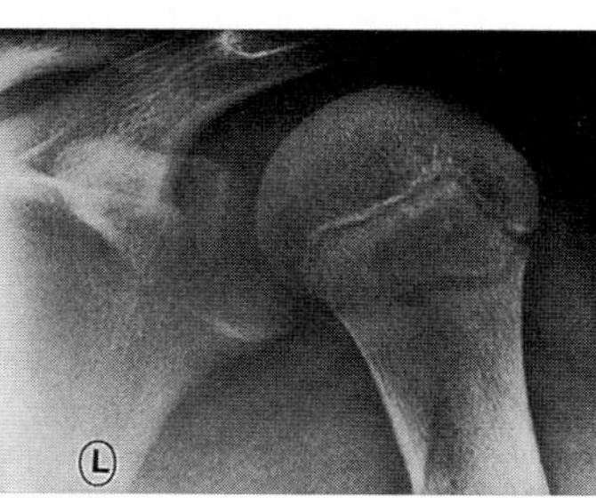

FIGURE 31-9. Widening of the growth plate on the right in this ballplayer. (From Busch M: Sports medicine. In Morrissey RT [ed]: Pediatric Orthopaedics, 3rd ed. Philadelphia, JB Lippincott, 1990.)

and to allow adequate periods of rest. No child or adolescent is aided by being told to work through the pain. In the upper extremity, the consequences of not resting an overused joint or of missing a fracture can be devastating.

REFERENCES

1. Barnett LS: Little league shoulder syndrome: Proximal humeral epiphysiolysis in adolescent baseball pitchers. JBJS 67A:495–496, 1985.
2. Brogdon BG, Crow NE: Little leaguer's elbow. AJR 83:671–685, 1960.
3. Garcia-Moral CA: Injuries to the hand and wrist. In Sullivan JA, Grana WA (eds): The Pediatric Athlete, Park Ridge, IL, American Academy of Orthopaedic Surgery, 1988.
4. Goldberg MJ: Gymnastic injuries. Orthop Clin North Am 11:717–726, 1980.
5. Graham TJ, Waters PM: Fractures and dislocations of the hand and carpus in children. In Rockwood and Wilken's Fractures in Children. Philadelphia, Lippincott Williams and Wilkens, 2001.
6. Green N: Fractures and dislocations about the elbow. In Green NE, Swiontkowski MF (eds): Skeletal Trauma in Children. Philadelphia, WB Saunders, 1994.
7. Gregg JR, Torg E: Upper extremity injuries in adolescent tennis players. Clin Sports Med 7: 371–385, 1988.
8. Henderson B, Letts M: Operative management of pediatric scaphoid fracture nonunion. J Pediatr Orthop 23(3):402–406, 2003.
9. Hovelius L: Anterior dislocation of the shoulder in teenagers and young adults: Five year prognosis. JBJS 69A:393–399, 1987.
10. Klingele KE, Kocher, MS: Little league elbow: Valgus overload injury in the paediatric athlete. Sports Med 32(15):1005–1015, 2002.
11. Lee SJ, Montgomery, K: Athletic hand injuries. Orthop Clin North Am 33:547–554, 2002.
12. Lyman S, Fleisig GS, Andrews JR: Effect of pitch type, pitch count, and pitching mechanics on risk of elbow and shoulder pain in youth baseball pitchers. Am J Sports Med 30:463–468, 2002.
13. Meyers JF: Injuries to the shoulder girdle and elbow in the pediatric athlete. In Sullivan JA, Frana WA (eds): The Pediatric Athlete. Park Ridge, IL, American Academy of Orthopaedic Surgeons, 1988.
14. Neer CS, Horowitz BS: Fractures of the proximal humeral epiphyseal plate. Clin Orthop 41:24–31, 1965.
15. Nofsinger CC, Wolfe SW: Common pediatric hand fractures. Curr Opin Pediatr 14(1):42–45, 2002.
16. Outerbridge AR, Micheli LJ: Overuse injuries in the young athlete. Clin Sports Med 14:503–516, 1995.
17. Perron AD, Brady WJ, Keats TE, Hersh RE: Orthopaedic pitfalls in the emergency department: Closed tendon injuries of the hand. Am J Emerg Med 19(1):76–80, 2001.
18. Rettig AC: Epidemiology of hand and wrist injuries in sports. Clin Sports Med 17:401–406, 1998.
19. Richardson AB, Jobe FW, Collins HR: The shoulder in competitive swimming. Am J Sports Med 8:159–163, 1980.
20. Roy S, Caine D, Singer KM: Stress changes of the distal radial epiphysis in young gymnasts. Am J Sports Med 13:301–308, 1985.
21. Simmons BP, Lovallo JL: Hand and wrist injuries in children. Clin Sports Med 7:495–512, 1988.
22. Snook GA: Injuries in women's gymnastics. Am J Sports Med 7:242–244, 1979.
23. Tibone JE: Shoulder problems of adolescents. Clin Sports Med 2:423–427, 1983.

32 The Spine

Gail S. Chorney

Spinal injuries, whether in the cervical, thoracic, or lumbar spine, are uncommon in children. The etiology of these injuries is age dependent. In the pediatric age group from years 5 to 15, the most common cause is motor vehicle accident. However, the second most common cause is recreational sports. Football is credited with the largest number of injuries, although gymnastics and wrestling also are associated with spinal injuries.[7] The number and severity of injuries can often be decreased with careful attention to training, supervision, and proper equipment.[1] The use of the trampoline, however, has a high association of catastrophic spinal injury (quadriplegia) that cannot be controlled by supervision or equipment. This has led to the recommendation that the trampoline be discouraged as a training device.[8]

This chapter is concerned with evaluation in the physician's office of back complaints in the pediatric patient. The care of the seriously injured patient with accompanying spinal cord injury on the playing field or ski slope is not dealt with here. In the office, a careful history and physical examination along with the appropriate radiographic studies can lead to a diagnosis and guidelines for treatments and further athletic participation.

HISTORY

Obtaining a history from the pediatric patient is always more difficult than in the adult patient. The type of athletic participation as well as the intensity of training can always be elicited from both child and parent. Many of the issues encountered in the physician's office are of a chronic nature. The child needs to be guided in the history taking to relate the complaints to the specific sport. Direct questions are asked about the location, nature, and timing of the pain. The timing of the pain should be established in relation to practice sessions, games, and the occurrence of the pain when not participating in sports. Does the pain occur during athletic participation or after the practice session/game is over? Obviously, any history of known injury must be obtained. In the older child, the patient can demonstrate which maneuvers in the sport reproduce the complaint. The child may minimize the complaint to prevent restriction of activity. The physician must still attempt to form an accurate picture of the child's impaired function, including deterioration in performance and changes in neurologic status.

PHYSICAL EVALUATION AND RADIOGRAPHY

The physical examination should be performed with the child undressed, with a hospital gown for modesty. Regardless of where the complaints are localized, the entire spine and the extremities need a complete evaluation. Again, the child will often minimize the complaints rather than exaggerate them in order to continue athletic participation.

As in every physical examination of a child, the general appearance should be noted. Does the child appear to be in pain or have difficulty rising up from the chair or getting onto the examination table? Is there difficulty in undressing?

Cervical Spine

The cervical spine should be observed for possible kyphosis. The range of motion of the cervical spine is determined as well as the presence of local tenderness in the midline. The cervical spine is more mobile in the young patient than in the adult because of increased ligamentous laxity in the pediatric age group. This increased motion accounts for the pseudo subluxation that can often be seen on a later radiograph. If there is a full, painless range of motion of the cervical spine, the physician need not be alarmed by the pseudo subluxation on the radiograph. The anterior translation is usually seen at C2–3 or C3–4. The presence of midline tenderness or restriction of motion in the cervical spine should alert the physician to the possibility of injury to the posterior ligamentous structures. Flexion and extension lateral radiographs of the cervical spine are the appropriate studies to obtain. Because initial radiographs may not be conclusive for instability, suspicion of this injury requires careful follow-up. Contact sports or diving need to be avoided. Minor injuries will resolve with time, with decreased tenderness and restoration of motion. However, persistent midline tenderness and continued loss of motion should alert the primary caregiver to refer the patient to a specialist for evaluation. Latent instability of the cervical spine requires posterior arthrodesis to protect the patient from possible neurologic injury.[6]

A short neck or a restriction of motion in the cervical spine that is not associated with tenderness may be an indication of congenital anomalies of the spine. Anterior–posterior and lateral views of the cervical spine should be obtained. Congenital anomalies of the cervical spine such as fusion of vertebral bodies is known as

Klippel-Feil syndrome. Again, participation in contact sports or diving should not be allowed for fear or neurologic injury. The physician must also investigate the child's cardiac and renal status because there is a high incidence of congenital problems in these organ systems associated with Klippel-Feil syndrome.

Thoracic Spine

The trunk is then inspected with regard to a possible increase in the thoracic kyphosis. A painless, round back in the pediatric patient is usually noted by the parent and not the child. On examination, the physician should view the patient from the front, back, and side to assess the presence of an increased kyphosis. An attempt should be made to passively correct the kyphosis. On a forward bend test, if there is rigidity to the kyphosis, the diagnosis of Scheuermann round back is suspected. There is frequently a complaint of mild pain. Tight hamstrings are often a physical finding. This diagnosis is confirmed on lateral radiographs of the thoraco-lumbar spine by the presence of wedging of three or more vertebral bodies (Figs. 32-1 and 32-2).

Scheuermann round back is a relatively common complaint in adolescent males. There is an increase in incidence in weight lifters, however. The treatment is bracing, which can decrease pain and prevent further deformity. Bracing may allow restoration of the height of the vertebral bodies in the skeletally immature skeleton and thus decrease the deformity. Weight lifting should probably be restricted during the treatment period.[6]

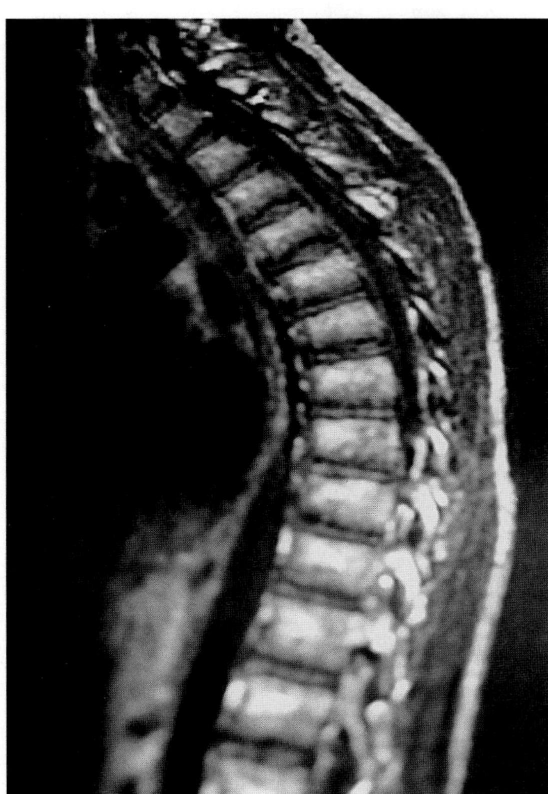

FIGURE 32-2. MRI of the spine of the same patient as in Figure 32-1, again showing the minor wedging of vertebral bodies resulting in a kyphosis.

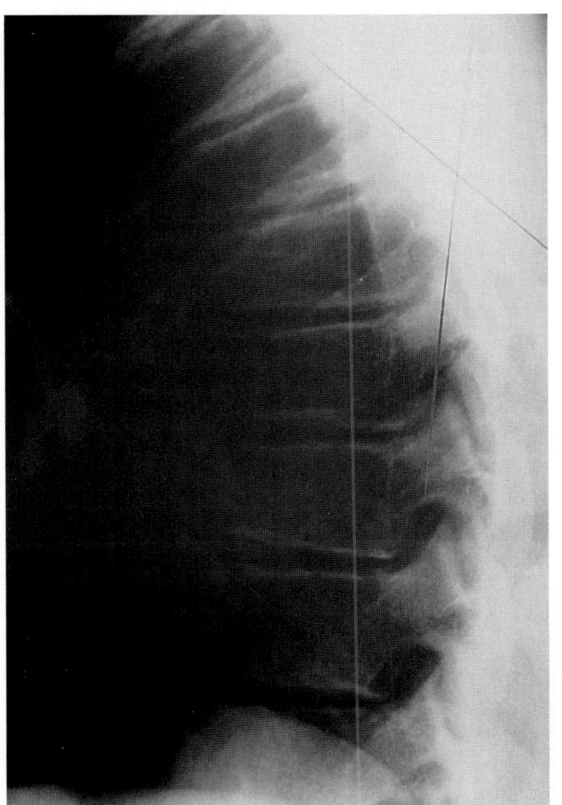

FIGURE 32-1. Lateral radiograph of thoracic spine showing minor wedging of three vertebral bodies characteristic of Scheuermann round back.

Lumbar Spine

An increase in the thoracic kyphosis is often accompanied by an increase in the lumbar lordosis. In addition, complaints of pain in the lumbar spine are probably the most common complaints of young athletes. Participation in recreational sports does not lead to an increase in mechanical back pain in young people, but it also does not decrease the incidence.[2] Before the diagnosis of mechanical back pain is made, the more serious diagnoses of spondylolysis and spondylolisthesis must be ruled out. Micheli has written extensively about these injuries in the gymnast.[5] These injuries should be suspected in young athletes participating in gymnastics or other sports involving repetitive hyperextension of the lumbar spine.

Spondylolisthesis is the slipping forward of one vertebral body on another. The usual location is L5 on S1 (Figs. 32-3 and 32-4). Spondylolysis is a disruption of the pars interarticularis. It may be unilateral or bilateral.

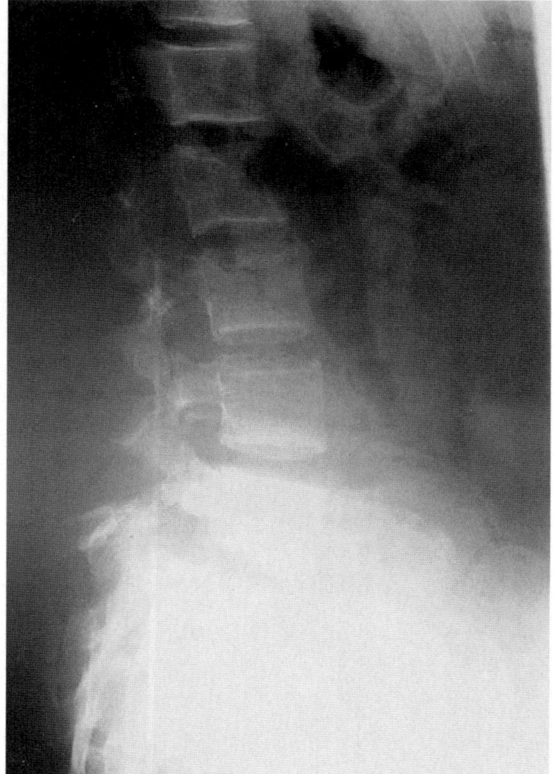

FIGURE 32-3. Lateral radiograph of the lumbar-sacral junction showing a Grade I spondylolisthesis of L5-S1.

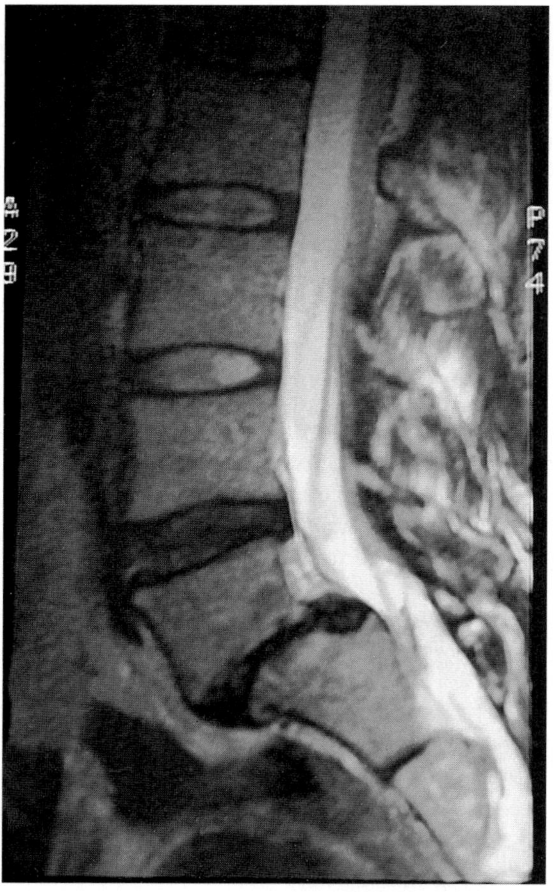

FIGURE 32-4. An MRI of the lateral lumbar spine shows the Grade I slippage more dramatically.

Slippage is not present (Fig. 32-5). There may be simply an elongation of the pars interarticularis rather than a fracture.[4] Congenital dysplasia may be a predisposing factor in addition to the athletic participation.

The physical examination for these injuries reveals an increase in the lumbar lordosis. The child may not be able to reverse the lordosis on forward bends. There may be midline tenderness to palpation over the lower lumbar spine. Paraspinal muscle spasms may be present if symptoms are severe enough. Forward flexion does not cause discomfort, but extension of the lumbar spine reproduces the symptoms. The child may have difficulty rising from a chair. Pain produced by standing on one leg is indicative of injury to the pars interarticularis on that side.

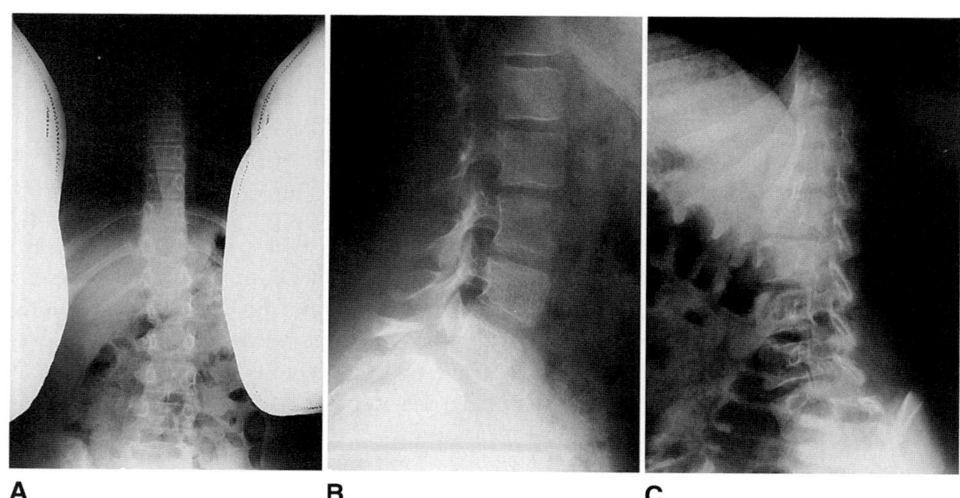

FIGURE 32-5. A, The AP radiograph of a patient with a spondylolysis shows a minor scoliosis that is secondary to the pain. **B,** The lateral radiograph shows elongation of the posterior element of L5. **C,** The oblique view also shows the defect in the pars interarticularis of L5.

Hamstring tightness is present. The examiner must bear in mind that children are more flexible than adults and that young athletes are probably even more flexible. Therefore, restrictions in motion may be subtle. The neurologic examination is normal.[3]

The radiographs to order are the usual standing anterior–posterior and lateral views. Oblique views are needed to demonstrate spondylolysis. However, radiographs may be negative for bony lesions, even the oblique views. A bone scan is often necessary to confirm the diagnosis.

The treatment of spondylolysis is bracing, which rapidly decreases the pain. The brace is a thoraco-lumbar orthosis. Casts have been used to increase compliance. Spondylolysis is a stable lesion, however, and thus continued participation in the sport during the healing process may be an issue. Guidelines for participation may be influenced by pain tolerance and the importance of competition to the young athlete. Usually avoidance of the specific maneuvers that reproduce the pain is suggested.[3,5]

Again, spondylolisthesis is the slippage of one vertebral body on the next lower one. Grading is based on the percentage of the lower body that is left uncovered. The child with a spondylolisthesis of greater than 50% will have a short trunk on physical examination and hamstring tightness. The hips may have a flexion contracture secondary to the tilt of the pelvis.

Progression of the slippage occurs early in the presentation. Therefore, a young child (younger than 10 years of age) with a spondylolisthesis should be followed with serial lateral radiographs. Lesions of greater than 50% are treated with a fusion. Any lesions that show progression of a slippage should also be treated with a fusion.

The asymptomatic athlete with less than a 25% spondylolisthesis may participate in sports without restriction. Those symptomatic patients with between 25% and 50% slippage are treated with a brace. The resolution of pain and no progression of slippage is criteria for returning to sports.

Down Syndrome

The athlete with Down syndrome must be carefully evaluated with respect to cervical instability at C2. Approximately 25% of individuals with Down syndrome demonstrate some level of instability. This instability is secondary to the generalized ligamentous laxity and common occurrence of hypoplasia of the dens or a defect in the posterior ring of C. These children are more difficult to evaluate because of the inability to obtain an accurate history and the increased mobility of their skeletons. In addition, it is much more difficult to obtain adequate flexion-extension lateral radiographs of the cervical spine because of lack of cooperation (Fig. 32-6).

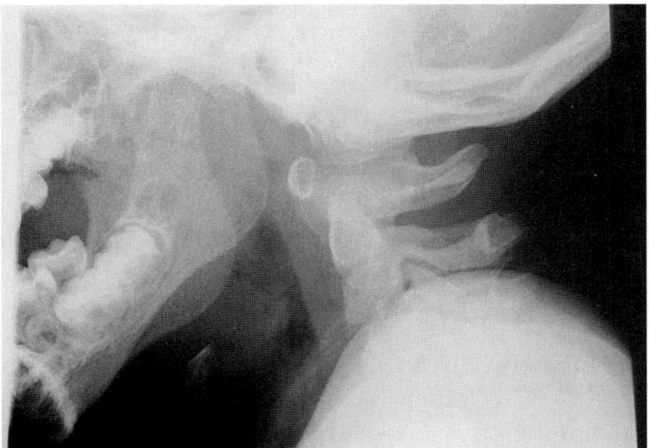

FIGURE 32-6. A hypoplastic dens in a patient with Down syndrome.

The child with Down syndrome definitely needs initial evaluation prior to athletic participation with a physical examination and radiographs. The child should be followed on a regular basis (every 6 to 12 months). There are no clear-cut guidelines for repeat radiographs. Any changes on clinical examinations should prompt the need for new imaging.

Accurate history taking from a parent or caretaker may elicit signs of atlantoaxial instability. Any signs of decrease in physical tolerance or regression in motor skills should be taken seriously. Changes in gait may represent ataxia.

On the lateral flexion and extension radiographs the atlanto-dens interval is measured. There is no need for concern when this interval is less than 5 mm. Over 9 mm of surgical fusion is necessary. The gray zone between these guidelines is where repeated examinations are a must. Changes in the neurologic examination would necessitate a fusion.

Uncommon Causes of Back Pain

When evaluating a young athlete for back pain, remember etiologies unrelated to sports participation. When tumor or infection presents as back pain in the pediatric patient, the child may relate the onset of symptoms to minor trauma received during some athletic event. The parents also may assume there is some correlation, particularly in a very active child. The clue to diagnosis is the physical presentation of the child. The child will appear more sickly than one would expect for an injury. The child may be pale and weak. The pain may be out of proportion to the minor injury and may not resolve within the expected time period. Screening radiographs of the spine are necessary. Multiple compression fractures would be indicative of a systemic illness such as leukemia. Destruction of a disc space would suggest infection.[7]

SUMMARY

The primary care physician can detect the more common spine injuries in the young athlete by paying attention to the type of athletic competition and having awareness of the injuries associated with various sports. A careful physical examination will lead to the proper imaging studies. Knowledge of the natural history of the more common problems will help establish guidelines for continued participation in sports.

REFERENCES

1. Blitzer CM, et al: Downhill skiing injuries in children. Am J Sports Med 12(2):142–147, 1984.
2. Burton AK, Tillotson KM: Does leisure sports activity influence lumbar mobility or the risk of low back trouble? J Spinal Disord 4(3):329–336, 1991.
3. Ciullo JV, Jackson DW: Pars interarticularis stress reaction, or: Spondylolysis and spondylolisthesis in gymnasts. Clin Sports Med 4(1):95–110, 1985.
4. Hardcastle P, et al: Spinal abnormalities in young fast bowlers. JBJS 74B:421–425, 1992.
5. Micheli LJ: Back injuries in gymnastics. Clin Sports Med 4(1):85–93, 1985.
6. Pizzutillo PD: Spinal considerations in the young athlete. Instructional Course Lect 42:463–472, 1993.
7. Sward L, et al: Vertebral ring apophysis injury in athletes is the etiology difference in the thoracic and lumbar spine. Am J Sports Med 21(6):841–846, 1993.
8. Torg JS, Das M: Trampoline and minitrampoline injuries to the cervical spine. Clin Sports Med 4(1):45–60, 1985.

VI

The Older Athlete

33 Medical Considerations for Sports and Exercise Participation in the Older Athlete

Anne R. Bass

The last century has seen a dramatic growth in the elderly U.S. population. The percentage of Americans over 65 has risen from 4.1% in 1900 to 12.4% in 2000, according to the U.S. Bureau of the Census. Individuals who reach the age of 65 currently have a life expectancy of an additional 17.9 years (19.2 years for women, 16.3 years for men). There are now 35 million Americans over the age of 65 and, as the "baby boom" generation ages, this number is expected to rise to 70 million by the year 2030 (Fig. 33-1).[55] Some of these elderly individuals will have maintained an active lifestyle including exercise and athletics from youth to old age. Others may decide to begin such activity later in life because of its benefits to health and quality of life.

In 1995, the Centers for Disease Control and Prevention and the American College of Sports Medicine recommended that all adults engage in at least 30 minutes of moderate intensity physical activity on most, and preferably all, days of the week.[41] Older adults participating in sports, whether for the first time or as veteran athletes, are more likely than their younger counterparts to have a chronic illness and to be on medications. They also have to adapt to an aging musculoskeletal system. The U.S. Department of Health and Human Services Administration on Aging reports that in the year 2000, 26% of individuals 65 to 74 years of age reported a limitation caused by a chronic condition, as did 45.1% of those over 75. These conditions included arthritis (49%), hypertension (36%), orthopedic impairments (30%), heart disease (27%), cataracts (17%), and diabetes (10%).[55]

This chapter will address the benefits and risks of exercise and sports participation in the elderly, the interaction between exercise and specific disease states, the effects of some medications on exercise, and the musculoskeletal effects of aging and their effect on sports participation. Sports injuries specific to elderly athletes will be discussed in the next chapter.

BENEFITS OF EXERCISE ON CARDIAC AND ALL-CAUSE MORTALITY

Epidemiological studies suggest that 12% of the 250,000 deaths per year in the United States are attributable to a lack of regular exercise.[41] Several longitudinal studies have demonstrated the association between physical activity and mortality in both men and women. Paffenbarger et al. studied alumni of the Harvard classes of 1916–1950. Questionnaires asking about level of physical activity, cigarette smoking, diseases, body size, and family history were sent to 10,269 alumni in 1962 or 1966, and again in 1977 (at which time the men were aged 45 to 84). Those with coronary heart disease in 1977 were excluded and the men were followed until 1985. There were 476 deaths between 1977 and 1985, 208 from cardiovascular disease, 156 from cancer. There was an inverse relationship between level of physical activity and risk of death. The relative risk of premature death was halved for those engaging in at least three hours of moderately vigorous physical activity compared to those who were sedentary. Vigorous activity in 1977 conferred survival advantage whether or not the individuals were physically active in the 1960s.[38] This study, along with an earlier analysis of the same alumni, demonstrated that participation in college athletics provided no survival advantage, neither in the period 1966–1978 nor in the period 1977–1985, unless that physical activity was maintained after graduation. Those individuals who took up an active lifestyle at a later date had the same low risk of death as classmates who exercised vigorously all along. Ex-varsity athletes who became inactive had the highest mortality of all.[38,39]

In the Iowa Women's Health Study, questionnaires were sent randomly to 99,826 postmenopausal women aged 55 to 69 in 1986. A total of 41,836 women responded. There were 2284 deaths documented during 7 years of follow-up, including 1101 due to cancer, 739 due to cardiovascular disease, and 150 due to respiratory disease. An increased level of physical activity was found to be associated with a decreased risk of death. Those who engaged in moderate physical activity at least five times per week had a relative risk of death of 0.59 compared to their sedentary peers after controlling for other risk factors. The relative risk of death for those exercising two to four times per week was 0.63. Even those exercising only once per week had a relative risk of death of 0.71 compared to those who did not exercise at all. The association between physical activity and decreased mortality was most dramatic for cardiovascular and respiratory causes of death.[28]

What level of physical activity is necessary to have an effect on health? The answer to this question is not entirely clear. A recent study of 73,763 women enrolled in The Women's Initiative Observational Study demonstrated similar benefits from walking as from vigorous exercise in reducing the risk of either cardiovascular

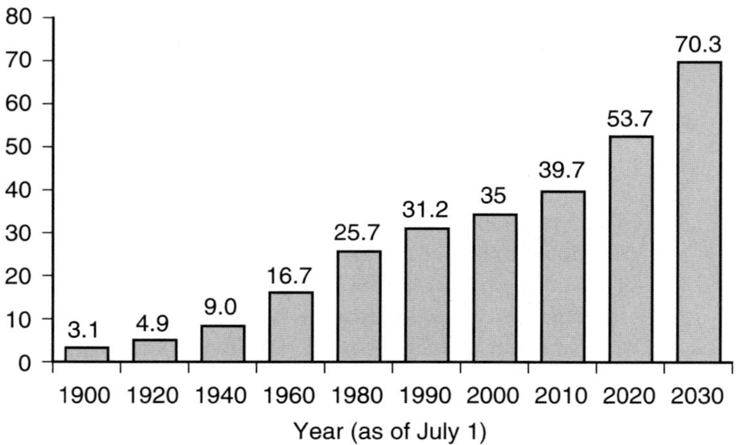

FIGURE 33-1. Data from the U.S. Bureau of the Census showing the number, in millions, of Americans over 65 years of age from 1900–2030. (From U.S. Department of Health and Human Services. A Profile of Older Americans: 2002. http:// www.aoa.dhhs.gov/aoa/STATS/profile/default.htm. Last modified 01/02/2003. Available at www.fedstats.gov.)

events or a newly diagnosed coronary artery disease. Engaging in either form of activity for at least 2.5 hours per week resulted in a 30% reduction in risk. There was a progressive reduction in risk associated with progressively higher weekly energy expenditure for either type of exercise.[31]

The Harvard Alumni Health Study, in contrast, demonstrated that vigorous exercise, but not light or moderate exercise was associated with decreased mortality, even when the same number of kilocalories per week was expended.[29] These differences may relate to the actual level of fitness (or lack thereof) in the "sedentary" populations studied, or conceivably to gender differences.

Studies based on individuals' reported level of physical activity are useful epidemiologically, but measures of fitness may be better predictors of mortality.7 Fitness is generally defined as maximal oxygen uptake ($\dot{V}O_{2max}$) measured during exercise testing. Exercise increases $\dot{V}O_{2max}$ by increasing maximum cardiac output and increasing the ability of muscle to extract and use oxygen from blood.[17] Fitness can also be approximated by exercise duration during exercise tolerance testing. Blair et al. followed 10,225 males and 3120 females for an average of 8 years. Baseline physical fitness (as measured by maximum time on the treadmill during exercise testing) correlated with mortality, particularly in those over 60 years of age. The relative risk of mortality from the least-fit to most-fit quintiles was 3.44 for men and 4.65 for women, with the most significant reduction in risk seen between the first and second quintile.[8] A later study by some of the same authors measured fitness at two time points, a mean of 4.9 years apart. Those unfit at baseline and follow-up had the highest mortality. Those unfit at baseline but fit at follow-up had intermediate mortality and those fit at both time points had the lowest mortality. Men over 60 years of age who improved their fitness had a 50% lower mortality than those who remained unfit (Fig. 33-2).[7]

THE EFFECT OF AGING ON FITNESS

Although increased fitness is associated with decreased mortality, fitness levels tend to decline with age. Maximum oxygen uptake falls 5% to 15% per decade between the ages of 20 and 80.[17] There are many reasons for this. Older individuals have lower cardiac stroke volumes, less left ventricular contractility during exercise, and higher blood pressure and systemic vascular resistance during maximal exercise.[2] Muscle mass and strength also decline with age and much of the decline in $\dot{V}O_{2max}$ associated with aging disappears when it is expressed relative to muscle mass. Is the lower level of fitness seen in older individuals the inevitable result of aging or does it reflect declining levels of exercise? Asked another way, can training minimize an individual's age-associated decline in fitness? The answer is, to some degree, yes. Intensive endurance training can increase

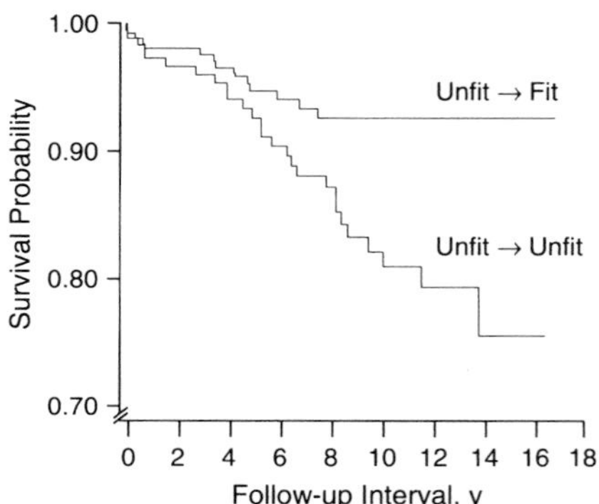

FIGURE 33-2. The lower line represents the survival curve for men in the least fit quintile. The upper line represents men who were in the least fit quintile at baseline but then become fit (quintiles 2–5) by the time of follow-up, an average of 4.9 years later. (From Blair SN, Kohl HW, Barlow CE: Changes in physical fitness and all-cause mortality. JAMA 273:1093–1098, 1995. Copyrighted 1995, American Medical Association. Reproduced with permission.)

$\dot{V}O_{2max}$ in those aged 60 to 70 to the same degree as younger individuals as long as it is done regularly, at a vigorous level, and for a prolonged period of time. Similarly, progressive endurance training over a 6-month period increases $\dot{V}O_{2max}$ by 22% in men and women aged 70 to 79. Resistance training, although it has been shown to increase strength by 18% over 6 months in those aged 70 to 79, has minimal if any impact on fitness as measured by $\dot{V}O_{2max}$.[22]

Although the decline in $\dot{V}O_{2max}$ seen over time in endurance-trained individuals (–5% per decade) is less than in their inactive counterparts (–9% per decade), there is still a decline. Is this due to aging or to a reduction in training? Pollock et al. studied 24 men aged 50 to 82 who had placed first through third in regional masters' competitions, mostly runners. They were tested in 1971–1974 and then again 10 years later. All the men maintained the same mileage per week, but one group was still actively training for competition at a pace within 30 seconds of their time 10 years before. The other group was no longer actively training and ran at a pace 90 seconds slower than the previous decade. The competitive group maintained $\dot{V}O_{2max}$ whereas the noncompetitive group did not.[44] Trappe and colleagues, on the other hand, studied aging over 22 years among elite long-distance runners. All men had a decline in $\dot{V}O_{2max}$. The loss was lower (–5.2%), however, in those who had maintained the highest level of training and competition than in those who no longer trained, or trained only for fitness (–16% and –15.5%, respectively). The subset of the oldest 10 runners, who were all over 60 years of age and trained only for fitness, had the greatest loss of $\dot{V}O_{2max}$ (–31.8%) and were the only group to lose lean body mass.[54] Thus it seems that even high-intensity exercise can lessen but not entirely eliminate the age-associated decline in $\dot{V}O_{2max}$.

RISKS OF EXERCISE

Although regular exercise reduces overall mortality, exercise can acutely increase the risk of sudden death. In the presence of coronary disease, exercise-related deaths are felt to be due to plaque rupture leading to myocardial infarction or arrhythmia.[18] A study of all exercise-related deaths in Rhode Island from 1975–1982 found that 88% were due to atherosclerotic heart disease.[45]

Two large studies published in 1993 demonstrated an association between strenuous activity and acute myocardial infarction. Willich et al. found the relative risk of having exercised strenuously at the onset of an acute myocardial infarction (MI) to be 2.1. The relative risk for those who normally exercised less than four times per week was 6.9 compared to 1.3 for those who exercised at least four times per week.[60] Mittleman et al. found the relative risk of MI in the hour after heavy exertion to be 5.9. In patients who rarely exerted themselves, the relative risk was 107 as compared to a relative risk of 2.4 for those who exercised vigorously at least five times per week.[36]

In the Physicians Health Study of 21,481 men without obvious cardiac disease, there were 122 episodes of sudden death from cardiac causes over 12 years of follow-up. Of these deaths, 13.9% occurred during exercise and 4.9% occurred within 30 minutes after exercise. The relative risk of sudden death during exercise was 16.9, but sudden death occurred in only 1/1.42 million person hours of vigorous exercise (versus 1/23 million person hours of nonexercise). Those who exercised rarely had a relative risk of sudden death during exercise of 74 whereas those who exercised at least five times per week had a relative risk of 10.9. Although there was an increased risk of sudden death during exercise, the overall risk of death from coronary artery disease was lower among men who participated in vigorous exercise at least once per week.[1]

Finally, a retrospective review of records from a large commercial fitness center found 71 fatal events in 182,307,244 workouts, 2 in nonmember guests. Of the 69 members who died, 34 exercised less than once per week at the center (including 10 who had made a total of only 0 to 2 visits) while only 3/69 fatalities were in members who worked out at least five times per week.[19]

Overall, the risk of death during exercise is felt to be 0.01 to 0.20/10,000 hours, while the risk of fatal and life-threatening events during exercise is 0.24/10,000 hours.[18] Reducing the risk of exercise-related death in older individuals involves screening for coronary artery risk factors such as diabetes, hypertension, hyperlipidemia, smoking, obesity, and family history of myocardial infarction, and performing exercise tolerance testing when such risk factors are present. In addition, careful questioning about cardiac symptoms is important not only in sedentary individuals about to begin an exercise program, but also in monitoring older individuals who are already established athletes. Members of this latter group often consider themselves to be immune to cardiac disease because of their lifestyle.[20] A British study of 51 cases of sudden death from coronary disease associated with playing squash found that 45 of 51 individuals had had at least one prodromal symptom within the week of their death and 9 had seen a physician. The symptoms included chest pain, fatigue, indigestion, shortness of breath, ear/neck pain, malaise, upper respiratory infection, dizziness/palpitations, and severe headache. The vast majority of these athletes were considered fit by their family but 32 of 51 had at least one cardiac risk factor.[37]

In summary, although exercise acutely increases the risk of sudden death, the absolute risk is low in properly screened individuals who exercise regularly. In addition, the increased risk of sudden death during exercise is offset by the overall reduced risk of cardiac death seen in those who are physically active. Elderly individuals embarking on exercise for the first time should follow a program that is progressive in both intensity and duration so that they can gradually increase their endurance. Activities like squash that require sudden, heavy exertion using both arms and legs are more highly associated with sudden cardiac death. Those at risk for sudden cardiac death should avoid highly competitive sports and games, as well as activities that require intermittent or prolonged high exertion levels, combined arm and leg exercise, or heavy weight lifting.[20]

HYPERTENSION

Aging is associated with changes in arterial structure, including intimal hyperplasia, disorganization of elastin in the media, and its replacement by less compliant collagen. All this results in increased arterial stiffness and decreased arterial compliance.[56] When sedentary older individuals participate in an aerobic exercise program (primarily walking) for 3 months, central arterial compliance can rise by 25%. In endurance-trained middle-aged and older men, central arterial compliance, as measured by carotid applantation tonometry, is 20% to 35% higher than in recreationally active men of the same age, and 40% higher than in those who are sedentary.[53]

As arterial compliance falls with age, systolic blood pressure and pulse pressure rise. Seals et al. showed that this age-related rise in systolic blood pressure occurs in sedentary women but not in endurance-trained women. This was linked to a lower prevalence of abdominal obesity and also to lower arterial stiffness in the endurance-trained women.[48]

Although blood pressure rises during exercise, blood pressure falls below baseline levels immediately after. This is due to a drop in cardiac output (due at least in part to decreased venous return) and a fall in systemic vascular resistance. This effect is particularly prominent in hypertensive individuals and can last up to 22 hours after exercise.[46] Regular endurance exercise lowers casual systolic and diastolic blood pressure in hypertensive individuals and this effect may be greater with moderate exercise than high-intensity exercise. Resistive strength training, although it markedly raises blood pressure acutely, also lowers resting blood pressure in the long term.[3]

Hypertensive individuals have an exaggerated rise in systolic blood pressure during aerobic and resistive exercise. Individuals with a blood pressure greater that 180/105 and those with left ventricular hypertrophy or other end-organ damage should be treated pharmacologically for their hypertension prior to starting an exercise program.[3]

DIABETES

According to the Centers for Disease Control and Prevention, there are 10.3 million Americans with diabetes and an estimated 5.4 million additional undiagnosed cases.[4] Physical activity increases insulin sensitivity and is inversely correlated with the development of diabetes, independent of its effect on body weight. Helmrich et al. studied 5990 University of Pennsylvania graduates aged 39 to 68 at baseline. The incidence of diabetes over the next 14 years was half in those with the highest level of activity compared to those with the lowest. They estimated that each additional hour of moderate activity performed weekly reduced the risk of diabetes by 6%. The protective effect of exercise was greatest in the group at highest risk for diabetes, namely those with a body mass index of at least 25, a history of hypertension, or a family history of diabetes.[24]

Patients who enter into diabetes treatment programs that include exercise as well as diet achieve greater weight loss than those that modify their diet alone.[10] The rate of oxygen consumption with exercise is lower in diabetics than in nondiabetics, however (and inversely related to glucose tolerance and glycemic control), and some diabetics cannot exercise at the level required for rapid weight loss. Weight loss can be achieved even in these individuals, however, if it is done at least five times per week and is continued long term, over a period of years.[4]

Diabetic end-organ damage can complicate exercise. Autonomic neuropathy can lead to postural hypotension, and an exaggerated fall in blood pressure after exercise. It may also limit maximum heart rate achieved with exercise (though resting heart rate may be higher than normal in these individuals). Peripheral neuropathy increases the risk of foot injury and in its presence only non–weight bearing exercise should be performed. Proper footwear will also help to prevent injury in affected individuals. Both diabetic nephropathy and retinopathy can be worsened by the high systolic blood pressures associated with high-intensity aerobic exercise and intense strength training. Patients with retinopathy should also avoid activities that involve jumping, exercise with the head down, or with the arms overhead.[4]

Elderly diabetics who plan to embark on an exercise program should undergo exercise tolerance testing and be assessed for the presence of hypertension, peripheral vascular disease, retinopathy, nephropathy, and autonomic neuropathy.[10] In addition to screening for ischemic heart disease, exercise testing will establish an individual's maximum heart rate (which may be lower than predicted in the presence of autonomic neuropathy). Diabetics should exercise at least three times per week at a moderate intensity (50% to 75% maximum heart rate, 40% to 70% $\dot{V}O_{2max}$). In patients with autonomic neuropathy, their own perceived level of exertion may be a better means of monitoring exercise intensity than heart rate. The duration of exercise should be gradually increased from 10 to 15 minutes to 30 minutes per session, but 60-minute sessions may be necessary if weight loss is a goal.[4]

PERIPHERAL VASCULAR DISEASE

Exercise has long been a mainstay of treatment for claudication, which affects 4% of the elderly population.[30] Patients with claudication use a higher percentage of $\dot{V}O_{2max}$ for a given amount of walking, but this percentage decreases after four months of exercise training.[50] A review of 10 trials of exercise for the treatment of claudication found that it significantly improved walking time in all studies and produced improvements comparable to those achieved by surgery.[30] A meta-analysis of exercise programs found a greater reduction in claudication associated with increased frequency and duration of exercise. Walking was more effective than a mix of exercises, and those programs that pushed patients to near maximal pain, rather than to the onset of pain had better outcomes.[21]

HYPERLIPIDEMIA

Although even low levels of exercise appear to have an effect on mortality, more intense exercise may be necessary to modify lipid levels. The National Runners Health Study found that elevation in HDL cholesterol after the initiation of a running program correlated with longer weekly distances run. The increase in HDL seen in these longer-distance runners, however, may have been due to their greater losses of body weight.[59]

A recent study of sedentary overweight individuals aged 40 to 65 entered into one of four exercise programs varying in frequency and intensity of exercise, found no effect of exercise on total cholesterol or LDL. It did, however, demonstrate a decline in the concentration of small LDL particles and an increase in the size of LDL particles with progressive amounts and intensity of exercise, even in the absence of significant weight loss.[27]

MEDICATIONS

Many elderly individuals take medications daily and some of these, particularly β-blockers, diuretics, and hypoglycemics, can have an impact on exercise.

β-Blockers

β-Blockers lower resting and maximum heart rate. They can also reduce maximum exercise capacity acutely. Endurance training (moderate-intensity exercise over a long duration) results in reduced sensitivity of β-receptors. Such training results in a lower heart rate for a given intensity of exercise. β-Blockers reduce heart rate by 20% to 30% and cardiac output by 5% to 23%. During moderately intense exercise, cardiac output is maintained by increasing stroke volume. Endurance-trained senior athletes may not tolerate β-blockade because they already have a reduced heart rate and increased stroke volume, and may not be able to compensate further.[23] Treatment with nonselective β-blockers such as propranolol can reduce jogging performance by 20% to 30%, compared to 10% with β_1-selective drugs. Nonselective β-blockers also cause more rapid falls in blood glucose level through interference with hepatic glycogenolysis, reduced hepatic gluconeogenesis, and a reduced supply of free fatty acids. In general, β_1-selective drugs, especially those that are in a controlled-release form, seem to have the least effect on endurance exercise capacity.[23]

Despite the effects of β-blockers on exercise performance, studies suggest that individuals on β-blockers can benefit from exercise training to the same degree as those not on them. Savin et al. studied sedentary men without coronary artery disease treated with either a β-blocker or placebo. All were entered into an intense 6-week program of daily exercise training. Peak oxygen consumption, peak work rate, and peak duration of work increased to the same degree in all groups, though maximum heart rates were 20% lower in the β-blocked men.[47] Studies have shown similar results in individuals with coronary artery disease. That is, patients who participate in cardiac rehabilitation programs can increase their level of fitness despite being on β-blockers.[47]

Diuretics

Diuretics reduce intravascular volume and cause renal losses of potassium and magnesium, both of which can interfere with exercise performance. Dorup et al. studied muscle biopsies from 25 patients on long-term diuretic therapy and 25 controls. Over half of the patients on diuretics had muscle potassium and magnesium levels less than two standard deviations below those of the controls, despite being on potassium supplements and having normal serum potassium and magnesium levels. There was also a decreased concentration of [Na/K] pumps in the muscles of the patients on diuretics.[14] Thus, adequate potassium and magnesium supplementation, as well as adequate hydration is important for optimizing the exercise performance of those on diuretics.

Medications for Diabetes

Exercise can have short-term effects on the blood glucose levels of diabetics that may require adjustments in medication. Light exercise for less than 10 minutes does not affect blood glucose. During the first 10 minutes of moderate to heavy exercise blood glucose will rise. Thereafter, hypoglycemia can develop the more vigorous and prolonged the exercise. Insulin injected before exercise will increase glucose uptake in the muscles and decrease hepatic glucose production. To avoid exercise-induced hypoglycemia, glucose should be measured before and after exercise and medication dosage adjusted accordingly. Insulin should be injected at least an hour prior to exercise in a nonexercising part of the body and the insulin dosage should initially be reduced by 50% for the period of planned exercise.[10]

Oral medications for diabetes, especially sulfonureas, can also produce postexercise hypoglycemia, particularly in nonobese individuals. Sulfonureas act by increasing pancreatic insulin secretion. Second-generation sulfonureas such as glyburide, glipizide, and glimepiride have effects for up to 24 hours and are usually dosed once or twice daily. Dosing should be timed so that peak effect does not coincide with exercise. Meglitinides (repaglinide), short-acting agents that stimulate pancreatic insulin secretion, and alpha-glucosidase inhibitors (acarbose and miglitol) which impair carbohydrate absorption, can cause exercise-induced hypoglycemia if exercise follows a meal. Biguanides (metformin) increase hepatic insulin sensitivity and can impair hepatic glucose production during exercise. Thiazolidinediones (troglitazone, pioglitazone, rosiglitazone) increase the insulin sensitivity of muscle and fat and enhance skeletal muscle glucose uptake.[10] By exercising not only daily but at the same time each day, diabetics can simplify any medication adjustments that need to be made to accommodate exercise.[4]

THE AGING MUSCULOSKELETAL SYSTEM

Aging has effects on muscle, bone, cartilage, and tendons that can affect elderly individuals' ability to maintain fitness and increase their risk of injury.

Muscle

There is a fall in lean muscle mass with aging in both sedentary and endurance-trained individuals. Structural changes in muscle that have been noted with age include a decrease in contractile elements, a fall in the number and size of type II (fast twitch) fibers, a loss of motor units, abnormal fiber grouping (suggestive of neuropathy), a decrease in the number and size of mitochondria, and a decrease in the activity of oxidative enzymes. It is difficult to know which of these changes are due to disuse atrophy and which to aging itself.[15]

Oxygen consumption during maximal exercise occurs largely in exercising muscles. Thus, the decline in fitness ($\dot{V}O_{2max}$) seen with age may simply be due to a selective loss of skeletal muscle mass. A cross-sectional analysis of participants in the Baltimore Longitudinal Study on Aging demonstrated a 23.4% loss of muscle mass (as measured by creatine excretion) in men, and a 22% loss of muscle mass in women between the ages of 30 to 70. After controlling for age, $\dot{V}O_{2max}$ correlated with muscle mass. Maximum oxygen uptake fell 39% for men and 30% for women between ages 30 and 70, but when this was normalized for muscle mass, the declines were only 18% and 14%, respectively.[16] This suggests that exercise regimens that help to maintain lean body mass will help to reduce the "age-associated" decline in fitness.

Bones

By age 70, women have a 20% loss in bone mineral density (BMD) at the spine and a 25% loss at the femoral neck, with much of the decline occurring after menopause. In men there is a small linear decline in proximal femur BMD starting in young adulthood, and only minimal loss of BMD at the spine.[32] In old age (after age 70) there is accelerated bone loss at the hip in both men and women.[57] Postmenopausal bone loss in women is due to an absence of estrogen, which leads to increased bone remodeling, perforated trabeculae, and architectural disruption. In men, trabecular connectivity is better maintained despite a decrease in the bone volume produced.[49]

Fat mass is correlated with BMD in women, possibly because of fat's ability to convert adrenal androgens to estrogen, but also because of the increased mechanical load on weight-bearing bones. Muscle strength and lean muscle mass are also associated with increased BMD, most likely because they reflect both overall physical activity levels, and because of the local effects of muscle contraction on bone.[51]

Physical activity levels are associated with increased BMD in both men and women.[42] Resistance training and weight-bearing exercise increase bone mass to a greater degree than other forms of exercise.[52] Sedentary postmenopausal women who undertake an exercise program over 9 months can increase bone density at the spine by 5.2%. This benefit is lost, however, if exercise is stopped.[12] Thus, physical activity is of benefit in maintaining bone density. At the same time, individuals with osteoporosis should avoid contact sports and sports associated with frequent falls (such as skiing) so as to lessen the likelihood of fracture.

Tendons and Ligaments

In contrast to the changes seen in bone structure, tendons and ligaments are less subject to age-related degeneration per se. Studies of cadaveric supraspinatous tendons from individuals over age 30 without a history of shoulder pain, for example, show no change in collagen weight or collagen synthesis with age.[6] The mode of ligament or tendon failure does, however, vary with age. In older individuals, anterior cruciate ligaments fail by bony avulsion more frequently than in the young. Similarly, in middle-aged and elderly women, Achilles tendon failure tends to occur because of bony avulsion. In middle-aged men, by contrast, Achilles tendons tend to fail because of tendon rupture. Experimental models suggest that the mode of failure relates to the density of the attached bone rather than to the characteristics of the tendons and ligaments themselves.[61]

At the shoulder, progressive weakness of the rotator cuff muscles with age can lead to tendon impingement and injury. There is a linear increase in the prevalence of grade 3 impingements at the shoulder after age 50; grade 3 impingements are present in 50% of subjects who are 60 to 69 years of age, and 80% of those aged 80 to 99.[33] Although most affected elderly individuals are asymptomatic, they will be prone to shoulder injury if they embark on upper extremity athletics without muscle strengthening beforehand.

Thus, although tendons and ligaments themselves may not degenerate with age, age-related changes in surrounding bone or muscle may increase the likelihood of injury to these soft-tissue structures.

Cartilage

The composition of articular cartilage changes with age. These changes include an increased concentration of noncollagenous proteins, a change in glycosaminoglycan composition, and an increase in hyaluronic acid production. Modification of articular proteins by reducing sugars (nonenzymatic glycosylation or NEG) also increases fifty-fold between the ages of 20 and 80.[13] At the same time, pyridinoline crosslinks, which are necessary for the structural integrity of cartilage, decline. Individuals over the age of 65 have a 50% reduction in the level of pyridinoline crosslinks in their vertebral disks, and a higher level of NEC as measured by pentosidine concentration. Higher levels of pentosidine also correlate with degenerative changes seen macroscopically.[43] Nonenzymatic glycosylation of cartilage results in a stiffer matrix and also interferes with cartilage proteoglycan production.[13] These changes may explain the high prevalence of osteoarthritis seen with advancing age.

OSTEOARTHRITIS

Twelve percent of individuals over 65 years of age are limited in their physical activity by arthritis.[35] Although there is a strong association between chronic or repetitive mechanical stress on joints and the development of osteoarthritis, animal and human studies do not support a cause and effect relationship between habitual exercise and arthritis in individuals with normal joints at baseline.[9] A study of long-term long-distance runners over age 50 failed to show a higher prevalence of osteoarthritis than in sedentary controls. The authors concluded that running "need not" be associated with premature degenerative change of the joints.[40] It is possible, however, that individuals prone to arthritis do not choose to or cannot maintain running as a long-term form of exercise.

Marginal osteophytes can develop in the joints of people who exercise vigorously lifelong, but this appears to be an adaptive strategy on the part of the body to distribute mechanical load over a larger surface area. It does not correlate with cartilage damage, nor is it predictive of the development of osteoarthritis.[9] In patients with joint instability or ligamentous or meniscal injury at baseline, however, repetitive joint impact or torsion can lead to the development of osteoarthritis. The time between injury and the development of degenerative arthritis is, in addition, shorter in the elderly than in younger individuals.[9]

Patients with osteoarthritis can benefit from exercise training to the same degree as those without arthritis. In the Seattle FICSIT trial, participants aged 68 to 85 with gait abnormalities were randomly assigned to strength and/or endurance training, while controls received routine care. Patients in all training groups improved their strength regardless of whether they had arthritis or not, and there was no change in arthritic complaints during the 6-month study in any of the exercise groups. Of note, the injury rate was 0.48/1000 hours of exercise.[11]

Joint motion is in fact chondroprotective, and patients with osteoarthritis are generally prescribed range of motion exercises, muscle strengthening, and some form of low-impact aerobic exercise.[34] An interventional study of patients with osteoarthritis of the knee demonstrated that an 8-week program of supervised fitness walking improved both functional status and measures of pain compared to routine care.[26]

Efforts should be made to protect the joints of patients with osteoarthritis during exercise. Approaches to this include choosing low-impact forms of exercise (such as walking, stationary cycling, swimming, or rowing), strengthening muscles so that they can both stabilize the joints and help to absorb impact stress, and wearing shoes with good shock absorption.[35] Viscoelastic insoles can reduce shock at the proximal tibia by 42%.[34] Some individuals will also benefit from orthotics.

BALANCE

Sixty-five percent of people over the age of 60 complain of dizziness or loss of balance. Balance is a response to somatosensory inputs from the proprioceptive, visual, and vestibular systems, and pressure sensors in the skin. The cerebellum and basal ganglia help mediate postural reflexes. Balance is optimal between the ages of 30 and 60. With aging there is a decrease in vestibular hair cells and vestibular neurons, a decrease in Purkinje and neuronal cells in the cerebellum, and degenerative changes in the sensory and motor systems, tendon receptors, and musculoskeletal system, all of which increase the likelihood of falls.[25] The elderly depend even more than the young on vision to compensate for degeneration in various neuromotor systems, but vision itself often declines with age.[58] Physical activity helps maintain strength and reaction times, lessening the likelihood of falls. At the same time, the decline in balance that occurs with age should be considered when choosing an exercise regimen for an elderly patient. Those who are veteran athletes in sports in which balance is particularly important, such as rock-climbing, skating, or downhill skiing, may need to modify their activities somewhat to accommodate these changes.

RECOMMENDATIONS FOR EXERCISE IN THE ELDERLY

In 1995 the Centers for Disease Control and Prevention and the American College of Sports Medicine (ACSM) jointly published guidelines for exercise. They recommended that every adult exercise for 30 minutes each day (which could be in 10-minute increments) at light to moderate intensity. Activities considered to be at this level included walking briskly (3 to 4 mph), cycling leisurely, swimming with moderate effort, table tennis, calisthenics, golf, canoeing slowly, house cleaning, lawn mowing, or home repair.[7] In a later position statement on exercise for older adults, however, the ACSM acknowledged that moderate- or high-intensity exercise might be required to elicit adaptations in the cardiovascular system and in cardiovascular disease risk factors.[2] Such activities include walking, cycling, or swimming at a faster pace and are estimated to require 50% to 70% of $\dot{V}O_{2max}$ (60% to 80% of maximum heart rate, calculated as 220 – age).

Patients with cardiovascular risk factors should undergo exercise tolerance testing prior to beginning an exercise program. Those with cardiac disease should be referred to a cardiologist for exercise prescription. Contraindications to exercise training or testing include recent EKG changes or myocardial infarction, unstable angina, uncontrolled arrhythmia, third-degree heart block, and acute congestive heart failure.[2]

Diabetics should be screened for the presence of autonomic and peripheral neuropathy, retinopathy, and nephropathy. Proper footwear should be prescribed for those with foot deformities or peripheral neuropathy. Patients with osteoarthritis of the hip or knee will tolerate non–weight bearing forms of exercise such as walking, stationary cycling, or swimming better than weight-bearing forms of exercise such as jogging. The addition of strength training to an aerobic exercise regimen will help to prevent injury and maintain bone density.

Exercise training should be gradually progressive in intensity and duration. Endurance training can include any activity that uses large muscle groups, is maintained continuously, and is rhythmical and aerobic in nature, such as walking, running, swimming, cycling, or rowing.[5] Elderly individuals who have previously been sedentary should begin endurance training at a low level (40% to 55% maximum heart rate, 30% to 40% $\dot{V}O_{2max}$) for 10 to 15 minutes, three times per week. After 4 to 6 weeks (up to 10 weeks if very unfit at baseline), effort can be gradually increased to a moderate level (50% to 70% maximum heart rate, 40% to 60% $\dot{V}O_{2max}$), and duration increased to 20 to 30 minutes per session. After six months, elderly individuals can begin to participate in sports and games but should continue endurance training to maintain fitness. A subset of individuals may be able to progress to higher intensity exercise (70% to 90% maximum heart rate, 60% to 80% $\dot{V}O_{2max}$), and to longer exercise duration (45 to 60 minutes). A warm-up consisting of flexibility exercises and lower level exercise should precede each session.[20] Elderly individuals who are already established athletes should continue to be monitored medically for the development of cardiac risk factors or symptoms.

REFERENCES

1. Albert CM, Mittleman MA, Chae CU, et al: Triggering of sudden death from cardiac causes by vigorous exertion. N Engl J Med 343:1355–1361, 2000.
2. American College of Sports Medicine position stand: Exercise and physical activity for older adults. Med Sci Sports Exerc 30:992–1008, 1998.
3. American College of Sports Medicine position stand: Physical activity, physical fitness, and hypertension. Med Sci Sports Exerc 25:i–x, 1993.
4. American College of Sports Medicine position stand: Exercise and type 2 diabetes. Med Sci Sports Exerc 32:1345–1360, 2000.
5. American College of Sports Medicine position stand: The recommended quantity and quality of exercise for developing and maintaining cardiorespiratory and muscular fitness in healthy adults. Med Sci Sports Exerc 22:265–274, 1990.
6. Bank RA, TeKoppele JM, Oostingh G, et al: Lysylhydroxylation and non-reducible crosslinking of human supraspinatus tendon collagen: Changes with age and in chronic rotator cuff tendinitis. Ann Rheum Dis 58:35–41, 1999.
7. Blair SN, Kohl HW, Barlow CE: Changes in physical fitness and all-cause mortality. JAMA 273: 1093–1098, 1995.
8. Blair SN, Kohl HW, Paffenbarger RS, et al: Physical fitness and all-cause mortality: A prospective study of healthy men and women. JAMA 262:2395–2401, 1989.
9. Buckwalter JA, Lane NE: Athletics and osteoarthritis. Am J Sports Med 25:873–881, 1997.
10. Chipkin SR, Klugh SA, Chasan-Taber L: Exercise in secondary prevention and cardiac rehabilitation. Cardiol Clin 19:489–505, 2001.
11. Coleman EA, Buchner DM, Cress ME, et al: The relationship of joint symptoms with exercise performance in older adults. J Am Geriatr Soc 44:14–21, 1996.

12. Dalsky GP, Stocke KS, Ehsani AA, et al: Weight-bearing exercise training and lumbar bone mineral content in postmenopausal women. Ann Intern Med 108:824–828, 1988.
13. DeGroot J, Verzijl M, Bank RA, et al: Age-related decrease in proteoglycan synthesis of human articular chondrocyes: The role of nonenzymatic glycation. Arthritis Rheum 42:1003–1009, 1999.
14. Dorup, I, Skajaa, K, Clausen, T et al: Reduced concentrations of potassium, magnesium, and sodium-potassium pumps in human skeletal muscle during treatment with diuretics. Br Med J 296:455–458, 1988.
15. Fiatarone MA, Evans WJ: The etiology and reversibility of muscle dysfunction in the aged. J Gerontol 48:77–83, 1993.
16. Fleg JL, Lakatta EG: Role of muscle loss in the age-associated reduction in VO_{2max}. J Appl Physiol 65:1147–1151, 1988.
17. Fletcher GF, Balady G, Blair SN, et al: Statement on exercise: Benefits and recommendations for physical activity programs for all Americans: A statement for health professionals by the Committee on Exercise and Cardiac Rehabilitation of the Council on Clinical Cardiology, American Heart Association. Circulation 94:857–862, 1996.
18. Foster C, Porcari JP: The risks of exercise training. J Cardiopulm Rehabil 21:347–352, 2001.
19. Franklin BA: Sporadic exercise: A trigger for acute cardiovascular events? Circulation 102:612, 2000.
20. Friedewald VE, Spence DW: Sudden cardiac death associated with exercise: The risk-benefit issue. Am J Cardiol 66:183–188, 1990.
21. Gardner AW, Poehlman ET: Exercise rehabilitation programs for the treatment of claudication pain. JAMA 274:975–980, 1995.
22. Hagberg JM, Graves JE, Limacher M, et al: Cardiovascular responses of 70- to 79-yr-old men and women to exercise training. J Appl Physiol 66: 2589–2594, 1989.
23. Head A: Exercise metabolism and beta-blocker therapy: An update. Sports Med 2:81–96, 1999.
24. Helmrich SP, Ragland DR, Leung RW, et al: Physical activity and reduced occurrence of non-insulin-dependent diabetes mellitus. N Engl J Med 325:147–152, 1991.
25. Hobeika CP: Equilibrium and balance in the elderly. Ear Nose Throat J 78:558–562, 1995.
26. Kovar PA, Allegrante JP, MacKenzie R, et al: Supervised fitness walking in patients with osteoarthritis of the knee. Ann Intern Med 116: 529–534, 1992.
27. Kraus WE, Houmard JA, Duscha BD, et al: Effects of the amount and intensity of exercise on plasma lipoproteins. N Engl J Med 347:1483–1492, 2002.
28. Kushi LH, Fee RM, Folsom AR, et al: Physical activity and mortality in postmenopausal women. JAMA 277:1287–1292, 1997.
29. Lee I, Hsieh C, Paffenbarger RS: Exercise intensity and longevity in men: The Harvard alumni study. JAMA 273:1179–1184, 1995.
30. Leng GC, Fowler B, Ernst E: Exercise for intermittent claudication (Cochrane Review). In The Cochrane Library 4, 2002, Oxford, Update Software.
31. Manson, JE, Greenland, P, LaCroix, AZ, et al: Walking compared with vigorous exercise for the prevention of cardiovascular events in women. N Engl J Med 347:716–725, 2002.
32. Mazess RB, Barden HS, Drinka PJ, et al: Influence of age and body weight on spine and femur bone mineral density in U.S. white men. J Bone Min Res 5:645–652, 1990.
33. Milgrom C, Schaffler M, Gilbert S, et al: Rotator-cuff changes in asymptomatic adults. J Bone Joint Surg [Br] 77–B:296–298, 1995,
34. Minor MA: Osteoarthritis. Rheum Dis Clin North Am 25:397–415, 1999.
35. Minor MA, Lane NE: Recreational exercise in arthritis. Rheum Dis Clin North Am 22:563–577, 1996.
36. Mittleman MA, Maclure M, Tofler G, et al: Triggering of acute myocardial infarction by heavy physical exertion—Protection against triggering by regular exertion. N Engl J Med 329:1677–1683, 1993.
37. Northcote RJ, Flannigan C, Ballantyne D: Sudden death and vigorous exercise—A study of 60 deaths associated with squash. Br Heart J 55:198–203, 1986.
38. Paffenbarger RS, Hyde RT, Wing AL, et al: The association of changes in physical-activity level and other lifestyle characteristics with mortality among men. N Engl J Med 328:538–554, 1993.
39. Paffenbarger RS, Hyde,RT, Wing AL, et al: A natural history of athleticism and cardiovascular health. JAMA 252:491–495, 1984.
40. Panush RS, Schmidt C, Caldwell JR, et al: Is running associated with degenerative joint disease? JAMA 255:1152–1154, 1986.
41. Pate RR, Pratt M, Blair SN, et al: Physical activity and public health: A recommendation from the Centers for Disease Control and Prevention and the American College of Sports Medicine. JAMA 273:402–407, 1995.
42. Pluijm SMF, Visser M, Smit JH, et al: Determinants of bone mineral density in older men and women: Body composition as mediator. J Bone Min Res 16: 2142–2151, 2001.
43. Pokharna HK, Phillips FM: Collagen crosslinks in human lumbar intervertebral disc aging. Spine 23:1645–1648, 1998.

44. Pollock ML Foster C, Knapp D, et al: Effect of age and training on aerobic capacity and body composition of master athletes. J Appl Physiol 62:725–731, 1987.
45. Ragosta M, Crabtree J, Sturner WQ, et al: Death during recreational exercise in the state of Rhode Island. Med Sci Sports Exerc 16:339–342, 1982.
46. Rondon MUPB, Alves MJNN, Braga AMFW, et al: Postexercise blood pressure reduction in elderly hypertensive patients. J Am Coll Cardiol 39: 676–682, 2002.
47. Savin WM, Gordon EP, Kaplan SM, et al: Exercise training during long-term beta-blockade treatment in healthy subjects. Am J Cardiol 55:101D–109D, 1985.
48. Seals DR, Stevenson ET, Jones PP, et al: Lack of age-associated elevations in 24-hour systolic and pulse pressures in women who exercise regularly. Am J Physiol 277:H947–H955, 1999.
49. Seeman E: Pathogenesis of bone fragility in women and men. Lancet 359:1841–1850, 2002.
50. Stewart KJ, Hiatt WR, Regensteiner JG, et al: Exercise training for claudication. N Engl J Med 347:1941–1951, 2002.
51. Taaffe DR, Cauley JA, Danielson M, et al: Race and sex effects on the association between muscle strength, soft tissue, and bone mineral density in healthy elders: The health, aging, and body composition study. J Bone Min Res 16:1343–1351, 2001.
52. Taaffe DR, Robinson TL, Snow CM, et al: High-impact exercise promotes bone gain in well-trained female athletes. J Bone Min Res 12:255–260, 1997.
53. Tanaka H, Dinenno FA, Monahan KD, et al: Aging, habitual exercise, and dynamic arterial compliance. Circulation 102:1270–1275, 2000.
54. Trappe SW, Costill DL, Vukovich MD, et al: Aging among elite distance runners: A 22-yr longitudinal study. J Appl Physiol 80:285–290, 1996.
55. U.S. Department of Health and Human Services. A Profile of Older Americans: 2002. http://www.aoa.dhhs.gov/aoa/STATS/profile/default.htm Last modified 01/02/2003. Available at www.fedstats.gov.
56. Vaitkevicius PV, Fleg JL, Engel JH, et al: Effects of age and aerobic capacity on arterial stiffness in healthy adults. Circulation 88:1456–1462, 1993.
57. Warming L, Hassager C, Christiansen C: Changes in bone mineral density with age in men and women: A longitudinal study. Osteoporos Int 13:105–112, 2002.
58. Whipple R, Wolfson L, Derby C: Altered sensory function and balance in older persons. J Gerontol 48:71–76, 1993.
59. Williams PT: High-density lipoprotein cholesterol and other risk factors for coronary heart disease in female runners. N Engl J Med 334:1298–1304, 1996.
60. Willich SN, Lewis M, Lowel H, et al: Physical exertion as a trigger of acute myocardial infarction. N Engl J Med 329:1684–1690, 1993.
61. Wren TAL, Yerby SA, Beaupre GS, et al: Influence of bone mineral density, age, and strain rate on the failure mode of human Achilles tendons. Clin Biomech 16:529–534, 2001.

34 Sports Medicine and Sports Injuries in the Older Population

Stuart B. Kahn and Nancy Kim

The enormous health benefits of exercise in the entire population are well documented. The health benefits of exercise in the elderly population, although equally important, are not without a host of general and specific risks for harm and injury. Many of these risks, although they do exist in the younger athletic population, are far greater in the elderly population. Generally speaking, risks of falls, joint injuries, fractures, and cardiorespiratory and vascular events are higher in the older athlete due to the aging process and the condition of the body as it ages.[21,23,44,50,94]

Despite these higher risks, the benefits of exercise and sports activity in the elderly population are significant, and if pursued with caution clearly outweigh the risks. To begin with, the psychologic and emotional benefits include improved quality of sleep, less risk of chronic depression, and improved cognitive function, which together can bring about a better sense of well-being for the patient.[8,20,37,40,43,54,70,73,79,84] Physiologically, several of the organ systems in the body show signs of improvement with exercise. The cardiovascular system responds to exercise with improvement in blood pressure, cardiac output, and decreased incidence of coronary artery disease. The respiratory system reveals increased VO_{2max}.[11,33,37,59,90] The skeletal system responds to exercise with a slower rate of bone loss and less osteoporosis in athletic postmenopausal women compared to nonathletic postmenopausal women.[24,37,38,57] The neuromuscular system, although the cause for improvement is not documented, reveals improvement in balance, which leads to fewer falls and fractures.[24,38,66] In general, diabetes is an illness that is seen less frequently in the older population that exercises, and those with diabetes have finer glucose control and sensitivity to insulin.[36,37,64] Patients with osteoarthritis report a lower level of pain.[10,51] There is some research that indicates that the risks for cancer are decreased in more active, athletic older people.[36,50]

To safely pursue a fitness program, it is recommended that patients pursuing sports activities for the first time in their older years seek medical care for clearance from a cardiovascular point of view prior to starting a program. In addition, patients who already have cardiovascular disease, degenerative arthritis, or history of stroke, respiratory illness, or neurological problems with a history of balance problems and falls should work closely with either a physical therapist or a certified athletic trainer to more safely begin a sports program.[21,23,37,44,47,50,94]

The remainder of this chapter will be dedicated to discussing common orthopedic and musculoskeletal sports injuries in the older population. It is necessary to point out that, although athletes of all ages are at risk for sports injuries, here we will discuss those injuries and conditions that are more common in the older population because of their age. When older patients present with a simple sports injury, one that may also be common in their younger counterparts, it may be more disabling and the healing process may be slower because of the physiologic changes that occur with aging.

Traumas from falls in general are epidemic among the elderly.[66] Although falls are less frequent in older athletic patients than in their age-matched contemporaries who are not athletic, this still represents a great concern for practitioners treating older athletes. In addition to the common strains, sprains, wounds, and fractures that occur when an athlete falls, the older athlete is more susceptible to traumatic brain injury and spinal cord injuries when they do fall.

HEAD AND NECK INJURIES

Falling is epidemic in the over-65 population. It is estimated that one-third of all people over 65 years of age experience one or more falls per year.[66] Falling is the most common cause of traumatic brain injury in people over 65 years of age. On impact of the cranium, because of atrophy, the older patient has greater movement of the brain relative to the dura and cranium. This allows for greater shearing and tearing, which can allow small vessels to rupture. If a sizeable vessel ruptures, a subdural hematoma is likely to ensue. Not only is the incident of subdural hematoma higher in falls in the elderly, but when they have subdural hematomas, the elderly are twice as likely to die from this injury than are their younger counterparts.[25,92] Serious disabling complications can occur, requiring prolonged inactivity and immobility and leading to further health deterioration. Long-term rehabilitation stays are necessary, as are alterations in lifestyle, depending on the degree of brain injury, if the patient does recover.

The older patient's cervical vertebral column and spinal cord also are at risk for injury. Nearly half of the cervical vertebral fractures that occur in the United States occur in the older population. According to statistics from emergency room admissions, the elderly are twice as likely to present with cervical spine injuries, and with serious sequelae from those injuries.[13,58]

For example, central cord syndrome is much more common in patients aged over 50 with cervical spondylosis and osteophytes than in younger people who fall. The mechanism of action is believed to be a hyperextension injury of the cervical spine with trauma to the cord from osteophytes. This can either be from hemorrhage or direct trauma to the spinal cord, with the corticospinal tract being the most likely to be involved.[19,30,45,67,76,78,93]

Statistically speaking, patients older than 50 years of age who do have these types of sports-related injuries are much more likely to have a poor outcome. Fifty-nine percent of spinal cord injuries in the elderly will not regain ambulation at all.[100]

As with all spinal cord injuries, these patients would be treated with a methylprednisolone protocol, and when stable, evaluated by MRI and a full spinal cord injury protocol including respiratory, bowel, and bladder support, skin protection, and functional restoration. ASIA (American Spinal Injury Association) classification is important in that it helps to determine the level of injury and allows the medical team to assess for progress and be better able to define the injury.[100]

Spinal cord injury is clearly the worst and most serious of the cervical injuries. Cervical radiculopathy and cervical pain syndromes are also quite common after falls, and with sports activities in which overhead activity, neck motion and rotation, and neck extension are involved.[80] The mechanism of action is believed to be extension and side bending or compression injuries to the nerve root in the spondylitic spine. Sports such as swimming, tennis, and golf are the main culprits because these sports require motion in the above-mentioned directions. It is well documented that the above-mentioned motions, such as extension and extension combined with rotation, narrow the central spinal canal and the foraminal exit of the nerve root. These movements can also load the zygapophyseal joints and the uncovertebral joints, creating a generalized neck pain syndrome.[12,15,51,72,80,81]

In evaluating older athletes for cervical injury, it is important to remember that scapular and upper thoracic pain is frequently a radicular symptom of the cervical roots. Arm pain, limb pain, limb weakness, and numbness in a dermatomal or myotomal distribution will also be seen frequently. It is important to carefully evaluate these patients with a physical examination, imaging studies, and, at times, electrodiagnostic studies. As shoulder pain syndromes are also common in the older athlete, it is important to include a good shoulder examination to rule out primary shoulder pain as mimicking cervical pain syndrome. Treatment can range from conservative care such as anti-inflammatory medication, rest, physical therapy, home exercise program, postural strengthening exercises, sport-specific training, and reeducating the patient on how to compensate for the lack of mobility in the cervical spine. If not successful, interventional techniques such as paravertebral nerve blocks, trigger point injections, epidural steroid injections, foraminal steroid injections, and zygapophyseal joint injections can be begun.[62] Surgery is reserved for intractable pain, progressive or nonimproving neurologic deficits, and of course for patients with a high risk of spinal cord injury or spinal cord compression. If surgery becomes necessary because of neurologic deficits, it is important to prepare the patient for the possibility that his or her pain will improve, but the weakness and sensory deficit may not improve.[49]

SHOULDER INJURIES

In the aging athlete, shoulder injuries represent one of the greatest incidences. It is even common for elderly who are asymptomatic to have rotator cuff tears. In one medical study of 25 asymptomatic patients who were arthroscoped, there were 28 rotator cuff tears seen in the bilateral shoulders.[31,91] Because of degenerative arthritis, impingement syndrome is commonly seen in the elderly, and this is believed to lead to rotator cuff injury as the patient becomes more active. As with all athletes, the anatomic type of acromion, shoulder instability, and repetitive microtrauma from overhead sports are all predisposing factors for this type of injury.[42,59,82,95,102,104]

Diagnosis is made by history, careful physical examination, diagnostic testing such as lidocaine impingement testing, and radiographic findings including plain x-rays and MRI with or without arthrography. As mentioned earlier in this chapter, there is an overlap with cervical injuries. Therefore, it is necessary to evaluate the cervical spine to rule out cervical radiculopathy as an underlying cause for shoulder pain.[34] It is equally necessary to rule out and evaluate for spontaneous adhesive capsulitis, subacromial bursitis, and labral tears. A physical examination, including positive impingement signs, is helpful. Weakness in abduction can be seen in multiple abnormalities of the shoulder. However, a simple lidocaine injection into the subacromial space can help determine if that weakness is due to guarding from pain or is true weakness related to a rotator cuff tear or underlying neurologic cause.

Labral tears are also more frequently seen in older athletes than in their younger counterparts because of the incidence of falls on an outstretched arm.[86] In addition, developmental joint laxity and arthropathy can lead to shoulder instability, which also predisposes a patient to labral tears. Patients often complain of a popping, clunking, or catching associated with shoulder motion. This is associated with a vague, constant ache that is worse with overhead and shoulder motion activity. Physical examination maneuvers including a clunk test and anterior glide test in which compression and rotation of the humeral head against the glenoid fossa are performed and will often bring about a clunk, pop, or painful sensation. One study found physical examination maneuvers to be 56% specific and 46% sensitive.[88] An MRI was only 42% sensitive, but had a high (92%) specificity rate.[88]

Bicipital tendinitis tends to be a condition that affects older patients in general. The mean age of diagnosis of bicipital tendinitis of all patients across the board is 55 years. It is often associated with rotator cuff tendinopathy. The risk factors are similar to those of rotator cuff tendinopathy and include overhead activities, sports, and recurrent subluxation of the bicipital tendon in its groove at the humeral head. This could be secondary to old trauma or a shallow groove. In addition, instability of the shoulder can also aggravate bicipital tendinitis.[65] Diagnosis is based on the history and physical examination, including severe bicipital tenderness in the bicipital groove, a positive Yergason test, and a positive speed test.[4]

Treatment of shoulder pathology in the elderly should remain nonoperative when at all possible. Rest, or relative rest from the activities that aggravate the pain, should be instituted. Range of motion must be instituted, as we do not want patients refraining from their sports activities to lose range that they will subsequently need for functional activities or return to sports. Anti-inflammatory medications, physical therapy, shoulder stabilization exercises, and cross-training are all helpful conservative measures. Corticosteroid injections used judiciously in tendinopathy can be very helpful in eliminating the pain. Indications for surgery in the older athlete should be intractable pain or substantial loss of function.[1]

ELBOW

Elbow pathology related to sports includes medial and lateral epicondylitis, as well as trauma. There does not appear to be a greater incidence of these conditions in the older athlete.[74] These conditions are treated with conservative management, including but not limited to rest, ice, anti-inflammatory medications, stretching, and physical therapy including ultrasound, electrical stimulation, iontophoresis, and strengthening. Tennis or golf elbow splints can be used. Activities should be modified. If conservative management fails, further diagnostic testing including an MRI can be performed. Surgery can be considered when conservative management has failed.[3,9,14,28,35,48,68,85,87,97,99]

WRIST AND HAND INJURIES

Scaphoid fractures occur in 4.5 out of 10,000 people over the age of 60.[39] The most common mechanism of injury is a fall on a dorsiflexed wrist. The torque of the fall creates a radial deviation. Because of the watershed area of blood supply in the scaphoid bone, this fracture has a high rate of avascular necrosis and nonunion.[26] With regard to wrist pain in the radial aspect after trauma, it is recommended to treat this as though it is a scaphoid fracture even if x-rays are initially negative. X-rays a week to 10 days later often better reveal a fracture. When in extreme doubt, an MRI, bone scan, or other diagnostic imaging should be used to rule out a fracture before determining that immobilization by casting can be discontinued.[29,75] Diagnosis is made by history, physical examination, and imaging studies. Patients most often present with a history of falls on a flexed wrist with pain, swelling, and ecchymosis over the radial aspect of the wrist with substantial pain in the anatomic snuffbox.[22] X-rays, as mentioned, should be repeated even if they are initially negative, because often a fracture line will not be visualized on the first set of films. Prognosis is good in patients in whom the fracture heals. In patients with nonunion of a scaphoid fracture, 100% will develop osteoarthritis of the wrist within 10 years.[26,75]

Another common wrist injury in older athletes, related to falls, is Colles fractures of the wrist. Sixteen percent of all women and 2.5% of all men over age 50 will sustain Colles fractures.[46,55]

LUMBOSACRAL

The incidence of spinal arthritis and spinal stenosis is generally high in the older population.[61] More and more elderly people are living active lifestyles. Spinal stenosis and pain related to the low back can be very limiting and can interfere with activity and sports in the older population. It is typical for patients who have spinal stenosis to find their symptoms to be worse when they are active in exercise, as well as with just walking. The anatomic changes that occur with aging of the spine, including hypertrophy of ligamentum flavum, hypertrophy of facet joints, and arthritic spurs that develop, can all lead to narrowing of the central spinal canal, the lateral recess, or the foraminal exit zone of the nerve root. As patients position themselves in an erect posture or twist and bend, their back pain and radicular pain can worsen. Pain can be mediated by either mechanical factors such as direct pressure on a nerve root and narrowing of the spinal canal that causes direct pressure on the nerve root, or chemical factors such as occur after an acute sports injury to the back in which the nerve root is inflamed and irritated.[7,52]

Acute radiculopathy from herniated discs can superimpose on an already arthritic spine. The diagnosis can be made by history, a careful physical examination, and diagnostic imaging studies. Special attention should be given to other causes of leg pain, such as degenerative arthropathy, vascular claudication, and peripheral neuropathy. Conservative management, including anti-inflammatory medications, pain medications (which may include those used for a neuropathic component of the radicular symptoms), lumbar stabilization exercises through physical therapy, and a home exercise program, should be instituted.[2] Dosing of narcotics and sedating medications must be done with extreme caution. Oversedation from build-up of metabolites, in combination with leg pain or weakness from the lumbar syndrome, can increase the risk of falls and injury. Further treatment with corticosteroid injections and surgery should be evaluated in the patient who fails conservative management.[5,6]

Unlike the cervical spine, there is not a high a risk for spinal cord injury in the lumbar spine. Cauda equina syndrome should be watched for because sports injury to an arthritic lumbar spine or compression fracture may cause enough narrowing to cause diffuse cauda equina and not just nerve root compression.[89]

It is important not to overlook the sacroiliac joint and the sacrum itself as a cause of low back and referred leg pain in the older athlete. Sacral insufficiency fractures due to trauma and sacroiliac joint strains are very common in the older athlete. Sacral insufficiency fractures due to osteoporosis are not uncommon and are very hard to diagnose. If x-rays are negative but suspicion is high, an MRI, CT scan, or bone scan can be helpful in diagnosis.[16,98,101] Compression fractures are common in the elderly population, with the most common underlying predisposing factor being osteoporosis.[41,53,60] Falls and exertion are common factors leading to compression fractures in this predisposed population.[17,41,60] Once diagnosis is made with imaging studies, a treatment course can be chosen. If the pain is manageable, most patients tend to improve and can overcome their disability with physical therapy.[17,77] If the pain is so excessive that the patient becomes immobile, one must consider interventions such as vertebroplasty and kyphoplasty because the risks of bedrest in the elderly are also high. These procedure are new and not without risks and complications. They should be done by someone with specific training and only after the patient understands the risks of spinal cord injury.[18,71]

Although it is not clearly documented, it is empiric that in the less flexible population, such as older athletes, lumbar strains from facet joint arthropathy, muscle strain, and tears may be more common than they are in younger athletes.

HIP AND PELVIS

Earlier in the chapter we noted that older patients who exercise fall less frequently in general and have potential benefits to their bone density. It has been calculated that fitness in the elderly accounts for a 6% lower risk factor in hip fractures compared with the inactive elderly.[27] That being said, however, the incidence of hip fracture in elderly patients that fall is clearly increased over the normal population.[96] Diagnosis is made by history, physical exam, and imaging studies. Severe pain experienced with hip trauma and inability to stand and ambulate combined with an externally rotated shortened leg can all help make the diagnosis. X-rays reveal fracture sites including the femoral neck, greater trochanter, and femoral head. Sacral and pelvic fractures and acetabular fractures need to be considered in the differential diagnosis. Most hip fractures are treated surgically to allow for early mobilization and rehabilitation.

Greater trochanteric bursitis can be extremely painful. It can mimic other pain syndromes. It can be present with underlying hip DJD, making the diagnosis even harder. Bursitis can be brought on by either trauma or overuse syndromes in the inflexible athlete. Greater trochanteric bursitis can be extremely painful and interfere with the patient's ability to perform exercise and ambulate. It is easily treated with corticosteroid injection. Resistant cases can be treated with stretching exercises, ultrasound, physical therapy, and gluteal strengthening.

KNEE

Many elderly patients who exercise have osteoarthritis and other forms of arthritis that predispose them to injuring the knee, in particular those patients with tricompartmental degenerative arthropathy of the knee. Elderly athletes are also at increased risk for meniscal injuries from even lower impact exercises than the normal population. The diagnosis of a meniscal injury in a patient with underlying degenerative arthropathy of the knee can be quite difficult on physical examination.[58] However, with imaging studies such as MRI, it can often be determined that there is a superimposed meniscal injury. Often, treating the meniscal injury arthroscopically, although this will have no affect on the underlying degenerative changes in the knee joint, will allow enough improvement for the patient to return to his or her preinjury baseline of athletic activity. It is important to explain to the patient in advance that the goal of intervention in that case is simply to eliminate some of the acute exacerbation of the pain and not to treat the underlying arthritic joint. If a patient has a substantial functional impediment despite interventions such as physical therapy, exercise training, injections, or arthroscopic surgery, a knee replacement can be considered.[69,83]

FOOT AND ANKLE INJURIES

There are no specific injuries to the foot and ankle that are inherently greater in older athletes than in their younger counterparts. Common complaints, however, include foot and ankle pain from underlying osteoarthritis. Metatarsalgia due to wasting of the metatarsal fat pad, heel spurs, plantar fasciitis, and tibialis posterior insufficiency and tendonopathy are all common. These conditions should be treated conservatively but aggressively with anti-inflammatory medication, stretches, physical therapy, and orthotics when needed.

CONCLUSION

Despite all of the potential injuries related to increased physical activities in the older population, the benefits outweigh the risks for the majority of patients. As the population ages and more patients pursue an active lifestyle, it is encumbent on the medical community to help prevent injuries through good patient education, preventive measures such as cardiovascular pulmonary function testing prior to entering fitness training, and recommendations of appropriate level of physical activities. Utilization of paraprofessionals such as certified athletic trainers with subspeciality training in geriatric populations could be utilized. Physical therapists are often needed in an injured or disabled population to help return patients to a more active lifestyle.

Treatment of sports injuries in the older population should be treated as aggressively as and considered as important as in younger athletes. All practitioners should aggressively treat new pain complaints, including those that are an exacerbation of a chronic pain condition. Often, older athletes will tolerate their baseline of pain, but be disabled from an exacerbation. Set realistic treatment goals for treatment of these exacerbations. Accepting improved function and less pain as opposed to becoming pain free may be preferable to offering patients aggressive surgical options with the risks that come with any surgery in the elderly. Older patients deserve the right to pursue their pleasurable sport activities for recreation, enjoyment, and health benefits.

REFERENCES

1. Almekinders LC: Impingement syndrome. Clin Sports Med 20(3):491–504, 2001.
2. Amundsen T, Weber H, Nordal HJ, et al: Lumbar spinal stenosis: conservative or surgical management? A prospective 10-year study. Spine 25(11):1424–1435; discussion 1435–1436, 2000.
3. Andrews, JR: Outcome of elbow surgery in professional baseball players. Am J Sports Med 23:407–413, 1995.
4 Bell RH: Biceps disorders. In Hawkins RJ, Misamore GW (eds): Shoulder Injuries in the Athlete. New York, Churchill Livingstone, 1996.
5. Botwin KP, Gruber RD, Bouchlas CG, et al: Fluoroscopically guided lumbar transformational epidural steroid injections in degenerative lumbar stenosis: an outcome study. Am J Phys Med Rehabil 81(12):898–905, 2002.
6. Botwin KP, Gruber RD: Lumbar epidural steroid injections in the patient with lumbar spinal stenosis. Phys Med Rehabil Clin N Am 14(1):121–141, 2003.
7. Bridwell KH: Lumbar spinal stenosis. Diagnosis, management, and treatment. Clin Geriatr Med 10(4):677–701, 1994.
8. Brisswalter J, Collardcau M, Rene A: Effects of acute physical exercise characteristics on cognitive performance. Sports Med 32(9):555–566, 2002.
9. Buchbinder R, Green S, Bell S, et al: Surgery for lateral elbow pain. Cochrane Database Syst Rev (1):CD003525, 2002.
10. Burkhart SS, Morgan CD, Kibler WB: Shoulder injuries in overhead athletes. The "dead arm" revisited. Clin Sports Med 19(1):125–158, 2000.
11. Campbell AJ, Reinken J, Allan BC, Martinez GS: Falls in old age: A study of frequency and related clinical factors. Age Ageing 10(4):264–270, 1981.
12. Collignon F, Martin D, Lenelle J, Stevenaert A: Acute traumatic central cord syndrome: Magnetic resonance imaging and clinical observations. J Neurosurg 96(1 Suppl):29–33, 2002.
13. Cotman CW, Engesser-Cesar C: Exercise enhances and protects brain function. Exerc Sport Sci Rev 30(2):75–79, 2002.
14. Crowther MA: A prospective, randomized study to compare extracorporeal shock-wave therapy and injection of steroid for the treatment of tennis elbow. J Bone Joint Surg Br 84:678–679, 2002.
15. Cummings SR, Nevitt MC, Browner WS, et al: Risk factors for hip fracture in white women. Study of Osteoporotic Fractures Research Group. N Engl J Med 332(12):767–773, 1995.
16. Dasgupta B, Shah N, Brown H, et al: Sacral insufficiency fractures: an unsuspected cause of low back pain. Br J Rheumatol 37(7):789–793, 1998.
17. Delmas PD: Treatment of postmenopausal osteoporosis. Lancet 359(9322):2018–2026, 2002.
18. Diamond TH, Champion B, Clark WA: Management of acute osteoporotic vertebral fractures: A nonrandomized trial comparing percutaneous vertebroplasty with conservative therapy. Am J Med 114(4):257–265, 2003.
19. Dunn AL, Trivedi MH, O'Neal HA: Physical activity dose-response effects on outcomes of depression and anxiety. Med Sci Sports Exerc 33(6 Suppl):S587–S597; discussion 609–610, 2001.
20. Ehara S, Shimamura T: Cervical spine injury in the elderly: Imaging features. Skeletal Radiol 30(1):1–7, 2001.
21. Elward K, Larson EB: Benefits of exercise for older adults. A review of existing evidence and current recommendations for the general population. Clin Geriatr Med 8(1):35–50, 1992.
22. Esberger DA: What value the scaphoid compression test? J Hand Surg (Br) 19(6):748–749, 1994.
23. Ettinger WH Jr, Burns R, Messier SP, et al: A randomized trial comparing aerobic exercise and resistance exercise with a health education program in older adults with knee osteoarthritis. The Fitness Arthritis and Seniors Trial (FAST). JAMA 277(1):25–31, 1997.
24. Fabre C, Chamari K, Mucci P, et al: Improvement of cognitive function by mental and/or individualized aerobic training in healthy elderly subjects. Int J Sports Med 23(6):415–421, 2002.

25. Farmer JC, Wisneski RJ: Cervical spine nerve root compression. An analysis of neuroforaminal pressures with varying head and arm positions. Spine 19(16):1850–1855, 1994.
26. Fernandez DL: Non-union of the scaphoid. J Bone Joint Surg (Am) 77A:883, 1995.
27. Feskanich D. Walking and leisure-time activity and risk of hip fracture in postmenopausal women. JAMA 288:2300–2306, 2002.
28. Fleisig GS: Kinetics of baseball pitching with implications about injury mechanisim. Am J Sports Med 23:233, 1995.
29. Fowler C: A comparison of bone scintigraphy and MRI in the early diagnosis of the occult scaphoid wrist fracture. Skeletal Radiol 27(12):683–687, 1998.
30. Fu FH, Harner CD, Klein AH: Shoulder impingement syndrome. A critical review. Clin Orthop (269):162–173, 1991.
31. Fuchs S, Chylarecki C, Langenbrinck A: Incidence and symptoms of clinically manifest rotator cuff lesions. Int J Sports Med 20(3):201–205, 1999.
32. Garrick JG: The frequency of injury, mechanism of injury, and epidemiology of ankle sprains. Am J Sports Med 5:241–242,1977.
33. Gill TJ, Melrvin E, Kocher MS, et al: The relative importance of acromial morphology and age with respect to rotator cuff pathology. J Shoulder Elbow Surg 11(4):327–330, 2002.
34. Gorski JM, Schwartz LH: Shoulder impingement presenting as neck pain. J Bone Joint Surg Am 85-A(4):635–638, 2003.
35. Grana W: Medial epicondylitis and cubital tunnel syndrome in the throwing athlete. Clin Sports Med 20(3):541–548, 2001.
36. Hamdy O, Goodyear LJ, Horton ES: Diet and exercise in type 2 diabetes mellitus. Endocrinol Metab Clin North Am 30(4):883–907, 2001.
37. Hardy AG: Cervical spinal cord injury without bony injury. Paraplegia 14(4):296–305, 1977.
38. Hoffman-Goetz L, Apter D, Demark-Wahnefried W, et al: Possible mechanisms mediating an association between physical activity and breast cancer. Cancer 83(3 Suppl):621–628, 1998.
39. Hove LM: Epidemiology of scaphoid fractures in Bergen, Norway. Scan J Plast Reconstr Surg II and Surg 33(4):423–426, 1999.
40. Inufusa A, An HS, Lim TH, et al: Anatomic changes of the spinal canal and intervertebral foramen associated with flexion-extension movement. Spine 21(21):2412–2420, 1996.
41. Johansson C, Mellstrom D, Rosengren K, Rundgren A: A community-based population study of vertebral fractures in 85-year-old men and women. Age Ageing 23(5):388–392, 1994.
42. Jolliffe JA, Rees K, Taylor RS, et al: Exercise-based rehabilitation for coronary heart disease. Cochrane Database Syst Rev (1):CD001800, 2001.
43. Kallinen M, Alen M: Sports-related injuries in elderly men still active in sports. Br J Sports Med 28(1):52–55, 1994.
44. Kannus P, Niittymaki S, Jarvinen M, Lehto M: Sports injuries in elderly athletes: A three-year prospective, controlled study. Age Ageing 18(4): 263–270, 1989.
45. Kannus, P: Preventing osteoporosis, falls, and fractures among elderly people. Promotion of lifelong physical activity is essential. BMJ 23:318(7178): 205–206, 1999.
46. Kanterewiez E: Association between Colles fracture and low bone mass:age based differences in postmenopausal women. Osteoporos Int 13:824–828, 2002.
47. Karin B, von Holst H: Cervical injuries in Sweden a national survey of patient data from 1987 to 1999. Injury Control and Safety Promotion 9(1):40–52, 2002.
48. Keizer SB: Botulinum toxin injection versus surgical treatment for tennis elbow: A randomized pilot study. Clin Orthop 401:125–131, 2002.
49. King AC, Oman RF, Brassington GS, et al: Moderate-intensity exercise and self-rated quality of sleep in older adults. A randomized controlled trial. JAMA 277(1):32–37, 1997.
50. Kohno K, Kumon Y, Oka Y, et al: Evaluation of prognostic factors following expansive laminoplasty for cervical spinal stenotic myelopathy. Surg Neurol 48(3):237–45, 1997.
51. Lane AM, Lovejoy DJ: The effects of exercise on mood changes: The moderating effect of depressed mood. J Sports Med Phys Fitness 41(4):539–545, 2001.
52. Lazaro L 4th, Quinet RJ: Low back pain: How to make the diagnosis in the older patient. Geriatrics 49(9):48–53, 1994.
53. Lee YL, Yip KM: The osteoporotic spine.Clin Orthop 323:91–97, 1996.
54. Leveille SG, Bean J, Bandeen-Roche K, et al: Musculoskeletal pain and risk for falls in older disabled women living in the community. J Am Geriatr Soc 50(4):671–678, 2002.
55. Lips P: Epidemiology and predictors of fractures associated with osteoporosis. Am J Med 103:3S–8S, 1997.
56. Lowery DW, Wald MM, Browne BJ, et al: Epidemiology of cervical spine injury victims. Ann Emerg Med 38(1):12–16, 2001.
57. Lucini D, Milani RV, Costantino G, et al: Effects of cardiac rehabilitation and exercise training on autonomic regulation in patients with coronary artery disease. Am Heart J 143(6):977–983, 2002.

58. Matheson GO, Macintyre JG, Taunton JE, et al: Musculoskeletal injuries associated with physical activity in older adults. Med Sci Sports Exerc 21(4):379–385, 1989.
59. McCann PD, Bigliani LU: Shoulder pain in tennis players. Sports Med 17(1):53–64, 1994.
60. Melton LJ 3rd, Kan SH, Frye MA, et al: Epidemiology of vertebral fractures in women. Am J Epidemiol 129(5):1000–1011, 1989.
61. Milhorat TH, Kotzen RM, Anzil AP: Stenosis of central canal of spinal cord in man: Incidence and pathological findings in 232 autopsy cases. J Neurosurg 80(4):716–722, 1994.
62. Mosenthal AC, Lavery RF, Addis M, et al: Isolated traumatic brain injury: age is an independent predictor of mortality and early outcome. J Trauma. 2002 52(5):907–911.
63. Motoyama M, Sunami Y, Kinoshita F, et al: Blood pressure lowering effect of low intensity aerobic training in elderly hypertensive patients. Med Sci Sports Exerc 30(6):818–823, 1998.
64. Muhle C, Resnick D, Ahn JM, Sudmeyer M, Heller M: In vivo changes in the neuroforaminal size at flexion-extension and axial rotation of the cervical spine in healthy persons examined using kinematic magnetic resonance imaging. Spine 26(13): E287–E293, 2001.
65. Murthi AM: Incidence of pathologic changes of the long head of the biceps tendon. J Shoulder Elbow Surg 9(5):382–385, 2000.
66. Nied RJ, Franklin B: Promoting and prescribing exercise for the elderly. Am Fam Phys 65(3): 419–426, 2002.
67. Nuckley DJ, Konodi MA, Raynak GC, et al: Neural space integrity of the lower cervical spine: Effect of normal range of motion. Spine 27(6):587–595, 2002.
68. O'Dwyer KJ: Medial epicondylitis of elbow. Int Orthop 19(2):69–71, 1995.
69. Paletta GA, Warren RF: Knee injuries and alpine skiing, treatment and rehabilitation. Sports Med 17(6):411–423, 1994.
70. Paluska SA, Schwenk TL: Physical activity and mental health: Current concepts. Sports Med 29(3):167–180, 2000.
71. Peh WC, Gelbart MS, Gilula LA, Peck DD: Percutaneous vertebroplasty: Treatment of painful vertebral compression fractures with intraosseous vacuum phenomena. Am J Roentgenol 180(5): 1411–1417, 2003.
72. Penrod LE, Hegde SK, Ditunno JF Jr: Age effect on prognosis for functional recovery in acute, traumatic central cord syndrome. Arch Phys Med Rehabil 71(12):963–968, 1990.
73. Radhakrishnan K, Litchy WJ, O'Fallon WM, Kurland LT: Epidemiology of cervical radiculopathy. A population-based study from Rochester, Minnesota, 1976 through 1990. Brain 117 (Pt 2): 325–335, 1994.
74. Roetert EP: The biomechanics of tennis elbow. An integrated approach. Clin Sports Med 14(1):47–57, 1995.
75. Roolker W: Diagnosis and treatment of scaphoid fractures, can non-union be prevented? Arch Orthop Trauma Surg 119(7–8):428–431, 1999.
76. Roth EJ, Lawler MH, Yarkony GM: Traumatic central cord syndrome: Clinical features and functional outcomes. Arch Phys Med Rehabil 71(1): 18–23, 1990.
77. Rutherford OM: Is there a role for exercise in the prevention of osteoporotic fractures? Br J Sports Med 33(6):378–386, 1999.
78. Saal JS, Saal JA, Yurth EF: Nonoperative management of herniated cervical intervertebral disc with radiculopathy. Spine 21(16):1877–1883, 1996.
79. Salmon P: Effects of physical exercise on anxiety, depression, and sensitivity to stress: A unifying theory. Clin Psychol Rev 21(1):33–61, 2001.
80. Sampath P, Bendebba M, Davis JD, Ducker T: Outcome in patients with cervical radiculopathy. Prospective, multicenter study with independent clinical review. Spine 24(6):591–597, 1999.
81. Scher AT: Hyperextension trauma in the elderly: an easily overlooked spinal injury. J Trauma 23(12): 1066–1068, 1983.
82. Schneider SII, Elouzi EB: The role of exercise in type II diabetes mellitus. Prev Cardiol 3(2):77–82, 2000.
83. Shelbourne KD, Patel DV, Adsit WS, Porter DA: Rehabilitation after meniscal repair. Clin Sports Med 15(3):595–612, 1996.
84. Sherrill DL, Kotchou K, Quan SP: Association of physical activity and human sleep disorders. Arch Intern Med 158(17):1894–1898, 1998.
85. Simunovic Z, Trobonjaca T, Trobonjaca Z: Treatment of medial and lateral epicondylitis–tennis and golfer's elbow–with low level laser therapy: A multicenter double blind, placebo-controlled clinical study on 324 patients. J Clin Laser Med Surg 16(3):145–151, 1998.
86. Snyder SJ: An Analysis of 140 injuries to the superior glenoid labrum. J Shoulder Elbow Surg 4(4): 243–248, 1995.
87. Stahl S: The efficacy of an injection of steroids for medial epicondyltis. A prospective study of sixty elbows. J Bone Joint Surg Am 79:1648–1652, 1997.
88. Stetson WB: The crank test, the O'brien test and routine magnetic resonance imaging in the diagnosis of labral tears. Am J Sports Med 30(6):806–809, 2002.

89. Storm PB, Chou D, Tamargo RJ: Lumbar spinal stenosis, cauda equina syndrome, and multiple lumbosacral radiculopathics. Phys Med Rehabil Clin N Am 13(3):713–733, ix, 2002.
90. Susman M, DiRusso SM, Sullivan T, et al: Traumatic brain injury in the elderly: Increased mortality and worse functional outcome at discharge despite lower injury severity. J Trauma 53(2):219–223, 2002.
91. Tempelhof S, Rupp S, Seil R: Age-related prevalence of rotator cuff tears in asymptomatic shoulders. J Shoulder Elbow Surg 8(4):296–299, 1999.
92. Thune I, Furberg AS: Physical activity and cancer risk: Dose-response and cancer, all sites and site-specific. Med Sci Sports Exerc 33(6 Suppl): S530–S550; discussion S609–S10, 2001.
93. Tow AM, Kong KH: Central cord syndrome: Functional outcome after rehabilitation. Spinal Cord 36(3):156–160, 1998.
94. Vad V, Hong HM, Zazzali M, et al: Exercise recommendations in athletes with early osteoarthritis of the knee. Sports Med 32(11):729–739, 2002.
95. Vad VB, Warren RF, Altchek DW, et al: Negative prognostic factors in managing massive rotator cuff tears. Clin J Sport Med 12(3):151–157, 2002.
96. van Schoor NM, Smit JH, Twisk JW, et al: Prevention of hip fractures by external hip protectors: A randomized controlled trial. JAMA 289(15):1957–1962, 2003.
97. Vangsness CT: Surgical Treatment of medial epicondylitis. Result in 35 elbows. J Bone Joint Surg Br 73(3):409–411, 1991.
98. Verhaegen MJ, Sauter AJ: Insufficiency fractures, an often unrecognized diagnosis. Arch Orthop Trauma Surg 119(1–2):115–116, 1999.
99. Wang CJ: Shock wave therapy for patients with lateral epicondylitis of the elbow: A one to two year follow up study. Am J Sports Med 30:422–425, 2002.
100. Weingarden SI, Graham PM: Falls resulting in spinal cord injury: patterns and outcomes in an older population. Paraplegia 27(6):423–427, 1989.
101. Wild A, Jaeger M, Haak H, Mehdian SH: Sacral insufficiency fracture, an unsuspected cause of low-back pain in elderly women. Arch Orthop Trauma Surg 122(I):58–60, 2002.
102. Winslow EB: Cardiac rehabilitation. JAMA 258(14):1937–1938, 1987.
103. Yamaguchi K, Tetro AM, Blam O, et al: Natural history of asymptomatic rotator cuff tears: A longitudinal analysis of asymptomatic tears detected sonographically. J Shoulder Elbow Surg 10(3): 199–203, 2000.
104. Yoo JU, Zou D, Edwards WT, et al: Effect of cervical spine motion on the neuroforaminal dimensions of human cervical spine. Spine 17(10): 1131–1136, 1992.

VII

Sport-Specific Injuries

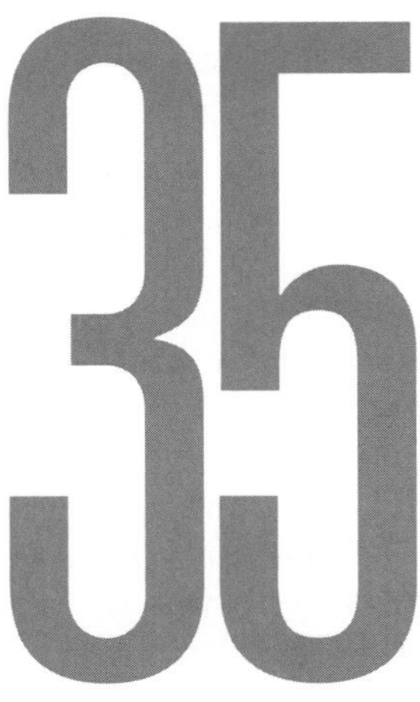

Basketball Injuries

Steven Arsht, Giles R. Scuderi, and Peter D. McCann

Modern day basketball has evolved over the past 25 years from an inadvertent contact sport to a highly physical game. Today's players are taller, stronger, and faster than ever before, adapting to the new style of play brought about by the addition of the "slam dunk" and three-point shot. Men and women of all ages and skill levels play basketball throughout the world. International competition is growing and basketball has become one of the most popular Olympic events. A sport once dominated by male participation has seen a dramatic rise in female athletes at the junior, collegiate, and professional levels in recent years.

Most injuries incurred by basketball players are minor and do not result in a significant loss of playing time. Injuries to the ankle, knee, finger, and face are most common. Players are more likely to be injured during a game rather than during a practice session. More serious injuries and injuries resulting in loss of playing time more commonly involve the lower limb than other body regions. At all levels of competition, the number and severity of knee injuries, including career-threatening anterior cruciate ligament (ACL) rupture, is greater in female athletes. A thorough understanding of the types of injuries sustained by the basketball player is necessary so that the medical staff can provide a rapid and accurate diagnosis, and administer the most appropriate treatment so that a more timely return to competition can be achieved.[6,17,19,25,28,29,43,46,49,54,67,70,71]

HEAD AND NECK

Facial lacerations, ocular trauma, orbital and nasal fractures, and dental trauma are the most commonly seen facial injuries. Basketball is second only to baseball in the number and severity of sports-related ocular[5] and oral trauma.[45] Depending on the severity of the injury and level of comfort of the treating physician, additional medical expertise can be received through consultation with an ophthalmologist, neurosurgeon, dentist, oral surgeon, otolaryngologist, or plastic surgeon. Significant neurotrauma is rare but should be aggressively evaluated if suspected.

Facial Lacerations

Lacerations are caused by direct contact with the floor or another player and often occur over bony prominences such as the chin, superior orbit, and zygomatic arch. These injuries are usually minor and can be treated with lavage, antibiotic ointment, and closure with steri-strips. Universal precautions should be practiced. 6.0 monofilament sutures can be used to close larger wounds, but should be removed within 5 days. Deep lacerations to the lip generally require copious lavage and a layered inside-out closure with absorbable suture. If the laceration was caused by contact with teeth, the risk of infection is elevated and oral antibiotics should be prescribed.[22]

Eye

The most common eye injuries are abrasions, lacerations, and contusions. Inadvertent contact with the fingers and elbows of other players during the course of rebounding or offensive play is the most common mechanism of injury. Eye injuries can be prevented by using goggles to protect the eye and dissipate impact force.[31,59,69] Corneal abrasions present with pain, photophobia, and a foreign body sensation. Fluorescein staining is diagnostic. Visual acuity and peripheral vision fields should always be assessed in a player with an eye injury. Most injuries can be treated conservatively with topical medications. NSAID drops may alleviate symptoms more quickly and allow for more timely return to the court.[11,33] A direct blow to the face by an elbow or finger can cause a blow-out fracture of the floor or medial wall of the orbit. This is a painful injury that may be accompanied by enopthalomos or diplopia. X-rays are often negative. CT scan is diagnostic. The player should be instructed to avoid the Valsalva maneuver, blowing the nose, or placing direct pressure upon the eye as this can cause air to enter the orbit and increase the intraocular pressure, putting the patient at risk for retinal ischemia and blindness. Management is controversial, and surgery is often required. Significant ocular injury such as retinal detachment or optic nerve avulsion can be missed on initial screening. Prompt ophthalmologic consultation should be strongly considered in players with persistent pain, diplopia, or decreased vision.[7,14]

Nasal Fracture

Nasal fractures are often caused by direct impact with the elbow or head of a player during the rebounding process.

Epistaxis is common. Marked deformity and crepitus and increased mobility of the fractured bones may be apparent on exam. Bleeding is initially controlled by direct compression. Packing the nose with epinephrine-impregnated pledgets may be helpful in refractory cases. Intranasal inspection is required to rule out septal hematoma, which can cause pressure necrosis and damage the cartilaginous septum, resulting in late cosmetic deformity. Nasal fractures can be managed by realignment under anesthesia if necessary. Return to play is possible before complete healing of the fracture if a nose protector is worn.[64]

Dental Trauma

Dental and oral soft-tissue injuries are often the result of contact with another player's hand, elbow, fist, shoulder, or head. Dental fractures and tooth avulsions are the most commonly reported injuries. Tooth fractures, commonly referred to as a "chipped tooth," involving the enamel do not require immediate medical attention, unless the tooth is sharp or is sensitive to changes in temperature. Fractures with exposed dentin are very sensitive. Temporary treatment with the direct application of zinc oxide and eugenol or petroleum jelly may alleviate pain and allow for the player's immediate return to the court. Postgame referral to a dentist is generally acceptable. Tooth avulsions from net entanglement or direct contact are more serious injuries and require immediate attention. If this occurs, the tooth should be gently rinsed in saline or tap water. Reimplantation may be possible. Viability decreases after 30 minutes, so the patient is transported to the dentist immediately. The tooth can be stored in the patient's mouth, in saline, or in milk. In all cases of dental trauma, a dentist should see the player as soon as possible. A more thorough clinical and radiographic assessment can be performed to ensure that more serious injury has not occurred. The use of custom-fitted plastic mouthguards has been shown to significantly reduce the morbidity and expense resulting from dental injuries in men's Division I college basketball, and their use should be encouraged for all players, regardless of age or skill level. Unfortunately, the rates of concussion and oral soft-tissue injuries were not affected by the use of mouthguards.[22,36,37,40,56]

CHEST

Most injuries to the chest are contusions that result from elbow impact. Rib fractures, pneumothorax, and manubriosternal joint subluxations have been reported but are not common. If suspected, radiographic evaluation is necessary before return to play is allowed. Breast contusions in female athletes can be a source of considerable pain. Conservative treatment is generally successful for most of these injuries, and athletes may return to play when comfortable enough to do so. Breast contusions should be treated with a well-fitting sports brassiere to provide compression and support in addition to cryotherapy.[66]

SPINE

Serious injuries to the spine are fortunately rare in the basketball player. Lumbar strains and contusions are most frequently seen and can be treated conservatively. Potentially debilitating injuries such as spine fractures, herniated discs, spondylolysis, and spinal stenosis are uncommon but should always be considered in the player who has sustained significant trauma or complains of persistent back pain or radicular symptoms. Skeletally immature athletes who complain of back pain should be evaluated for a stress fracture of the pars interarticularis or spondylolysis. Stress on the bony architecture of the spine that occurs with repetitive jumping and extension, such as when forwards and centers "post up," puts the player at risk for this injury. Examination reveals low back pain that is exacerbated by twisting and hyperextension, and hamstring tightness. X-rays should be obtained. If negative, single-photon emission computed tomography (SPECT) scan could be diagnostic. Initial treatment is with rest and avoidance of hyperextension activities. Sometimes, a lumbosacral orthosis that limits hyperextension may be necessary. If the condition fails to improve with conservative treatment, surgical repair may be indicated. Players that sustain significant trauma, have unremitting pain, or report radicular symptoms should undergo MRI evaluation.[26]

UPPER EXTREMITY

Injuries to the upper extremity in basketball players commonly involve the hand and wrist and are often the result of falling to the ground and direct impact with the ball. The player may give a history of "jamming" a finger, being undercut while in the act of shooting or rebounding, or being tripped and falling down. Most hand injuries involve the fingers, particularly at the proximal interphalangeal and metacarpal phalangeal joints.[58] Shoulder and elbow injuries are less common and are usually associated with high-speed collisions with other players or falls.[7]

Finger Injuries

Most hand injuries involve the fingers of the dominant hand. PIP and MCP joint sprains are responsible for 90% of all basketball injuries.[58,65,67] Swelling around the joint is typical, along with tenderness over the collateral ligaments. Range of motion and stability should be assessed. X-rays should always be taken to rule out a fracture. Conservative treatment is sufficient. Buddy taping of the fingers is helpful for mild sprains and return to play is dependent on level of comfort and the player's ability to be competitive. More severe injuries may require immobilization or surgical reconstruction.

Tendon injuries to the finger must be accurately diagnosed and treated to prevent late functional impairment. Avulsion of the extensor tendon off the distal phalanx can result in a mallet finger, and disruption of the central slip of the extensor tendon at the middle phalanx can result in a boutonniere deformity. Mallet finger commonly occurs when the basketball impacts and forcefully flexes the extended DIP joint. There is a flexion deformity of the fingertip and the player cannot actively extend the joint, which is tender to the touch and swollen. A lateral x-ray is necessary to rule out fracture. The DIP joint is immobilized in full extension with a Stack splint for 6 weeks. An acute injury to the central slip of the extensor tendon is often missed in the acute setting and is made apparent only when the player presents with a late deformity. The player is often unable to fully extend the PIP joint. Motion at the joint is often painful. A digital block can be helpful in determining loss of motion due to pain or extensor tendon insufficiency. Early and accurate diagnosis is imperative to avoid late deformity and diminished function. Conservative treatment with immobilization of the PIP joint in full extension for 6 weeks is recommended.[55]

Axial loading of the PIP joint that occurs with direct ball impact or collision with a player can result in a dorsal dislocation of the middle phalanx. An obvious deformity will be present on exam. Closed reduction should be performed by exaggerating the deformity and applying longitudinal traction. Interposed joint capsule, collateral ligaments, flexor tendons, or volar plate may prevent reduction. X-rays should be taken to rule out a fracture. Treatment is conservative and includes a period of splinting and buddy taping. Unrecognized volar plate injury may result in a pseudoboutonniere deformity.[41]

Phalangeal fractures present with pain, swelling, crepitus, and limited digital motion. X-rays should always be taken to rule out a fracture. Treatment depends on the fracture type and location. Most can be treated conservatively with early return to competition. Distal phalanx fractures can be managed with DIP joint splinting, and nondisplaced fractures of the proximal phalanx can be treated with buddy taping. Middle phalanx fractures are often unstable and surgical treatment may be necessary if acceptable alignment cannot be maintained. Fractures involving the joint that demonstrate articular incongruity and subluxation may also require operative intervention.[23]

Wrist Injuries

Players with wrist injuries will often give a history of falling forcefully to the ground. The injured hand or wrist has been used to break the fall. Wrist pain should be aggressively evaluated. Patients diagnosed with wrist sprains may have sustained a serious bony or ligamentous injury, such as a scaphoid fracture, perilunate dislocation, or scapholunate dissociation. Scapholunate dissociation is the most common ligamentous injury of the wrist and, if unrecognized, can lead to extensive loss of playing time and disability. There is often exquisite tenderness to palpation over the midwrist and scapholunate interval, and carpal instability may be detected. Perilunate dislocation presents with severe wrist pain and swelling. Players with radial-sided wrist pain and tenderness over the anatomic snuffbox may have a scaphoid fracture; ulnar-sided pain may be indicative of a TFCC tear. If serious injury to the wrist is suspected, the wrist should be immobilized. X-rays of the wrist should always be obtained. Scapholunate dissociation is best seen with the clenched fist PA view. MRI is helpful in defining the extent of ligamentous injury to the carpal bones. Perilunate dislocation is best seen on the lateral view, but is often misdiagnosed. Initial x-rays are normal in 5% to 15% of scaphoid fractures. A PA view of the wrist in ulnar deviation may be helpful in identifying a scaphoid fracture. If there is a high index of suspicion and rapid diagnosis is required, MRI or CT scan can be obtained. Although many scaphoid fractures can be treated nonoperatively, surgical intervention is sometimes necessary.

LOWER EXTREMITY

Overuse Injuries

The most common overuse injuries seen in basketball players are patellar tendonitis or jumper's knee, Achilles tendonitis, shin splints or medial tibial stress syndrome, and peroneal tendonitis.[48] These conditions have been discussed in detail elsewhere in this book. Many of these injuries are seen early in the season and result from poor off-season conditioning. The quick pace of the sport, which demands rapid acceleration and deceleration, along with repetitive cutting, pivoting, and jumping, predisposes players to overuse injuries. If diagnosed early, these injuries often can be treated conservatively and result in little loss of playing time. Unfortunately, many players try to play through the pain and report symptoms only after considerable time has passed and more significant injuries occurred.

Patellar Tendonitis. Acute patellar tendonitis or "jumper's knee" refers to inflammation of the patellar tendon. Repetitive eccentric loading of the knee during the landing phase of a jump may precipitate this condition. The player will complain of anterior knee pain inferior to the patella that is most pronounced when competing, running, and jumping.[21,48,50] Symptoms will often resolve with a period of rest. On examination, there is tenderness over the inferior pole of the patella, proximal and middle thirds of the tendon, or, less frequently, at the tendon's insertion to the tibial tubercle. Exacerbation of symptoms can be seen with resisted knee extension. The patellar tendon may feel thickened or swollen. Hamstring tightness and hip flexor weakness may also be seen.[21,50] Conservative treatment is generally sufficient and should focus on quadriceps, hamstring, and hip flexor strengthening. Relative rest and modalities including ice and ultrasound, and iontophoresis or phonophoresis can be helpful. A short course of nonsteroidal anti-inflammatory medication can be prescribed. Steroid injections should never be given. X-rays should be obtained in the initial evaluation of players with patellar tendonitis. Although frequently negative, x-rays may demonstrate an osteophyte at the inferior pole of the patella ("tooth sign"), proximal tendon calcification, or an unresolved ossicle in the distal portion of the tendon in a patient with prior Osgood-Schlatter disease. MRI is recommended for evaluation of chronic symptoms and can be helpful in differentiating patellar tendonitis from a partial tear.[44,52,68] Chronic tendonitis with pathologic changes within the tendon evident on MRI may respond to surgical treatment.[21,52,68] Players with an "unresolved ossicle" within the inferior portion of the tendon may be candidates for surgical excision.[47,51]

Achilles Tendonitis. Players with Achilles tendonitis complain of pain over the posterior ankle that is worse with running and jumping. Examination may reveal tenderness over the tendon in the watershed area 4-6 cm above the os calcis, with increased warmth, swelling, and crepitus. Tenderness at the posterior heel may indicate insert ional tendonitis or retrocalcaneal bursitis. An antalgic gait, painful single-toe rise, and variable gastrocnemius-soleus weakness can also be seen. Chronic symptoms may be indicative of tendon degeneration. Longitudinal tears have been reported in basketball players. Acute, complete ruptures are less common but can occur and are usually associated with a pop, extreme pain and swelling, a palpable defect, and a positive Thompson test. X-rays should be obtained in all cases. MRI can be helpful in defining the extent of the athlete's injury. Relative rest, ice, stretching, NSAIDs, ultrasound, heel lifts, and orthotics are the mainstay of treatment.[2] A period of immobilization may be helpful in difficult cases. Players with MRI evidence of Achilles tendonitis that have failed an adequate course of immobilization may require exploration of the degenerative tendon. It is recommended that elite athletes with Achilles tendon rupture undergo acute surgical reconstruction.[12,63]

Medial Tibial Stress Syndrome. Medial tibial stress syndrome or "shin splints" presents with pain over the distal third of the medial aspect of the tibia that is worse with running and jumping. Inflammation of the periostial insertion of the soleus and posterior tibialis fascia on the posteromedial tibia is the proposed location of injury. Players will have moderate tenderness over the medial tibia. Radiographs are often negative. Bone scan and MRI can be diagnostic and helpful in differentiating MTSS from a tibial stress fracture. Treatment is conservative and consists of a period of relative rest, ice, activity modification, NSAIDs, and stretching of the gastroc-soleus complex. Local modalities such as ultrasound and iontophoresis may also be helpful in returning the athlete to play. Orthotics may be useful if excessive pronation of the foot has been identified as a causative factor. In rare instances, conditions that are refractory to standard conservative treatment protocols may require operative intervention.[1,4]

Peroneal Tendonitis. Peroneal tendonitis presents with lateral ankle pain. Differentiation among tendonitis, partial longitudinal tearing of the peroneus brevis, lateral gutter synovial impingement, and peroneal tendon subluxation must be made. A history of subjective ankle instability, weakness, popping, and swelling may be elicited. Players may have an antalgic gait, tenderness in the lateral retromalleolar groove, swelling, crepitus, and pain with passive inversion of the subtalar joint. MRI is helpful in defining the extent of tendon injury. The mainstay of treatment of peroneal tenosynovitis is rest, ice, NSAIDs, and physical therapy. The use of a lateral heel wedge may also be used. A period of immobilization is helpful in cases that are slow to respond. Recalcitrant cases with MRI evidence of tearing of the peroneal tendons may benefit from surgical exploration and repair. Occult ankle instability may be associated with these injuries and should be assessed.

Knee Injuries

Knee injuries are common in basketball players of all ages and levels of competition. Patellofemoral syndrome, acute and chronic patellar or quadriceps tendonitis, and Osgood-Schlatter's disease, with or without an unresolved ossicle can be a source of anterior knee pain in the athlete. Acute partial or complete rupture of the patellar tendon and injury to the articular cartilage, meniscus, and supporting ligamentous structures of the knee may occur during the course of play, resulting in pain, swelling, and the inability to continue the game. A comprehensive history and physical examination is mandatory, and x-rays and MRI evaluation can be helpful in confirming a diagnosis. Of these injuries, anterior cruciate ligament disruption has been occurring with increasing frequency in basketball players, and can result in considerable disability and loss of playing time for the young athlete.[3,9,19,20,25,43,57,70]

High-intensity running, cutting, pivoting, jumping, and rapid deceleration movements required of the basketball player during competition place the anterior cruciate ligament under constant stress and at risk for injury.[9] Women basketball players are more likely to sustain an ACL injury than are their male counterparts.[3] In the male basketball player, ACL injuries more commonly result from mechanisms involving contact, such as a direct blow to the knee or the force of landing after jumping up to grab a rebound.[3] A direct blow to the lateral aspect of the knee imparts a combined valgus and rotational stress on the ACL, whereas the combination of hyperextension, varus stress, and eccentric contraction of the quadriceps that occurs with landing puts the ligament under excessive tension which can result in failure.[9] Female athletes are more likely to sustain a noncontact injury that results in ligamentous disruption. The most common noncontact mechanism is rapid deceleration and a change in direction (either internal or external rotation). No clearly defined or scientifically proven explanation for the differences in injury rate between men and women has been established. Training deficiencies and abnormal hamstring–quadriceps ratio, skill level, shoe modification, femoral notch width, and circulating levels of estrogen that vary with the menstrual cycle have been examined as potential causes, however, further study is necessary to truly understand these differences.[20]

Treatment of the ACL-deficient knee in a basketball player who would like to continue playing at competitive level is based on surgical reconstruction. A structured rehabilitation program emphasizing strengthening of the quadriceps and hamstrings in conjunction with proprioceptive retraining is essential to improve dynamic stabilization of the knee joint and should begin in the early postoperative period. Return to play can be expected roughly 6 months from the time of surgery.[57]

Foot and Ankle

Ankle Sprain. Ankle ligament injuries are the most common injuries in sports. The lateral ankle ligaments are the most frequently injured structures and account for the vast majority of injuries sustained by basketball players today.[42,46,49,54] Isolated injury of the anterior talofibular ligament accounts for two-thirds of all sprains. Combined anterior talofibular and calcaneofibular injuries occur 20% of the time. Deltoid and syndesmotic injuries are much less common.

A recent study of ankle injuries in basketball players identified three risk factors for ankle injury. Players with a prior history of ankle injury, those wearing shoes with air cells in the heel, and those who did not stretch before the game were more likely to sustain an ankle injury.[42] Preperformance taping of the ankle may improve stability and decrease the likelihood of injury.[34,53]

Sudden and uncontrolled inversion of the foot and ankle or "rolling" the ankle that occurs when a player steps awkwardly results in injury to the lateral supporting structures. This most commonly occurs when the player is in the act of landing. Injury is often accompanied by anterolateral ankle pain and swelling. The athlete may have difficulty bearing weight. There is tenderness over the lateral aspect of the ankle. A thorough examination is required to rule out bony and tendinous injuries. Fractures of the fibula, fifth metatarsal, acute traumatic peroneal tendon dislocation, and osteochondral injuries can occur and should be considered in the differential diagnosis. X-rays should be obtained to confirm the presence or absence of associated pathology. Stress views may be helpful once the acute period of injury has subsided to objectively document ankle stability.

The treatment is conservative.[53] A rehabilitation program should be started as soon as possible to work on proprioception and general strengthening and conditioning of the musculature of the foot and ankle. This is critical in reducing the incidence of symptomatic instability, pain, and recurrent ankle sprains in the future.[30,60] Chronic lateral ankle pain in the athlete who has previously sustained an ankle sprain could be a result of incomplete rehabilitation, lateral talar exostosis, interosseus ligament tears, unrecognized syndesmosis sprain, subtalar instability, meniscoid lesion, anterior tibiotalar impingement, or lateral gutter synovial impingement, and evaluation should proceed accordingly. Arthroscopy can be useful in the diagnosis and treatment of these disorders.[8,13,15,27,38,60] Surgical reconstruction can be successful in appropriately selected patients with chronic lateral ankle instability.[16,39]

Impingement Syndromes. Anterior tibiotalar joint impingement is not uncommon in basketball players with a history of recurrent ankle sprains. Osteophytes may form on the anterior lip of the tibia and the talar neck. Players will complain of anterior ankle pain with jumping. Diagnosis is confirmed by limited active and passive dorsiflexion, painful forced dorsiflexion, and osteophyte formation seen on the lateral ankle x-ray. Conservative treatment should be tried initially. Heel lifts, NSAIDs, and avoidance of excessive dorsiflexion may be helpful. If conservative treatment fails, surgical excision may be required.

Anterolateral soft-tissue impingement of the ankle is commonly seen as a result of repetitive ankle injury. A hyalinized connective tissue "meniscoid lesion" can form in the anterolateral gutter, causing pain and the feeling of instability. A high success rate has been reported with arthroscopic excision.[8,38]

Navicular Stress Fractures. Navicular stress fractures present with the insidious onset of forefoot pain that is worse with activity. The symptoms are vague and physical findings often nonspecific. A delay in diagnosis is not uncommon and players are often misdiagnosed with a forefoot sprain and treated inappropriately for an extended period of time before an accurate diagnosis is obtained. If the diagnosis is suspected and plain radiographs are equivocal, MRI or CT scan can be ordered to confirm the diagnosis. The treatment for early, incomplete, nondisplaced fractures requires the athlete to be immobilized in a short leg cast and prohibited from bearing weight for six weeks, followed by gradual resumption of activity over the next six weeks. A CT scan can be repeated to confirm healing. If progressive healing is evident, return to play may be expected within 12 to 18 weeks from the time treatment was initiated. If there is displacement, delayed union, or nonunion, then surgical treatment will be necessary.[35,62]

Fifth Metatarsal Fractures. Fractures of the proximal third of the fifth metatarsal are common in sports that involve significant amounts of running and jumping.[61] Players may present with the insidious onset of a vague, dull ache along the lateral border of the foot that is exacerbated during play and relieved with rest, or with the acute onset of pain along the fifth metatarsal. X-rays may demonstrate an obvious fracture with sclerosis indicating the chronicity of the problem. Typically, a history of prodromal symptoms combined with intramedullary sclerosis and a widened fracture line is indicative of a preexisting stress fracture. Conservative treatment with casting and strict non–weight bearing has been successful;[10,32] however, there is an increased risk of delayed union, nonunion, and hindfoot stiffness with this treatment. Primary surgical management with intramedullary screw fixation is the treatment of choice in competitive athletes and serves as a more reliable and predictable treatment option that allows for a more timely return to competition.[10]

Medial Subtalar Joint Dislocation. A medial subtalar joint dislocation results from a high-energy force applied to the inverted foot. Grantham coined the term *basketball foot* to describe this entity because four of his five patients sustained this injury in falls on the basketball court.[18] The player with this injury is in excruciating pain and cannot bear weight. There is significant deformity and distortion of the soft tissues, with tenting of the skin over the prominent talar head. Extreme swelling occurs rapidly and may obscure the bony deformity. The injury has also been referred to as having the appearance of an "acquired clubfoot." X-rays of both the ankle and the foot are mandatory. The talus lies in a normal relationship to the tibia and fibula on all views, while the talonavicular joint dislocation is readily apparent on the AP view of the foot. Prompt and gentle closed reduction under spinal or general anesthesia is suggested to avoid additional osteochondral injury. Approximately 10% of medial subtalar joint dislocations cannot be reduced by closed means and require operative intervention. Initial immobilization in a short leg posterior splint is recommended. Immobilization for four weeks in a short leg cast followed by an active exercise program to regain subtalar and midtarsal joint motion typically results in minimal long-term loss of function.[24]

CONCLUSION

Most injuries incurred by basketball players are minor and do not result in a significant loss of playing time. Injuries to the ankle, knee, finger, and face are most common. At all levels of competition, the number and severity of knee injuries, including career-threatening ACL rupture, is greater in female athletes. Injuries involving the lower limb are more likely to result in a loss of playing time than injuries involving other body regions. Adherence to strict preseason and in-season conditioning programs, the use of mouthguards, and appropriate rehabilitation after an injury has occurred is helpful in preventing serious or recurrent injury. A thorough understanding of the types of injuries sustained by the basketball player is necessary so that the medical staff can provide a rapid and accurate diagnosis, and administer the most appropriate treatment so that a more timely return to competition can be achieved.

REFERENCES

1. Abramowitz A, Schepsis A, McArthur C: The medial tibial stress syndrome: The role of surgery. Orthop Rev 23:875–881, 1999.
2. Angermann P, Hovgaard D: Chronic Achilles tendonopathy in athletic individuals: Results of nonsurgical treatment. Foot Ankle Int 20:304–306, 1999.
3. Arendt E, Dick R: Knee injury patterns among men and women in collegiate basketball and soccer. Am J Sports Med 23:694–701, 1995.
4. Beck B, Osternig L: Medial tibial stress syndrome: The location of muscles in the leg in relation to symptoms. J Bone Joint Surg 76A:1057–1061, 1994.
5. Castaldi C: Sports related oral and facial injuries in the young athlete: A new challenge for the pediatric dentist. Pediatr Dent 8:311–314, 1986.
6. Chandy T, Grana W: Secondary school athletic injury in boys and girls: A three year study. Phys Sports Med 13:106–111, 1985.
7. Delaney J, Cross S, Piacentini M: Orbital emphysema in a collegiate basketball player. Clin J Sport Med 8:310–312, 1998.
8. Dixon D, Monroe M, Gabel S, et al: Excrescent lesion: A diagnosis of lateral talar exostosis in chronically symptomatic sprained ankles. Foot Ankle Int 20:331–336, 1999.
9. Emerson R: Basketball knee injuries and the anterior cruciate ligament. Clin Sports Med 12:317–328, 1993.

10. Fairen M: Fracture of the fifth metatarsal in basketball players. Knee Surg Sports Traumatol Arthrosc 7:373–377, 1999.
11. Flynn C, D'Amico F, Smith G: Should we patch corneal abrasions? A metanalysis. J Fam Pract 48:8–9, 1998.
12. Frey C, Feder K: Foot and ankle injuries in sports. In Arendt E (ed): OKU Sports Medicine. Rosemont, IL, American Academy of Orthopaedic Surgeons, 1999, pp 379–394.
13. Frey C, Feder K, DiGiovanni C: Arthroscopic evaluation of the subtalar joint: Does sinus tarsi syndrome exist? Foot Ankle Int 20:185–191, 1999.
14. Friedman S: Optic nerve avulsion secondary to basketball injury. Ophthalmic Surg Lasers 30:676–677, 1999.
15. Gerber J, Williams G, Scoville C, et al: Persistent disability associated with ankle sprains: A prospective evaluation of an athletic population. Foot Ankle Int 19:653–660, 1998.
16. Girard P, Anderson R, Davis W, et al: Clinical evaluation of the modified Brostrom-Evans procedure to restore ankle stability. Foot Ankle Int 20:246–252, 1999.
17. Gomez E, DeLee J, Farney W: Incidence of injury in Texas girl's high school basketball. Am J Sports Med 24:684–687, 1996.
18. Grantham S: Medial subtalar dislocation: Five cases with a common etiology. J Trauma 4:845–849, 1964.
19. Gray J: A survey of injuries to the anterior cruciate ligament of the knee in female basketball players. Int J Sports Med 6:314–316, 1985.
20. Griffin L, Agel J, Albohm M, et al: Noncontact anterior cruciate ligament cruciate injuries: Risk factors and prevention strategies. J Am Acad Orthop Surg 8:141–150, 2000.
21. Griffiths G, Selesnick F: Operative treatment and arthroscopic findings in chronic patellar tendonitis. Arthroscopy 14:836–839, 1998.
22. Guyette R: Facial injuries in basketball players. Clin Sports Med 12:247–264, 1993.
23. Hankin F, Peel S: Sports-related fractures and dislocations of the hand. Hand Clin 6:429–444, 1990.
24. Heckman J: Fractures and dislocations of the foot. In Rockwood C, Green D, Bucholz R, Heckman J (eds): Fractures in Adults, 4th ed. Philadelphia, Lippincott-Raven, 1996, pp 2267–2405.
25. Henry J, Lauear B, Neigut D: The injury rate in professional basketball. Am J Sports Med 1:16–18, 1982.
26. Herskowitz A, Selesnick H: Back injuries in basketball players. Clin Sports Med 12:293–306, 1993.
27. Hertel J, Denegar C, Monroe M, et al: Talocrural and subtalar joint instability after lateral ankle sprain. Med Sci Sports Exerc 31:1501–1508, 1999.
28. Hickey G, Fricker P, McDonald W: Injuries to young elite female basketball players over a six-year period. Clin J Sports Med 7:252–256, 1997.
29. Hippe M, Flint A, Lee R: University basketball injuries: A five year study of women's and men's varsity teams. Scand J Med Sci Sports 3:117–121, 1993.
30. Johnson K, Teasdale R: Sprained ankles as they relate to the basketball player. Clin Sports Med 12:363–371, 1993.
31. Jones N: Eye injury in sports. Sports Med 7:163–175, 1989.
32. Josefsson P: Closed treatment of Jones Fractures: good results in 40 cases after 11-26 years. Acta Orthop Scand 65:545–547, 1994.
33. Kaiser P, Pineda R: A study of topical non-steroidal anti-inflammatory drops and no pressure patching in treatment of corneal abrasions. Ophthalmology 104:1353–1359, 1997.
34. Karlsson J, Sward L, Andreasson G: The effect of taping on ankle stability: Practical implications. Sports Med 16:210–215, 1993.
35. Khan K: Outcome of conservative and surgical management of navicular stress fractures in athletes. Am J Sports Med 20:657–665, 1992.
36. Kumamoto D: Tooth avulsions resulting from basketball net entanglement. J Am Dent Assoc 128:1273–1275, 1997.
37. Labella C, Smith B, Sigurdsson A: Effect of mouthguards on dental injuries and concussions in college basketball. Med Sci Sports Exerc 34(1):41–44, 2002.
38. Lahm A, Erggelet C, Reichelt A: Ankle joint arthroscopy for meniscoid lesions in athletes. Arthroscopy 14:572–575, 1998.
39. Liu S, Baker C: Comparison of lateral ankle ligamentous reconstruction procedures. Am J Sports Med 22:313–317, 1994.
40. Maestrello-deMoya M, Primosch R: Orofacial trauma and mouth protector wear among high school varsity basketball players. J Dent Child 56:36–39, 1989.
41. McCue F: Pseudo-boutonniere deformity. Hand 7:166–169, 1975.
42. McKay G, Goldie P, Payne W, et al: Ankle injuries in basketball: Injury rate and risk factors. Br J Sports Med 35(2):103–108, 2001.
43. McKay GD, Goldie PA, Payne WR, et al: A prospective study of injuries in basketball: A total profile and comparison by gender and standard of competition. J Sci Med Sport 4(2):196–211, 2001.
44. McLoughin, R, Raber E, Vellet A: Patellar tendonitis: MR imaging features with suggested pathogenesis and proposed classification. Radiology 197:843–848, 1995.

45. McNutt T: Oral trauma and the adolescent athlete: A study on mouth protectors. Pediatr Dent 11:209–213, 1989.
46. Messina D, Farney W, DeLee J: The incidence of injury in Texas high school basketball: A prospective study among male and female athletes. Am J Sports Med 27:294–299, 1999.
47. Mital M, Matza R, Cohen J: The so-called unresolved Osgood-Schlatter lesion: A concept based on fifteen surgically treated lesions. J Bone Joint Surg 62(5):732–739, 1980.
48. Molnar T, Fox J: Overuse injuries of the knee in basketball. Clin Sports Med 12(2):349–362, 1993.
49. Moretz A, Grana W: High school basketball injuries. Phys Sports Med 6:91–95, 1978.
50. Nichols C: Patellar tendon injuries. Clin Sports Med 11:807–813, 1992.
51. Orava S, Malinen L, Karpakka J, et al: Results of surgical treatment of unresolved Osgood-Schlatter lesion. Ann Chir Gynaecol 89(4):298–302, 2000.
52. Popp J, Yu J, Kaeding C: Recalcitrant patellar tendonitis: Magnetic resonance imaging, histologic evaluation, and surgical treatment. Am J Sports Med 25:218–222, 1997.
53. Povacz P, Unger S, Miller W, et al: A randomized prospective study of operative and nonoperative treatment of injuries of the fibular collateral ligaments of the ankle. J Bone Joint Surg Am 80:345–351, 1998.
54. Prebble T: Basketball injuries in a rural area. Wisc Med J 98:22–25, 1999.
55. Rettig A: Closed tendon injuries of the hand and wrist in athletes. Clin Sports Med 11:77–79, 1992.
56. Sane J: Comparison of maxillofacial and dental injuries in four contact team sports. Am J Sports Med 16:647–652, 1988.
57. Shelbourne K, Gray T: Anterior cruciate ligament reconstruction with autogenous patellar tendon graft followed by accelerated rehabilitation: A 2-9 year follow-up. Am J Sports Med 25:786–795, 1997.
58. Sonzogni J, Gross M: Assessment and treatment of basketball injuries. Clin Sports Med 12:221–237, 1993.
59. Stock J, Cornell F: Prevention of sports related eye trauma. Am Fam Physician 44:515–520, 1991.
60. Thacker S, Stroup D, Branche C, et al: The prevention of ankle sprains in sports: A systematic review of the literature. Am J Sports Med 27:753–760, 1999.
61. Torg J: Fractures of the base of the fifth metatarsal distal to the tuberosity: Classification and guidelines for non-surgical and surgical management. J Bone Joint Surg Am 66:209–214, 1984.
62. Torg J: Stress fractures of the tarsal navicular. J Bone Joint Surg 64:700–712, 1982.
63. Traina S, Yonezuka N, Zinis Y: Achilles tendon injury in a professional basketball player. Orthopaedics 22:625–626, 1999.
64. Tucker C: Management of early nasal injuries with long-term follow-up. Rhinology 22:45–53, 1984.
65. Wilson R, McGinty L: Common hand and wrist injuries in basketball players. Clin Sports Med 12:265–291, 1993.
66. Woo C: Traumatic manubriosternal joint subluxations in two basketball players. J Manipulative Physiol Ther 11:433–437, 1988.
67. Yde J, Nielsen A: Sports injuries in adolescents' ball games: Soccer, handball, and basketball. Br J Sports Med 24:51–54, 1990.
68. Yu J, Popp J, Kaeding C, et al: Correlation of MR imaging and pathologic findings in athletes undergoing surgery for chronic patellar tendonitis. Am J Roentgenol 165:115–118, 1995.
69. Zagelbaum B: The national basketball association eye injury study. Arch Ophthamol 113:749–752, 1995.
70. Zelisko J, Noble H, Proter M: A comparison of men's and women's professional basketball injuries. Am J Sports Med 10:297–299, 1982.
71. Zilmer D, Powell J, Albright J: Gender-specific injury patterns in high school varsity basketball. J Women's Health 1:69–76, 1992.

36 Baseball Injuries

Steven Arsht, Giles R. Scuderi, and Peter D. McCann

Baseball is considered America's national pastime. Millions of players of all ages and skill levels enjoy the sport. Baseball is a noncontact sport that requires minimal protective gear and is therefore considered to be relatively safe. The relative incidence of injury ranks last among competitive team sports, but because of the large number of participants worldwide, is second only to football in total number of injuries and fatalities annually reported. Injury demographics vary between Little League and the collegiate and professional players. At the Little League level, the impact of the ball is responsible for the greatest number of injuries, accounting for almost 60% of the injuries reported in one study. Facial injuries appear to be most common, followed by the hand and fingers and shoulder. Overuse injuries are also common in this age group. Injuries sustained by impact with the ball were common on defense (68%). In contrast, at the collegiate level, 58% of the injuries occurred in the shoulder region, with rotator cuff tendinitis being the most frequent complaint. At this level, strains (23%), sprains (19%), and contusions (17%) account for the majority of injuries.[22,44,50,57,77]

SHOULDER

Injuries to the shoulder are most commonly due to the accumulation of microtrauma from the repetitive throwing motion, and account for the majority of injuries seen in baseball players today.[2,6,16,21,40,63,70,74] The differential diagnosis of shoulder pain in the baseball player is extensive (Table 36-1). A thorough understanding of shoulder anatomy and the biomechanics of throwing are essential to the recognition, diagnosis, and treatment of these injuries. The biomechanics of throwing a baseball has been extensively studied and has been divided into five phases: wind-up, cocking, acceleration, deceleration, and follow-through. In caring for throwing athletes, it is critical to understand the phases of throwing because this offers a framework to sort out the athlete's symptoms and arrive at a diagnosis.[12,29,47,75]

Evaluation

A detailed history, including the review of available medical records and past history of shoulder problems and treatment rendered, is necessary. The athlete is often vague about time of onset of symptoms or inciting event. Loss of velocity, accuracy, and distance usually alert the thrower that the injury is more serious than just the usual aches and pains. Recent changes in the mechanics of throwing such as the introduction of a new type of pitch (curve ball) or delivery (side arm), or a change in the velocity, duration, distance, intensity, or amount of throwing must be noted. Any perceived or objectively observed decrease in velocity or accuracy is important. Knowledge of the location and character of the pain, the presence of night pain, duration of symptoms, alleviating and exacerbating factors, and analgesic requirements should be considered. The timing of symptom development relative to the number of pitches thrown or innings completed and the timing during the throwing cycle that symptoms are greatest is useful. It is important to establish a temporal relationship, if possible, between the phase of throwing and arm position and the onset of symptoms. Players with anterior shoulder instability may report anterior shoulder pain during the cocking phase, and those with posterior instability report posterior shoulder pain during the follow-through phase. Posterior shoulder pain during the late cocking and early acceleration phase may be indicative of internal impingement, or a Bennet's lesion, but players with subacromial impingement and rotator cuff tendinitis may report anterior shoulder pain during the acceleration phase. Pain at the inferomedial border of the scapula during late cocking and acceleration is seen with scapulothoracic bursitis. Persistent night pain may be a sign of a rotator cuff tear.[62]

Evaluation of the injured shoulder includes a thorough musculoskeletal, neurologic, and vascular examination. Assessment of the cervical spine and contralateral shoulder is mandatory. The player's posture and shoulder girdle symmetry is observed in the standing position. Wasting or atrophy of the supraspinatus and/or infraspinatus muscles may be a sign of suprascapular neuropathy. Range of motion in the sitting and supine position is recorded. Overdevelopment of the dominant extremity is common. The musculature of the throwing arm is often hypertrophied and the scapula may be slightly displaced inferiorly. Asymmetric loss of internal rotation and an increase in external rotation of the throwing arm is typical. There is some degree of asymmetric joint laxity that exists in the normal shoulder of the throwing athlete. This is often more pronounced in pitchers compared to position players. The examiner must be able

TABLE 36-1 Shoulder Pain

Shoulder Pain
Rotator Cuff
1. Tendinitis
a. Edema and hemorrhage
b. Inflammation and fibrosis
2. Tears
a. Partial thickness
b. Full thickness
Glenohumeral Joint Instability
1. Anterior
2. Posterior
3. Multidirectional
4. Labral tears
Biceps
1. Tendinitis
2. Subluxation
3. SLAP tear
Humeral Fracture
1. Microfracture (stress)
a. Adult vs. pediatric
b. Macrofracture (overt)
Neurovascular
1. Thoracic outlet syndrome
2. "Effort" thrombosis
3. Suprascapular neuropathy
4. Quadrilateral space syndrome
5. Cervical radiculopathy
Glenohumeral Joint Arthritis
Acromioclavicular Joint Arthritis
Scapulothoracic Bursitis
Bennet's Exostosis

to differentiate between physiologic and pathologic laxity. Posterior capsular tightness and anterior capsular laxity is not unusual. Occult anterior glenohumeral joint instability may potentiate rotator cuff disease and is often overlooked as a contributing factor. Manual strength testing to evaluate the rotator cuff is necessary. The examiner must differentiate shoulder weakness due to rotator cuff deficiency from pain due to inflammation and recent injury. A subacromial injection of 1% lidocaine can be helpful. If the patient has complete relief of pain and the shoulder remains weak, then significant rotator cuff injury must be suspected. Isokinetic testing can be performed to objectively document strength.[3,10,49,62]

Diagnostic Tests

Radiographic evaluation of the shoulder should include AP view in neutral, internal, and external rotation, along with axillary, and supraspinatus outlet views. MRI with or without intraarticular gadolinium is valuable for evaluation of the rotator cuff[40,61] and labrum.[39] Comparison with prior studies, if available, is recommended. If a neurologic injury is suspected, EMG and nerve conduction velocity testing may be diagnostic. Radiographs and MRI of the cervical spine may also be obtained if the player has radicular symptoms. Duplex ultrasonography and venography should be included if upper extremity vascular occlusion is suspected.

Treatment

The majority of shoulder injuries respond to conservative management. The treatment plan aims to eliminate pain and decrease inflammation, restore motion, correct strength deficits, regain normal, synchronous muscle activity, and return the athlete to his pre-injury level of function in a timely manner.[62,97,98]

Initial measures to decrease pain are rest, avoidance of aggravating activities, NSAIDs, cryotherapy, and other modalities. Occasional subacromial injection of corticosteroid for an athlete who is not responding to initial treatment is not unreasonable. Proper rehabilitation of the rotator cuff is essential for full recovery from shoulder injury. A conditioning program focused on the strengthening and conditioning of the rotator cuff and scapular stabilizers is essential in restoring dynamic stability to the joint. Posterior capsular stretching to eliminate posterior capsular contracture is also helpful. A gradual return to throwing may begin once normal isokinetic profiles for the rehabbed shoulder have been established.[62,97,98] Failure of nonoperative treatment is defined as lack of definitive progress after a minimum of three months and the inability of the athlete to return asymptomatically to a competitive level of function by six months.[62]

Rotator Cuff Injuries

Etiology of rotator cuff tendon injury is multifactorial. Throwing a baseball subjects the rotator cuff to repetitive microtrauma, which can result in a gradual failure of the tendon fibers over time. Full thickness rotator cuff tears in players under the age of 35 are rare and carry a poor prognosis. Partial thickness tears, tendinopathy, bursitis, and muscle fatigue predominate in younger athletes. Muscle fatigue can lead to abnormal shoulder kinematics and instability, which can precipitate or accentuate glenohumeral translation and subluxation, placing the player at risk for secondary impingement and tensile failure of the rotator cuff. The key to successful treatment of rotator cuff injury is the recognition and treatment of all factors that may contribute to the development of injury. The presence of underlying instability must be considered in the evaluation of the baseball player with rotator cuff pathology.[16,21,53,91]

Impingement. Players with subacromial impingement complain of pain in the anterior shoulder during the acceleration phase of throwing, and sometimes during follow-through. There is pain with overhead activity and when the arm is in a position of forward flexion and internal rotation. Tenderness to palpation over the anterior acromion and greater tuberosity and a positive impingement sign and test can be elicited.

It is necessary to distinguish primary from secondary impingement, which is related to glenohumeral joint instability. Occult subluxation of the glenhumeral joint has been implicated as the underlying cause for impingement syndrome in the young overhead athlete. This may be accentuated by the presence of posterior capsular tightness, anterior capsuloligamentous insufficiency, type 2 SLAP lesion, and early fatigue of the dynamic stabilizers of the shoulder. X-rays may demonstrate a curved or hooked acromion. MRI should be reviewed to assess integrity of the rotator cuff, biceps, and capsulolabral complex. Treatment is conservative. Return to play and success of treatment is dependent on the stage of the disease as described by Neer,[67] and the correction of instability, if present. The presence of symptoms for less than four weeks and a flat acromion are favorable prognostic signs. The administration of one to two cortisone injections may increase the likelihood of success with nonoperative treatment.

Internal Impingement. Players complain of pain in the posterior aspect of the shoulder during the late cocking and early acceleration phases of throwing, when the deep surface of the supraspinatus contacts the posterior glenoid rim. Symptoms can be reproduced on exam by placing the arm in maximum abduction and external rotation. Intraarticular injection of 1% lidocaine may be helpful in differentiating internal impingement from primary subacromial impingement. This condition may be exacerbated by occult glenohumeral joint instability or the presence of a Bennet's lesion and accounts for a significant percentage of the articular-sided cuff tears and posterosuperior labral tears observed in the throwing shoulder. MR arthrography with traction and abduction–external rotation views is the most helpful imaging study. Blunting of the posterior labrum and undersurface rotator cuff abnormalities can be seen. If conservative treatment fails, successful treatment with arthroscopic debridement is possible. Correction of underlying instability, if present, is mandatory for the successful treatment of this condition.[5,40,73,95]

Primary and Secondary Tensile Failure of the Rotator Cuff. The repetitive tensile forces acting on the rotator cuff during ball release and follow-through can result in serious injury. This may occur due to incomplete conditioning in the off-season, insufficient between-game workouts, or insufficient pregame warm-up. Early in the season, players may demonstrate acute tendinitis; however, late in the season, they may experience chronic overload cuff failure. Secondary tensile failure of the rotator cuff is precipitated by shoulder instability, causing the dynamic stabilizers to fatigue and be more susceptible to injury. The spectrum of injury ranges from tendinitis to complete tear.[21]

Treatment. The treatment of the majority of rotator cuff injuries in the throwing athlete is conservative. Isolated surgical treatment of chronic tendinitis and tears of the labrum and rotator cuff in the throwing athlete has not yielded consistently favorable outcomes, which is likely due to the failure to diagnose and correct all factors that contribute to the pathology. Full-thickness rotator cuff tears have a poor prognosis. Surgical repair in competitive athletes has had disappointing results. In a recent study, only 56% returned to formal competitive level after repair and only 32% of throwers were able to return to collegiate or professional sports at the same level.[83,91,92]

Shoulder Instability

Anterior Instability. Frank anterior shoulder instability is rare. Differentiation between physiologic laxity and pathologic instability must be made. Attenuation of anterior capsular supporting structures can occur with repetitive throwing. Elite throwers may have posterior capsular contracture that predisposes to anterior humeral head translation. Type 2 SLAP tears and rotator cuff weakness may play a role. The diagnosis of occult instability can be difficult, and the clinician must have a high index of suspicion. The pitcher may report anterior shoulder pain, numbness, tingling, early fatigue, or experience a "dead arm" while throwing. The apprehension test and Jobe relocation test may be positive. X-rays are often negative. MRI is useful in showing labral pathology. Accurate identification of the cause of the instability is necessary. Most patients can be treated successfully with physical therapy. Patients with type 2 SLAP tears may benefit from surgical repair.[5,16,21,53,63]

Posterior Instability. Posterior instability is often unrecognized in throwing athletes. Throwers complain of posterior shoulder pain during follow-through. The pain can radiate to the scapula. There is pain with forward flexion, adduction, and internal rotation on exam. Occasionally posterior instability can be detected. Conservative treatment is generally successful, with symptomatic improvement seen in up to two-thirds of players.[16,21]

Other Shoulder Injuries

SLAP Tears. Players give a history of anterior shoulder pain with throwing and with overhead activities.

A "catching" or "popping" sensation may also be reported, and may be a sign of biceps tendinitis or subluxation. Numerous tests for tears of the superior labrum have been described, but many clinicians find it difficult to make an accurate diagnosis by physical exam alone. MRI with intraarticular gadolinium is the most sensitive and specific test for the diagnosis for labral pathology. Surgical treatment can be successful in alleviating pain and returning athletes to play. Labral lesions that destabilize the biceps anchor can potentiate anterior glenohumeral joint instability and may benefit from repair.[5,9,16,35,63,66,71]

Bennet's Lesion or Thrower's Exostosis. Players are asymptomatic with light throwing, but typically develop posterior shoulder pain after two to three innings of hard throwing. There is localized tenderness over the posterior aspect of the shoulder. X-rays may show extraarticular ossification in close proximity to the posterior band of IGHL. There is an association with posterior labral injury and undersurface rotator cuff tears and internal impingement. Initial treatment is nonoperative. Success depends on the amount of intraarticular pathology. If conservative management fails, then removal of the exostosis and treatment of associated intraarticular pathology is necessary.[32,60]

Scapulothoracic Bursitis. There is the insidious onset of painless crepitus with elevation of the arm, and as inflammation increases, players develop posterior shoulder pain that can be localized to the inferomedial angle of the scapula during the late cocking and acceleration phases of throwing. A palpable or audible grinding at the superior or inferior angle of the scapula is consistently present on exam. There is tenderness at the inferomedial border of the scapula, and occasionally, a small mass representing inflamed bursal tissue can be felt. X-rays, MRI, and CT scan are typically normal, but should be obtained to rule out a bony cause. The treatment is conservative, and with time, the pain resolves. The crepitus often remains, however. If pain continues and the player cannot compete, then surgery may be necessary.[51,86]

Suprascapular Nerve Palsy. Entrapment of the suprascapular nerve is a well-recognized cause of supraspinatus and infraspinatus muscular dysfunction. This can be caused by ganglion cyst, tumor, and entrapment at the suprascapular or spinoglenoid notch. Players report a progressive, vague pain over the posterolateral shoulder during the acceleration phase of throwing that may even radiate to neck and chest. The onset is insidious and there can be a slow decline in function. Symptoms are often present for a long time before a diagnosis is made. The most common sign is atrophy of the supraspinatus or infraspinatus.

Early examination may be unremarkable. There may be discomfort with compression of the spinoglenoid or suprascapular notch, weakness, posterolateral shoulder pain, a varying degree of wasting of supraspinatus and infraspinatus, and possible reduction in external rotation power. Diagnostic evaluation includes EMG and NCV and MRI. A diagnostic injection with local anesthetic at the suprascapular or spinoglenoid notch may be helpful.

In the absence of a ganglion or space-occupying lesion, most players respond to nonoperative treatment. Rotator cuff and periscapular strengthening and improvement in external rotation strength are helpful. If no improvement is seen after 3 to 6 months, surgical decompression may be indicated.

Isolated infraspinatus involvement with loss of external rotation strength and asymmetry of the shoulder girdle is unique to the throwing athlete. During the late cocking and follow-through phase of throwing, the terminal branches of the nerve to the infraspinatus are shifted medially and tension is placed on the nerve as it crosses the lateral edge of scapula. A consistent pattern of progressive worsening and denervation can occur with continued throwing, which is reversible with rest.[1,15,30,59,81]

Quadrilateral Space Syndrome. The axillary nerve is at risk for entrapment by the fibrous bands of the quadrilateral space when the arm is positioned in maximum abduction and external rotation. Players report posterior shoulder pain during the late cocking phase. There may be tenderness around the teres minor and quadrilateral space. Muscle atrophy is not typically seen on gross examination, but may be evident by MRI. EMG and nerve conduction velocity studies are nondiagnostic. If conservative treatment fails, surgical decompression may be necessary.[1,17,33,80]

Vascular Injuries. Upper extremity vascular injuries are uncommon in the elite throwing athlete and are often precipitated by repeated compression of the subclavian vasculature between the first rib or scalene muscles that occurs with extreme shoulder abduction and external rotation during throwing.[28,79] Axillary artery thrombosis or aneurysm, subclavian vein and artery thrombosis ("effort thrombosis"), and thoracic outlet syndrome have been described. The symptoms are vague and the physical findings are subtle, making diagnosis difficult. Pitchers report a variety of symptoms such as forearm pain, early fatigue, diminished endurance and velocity, and throwing arm "heaviness." Duplex ultrasonography and contrast venography are helpful in making the diagnosis. MRI is also useful. In the absence of clot or aneurysm, the treatment is conservative. If vascular thrombosis is detected, a more aggressive approach is warranted, which would include surgical decompression or pharmacological thrombolysis, and systemic anticoagulation.

The symptoms are vague in the case of thoracic outlet syndrome and a diagnosis is often difficult to make. Thoracic outlet syndrome is rare in the throwing athlete.

Players may report parasthesias and pain that radiates down the lateral side of the neck to the shoulder, medial arm, and ring and small fingers of the hand with throwing. Conservative treatment is generally successful.

Little Leaguer's Shoulder. A stress fracture of proximal humeral physis can develop in the skeletally immature pitcher. Athletes between the ages of 13 and 16 are at greatest risk. Players complain of posterolateral shoulder pain at the end of a hard throw. The pain does not usually stop the pitcher from throwing. Tenderness over the lateral proximal humeral physis is noted.

X-rays demonstrate uniform widening proximal to the humeral epiphysis. Simple bone cysts are common in this age group and should be ruled out in any young player with shoulder pain. X-rays of the opposite shoulder should be reviewed for comparison. This is usually a benign, self-limiting condition that resolves with rest. Healing may take up to three months. A gradual return to throwing with strict adherence to pitch count and avoidance of breaking pitches is recommended.[7,19]

Humeral Stress Fractures. The humerus is subject to enormous force during throwing, which can result in stress fractures or overt fractures. A thrower complaining of proximal arm pain should be evaluated for stress fracture. If x-rays are negative, MRI should be obtained. The treatment of stress fractures is conservative. Serial MRIs will show healing of the fracture and will help determine return to play.

Rotatory tensile overload in the acceleration phase of throwing can precipitate an overt humerus fracture, which most commonly presents as a spiral fracture in the diaphysis around the junction of the middle and distal thirds. Professional and collegiate players seem protected from these injuries because of adaptive cortical remodeling that occurs over time with increased amounts of conditioning and play. Treatment is conservative, with a functional fracture brace.[13,14,54,72]

ELBOW INJURIES

Baseball pitchers are particularly susceptible to elbow injuries due to the high angular velocity and force placed across the elbow during throwing. The culmination of these forces can lead to a variety of conditions that can cause pain and disability, affect performance, and keep the athlete from competition. Medial elbow symptoms account for the majority of elbow complaints in pitchers, and occur as a result of the valgus force across the elbow during the late cocking and early acceleration phases of throwing. Although acute, traumatic injuries to the bony, musculotendinous, and ligamentous structures about the elbow can occur, the majority of injuries are chronic overuse injuries resulting from repetitive intrinsic and extrinsic overload. The differential diagnosis of elbow pain in the baseball player is extensive (Table 36-2).

TABLE 36-2 Elbow Pain

Elbow Pain
Medial Pain
UCL injuries
Ulnar nerve symptoms
Medial flexor mass injuries and tendinitis
Olecranon stress fractures
Medial epicondyle apophyseal injuries
Medial epicondylitis
Posteromedial olecranon osteophytes with valgus extension overload syndrome
Medial subluxation of triceps tendon
Lateral Pain
Radiocapitellar disorders, osteochondritis dissecans, chondromalacia, lateral epicondylitis
Posterior Pain
Valgus extension overload
Impingement
Triceps tendinitis
Anterior Pain
Not common: biceps tendinitis, anterior capsular strain, anterior impingement from coronoid osteophyte

A thorough understanding of functional elbow anatomy and the biomechanics of throwing are essential to the recognition, diagnosis, and treatment of these injuries.[18,20,29,36,37,41,45,46,64,85,99]

General Evaluation

A thorough history should be obtained from the patient, coaching staff, and trainer. The acute onset of elbow pain while throwing may indicate UCL rupture, medial epicondyle avulsion, biceps or triceps tendon rupture, loose body, or acute subluxation of ulnar nerve. It is more common, however, for the athlete to complain of a chronic, progressive elbow pain. Recent changes in the mechanics of throwing, such as the introduction of a new type of pitch (curve ball) or delivery (side arm), or a change in the velocity, duration, distance, intensity, or amount of throwing must be noted. Any perceived or objectively observed decrease in velocity or accuracy is important. Knowledge of the location of the pain, timing of onset relative to number of pitches thrown or innings completed, duration of symptoms, alleviating and exacerbating factors, and the timing during the throwing cycle that symptoms occur is useful. Medial injuries such as ulnar collateral ligament insufficiency and medial epicondylitis are most pronounced during the late cocking and early acceleration phases of throwing, whereas posterior impingement is most noticeable during late acceleration and follow-through.[18,20,36,37,41,45,46,64,85,99]

Ulnar Collateral Ligament Injuries

The primary stabilizer of the elbow to valgus stress is the anterior band of the UCL, and the demands placed on it during throwing can approximate or exceed its ultimate tensile strength. Prolonged exposure to the repetitive stress of throwing can cause inflammation and micro-tearing of the UCL, resulting in attenuation and eventual rupture.

Improper throwing mechanics, poor flexibility, and inadequate conditioning may potentiate this problem. With acute ruptures, pitchers report sudden onset of pain after throwing, with or without a popping sensation, and are unable to continue throwing. In chronic conditions, the athlete will report medial elbow pain during late cocking and early acceleration. Accuracy, pitch count, and velocity are often diminished. Ulnar nerve symptoms are not uncommon. There is tenderness just distal to the medial epicondyle. The absence of pain with wrist flexion coupled with pain localized slightly posterior to common flexor origin helps to differentiate UCL injury from flexor pronator muscle injury. A flexion contracture and a positive Tinel's sign are frequent findings. The loss of a firm endpoint with valgus stress testing may be indicative of an incompetent UCL, although clinical laxity with valgus stress is noted in only 25% of cases.[4,18,46,48,69,85]

Imaging Studies. Standard radiographs of the elbow, including valgus stress views, are recommended. Calcification of the ligament may be seen. Stress radiographs exhibiting medial joint widening greater than 3 mm may be consistent with instability, however, this study has not demonstrated predictable objective reliability, and recent studies have found it difficult to determine pathologic laxity from the normal degree of laxity seen in the dominant arms of elite throwers. Contrast MRI and CT arthrography can be helpful in evaluating the soft-tissue anatomy of the elbow.[31,93]

Treatment. Treatment depends on the integrity of UCL and the degree of instability. Nonoperative management instituted at an early stage has been shown to arrest the progression of instability and functional impairment with up to 50% of athletes able to return to their preinjury level of throwing. Strengthening and conditioning of the flexor pronator mass may increase dynamic elbow stability and enhance valgus stability of the elbow.

A supervised throwing and conditioning program begins at three months once athlete regains full range of motion and strength. Surgical intervention is recommended for competitive athletes with acute complete ruptures or chronic symptoms secondary to instability that have not significantly improved after 3-6 months of rehabilitation. If UCL reconstruction is performed, a return to previous level of sport activity can be expected in roughly 80% of patients. One year of recovery is typically necessary for overhead athletes.[4,23,26,41]

Medial Epicondylitis

Medial epicondylitis is an overuse syndrome of the flexor pronator mass. A combination of valgus stress and intrinsic muscular contractions that occurs during throwing predisposes the pronator teres and flexor carpi radialis to inflammation and injury. Pitchers will complain of the insidious onset of medial elbow pain that worsens with continued throwing. Activities that involve resisted wrist flexion or pronation may exacerbate the symptoms. The point of maximum tenderness is over the flexor pronator origin 5 mm distal and anterior to the medial epicondyle. Symptoms are exacerbated by resisted wrist flexion and forearm pronation. A flexion contracture may be present. The examiner must assess elbow stability, because flexor pronator overuse may predispose to medial ligamentous injury or valgus instability.[21] A high incidence of ulnar neuropraxia is seen with medial epicondylitis, so it is important to evaluate for concurrent ulnar neuropathy.[26,34,45,52,87,94]

Imaging. X-rays may be entirely normal or reveal calcification adjacent to the medial epicondyle or a traction spur, which can be evidence of a chronic UCL injury. An MRI may reveal increased signal in musculotendinous structures and be helpful in the recalcitrant case by further delineating the underlying pathoanatomy. Full-thickness tears of the flexor pronator mass carry a poor prognosis and may benefit from operative intervention.

Treatment. Nonoperative treatment of medial epicondylitis is generally successful. Initial treatment consists of rest, ice, NSAIDs, and local modalities. Although corticosteroid injections deep to the flexor pronator mass may provide good short-term symptomatic relief, long-term results are no different than in treatment with physical therapy and oral anti-inflammatory medication alone, and should be used cautiously because of the associated risk of tendon attenuation and rupture with repeated injections. Surgical treatment is reserved for patients with persistent symptoms after six months of supervised physical therapy. Patients who do not respond to conservative treatment often have full-thickness tendon tears that are amenable to surgical repair.[34,52,87,94]

Flexor–Pronator Injuries

The flexor–pronator musculature provides dynamic stability to the medial elbow and may be injured with repetitive valgus stress. Tendinitis, partial tears, and complete tears can be seen. Throwers will report pain and swelling along the medial aspect of the elbow, which is most evident during acceleration and follow-through. On examination, there is tenderness at the medial epicondylar origin and increased pain with resisted wrist flexion and elbow extension. Evaluation for concurrent UCL insufficiency is mandatory. Minor partial injuries can be treated with rest, ice, and oral anti-inflammatory medication. More severe injuies and complete ruptures that compromise elbow stability require surgical attention.[26,36,41,69,85]

Pronator Syndrome. Hypertrophy of the pronator teres can cause compression of the median nerve in the forearm. Throwers report a fatiguelike pain in the proximal volar aspect of the forearm that gradually worsens with throwing and is exacerbated by resisted forearm pronation and wrist flexion. Surgical exploration and decompression of the median nerve is sometimes necessary.

Exertional Compartment Syndrome. Hypertrophy of the flexor pronator musculature can result in a type of exertional compartment syndrome of the forearm. Pitchers will report pain about the medial elbow and proximal forearm that becomes more intense and disabling with throwing, causing the pitcher to stop throwing after only a few innings. Adequate pregame warm-up and proper timing of pitching can prevent this condition so that sufficient rest is achieved between hard throwing sessions.[64]

Ulnar Neuritis

Ulnar neuropathy is a common finding that may be related to traction, friction, and compression of the ulnar nerve during the throwing cycle. More than 40% of athletes with valgus instability develop ulnar neuritis secondary to irritation from inflammation of UCL, and up to 60% of throwers with medial epicondylitis have concomitant ulnar nerve symptoms. Players complain of intermittent medial elbow pain that may radiate down the ulnar side of the forearm to the hand. Symptoms are generally exacerbated by throwing and resolve with rest. A clumsiness or heaviness in the fingers along with numbness and paresthesias in the small and ring fingers may be reported. A painful popping or snapping sensation at the elbow accompanied by parasthesias during throwing is seen with recurrent nerve subluxations or dislocations.

A careful neurologic examination of neck and upper extremity to rule out more proximal causes of neuropathy is required, along with a complete examination of the elbow to evaluate for associated injuries.

The initial treatment is conservative, and begins with rest, ice, activity modification, cessation of throwing, and anti-inflammatory medication. Local steroid injections are not recommended. A brief period of immobilization may be helpful, particularly when treating ulnar nerve subluxation or dislocation. Although this approach has been successful in treating the general population, many pitchers, particularly those with concomitant valgus instability, experience recurrent symptoms with throwing and may require surgery. Indications include failed nonoperative management, persistent ulnar nerve subluxation, symptomatic tension neuropraxia, and concomitant medial elbow problems requiring surgery.[23,27,37,82]

Posterior Impaction Injuries

Posterior impaction injuries occur primarily during the deceleration phase of throwing. Repeated impaction of the posteromedial olecranon in the olecranon fossa leads to synovitis, chondromalacia, hypertrophic spur, and osteophyte formation, especially on the medial aspect of ulnar notch. Posteromedial impingement by osteophytes and scar tissue results in pain during late acceleration and follow-through. Mechanical symptoms such as catching and locking are indicative of intraarticular loose bodies. The coaching staff may notice a shortened pitch count along with diminished accuracy and velocity. The pitcher may demonstrate early ball release, allowing the ball to be thrown high and out of the strike zone. A loss of terminal extension, tenderness along the posterior and posteromedial aspect of the olecranon, and pain with forced extension may be seen on exam. X-rays of the elbow, including an axial view, are generally sufficient and may reveal posteromedial osteophytes. MRI and CT scan may be helpful.

Treatment. Conservative management aimed at decreasing pain and swelling and restoring elbow motion is necessary. Functional strengthening of the elbow and forearm musculature helps to minimize injury related to forceful elbow extension that occurs during the deceleration phase of pitching. Chronic posterior impingement and persistent mechanical symptoms usually necessitate arthroscopic removal of spurs and loose bodies, which is favored over open procedures because it involves less soft-tissue dissection and allows earlier and more aggressive rehabilitation.[41,64,99]

Lateral Epicondylitis

Rapid forearm pronation during the acceleration phase of throwing puts tension on the lateral musculotendinous origin. Repeated stress may induce a lateral epicondylitis. The pitcher may have lateral elbow pain during the acceleration phase of throwing, with handshake, or when grasping objects. Tenderness to palpation is elicited over the lateral epicondyle 5 mm distal and anterior to the midpoint of the condyle. Symptoms are exacerbated by resisted wrist dorsiflexion and forearm supination. Plain radiographs are typically normal. Occasionally, calcific tendinitis may be seen. MRI may demonstrate tendon thickening, but is generally not needed. Conservative treatment with physical therapy, ultrasound, iontophoresis, electrical stimulation, ice, stretching and strengthening, augmented soft-tissue mobilization, and friction massage, along with early local corticosteroid injection, can be helpful. Recalcitrant cases may be amenable to surgical treatment.[11,42,45]

Stress Fractures

Stress fractures of the olecranon and stress related injury to the proximal posteromedial ulna have been reported. Players with olecranon stress fractures present with the insidious onset of vague posterior or posterolateral elbow pain that is exacerbated by throwing and relieved by rest. There is tenderness over the olecranon, which can be confused with triceps tendinitis. Players with proximal posteromedial stress injury will report posteromedial elbow pain during acceleration and follow-through phases of throwing. Pain is reproduced with the application of a valgus stress, forced hyperextension of the elbow, or percussion of the posteromedial olecranon.

X-rays are typically unremarkable. Views of the contralateral elbow are useful for comparison, particularly in the skeletally immature athlete. If the fracture is not readily apparent, MRI is helpful in making the diagnosis.

Fractures of the body of the olecranon tend to heal with conservative management over an 8- to 12-week period of time. The athlete should be kept from throwing. Return to full activity may require 3 to 6 months. Surgical intervention may be undertaken for fractures of the olecranon tip because these are prone to nonunion, and for fractures of the body that fail to heal with conservative treatment. Some athletes may undergo immediate surgical treatment if a more timely return to competition is desired.[14,84,90]

Little Leaguer's Elbow

Injury to the medial epicondylar physis can be attributed to repeated valgus stress or repetitive violent forearm flexor–pronator muscle contractions that occur with throwing. A history of an increased amount of recent throwing is often given. The athlete will typically complain of medial elbow pain with throwing, which, over time, results in decreased effectiveness, accuracy, velocity, and throwing distance. Examination reveals tenderness over the medial epicondyle and pain with valgus stress. Soft-tissue swelling, restricted range of motion, and a flexion contracture may be evident, depending on the chronicity of the symptoms. X-rays reveal a widened or fragmented epicondylar physis. Because findings may be subtle and difficult to appreciate, comparison views of the contralateral elbow can be helpful in detecting abnormal anatomy. The degree of displacement must be noted, because late laxity of the UCL can develop in the throwing athlete, and early surgical intervention may therefore be necessary. Nonoperative treatment is generally sufficient. A 2- to 3-month break from throwing is sometimes necessary. A pitcher may switch to a position in the field that requires less throwing to rest the elbow.

If a more vigorous valgus stress is absorbed, an avulsion fracture of the medial epicondyle can occur, which presents with sudden medial pain, exquisite tenderness over the medial epicondyle, and a flexion contracture. Treatment depends on the stability and displacement of the fracture. If the fragment is stable, then immobilization is sufficient treatment. Healing may occur as early as 6 to 8 weeks, but can take up to 10 to 12 weeks. If the fragment is unstable and mobile and the elbow itself is unstable, then early surgical treatment is necessary.[56,76]

Osteochondritis Dissecans

Osteochondritis dissecans of the capitellum occurs in young athletes between the ages of 13 and 16 and results from a combination of valgus extension overload and shear forces related to the repetitive motion of throwing. Throwers complain of a dull, achy pain over the lateral elbow that may be associated with a slight flexion contracture and occasional locking. Loss of extension and a joint effusion may be seen on exam. Standard radiographs of the elbow are generally sufficient in the initial evaluation and may demonstrate a focal island of subchondral bone demarcated by a rarefied zone. Loose bodies may or may not be seen. Imaging of the contralateral elbow is always helpful in the skeletally immature patient. MRI and CT scanning can be helpful when plain x-rays are negative or when further definition of the extent of the lesion is necessary.

Treatment is based on several factors, such as the size and location of the lesion, condition of the articular cartilage, whether the fragment is attached or loose, and the age of the patient. If the articular cartilage is intact, then activity modification and relative rest for 8 to 12 weeks is recommended. In the absence of symptoms, athletes may return to sporting activity after 3 to 6 months. If, however, the athlete presents with a very painful and swollen elbow with a history of mechanical symptoms such as catching and locking, this is highly suggestive of a partially or completely detached articular fragment that warrants surgical attention.[8,76,78]

OTHER INJURIES

Finger Pain

Circulatory disturbances in the fingers of the pitcher's throwing hand have also been reported and are thought to be caused by compression of the digital artery beneath

Cleland's ligament. Pitchers may complain of finger pain, and signs of digital ischemia, cyanosis, pallor, and ulceration may be evident. Surgical release of Cleland's ligament in the affected fingers is often successful in alleviating symptoms.[43,55,89]

Blunt Chest Trauma

Serious injury, ranging from transient apneic episodes to fatal arrhythmia, can be caused by the baseball's impact on the chest wall. Commotio cordis or nonstructural injury to the heart is precipitated by chest trauma that alters the heart's electrophysiological and hemodynamic status, which can lead to fatal ventricular arrhythmia. Myocardial contusion can lead to ischemic necrosis and hemorrhage. Arrhythmias can occur shortly after trauma, but have been found to develop as late as one week after injury. CPK, ECG, and echocardiography can be helpful in diagnosis. Exercise stress testing is recommended before return to play.[25,58,65]

Head and Neck

Numerous studies have found baseball to be the leading cause of youth sports-related head injuries. Direct ball impact, collision trauma, and sliding accidents are frequently responsible. Head injuries are especially common in the 5- to 14-year-old age group, accounting for 40% of all baseball injuries. Approximately half of baseball fatalities are the result of head and neck trauma. Between 40% and 70% of baseball-related youth eye injuries occur from being hit by a pitch while batting. Injuries to the teeth, jaw, facial bones, nose, orbit, and skull can occur. Ocular injuries such as lid lacerations, foreign bodies, hyphema, vitreous hemorrhage, retinal detachment, optic nerve damage, and blindness have all been reported. Collisions that occur when sliding headfirst can result in neck hyperflexion and quadriplegia. Concussions, skull fractures, epidural and subdural hematomas, and cervical spine injury must always be considered. A thorough head and neck examination is mandatory. Any loss of consciousness, sensory change, motor deficit, neck stiffness, or altered mental status other than a transient concussion with rapid recovery of all senses should be aggressively evaluated. A complete ophthalmologic and neurologic assessment is required and rigid immobilization of the cervical spine is necessary until a more formal assessment can be made.[57,68]

Lumbar Spine

Injury to the lower back and lumbar spine can adversely affect the player's ability to field, hit, and pitch the ball. Trunk stabilization is a key element in both throwing and hitting a baseball. Pain alters the biomechanics necessary to perform these activities properly, leading to poor functional performance and further injury. Pitchers may demonstrate poor mechanics with diminished accuracy and loss of velocity. Batters may demonstrate lack of power in the swing and poor timing. A recent survey of a college baseball team found that roughly 15% of reported injuries involved the lower back. Lumbar strains and spondylolysis were most common, and more than 50% of these players spent time on the injured reserve list. Back injuries are less common in the Little League population, and typically involve muscular strains or spondylolisthesis.

Diagnosis is made by careful physical exam. X-rays may be helpful and MRI may be necessary, particularly if there is a history of trauma or radicular symptoms.

The treatment of low back pain is conservative and focuses on general strengthening and conditioning of the trunk musculature. Maintaining proper mechanics in both pitching and hitting, with emphasis on strengthening of the trunk, erector spinae, and abdominal oblique muscle groups are important in preventing injuries to the lower back.[57,96]

ACTIVITY-SPECIFIC INJURIES

Hitting

Most batting injuries result from being hit by a pitch. Deep contusions and fractures at the site of impact are possible. Fouling a pitch off the lead foot and ankle can also result in injury. Most major league ball players wear protective gear to minimize this problem. Dislocation of the patella of the trailing leg during a full, uncontrolled swing has been reported. Treatment is conservative, with a period of immobilization and quadriceps strengthening. Some authors advocate early surgical reconstruction to minimize the likelihood of recurrence. Direct impact with the bat handle can cause a hook of hamate fracture. This is typically seen in the left hand of a right-handed batter or vice versa. Players will complain of a dull, aching pain over the palmar and ulnar aspect of the wrist that worsens with active or passive wrist extension. There is tenderness over the hamate and grip strength is diminished. A carpal tunnel or oblique view of the supinated wrist is likely to show the fracture. If not readily apparent, bone scan, MRI, or CT scan of the wrist can make the diagnosis. A 4- to 6-week period of immobilization is necessary. However, to avoid the chance of painful nonunion, some authors advocate early hook excision, which can return the player to competition in a more timely fashion.[38,88]

Sliding

Sliding is responsible for a large proportion of injuries in baseball and softball. It is estimated that up to 71% of reported softball injuries occur while sliding. Most injuries occur during the landing phase, in which significant forces are acting on the body during impact with the

TABLE 36-3 Comparison of Feet-First Versus Head-First Sliding Injuries

Phase	Feet First	Head First
Sprinting	Hamstring strains and ankle sprains	Hamstring strains and ankle sprains
Sliding position	Ankle sprains	Ankle sprains
Airborne position		
Landing	Lower extremity abrasions, contusions, fractures, ankle and knee sprains	Upper extremity abrasions, contusions, head, cervical spine, oro-maxillofacial injuries, upper extremity fractures, finger, wrist, elbow sprains

ground, base, or opposing player. Shear forces acting on the body while sliding along the ground can produce abrasions and contusions, and direct impact and rapid deceleration against a potentially stationary bag or opposing player can result in ankle, knee, or hand and wrist sprains or fractures. Hamstring strains are common and result from rapid acceleration from a standing position during the sprint phase of base running. Feet-first sliding tends to result in lower extremity injuries, and head-first sliding tends to produce head, neck, and upper extremity injuries (Table 36-3). Although it is difficult to determine whether feet-first sliding or head-first sliding results in a greater percentage of injuries, it is clear that head-first sliding injuries are potentially more severe. The use of base running helmets, face guards, mouthguards, adherence to proper sliding techniques, musculoskeletal conditioning, and recessed or breakaway bases can decrease the chance of injury to the base runner.[24,57]

POSITION-SPECIFIC INJURIES

Catcher

The position of catcher is physically demanding. The player is constantly receiving pitches, making throws, getting up and down from a squatting position, sprinting to get foul balls and passed balls, and avoiding collisions with the ball, bat, and base runner. Chronic repetitive catching impact can cause digital ischemia and finger pain in the gloved hand. Acute collisions with the ball, bat, or base runner can result in head injuries, fractures, and sprains. The direct impact of a foul ball off the tip of a finger could result in mallet finger. Loss of DIP joint extension is diagnostic. Constant squatting and pivoting required to play the position may lead to knee pain or meniscal tear in older athletes. The use of a well-padded mitt, protective gear, shielding of the noncatching hand, and proper instruction on catching technique can reduce the incidence of injuries to the catcher.

Fielding

Injuries to position players in the field can result from collision with other players or the ballpark fence, ball trauma from uncaught balls, and rapid acceleration or explosive bursts of muscle activity required to quickly retrieve the batted ball. Head and neck injuries, fractures, sprains, and hamstring strains are not unusual. In-season conditioning programs, stretching exercises, good communications between players to avoid collision, and warning tracks around the perimeter of the playing field to avoid wall collisions can be helpful in decreasing the incidence of injury to position players.

SUMMARY

The vast majority of injuries that occur while playing baseball are minor and do not result in a significant loss of playing time. Most injuries to the shoulder and elbow are the result of chronic repetitive microtrauma associated with throwing a baseball. Over time, this can lead to a variety of conditions that can cause pain and disability, affect performance, and keep the athlete from competition. A thorough understanding of functional anatomy of the shoulder and elbow and the biomechanics of throwing is essential to the recognition, diagnosis, and treatment of these injuries. Most injuries respond to conservative management, although surgical intervention is sometimes necessary. Learning proper pitching mechanics as early in the career as possible, building strength as the body matures, and strict adherence to pitch count and the avoidance of breaking pitches in young throwers can decrease the risk of repetitive stress injuries. The early recognition and treatment of the injured baseball player is necessary to prevent further injury from occurring and allow for a more timely return to competition.

REFERENCES

1. Altchek D, Dines D: Shoulder injuries in the throwing athlete. J Am Acad Orthop Surg 3:159–165,1995.
2. Andrews J, Fleisig G: Preventing throwing injuries. J Orthop Sports Phys Ther 27:187–188, 1998.
3. Arroyo J, Hershon S, Bigliani L: Special considerations in the athletic throwing shoulder. Orthop Clin North Am 28:69–78, 1997.

4. Azar F, Andrews J, Wlik K, et al: Operative treatment of ulnar collateral ligament injuries of the elbow in athletes. Am J Sports Med 28:16–23, 2000.
5. Barber F, Morgan C, Burkhart, Jobe C: Labrum/biceps/cuff dysfunction in the throwing athlete. Arthroscopy 15:852–857, 1999.
6. Barnes D, Tullus H: An analysis of 100 symptomatic baseball players. Am J Sports Med 6:63–67, 1978.
7. Barnett L: Little League shoulder syndrome: Proximal humeral epiphyseolysis in adolescent baseball pitchers. A case report. J Bone Joint Surg 67A:495–496, 1985.
8. Baumgarten T, Andrews J, Satterwhite Y: The arthroscopic classification and treatment of osteochondritis dissecans of the capitellum. Am J Sports Med 26:520–523, 1999.
9. Bey M, Elders G, Huston L, et al: The mechanism of creation of superior labrum, anterior, and posterior lesions in a dynamic biomechanical model of the shoulder: The role of inferior subluxation. J Shoulder Elbow Surg 7:397–401, 1998.
10. Bigliani L, Codd T, Connor P, et al: Shoulder motion and laxity in the professional baseball player. Am J Sports Med 25:609–613, 1997.
11. Boyer M, Hastings H III: Lateral tennis elbow: "Is there any science out there?" J Shoulder Elbow Surg 8:481–491, 1999.
12. Bradley J, Perry J, Jobe F: The biomechanics of the throwing shoulder. Perspec Orthop Surg 1:49–59, 1990.
13. Branch T, Partin C, Chamberlain P, et al: Spontaneous fractures of the humerus during pitching: A series of 12 cases. Am J Sports Med 20:468–470, 1992.
14. Brukner P: Stress fractures of the upper limb. Sports Med 26:415–424, 1998.
15. Bryan W, Wild J Jr: Isolated infraspinatus atrophy. A common cause of posterior shoulder pain and weakness in athletes? Am J Sports Med 17:130–131, 1989.
16. Burkhart S, Morgan C, Kibler W: Shoulder injuries in overhead athletes: The "dead-arm" revisited. Clin Sports Med 19:125–158, 2000.
17. Cahill B: Quadrilateral space syndrome. J Hand Surg 8A:65–69, 1983.
18. Callaway G, Field L, Deng X, et al: Biomechanical evaluation of the medial collateral ligament of the elbow. J Bone Joint Surg Am 79:1223–1231, 1997.
19. Carson W, Gasser S: Little Leaguer's shoulder. A report of 23 cases. Am J Sports Med 26:575–580, 1998.
20. Chen F, Rokito A, Jobe F: Medial elbow problems in the overhead-throwing athlete. J Acad Orthop Surg 9(2):99–113, 2001.
21. Cleeman E, Flatow E: Classification and diagnosis of impingement and rotator cuff lesions in athletes. Sports Med Arthrosc Rev 8:141–157, 2000.
22. Collins H, Lund D: Baseball injuries. In Schneider R, Kennedy J, Plant M (eds): Sports Injuries: Mechanisms, Prevention, and Treatment. Baltimore, Williams and Wilkins, 1986, pp 64–77.
23. Conway J, Jobe F, Glousman R, et al: Medial instability of the elbow in throwing athletes: Treatment by repair or reconstruction of the ulnar collateral ligament. J Bone Joint Surg Am 74:67–83, 1992.
24. Corzatt R: The biomechanics of head-first versus feet-first sliding. Am J Sports Med 12:229–232, 1984.
25. Curfman G: Fatal impact-concussion of the heart. N Engl J Med 338:1841–1843, 1998.
26. Davidson P, Pink M, Perry J, et al: Functional anatomy of the flexor pronator muscle group in relation to the medial collateral ligament of the elbow. Am J Sports Med 23:245–250, 1995.
27. Del Pizzo W, Jobe F, Norwood L: Ulnar nerve entrapment syndrome in baseball players. Am J Sports Med 5:182, 1977.
28. DiFelice G, Paletta G, Phillips B, et al: Effort thrombosis in the elite throwing athlete. Am J Sports Med 30:708–712, 2002.
29. DiGiovine N, Jobe F, Pink M, Perry J: An electromyographic analysis of the upper extremity in pitching. J Shoulder Elbow Surg 1:15–25, 1992.
30. Drez D Jr: Suprascapular neuropathy in the differential diagnosis of rotator cuff injuries. Am J Sports Med 4:43–45, 1976.
31. Ellenbecker T, Mattalino A, Elam E, et al: Medial elbow joint laxity in professional baseball pitchers: A bilateral comparison using stress radiography. Am J Sports Med 26:420–424, 1998.
32. Ferrari J, Ferrari D, Coumas J, et al: Posterior ossification of the shoulder: The Bennett lesion. Etiology, diagnosis, and treatment. Am J Sports Med 22:171–176, 1994.
33. Francel T, Dellon A, Campbell J: Quadrilateral space syndrome: Diagnosis and operative decompression technique. Plast Reconstr Surg 87:911–916, 1991.
34. Gabel G, Morrey B: Operative treatment of medial epicondylitis: Influence of concomitant ulnar neuropathy at the elbow. J Bone Joint Surg Am 77: 1065–1069, 1995.
35. Gartsman G, Hammerman S: Superior labrum, anterior and posterior lesions: When and how to treat them. Clin Sports Med 19:115–124, 2000.
36. Glousman R, Barron J, Jobe F, et al: An electromyographic analysis of the elbow in normal and injured pitchers with medial collateral ligament insufficiency. Am J Sports Med 20:311–317, 1992.
37. Glousman R: Ulnar nerve problems in the athlete's elbow. Clin Sports Med 9:365–377, 1990.
38. Gross R: Acute dislocation of the patella: The Mudville mystery. J Bone Joint Surg Am 68:780–781, 1986.

39. Gusmer P, Potter H, Schatz J, et al: Labral injuries: Accuracy of detection with unenhanced MR imaging of the shoulder. Radiology 200:519–524, 1996.
40. Halbrecht J, Tirman P, Atkin D: Internal impingement of the shoulder: Comparison of findings between the throwing and nonthrowing shoulders of college baseball players. Arthroscopy 15:253–258, 1999.
41. Hamilton C, Glousman R, Jobe F, et al: Dynamic stability of the elbow: Electromyographic analysis of the flexor pronator group and the extensor group in pitchers with valgus instability. J Shoulder Elbow Surg 5:347–354, 1996.
42. Hay E, Paterson S, Lewis M, et al: Pragmatic randomized controlled trial of local corticosteroid injection and naproxen for treatment of lateral epicondylitis of elbow in primary care. Br Med J 319:964–968, 1999.
43. Itoh Y: Circulatory disturbances in the throwing hand of baseball pitchers. Am J Sports Med 15: 264–269, 1987.
44. Janda D: Softball sliding injuries: A prospective study comparing standard and modified bases. JAMA 259:1848–1850, 1988.
45. Jobe F, Ciccotti M: Lateral and medial epicondylitis of the elbow. J Am Acad Orthop Surg 2:1–8, 1994.
46. Jobe F, Kvitne R: Elbow instability in the athlete. Instr Course Lect 40:17–23, 1991.
47. Jobe F, Moynes D, Tibone J, Perry J: An EMG analysis of the shoulder in pitching: A second report. Am J Sports Med 12:218–220, 1984.
48. Jobe F, Stark H, Lombardo S: Reconstruction of the ulnar collateral ligament in athletes. J Bone Joint Surg Am 68:1158–1163, 1986.
49. King J, Brelsford H, Tullos H: Analysis of the pitching arm of the professional baseball pitcher. Clin Orthop 67:116–123, 1969.
50. Kraus J, Conroy C: Mortality and morbidity from injuries in sports and recreation. Annu Rev Public Health 5:163–192, 1984.
51. Kuhn J, Plancher K, Hawkins R: Symptomatic scapulothoracic crepitus and bursitis. J Am Acad Orthop Surg 6:267–273, 1998.
52. Kurvers H, Verhaar J: The results of operative treatment of medial epicondylitis. J Bone Joint Surg Am 77:1374–1379, 1995.
53. Kvitne R, Jobe F, Jobe C: Shoulder instability in the overhand athlete. Clin Sports Med 14:917–935, 1995.
54. Linn R, Kreigshauer L: Ball thrower's fracture of the humerus. Am J Sports Med 19:194–197, 1991.
55. Lowrey C, Chadwick R, Waltman E: Digital vessel trauma from repetitive impact in baseball pitchers. J Hand Surg 1:236–238, 1976.
56. Lyman S, Flesig G, Andrews J, et al: Effect of pitch type, pitch count, and pitching mechanics on risk of elbow and shoulder pain in youth baseball pitchers. Am J Sports Med 30:463–468, 2002.
57. MacFarland E, Waswik M: Collegiate baseball injuries. Clin J Sports Med 8:10–13, 1998.
58. Maron B, Poliac L, Kaplan J, et al: Blunt impact to the chest leading to sudden death from cardiac arrest during sporting activities. N Engl J Med 333: 337–342, 1995.
59. Martin S, Warren R, Martin T, et al: Suprascapular neuropathy. Results of nonoperative treatment. J Bone Joint Surg Am 79A:1159–1165, 1997.
60. Meister K, Andrews J, Batts J, et al: Symptomatic thrower's exostosis. Arthroscopic evaluation and treatment. Am J Sports Med 27:133–136, 1999.
61. Meister K, Walczak S, Fontenot W, et al: Evaluation of partial undersurface tears of the rotator cuff in the overhand athlete: MRI arthrography versus arthroscopy. Arthroscopy 14:451–458, 1999.
62. Meister K: Current concepts: Injuries to the shoulder in the throwing athlete. Part two: Evaluation and treatment. Am J Sports Med 28:587–601, 2000.
63. Mileski R, Snyder S: Superior labral lesions in the shoulder: Pathoanatomy and surgical management. J Am Acad Orthop Surg 6:121–131, 1998.
64. Miller C, Savoie F III: Valgus extension injuries of the elbow in the throwing athlete. J Am Acad Orthop Surg 2:261–269, 1994.
65. Morikawa M: Myocardial contusion caused by baseball. Clin Cardiol 19:831–833, 1996.
66. Musgrave D, Rodosky M: SLAP lesions: Current concepts. Am J Orthop 30:29–38, 2001.
67. Neer C: Impingement lesions. Clin Orthop 173:70–77, 1983.
68. Nelson L, Wilson T, Jeffers J: Eye injuries in childhood: Demography, etiology, and prevention. Pediatrics 84:438–441, 1989.
69. Norwood L, Shook J, Andrews J: Acute medial elbow ruptures. Am J Sports Med 9:16–19, 1981.
70. Oberlander M, Chisar M, Campbell B: Epidemiology of shoulder injuries in throwing and overhead athletes. Sports Med Arthrosc Rev 8:115–123, 2000.
71. O'Donoghue D: Subluxing biceps tendon in the athlete. Am J Sports Med 1:20, 1973.
72. Ogawa K, Yolshida A: Throwing fracture of the humeral shaft: An analysis of 90 patients. Am J Sports Med 26:242–246, 1998.
73. Paley K, Jobe F, Pink M, et al: Arthroscopic findings in the overhand throwing athlete: Evidence for posterior internal impingement of the rotator cuff. Arthroscopy 16:35–40, 2000.
74. Pappas A, Zawacki R, McCarthy C: Rehabilitation of the pitching shoulder. Am J Sports Med 13:223–235, 1985.
75. Pappas A, Zawacki R, Sullivan T: Biomechanics of baseball pitching: A preliminary report. Am J Sports Med 13:216–222, 1985.

76. Pappas A: Elbow problems associated with baseball during childhood and adolescence. Clin Orthop 701:84–90, 1986.
77. Pasternack J, Veenema K, Callahan C: Baseball injuries: A Little League survey. Pediatrics 98: 445–448, 1996.
78. Peterson R, Savoie F III, Field L: Osteochondritis dissecans of the elbow. Instr Course Lect 48: 393–398, 1999.
79. Rayan G: Thoracic outlet syndrome. J Shoulder Elbow Surg 7:440–451, 1998.
80. Redler M, Ruland J, McCue F: Quadrilateral space syndrome in the throwing athlete. Am J Sports Med 14:511–513, 1986.
81. Ringel S, Treihaft M, Carry M, et al: Suprascapular neuropathy in pitchers. Am J Sports Med 18:80–86, 1990.
82. Rokito A, McMahon P, Jobe F: Cubital tunnel syndrome. Op Tech Sports Med 4:15–20, 1996.
83. Roye R, Grana W, Yates C: Arthroscopic subacromial decompression: Two to seven year follow-up. Arthroscopy 11:301–306, 1995.
84. Schickendantz M, Ho C, Koh J: Stress injury of the proximal ulna in professional baseball players. Am J Sports Med 30:737–741, 2002.
85. Sisto D, Jobe F, Moynes D, et al: An electromyographic analysis of the elbow in pitching. Am J Sports Med 15:260–263, 1987.
86. Sisto D, Jobe F: The operative treatment of scapulothoracic bursitis in professional pitchers. Am J Sports Med 14:192–194, 1986.
87. Stahl S, Kaufman T: The efficacy of an injection of steroids for medial epicondylitis: A prosepective study of sixty elbows. J Bone Joint Surg Am 79:1648–1652, 1997.
88. Stark H: Fracture of the hood of the hamate. J Bone Joint Surg Am 71:1202–1207, 1989.
89. Sugawara M: Digital ischemia in baseball players. Am J Sports Med 14:329–334, 1986.
90. Suzucki K, Minami A, Suennaga N, et al: Oblique stress fractures of the olecranon in baseball pitchers. J Shoulder Elbow Surg 6:491–494, 1997.
91. Tibone J, Elrod B, Jobe F, et al: Surgical management of tears of the rotator cuff in athletes. J Bone Joint Surg Am 68:887–891, 1986.
92. Tibone J, Jobe F, Kerlan R, et al: Shoulder impingement syndrome in athletes treated by an anterior acromioplasty. Clin Orthop 198:134–140, 1985.
93. Timmerman L, Schwartz M, Andrews J: Preoperative evaluation of the ulnar collateral ligament by magnetic resonance imaging and computed tomagraphy arthrography. Evaluation in 25 baseball pitchers with surgical confirmation. Am J Sports Med 22:26–32, 1994.
94. Vangsness C, Jobe F: Surgical treatment of medial epicondylitis: Results in 35 elbows. J Bone Joint Surg Br 73:409–411, 1991.
95. Walch G, Boileau P, Noel E, et al: Impingement of the deep surface of the supraspinatus tendon on the posterosuperior glenoid rim: An arthroscopic study. J Shoulder Elbow Surg 1:238–245, 1992.
96. Watkins R: Baseball. In Watkins R (ed): The Spine in Sports. St. Louis, Mosby, 1996, pp 436–455.
97. Wilk K, Arrigo C: Current concepts in the rehabilitation of the athletic shoulder. J Orthop Sports Phys Ther 18:365–378, 1993.
98. Wilk K, Meister K, Andrews J: Current concepts in the rehabilitation of the overhead throwing athlete. Am J Sports Med 30(1):136–151, 2001.
99. Wilson F, Andrews J, Blackburn T, et al: Valgus extension overload in the pitching elbow. Am J Sports Med 11:83–88, 1983.

37 Football Injuries

Andrew L. Rosen, Giles R. Scuderi, and Peter D. McCann

Football represents a very popular sport for much of the American public. Participation at all levels, from elementary school to professional leagues, remains very high today. Elements of high speed and forceful contact between players interact to produce a high level of injuries in the sport. The wide variety of possible mechanisms for injury creates an incredibly diverse catalog of injuries that are commonly sustained.

EPIDEMIOLOGY

Numerous studies have sought to define the overall incidence of injuries sustained in many levels of American football. DeLee and Farney studied high school athletes and found an incidence of 0.506 injuries per year. Severe injuries occurred at a rate of 0.031 injuries per year.[7] However, variations in the definitions of injuries and the methods of collecting injury event data make precise determination of rates difficult.

Comparisons between other sports are also difficult. A study by Radelet et al. has shown similar injury rates between baseball, soccer, and football in children age 7 to 13 (1.5 injuries per 100 athlete events).[15] Powell et al. examined head injuries in high school varsity athletes and found dramatically higher rates of mild traumatic brain injuries in football compared to other sports (3.66 head injuries per 100 player years for football, compared to 1.58–0.14 for other sports).[13]

The location of injuries has been studied extensively with more success. The knee and ankle have been shown to be the most commonly injured joints. Many other areas show significant levels of injury, but less commonly.[7]

PREVENTION

Turbeville et al. have examined risk factors for middle school players (age 10 to 15) and concluded that few physical characteristics of players are associated with injuries. Only increased playing experience correlated with injury risk. Conditioning, player position, height, and weight did not affect the risk of injury.[20]

Changes in helmet design and rule changes have led to decreased incidence of brain-related fatalities. In 1976 a rule was established that prohibited use of the head and face in the initial contact involved in tackling. Player education and enforcement of this rule has been credited with a dramatic decrease in head and cervical spine injuries.[10] A new national helmet standard was enacted in 1980 which has had a similar effect on the decline of brain injuries.[3]

Proper fitting and maintenance of equipment is crucial to injury prevention. Older equipment, damaged by successive seasons of abuse, will potentially fail to successfully protect a player from a significant force. Care should be taken on all teams to fit and inspect all equipment carefully for all players.

HEAD TRAUMA

Traumatic brain injuries (TBIs) are common and potentially serious injuries sustained in football play. These events can range from mild, transient changes in mental status to complete loss of consciousness and death. Overall, head injuries represent the most common cause of mortality for participation in football (61% of fatalities).[3] Most injuries are mild and are often labeled concussions. Several grading scales exist to attempt to quantify severity of neurologic changes.

The overall effect of even mild brain injuries is still unclear. Several studies have shown links between concussions and lowered neuropsychological testing, suggesting that even seemingly benign injuries may have long-term effects.[6] Postconcussive syndrome can manifest itself as memory loss, lethargy, headaches, and labile emotions which can severely affect the lives of affected athletes.[22]

The “second impact syndrome” concept has been proposed to explain sudden deaths sustained from relatively mild, repeated head injuries. Although the definitive pathophysiology of these events is still unclear, this concept has serious implication for the treatment and future sports play of injured players.[2]

Return to Game

One of the most difficult decisions in the treatment of football players involves deciding when a player can return to play following a traumatic brain injury. Although numerous guidelines exist for use, no definitive data exist to validate any technique as absolutely safe and reliable. Consideration of each player and injury individually is necessary to determine proper treatment. In general, players with mild concussions with no loss of consciousness can return to play if neurologic and cognitive status is normal after a brief period of sideline evaluation.[12]

Any loss of consciousness is an indication for removal from play and hospital evaluation. With the potential danger of the second impact syndrome, the team physician should generally be very cautious when allowing players back into the game. Players with repeated traumatic brain injuries should be evaluated by a neurologist for discussions regarding future play.

NECK AND SPINE TRAUMA

Changes in football tackling technique have markedly reduced the number of spinal cord injuries in the last two decades. However, uncontrolled contact still places the player at risk for both transient and permanent spinal damage. Axial loading of the neck appears to be the predominant mechanism of serious injury in most game play.

An entity called transient quadriparesis has been described. This injury consists of temporary motor and/or sensory neurological changes with complete recovery within minutes or two days. Because a very large proportion of permanently injured players have sustained previous transient symptoms, any player sustaining a cord neuropraxia should be evaluated by an MRI study. The presence of cord deformity, edema, or ligamentous instability represents contraindications to future play.[10,19]

"Spear tackler's spine" is a radiographic condition seen in players that have used axial-loading tackling techniques. Players with developmental narrowing of the cervical canal width and reversal of normal cervical lordotic curves are at high risk for complete neurologic damage and are prohibited from collision sports.[19]

UNCONSCIOUS PLAYERS

The management of a player found unconscious at the end of a play can be one of the most frightening scenerios in a team physician's duties. Planning a careful approach to an injured player is important for proper treatment. The most important principle is that a spinal cord injury should be assumed in the unconscious player until proven otherwise. This affects many aspects of the player's care. An assistant should be directed immediately to call EMS and request ambulance assistance. Directions to the game site should be prepared carefully before the start of the game to assist if there is need.

The first stage in treatment is to assess the standard emergency ABCs: airway, breathing, and circulation. The athlete should not be repositioned unless these are compromised. A logroll maneuver with axial traction and control of the head is essential if necessary to perform CPR. This should be accomplished with as many assistants as possible (preferably five to six).

The helmet and shoulder pads should be left in place on all unconscious players, if possible. Removal of either equipment can force the cervical spine into either hyperextension or hyperflexion when immobilized on a long spine board.[8] The face mask should be removed quickly if there is need to perform resuscitation. Face mask removal tools are sold for this purpose, or a sharp box-cutter can function as well. Assistants must hold the helmet in place while the face-mask attachment points are severed.[21] In the emergency room, under controlled conditions, the equipment can be carefully removed for proper imaging.

STINGERS

Traction injuries to the brachial plexus are commonly sustained in football play. One study has shown these injuries occur in 7.7% of players in college sports.[4] Although the injury mechanism is unclear in many cases, these injuries present with complaints of burning pain from the shoulder to the hand after contact is sustained. Most patients have only transient symptoms and are quick to recover.[23] Return to play can be allowed if all symptoms have cleared and full, painless range of motion of the shoulder is observed.

Some players have been shown to have multiple episodes in each season. These players with recurrent symptoms may benefit from modification of pads and technique adaptation. Players with smaller cervical spinal canal diameters may have increased risk of recurrent symptoms.[4]

AC JOINT DISLOCATIONS

Direct impacts of the shoulder into the ground are a common mechanism for acromiclavicular joint injuries in football players. Football pads often fail to protect against direct blows into the unyielding play surface. Treatment for these injuries in football players follows usual protocols, including nonoperative treatment for minimally displaced injuries and operative treatment for wide joint disruptions. Treatment of the "in-between" AC joint separations, so-called Type III injuries, remains controversial, with some advocates for both conservative and operative methods.

SHOULDER DISLOCATIONS AND INSTABILITY

Injuries to players with an arm in an abducted position can result in an acute shoulder dislocation. Most of these injuries are anterior in direction, although complex collisions can create posterior dislocations. Initial treatment consists of reduction of the shoulder and early protected range of motion and rehabilitation. Many of these younger athletes will go on to develop instability and recurrent dislocations. Surgical reconstruction is required to return these players to effective game play.

ELBOW INJURIES

No specific common injury patterns occur in injuries to the elbow in football. Sprains, dislocations, and medial collateral ligament injuries are uncommon but are seen with falls to an outstretched arm. Fractures are seen fairly uncommonly.[9] These injuries are typically treated with reduction, early mobilization, and reconstruction if instability develops.

HAND INJURIES

In contrast to the well-padded body, the distal extremities are relatively vulnerable to injury in the course of game play. The hand is an integral part of throwing, blocking, and tackling and is commonly injured in football play. Fractures of metacarpals and scaphoid bones are seen frequently, with operative treatment indicated for many displaced fractures. Occult scaphoid fractures can occur and should be suspected for tenderness in the anatomic snuffbox.

Ulnar collateral ligament injuries to the thumb are also common in football. "Skier's" or "gamekeeper's" thumb is an injury involving forced abduction of the thumb which tears the ulnar collateral ligament of the thumb. Complete injuries with instability demonstrated on exam or stress radiographs generally require operative repair.

Injury to the flexor digitorum profundis (FDP) has been termed "jersey finger." These digits are injured when a player grabs an opponent's jersey, avulsing the terminal portion of the flexor tendon. Presentation of an inability to flex the distal interphalangeal joint (DIP) generally requires operative repair.

HIP INJURIES

Most injuries to the hip in football are simple contusions, described as "hip pointers" when they occur over the iliac crest. Most of these injuries are managed with conservative modalities of ice, rest, and protective padding. Avulsion fractures can also occur in multiple areas of the ilium and are generally treated conservatively.

Dislocations and subluxations of the femoral head are quite rare but can occur in high-impact football injuries. Acute dislocations must be reduced emergently to avoid the complication of avascular necrosis.[17] Traumatic posterior subluxation is an injury that can be difficult to recognize. Characteristic MRI findings of posterior acetabular lip fractures and joint hemarthrosis can help establish the diagnosis. Treatment consists of protected weight bearing and restriction from play for at least six weeks. Even subluxation can pose some risk of subsequent avascular necrosis and must be observed carefully.[11]

THIGH INJURIES

Direct impacts to the quadriceps muscle can create significant contusions and hematoma within the large muscle. These injuries can be quite painful, resulting in a loss of weeks of playing and practice time. The potential for loss of motion and the development of myositis ossificans in the traumatized area is significant and can be influenced by proper treatment. This heterotopic ossification can develop in as many as 9% of patients. Treatment is based on early treatment emphasizing knee flexion. Wrapping of the leg in a hyperflexed position as early as possible can be effective in preventing loss of motion.[16] In contrast to most injuries, early aggressive physical therapy can be harmful to the player and should be avoided. Resting of the knee in flexion is more effective.

KNEE INJURIES

Several studies have shown the knee to be the most injured body part in American football.[7] Both contact injuries and twisting forces during running and cutting maneuvers place the knee at significant risk. The most commonly injured structure is the medial collateral ligament (MCL). Typically caused by direct trauma of tackling against the lateral aspect of the knee, these injuries, when isolated, typically recover well with bracing and physical therapy.

Twisting or deceleration mechanisms can injure the menisci or anterior cruciate ligaments (ACL). ACL disruptions are suspected in patients with large traumatic effusions and a history of an audible "pop" at the time of injury. These are generally confirmed with MRI evaluation. Although some patients with ACL tears can be treated conservatively, most of these injuries will require operative reconstruction for a player to return to football play.

Tears of the medial and lateral menisci are common in football and can occur alone or with injuries to the ACL or MCL. Symptoms of pain with knee flexion, locking, and catching are suggestive of these tears. A knee arthroscopy with either partial menisectomy or meniscal repair is generally required for treatment.

ANKLE INJURIES

Twisting injuries to the ankle occur commonly with the cutting and turning motions required for aggressive football play. Most of these injuries are simple ankle sprains. X-rays are necessary in most of these players to rule out fractures and severe ligament disruptions.[14] Described as "high" ankle sprains, injuries to the syndesmosis of the ankle can be severe, requiring lengthy rehabilitation and even surgical fixation in many cases. Careful examination of the syndesmotic width on x-ray is important to avoid neglecting these injuries.[1]

Simple ankle sprains can be either very benign or quite severe. Most are treated with rest, ice, and stirrup ankle braces. Return to play is dependent on improvement in pain and strength. Protective braces, taping, and shoes can all be helpful for players returning football play. Players with recurrent episodes of ankle sprains should be treated with physical therapy for strengthening and proprioception. Some players with instability and recurrent sprains will require surgical reconstruction if symptoms fail to respond to conservative means.

TURF TOE

Injury to the metatarsal phalangeal (MTP) joint of the great toe has been described with the use of flexible shoes on hard artificial playing surfaces and has been described as "turf toe." Forced hyperflexion of the toe can cause a tear of the plantar MTP joint capsule, which results in pain and swelling in the great toe.[18] Treatment generally consists of rest, ice, taping, and use of a firm shoe insert. These injuries can result in long-term, persistent symptoms in as many as 50% of significant injuries and should be treated carefully on initial presentation.[5]

REFERENCES

1. Boytim, MJ, Fischer DA, Neumann L: Syndesmotic ankle sprains. Am J Sports Med 19(3):294–298, 1991.
2. Cantu RC: Second-impact syndrome. Clin Sports Med 17(1):37–44, 1998.
3. Cantu RC, Mueller FO: Brain injury–related fatalities in American football, 1945–1999. Neurosurgery 52(4):846–852; discussion 852–853, 2003.
4. Castro FP Jr, et al: Stingers, the Torg ratio, and the cervical spine. Am J Sports Med 25(5):603–608, 1997.
5. Clanton TO, Ford JJ: Turf toe injury. Clin Sports Med 13(4):731–736, 1994.
6. Collins MW, et al: Relationship between concussion and neuropsychological performance in college football players. JAMA 282(10):964–970, 1999.
7. DeLee JC, Farney WC: Incidence of injury in Texas high school football. Am J Sports Med 20(5):575–580, 1992.
8. Gastel JA, et al: Emergency removal of football equipment: A cadaveric cervical spine injury model. Ann Emerg Med 32(4):411–417, 1998.
9. Kenter K, et al: Acute elbow injuries in the National Football League. J Shoulder Elbow Surg 9(1):1–5, 2000.
10. Kim DH, Vaccaro AR, and Berta SC: Acute sports-related spinal cord injury: contemporary management principles. Clin Sports Med 22(3):501–512, 2003.
11. Moorman CT, 3rd, et al: Traumatic posterior hip subluxation in American football. J Bone Joint Surg Am 85-A(7):1190-1196, 2003.
12. Nicholas JA, Hershman EB: The Lower Extremity and Spine in Sports Medicine, 2nd ed. St. Louis, Mosby, 1995, vol 2, pp xxvii, 1576, 1578.
13. Powell JW, Barber-Foss KD: Traumatic brain injury in high school athletes. JAMA 282(10):958–963, 1999.
14. Puffer JC: The sprained ankle. Clin Cornerstone 3(5):38–49, 2001.
15. Radelet MA, et al: Survey of the injury rate for children in community sports. Pediatrics 110(3):e28, 2002.
16. Ryan JB, et al: Quadriceps contusions: West Point update. Am J Sports Med 19(3):299–304, 1991.
17. Scopp JM, Moorman CT 3rd: Acute athletic trauma to the hip and pelvis. Orthop Clin North Am 33(3):555–563, 2002.
18. Tewes DP, et al: MRI findings of acute turf toe. A case report and review of anatomy. Clin Orthop 304:200–203, 1994.
19. Torg JS, Guille JT, Jaffe S: Injuries to the cervical spine in American football players. J Bone Joint Surg Am 84-A(1):112–122, 2002.
20. Turbeville SD, et al: Risk factors for injury in middle school football players. Am J Sports Med 31(2):276–281, 2003.
21. University of Georgia Sports Medicine Suspected Spinal Injury Protocol. 11/12/01.
22. Vastag B: Football brain injuries draw increased scrutiny. JAMA 287(4):437–439, 2002.
23. Weinberg J, Rokito S, Silber JS: Etiology, treatment, and prevention of athletic "stingers." Clin Sports Med 22(3):493–500, viii, 2003.

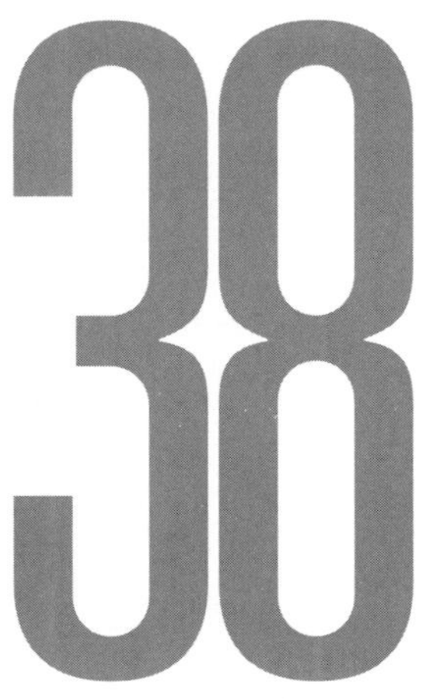

Running Injuries

Andrew L. Rosen, Giles R. Scuderi, and Peter D. McCann

Running has become one of the prominent exercise activities in the world. A basic pair of athletic shoes and a safe route are all that are needed to acquire aerobic conditioning, lower extremity strengthening, weight loss, and cardiovascular benefits. Improvements in the quality and availability of treadmills continue to expand running activities into the winter months. With an estimated 30 million runners in the United States alone, running represents a significant portion of all exercise activities.[32]

Although there are significant benefits to be derived from running, the act of running is associated with a reasonably high injury rate. Between 37% and 56% of all regular runners will sustain at least one injury annually. These injuries will affect exercise and sports activities, as well as regular activities of daily living. Although the rates of injury are comparatively less than many other sports, running injuries represent a significant number of physician visits.

MECHANISMS OF INJURY

The majority of running disorders affect the lower extremities and are a factor of tremendous repetitive forces placed on the body in the course of activity. Joint reactive force can approach six times body weight with each step.[9] With about 1000 foot-strikes estimated per mile, it is clear that running puts fairly extreme stresses on the lower extremities.[19] Although acute trauma can occur during running, most injuries sustained in recreational running are classified as overuse syndromes. Understanding of the conceptual reason for most of these injuries is crucial to successful diagnosis, treatment, and prevention.

A useful framework for analysis is the theory of an "envelope of function," described by Scott Dye.[8] His theory, which is easily applied to running injuries, is that the human body can withstand a certain level of repetitive stress before injury occurs. Activities below this "threshold" level will not disrupt the homeostasis between injury and repair. Repetitive loads above the threshold level result in homeostatic failure and injury. Genetic factors and good conditioning can act to raise this level for individuals, but illness, age, and injury will lower the threshold level. Use of this conceptual theory is valuable in considering the underlying causes of an injury to a specific patient.

STRESS FRACTURES

Running injuries that result from the chronic overload of bone that surpasses its own remodeling capacity result in stress fractures.[15] These lesions are more common in females and can be a part of a triad including eating disorders and irregular menses.[3] Although these injuries are still relatively uncommon, a high index of suspicion should always be present. Progression of an insufficiency fracture to a complete fracture carries higher morbidity and need for operative treatment. The initial evaluation of many running injuries is focused on ruling out these lesions to prevent the consequences of a missed stress fracture.

Plain film radiographs and computed tomography (CT) can show these lesions if they have progressed to substantial compromise of the bone, but they are often normal in many patients. Technetium bone scans are very sensitive for stress fractures, but they are less than 100% sensitive and they also can be positive in other conditions such as medial tibial stress syndrome (MTSS).[1] Magnetic resonance imaging (MRI) is currently the most effective method of diagnosing an early insufficiency fracture and allows precise definition of location and the extent of injury.[29]

Common locations for athletic stress fractures, studied by Matheson et al., include the tibia (49.1%), tarsals (25.3%), metatarsals (8.8%), femur (7.2%), fibula (6.6%), pelvis (1.6%), sesamoids (0.9%), and spine (0.6%).[20]

Treatment of these lesions is individualized to the specific bone involved, but generally requires a complete cessation of running, possible protection with non weight-bearing ambulation, and even prophylactic fixation for some lesions. Full evaluation of nutritional status is also important once the diagnosis of an insufficiency fracture is established.

RELATION TO OSTEOARTHRITIS

Although some animal experiments suggest that excessive running may lead to early arthritis,[30] no studies exist which prove that regular running activity in humans advances osteoarthritis in any joint. Several studies exist that show no correlation between a long lifetime history of regular running and the development of joint arthrosis.[16] Lane et al. showed no difference in the development of arthritis in active runners aged between 60 and 77 years and less disability and loss of functional capacity than in nonrunning individuals.[17] Fries et al. concluded that older patients engaging in running activities have no increased arthritis and decreased overall disability.[10] Although definitive evidence does not exist to define the exact risk of running activities, it is fairly clear that running activities are not regularly detrimental to individuals without existing arthritic changes.

PREVENTION OF INJURY

The same theory provides the framework for prevention of running injuries. The key to avoidance of running injury is careful increases in mileage that stay below the threshold level of homeostasis. Increased training mileage per week has emerged as an important clear risk factor for running-related injuries.[34] Such "errors" in training include excessively high increases in distance per run, total miles per week, and overall training intensity. Gradual increases in mileage and intensity are crucial for successful training.

The use of muscular stretching prior to running remains controversial. Many studies have shown little or no benefits to this activity,[12] yet for some areas, such as the Achilles tendon, it seems to be a useful method of injury prevention.[21,26] Overall, prerun stretching, if performed correctly, seems to have some potential benefits, few disadvantages, and is generally recommended.

THE RUNNING HISTORY

Treatment of a runner with a specific running-related injury must begin with a careful history of running activities. Although evaluation of the specific body part injured is primary to diagnosis and treatment, a general history of the runner's activities is also vital to successful diagnosis and treatment.

Assessment of weekly running mileage, mileage of long runs, and weekly increases is the primary focus of the running history. Examination of the runner's training history often gives information regarding the etiology and the severity of a particular injury. Mileage of greater than 20 miles per week has been shown in several studies to result in higher rates of injury.[11] However, it should be recognized that, although very uncommon, serious injuries can occur at relatively low levels of weekly distance.

History of previous injuries, amount and type of stretching, and assessment of other athletic activities can also provide useful information. Other factors for consideration include surface and terrain of running activities, type and age of running shoes, weight loss, and menstruation.[31] Table 38-1 summarizes a basic running history.

TABLE 38-1 Basic Components of the Running History

Important Elements	Variable Elements
Weekly running mileage	Cross-training
Mileage of long runs	Terrain, surface
Weekly increases in mileage	Stretching used
History of previous injuries	Running shoes: type, age
Weight loss	
Menstruation	

Treatment

Activity Modification. Although specific treatment varies depending on the type of injury, the basic principle of reducing activity levels remains paramount to overcoming overuse injuries. This concept of "rest" is often ignored by runners, who often try to "run through" an injury. It is important for the treating physician to educate patients to the concept of overuse injuries to overcome their unwillingness to reduce their activity.

Returning to Dye's threshold theory, injury causes a lowering of the homeostatic threshold. The amount of this decrease is directly dependent on the severity of the injury. Recovery from a running overuse injury requires decreasing activity to a weekly mileage level that is below the new threshold. For a severe injury, complete cessation of running activities may be necessary to stay within tissue homeostasis. It is necessary to convince patients that the old adage of "no pain, no gain" is no longer valid once an injury occurs. Recovery should focus on a gradual, relatively pain-free increase in activity while the patient's homeostatic threshold improves. Recurrence rates for running-related injury are very high and are often related to failure to allow adequate time for recovery.[32]

Cross-training can allow general maintenance of cardiovascular fitness and endurance, while preventing further overuse injury. Low-impact activities such as bicycling, swimming, and elliptical machines can be an effective substitutes while recovery commences.

Physical Therapy. Functional rehabilitation can be effective in enhancing the recovery from many overuse injuries. Traditional measures of rest, ice, compression, and elevation (RICE) are useful in the initial period of treatment. Other local modalities including ultrasound, electrical stimulation, deep tissue massage, iontophoresis, and extracorporeal shock wave treatments can be effective for many running injuries. A well-organized functional rehabilitation program can give structure to a patient's efforts at overcoming a running injury.

Footwear Modification. Subtle malalignments of the lower extremity can create abnormal stresses within the lower extremity during running activities and contribute to the development of overuse syndromes. A change in running shoes to a different type can sometimes be useful in addressing these problems. Although sometimes expensive to the runner, simply buying new running shoes can sometimes be effective in allowing recovery and prevention of future injury.

Custom-Fit Orthotics. These devices are commonly prescribed for treatment of runners with injuries related to limb malalignment. Control of excessive foot pronation is the most common use of orthotics for runners and can be useful in the treatment and prevention of several disorders. However, the efficacy of these devices has not been well-proven in clinical studies, and is still relatively controversial.[27] Furthermore, these devices can be relatively expensive and sometimes uncomfortable and should be generally reserved for secondary treatments of running injuries.

HIP AND GROIN PAIN

Stress Fractures of the Hip

Although less common than other sites of stress fractures, insufficiency fracture of the femoral neck represents one of the few running injuries with a high potential for permanent and severe disability. These rare injuries typically present with an insidious onset of groin pain that manifests during running and decreases following cessation of activity. As it progresses, the pain often prevents running and causes a noticeable limp. Early diagnosis with plain radiographs and a MRI evaluation is critical to prevention of serious complications. Completion of a femoral neck stress fracture carries with it a 50% rate of complications, including osteonecrosis, refracture, and malunion.[14]

Anatomically, these fractures can begin on both the superior (tension-side) and inferior (compression-side) of the hip.[7] Tension-sided lesions and compression-sided lesions occupying greater than 50% of the femoral neck carry a much higher potential for progression to complete fracture. For these fractures, prophylactic percutaneous internal fixation is indicated to prevent displacement.

Treatment for compression-sided fractures includes non-weight-bearing protection until no pain is felt with range of motion and partial weight bearing (generally several weeks). Complete cessation of all running is required for all patients with a femoral neck fracture for a period of about 4 to 6 months. A second MRI is often helpful to make the diagnosis.

Iliac Apophysitis

Seen in adolescent middle- and long-distance runners, increased shear at the attachment sites of the external oblique and abdominal oblique muscles can cause pain. It is more commonly seen in cross-country runners who run on irregular surfaces. Most cases will resolve with 4 to 6 weeks of complete cessation of running.[6]

Osteitis Pubis

A stress phenomenon involving the pubic symphysis, osteitis pubis causes activity-related pain located in the midline of the pelvis, directly over the pubic symphysis. Although the origin of the disorder is unclear, tension in the adductor and rectus abdominus muscles appears to be involved. Diagnosis is made by plain film radiographs demonstrating sclerosis of the symphysis or by positive uptake on bone scan. Rest, moist heat, and nonsteroidal anti-inflammatory agents (NSAIDs) represent the focus of treatment. Most symptoms resolve within three months with conservative measures but can occasionally persist for up to a year.

KNEE PAIN

Patellofemoral Pain

Anterior knee pain represents the most common type of running injury, ranging from 15% to 28% of all injuries.[32] The term "runner's knee" has been used in the past to describe this disorder. Full evaluation and treatment of this disorder has been discussed at length in previous chapters. Treatment of this disorder in a running individual should focus on the usual modalities of quadriceps strengthening but should also include a focus evaluation of limb alignment. Patients with excessive pronation may be improved by the use of a custom shoe orthotic.

Iliotibial Band Syndrome

Iliotibial band friction syndrome (ITBS) is another common overuse injury seen in the running population. It is characterized by pain on the lateral aspect of the knee, but the pain is often somewhat poorly localized. It is typically more severe when running downhill.[24] On physical exam, there may be tenderness over the lateral femoral condylar region, with swelling present in some patients. Malalignment factors including genu varum, heel varus, and compensatory pronation have been implicated in ITBS. Hip abductor weakness may also play a role in tightening the ITB. Increased friction between the ITB and the lateral femoral condyle results in a synovitis which causes pain. Diagnosis is aided by Ober's test of ITB tightness, which is performed by placing the patient on their side with the affected limb up.

Treatment is directed toward activity modification, ITB stretching, and local modalities including corticosteroid injections, ultrasound, cryotherapy, and iontophoresis. Surgical release of the posterior portion of the ITB is rarely indicated for failure of conservative modalities.[13]

Meniscal Tears

Although tears of the meniscal cartilage are relatively rare in the younger running population, middle-aged and older runners may suffer from a chronic degenerative meniscal tear. As running becomes more popular with older generations, these injuries may become more common in the running population. These tears may not be directly related to the running activity or training errors, but may be made symptomatic by running activities. Diagnosis of meniscal tears can be suggested by the presence of effusions and joint line tenderness. MRI is used to confirm the diagnosis.

LOWER LEG PAIN

Stress Fractures of the Tibia

These lesions present with activity-related pain that increases with mileage. Tibial stress fractures are commonly located in the proximal one-third of the tibial shaft, but they can occur in any portion of the bone. Unlike femoral neck lesions, stress fractures of the tibial shaft carry minimal risk of complete fracture. Most fractures in runners occur along the posterior or compression side of the tibia. The more troublesome anterior (tension) stress fractures are more commonly seen in jumping sports such as basketball.

Plain film radiographs are typically normal in runners' tibial stress fractures. The "dreaded black line" seen with anterior (tension) fractures is typically absent in most runners. MRI is best suited for diagnosis of these fractures and can differentiate them from other conditions affecting the lower leg. Bone scan is less effective, as increased uptake along the tibia is common with other benign conditions such as MTSS.

Treatment for these fractures consists primarily of discontinuation of running until all pain with weight bearing has subsided. Between 3 and 6 weeks is generally required for most patients, but some will require longer for more severe lesions.[4] Use of a pneumatic tibial brace may also assist in decreasing the time for recovery.

Medial Tibial Stress Syndrome (MTSS)

A relatively common disorder affecting runners, often nicknamed "shin splints," MTSS represents pain located along the anteromedial border of the distal third of the tibia. This pain typically begins during a run, but does not increase dramatically as the exercise continues. Although the etiology of this disorder is still unclear, the periosteal origin of the soleus along the anteromedial tibia appears to be the anatomic site of injury.[22] Excessive pronation of the foot also has been implicated as causative factor.

Physical exam exhibits a characteristic tenderness directly along the anteromedial border of the distal third of the tibia. Radiographs of the tibia often reveal thickening of the anteromedial tibial cortex in long-standing cases. Bone scan may show increased uptake in the distal tibia which can sometimes be difficult to distinguish from stress fractures. MRI is often necessary to differentiate MTSS from tibial stress fractures. Increased signal along the tibial periosteum, in the absence of bony cortical signal changes, is characteristic for MTSS.

Treatment begins, as in most running disorders, with simple decreases in mileage and cross-training. Complete cessation of running may be necessary for a few weeks in difficult cases. Local modalities such as ultrasound, iontophoresis, and cryotherapy may be helpful in recovery. Stretching of the gastroc-soleus complex has also been described as a treatment addition. Very rarely, failure of conservative treatment may require a surgical release of the anteromedial fascia. Although this disorder typically possesses little risk of permanent disability, it can be quite difficult for runners in a structured training program.

Chronic Compartment Syndrome

Another cause of lower leg pain in the active runner occurs as a result of increased pressure that develops within the muscular compartments of the lower leg. This disorder presents with complaints of a general feeling of leg tightness and pain that begins typically at a predictable running mileage. Some weakness and mild paresthesias also are not uncommon. The anterior and anterolateral compartments are most commonly involved.

Diagnosis is confirmed with compartment pressures measured with a slit-catheter inserted in the anterior and anterolateral compartments. Pedowitz developed a criteria that is generally followed for the diagnosis. Pressure measurements that are considered positive are as follows: more than 15 mm Hg before exercise, more than 30 mm Hg at 1 minute after exercise, and more than 20 mm Hg at 5 minutes after exercise.[25] MRI has also been described as a diagnostic tool that avoids painful needle insertions; however, its accuracy is unproven.[33]

In contrast to most other running injuries, conservative treatment of runners with chronic compartment syndrome is typically unsuccessful. Attempts to return to previous levels of mileage and performance commonly result in increased pain and disability.[23] For most patients who desire a return to running, surgical release of the anterior compartment is indicated. Results of fasciotomy for exertional compartment syndrome are good, but some patients are unable to fully return to preinjury exercise levels with complete pain relief.[28] A recently described endoscopic method may provide less morbidity for this procedure, but this technique has not been fully studied.[18]

FOOT AND ANKLE PAIN

Stress Fractures

Stress fractures involving the metatarsals typically have an insidious onset of pain. Forefoot discomfort increases as run progresses, often with improvement upon ending a run. Training errors, poorly cushioned shoes, and hard surface running have all been implicated as possible causative factors.

Plain film radiographs are typically normal for the first 3 to 4 weeks of the patient's symptoms. A radiolucent line and callus formation can be evident if the fracture progresses. Bone scan or MRI is useful in evaluating early symptoms in an active runner and can differentiate these from benign metatarsalgia.

Reduction of activity is the focus of treatment for these fractures. Limitation of weight bearing or cast immobilization is seldom necessary unless a lesion persists despite complete cessation of running.[2]

Plantar Fasciitis

A common disorder in runners, heel pain can range from a mere annoyance to a disabiling condition. Plantar fasciitis arises with chronic inflammation of the plantar fascia as it arises from the medial tubercle of the calcaneus. Patients have a history of severe pain with the first step out of bed in the morning. Pain typically improves with walking, but becomes worse with running. Hill climbing and sprinting can exacerbate the symptoms considerably. Physical exam is fairly benign, with patients exhibiting tenderness along the plantar fascia, especially at the proximal origin. Dorsiflexion of the ankle is usually decreased and forced dorsiflexion typically elicits increased discomfort. Radiographic studies are typically normal.

Initial treatment of plantar fasciitis consists of activity modification, anti-inflammatory medications, and aggressive stretching program. If symptoms persist, dorsiflexion night splints may be useful, and referral to a physical therapist for local modalities may be necessary. Use of extracorporeal shock wave (ECSW) therapy may be another method of successful treatment but its efficacy is still contested in the medical literature.[5,35] Although it occurs rarely, recurrent or recalcitrant pain may require a partial plantar fascia release if symptoms warrant.

Entrapment of the lateral plantar nerve by the abductor hallucis is another cause of heel pain and should be considered in the differential diagnosis for patients who do not present with the classic pattern of plantar fasciitis. Plantar nerve entrapment typically produces pain that is of a burning quality with increased radiation of the pain both proximally and distally. Surgical decompression is indicated for symptoms that do not respond to conservative treatment.

Ankle Sprain

Sprains of the lateral ligamentous complex of the ankle are one of the few traumatic, nonoveruse injuries seen commonly in runners. Irregular terrain such as in cross-country or trail running is often implicated in these injuries. Typical ankle sprains represent disruptions of the lateral talofibular ligament and can range from very mild to quite severe injuries. More severe sprains can also disrupt the interosseous membrane, resulting in the "high ankle sprain" pattern that can result in weeks of disability.

Rest, ice, and stirrup ankle brace immobilization are all useful in the initial period of recovery. Involvement in a physical therapy program consisting of peroneal strengthening exercises and proprioceptive development can be useful in prevention of recurrent sprains.

Achilles Tendonitis

Representing a spectrum of pathologic changes, disorders of the achilles tendon are quite common and affect many active runners. Injury begins with simple inflammatory changes of the peritendinous structures and progresses to tendinosis. Pain is located on the posterior aspect of the lower leg and is commonly worse at the beginning of a run and in the mornings. Uphill running also tends to produce more severe symptoms. Active stretching programs have been shown to be protective against these injuries.

These injuries can be located in the proximal (noninsertional) area of the Achilles tendon, or in the distal (insertional) region. Noninsertional tendonitis is much more common with typical running injuries and is generally easier to treat. Conservative treatment is typically effective in these patients and consists of rest, ice, anti-inflammatory agents, and progressive stretching. Use of a heel lift for both running and daily wear can also aid in decreasing tendon strain. If conservative measures fail after several months, surgical debridement and repair of the Achilles tendon may be indicated.

Posterior Tibial Tendonitis

Inflammation of the posterior tibialis tendon produces pain localized to the medial aspect of the ankle, typically slightly posterior and distal to the medial malleolus. A spectrum of pathology exists, beginning with simple inflammation and progressing to degenerative changes and tears. Typical conservative measures of rest and anti-inflammatory agents are effective for mild disorders. For patients that do not respond to basic treatments, immobilization of 4 to 6 weeks in a cast or cam walker brace can be necessary. Severe cases may require tenosynovectomy, debridement, and tendon repair to alleviate symptoms.

Peroneal Tendonitis

Pain on the lateral side of the ankle may represent disorders of the peroneal tendons. Symptoms occur over the posterior aspect of the distal fibula, with some radiation proximally. Forced supination of the foot will elicit pain on physical exam. Tendon subluxation may also be a component of pain and can be evaluated on physical exam with palpation of the tendons during active eversion against resistance.

Most of these disorders are mild and respond to rest and local modalities. More severe or recurrent injuries may require exploration of the tendons, tendon repair, or debridement. Recurrent symptomatic subluxation may require reconstruction of the lateral retinaculum.

CONCLUSIONS

Although injuries are common in active runners, most are simple overuse injuries that respond to the basic principle of rest. Unfortunately, most runners are resistant to decreasing activity and some participants in marathon training programs may be highly opposed to such suggestions. The duty of the treating physician is to explain the rationale behind these treatment principles so that the patient can make informed choices regarding activities.

For many injuries, it is important to exclude the possibility of a stress fracture before starting conservative management. For some areas, such as the hip, an MRI should be obtained early to prevent possible catastrophic fracture. The orthopedic disorders that affect most runners are benign, but it is important not to delay treatment in the few dangerous problems.

REFERENCES

1. Bal BS, Sandow T: Bilateral femoral neck fractures with negative bone scans. Orthopaedics 19:974–976, 1996.
2. Baxter D, Zingas C: The foot in running. J Am Acad Orthop Surg 3:136–145, 1995.
3. Bennell KL, Malcolm SA, Thomas SA, et al: Risk factors for stress fractures in female track-and-field athletes: A retrospective analysis. Clin J Sport Med 5:229–235, 1995.
4. Boden B, Oshahr D: High-risk stress fractures: Evaluation and treatment. J Am Acad Orthop Surg 8:344–353, 2000.
5. Buchbinder R, Ptasznik R, Gordon J: Ultrasound-guided extracorporeal shock wave therapy for plantar fasciitis: a randomized controlled trial. JAMA 288(11):1364–1372, 2002.
6. Clancy WG Jr, Foltz AS: Iliac apophysitis and stress fractures in adolescent runners. Am J Sports Med 4:214–218, 1976.
7. Devas MB: Stress fractures of the femoral neck. J Bone Joint Surg 47B:728–738, 1965.
8. Dye SF: The knee as a biologic transmission with an envelope of function: A theory. Clin Orthop 325:10–18, 1996.
9. Flynn TW, Soutas-Little RW: Patellofemoral joint compressive forces in forward and backward running. J Orthop Sports Phys Ther 21(5):277–282, 1995.
10. Fries JF, et al: Running and the development of disability with age. Ann Intern Med 121(7):502–509, 1994.
11. Hootman JM, Macera CA, Ainsworth BE, et al: Predictors of lower extremity injury among recreationally active adults. Clin J Sport Med 12(2): 99–106, 2002.
12. Jacobs SJ, Berson BL: Injuries to runners: A study of entrants to a 10,000 meter race. Am J Sports Med 14:151–155, 1986.
13. James S: Running injuries to the knee. J Am Acad Orthop Surg 3:309–318, 1995.
14. Johansson C, Ekenman I, Tornkvist H, Eriksson E: Stress fractures of the femoral neck in athletes. The consequence of a delay in diagnosis. Am J Sports Med 18:524–528, 1990.
15. Knapp TP, Garrett WE Jr: Stress fractures, general concepts. Clin Sports Med 15:339–356, 1997.
16. Konradsen L, Hansen EM, Sondergaard: Long distance running and osteoarthrosis. Am J Sports Med 18:379–381, 1990.
17. Lane NE, Oehlert JW, Bloch DA, Fries JF: The relationship of running to osteoarthritis of the knee and hip and bone mineral density of the lumbar spine: A 9 year longitudinal study. J Rheumatol 25(2):334–412, 1998.
18. Leversedge FJ, et al: Endoscopically assisted fasciotomy: Description of technique and in vitro assessment of lower-leg compartment decompression. Am J Sports Med 30:272–278, 2002.
19. Mann RA, Baxter DE, Lutter LD: Running symposium. Foot Ankle 1:190–224, 1981.
20. Matheson GO, Clement DB, McKenzie WD, et al: Stress fractures in athletes. A study of 320 cases. Am J Sports Med 15: 46–58, 1987.
21. McCrory JL, Martin DF, Lowery RB, et al: Etiologic factors associated with Achilles tendinitis in runners. Med Sci Sports Exerc 31(10):1374–1381, 1999.
22. Michael RH, Holder LE: The soleus syndrome. A cause of medial tibial stress (shin splints). Am J Sports Med 13(2):87–94, 1985.
23. Moeyersoons JP, Martens M: Chronic compartment syndrome: Diagnosis and management. Acta Orthop Belg 58(1):23–27, 1992.
24. Noble CA: Iliotibial band friction syndrome in runners. Am J Sports Med 8:232–234, 1980.

25. Pedowitz RA, Hargens AR, Mubarak SJ, et al: Modified criteria for the objective diagnosis of chronic compartment syndrome of the leg. Am J Sports Med 18:35–40, 1990.
26. Porter D, Barrill E, Oneacre K, May BD: The effects of duration and frequency of Achilles tendon stretching on dorsiflexion and outcome in painful heel syndrome: A randomized, blinded, control study. Foot Ankle Int 23(7):619–624, 2002.
27. Razeghi M, Batt ME: Biomechanical analysis of the effect of orthotic shoe inserts: A review of the literature. Sports Med 29(6):425–438, 2000.
28. Slimmon D, Bennell K, Brukner P: long-term outcome of fasciotomy with partial fasciectomy for chronic exertional compartment syndrome of the lower leg. Am J Sports Med 30(4):581–588, 2002.
29. Spitz DJ, Newberg AH: Imaging of stress fractures in the athlete. Radiol Clin North Am 40(2):313–331, 2002.
30. Takasu N: [Experimental study on the effect of forced running on occurrence of osteoarthritis in the knee of C 57 BL mice]. Nippon Seikeigeka Gakkai Zasshi 66(11):1165–1175, 1992.
31. Taunton JE, Ryan MB, Clement DB, et al: A retrospective case-control analysis of 2002 running injuries. Br J Sports Med 36:95–101, 2002.
32. Van Mechelen W: Running injuries: A review of the epidemiological literature. Sports Med 14: 320, 1992.
33. Verleisdonk EJ, van Gils A, van der Werken C: The diagnostic value of MRI scans for the diagnosis of chronic exertional compartment syndrome of the lower leg. Skeletal Radiol 30(6):321–325, 2001.
34. Walter SD, Hart LE, McIntosh JM, Sutton JR: The Ontario cohort study of running-related injuries. Arch Intern Med 149(11):2561–2564, 1989.
35. Weil LS Jr, Roukis TS, Weil LS, Borrelli AH: Extracorporeal shock wave therapy for the treatment of chronic plantar fasciitis: Indications, protocol, intermediate results, and a comparison of results to fasciotomy. J Foot Ankle Surg 41(3):166–172, 2002.

39 Soccer Injuries

Steven Arsht, Giles R. Scuderi, and Peter D. McCann

Soccer is the most popular sport in the world and is the fastest growing team sport in the United States. Because soccer is a contact sport, players are at risk for a number of types of injuries. The average incidence of injury is 10 to 15 per 1000 playing hours. The incidence and severity of injury appears to increase with advancing age, level of play, and frequency of competition. Injuries in young players, however, especially those under the age of 12, are uncommon, and typically do not result in significant lost playing time. Most injuries are caused by direct trauma related to physical contact between players, and up to a third are associated with foul play. Overuse injuries account for 9% to 34% of injuries. Injuries in soccer players most commonly involve the lower extremity, and predominantly affect the ankle and knee, and the muscles of the thigh and calf. Players are more likely to sustain an injury during a game rather than in practice. Center forwards and midfielders have the highest injury rates and goalkeepers are the most likely to sustain upper extremity injuries. Contusions, ligament sprains, and muscle strains account for about 75% of all injuries. Serious, permanently disabling injuries are rare and account for less than 0.1% of injuries at all levels. Female soccer players seem to be more likely than males to be injured in the younger age groups. This difference disappears after puberty, with the exception that knee injuries are about twice as common in women players than in men of the same age and playing level. At all levels of competition, the number and severity of knee injuries, including career-threatening ACL rupture, is greater in female athletes. Knee injuries usually result in the most time lost from participation and are the most common cause for surgery in the soccer player. A thorough understanding of the types of injuries sustained by the soccer player is necessary so that the medical staff can provide a rapid and accurate diagnosis and administer the most appropriate treatment so that a more timely return to competition can be achieved.[3,6,10,14–16,20,26,28,30,31,35–37,41,43,50,52,56,59,68,71,73]

HEAD AND NECK

A unique aspect of soccer is the purposeful use of the head for advancing and controlling the ball. Because heading the ball is an integral part of soccer, injuries may occur when competing for the airborne ball. Injuries to the head, face, and neck account for between 4% and 22% of all soccer injuries. Most of these injuries are abrasions, minor lacerations, and contusions. More serious injuries such as skull fractures, concussions, epidural hematoma, and cervical spine trauma have been reported. With increasing exposure to the game, the risk and incidence of head injury increases. Accidental blows to the head may occur during the course of competition. Concussions account for roughly 2% to 3% of all soccer injuries, but are probably more common than previously reported. These injuries typically result from a collision with other players, the ground, or the goalpost, and not from intentional heading of the ball. Dental injuries are uncommon, and their occurrence can be diminished by the use of protective mouthguards. Eye injuries such as hyphema, retinal edema, vitreous and retinal hemorrhage, corneal abrasion, traumatic iritis, and retinal tears have all been reported. Prompt ophthalmologic consultation should be strongly considered in players with persistent pain, diplopia, or decreased vision. A comprehensive physical examination of the head and neck is mandatory. If cervical spine injury is suspected, immediate immobilization is required. Depending on the severity of the injury and level of comfort of the treating physician, additional medical expertise can be received through consultation with an ophthalmologist, neurosurgeon, dentist, oral surgeon, otolaryngologist, or plastic surgeon.

Significant neurotrauma is rare but should be aggressively evaluated if suspected. If a player has experienced a loss of consciousness, immediate transport to the hospital for a comprehensive neurologic examination, including advanced imaging studies such as a CT scan or MRI, is recommended. Concerns have been raised about the cumulative effects of heading and its relation to brain injury in soccer players. Although some authors attributed neuropsychologic deficits in soccer players to the cumulative effects of heading the ball, other investigators have failed to show any correlation between career heading exposure and the development of a chronic encephalopathy. It is likely that long-term encephalopathic changes result from a combination of acute and chronic injuries, rather than heading the soccer ball.[7,8,12,22,25,33,45,46,68,69,70,73]

BACK, TRUNK, AND PELVIS

Injuries to the back, trunk, and pelvis are uncommon in soccer and account for less than 10% of all injuries resulting in lost playing time. Complaints of lower back pain are often the result of muscle strains or ligament sprains and typically respond well to conservative treatment. Spondylolysis may be seen in goalkeepers because of the repetitive lumbar hyperextension required in diving saves. Degenerative disc disease and disc herniation are rare. Persistent or recurrent back pain or radicular symptoms should alert the physician that additional diagnostic evaluation is necessary. X-rays, along with advanced imaging studies such as MRI and SPECT scan, are useful.[20,68,73]

CHRONIC GROIN PAIN

Soccer places repetitive stresses on the hip, inner thigh, and lower abdominal musculature, making both acute and chronic injuries in these areas quite common. Recurrent adductor, abdominal, and iliopsoas strains, tendinitis, osteitis pubis, and osteoarthritis are all frequent sources of groin pain in the athlete. Inguinal and femoral hernias and genitourinary and visceral pathology should also be considered in the clinician's differential diagnosis. Consultation with a general surgeon is often helpful when evaluating an athlete with groin pain.

Athletic pubalgia refers to a chronic inguinal or pubica area pain in athletes, which is noted on exertion. The pain appears to be related to weakness in the pelvic floor musculature between the inguinal canal and rectus abdominus insertion. The condition may begin insidiously, however, many athletes describe a hyperextension injury in association with hyperabduction of the thigh, followed by groin pain that is progressive, exacerbated by exertion such as running, and lasting several hours or days afterward. The pain is primarily felt in the inguinal region but can radiate posteriorly to the ischium or superiorly to the lower abdomen. The symptoms are clearly aggravated by activity and relieved by rest. Sit-ups can be painful. In the majority of athletes, the pain causes them to stop competing in sports. On physical exam, pain can be reproduced with active hip flexion, adduction, and internal rotation against resistance. A small percentage of patients will have point tenderness in the inguinal region near the anterior pelvic tubercle or along the adductor tendons near the pubis. The acute management of groin pain is conservative and includes rest, ice, compression, NSAIDs, and massage. If the pain continues for several months and prevents the athlete from competing, then surgical treatment may be considered.[14,20,28,30,49,68,71]

UPPER EXTREMITY INJURIES

Upper extremity injuries account for 5% to 15% of all soccer injuries, and rarely result in lost playing time. These injuries are more common in goalkeepers and typically occur as a result of contact with the ball. Injuries to the hand are usually caused by player collision, ground contact, foul play in field players, and by direct or indirect trauma in goalkeepers. Indirect noncontact injuries occur when a player falls on the outstretched hand or onto the point of the shoulder. Finger fractures, dislocations, and mallet fingers can occur from ball impacts on the ends of fingers. Forearm fractures, wrist fractures, or sprains may also occur as the goalkeeper attempts to stop oncoming shots. Fractures of the scaphoid or injury to the scapholunate ligament can occur when forced dorsiflexion of the hand and wrist is encountered when the player falls on the outstretched hand or when the goalkeeper attempts to block a shot. If a bony or ligamentous injury is suspected, radiographic and magnetic resonance imaging evaluation is necessary. Acromioclavicular joint separations should be suspected in field players with shoulder pain who give a history of falling onto the point of the shoulder.[11,14,20,43,50,68]

LOWER EXTREMITY INJURIES

Injuries in soccer players most commonly involve the lower extremity, and predominantly affect the ankle and knee and the muscles of the thigh and calf. Overuse injuries such as stress fractures and tendinitis of the leg, ankle, and foot are frequently encountered. The occurrence of foul play puts players at increased risk of serious injury and is directly responsible for approximately 22% to 33% of all soccer injuries.[3,6,10,16,20,28,30,41,56,68,71]

Contusions

Contusions to the thigh and calf are common but rarely result in lost playing time. Contusions of the thigh represent one of the most common contact injuries in soccer, especially in young players. Partial ruptures of the quadriceps muscle can occur as a result of impact against the contracted muscle, such as can occur when one player's knee hits an opposing player's thigh. Another cause of quadriceps muscle strains or partial rupture is noncontact overload, such as occurs during sudden explosive contractions in a fast start or sprint. Deep muscle contusions can be disabling and lead to complications such as acute compartment syndrome or myositis ossificans. Myositis ossificans can develop after a deep muscle contusion, particularly in the anterior thigh. Examination reveals a tender, erythematous, firm mass. X-rays demonstrate a fluffy opacity with increased peripheral density. Treatment of deep thigh contusion is conservative, with rest, ice, and anti-inflammatory medication. Massage should be avoided. Passive range of motion and whirlpool therapy can help maintain mobility and should be initiated as early as possible. The use of shin guards reduces the frequency of leg contusions and season-ending tibia fractures, and are now required in many leagues.[20,30,68]

Muscle Strains

Strains of the hamstrings, adductors, and quadriceps are common in soccer players and can result in extended periods of lost playing time. Frequently overlooked as minor injuries, these strains can become chronic, recurrent injuries that have a great effect on the player's ability to compete. The treatment is conservative, with rest, ice, compression, and elevation in the first 24 hours to help minimize bleeding and edema. Anti-inflammatory medication can also be helpful. Gentle passive range of motion should be started as soon after the injury as possible, followed by active motion, stretching, and strengthening as soon as tolerated. Soccer players with increased tightness of the hamstring or quadriceps muscles are at increased risk for injury. Players at risk can be identified through formal flexibility testing. Preseason hamstring and quadriceps muscle conditioning, proper warm-up, and pregame stretching can limit the frequency and severity of muscle strains and injuries.[3,6,10,14,16,20,28,30,41,56,68,71]

Knee Injuries

Knee injuries are the most common reason for surgeries in soccer players and can result in significant physical disability and lost playing time. Meniscal tears and ligament injuries in soccer typically result from pivoting or sudden deceleration stresses rather than from direct contact. Articular cartilage or osteochondral injuries are not uncommon and may result from hyperextension loading of the strong shot or kick. Such lesions typically occur in the femoral condyle and should be suspected when a persistent effusion develops in the absence of discrete point tenderness or instability. Isolated posterior cruciate ligament rupture can occur if a player is struck directly against the proximal anterior tibia. Tears of the ACL are generally the most disabling of knee injuries for the soccer player and account for the majority of time lost due to knee injuries. The rate of ACL injuries in women is much higher than in their male counterparts. The majority of cases are traumatic noncontact injuries. These injuries are often a result of overuse, fatigue, physical overload, or inadequate training. Reduced muscle strength may predispose players to noncontact injuries of the knee, especially in youth and lower-skill players.

Conditioning and strength training may play an important role in reducing the incidence of knee injuries. A history of prior injury and instability of the knee may predispose soccer players to subsequent major knee injury. The severity of knee injuries increases with age. Contact with opposing players and foul play, such as tackling and kicking, represent additional factors predisposing players to ACL injury. Few soccer players are able to remain competitive with an ACL-deficient knee despite strengthening and bracing. Surgical reconstruction should be recommended for all patients who wish to continue playing competitive soccer. The diagnosis and management of knee injuries is discussed in detail elsewhere in this book.[3,4,6,14,20,23,30,41,50,56,61,62,63,68]

Overuse Syndromes of the Knee

Iliotibial band friction syndrome, popliteus tendinitis, patellar tendinitis, pes anserine bursitis, and irritation of synovial plicae are common overuse syndromes of the knee seen in soccer players. Subluxing biceps femoris tendons have been reported as a cause of lateral knee pain in soccer players. Iliotibial band syndrome is caused by excessive friction between the iliotibial band and lateral femoral condyle. Players report lateral knee pain that progressively worsens with running after a pain-free start. There is tenderness over the ITB at the lateral femoral condyle. Symptoms may be reproduced with a single-leg squat. Excessive iliotibial band tightness can be determined by the Ober test. Treatment is conservative and consists of relative rest, ice, NSAIDs, ITB stretching, ultrasound, and other local modalities. An occasional bursal injection of corticosteroid may be helpful in chronic cases. In refractory cases, surgical treatment may be necessary.

Patellar tendinitis develops from cyclic overloading of the extensor mechanism during jumping and kicking. The player will complain of anterior knee pain inferior to the patella that is most pronounced when competing, running, and kicking. Symptoms will often resolve with a period of rest. On examination, there is tenderness over the inferior pole of the patella. Exacerbation of symptoms can be seen with resisted knee extension. The patellar tendon may feel thickened or swollen. Hamstring tightness and hip flexor weakness may also be seen. Conservative treatment is generally sufficient and should focus on quadriceps, hamstring, and hip flexor strengthening. Relative rest and modalities including ice, ultrasound, and iontophoresis or phonophoresis can be helpful. A short course of nonsteroidal anti-inflammatory medication can be prescribed. Steroid injections should never be given. X-rays should be obtained in the initial evaluation of players with patellar tendinitis. MRI is recommended for evaluation of chronic symptoms and can be helpful in differentiating patellar tendinitis from a partial tear. Chronic tendinitis with pathologic changes within the tendon evident on MRI may respond to surgical treatment.[1,24,51,55,57,74]

Tibia Fractures

A direct kick to the anterior leg is common in soccer and may result in a tibia fracture. Shin guards are helpful in decreasing the incidence of tibia fractures and are effective at decreasing soft-tissue trauma. A fracture should be strongly suspected if an injured player is unable to bear weight and complains of shin pain. Prompt radiographic evaluation is mandatory. Nondisplaced fractures can be treated with a functional fracture brace and progressive weight bearing. Displaced or comminuted fractures may require intramedullary nailing. Return to play can be expected after several months.

Stress fractures of the tibia can also occur and result in a significant loss of playing time. This condition should be considered in the differential diagnosis when evaluating an athlete with leg pain. The diagnosis and management of tibial stress fractures are discussed elsewhere in this book.[5,17]

Chronic Exertional Compartment Syndrome

Chronic exertional compartment syndrome presents as activity-related leg pain. The anterior compartment is most commonly affected, although the lateral and deep posterior compartments can also be involved. The differential diagnosis includes tibial stress fracture, venous thrombosis, and medial tibial stress syndrome or shin splints. Typically, the athlete will complain of pain during and immediately after exercise, particularly running. The pain is described as aching or cramping, increases with the intensity of exercise, and improves with rest. Symptoms resolve quickly after stopping exercise and are not present during normal activities of daily living. Players may not be able to play through the pain and often will take themselves out of the game. On physical exam, tenderness may be localized to the involved compartment or may be absent, especially if considerable time has lapsed since the exercise session. Examination performed immediately after exercise may reveal a tense, tender area localized near the involved compartment. Fascial herniations may also be noted. Radiographic evaluation is useful in ruling out conditions such as stress fractures, tumors, or periostitis. Pre- and postexercise intracompartmental pressure measurements are diagnostic. Treatment is surgical release of the involved muscle compartment.[1]

Ankle Sprains

Ankle sprains are the most common injuries accounting for lost playing time at all age levels and levels of competition in soccer. The lateral ankle ligaments are the most frequently injured structures and account for the vast majority of injuries sustained by soccer players today. Deltoid and syndesmotic injuries are less common. Sudden and uncontrolled inversion and plantarflexion of the foot and ankle or "rolling" of the ankle that occurs when a player steps awkwardly can result in injury to the lateral supporting structures. Injury is often accompanied by anterolateral ankle pain and swelling. The athlete may have difficulty bearing weight. There is tenderness over the lateral aspect of the ankle. A thorough examination is required to rule out bony and tendinous injuries. Fractures of the fibula, fifth metatarsal, acute traumatic peroneal tendon dislocation or rupture, and osteochondral injuries can occur and should be considered in the differential diagnosis. X-rays should be obtained to confirm the presence or absence of associated pathology. Stress views may be helpful once the acute period of injury has subsided to objectively document ankle stability.

The treatment is conservative and a rehabilitation program should be started as soon as possible to work on proprioception and general strengthening and conditioning of the musculature of the foot and ankle. A soccer player's ball control depends heavily on ankle and foot coordination. This rehabilitation is critical in reducing the incidence of symptomatic instability, pain, and recurrent ankle sprains in the future. Inadequate treatment and rehabilitation of ankle sprains increases a player's predisposition to reinjury.

It is not unusual for a player to experience persistent pain and swelling for many months after a severe ankle sprain. Players with a history of repeated ankle sprains and residual joint laxity may benefit from taping or bracing. Chronic lateral ankle pain in the athlete who has previously sustained an ankle sprain could be a result of incomplete rehabilitation, lateral talar exostosis, interosseus ligament tears, unrecognized syndesmosis sprain, subtalar instability, meniscoid lesion, anterior tibiotalar impingement, or lateral gutter synovial impingement and evaluation should proceed accordingly. Arthroscopy can be useful in the diagnosis and treatment of these disorders. Players with chronic recurrent ankle sprains and functional instability may be candidates for surgical reconstruction.[9,13,14,16,18–21,29,38,40–42,47,53,58,64,68]

Athletes with a syndesmotic injury or "high ankle sprain" take longer to return to full activity than those with a typical anterolateral ankle sprain. Athletes describe the foot moving in external rotation and dorsiflexion at the time of injury. Most players immediately recognize that this injury is different from a common ankle sprain. On physical exam, there is less swelling than that seen with a lateral ligament injury. Ecchymosis may be present proximal to the ankle joint. There is tenderness along the lateral aspect of the distal tibia and a positive squeeze test and external rotation stress test. Widening of the syndesmosis on x-ray is diagnostic. Mild sprains can be treated conservatively with ice, elevation, compression, and crutches to minimize weight-bearing activity. Early mobilization is permitted and return to play is possible when the player is comfortable. Return to play can take up to six weeks. Moderate sprains are immobilized and weight bearing is restricted for several weeks. Athletes can be expected to return to sport within 8 to 10 weeks. Severe sprains with syndesmotic diastasis require surgical treatment. Return to sport may take 5 to 6 months. Chronic pain after syndesmotic injury may indicate subtle instability, heterotopic ossification, or soft-tissue impingement.[47]

Peroneal Tendon Subluxation or Dislocation

Acute peroneal tendon dislocations are rare injuries that are frequently misdiagnosed as lateral ankle sprains. Subluxation or dislocation of the peroneal tendons can be a cause of chronic lateral ankle pain. The injury occurs with forceful ankle dorsiflexion and inversion, causing the superior peroneal retinaculum to tear and the preoneus brevis to dislocate anteriorly. A split-tear in the tendon may occur at the time of injury. Traumatic rupture of both peroneal tendons has been described in soccer players. Symptoms include swelling and tenderness in the lateral retromalleolar region over the peroneal tendons. Having the player actively evert the foot or roll the foot in circles may allow for the tendons to be observed subluxing. Maximal tenderness and swelling are along the posterior aspect of the distal fibula, and the player will be unable or reluctant to dorsiflex and evert against resistance. A "rim" fracture from the lateral ridge of the distal fibula may occasionally be seen on radiographs indicating avulsion of the superior peroneal retinaculum. MRI is useful to evaluate the retinaculum and to assess the integrity of the tendons. Conservative treatment includes the use of a non–weight bearing short leg cast for four weeks. Symptomatic chronic peroneal tendon subluxation is an indication for surgical reconstruction.[9,47]

Achilles Tendonopathy and Rupture

Players with Achilles tendinitis complain of pain over the posterior ankle that is worse with running and jumping. Examination may reveal tenderness over the tendon in the watershed area 4 to 6 cm above the os calcis, with increased warmth, swelling, and crepitus. Tenderness at the posterior heel may indicate insertional tendinitis or retrocalcaneal bursitis. An antalgic gait, painful single toe rise, and variable gastrocnimeus-soleus weakness can also be seen. Chronic symptoms may be indicative of tendon degeneration. Acute, complete ruptures are less common but can occur and are usually associated with a pop, extreme pain and swelling, a palpable defect, and a positive Thompson test. X-rays should be obtained in all cases. MRI can be helpful in defining the extent of the athlete's injury. Relative rest, ice, stretching, NSAIDs, ultrasound, heel lifts, and orthotics are the mainstay of treatment. A period of immobilization may be helpful in difficult cases. Players with MRI evidence of Achilles tendinosis that has failed an adequate course of immobilization may require exploration of the degenerative tendon. Athletes with chronic partial tears do poorly with conservative treatment and most are unable to return to their preinjury level of competition. Surgical treatment is often successful. It is recommended that elite athletes with Achilles tendon rupture undergo acute surgical reconstruction.[2,18]

Ankle Impingement Syndromes

Anterior Ankle Impingement Syndrome. Impingement syndromes of the foot and ankle are extremely common in soccer players but remain a diagnostic and therapeutic challenge to the clinician.

The formation of tibiotalar osteophytes at the anterior part of ankle joint is a common cause of chronic anterior ankle pain in soccer players. In 1950, McMurray[48] named the condition "footballer's ankle," a condition that is now commonly referred to as anterior ankle impingement syndrome. It has been suggested that this is an overuse type of injury, and that spur formation is related to recurrent ball impact and chronic repetitive microtrauma to the anteromedial aspect of the ankle. Players will complain of anterior ankle pain, particularly with jumping. Diagnosis is confirmed with the findings of limited active and passive dorsiflexion, pain with forced dorsiflexion, and radiographic evidence of spur formation, which is best seen on the lateral ankle x-ray. The initial treatment is conservative. Heel lifts, NSAIDs, and avoidance of excessive dorsiflexion can be helpful. If symptoms persist and the player cannot compete, then surgical excision may be beneficial.[14,44,48,54,65,68]

Anterolateral Soft-Tissue Impingement. Anterolateral soft-tissue impingement of the ankle is commonly seen as a result of repetitive ankle injury. A hyalinized connective tissue lesion can form in the anterolateral gutter and result in pain and the feeling of instability. A high success rate has been reported with arthroscopic treatment.[40]

Posterior Impingement Syndrome. Posterior impingement syndrome, also called os trigonum syndrome, involves impaction of the os trigonum and/or the posterior capsular structures between the tibia and calcaneus. Players complain of a vague posterior ankle pain that is worsened by kicking or passive ankle dorsiflexion. Retrocalcaneal tenderness is evident on exam. X-rays are typically negative, but may show a fracture of the posterior talar process. MRI is useful in defining additional pathology, such as a flexor hallucis longus tendinitis. The differential diagnosis of a soccer player with posterior ankle pain should include Achilles tendinitis, retrocalcaneal bursitis, flexor hallucis longus tendinitis, and stress fracture. Chronic posterior impingement of the talocalcaneal joint during instep kicking may result in failure of the synchondrosis to ossify or lead to stress fracture of the posterior talar process. Symptomatic os trigona are treated conservatively. Persistent symptoms may warrant surgical excision.[72]

Peroneal Tendinitis

Attritional tears of the peroneus longus and brevis tendons can occur in the soccer player. More commonly, however, the athlete will experience an acute tendinitis or traumatic subluxation of the tendons. Peroneal tendinitis presents with diffuse lateral retromalleolar pain. Differentiation between tendinitis, partial longitudinal tearing of the peroneus brevis, lateral gutter synovial impingement, and peroneal tendon subluxation must be made. A history of subjective ankle instability, weakness, popping, and swelling may be elicited. Players may have an antalgic gait, tenderness in the lateral retromalleolar groove, swelling, crepitus, and pain with passive inversion of the subtalar joint. X-rays are typically negative. MRI is helpful in defining the extent of tendon injury and facilitating surgical planning. The mainstay of treatment of peroneal tendinitis is rest, ice, NSAIDs, and physical therapy. A lateral heel wedge and stirrup brace may also be used. A period of immobilization is helpful in cases that are slow to respond. Recalcitrant cases with MRI evidence of tearing of the peroneal tendons may benefit from surgical exploration and repair. Occult ankle instability may be associated with these injuries and should be assessed.[18]

Flexor Hallucis Longus Tendinitis

Flexor hallucis longus (FHL) tendinitis presents as a medial retromalleolar ankle pain, and develops as a result of repetitive hyperplantarflexion of the ankle during kicking. It can be seen alone or in combination with posterior ankle impingement. On examination, with the ankle dorsiflexed, there is limited dorsiflexion of the great toe and pain. With subsequent plantarflexion of the ankle, there is increased dorsiflexion of the great toe with less discomfort. A local injection of 1% lidocaine that eliminates pain with forced plantarflexion confirms the diagnosis. The physician must differentiate flexor hallucis longus tendinitis from posterior tibial tendinitis, Achilles tendinitis, and retrocalcaneal bursitis. Early treatment of FHL tendinitis is conservative, with NSAIDs, rest, and early restrictive taping of the ankle and first MTP joint. A brief period of immobilization may be required. In refractory cases, surgical debridement may be necessary.[18]

FOOT INJURIES

Midfoot Sprains

Sprains of the midfoot can occur as isolated injuries but are usually associated with tarsal or tarsometatarsal fractures. A common mechanism of injury in soccer players occurs when a plantarflexed foot is planted on the ground and is struck from behind by another player. Swelling of the midfoot and inability to bear weight is highly suggestive of a tarsometatarsal joint injury. On examination, there is marked pain with palpation of the midfoot, particularly over the second MTP joint, in conjunction with provocative side-to-side midfoot compression and dorsi-plantar stress of the first and second metatarsal joints. Weight-bearing radiographs are helpful in assessing tarsal alignment. Excessive pain may prohibit weight-bearing x-ray, in which case a bone scan or CT scan helpful diagnostic studies. Diastasis of the first or second tarsometatarsal joints more than 2 mm requires surgical treatment. In the absence of diastasis, conservative treatment is appropriate and consists of immobilization and restricted weight bearing for 4 to 6 weeks. Medial midfoot sprains take much longer to heal than lateral sprains and return to competition can take up to several months.[27,47]

Plantar Fasciitis

The most common cause of hindfoot pain in sports is plantar fasciitis. Repetitive microtrauma during bursts of sprinting can lead to significant damage to the plantar fascia in soccer players and cause arch or heel pain. It is characterized by the insidious onset of medial plantar heel pain that is worse when getting out of bed in the morning or after sitting for a period of time. Physical exam shows point tenderness at the medial origin of the plantar fascia or distally along the medial longitudinal arch. Heel or plantar arch pain can be reproduced by passively dorsiflexing the toes of the foot. Achilles tendon contracture may be present. X-rays are often negative but may show calcaneal traction spur. Nonsurgical treatment is successful in nearly all cases. A regimen of Achilles tendon and plantar fascia stretching combined with activity modification, NSAIDs, heel cushions or arch supports, a dorsiflexion night splint, and corticosteroid injection may be successful in the majority of players. Recalcitrant cases may benefit from immobilization for several weeks. If symptoms persist beyond 6 to 9 months of appropriate conservative treatment, then surgical release may be indicated.[18]

Fifth Metatarsal Fractures

Fractures of the proximal third of the fifth metatarsal are common in sports that involve significant amounts of running and jumping. Players may present with the insidious onset of a vague, dull ache along the lateral border of the foot that is exacerbated during play and relieved with rest, or with the acute onset of pain along the fifth metatarsal. X-rays may demonstrate an obvious fracture with sclerosis indicating the chronicity of the problem. Typically, a history of prodromal symptoms combined with intramedullary sclerosis and a widened fracture line is indicative of a preexisting stress fracture. Conservative treatment with casting and strict non–weight bearing has been successful; however, there is an increased risk of delayed union, nonunion, and hindfoot stiffness with this treatment. Primary surgical management with intramedullary screw fixation is the treatment of choice in competitive athletes and serves as a more reliable and predictable treatment option that allows for a more timely return to competition.

Forced inversion of the foot and ankle during competition can result in acute, traumatic fractures of the diaphysis of the fifth metatarsal. Fractures involving the base of the metatarsal can be confused with an ankle sprain, and moderate tenderness along the lateral border of the foot should alert the medical staff that x-ray evaluation is necessary. Conservative treatment is generally sufficient and players may return to competition in six weeks or when comfortable enough to do so.[27,34,66]

Digital Fractures

Contusions to the toes are so common in soccer players that many fractures tend to go unnoticed. Fractures are typically caused by direct trauma from ball strike or contact with another player. Discrete tenderness, swelling, and crepitus discovered while examining the toes should alert the physician to fracture. X-rays are taken to confirm the diagnosis. Phalangeal fractures rarely require surgical intervention, with the great toe being the rare exception. Some phalangeal fractures can be loosely buddy taped to adjacent toes for comfort or simply left alone in a shoe with a wide toe box or stiff sole. Early weight bearing can improve outcome and healing times. Athletes should return to play when comfortable enough to appropriately compete.[27]

Stress Fractures

Stress fractures of the foot and ankle in soccer are most typically seen in elite or professional players with heavy daily training and game schedules. Stress fractures in the forefoot usually involve the second and third metatarsal shafts. Stress fractures of the fourth and fifth metatarsals are less common. Physical exam may demonstrate swelling, tenderness, and pain on passive motion of the involved toe. X-rays may show periosteal reaction in diaphyseal stress fracture but can be negative. Bone scan or MRI can be diagnostic. Conservative treatment with relative rest and avoidance of pain-producing activity is generally successful. Immobilization is rarely necessary. Custom-molded rigid pedal orthosis may be used by the player, who may return to play when comfortable. Refractory cases or those involving the proximal fifth metatarsal may require surgical treatment.[18,27]

Navicular Stress Fractures

Navicular stress fractures present with the insidious onset of forefoot pain that is worse with activity. Players frequently complain of diffuse ankle and midfoot pain during running and kicking. The symptoms are vague and physical findings often are nonspecific. A delay in diagnosis is not uncommon and players are often misdiagnosed with a forefoot sprain and treated inappropriately for an extended period of time before an accurate diagnosis is obtained. If the diagnosis is suspected and plain radiographs are equivocal, MRI or CT scan can be ordered to confirm the diagnosis. The treatment for early, incomplete, nondisplaced fractures requires the athlete to be immobilized in a short leg cast and prohibited from bearing weight for six weeks, followed by gradual resumption of activity over the next six weeks. A CT scan can be repeated to confirm healing. If progressive healing is evident, return to play may be expected within 12 to 18 weeks from the time treatment was initiated. If there is displacement, delayed union, or nonunion, then surgical treatment will be necessary.[18,27,39,67]

Calcaneal Stress Fractures

Calcaneal stress fractures are infrequent but remain part of the differential diagnosis of heel pain in soccer players. Players may complain of vague symptoms and are often misdiagnosed as having plantar fasciitis, os trigonum, retrocalcaneal bursitis, or Achilles tendinosis. A dense sclerotic line may be seen on x-ray. Bone scan or CT scan will confirm the diagnosis. Stress fractures of the os calcis require at least six weeks of rest. The athlete is instructed to participate in activities, staying below the level of pain. A walking boot can be used and removed to work on range of motion so hindfoot stiffness can be minimized.[18,27]

Malleolar Stress Fractures

Stress fractures involving the medial and lateral malleoli should be considered in soccer players complaining of persistent ankle pain, especially in the setting of recurrent ankle sprains. Distal fibula stress fractures can be confused with ankle sprains or peroneal tenosynovitis. Exquisite point tenderness over the distal fibula or anteromedial tibia is highly suggestive of a stress fracture. X-rays are often negative and MRI or bone scan can be diagnostic. Medial malleoli stress fractures are potentially unstable and are at risk of nonunion. If the fracture is not displaced, then treatment consisting of immobilization and non–weight bearing may suffice; however, if the fracture should displace or be slow to heal, then surgical treatment is recommended. Lateral malleoli stress fractures are more stable and generally heal with conservative treatment.[18,27]

Sesamoiditis and Sesamoid Fractures

Injury to the hallucal sesamoids is common among soccer players. Repetitive microtrauma during loading cycles at the great toe during soccer may lead to stress fractures or avascular necrosis. The presence of a metal stud or cleat directly beneath the first MTP joint on nearly all soccer shoes aggravates this problem by increasing local stresses, particularly during the push-off phase of running. Over time, this may lead to increased local ischemia and avascular necrosis with fragmentation of the sesamoid. Stress fractures involving the medial sesamoid are most common and the risk of nonunion is high. There is localized tenderness over the sesamoid that is exacerbated by passive dorsiflexion of the great toe. A local lidocaine injection that results in complete symptomatic relief is diagnostic. Axial radiographs are useful and a bone scan or MRI can provide additional diagnostic support. Treatment is symptomatic, with ice, NSAIDs, and a custom-molded foot othosis. Immobilization is helpful in cases slow to respond. Surgical excision may be considered in recalcitrant cases.[18,32,60]

Turf Toe

Injury to the plantar capsule of the first MTP joint is commonly referred to as "turf toe." Partial tearing of the plantar capsule of the hallucal MTP joint occurs with repetitive forced hyperdorsiflexion, which may occur during the push-off phase of running in a player wearing a soft and flexible shoe. In chronic cases, the condition is aggravated by push-off and cutting. The severity of the injury may vary, however, and more acute injuries are extremely painful and the player is often too uncomfortable to continue in the game. On examination, there is exquisite tenderness over the plantar aspect of the first MTP joint and the pain is made worse with passive dorsiflexion. Moderate swelling may also be seen. Conservative treatment is generally sufficient, and taping of the toe to prevent excessive dorsiflexion is helpful. A thin steel prefabricated insole or a custom orthosis can also be used. A high incidence of chronic problems are associated with turf toe, such as hallux valgus, hallux rigidis, and chronic pain, reflecting the potential severity and disability resulting from this injury.[18]

Reverse Turf Toe (Soccer Toe)

Acute and chronic capsular damage to the dorsal aspect of the hallucal MTP joint can be seen in soccer players. This typically results from repetitive forced hyperplantarflexion of the joint, especially during instep ball strike, because of the supple nature of the toe box. Significant functional disability can result from the injury, which can compromise push-off, forward drive, running, and jumping. Diagnosis is confirmed by physical exam. There is swelling and tenderness over the hallucal MTP joint and the pain is exacerbated by passive plantarflexion of the joint. Soccer toe responds well to conservative management, which consists of taping, anti-inflammatory medication, ice, and rest, along with a toe strengthening program. Taping to prevent MTP plantarflexion is helpful. A prolonged recovery can be seen and players may be unable to compete for some time, particularly if the great toe of the dominant foot is involved. Some athletes may experience chronic pain, loss of dorsiflexion, and hallux rigidis.[18]

Hallux Rigidis

Hallux rigidis is a progressive degenerative disorder of the first metatarsalphalangeal joint associated with localized pain, limited motion, and prominent dorsal osteophytes. Post-traumatic arthritis of the hallucal MTP joint can occur as a result of previous fracture, osteochondritis, avascular necrosis, turf toe, or soccer toe. Athletes complain of pain and stiffness in the great toe, which is particularly noticeable while cutting or pushing off. A chronically stiff and tender first MTP joint is found on examination. The pain is exacerbated by forced dorsiflexion of the first MTP joint. X-rays demonstrate dorsal osteophytes and first MTP joint space narrowing. The initial treatment is conservative and consists of rest, NSAIDs, and a custom orthosis or carbon footplate insert. Intraarticular corticosteroid injections may be helpful, but the results are often unpredictable. A cheilectomy or arthrodesis may be necessary in recalcitrant cases. A first MTP joint arthrodesis is recommended for advanced disease in soccer players because of the need for strong push-off during running.[18]

Subungual Hematoma

Most soccer players will sustain numerus subungual hematomas during their careers. These injuries generally involve the great toe as a result of a direct crush by the foot of another player or from the shear stresses of sudden stops and starts as the toe impacts the toe box. For many players, the toenail becomes dystrophic due to the repeated damage to the nail bed. An acute subungual hematoma can be quite painful and the initial treatment should involve releasing the pressure of the blood collected beneath the nail. The nail should be left intact even if it is detached from the nail bed.[18]

CONCLUSION

Most injuries are caused by direct trauma related to physical contact between players. The occurrence of foul play puts players at increased risk for serious injury and is directly responsible for approximately one-third of all soccer injuries. The incidence and severity of injury appears to increase with advancing age, level of play, and frequency of competition. Injuries in soccer players most commonly involve the lower extremity, and predominantly affect the ankle and knee and the muscles of the thigh and calf. Players are more likely to sustain an injury during a game rather than in practice. Contusions, ligament sprains, and muscle strains account for about 75%

of all injuries. Serious, permanently disabling injuries are rare and account for less than 0.1% of injuries at all levels. At all levels of competition, the number and severity of knee injuries, including career-threatening ACL rupture, is greater in female athletes. Knee injuries usually result in the most time lost from participation and are the most common cause for surgery in the soccer player. Mild head injuries, including lacerations of the scalp, dental, ophthalmologic, and closed head trauma, also represent a significant cause of morbidity. Concussions account for roughly 2% to 3% of all soccer injuries, but are probably more common than previously reported. These injuries typically result from a collision with other players, the ground, or the goalpost, and not from intentional heading of the ball.

The development of injury prevention programs and continuing education by the coaching staff in techniques and skills may reduce the incidence of injuries in soccer players over time. Appropriate sport-specific preseason conditioning is helpful in minimizing injuries during the season. It is well known that soccer players with increased tightness of the hamstring or quadriceps muscles are at increased risk for injury. Preseason muscle flexibility testing can identify players at risk so that amendments to the players' conditioning program can be made and the potential risk of in-season injury reduced. Other factors such as a pregame warm-up with emphasis on stretching, particularly of the adductors, quadriceps, and hamstring muscle groups; a regular cool-down period after training; adequate rehabilitation of specific injuries with sufficient recovery time, including proprioceptive training; the use of protective equipment, such as mouthguards and shin guards; good playing field conditions; and adherence to existing rules and avoidance of foul play, are helpful in minimizing serious injury that could keep the athlete from competition.[10,15,28,37,71]

REFERENCES

1. Amendola A, Clatworthy M, Magnes S: Overuse injuries of the lower extremity. In Arendt E (ed): OKU Sports Medicine. Rosemont, IL, American Academy of Orthopaedic Surgeons, 1999, pp 365–372.
2. Angermann P, Hovgaard D: Chronic Achilles tendonopathy in athletic individuals: Results of nonsurgical treatment. Foot Ankle Int 20:304–306, 1999.
3. Arendt E, Dick R: Knee injury patterns among men and women in collegiate basketball and soccer. Am J Sports Med 23:694–701, 1995.
4. Bach B, Minihane K: Subluxating biceps femoris tendon: An unusual cause of lateral knee pain in a soccer athlete: A case report. Am J Sports Med 29:93–95, 2001.
5. Bir C, Cassatta S, Janda D: An analysis and comparison of soccer shin guards. Clin J Sports Med 5:95–99, 1995.
6. Bjordal J, Arnoy F, Hannestad B, et al: Epidemiology of anterior cruciate ligament injuries in soccer. Am J Sports Med 25:341–345, 1997.
7. Boden B, Kirkendall D, Garrett W Jr: Concussion incidence in elite college soccer players. Am J Sports Med 26:238–241, 1998.
8. Bruzzone E, Cocito L, Pisani R: Intracranial delayed epidural hematoma in a soccer player: A case report. Am J Sports Med 28:901–903, 2000.
9. Cees C, Verheyen M, Bras J, et al: Rupture of both peroneal tendons in a professional athlete: A case report. Am J Sports Med 28:897–900, 2000.
10. Chomiak J, Junge A, Peterson L, et al: Severe injuries in football players: Influencing factors. Am J Sports Med 28(Suppl 5):S38–S58, 2000.
11. Curtin J, Kay N: Hand injuries due to soccer. Hand 8:93–95, 1976.
12. Daily S, Barsan W: Head injuries in soccer. A case for protective headgear. Physician Sports Med 20:79–85, 1992.
13. Dixon D, Monroe M, Gabel S, et al: Excrescent lesion: A diagnosis of lateral talar exostosis in chronically symptomatic sprained ankles. Foot Ankle Int 20:331–336, 1999.
14. Dvorak J, Junge A: Football injuries and physical symptoms: A review of the literature. Am J Sports Med 28(Suppl):S1–S14, 2000.
15. Dvorak J, Junge A, Chomiak J, et al: Risk factor analysis for injuries in football players: Possibilities for a prevention program. Am J Sports Med 28:S69–S79, 2000.
16. Ekstrand J, Tropp H: The incidence of ankle sprains in soccer. Foot Ankle 11:41–44, 1990.
17. Francisco A, Nightingale R, Guilak F, et al: Comparison of soccer shin guards in preventing tibia fracture. Am J Sports Med 28:227–233, 2000.
18. Frey C, Feder K: Foot and ankle injuries in sports. In Arendt E (ed): OKU Sports Medicine. Rosemont, IL, American Academy of Orthopaedic Surgeons, 1999, pp 379–394.
19. Frey C, Feder K, DiGiovanni C: Arthroscopic evaluation of the subtalar joint: Does sinus tarsi syndrome exist? Foot Ankle Int 20:185–191, 1999.
20. Fried T, Lloyd G: An overview of common soccer injuries: Management and prevention. Sports Med 14:269–275, 1992.
21. Gerber J, Williams G, Scoville C, et al. Persistent disability associated with ankle sprains: A prospective evaluation of an athletic population. Foot Ankle Int 19:653-660, 1998.
22. Green G, Jordan S: Are brain injuries a significant problem in soccer? Clin Sports Med 17:795–809, 1998.

23. Griffin L, Agel J, Albohm M, et al: Noncontact anterior cruciate ligament injuries: Risk factors and prevention strategies. J Am Acad Orthop Surg 8:141–150, 2000.
24. Griffiths G, Selesnick F: Operative treatment and arthroscopic findings in chronic patellar tendonitis. Arthroscopy 14:836–839, 1998.
25. Guskiewicz K, Marshall S, Broglio S, et al: No evidence of impaired neurocognitive performance in collegiate soccer players. Am J Sports Med 30:157–162, 2002.
26. Hawkins R, Fuller C: An examination of the frequency and severity of injuries and incidents at three levels of professional football. Br J Sports Med 32:326–332, 1998.
27. Heckman J: Fractures and dislocations of the foot. In Rockwood C, Green D, Bucholz R, Heckman J (ed): Fractures in Adults, 4th ed. Philadelphia, Lippincott-Raven, 1996, pp 2267–2405.
28. Heidt R, Sweeterman L, Carlonas R, et al: Avoidance of soccer injuries with preseason conditioning. Am J Sports Med 28:659–662, 2000.
29. Hertel J, Denegar C, Monroe M, et al: Talocrural and subtalar joint instability after lateral ankle sprain. Med Sci Sports Exerc 31:1501–1508, 1999.
30. Inklaar H: Soccer injuries I: Incidence and severity. Sports Med 18:55–73, 1994.
31. Inklaar H: Soccer injuries II: Aetiology and prevention. Sports Med 18:81–93, 1994.
32. Jahss M: The sesamoids of the hallux. Clin Orthop 157:88–96, 1981.
33. Jordan S, Green G, Galanty S, et al: Acute and chronic brain injury in United States national team soccer players. Am J Sports Med 24:205–210, 1996.
34. Josefsson P: Closed treatment of Jones fractures: Good results in 40 cases after 11–26 years. Acta Orthop Scand 65:545–547, 1994.
35. Junge A, Chomiak J, Dvorak J: Incidence of football injuries in youth players: Comparison of players from two European regions. Am J Sports Med 28(Suppl 5):S47, 2000.
36. Junge A, Dvorak J: Influence of definition and data collection on the incidence of injuries in football. Am J Sports Med 28(Suppl):S40–S46, 2000.
37. Junge A, Rosch D, Peterson L, et al: Prevention of soccer injuries: A prospective intervention study in youth amateur players. Am J Sports Med 30:652–659, 2002.
38. Karlsson J Sward L, Andreasson G: The effect of taping on ankle stability: Practical implications. Sports Med 16:210–215, 1993.
39. Khan K: Outcome of conservative and surgical management of navicular stress fractures in athletes. Am J Sports Med 20:657–665, 1992.
40. Lahm A, Erggelet C, Reichelt A: Ankle joint arthroscopy for meniscoid lesions in athletes. Arthroscopy 14:572–575, 1998.
41. Larson E, Jensen P, Jensen P: Long-term outcome of knee and ankle injuries in elite football. Scand J Med Sci Sports 9:285–289, 1999.
42. Liu S, Baker C: Comparison of lateral ankle ligamentous reconstruction procedures. Am J Sports Med 22:313–317, 1994.
43. Luthje P, Nurmi I, Kataja M, et al: Epidemiology and traumatology of injuries in soccer: A prospective study in Finland. Scand J Med Sci Sports 6:180–185, 1996.
44. Massada J: Ankle overuse injuries in soccer players: Morphological adaptation of the talus in the anterior impingement. J Sports Med Phys Fitness 31: 447–451, 1991.
45. Matser J, Kessels A, Jordan B, et al: Chronic traumatic brain injury in professional soccer players. Neurology 51:791–796, 1998.
46. Matser J, Kessels A, Lezak M, et al: Neuropsychological impairment in amateur soccer players. JAMA 282:971–973, 1999.
47. Mazur D, Bartolozzi A: Ankle soft-tissue injuries. In Arendt E (ed): OKU Sports Medicine. Rosemont, IL, American Academy of Orthopaedic Surgeons, 1999, pp 373–378.
48. McMurray T: Footballer's ankle. J Bone Joint Surg 32B:68–69, 1950.
49. Meyers W, Ricciardi R, Busconi B, et al: Groin pain in the athlete. In Arendt E (ed): OKU Sports Medicine. Rosemont, IL, American Academy of Orthopaedic Surgeons, 1999, pp 281–290.
50. Morgan B, Oberlander M: An examination of injuries in major league soccer: The inaugural season. Am J Sports Med 29:426–430, 2001.
51. Nichols C: Patellar tendon injuries. Clin Sports Med 11:807–813, 1992.
52. Nielsen A, Yde J: Epidemiology and traumatology of injuries in soccer. Am J Sports Med 17:803–807, 1989.
53. Noakes T, et al: A fivefold reduction in the incidence of recurrent ankle sprains in soccer players using the Sport-Stirrup orthosis. Am J Sports Med 22:601–606, 1994.
54. Ogilvie-Harris D, Mahomed N, Demaziere A: Anterior impingement of the ankle treated by arthroscopic removal of bony spurs. J Bone Joint Surg 75B:437–440, 1993.
55. Orava S, Malinen L, Karpakka J, et al: Results of surgical treatment of unresolved Osgood-Schlatter lesion. Ann Chir Gynaecol 89(4):298–302, 2000.
56. Peterson L, Junge A, Chomiak J, et al: Incidence of football injuries and complaints in different age groups and skill-level groups. Am J Sports Med 28(Suppl 5):51–61, 2000.

57. Popp J, Yu J, Kaeding C: Recalcitrant patellar tendonitis: Magnetic resonance imaging, histologic evaluation, and surgical treatment. Am J Sports Med 25:218–222, 1997.
58. Povacz P, Unger S, Miller W, et al: A randomized prospective study of operative and nonoperative treatment of injuries of the fibular collateral ligaments of the ankle. J Bone Joint Surg Am 80:345–351, 1998.
59. Powell J, Barber-Foss K: Sex-related injury patterns among selected high school sports. Am J Sports Med 28:385–391, 2000.
60. Richardsom E: Injuries to the hallucal sesamoids in the athlete. Foot Ankle 7:229–244, 1987.
61. Roos H, Ornell M, Gardsell P, et al: Soccer after anterior cruciate ligament injury: An incompatible combination? A national survey of incidence and risk factors and a 7-year follow-up of 310 players. Acta Orthop Scand 66:107–112, 1995.
62. Rozzi S, Lephart S, Gear W, et al: Knee joint laxity and neuromuscular characteristics of male and female soccer and basketball players. Am J Sports Med 27:312–319, 1999.
63. Shelbourne K, Gray T: Anterior cruciate ligament reconstruction with autogenous patellar tendon graft followed by accelerated rehabilitation: A 2–9 year follow-up. Am J Sports Med 25:786–795, 1997.
64. Thacker S, Stroup D, Branche C, et al: The prevention of ankle sprains in sports: A systematic review of the literature. Am J Sports Med 27:753–760, 1999.
65. Tol J, Slim E, van Soest A, et al: The relationship of the kicking action in soccer and anterior ankle impingement syndrome: A biomechanical analysis. Am J Sports Med 30:45–50, 2002.
66. Torg J: Fractures of the base of the fifth metatarsal distal to the tuberosity: classification and guidelines for non-surgical and surgical management. J Bone Joint Surg Am 66:209–214, 1984.
67. Torg J: Stress fractures of the tarsal navicular. J Bone Joint Surg 64:700–712, 1982.
68. Tucker A: Common soccer injuries: Diagnosis, treatment, and rehabilitation. Sports Med 23:21-32, 1997.
69. Tysvaer A: Head and neck injuries in soccer. Impact of minor trauma. Sports Med 14:200–213, 1992.
70. Tysvaer A, Locher E: Soccer injuries to the brain: A neuropsychologic study of former soccer players. Am J Sports Med 19:56–60, 1991.
71. Witvrouw E, Danneels L, Asselman P, et al: Muscle flexibility as a risk factor for developing muscle injuries in male professional soccer players: A prospective study. Am J Sports Med 31:41–46, 2003.
72. Wredemark T, Carlstedt C, Bauer H, et al: Os trigonum syndrome: A clinical entity in ballet dancers. Foot Ankle 11:404–406, 1991.
73. Yde J, Nielsen A: Sports injuries in adolescents' ball games: Soccer, handball, and basketball. Br J Sports Med 24:51–54, 1990.
74. Yu J, Popp J, Kaeding C, et al: Correlation of MR imaging and pathologic findings in athletes undergoing surgery for chronic patellar tendonitis. Am J Roentgenol 165:115–118, 1995.

40 Injuries in Alpine Skiing

Andrew L. Rosen, Giles R. Scuderi, and Peter D. McCann

Alpine sports continue to be a significant form of winter recreation for many people worldwide. Technological advances in mountain development, snowmaking, clothing, and equipment have made snow sports more attractive to the general public. Participation grows annually, with an estimated 15 million participants in the United States in the year 2001. Elements of the sport that attract many individuals include the thrill of high speeds, jumping, steep slopes, tree runs, and deep powder. Unfortunately, many of these same activities are also dangerous.

Significant injuries sustained in snow sports are relatively common and estimated to occur at a rate of two to three per 1000 skier days. Fortunately, these rates have decreased from the 1970s, when rates of five to eight injuries per 1000 skier days were reported. Changes in equipment and participant behavior are likely responsible for this improvement.[13]

Equipment design has also advanced dramatically in the last 30 years. Evolution of alpine sports has split into two distinct groups: skiing and snowboarding. Although many variations of each group exist, the types of injuries described in the two sports differ dramatically.

MECHANISMS OF INJURY

Most injuries sustained in alpine sports arise from direct trauma forces. Although overuse injuries can occur in any sport, most ski and snowboard injuries occur through trauma. The simplest mechanism is that of a fall, resulting in direct contact with the snow or ice. Angle of slope, firmness of the snow, and fall direction all influence the magnitude of injury seen with this mechanism. A second type of injury cause is that of skier-to-object collisions. Trees, rocks, lift poles, and other man-made and natural objects are numerous on a ski slope and can be sources of significant injury. Ski resorts attempt to minimize the risk of these objects as much as possible, but such injuries still occur as an inherent risk of the sport. A final mechanism is the result of a collision between two snow sport participants. Poor visibility, lack of control, and crowding on the slopes act to increase the risk of these injuries.

Speed often plays a significant role in almost any type of injury. Increased velocity creates increased force with any collision on a ski slope and typically plays the largest role in predicting the morbidity of any injury. Most skier safety initiatives focus on increasing the awareness of the need to ski under control and at a reasonable speed for the terrain involved.

RISK OF DEATH

Despite the reputation of snow sports as dangerous activities, very few fatal accidents occur on a ski slope. Only an estimated 24 deaths per year occurred in the United States from 1990–1997. Despite the deaths of two celebrities in the 1997–1998 ski season, which raised public awareness of ski risks, most injuries sustained in snow sports are not life-threatening. Fifty-eight percent of these injuries were the result of head injuries, and most of these occurred during a collision with a stationary object.[5] Most fatalities occur in male experienced skiers who are skiing at high velocity and sustain blunt trauma injuries.[26]

Avalanche deaths in the United States occur also, although the risk to visitors to established mountain resorts is quite minimal. About 10 deaths annually are attributed to avalanches, although in-bounds resort skiers represent only 5% of these fatalities. Backcountry and out-of-bounds skiers reflect approximately 26% of these deaths.[21]

SKIING VERSUS SNOWBOARDING

Snowboarding arose in the 1970s and has become an established sport in the alpine industry, gaining worldwide acceptance with its inclusion in the Olympic games. Snowboarding enjoyed a phenomenal rise in the 1990s and has now plateaued at about a quarter of all visitors to mountain resorts. The sport distinguishes itself from skiing with use of a single wide board, with nonreleasable bindings that are mounted toward the side of the board. The technique varies dramatically from skiing, with emphasis on wide turns, jumping, and spins. Snowboard riding has inherently less stability in relation to forward or backwards falls, which also affects the risk and types of injuries sustained.

Most studies have shown a much higher overall risk of injury associated with snowboard use. Ronning et al. found snowboarding to possess three to four times the risk of injury requiring hospital treatment.[24] Langran et al. demonstrated a higher overall injury rate and a higher risk of fractures in a snowboarding population.[14]

Levy et al. showed snowboarders to be at three times higher risk of sustaining a head injury than skiers.[15]

Some of these patterns may be the result of the sport's appeal to beginners and the frequent lack of proper instruction. Beginner snowboarders have shown a much higher injury rate than beginner skiers.[6] Demographic patterns of younger participants who may possess more inherent risk-taking behavior may be more of a factor than the inherent risks involved in the sport. The boxes list common actions that can help prevent injuries in each of the two sports.

PREVENTION OF INJURY

Role of Technique and Experience

Development of good form and experience in alpine sports can be protective against injury. Higher rates of injury are seen in first-time participants of both skiing and snowboarding. Langran et al. showed decreased injury rates in participants with greater than 5 days experience in season and greater than 7 days total experience.[14] Jorgensen et al. demonstrated reduction in injury rates with the use of a fall technique instructional video.[10]

Role of Conditioning

Participating with good physical conditioning is also important for avoidance of injury. Increased injury rates are seen later in the afternoon, suggesting that fatigue plays a role in many ski and snowboard accidents.[18] Consumption of alcohol either before or during alpine sports may also play a role in increasing injury rates. Intoxication or hangovers can reduce balance and coordination, and should be minimized to reduce injury risk.[4]

Hydration can be very important in an athletic activity performed at a high-altitude environment. Prevention of acute mountain sickness (AMS) can often be accomplished by maintaining good hydration status.

Helmet Use

The use of helmets for reduction of injuries to the head has widespread acceptance in many other sports (bicycling, climbing, kayaking), but their penetration into the ski market remains small. There are relatively few studies directly addressing the effectiveness and need for helmets in skiing and snowboarding. Macnab et al. showed a decrease in head injuries with no increase in cervical spine injuries in skiers and snowboarders under the age of 13 who used helmets.[17]

A report of the Consumer Product Safety Commission (CPSC) in 1999 found that 44%, or 7,700 injuries per year, could be addressed by helmet use. In children under the age of 15, 53% of injuries could be prevented. The report also concluded that approximately 11 deaths per year could be prevented.[5] Although the report recommends the use of helmets, the relative risk of head injuries (7,700 injuries in 15 million participants) is quite low.

The decision to wear a helmet is also affected by issues of comfort and expense. Helmets are not yet mandatory at any ski area, and will probably be most beneficial to a high-risk population of very aggressive skiers and beginner snowboarders.

CHECKLIST

Tips for Prevention of Skiing Injuries

- Have bindings adjusted regularly
- Use modern poles without top or bottom platforms
- Take lessons to develop good technique
- Maintain good conditioning and hydration
- Use a helmet

CHECKLIST

Tips for Prevention of Snowboarding Injuries

- Wear protective gloves with wrist guards
- All beginners should take lessons
- Avoid hard boots for beginners
- Use a helmet

The Role of Bindings

Automatic release of the binding from its attachment to the ski is a crucial mechanism to prevent injuries. Retention of the ski at the time of fall can create high rotational forces across the lower extremity, which can lead to knee and other lower extremity injuries. Several studies have shown high rates of nonrelease of skis during ski injuries.[3] Proper adjustment of bindings is a complex function that can be crucial in attaining proper release. Regular maintenance and readjustment is important to prevention of injury.

Better binding designs may also help to reduce injury risk. New designs of ski bindings and boots are emerging which are better designed to allow multidirectional release of skis. These designs have not been studied but may be effective in reducing risks.

COMMON SKIING INJURIES

Hip and Femur Injuries

Lateral falls on a ski slope can result in a direct blow to the hip or a twisting injury to the leg. In an older skier with osteoporotic bone, a fracture of the hip or femur can occur. Although these are fairly rare injuries, they may become more common as the ranks of older skiers increase.

Younger patients involved in high-speed collisions and falls can also sustain hip dislocations or fractures of the hip and femur. Most of these injuries require prompt reduction and internal fixation.

Knee Injuries

The knee represents the most common area of injury in ski accidents, encompassing up to 25% to 30% of all ski injuries. High- and low-velocity mechanisms can result in significant damage to the skier's knee.

The anterior cruciate ligament is a particularly vulnerable structure that is commonly torn in skiers. Ski boots act to connect the leg to the rigid structure of the ski. The long lever arm imparted by twisting of the ski creates excessive torsional forces around the knee. Although bindings are designed to release and protect the knee, much force can be transmitted before binding release. Poorly fitted bindings further increase the risk of injury. A history of a knee injury with an audible "pop" and immediate knee swelling is highly suggestive of an ACL tear and should be investigated with a MRI evaluation in most cases. Although both conservative and surgical options exist for skiers with ACL tears, most patients will benefit from ACL reconstruction procedures. Injuries to other soft-tissue structures such as the MCL and menisci are also common in ski accidents, either in association with or separate from ACL tears.

High-speed mechanisms can also produce more severe injuries. Tears of the posterior cruciate ligament (PCL) are rare, but can occur with direct blows to the knee. Severe angular stress to the knee can also produce tibial plateau fractures in high-energy trauma.

Tibia Fractures

Changes in boot design have dramatically reduced the incidence of tibial fractures in the last 20 years. Lower-cut boots place an extreme amount of stress on the relatively weak bone of the distal tibia. A change to modern, higher boots shifted the location of injury to the stronger midshaft tibial bone. These boots have virtually eliminated lower tibia and ankle injuries on the ski slope. Although these "boot-top" fractures in adults have decreased in incidence, tibia fractures are still common in the pediatric skiing population. These fractures are a result of rotational forces across the bone and typically are in a spiral-type pattern.[2] Treatment of all tibia fractures depends on the age of the patient, nature of the fracture, and medical condition of the patient. Many of these fractures require operative intervention.

Shoulder Injuries

Injuries to the shoulder have been estimated to represent 11.4% of skiing injuries and 39.1% of upper extremity injuries, although this may be understated due to lack of reporting of these injuries at mountain sites. Many patients sustaining shoulder injuries are able to ski down the mountain and do not seek immediate medical care.

Most of these fractures are due to falls resulting in either trauma through an outstretched arm or directly to the shoulder. Virtually any traumatic injury can be the result of a ski fall. Rotator cuff strains, shoulder dislocations, acromioclavicular separations, and clavicle fractures are most common.[12] The treatment of each disorder is based on a multitude of factors related to the patient and severity of injury.

Skier's Thumb

Injury to the ulnar collateral ligament (UCL) of the thumb metacarpophalengeal joint may be the most common upper extremity injury in a skiing population and has been described as *skier's thumb*.[25] Also known as *gamekeeper's thumb*, this injury is the result of a ski pole forcing the thumb into an abducted and extended position. Use of ski poles with conforming grips and top plates have been shown to have an increased incidence of these injuries.[7] Most modern poles do not follow this design. Use of pole straps has not been shown to increase or decrease the incidence of UCL injuries.[7]

Diagnosis of UCL tears is suggested by tenderness and ecchymosis over the medial aspect of the MCP joint and confirmed by instability to radial stress in full extension. A MRI evaluation can also be helpful in confirming the location and severity of injury. Mild sprains typically respond well to splint immobilization if recognized and treated early. More severe ruptures with complete instability or bony avulsion fragments generally require early open repair.[8]

COMMON SNOWBOARDING INJURIES

Basic Demographics

The pattern of injuries seen in snowboarding is distributed more toward upper extremities than are injuries in skiers. Snowboarders possess somewhat limited vertical stability. Failure to balance on an uneven slope creates a natural tendency to fall directly forward or backwards. Beginner snowboarders typically injure the wrist and hand, and more experienced riders sustain trauma to the ankle and shoulder.[27]

Head Injuries

Although head injuries are still uncommon in snowboarding (6.5 per 100,000 skier visits), they occur more frequently than in skiers (3.8 per 100,000 skier visits) and with a mechanism requiring less velocity.[19] The predominant mechanism of serious head injury in snowboarding is related to a backwards fall resulting in the contact of the occiput with the snow slope. Many of these occur on beginner slopes at low speed.[20] The use of helmets has been discussed previously and should be considered strongly by all snowboarders.

Hand and Wrist Injuries

Forward falls to the slope are extremely common in snowboarding due to the careful balance required to stay upright while riding on uneven slopes. Injuries to the wrist are the most common snowboarding injury, representing over 30% of all reported injuries.[16] Most of these injuries occur during a backwards fall to an outstretched arm.[6] Other injuries to the hand such as ligament tears, metacarpal fractures, and finger dislocations, have been reported but are relatively uncommon. Fractures of the distal radius are seen frequently, with beginners being more prone to these injuries.[9] Most of these fractures require reduction and many require operative treatment.

The use of wrist protectors has been shown to be highly protective in several studies and is highly recommended for all snowboarders, especially beginners. Although fractures can occur even while using protective wrist guards, there has been shown to be a two to four times reduction in wrist fractures associated with their use.[16,23]

Foot and Ankle Injuries

High torsional forces combined with impacts from hard landings create a high incidence of foot and ankle injuries in snowboarders. Estimated to represent about 17% of injuries, foot and ankle trauma can create a wide variety of sprains and fractures. These fractures are more common in intermediate rather than beginner snowboarders, which is likely reflective of jumping as an underlying mechanism.[6]

Fractures of the lateral process of the talus are relatively common (up to 15% of all snowboarding ankle injuries) and difficult to diagnose. These fractures occur from forced ankle dorsiflexion with hindfoot inversion and are especially rare as non-snowboarding injuries. Pain and swelling over the lateral aspect of the ankle can be easily misdiagnosed as a simple ankle sprain. Plain film radiographs are often negative. CT imaging is recommended for diagnosis and assessment of these fractures. Nondisplaced fractures are treated with cast immobilization, but displaced fractures may require open reduction and internal fixation. Failure to recognize these injuries can result in persistent ankle pain.[22]

Numerous types of boots (soft, hard) and bindings (buckles, sole-mount) exist for snowboards; however, none have been shown to influence the rate of foot and ankle injury.[11] Use of hard-shell boots by novice riders has shown some increase in tibia and knee fractures and is generally not recommended.[1]

REFERENCES

1. Bladin C, Giddings P, Robinson M: Australian snowboard injury data base study. A four-year prospective study. Am J Sports Med 21(5):701–704, 1993.
2. Blitzer CM, et al: Downhill skiing injuries in children. Am J Sports Med12(2):142–147, 1984.
3. Bouter LM, Knipschild PG, Volovics A: Binding function in relation to injury risk in downhill skiing. Am J Sports Med 17(2):226–233, 1989.
4. Cherpitel CJ, Meyers AR, Perrine MW: Alcohol consumption, sensation seeking and ski injury: A case-control study. J Stud Alcohol 59(2): 216–221, 1998.
5. Commission, U.C.P.S: Skiing Helmets: An Evaluation of the Potential to Reduce Head Injury. Washington, DC, 1999.
6. Davidson TM, Laliotis AT: Snowboarding injuries, a four-year study with comparison with alpine ski injuries. West J Med 164(3):231–237, 1996.
7. Engkvist O, Balkfors B, Lindsjo U: Thumb injuries in downhill skiing. Int J Sports Med 3(1):50–55, 1982.
8. Fricker R, Hintermann B: Skier's thumb. Treatment, prevention and recommendations. Sports Med 19(1):73–79, 1995.
9. Idzikowski JR, Janes PC, Abbott PJ: Upper extremity snowboarding injuries. Ten-year results from the Colorado snowboard injury survey. Am J Sports Med 28(6):825–832, 2000.
10. Jorgensen UFT, Haraszuk JP, et al: Reduction of injuries in downhill skiing by use of an instructional ski-video: A prospective randomized intervention study. Knee Surg Sports Traumatol Arthrosc 6:194–200, 1998.
11. Kirkpatrick DP, et al: The snowboarder's foot and ankle. Am J Sports Med 26(2):271–277, 1998.
12. Kocher MS, Feagin JA Jr: Shoulder injuries during alpine skiing. Am J Sports Med 24(5):665–669, 1996.
13. Koehle MS, Lloyd-Smith R, Taunton JE: Alpine ski injuries and their prevention. Sports Med 32(12):785–793, 2002.
14. Langran M, Selvaraj S: Snow sports injuries in Scotland: A case-control study. Br J Sports Med 36(2):135–140, 2002.
15. Levy AS, et al: An analysis of head injuries among skiers and snowboarders. J Trauma 53(4):695–704, 2002.
16. Machold W, et al: Risk of injury through snowboarding. J Trauma 48(6):1109–1114, 2000.
17. Macnab AJ, et al: Effect of helmet wear on the incidence of head/face and cervical spine injuries in young skiers and snowboarders. Injury Prev 8(4):324–327, 2002.

18. Morrow PL, Adesina A: Ski fatalities in Vermont. J Trauma 31(1):150, 1991.
19. Nakaguchi H, et al: Snowboard head injury: Prospective study in Chino, Nagano, for two seasons from 1995 to 1997. J Trauma 46(6):1066–1069, 1999.
20. Nakaguchi H, Tsutsumi K: Mechanisms of snowboarding-related severe head injury: Shear strain induced by the opposite-edge phenomenon. J Neurosurg 97(3):542–548, 2002.
21. Page CE, et al: Avalanche deaths in the United States: A 45-year analysis. Wilderness Environ Med 10(3):146–151, 1999.
22. Platz A, Sommer C: [A typical snowboarding injury—Fracture of the processus lateralis tali]. Ther Umsch 57(12):756–759, 2000.
23. Ronning R, et al: The efficacy of wrist protectors in preventing snowboarding injuries. Am J Sports Med 29(5):581–585, 2001.
24. Ronning R, Gerner T, Engebretsen L: Risk of injury during alpine and telemark skiing and snowboarding. The equipment-specific distance-correlated injury index. Am J Sports Med 28(4):506–508, 2000.
25. Shephard GJ, Saab M, Ali KH: Upper limb injuries in dry ski slope skiing—A continuing problem. Eur J Emerg Med 7(1):31–34, 2000.
26. Tough SC, Butt JC: A review of fatal injuries associated with downhill skiing. Am J Forensic Med Pathol 14(1):12–16, 1993.
27. Zollinger H, Gorschewsky O, Cathrein P: [Injuries in snowboarding—a prospective study]. Sportverletz Sportschaden 8(1):31–37, 1994.

41 Swimming Injuries

Steven Arsht, Giles R. Scuderi, and Peter D. McCann

It is estimated that more than 100 million Americans of all ages participate in the sport of swimming. The increasing popularity of masters swimming and triathlon competition has played an important role in the sport's continued growth. Many who swim are competitive athletes, but others swim simply for fitness or recreation. Although the vast majority of injuries incurred by the swimmer involve the shoulder, injury to the elbow, knee, foot and ankle, and lumbar spine also can occur and result in varying degrees of disability that may prevent the athlete from competing.[8,11,14]

THE SHOULDER

Shoulder injuries are not uncommon in swimming athletes and have been reported to occur in 15% to 80% of competitive swimmers over the course of a career and at all levels of participation.[2,22] Shoulder problems in swimmers appear to be more prevalent than in other athletes who routinely perform overhead activity as part of their sport. In a study of elite athletes, shoulder problems were reported in 66% of swimmers, compared to only 57% of professional baseball pitchers, 44% of collegiate volleyball players, and 29% of collegiate javelin throwers.[11] Although swimming is essentially a nonimpact activity with few inherent risks, the repetitive motions required to propel the body through the water predispose the athlete to overuse problems.[3,6,9,13,22,27,28] Unlike other sports, the swimmer's shoulder functions in a continuous fashion, in sequence, and without time for the shoulder girdle musculature to rest and recover. Furthermore, it has been estimated that 90% of the propulsive force in swimming is generated by the upper extremity.[5] Swimmers at the elite level generally practice 20 to 30 hours a week, and competitive athletes may swim 10,000 to 14,000 meters a day, 6 to 7 days a week. To accomplish this, roughly 2500 shoulder revolutions a day and 16,000 revolutions a week are performed. During a year's time, the average top-level swimmer will perform more than 500,000 stroke revolutions per arm. This may be doubled in those who swim for distance. This continuous movement puts a great deal of stress on the shoulder and can lead to muscular fatigue, inefficient and faulty stroke mechanics, and injury to the soft tissues from repetitive microtrauma. Shoulder pain in the swimming athlete can be especially problematic when it interferes with training progress and hinders performance.[3,6,9,13,22,27,28]

The innumerable repetitions required of the shoulder over many years of hard training combined with an increasing muscular imbalance around the shoulder girdle appear to be the main etiologic factors in the development of the overuse syndrome known as "swimmer's shoulder." Swimmer's shoulder was first described by Kennedy and Hawkins in 1974, and was regarded as an outlet impingement syndrome that resulted in a tendinitis of the musculotendinous cuff or biceps tendon due to repeated impingement under the coracoacromial arch,[13] and for many years, shoulder pain in swimming athletes has been considered to be synonymous with coracoacromial impingement. More recently, however, it has been proposed that swimmers may not have a true outlet impingement, but an impingement that occurs because of abnormal glenohumeral laxity, which places stress upon the tendons of the rotator cuff.[1,3,9,10,17,18,21,28–31,33] Furthermore, periscapular muscle fatigue and dysfunction result in an abnormal scapular humeral rhythm that causes a malpositioning of the glenoid platform during the swimmer's stroke.[16] This dynamic anatomic alteration creates increased stress and strain on the anterior capsular structures, which can lead to increased laxity and excessive anterior glenohumeral translation with secondary impingement of the rotator cuff. As all of this continues over time, injury to the rotator cuff, biceps tendon, and anterior capsulolabral complex can develop.[1,3,9,10,17,18,21,28–31,33] If allowed to progress without treatment, the athlete may develop diffuse and debilitating shoulder pain and be at increased risk for irreversible structural damage to the shoulder. Internal impingement of the rotator cuff on the posterosuperior glenoid rim and a strength imbalance between the internal and external rotators of the shoulder may also be contributing factors in the development of swimmer's shoulder.[19,20,23,26,34,35]

DIAGNOSIS

History

The swimmer with a painful shoulder often does not recall a specific traumatic event. The progression of symptoms is rather insidious, and the swimmer often mistakes a true injury for general activity-related muscle soreness, and may try to swim through the pain. A gradual reduction in shoulder range of motion can occur as the inflammation progresses, and the swimmer will attempt to compensate for the injury by avoiding painful positions that aggravate the symptoms. Subtle changes in stroke mechanics such as the swimmer's hand entering the water wide and flat, an excessive trunk roll leading into an early hand exit, or a dropped elbow in the recovery phase may be detected by a vigilant coaching staff and can be indicative of an underlying injury. The careful observer might also notice that the swimmer's pull may be slightly asymmetric because the painful shoulder cannot generate a propulsive force comparable to the contralateral side. As a result, the swimmer may have some difficulty remaining in the center of the lane, and a gradual decrease in velocity with longer finishing times may also be observed.[28]

Swimmers will frequently localize their pain to the antero-superior aspect of the shoulder. However, as the inflammation worsens, a more diffuse soreness about the shoulder is reported and is often a sign of a chronic, ongoing process with a higher likelihood of structural damage to the rotator cuff, biceps tendon, or anterior capsulolabral complex. The most painful phase of the freestyle stroke, and the phase in which the vast majority of symptoms occur, is the first half of pull-through, when the greatest propulsive force is generated and the arm unilaterally pulls the body through the water. Symptoms are also reported to a lesser degree around mid-recovery, when humeral hyperextension can aggravate conditions related to anterior impingement, capsular inflammation, and labral damage.[22,28,35] The swimmer may also report that the shoulder pain is exacerbated by increasing the intensity of a workout and by swimming longer distances.[35]

Examination

The shoulder is typically normal in appearance. Anterior or antero-lateral shoulder tenderness is often present. Tenderness over the biceps tendon in the intertubercular groove and positive Speed's test is suggestive of biceps tendinopathy. Tenderness over the supraspinatus tendon at its insertion to the greater tuberosity and a positive impingement sign/test is indicative of rotator cuff tendinitis and subacromial bursitis. The presence of scapular dyskinesia, winging, and early and excessive scapular motion or lateral scapular slide can be indicative of a weak serratus anterior muscle and periscapular muscular dysfunction.[16] Deficits in external rotation strength should be noted. A thorough musculoskeletal evaluation for the presence of generalized ligamentous laxity should be performed. Increased glenohumeral translation in the antero-inferior direction may be present. Frank anterior or posterior instability is generally not a problem.

Imaging Studies

X-rays of the shoulder are typically normal but should be reviewed to ensure that an unusual anatomic variant is not present. Magnetic resonance imaging is of little diagnostic yield and, in general, is not beneficial in the evaluation of a swimmer's shoulder. Although signal changes within the musculotendinous cuff are not uncommon, clinically significant partial thickness and full-thickness tears are rarely seen in young competitive swimmers. A greater degree of rotator cuff and biceps tendon pathology may be seen, however, in the middle-aged and more senior swimmers. A gadolinium-enhanced MRI may be useful in evaluating anterior capsulolabral damage in a swimmer who routinely performs the backstroke, because this subgroup is more prone to injury in this region.

Treatment

The vast majority of shoulder problems in the swimmer are amenable to conservative treatment. The timely reporting of shoulder pain allows for a more specific diagnosis to be made and a more directed treatment plan to be devised. Conservative treatment is likely to be more effective if intervention occurs early. A delay in reporting allows for the inflammation and structural damage to progress. The condition is then more difficult to treat, takes the athlete longer to recover from, and is perhaps responsible for the high rate of recurrence of shoulder injuries in swimmers.[35] A supervised course of physical therapy focusing on general strengthening and conditioning of the musculature of the shoulder girdle is critical. Maintenance of flexibility and restoration of strength, endurance, and scapulohumeral rhythm are essential. Any imbalance in muscle strength or specific muscle group weakness should be noted and an appropriate exercise program instituted. Particular attention should be given to the conditioning of the serratus anterior and subscapularis muscles because they are prone to fatigue and play an important role in normal shoulder function.[3,16,23,34,35] Fatigue and weakness of these muscles can lead to muscle imbalance and altered stroke mechanics that put the swimmer at risk for further injury.[1–3,21]

An important component to the swimmer's recovery is the timely elimination of the painful, and often debilitating, inflammatory process. Relative rest, avoidance of activities or positions that cause pain in the shoulder, and oral anti-inflammatory medication are important in the acute convalescent period. Other modalities such as cryotherapy, ultrasound, and electrostimulation are useful adjuncts. If it is not painful to do so, the patient may swim provided that the strokes performed do not exacerbate symptoms. Heavy-resistance overhead weight training and the use of hand paddles should be avoided. Legwork should be emphasized. Kickboards may put the shoulder in a pain-provoking position and should be used cautiously. Out-of-water cross-training should be encouraged. Running, cycling, or the use of an elliptical machine can maintain cardiovascular status and augment a limited swimming workout. A subacromial injection of corticosteroid can be helpful in decreasing the local inflammatory process. To receive the maximal benefit of this medication, the athlete should refrain from swimming for 2 to 3 weeks after the injection is administered. These medications should never be used routinely. In the presence of rotator cuff pathology and persistent inflammation, surgical intervention may be necessary. In refractory cases, the athlete may have to consider changing the stroke or retiring from the sport. A successful rehabilitation program should allow for the gradual return to a full training schedule without pain or alteration in stroke mechanics. Restoration of the athlete's preinjury level of function and return to competition should be achieved in a timely fashion. Once the athlete returns to swimming, a training program emphasizing balanced muscle strengthening, flexibility, and avoidance of overwork, along with careful surveillance by the coaching staff, ongoing stroke analysis, and technique modification to ensure proper stroke mechanics is necessary to minimize the chance of recurrent injury.[7]

ELBOW

The high elbow position used by competitive swimmers during the arm-pull phase can place excessive stress on the elbow over time. Swimmers performing the butterfly and breaststrokes are more commonly afflicted than those swimming freestyle. The repetition of the stroke can result in excessive muscle contractions and extrinsic overload, resulting in fatigue and inflammation of the extensor carpi radialis brevis and the extensor communis. The swimmer typically complains of a burning lateral elbow pain. Tenderness is present over the lateral epicondyle approximately 5 mm distal and anterior to the midpoint of the condyle. Symptoms are exacerbated by resisted wrist and long finger dorsiflexion with the elbow extended and the forearm flexed. Plain radiographs are often negative but should be obtained to rule out other pathology. MRI can demonstrate tendon thickening and further delineate the underlying pathoanatomy in chronic cases, but typically is not indicated. The differential diagnosis includes posterior interosseus nerve intrapment, osteochondritis dissecans of the capitellum, injury to the radial head, and cervical radiculopathy, and should be considered when evaluating the athlete for lateral elbow pain.

Lateral epicondylitis in the swimmer is treated with rest, ice, anti-inflammatory medicine, ultrasound, and physical therapy, with particular attention paid to forearm extensor power, flexibility, and endurance. Local corticosteroid injection may be necessary in cases that are slow to respond. Surgical intervention may be required in recalcitrant cases, but only after all other conservative measures have been exhausted.[4,25]

KNEE PAIN

Knee pain in the swimmer is generally localized to the medial side and often attributed to medial collateral ligament stress syndrome, synovitis, with or without a hypertrophic medial synovial plica, and patellofemoral syndrome.[8,12,14,15] A relationship between the development of medial knee pain and advancing age, increased years of competition, increased training distance, and decreased warm-up distance has been established.[12,15] Knee pain is most commonly seen in those who perform the breaststroke and use the whip kick. The whip kick serves as the most efficient kick to the swimmer for speed and propulsion; however, it subjects the knee to an unnatural motion with high angular velocity at the hip and knee and excessive outward rotation of the tibia relative to the femur, and places increased stress on the knee, resulting in injury. Limited internal rotation at the hip joint and abnormal hip abduction angles at the time of kick initiation may also play a role.[15]

Medial collateral ligament stress syndrome[12] is a common cause of pain in the elite breaststroker and examination will typically demonstrate tenderness to palpation along the course of the MCL, particularly at medial femoral epicondyle and distally where the superficial fibers cross the upper tibia. Pain also may be reproduced along the medial aspect of the knee when a valgus stress is applied with the knee in 20–30° of flexion.

Medial synovitis and medial synovial plica syndrome is not uncommon and has been detected by clinical exam and observed arthroscopically in swimmers with knee pain. The repetitive flexion and extension motion of the knee during the whip kick causes friction between the plica and the medial femoral condyle, precipitating inflammation and pain. The diagnosis is confirmed by palpating the thickened synovial shelf and reproducing the patient's painful symptoms when direct pressure is applied to the area.[15,32]

Patellofemoral syndrome, hypermobility, or instability of the patellofemoral joint can be a cause of knee pain in swimmers. Patella alta, tenderness over the patellar facets or lateral trochlear margin, pain with patellar compression, excessive patellar glide or hypermobility, and apprehension when a laterally directed force is applied to the patella with the knee in extension can be seen on physical exam and are helpful in making the diagnosis.

Treatment

Once the swimmer complains of knee pain, early intervention is mandatory. A thorough evaluation of stroke mechanics is imperative because the timely correction of faulty whip kick technique can lead to resolution of symptoms before excessive inflammation or structural changes occur. A detailed history and physical exam should be performed. Anatomic factors such as ligamentous insufficiency or patellofemoral instability may render the knee incapable of withstanding the stresses of the whip kick, and the swimmer may simply need to find a more suitable stroke.

Reducing or eliminating breaststroke training distance along with an alteration in the swimmer's kick technique should be the first step in treating knee pain.[12,15,32,36] A supervised course of physical therapy to work on general strengthening and conditioning of the musculature of the hips and knees should be undertaken. Stretching exercises to increase hip rotation are also helpful. Cryotherapy, ultrasound, and anti-inflammatory medication are useful adjuncts. Corticosteroid injections should be used sparingly and may have some role in the treatment of a pathologic, hypertrophic synovial plica.[32]

The breaststroke training distance should be increased gradually in the early season, and warm-up distance should be adequate to help minimize the occurrence of breaststroker's knee. If an injury should develop, the stroke may be reintroduced slowly, after an adequate period of rest, closely monitored by the coaching staff or trainer to prevent recurrence.[12,15,32,36]

Although these conditions are the most commonly observed, knee pain in the swimmer can be multifactorial and the physician is obligated to evaluate for and rule out the possibility of other potential causes such as meniscal or chondral injury and ligamentous insufficiency.

FOOT AND ANKLE

Tendinopathy of the extensor tendons of the foot and ankle is a common cause of pain in the swimmer.[8,14] These tendons are bound dorsally by the extensor retinaculum, enclosed in sheaths, and susceptible to irritation, particularly with the repetitive motion seen with the flutter and dolphin kicks, rapidly alternating the foot between the positions of extreme plantarflexion and neutral. Local irritation of the tendons precipitates a cycle of inflammation and edema, which leads to additional painful impingement on the retinaculum when the swimmer kicks.

Swimmers will complain of pain with kicking and with active dorsiflexion of the foot. Palpable, and even audible, crepitus may be appreciated when the foot is passively brought from plantarflexion to dorsiflexion.

Prevention should be stressed, with emphasis on routine extensor tendon stretching before swimming. Swimming can continue with diminished or no kicking, and the swimmer may gauge the amount based upon the presence or absence of symptoms. Rest, cryotherapy, anti-inflammatory medication, physical therapy, and ultrasound are helpful in treating this disorder. A walking boot may be applied in severe or refractory cases. A gradual return to normal kicking, with the swimmer staying below the level of pain, is recommended.

BACK

Swimmers performing the breast and butterfly strokes have a tendency to accentuate the lordotic posture of the lumbar spine, which places additional and abnormal stress on the lumbar spine. This repetitive hyperextension can lead to a variety of low back problems such as a stress fracture of the pars interarticularis or even a frank spondylolisthesis.[24,37] Typically, however, it is the exacerbation of a mildly symptomatic spondylolisthesis or posterior facet irritation causing mechanical low back pain that is sufficiently problematic to curtail the swimmer's training. The differential diagnosis of low back pain in swimmers should include muscle and ligament sprains, facet joint injury, herniated disc, spondylolysis, Scheuerman disease, infection, and tumor.

Findings on examination suggestive of a spondylolisthesis include hamstring tightness, a palpable step-off at the L5-S1 junction, and an abnormal gait with a posterior pelvic tilt. The diagnosis is confirmed by x-ray, but if no obvious fracture or deformity is seen, a bone scan or MRI is helpful to identify a pars interarticularis stress fracture and to rule out the possibility of a herniated nucleus propulsus, a condition seen more frequently in older swimmers.

If a stress fracture is identified, the mainstay of treatment is activity modification and rest. Bracing is not necessary. Management of a spondylolisthesis is symptomatic and depends on the degree of deformity and the severity of the complaints. A supervised course of physical therapy to work on general strengthening and conditioning of the trunk muscles, with particular attention to abdominal strengthening and hamstring stretching, is critical. If the source of pain is related to posterior facet irritation or paraspinal muscle spasm, a similar rehabilitation program should be followed. Additional modalities such as cryotherapy, ultrasound, transcutaneous nerve stimulation, and oral anti-inflammatory medicines are useful adjuncts. A corticosteroid injection of an inflamed facet joint may be required for pain relief in recalcitrant cases.[24,37]

SUMMARY

Many of the injuries seen in swimmers are overuse syndromes related to repetitive microtrauma. A vigilant coaching staff that can provide ongoing stroke analysis and correct faulty stroke mechanics or recognize the early stages of injury is important. Once a swimmer complains of pain or an injury is evident, a thorough diagnostic evaluation is mandatory. Conservative management is generally sufficient to treat the majority of injuries that occur. Early recognition of injury, adherence to a structured rehabilitation program, and communication among physician, patient, coaching staff, and therapist are essential in allowing swimmers to overcome injury and return to their preinjury level of function in a timely fashion.

REFERENCES

1. Bak K: Nontraumatic glenohumeral instability and coracoacromial impingement in swimmers. Scand J Med Sci Sports 6(3):132–144, 1996.
2. Bak K, Faunl P: Clinical findings in competitive swimmers with shoulder pain. Am J Sports Med 25:254–260, 1997.
3. Bak K, and Magnusson SP. Shoulder strength and range of motion in symptomatic and pain-free elite swimmers. Am J Sports Med 25:454–459, 1997.
4. Ciccotti MG. Epicondylitis in the athlete. Instruct Course Lect 48:375–381, 1999.
5. Councilman JE: Swimming power. Swimming World and Junior Swimmer 18:30, 1977.
6. Fowler PJ: Shoulder injuries in the mature athlete. Adv Sports Med Fitness 1:225–238, 1988.
7. Fowler PJ: Swimming. In Fu F, Stone D (ed): Sports Injuries: Mechanism, Prevention, and Treatment, 2nd ed. Philadelphia, Lippincott Williams and Wilkins, 2001, pp 733–734.
8. Fowler PJ, Regan WD: Swimming injuries of the knee, foot and ankle, elbow, and back. Clin Sports Med 5:139, 1986.
9. Fowler PJ, Webster MS: Shoulder pain in highly competitive swimmers. Orthop Trans 7:170, 1983.
10. Jobe CM, Pink MM, Jobe FW, et al: Anterior shoulder instability, impingement, and rotator cuff tear: Theories and concepts. In Jobe FW (ed): Operative Techniques in Upper Extremity Sports Injuries. St. Louis, Mosby-Year Book, 1996, pp 164–176.
11. Johnson D: Swimming, shoulder the burden. Sportcare Fitness May/June:24–30, 1988.
12. Kennedy JC, Hawkins RJ: Breaststroker's knee. Phys Sports Med 2:33, 1974.
13. Kennedy JC, Hawkins RJ: Swimmer's shoulder. Phys Sports Med 2:35, 1974.
14. Kennedy JC, Hawkins RJ, Krissoff WB: Orthopaedic manifestations of swimming. Am J Sports Med 6:309–322, 1978.
15. Keskinen K, Eriksson E, Komi P: Breaststroke swimmer's knee. A biomechanical and arthroscopic study. Am J Sports Med 8:228–231, 1980.
16. Kibler WB: The role of the scapula in athletic shoulder function. Am J Sports Med 26(2):325–337, 1998.
17. McMaster WC: Anterior glenoid damage: A painful lesion in swimmers. Am J Sports Med 14:383–387, 1986.
18. McMaster WC: Painful shoulder in swimmers: A diagnostic challenge. Phys Sports Med 12:108–122, 1986.
19. McMaster WC, Long SC, Caiozzo VJ: Isokinetic torque imbalances in the rotator cuff of the elite water polo player. Am J Sports Med 19:72–75, 1991.
20. McMaster WC, Long SC, Caiozzo VJ: Shoulder torque in the swimming athlete. Am J Sports Med 20:323–327, 1992.
21. McMaster WC, Roberts A, Stoddard T: A correlation between shoulder laxity and interfereing pain in competitive swimmers. Am J Sports Med 26(1):83–86, 1998.
22. McMaster WC, Troup J: A survey of interfering shoulder pain in United States competitive swimmers. Am J Sports Med 21:67–70, 1993.
23. Nuber GW, Jobe FW, Perry J, et al: Fine wire electromyography analysis of muscles of the shoulder during swimming. Am J Sports Med 14:7–11, 1986.
24. Nyska M, Constantin, N, Cale-Benzoor M, et al: Spondylolysis as a cause of low back pain in swimmers. Int J Sports Med 21(5):375–379, 2000.
25. Peters T, Baker CL: Lateral epicondylitis. Clin Sports Med 20(3):549–563, 2001.
26. Pink M, Perry J, Browne A, et al: The normal freestyle swimming: An electromyographic and cinematographic analysis of twelve muscles. Am J Sports Med 19:569–576, 1991.
27. Pink MM, Jobe FW: Biomechanics of swimming. In Zachazewski JE, Magee DJ, Quillen WS (eds): Athletic Injuries and Rehabilitation. Philadelphia, WB Saunders, 1996, pp 317–331.
28. Pink MM Tibone J: The painful shoulder in the swimming athlete. Orthop Clin North Am 31(2): 247–261, 2000.
29. Richardson AB: The biomechanics of swimming. The knee and shoulder. Clin Sports Med 5:103–113, 1986.
30. Richardson AB: Overuse syndromes in baseball, tennis, gymnastics, and swimming. Clin Sports Med 2:379–390, 1983.
31. Richardson AB, Jobe FW, Collins WR: The shoulder in competitive swimming. Am J Sports Med 8:159–163, 1980.
32. Rovere GD and Nichols AW: Frequency, associated factors, and treatment of breaststroker's knee in competitive swimmers. Am J Sports Med13:99–104, 1985.
33. Rupp S, Berninger K, Hopf T: Shoulder problems in high level swimmers: Impingement, anterior

instability, muscular imbalance? Int J Sports Med 16:557–562, 1995.

34. Scovazzo ML, Browne A, Pink M, et al: The painful shoulder during freestyle swimming: An electromyographic and cinematographic analysis of twelve muscles. Am J Sports Med 19:577–582, 1991.
35. Stocker D, Pink MM, Jobe FW: Comparison of shoulder injury in collegiate and master's-level swimmers. Clin J Sports Med 5:4–8, 1995.
36. Vizsolyi P, Taunton J, Robertson G, et al: Breaststroker's knee. An analysis of epidemiologic and biomechanical factors. Am J Sports Med 15:63–71, 1987.
37. Wilson FD, Linseth RE: The adolescent swimmer's back. Am J Sports Med 10:174–176, 1982.

42 Racquet Sports Injuries

Andrew L. Rosen, Giles R. Scuderi, and Peter D. McCann

The different varieties of sports employing racquets are very popular across the world and are enjoyed by many age groups. Unlike many sports, racquet sports can be played by much older individuals who continue their play well into their geriatric years. Tennis, racquetball, squash, and badminton share similar rules and mechanics of play. Injuries sustained in these sports are also the result of similar mechanisms.

These sports are noncontact-type activities involving rapid motions of the body and repetitive motion of the upper extremity during a racquet swing. These mechanisms result in both acute injuries and chronic overuse syndromes in both upper and lower extremities. Younger players are more prone to explosive motions and diving racquet swings and sustain more traumatic injuries. Older players are more susceptible to chronic stress-related disorders. As these sports enjoy participation by both men and women players, some gender-related differences may play a role in racquet sports injuries.

SPECIFIC SPORTS

Tennis is played on a large court (78 feet × 27 or 36 feet) constructed of hard court, clay, or grass. Large distances involved in the sport require forceful swings and large rotational movements of the torso to generate the power and spin required to create effective shots. Singles tennis (two players against each other) generally requires greater effort with longer distances traveled to reach shots. Doubles (two teams of two players) tennis allows less exertion as players share the coverage of the court and balls returned.

Badminton shares similar characteristics to tennis with an individual area of play for each player (total court size 44 feet × 20 feet) and long racquets. The game originated in England and spread worldwide. Although competitive badminton is uncommonly played in the United States, it is very popular in some countries in Asia and Europe. Because the play typically involves long volleying periods, there are greater numbers of racquet swings and greater distances traveled on the court. This may predispose players to greater numbers of overuse-type injuries.[7] Achilles tendinitis and lateral epicondylitis are the most common injuries seen in badminton players.[8]

Racquetball and squash share similar court configurations and play dynamics. The courts measure 40 feet by 20 feet for racquetball and 32 feet by 16½ feet for squash. Unlike tennis and badminton, the margins of the court are lined with walls that are used during play. Another important difference is that both players stay on the same side of the court during squash and racquetball play, alternating shots. These differences create more opportunities for direct traumatic injuries. Players are in close proximity to each other and to the unforgiving side walls of the court. This can lead to inadvertent contact and injury. Head and facial injuries are much more common than in the other sports. The fast speed and unpredictable nature of the ball striking the sidewalls also leads to greater potential for eye injuries.[18]

PREVENTION

The most important factor in avoidance of the most common racquet sports injuries is adherence to basic principles for preventing overuse injuries. Most injuries occur in players who play infrequent matches or practice for long durations. Gradually increasing the duration and frequency of play is critical to avoid repetitive stress injuries.[2] Older players are especially at risk for injury sustained by failure to slowly increase activities.

Improvements in flexibility are helpful in injury prevention. A short stretching period prior to play can help avoid muscular strains common in the ballistic motions required to play racquet sports. In particular, hamstring, shoulder, and lower back stretches are most important. Participating in a reasonable warm-up period prior to aggressive play also is a good practice.

Proper muscular and cardiovascular conditioning can also be important in prevention of injuries in physically demanding racquet sports. A program emphasizing fitness, endurance, and strengthening can be helpful at both recreational and competitive levels.[3]

Another factor in injury avoidance is prevention and correction of technique errors in the racquet sport. Abnormalities in racquet swing mechanics can lead to disorders such as lateral epicondylitis. Sport-specific instruction addressing proper techniques for the grip and stroke can act to prevent and treat such injuries. In racquetball and squash, it is important to learn proper court position to avoid contact with the ball and other players. Instruction in some basic techniques can play a role in prevention of acute traumatic injuries.

The use of proper equipment also can be important in prevention of racquet sports injuries. The use of an improperly sized racquet grip can lead to the need for excessive grip tension, which can create an overuse injury in the arm. Lighter racquets with less string tension can also reduce the amount of force required to swing and reduce the stress to the upper extremity. Use of shoes designed for the lateral motions and cutting maneuvers required in racquet sports can also help to avoid injuries to the foot and ankle.

Court surfaces that act to lower the speed of the ball, such as clay and grass, may also reduce stroke force and help avoid overuse injuries.[6] Players can also become acclimated to specific surfaces. A slow introduction to new court surfaces can prevent injuries that can develop while the player adapts to new biomechanical forces.[2]

SHOULDER

A racquet swing requires complex interactions of numerous muscular units to create a controlled motion of the ball. Repetitive motions of the shoulder, each generating strong biomechanical forces, are required for the play of racquet sports. These activities can lead to repetitive microtrauma and overuse injuries to the shoulder. These injuries to the shoulder are well described in overhead throwing athletes. Although the specific mechanism of shoulder dysfunction is multifactorial in many patients, subacromial impingement, capsular laxity, internal impingement, and scapular imbalance represent the basic causes of shoulder disorders.[16]

Rotator cuff pathology is common in racquet sports participants. Inflammation of the cuff and bursal covering can occur as a result of the frequent amount of overhead activity required in serving and overhead volleys. This process can progress to degeneration of the tendon resulting in partial and full-thickness tears of the rotator cuff. Conservative treatment is often successful in patients with both impingement and small tears. Successful treatment is designed to decrease the inflammatory component of the pathology and restore strength and motion to the shoulder.[11] Subacromial steroid injections, anti-inflammatory agents, and physical therapy are the common methods for initial treatment.

Degeneration of the rotator cuff tissue can be a component of pain for older athletes. Full-thickness tears, while uncommon in young players, are more common in patients older than 50 years. Although conservative treatment is successful in many patients, some will require operative repair of the rotator cuff. Approached with either complete arthroscopic or arthroscopically assisted mini-open repairs, the majority of players are able to return to racquet sports following repairs.[1,19]

In younger players, shoulder pain is frequently related to laxity of the glenohumeral joint. Laxity of the glenohumeral capsule can allow abnormal translation and resulting pain. This subluxation of the shoulder can also create contact between the posterosuperior glenoid rim and the rotator cuff undersurface, described as "internal impingement."[14] Proper treatment should consist of physical therapy that addresses the underlying instability. Individuals who fail to respond to conservative treatment may require rotator cuff repair and surgical stabilization procedures.

Although traumatic injuries are rare in tennis and badminton, they occur more commonly in both racquetball and squash. Contact with court walls can result in acute injuries such as acromioclavicular separations and glenohumeral dislocations.

ELBOW

Epicondylitis, seen both laterally and medially, is a common elbow disorder seen in racquet sports players. Lateral epicondylitis, "tennis elbow," is more commonly seen with these activities. The swing of a racquet requires strong effort from the muscles used to stabilize the wrist.[12] These include the extensor carpi radialis brevis (ECRB), extensor carpi radialis longus (ECRL), and the extensor digitorum comminus (EDC). Microtears of the origin of the ECRB have been implicated in the onset of this disorder. Symptoms consist of pain over the lateral aspect of the dominant elbow that is exacerbated by use of the wrist and hand. Tenderness over the extensor origin on the lateral epicondyle and pain with resisted wrist extension are common physical exam findings.

Nonsurgical treatment consists of two phases, relief of pain and inflammation and tissue healing. Pain relief is accomplished with rest, ice, nonsteroidal anti-inflammatory agents, and steroid injections. Tissue healing occurs with careful, slow return to racquet swings and guided stretching and strengthening programs.[6] Counterforce "tennis elbow strap" and wrist extension bracing also can be used. Correction of grip and technique errors is important. Surgical treatment of lateral epicondylitis is uncommonly required and is reserved for players who have failed lengthy courses of conservative management.

Medial epicondylitis, "golfer's elbow," is rare in tennis players and describes similar symptoms and pathology on the medial aspect of the elbow. An injury involving stress of the flexor pronator origin, medial epicondylitis shares common characteristics with overuse injuries. Tenderness over the medial aspect of the elbow and pain with resisted wrist flexion and pronation are typical on physical exam. Treatment principles are similar to the lateral side, emphasizing anti-inflammatory treatment and guided rehabilitation.[6]

WRIST AND HAND

Pain in the hands and wrist is fairly common in racquet sports due to the grip intensity and wrist motion required to produce a swing. The dominant arm is typically affected. However, in players with a two-handed backhand swing, injury to the nondominant arm may occur. Most injuries are overuse injuries involving the extensors and flexors (less commonly) of the wrist. Treatment of tendinitis is directed toward the usual pattern of rest, ice, and anti-inflammatory treatment. Identification of the specific tendon involved can assist with directed treatment.[13]

Many other uncommon wrist disorders have been described in tennis players. These include fractures of the hook of the hamate, tears of the triangular fibrocartilage complex (TFCC), ulnar nerve compression, and ganglion cysts.[9] Traumatic injuries such as wrist and hand fractures are more common in racquetball and squash.

BACK

Disorders of the upper and lower back are common in frequent participants in racquet sports. A survey estimated 38% of competitive players missed at least one match because of pain in the lower back.[10] Repetitive rotational motions of the trunk may predispose players to overuse injuries of the muscles and spine. Although a single injury type is not defined, muscular overuse, mechanical low back pain, and lumbar disc disease have been described with racquet sports.[4] Treatment is typically conservative. Identification of the involved pathology and directed physical therapy represent the most common treatments.

HIP AND THIGH

Injuries to the hip and upper leg can occur from both overuse and acute strains. Injuries to the hip adductors and hamstrings are common from accidental motions sustained in slipping while reaching for a ball. These disorders are treated conservatively with rest, ice, and compression. Careful stretching and warm-up can help prevent these injuries.

KNEE

Racquet sports generally require some element of explosive motion of the body to reach shots and play competitively. These motions require significant twisting and flexion of the knees. Both overuse injuries and acute trauma are common in these sports. Patellofemoral pain syndrome and quadriceps and patellar tendinitis occur commonly in younger players and are generally treated with conservative treatment.[5] A change of play surface to a low-friction type such as clay can help treat and prevent some of these disorders. Hard concrete surfaces are more fatiguing and create greater forces with deceleration than softer types.[15]

Significant abrupt forces can create medial collateral ligament strains, meniscal tears, and, less commonly, anterior cruciate ligament injuries. Older players may develop degenerative meniscal and articular cartilage damage through racquet sport play. Many of these injuries require operative treatment.

FOOT AND ANKLE

Achilles tendinitis presents as pain in the posterior aspect of the calf and upper heel with play and, later, ambulation. These overuse injuries can be quite painful and are more common in older athletes. Treatment of tendinopathy consists of limitation of activity, ice, heel lifts, and a stretching program. Achilles tendon ruptures can occur with the sudden deceleration forces involved in racquet sports.[17]

Ankle sprains are very common due to the rapid pivoting and direction changes required in racquet sports.[2] Most are simple lateral ankle sprains which respond well to rest and bracing. Recurrent sprains often require physical therapy for strengthening and restoration of ankle proprioception. Taping and sports-type ankle braces can be effective in early return to sports.

"Tennis toe" is a disorder that is created by the severe deceleration motion required in racquet sports. A quick stop when traveling in a forward direction can result in sliding of the foot forward in the shoe, striking the distal portion. Injury to the nail bed and interphalangeal joints is common, resulting in subungual hematomas and painful toes. Changing tennis shoes and court surfaces can be effective in prevention of these injuries.

REFERENCES

1. Bigiliani LU, et al: Repair of rotator cuff tears in tennis players. Am J Sports Med 20(2):112–117, 1992.
2. Bylak J, Hutchinson MR: Common sports injuries in young tennis players. Sports Med 26(2):119–132, 1998.
3. Chandler TJ: Exercise training for tennis. Clin Sports Med 14(1):33–46, 1995.
4. Hainline B: Low back injury. Clin Sports Med 14(1):241–265, 1995.
5. Host JV, Craig R, Lehman RC: Patellofemoral dysfunction in tennis players: A dynamic problem. Clin Sports Med 14(1):177–203, 1995.
6. Jobe FW, Ciccotti MG: Lateral and medial epicondylitis of the elbow. J Am Acad Orthop Surg 2(1):1–8, 1994.
7. Jorgensen U, Winge S: Epidemiology of badminton injuries. Int J Sports Med 8(6):379–382, 1987.
8. Jorgensen U, Winge S: Injuries in badminton. Sports Med 10(1):P59–64, 1990.
9. Kulund DN, et al: Tennis injuries: Prevention and treatment: A review. Am J Sports Med 7(4):249–253, 1979.

10. Marks MR, Haas SS, Wiesel SW: Low back pain in the competitive tennis player. Clin Sports Med 7(2):277–287, 1988.
11. McCann PD, Bigliani LU: Shoulder pain in tennis players. Sports Med 17(1):53–64, 1994.
12. Morris M, et al: Electromyographic analysis of elbow function in tennis players. Am J Sports Med 17(2):241–247, 1989.
13. Osterman AL, Moskow L, Low DW: Soft-tissue injuries of the hand and wrist in racquet sports. Clin Sports Med 7(2):329–348, 1988.
14. Paley KJ, et al: Arthroscopic findings in the overhand throwing athlete: Evidence for posterior internal impingement of the rotator cuff. Arthroscopy 16(1):35–40, 2000.
15. Renstrom AF: Knee pain in tennis players. Clin Sports Med 14(1):163–175, 1995.
16. Ruotolo C, et al: Shoulder pain and the overhand athlete. Am J Orthop 32(5):248–258, 2003.
17. Saltzman CL, Tearse DS: Achilles tendon injuries. J Am Acad Orthop Surg 6(5):316–325, 1998.
18. Soderstrom CA, Doxanas MT: Racquetball. A game with preventable injuries. Am J Sports Med 10(3): 180–183, 1982.
19. Sonnery-Cottet B, et al: Rotator cuff tears in middle-aged tennis players: Results of surgical treatment. Am J Sports Med 30(4):558–564, 2002.

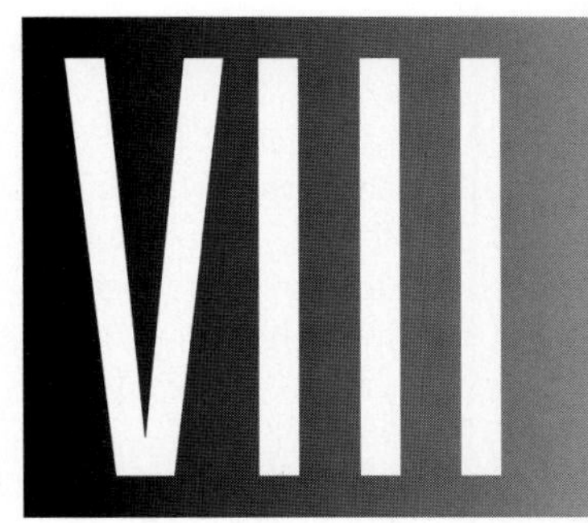

Rehabilitation

43 Rehabilitation Techniques and Therapeutic Modalities

David A. Gold, Michael Saunders, and Gordon Huie

In this chapter, the basic principles for various common techniques and therapeutic modalities in the rehabilitation of a sports medicine patient are discussed. The basic application of these modalities is also described.

In general, after a sports-related injury, the goal of the postinjury therapeutic period is to address pain, inflammation, stiffness, muscle weakness, and muscle spasm. These elements of the injured state can exist individually, but more commonly they are interrelated. Injury causes tissue inflammation, which in turn leads to pain, which may cause muscle spasm and joint stiffness.

Breaking this inflammation-pain-spasm cycle is crucial to a patient's early return to activities. There are certain treatment techniques and therapeutic modalities that can make it a smoother transition. Selection of the appropriate technique or modality is determined by the type of injury, its severity, and the goals of the patient.

The commonly performed treatment techniques available to the patient and therapist are immobilization, mechanical modalities, stretching, and continuous passive motion. The readily available therapeutic strategies are thermotherapy (heat treatments), cryotherapy (cold treatments), and electrical stimulation.

Each of these techniques and modalities is addressed in this chapter. Muscle physiology, exact rehabilitation protocols, the specifics of exercise regimens, and the pharmacology of rehabilitation are covered elsewhere in the text.

TREATMENT TECHNIQUES IN REHABILITATION

Immobilization

In sports, as well as in many activities of daily living, injuries to the extremities are quite common. Soft-tissue trauma, muscle strains, ligamentous injuries, cartilage damage, and bony fractures are frequently encountered. Immobilization of the affected extremity not only reduces pain, but also prevents further insult until a definitive diagnosis and treatment plan are established. Immobilization can be used to rest an injured or postoperative extremity during the healing phase because it assists in the resolution of swelling and in holding proximate injured tissues still during healing.

In the primary care setting, immobilization is most useful when treating an acutely injured extremity. Depending on the age of the patient, the extremity injured, the tissue involved, and the degree of injury, the use of immobilization will be applied differently.

Immobilization for Specific Types of Injuries. In acute soft-tissue contusions, there often is muscular injury as well as hematoma formation. Depending on the extent of the injury, extremity immobilization may play a role in the healing process. In a recent study of quadriceps muscle contusions, the authors found that a short course of early immobilization of the knee in flexion assists in returning patients to activity earlier.[2] Most clinicians agree, however, that after a short course of initial immobilization, early motion is essential to avoiding atrophy and joint stiffness.

Muscle strains most often are treated with rest, ice, compression, and elevation in the early periods after an injury. This is usually followed by modalities to reduce pain and swelling, and range of motion and strengthening exercises. Immobilization usually is not necessary for this type of injury.

In ligamentous injuries such as ankle sprains, the use of immobilization is based on the extent of injury. The goal of immobilization in ligamentous injuries is to assist with pain control and swelling, and to prevent additional injury. A padded stirrup-type splint (Fig. 43-1) is useful in treating these injuries. This type of immobilization protects the sprained lateral ligaments but allows for other motions that do not adversely affect the injured tissues (i.e., ankle dorsiflexion and plantar flexion). The immobilization allows for weight-bearing functional rehabilitation without the loss of joint range of motion.

Ligament injuries heal at variable rates and immobilization is prescribed accordingly. The typical healing time required for basic ligamentous sprains varies from three days for minor ankle sprains to eight weeks for moderate to severe sprains.[67]

Immobilization can be used in treating certain types of cartilage injuries. Salter fractures in children affect the growing physeal cartilage in varying degrees. Anatomic positioning is vital for appropriate healing. Splints or casts can help in maintaining such positioning during the healing phase.

Immobilization can play a role in treating other cartilaginous injuries such as osteochondral fractures. After surgical treatment of these injuries, a period of immobilization is usually necessary to help facilitate early healing.

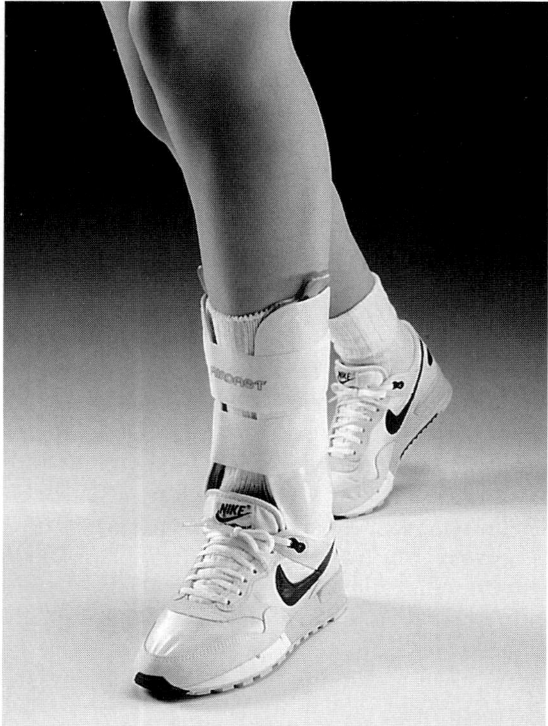

FIGURE 43-1. A padded prefabricated ankle stirrup splint. (Courtesy of Aircast, Inc.)

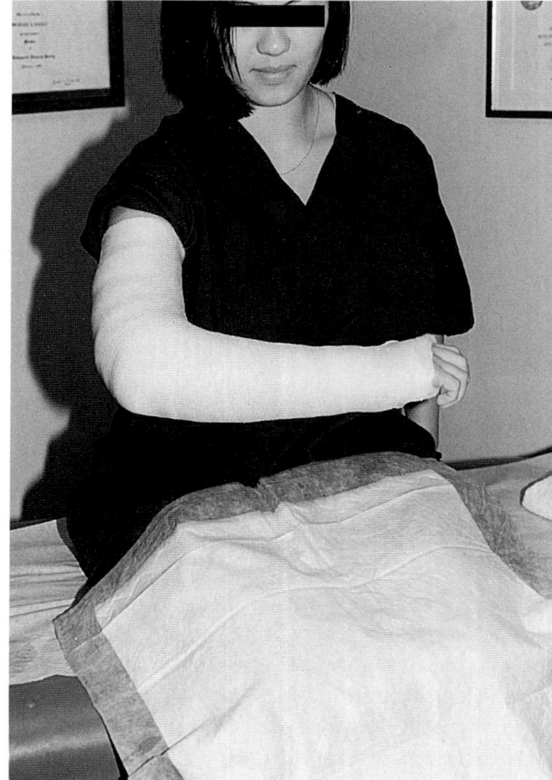

FIGURE 43-2. A long arm plaster cast.

The most notable use of immobilization is the use of casts (Fig. 43-2) for fractures. In general, a period of immobilization is required to maintain alignment and allow for direct bone healing and the formation of fracture callus. The age of the patient, the specific bone fractured, the extent of concomitant soft-tissue injury, the need for surgical intervention, and several other factors measure into the type and length of immobilization necessary.

Specific Types of Immobilization. Splinting is similar to cast immobilization except that it is not applied circumferentially. A splint is a rigid device that is applied to one part of an extremity and held in place around the extremity with straps. This allows for easy removal for wound care and other purposes. A splint is usually used for more minor injuries or as an intermediate device between a cast and no immobilization.

A brace is a splinting device that spans and stabilizes a joint but may allow for motion of the joint. There are many types of braces available. Braces for the upper extremities include thumb cone splints, wrist splints, elbow immobilizers, and shoulder immobilizers. The spine can be immobilized or protected using thoracolumbar-sacral orthoses or lumbosacral corsets. Lower extremity braces include hip spica orthoses and various types of knee and ankle splints. Because braces are most commonly used for the knee joint, the following is a discussion of the different types of knee braces.

Knee braces can be classified as either prophylactic, functional, or rehabilitative.[76] A prophylactic knee brace is designed to protect the knee against or reduce the severity of a sports injury. There is currently no consensus as to whether or not these braces actually achieve this goal. Most of the clinical data on this subject come from studying college athletes.[23,52,63,65] Conflicting conclusions abound, with some studies reporting a protective value for the brace,[63] some studies showing no difference in ligament injury between braced and unbraced players,[23] and some studies suggesting an actual increase in the injury rate among the braced players.[52,65] Teitz and others, for instance, found that braced players had an injury rate of 10.2% compared to 6.2% in the unbraced group.[65] A study by Hewson and others, however, showed no significant difference in the rate of injury between their two groups.[23] Thus the routine use of prophylactic knee braces is limited at this time.[76]

A functional knee brace (Fig. 43-3) is designed to provide stability to an unstable knee. These braces, some of which are also called derotational braces, come in several varieties. Functional knee braces are commonly used for anterior cruciate ligament (ACL)–deficient knees, and for some knees after ACL reconstruction, to protect the reconstructed ligament if some level of residual

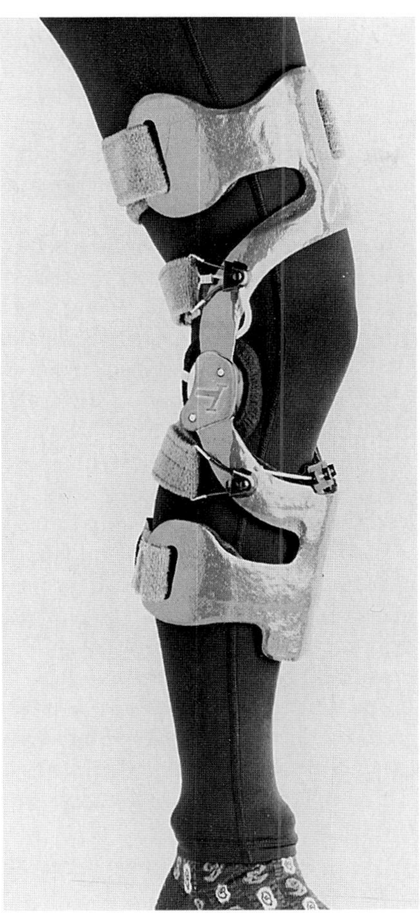

FIGURE 43-3. A functional (derotational) knee brace. (Courtesy of Sutter Corporation.)

instability persists. The braces are used also during the graft maturation phase of healing, especially in high-profile competitive athletes. A study examining the efficacy of functional knee braces in a group of patients with ACL-deficient knees revealed subjective improvement in 90% and a global improvement of at least one grade of instability when compared to the same knee unbraced.[7] Many other investigators point out, however, that the force applied in objective ligament testing is a fraction of the force applied in normal knee function and in sports participation.[44] It is important to realize that a functional knee brace, although providing some level of added cruciate and collateral ligament stability, is not a reliable substitute for intact ACL.[76] Activity modification, surgical intervention, and a focused physical therapy regimen also play an important role in managing the unstable knee.

The rehabilitative knee brace (Fig. 43-4) is a brace with a simple design that protects the injured or postoperative patient from the excesses of motion. It is usually hinged at the joint line with changeable stops to control the extents of flexion and extension. These braces are commonly used after injury or surgery to provide support

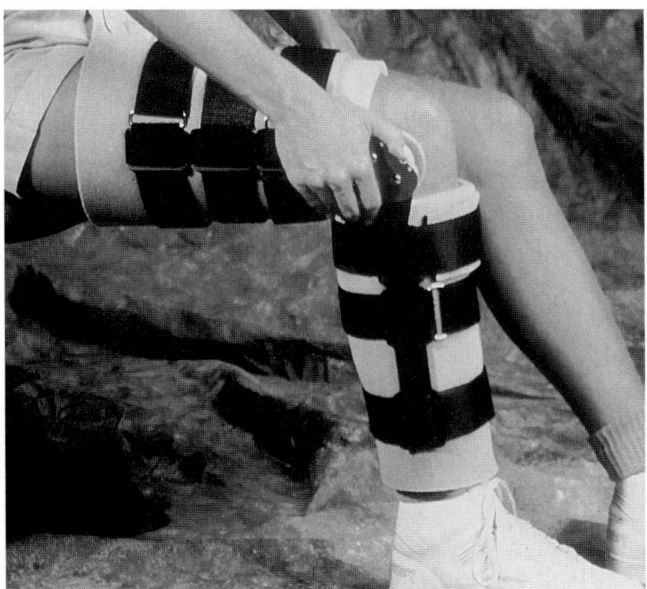

FIGURE 43-4. A rehabilitative knee brace. (Courtesy of Sutter Corporation.)

and stability. Also, the brace allows a protected range of motion to help prevent postinjury or postoperative joint stiffness. Smaller, lower-profile models of rehabilitative knee braces are the hinged knee braces designed for protection of collateral ligament injuries.

Patella cut-out neoprene sleeves (Fig. 43-5) provide gentle elastic compression around the knee, theoretically

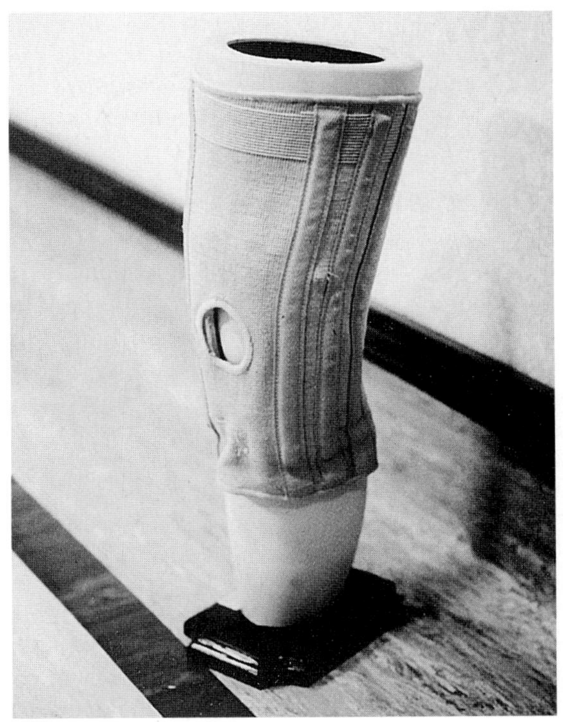

FIGURE 43-5. A patella cut-out knee sleeve.

to help maintain normal patellar tracking and to provide some proprioceptive feedback and the sensation of additional stability. Some are hinged and some have lateral struts for additional varus–valgus support. The theory that they function to help stabilize the patella throughout the knee range of motion is debatable. A recent study evaluated the effect of a new patellar realignment brace on patellofemoral displacement, using an active-movement kinematic magnetic resonance imager.[56] The study showed that a brace consisting of a neoprene sleeve with a circular silicone and plastic insert to stabilize the patella provided some level of patellofemoral displacement correction in 76% of the knees studied. The radiographic results, however, were not correlated with any clinical data.[56]

Another study compared the effectiveness of a simple elastic knee sleeve, one with a silicone patellar ring, and no brace at all in a population of military recruits with overuse patellofemoral pain.[15] The study concluded that the simple elastic knee sleeve was no more effective than no treatment at all but that it was better than the knee sleeve with the silicone patellar ring.[15]

It is important to remember that immobilization causes some possible deleterious effects to the immobilized tissues. Immobilization can result in muscle atrophy, ligamentous and tendinous stiffening, cartilage dehydration, and osteoporosis.[48] A recent study showed that only nine days of wrist immobilization caused forearm cross-sectional area to decrease by 4.1% and that muscle strength decreased by 29.3% for wrist flexion and 32.5% for extension.[40]

The goal of treatment is to return a patient to the preinjury level of function. It is imperative to take note of potential complications of immobilization so as to most effectively treat a patient. There is a delicate balance between too much and too little immobilization.

Mechanical Modalities

There are several rehabilitation modalities that rely on the mechanical manipulation of tissues. The most commonly used of these are traction and massage.

Traction is used most effectively and efficiently for muscle spasm in the neck or low back, and for some spinal nerve impingement conditions.[41] The traction is usually applied in either a continuous mode over the course of 30 to 120 minutes or in an intermittent mode in which the traction is cycled on for 15 to 30 seconds and then released for 5 to 10 seconds. Traction is typically used as an adjunct treatment to other therapeutic modalities.

A recent review of the literature on the efficacy of traction for back and neck pain concluded that most studies are flawed in their design; therefore it remains questionable whether or not traction offers any statistically significant advantage in the management of these conditions.[66] Nonetheless, traction is a commonly employed and popular therapeutic modality.

Massage (Fig. 43-6) is another mechanical modality designed to manually manipulate soft tissues. Most people agree that massage is relaxing and that it feels good, but there is also some science behind its effectiveness. Massage increases local blood circulation, relaxes muscles, and mobilizes and stretches scar tissue.[41] Massage also has been found to reduce levels of creatinine kinase, circulating neutrophil count, and delayed-onset muscle soreness after eccentric exercise, theoretically by interrupting the inflammatory response.[59] Another recent study, however, showed no statistical difference between massage, electrical stimulation, ergometry, and simple rest in reducing delayed-onset muscle soreness after exercise.[72] Similarly, Pope in a prospective randomized study, showed that their massage group scored the greatest improvement in extension effort and fatigue time, but that massage offered no significant difference in physical outcome measures, when compared to electrical stimulation or chiropractic spinal manipulation,[49] in treating subacute low back pain. Koes and others found that manual therapy and physiotherapy were effective methods of reducing pain and restoring function in patients with nonspecific back and neck complaints, but they conjectured that much of the improvement was likely due to placebo effects.[28]

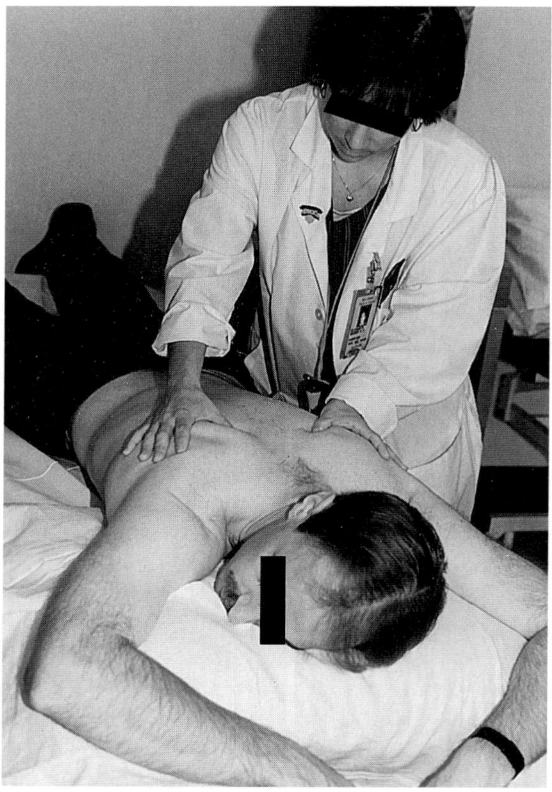

FIGURE 43-6. Massage.

Stretching

Stretching is a therapeutic modality usually employed by athletes on their own. Stretching is used to achieve and maintain maximal joint range of motion and soft tissue excursion. It is most commonly used before participating in sports in the warming-up period, and after an injury or surgery to regain passive and active joint range of motion.

The three major types of stretching techniques are static, ballistic, and proprioceptive neuromuscular facilitation (PNF).[68] Static stretching (Fig. 43-7), using a slow and progressive stretch for a period of 10 to 30 seconds, is the most common type used.

Ballistic stretching employs repetitive forceful motions to stretch tissues. An example of ballistic stretching is bouncing forward lunges, with one heel on the ground, designed to stretch the gastrocnemius-soleus-Achilles complex. This technique is less popular than static stretching because it requires more energy and puts the tissues at a higher risk for injury. A recent study comparing static and ballistic stretching found these two techniques to be similar in their ability to increase flexibility.[70]

PNF has been shown to increase the ease and range of extremity motion because it involves alternating muscle contraction with relaxation. Typically, PNF is performed with a therapist, who passively stretches a muscle to its greatest length. The patient then exerts a maximal contraction against resistance, which is followed by additional passive stretching by the therapist.[64] How PNF compares to other stretching techniques remains debatable.[47]

For effectiveness, it is recommended that the local temperature of the tissues be raised before stretching.[68] This can be achieved by some form of light exercise or by the application of heat. Raising the temperature of the soft tissues increases elasticity and optimizes muscle contractions and nerve impulse conductions.[68] A recent study compared passive stretching to no stretching in a small group of patients with short hamstrings. It was found that four weeks of daily home hamstring stretching produced a significant increase in the extensibility and stretching moment tolerated by the hamstrings but that the stretching program did not actually lengthen the muscles nor significantly alter their elasticity.[19]

Continuous Passive Motion

Continuous passive motion (CPM) is a technique designed to provide pure external passive movement to a joint (Fig. 43-8). It was first introduced as a concept in the early 1970s and has since been elaborated and refined. Basic science and clinical studies have validated its use.[42,53] In addition to playing a role in cartilage, tendon, and ligament healing after injury or surgery,[46,54,75] CPM has been found to increase knee range of motion,[26,35] decrease postoperative swelling,[35] decrease the length of hospital stay,[8,26,71] and decrease the use of narcotic analgesics[8,69] after total knee replacement. Other studies of patients with knee replacements dispute some of these findings.[50]

In animal studies comparing CPM to immobilization, CPM has been shown to increase muscle mass,[17] maintain normal biomechanical properties of tendons,[33] improve joint nutrition,[34,54,58] and prevent joint stiffness.

CPM is commonly used in sports rehabilitation after joint or extremity injury or after surgery when potential stiffness is a major concern. After ACL reconstruction, CPM often is used in the early postoperative period for several reasons: it helps to maintain knee joint nutrition, promotes healing by increasing collagen formation and organization, reduces pain and swelling, and helps achieve and maintain knee range of motion.[20]

THERAPEUTIC MODALITIES IN REHABILITATION

Thermotherapy

Thermotherapy, or heat treatment, has several applications. It is used for pain relief, to improve soft-tissue

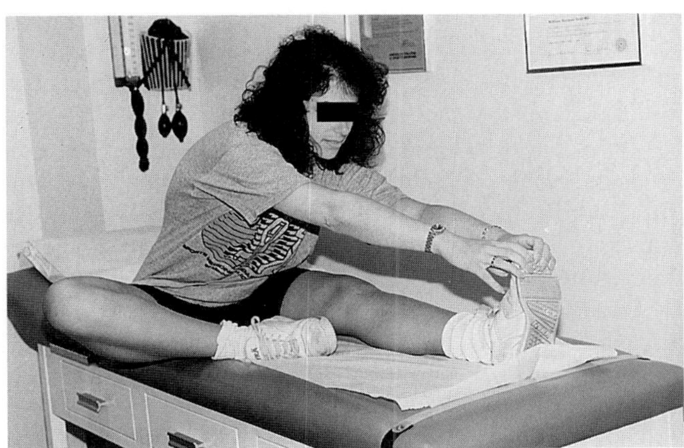

FIGURE 43-7. Static stretching of the hamstrings.

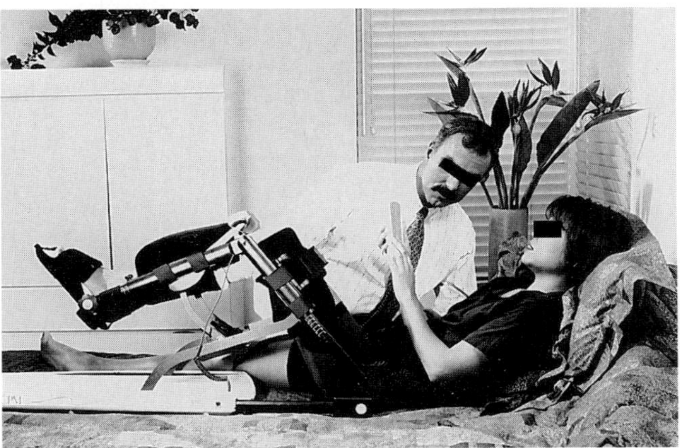

FIGURE 43-8. A continuous passive motion machine. (Courtesy of Sutter Corporation.)

stretching, and to raise the metabolic rate of local tissues. Although the science behind thermotherapy is not fully understood, it is known that heat applied to tissues causes local vasodilatation, which in turn causes analgesia through a variety of mechanisms that serve to raise the pain threshold, decrease muscle spindle activity, and increase local oxygen and other cellular nutrients.[51] It is to be avoided in the treatment of acute injuries, near the eyes, and in areas of abnormal sensation.

There are several ways to apply thermotherapy. Superficial techniques include hydrocollator packs, whirlpool, fluidotherapy, paraffin baths, and infrared heat lamps. Deep techniques include diathermy and ultrasound. Each of these techniques will be reviewed individually.

Hydrocollator packs (Fig. 43-9) are used to apply moist heat. These are composed of a silicone gel wrapped in canvas containers. They are heated in hot water tanks and are able to absorb large amounts of the surrounding heat. They are wrapped in towels before being applied to the affected area to protect the underlying skin from thermal injury. Hydrocollator packs are used primarily for chronic soft-tissue maladies such as muscle spasms, cramps, contusions, and strains. The recommended time of treatment is 15 to 20 minutes.[51]

Whirlpool (Fig. 43-10) is one of the most commonly used therapeutic modalities for applying heat. A whirlpool bath is effective in raising the temperature of the skin and subcutaneous tissues and providing gentle fluid massage to the portion of the body immersed in the bath. These effects combine to provide muscle relaxation, increased blood flow, and pain relief. Some of the effects of whirlpool therapy can be augmented by the patient's performing gentle exercises during the treatment.[51] Whirlpool is used primarily for increasing joint range of motion and for treating soft-tissue trauma.

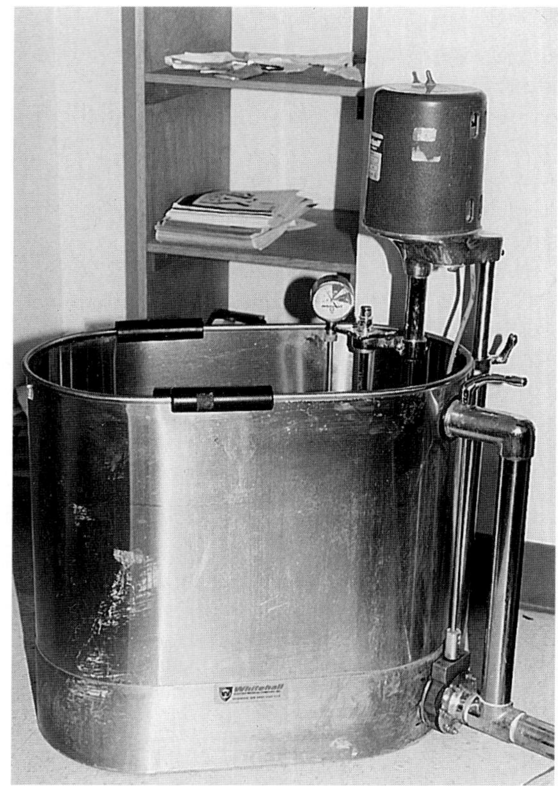

FIGURE 43-10. A whirlpool bath.

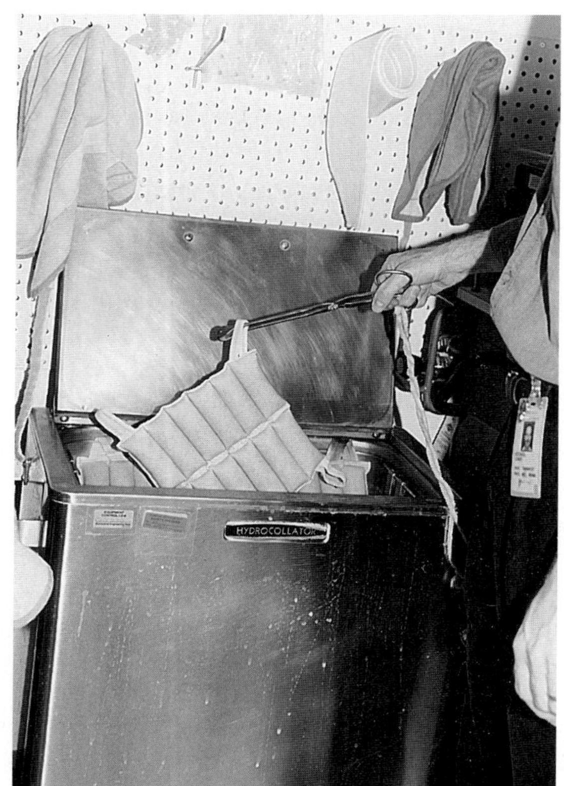

FIGURE 43-9. A hydrocollator pack.

Fluidotherapy (Fig. 43-11) is a method of applying heat and massage that involves circulating small solid particles (usually cellulose) in a heated air unit. It compares favorably to other superficial thermotherapy modalities in its effectiveness in elevating tissue temperatures.[4] Typically, the affected extremity is exercised in the fluidotherapy unit in an attempt to increase range of motion. There are also units that are designed to treat back problems. A fluidotherapy unit can vary temperature and the agitation of the air. It is used to treat muscle spasms, painful soft tissue injuries, and to assist in increasing the range of motion of stiff or injured joints.

Paraffin baths are a very effective way of providing thermotherapy to injured or arthritic hands and feet. This thermotherapy involves immersing the affected extremity into a heated mixture of mineral oil and paraffin wax for a few seconds. After the extremity is removed and the paraffin hardens, the process is repeated several

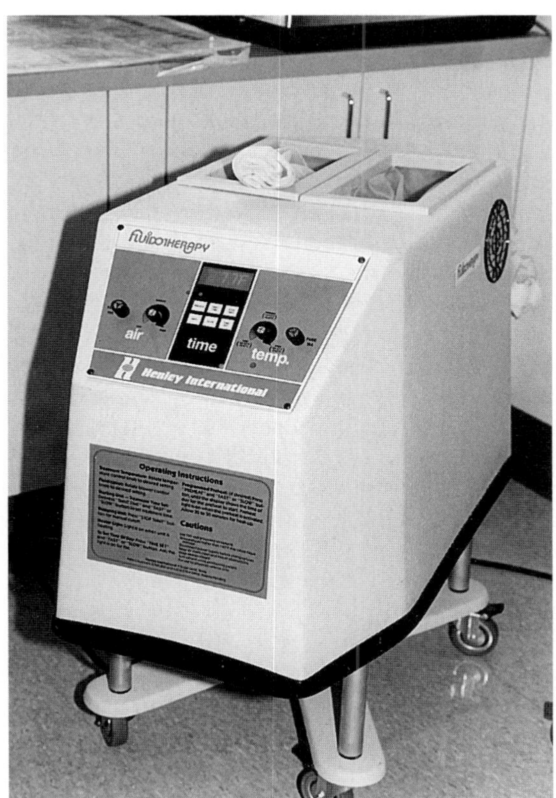

FIGURE 43-11. A fluidotherapy unit.

times to form a thick layer. The extremity is then typically soaked in the heated paraffin for about 20 minutes. Another method involves several repetitions of the immersing–hardening cycle followed by wrapping the extremity in a plastic bag and several towels to insulate the heat. The extremity typically is elevated for about 20 minutes and then is exercised. It is important to monitor the patient closely during paraffin treatments because the risk of burns is significantly greater than with other types of thermotherapy.[51] Paraffin baths should not be used for patients with open wounds.

Infrared heat lamps are a relatively inexpensive and simple method of applying superficial heat to a body area. Heat lamps provide a more rapid superficial temperature rise than hydrocollator packs.[51] Surrounding regions not being treated usually are draped off with towels. It is recommended that the treatment area be situated 20 inches from the lamp and that heat be applied for approximately 20 minutes.

Diathermy is a method of applying deep thermotherapy. Diathermy takes advantage of the fact that applying high-frequency electromagnetic current to the skin produces a rise in temperature of deeper tissues. This causes an increase in deep tissue circulation and metabolism and a decrease in muscle spasm and pain.[55] Since it is difficult to control and monitor tissue temperature,[1] and since there is a significant degree of variability in the heating patterns produced by different units,[30] diathermy should be applied only by a therapist with expertise in its use. Indications for diathermy include painful inflammatory conditions and osteoarthritis, muscle strains, ligament sprains, tendinopathies, and hematomas.

Diathermy can be applied using shortwave or microwave units. Shortwave diathermy uses radio waves as its power source. It has been shown to be effective in managing pain and swelling, muscle spasm, and joint stiffness,[18] as well as in accelerating wound healing and resolving hematomas.[55] In a recent critical evaluation of the most common physical therapy modalities used for controlling musculoskeletal pain, shortwave diathermy was found to be the one type of heat therapy that had reasonable scientific evidence to support its use.[5]

Microwave diathermy uses higher-frequency electromagnetic waves than shortwave diathermy, which makes it somewhat more efficient in its energy transmission. Microwave diathermy has been shown to be effective for managing muscle contractures and tenosynovitis,[1] and for resolving hematomas.[29]

Ultrasound (Fig. 43-12) is a therapeutic modality that uses high-frequency sound waves to elevate soft-tissue temperature. Like other deep-heat modalities, ultrasound increases local blood circulation and tissue metabolism. Ultrasound also has been shown to increase cortisol levels in peripheral nerves, which may account for some of its analgesic properties.[55] It is used primarily to treat muscle spasm and pain and, like other forms of heat therapy, is usually avoided in the acute trauma setting. The ultrasound probe is applied to the skin and a glycerin or mineral oil conductive medium is used to facilitate energy transfer. The probe is moved in a circular fashion to prevent any one specific area from being heated too much. Ultrasound has been used successfully to treat numerous maladies including soft-tissue pain, muscle spasms, tendon injuries,[51] and back pain.[45,55]

Pulsed ultrasound is a technique that causes primarily nonthermal effects on the treatment tissues, which result

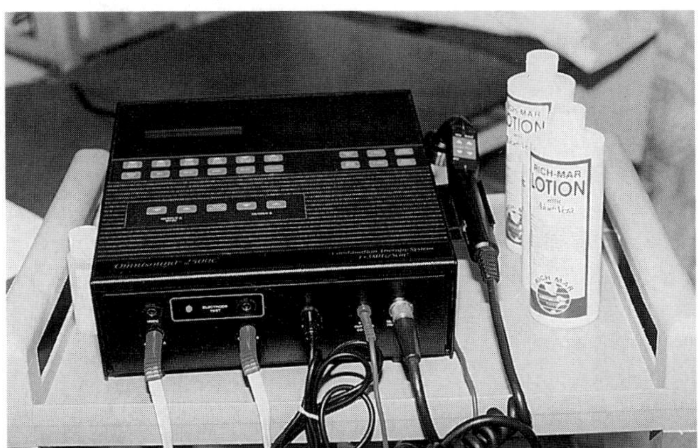

FIGURE 43-12. An ultrasound machine and probe.

in the relief of pain and inflammation. Because there is no significant thermal effect, pulsed ultrasound is sometimes applied in the acute injury setting.[51]

Another application of ultrasound is phonophoresis. Phonophoresis is a method of delivering analgesic and anti-inflammatory medication (usually hydrocortisone, lidocaine, or aspirin cream) to local tissues by the use of ultrasound.[51] Cooling the area with ice or heating the area with a hydrocollator pack before phonophoresis have both been shown to improve the absorption and distribution of the applied medicine.[31]

Cryotherapy

Cryotherapy is a commonly employed physical therapy modality that uses the application of cold temperature for treating tissue injuries. Although the science behind cryotherapy is not fully understood, it is believed to provide its beneficial effects through mechanisms of vasoconstriction followed by vasodilation, which blocks pain sensory transmission and decreases muscle spasm.

Cryotherapy is particularly useful in the early postinjury period in reducing inflammation, pain, swelling, and muscle spasm.[36,51] Hocutt compared early cryotherapy, late cryotherapy, and heat therapy in the treatment of ankle sprains and found that early cryotherapy was the superior method.[24] As the main component of "RICE" therapy (rest, ice, compression, elevation), ice is used to treat acute musculoskeletal injuries such as sprains, strains, and contusions. Ice decreases swelling, pain, and tissue metabolism, which, in turn, decreases the patient's "down time."

Cryotherapy is commonly used after surgical procedures. Scientific evidence is unclear as to its effectiveness in this setting. Cohn showed that patients receiving cold therapy after anterior cruciate ligament reconstruction required less postoperative pain medication and were converted from injectable to oral pain medication faster than patients not receiving cold therapy.[6] Another study of ACL reconstruction patients, however, showed no difference between those treated and those not treated with cryotherapy with respect to the use of pain medication, length of hospital stay, perceived pain, knee girth, and range of motion.[9] Studies of total knee arthroplasty patients have shown that those given cold compression therapy had significantly less postoperative blood loss, mild improvement in early return of range of motion, and lower pain medication requirements than those not receiving cold therapy.[32] A similar study, however, showed no appreciable advantage to a cold compression dressing with respect to range of motion, swelling, wound drainage, or narcotic requirements after total knee arthroplasty.[22]

It has been postulated that the analgesic effect of cryotherapy is probably due to many factors, including an antinociceptive effect on the gate control of pain—a theoretical effect of eliminating or reducing spasm and edema, and of decreasing sensory nerve conduction.[13]

Cold therapy also is useful in the later rehabilitative phase after tissue injury. As in the acute postinjury phase, cooling reduces muscle spasm and sensory nerve conduction in the later rehabilitative phase, which can provide pain relief. Also in the rehabilitative phase, cryotherapy has been shown to be helpful used in conjunction with exercises (cryokinetics).[27]

There are several important contraindications to the use of cold therapy. Absolute contraindications include Raynaud's phenomenon, cardiovascular disease, cryoglobulinemia, and paroxysmal cold hemoglobinuria. Relative contraindications include cold allergy, sensory impairment, and arthritic conditions.[51] Complications of cold therapy include ice burns, frostbite, and nerve palsy.[10]

As in thermotherapy, there are many different ways of applying cryotherapy. These include ice packs, refreezable gel cold packs, chemical cold packs, ice massage, cold compression devices, cold hydrotherapy, and evaporative vapocoolant sprays. In the following paragraphs we review each of these techniques individually.

Ice packs are plastic bags filled with ice. They are inexpensive, readily available, and simple to use. When compared to gel cold packs, chemical cold packs, and a refrigerant gas bladder, ice packs were shown to be superior in their ability to cool deep soft tissues.[37] An ice pack is either simply placed on the affected area or held there with a compressive elastic bandage and the area is elevated. It is recommended that a moist cloth barrier, such as a terry cloth towel, be used between the ice bag and the skin to prevent any unwanted "burning" skin reaction. Treatment usually lasts for 15 to 30 minutes.

Refreezable gel cold packs (Fig. 43-13) provide another simple and effective method of applying local cold therapy. They are thin plastic bags containing a flexible refreezable gel. For hygiene reasons, it is recommended that gel cold packs be wrapped in a towel before application to the skin. Like ice packs, refreezable gel cold

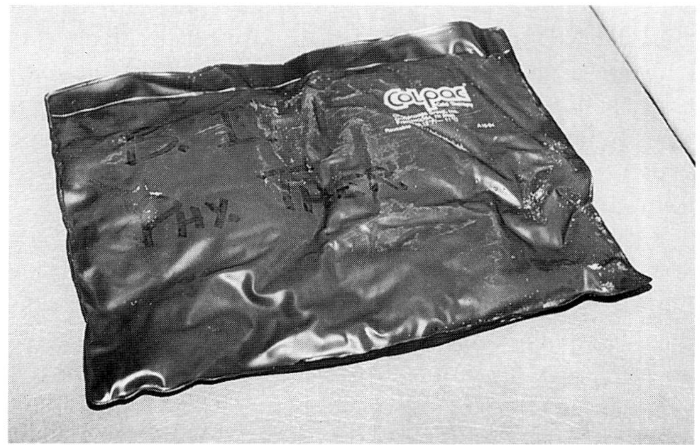

FIGURE 43-13. A refreezable gel cold pack.

packs are often applied in conjunction with compression and elevation and are usually applied for 15 to 30 minutes.

Chemical cold packs involve the mixing of two chemicals to produce an endothermic cooling reaction. These packs are less commonly used because they cool in an inconsistent manner, are relatively expensive, are not reusable, and can cause a chemical burn if the packs leak their contents.[41]

Ice massage involves freezing a paper or Styrofoam cup full of water and then removing the block of ice from the cup and directly massaging it into the treatment area. Massage is usually done for approximately 5 to 10 minutes, until analgesia is achieved. It is most commonly used for back pain and painful inflammatory conditions such as tendinitis. Ice massage compares favorably with electrical stimulation in the treatment of low back pain.[38]

A cold compression device (Fig. 43-14) is a commercially manufactured unit composed of a cold substance that is circulated into a sleeve covering and compressing the treatment area. It is an effective method of cooling tissues to assist in pain and edema control. There is conflicting evidence as to its usefulness after knee replacement or ligament reconstruction.[6,9,22,32]

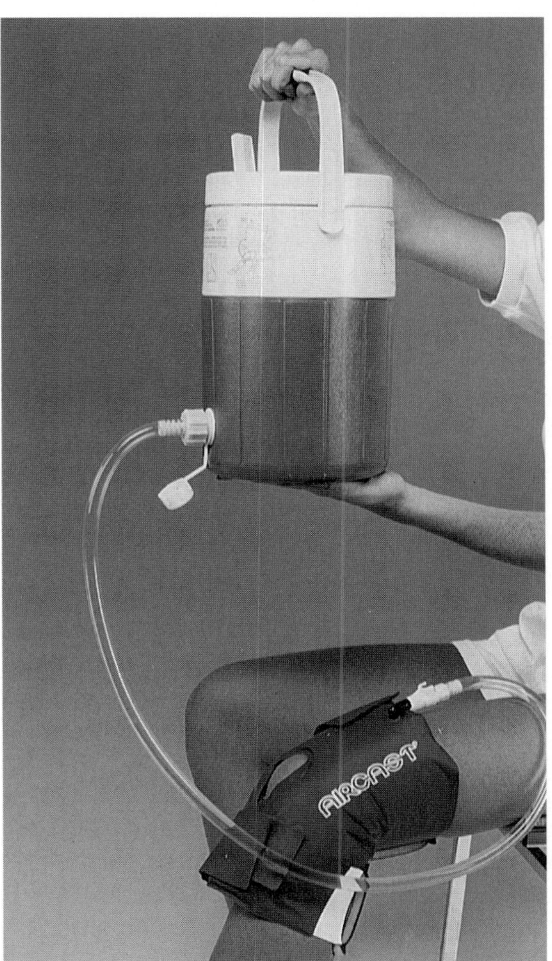

FIGURE 43-14. A knee cold compression unit.

Cold hydrotherapy is low-temperature whirlpool treatment, usually in the 55° F to 65° F range. Cold hydrotherapy provides excellent contact with and cooling of an affected extremity. It is used most commonly for upper and lower extremity injuries. Cold hydrotherapy is usually avoided in patients with acute postinjury edema because the extremity must be placed in a dependent position in the unit.

Evaporative vapocoolant sprays cool the skin on contact by the rapid evaporation of methyl fluoride or ethyl chloride. They are most commonly used in combination with other therapies to treat myofascial disorders, and to stretch out areas of pain, muscle spasm, and joint stiffness. Typically, the coolant is sprayed onto the affected area and then stretching or massage is begun. It is important to avoid inhaling the vapors and to avoid inducing frostbite.

Electrical Stimulation

Electrical stimulation is used as a rehabilitative therapeutic modality primarily to reduce pain and to assist in muscle strengthening. Although the specific mechanisms of its action have not been entirely made clear, electrical stimulation has been found to be effective in various clinical situations.

In this section, the basic principles behind electrical stimulation as a therapeutic modality are discussed and the most common applications of this technique are described.

Principles of Electrical Stimulation. It has been known since the 18th century that an electric current can cause a muscle to contract. This action involves the depolarization of nerve fibers in response to an electrical impulse placed on the surface of the skin. Biologic tissues offer both resistance and variability to current flow because of their nonhomogenous nature. Other determinants of current flow are its wave amplitude, frequency, and wave form.

Electrical stimulation gives the clinician the opportunity to alter the normal electrical characteristics and thus the cellular environment of biologic tissues. Because all tissues contain positively and negatively charged ions, applying electricity can cause these ions to move in such a way as to increase the cellular activity of the tissues. The resulting change in cellular activity can be associated with pain control, involuntary muscle contraction, and injured tissue healing.

For rehabilitative purposes, the electrical current is most commonly applied through surface electrodes connected to an alternating current source. Most current sources offer the clinician the option of varying wave form, pulse width and amplitude, and frequency. These parameters are manipulated to obtain the desired clinical effect.

Electrical Stimulation for Pain Control. Upon the description of the gate theory of pain in 1965,[39] scientists began experimenting with electrical stimulation in an attempt to modulate a patient's perception of pain by "closing" the pain "gate." This gave rise to the development of the transcutaneous electric nerve stimulation (TENS) unit (Fig. 43-15).

Although studies have documented the effectiveness of TENS for pain control, there is little agreement as to the way it works. In fact, although many different types of units exist with the ability to vary multiple parameters, no one particular type of unit or regimen has emerged as being more effective than any other.[25] Nonetheless, several theories have been proposed, including the stimulation of endorphin and enkephalin release,[3] the electrical blocking of afferent pain impulses,[3] and the triggering of a central pain inhibition center.[62]

TENS applies an electrical stimulus in such a way as to inhibit pain fiber nerve transmission and, at the same time, stimulates large afferent fibers, which also theoretically assists in "closing the gate" to pain transmission. Another way of using TENS is to alter the frequency of electrical current to induce the release of endogenous opiates, thus helping to control pain.[12]

Although it is difficult to measure the effectiveness of any type of pain control regimen because of the inherent subjectivity involved, there are studies that support the use of TENS for pain control.[61] Although TENS has been used for nearly all types of pain, it is most commonly used as an adjunct treatment for pain that arises from acute trauma and surgical procedures. It has been shown to be effective in improving acute as well as chronic low back pain.[14,55] It is usually applied once daily for 20 minutes for several days' duration, but particular protocols vary depending on the type and location of pain.

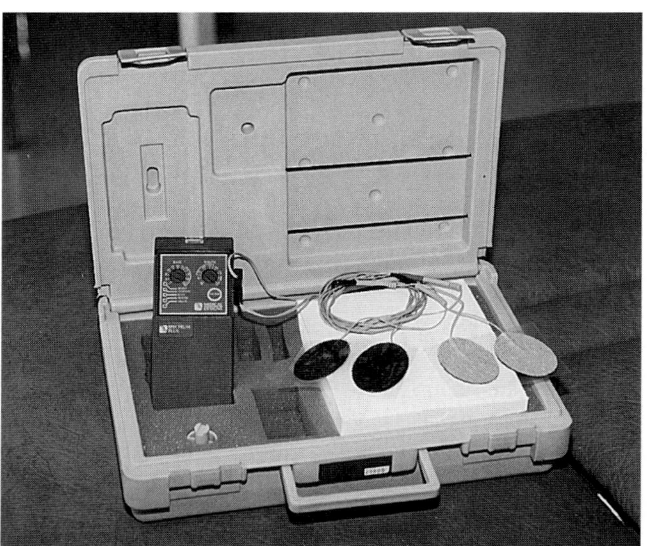

FIGURE 43-15. A transcutaneous electric nerve stimulation (TENS) unit.

TENS is also useful as adjunct therapy when pain is limiting the progression of a global rehabilitation protocol (i.e., ACL reconstruction rehabilitation, shoulder capsular reconstruction rehabilitation). In these situations, especially in the early postoperative period when oral analgesic medication is only partially effective, TENS can provide an additional method of pain control to allow specific rehabilitation goals to be achieved.

Although TENS has been applied in many conditions, few scientific data to support its use in controlling chronic pain syndromes exist.[16] It is also important to remember that there are known contraindications to the use of TENS for pain control.[43] TENS should be avoided in patients with cardiac pacemakers, in those who are pregnant, and in patients with an unclear etiology of pain. TENS applied to the head theoretically can affect seizure threshold and vascular activity and is not recommended. TENS also can be dangerous when applied in the region of the carotid sinus because it can elicit reflex hypotension; thus it is not recommended. TENS should be avoided in an anterior to posterior plane in the transthoracic region because of the possibility of inducing a cardiac arrhythmia.[43]

In general, TENS remains somewhat of an enigma. It is difficult to discern from available scientific data its applicability to any given pain situation. It also remains difficult to pinpoint its actual mechanism of pain modulation. Nonetheless, TENS is commonly and effectively used for acute and postoperative pain and as an adjunct therapy to a rehabilitation protocol that is being slowed by pain.

Another application of electrical stimulation for pain control is the point stimulator. The point stimulator elicits a brain stem response to inhibit pain by a focused, high-intensity, low-frequency current. This type of electrical analgesia has been likened to acupuncture.[41]

Electrical Stimulation for Muscle Strengthening. Since it is known that surface electrical stimulation can elicit muscle contractions, this modality has been used in the rehabilitative strengthening of muscles in the postoperative and postinjury periods when voluntary muscle contraction may be limited. It has also been applied to the strengthening of otherwise normal muscles.

In the postoperative or postinjury patient population, electrical stimulation can be used to rehabilitate muscles. In general, electrodes are placed in such a way as to excite the motor nerve to the muscle or group of muscles being stimulated. A tetanic muscle contraction is induced and maintained for a period of seconds.

This has been reported to be useful, when combined with a regimen of strengthening exercises, in preventing muscle atrophy and loss of strength after major knee ligament surgery.[11,74] Snyder-Mackler and others found that patients who received electrical stimulation after ACL reconstruction had stronger quadriceps and a more normal gait pattern than those who did not.[60] There are other articles in the literature, however, that show no significant difference in long-lasting strength gains and/or muscle mass when comparing an exercise group with an exercise plus electrical stimulation group.[57] It also has been suggested that many of the gains made by electrical stimulation are lost after a period of time.

Electrical stimulation has been applied to normal muscles with hopes of building both strength and muscle mass. The main problem encountered in this application is that, typically, the muscle contraction elicited by electrical stimulation is not as strong as the contraction produced by a patient's own maximal voluntary effort. Because strength gains are directly proportional to the ability to contract muscles as strongly as possible, electrical stimulation has only a theoretical role at this time.

Other Applications of Electrical Stimulation. Electrical current can be used to help deliver certain medications to the tissues beneath the skin. This process, called iontophoresis, takes advantage of the ionized nature of certain medications (most commonly salicylates and hydrocortisone). When electrodes are positioned in the appropriate fashion, low-voltage electrical stimulation can actually repel the medication away from the electric source and drive it into the symptomatic tissues. Iontophoresis is most commonly used as an adjunct treatment for acute soft-tissue conditions such as muscle strains and contusions, bursitis, and tendinitis. It has also been shown to be useful in treating traumatic myositis ossificans.[73] A recent study showed that dexamethasone iontophoresis significantly decreased the perception of muscle soreness but did not significantly alter maximal muscle contraction, peak torque, or work.[21]

Interferential electrical stimulation is similar to other types of electrical analgesia except in the configuration and type of electrodes used. Essentially, paired biphasic electrodes are used in concert to deliver the current, which allows the current intensity to be lessened but still provide as good or even better therapeutic response.

Electrical stimulation has been studied to assess its applicability to soft-tissue healing. Although animal studies have been performed, few methods are applicable to human subjects. One clinical study assessing the use of electrical stimulation in ankle sprains showed no significant difference between ankles treated with electrical stimulation and those that were not.[1] The applicability for the routine use of electrical stimulation for soft tissue healing has yet to be determined.

REFERENCES

1. American Academy of Orthopaedic Surgeons: Therapeutic modalities in sports medicine. In Griffin LY (ed): Orthopaedic Knowledge Update: Sports Medicine. Rosemont, IL, AAOS, 1994.
2. Aronen JA, Chronister R, Ove P, McDevitt ER: Thigh contusions: Minimizing the length of time before return to full athletic activities with early immobilization in 120 degrees of knee flexion. Presented at the American Orthopaedic Society for Sports Medicine Annual Meeting, July 16–19, 1990, Sun Valley, Idaho.
3. Bishop B: Pain: Its physiology and rationale for management. Phys Ther 60:13–37, 1980.
4. Borrell RM, Parker R, Henley EJ, Masley D, Repinecz M: Comparison of in vivo temperatures produced by hydrotherapy, paraffin wax treatment, and fluidotherapy. Phys Ther 60:1273–1276, 1980.
5. Chapman CE: Can the use of physical modalities for pain control be rationalized by the research evidence? Can J Physiol Pharmacol 69:704–712, 1991.
6. Cohn BT, Draeger RI, Jackson DW: The effects of cold therapy in the postoperative management of pain in patients undergoing anterior cruciate ligament reconstruction. Am J Sports Med 17:344–349, 1989.
7. Colville MR, Lee CL, Ciullo JV: The Lenox Hill Brace: An evaluation of effectiveness in treating knee instability. Am J Sports Med 14:257–261, 1986.
8. Colwell CW Jr, Morris BA: The influence of continuous passive motion on the results of total knee arthroplasty. Clin Orthop 276:225–228, 1992.
9. Daniel DM, Stone ML, Arendt DL: The effect of cold therapy on pain, swelling, and range of motion after anterior cruciate ligament reconstructive surgery. Arthroscopy 10:530–533, 1994.
10. Drez D, Faust DC, Evans JP: Cryotherapy and nerve palsy. Am J Sports Med 9:256–257, 1981.
11. Eriksson E, Haggmark T: Comparison of isometric muscle training and electrical stimulation supplementing isometric muscle training in the recovery after major knee ligament surgery: A preliminary report. Am J Sports Med 7:169–171, 1979.
12. Eriksson MBE, Sjolund BH, Nielzen S: Long term results of peripheral conditioning stimulation as an analgesic measure in chronic pain. Pain 6:335–347, 1979.
13. Ernst E, Fialka V: Ice freezes pain? A review of the clinical effectiveness of analgesic cold therapy. J Pain Symptom Manage 9:56–59, 1994.
14. Ersek RA: Low-back pain: Prompt relief with transcutaneous neurostimulation. Orthop Rev 5:12–16, 1976.
15. Finestone A, Radin EL, Lev B, Shlamkovitch N, et al: Treatment of overuse patellofemoral pain: Prospective randomized controlled clinical trial in a military setting. Clin Orthop 293:208–210, 1993.
16. Fried T, Johnson R, McCracken W: Transcutaneous electrical nerve stimulation: Its role in the control of chronic pain. Arch Phys Med Rehabil 65:228–231, 1984.

17. Gebhard JS, Kabo JM, Meals RA: Passive motion: The dose effects on joint stiffness, muscle mass, bone density, and regional swelling. A study in an experimental model following intra-articular injury. J Bone Joint Surg 75:1636–1647, 1993.
18. Goats GC: Continuous short-wave (radio-frequency) diathermy. Br J Sports Med 23:123–127, 1989.
19. Halberstan JP, Goeken LN: Stretching exercises: Effect on passive extensibility and stiffness in short hamstrings of healthy subjects. Arch Phys Med Rehabil 75:976–981, 1994.
20. Halling AH, Howard ME, Cawley PW: Rehabilitation of anterior cruciate ligament injuries. Clin Sports Med 12:329–348, 1993.
21. Hasson SM, Wible CL, Reich M: Dexamethasone iontophoresis: Effect on delayed muscle soreness and muscle function. Can J Sports Sci 17:8–13, 1992.
22. Healy WL, Seidman J, Pfeifer BA, Brown DG: Cold compressive dressing after total knee arthroplasty. Clin Orthop 229:143–146, 1994.
23. Hewson GR Jr, Mendini RA, Wong JB: Prophylactic knee bracing in college football. Am J Sports Med 14:262–266, 1986.
24. Hocutt JE Jr, Jaffe R, Rylander CR, Beebe JK: Cryotherapy in ankle sprains. Am J Sports Med 10:316–319, 1982.
25. Jensen JE, Etheridge GL, Hazelrigg G: Effectiveness of transcutaneous electrical neural stimulation in the treatment of pain. Recommendations for use in the treatment of sports injuries. Sports Med 3:79–88, 1986.
26. Johnson DP: The effect of continuous passive motion on wound-healing and joint mobility after knee arthroplasty. J Bone Joint Surg 72:421–426, 1990.
27. Knight KL Londeree BR: Comparison of blood flow in the ankle of uninjured subjects during therapeutic applications of heat, cold, and exercise. Med Sci Sports Exerc 12:76–80, 1980.
28. Koes BW, Bouter LM, van Mameren H, et al: The effectiveness of manual therapy, physiotherapy, and treatment by the general practitioner for nonspecific back and neck complaints. A randomized clinical trial. Spine 17:28–35, 1992.
29. Lehmann JF, Dundore DE, Esselman PC, Nelp WB: Microwave diathermy: Effects on experimental muscle hematoma resolution. Arch Phys Med Rehabil 64:127–129, 1983.
30. Lehmann JF, McDougall JA, Guy AW, et al.: Heating patterns produced by shortwave diathermy applicators in tissue substitute models. Arch Phys Med Rehabil 64:575–577, 1983.
31. Lehman JF, Warren CG, Scham SM: Therapeutic heat and cold. Clin Orthop 99:207–245, 1974.
32. Levy AS, Marmar E: The role of cold compression dressings in the postoperative treatment of total knee arthroplasty. Clin Orthop 297:174–178, 1993.
33. Loitz BJ, Zernicke RF, Vailas AC, Kody MH, Meals RA: Effect of short-term immobilization versus continuous passive motion on the biomechanical and biochemical properties of the rabbit tendon. Clin Orthop 244:265–271, 1989.
34. McDonough AL: Effects of immobilization and exercise on articular cartilage—A review of literature. J Orthop Sports Phys Ther 3:2–4, 1981.
35. McInnes J, Larson MG, Daltroy LH: A controlled evaluation of continuous passive motion in patients undergoing total knee arthroplasty. JAMA 268:1423–1428, 1992.
36. McMaster WC: A literary review on ice therapy in injuries. Am J Sports Med 5:124–126, 1977.
37. McMaster WC, Liddle S, Waugh TR: Laboratory evaluation of various cold therapy modalities. Am J Sports Med 6:291–294, 1978.
38. Melzack R, Jeans ME, Stratford JG, Monks RC: Ice massage and transcutaneous electrical stimulation: Comparison of treatment for low-back pain. Pain 9:209–217, 1980.
39. Melzack R, Wall PD: Pain mechanisms: A new theory. Science 150:971–979, 1965.
40. Miles MP, Clarkson PM, Bean M: Muscle function at the wrist following nine days of immobilization and suspension. Med Sci Sports Exerc 26:615–623, 1994.
41. American Academy of Orthopaedic Surgeons: Modalities. In Athletic Training and Sports Medicine, 2nd ed. Rosemont, IL, The Academy, 1991.
42. Namba RS, Kabo JM, Dorey FJ, Meals RA: Continuous passive motion versus immobilization. The effect on post-traumatic joint stiffness. Clin Orthop 267:218–223, 1991.
43. Neuromuscular stimulation. Presented at The International Academy of Physio Therapeutics, Electrotherapy and Ultrasound Update, November 19–20, 1994.
44. Noyes FR, Grood ES, Butler DL, Malek M: Clinical laxity tests and functional stability of the knee: Biomechanical concepts. Clin Orthop 146:84–89, 1980.
45. Nwuga VC: Ultrasound in the treatment of back pain resulting from prolapsed intervertebral disc. Arth Phys Med Rehabil 64:88–89, 1983.
46. O'Driscoll SW, Salter RB: The induction of neochondrogenesis in free intraarticular periosteal autografts under the influence of continuous passive motion. J Bone Joint Surg 66:1248–1257, 1984.
47. Osternig LR, Robertson R, Troxel R, Hansen P: Muscle activation during proprioceptive neuromuscular facilitation stretching techniques. Am J Phys Med 66:298–307, 1987.
48. Paulos LE, Grauer JD: Exercise. In DeLee JC, Drez D (eds): Orthopaedic Sports Medicine: Principles and Practice. Philadelphia, WB Saunders, 1994.

49. Pope MH, Phillips RB, Haugh LD: A prospective randomized three-week trial of spinal manipulation, transcutaneous muscle stimulation, massage and corset in the treatment of subacute low back pain. Spine 19:2571–2577, 1994.
50. Ritter MA, Gandolf VS, Holston KS: Continuous passive motion versus physical therapy in total knee arthroplasty. Clin Orthop 244:239–243, 1989.
51. Rivenburgh DW: Physical modalities in the treatment of tendon injuries. Clin Sports Med 11: 645–659, 1992.
52. Rovere GD, Haupt HA, Yates CS: Prophylactic knee bracing in college football. Am J Sports Med 15: 111–116, 1987.
53. Salter RB: The biologic concept of continuous passive motion of synovial joints. The first 18 years of basic research and its clinical application. Clin Orthop 242:12–25, 1989.
54. Salter RB, Simmonds DF, Malcolm BW, et al: The biological effect of continuous passive motion on the healing of full thickness defects in articular cartilage. J Bone Joint Surg 62:1232–1251, 1980.
55. Santiesteban AJ: The role of physical agents in the treatment of spine pain. Clin Orthop 179:24–30, 1983.
56. Shellock FG, Mink JH, Deutsch AL: Effect of a patellar realignment brace on patellofemoral relationships: Evaluation with kinematic MR imaging. J Magn Reson Imaging 4:590–594, 1994.
57. Sisk TD, Stalka SW, Deering MB, Griffen JW: Effect of electrical stimulation on quadriceps strength after reconstructive surgery of the anterior cruciate ligament. Am J Sports Med 13:215–220, 1985.
58. Skyhar MJ, Danzig LA, Hargens AR, Akeson WH: Nutrition of the anterior cruciate ligament. Effects of continuous passive motion. Am J Sports Med 13:415–418, 1985.
59. Smith LL, Keating MN, Holbert D: The effects of athletic massage on delayed onset muscle soreness, creatinine kinase, and neutrophil count: A preliminary report. J Orthop Sports Phys Ther 19:93–99, 1994.
60. Snyder-Mackler L, Ladin Z, Schepsis AA, Young JC: Electrical stimulation of the thigh muscles after reconstruction of the anterior cruciate ligament. J Bone Joint Surg 73:1025–1036, 1991.
61. Solomon RA, Vienstein MC, Long DM: Reduction of postoperative pain and narcotic use by transcutaneous electrical nerve stimulation. Surgery 87:142–146, 1980.
62. Soric R, Devlin M: Transcutaneous electrical nerve stimulation: Practical aspects and applications. Postgrad Med 78:101–107, 1985.
63. Taft TN, Hunter S, Fundurbeck CH Jr: Preventative lateral knee bracing in football. Presented at the American Orthopaedic Society for Sports Medicine Annual Meeting, July 2, 1985, Nashville, Tennessee.
64. Tanigawa MC: Comparison of the hold-relax procedure and passive mobilization on increasing muscle length. Phys Ther 52:725–735, 1972.
65. Teitz CC, Hermanson BK, Kronmal RA, Diehr PH: Evaluation of the use of braces to prevent injury to the knee in collegiate football players. J Bone Joint Surg 69:2–9, 1987.
66. van der Heijden GJ, Beurskens AJ, Koes BW: The efficacy of traction for back and neck pain: A systematic, blinded review of randomized clinical trial methods. Phys Ther 75:93–104, 1995.
67. Vegso JJ: Ankle sprain: Nonoperative management. In Torg JS, Shephard RJ (eds): Current Therapy in Sports Medicine, 3rd ed. St. Louis, Mosby–Year Book, 1995.
68. Vegso JJ: Principles of stretching. In Torg JS, Shephard RJ (eds): Current Therapy in Sports Medicine, 3rd ed. St. Louis, Mosby–Year Book, 1995.
69. Walker RH, Morris BA, Angulo DL: Postoperative use of continuous passive motion, transcutaneous electrical nerve stimulation, and continuous cooling pad following total knee arthroplasty. J Arthroplasty 6:151–156, 1991.
70. Wallin D, Ekblom B, Graham R, Nordenborg T: Improvement of muscle flexibility: A comparison between two techniques. Am J Sports Med 13:263–268, 1985.
71. Wasilewski SA, Woods LC, Togerson WR Jr, Healy WL: Value of continuous passive motion in total knee arthroplasty. Orthopaedics 13:291–295, 1990.
72. Weber MD, Servedio FJ, Woodall WR: The effects of three modalities on delayed onset muscle soreness. J Orthop Sports Phys Ther 20:236–242, 1994.
73. Wieder DL: Treatment of traumatic myositis ossificans with acetic acid iontophoresis. Phys Ther 72:133–137, 1992.
74. Wigerstad-Lossing I, Grimby G, Jonsson T: Effects of electrical muscle stimulation combined with voluntary contractions after knee ligament surgery. Med Sci Sports Exerc 20:93–98, 1988.
75. Williams JM, Moran M, Thonar EJ, Salter RB: Continuous passive motion stimulates repair of rabbit knee articular cartilage after matrix proteoglycan loss. Clin Orthop 304:252–262, 1994.
76. Wirth MA, DeLee JC: The history and classification of knee braces. Clin Sports Med 9:731–741, 1990.

44 The Lower Extremity

Robert S. Gotlin

Participation in aerobic and physical activities continues to increase across the ages. The era of improved health and physical fitness, while successfully improving longevity and medical morbidity, has lead to significant numbers of lower extremity injuries. Work and everyday demands exert considerable stresses along and through the lower extremities and awareness of preventive and therapeutic measures are necessary. The appendicular and axial skeletons are the lattices that maintain the stability of our upright posture. Through the highly sophisticated coordination of the neuromusculoskeletal system, the appendicular skeleton, comprising the upper and lower extremities, and the axial skeleton, comprising the vertebral column and pelvis, form the biomechanical structures that allow purposeful movement. Every one of our actions is a process of patterned, programmed, and skillfully regulated information processed through the central nervous system. A delicate blend of force production and absorption allows our lower extremity muscles to propel our bodies.

Particularly vulnerable to injury, the lower extremities constantly accept forces from the environment. Just as the body produces a force as a person makes foot-to-floor contact, an equal force is produced by the surface (ground reactive) onto the body above. Rehabilitation programs must include both force production (acceleration) and force absorption (deceleration) strategies. The lower extremities—hip, thigh, knee, leg, ankle, and feet—are closely related in functional activities and all must be considered when we focus on a specific disability. Although the emphasis in treating injuries of the lower extremities initially is on the particular joint or region involved, the ultimate rehabilitation program must emphasize training the entire lower limb. Our obligation as clinicians is not merely to treat dysfunction but also to determine its etiology. A thorough biomechanical analysis of the specific motions required of an injured athlete's sport is essential when customizing a rehabilitation program. In all training paradigms, the development of skill is the driving force behind goal setting. Skill defines excellence of performance and when choreographing rehabilitation strategies, four essential components of skill training must be stressed.

Coordination, stability (balance), force production, and force absorption are four key elements for skill and serve as the backbone for mastering a task. All play an important role in various levels of activities, and each must be addressed as part of skill training. It is our experience that success is not fully appreciated unless this is accomplished.

Coordination, as described in motor learning, integrates the nervous system's ability to regulate the interaction of agonist and antagonist muscles.[22] The ordered firing of motor units on the cellular level, in synchrony with the actions of the muscles of the body on the macro level, lays the foundation for purposeful movement. The ability of a torso muscle to contract and stabilize the trunk while a seemingly unassociated limb muscle contracts to produce a movement is an example of this. Without the coordinated contraction of the torso muscle group, the action carried out by the lower limb muscle group would likely be off balance, inefficient, and not purposeful. Rehabilitating a specific part of a lower limb actually encompasses a much broader scope of training than merely focusing on the isolated injured area.

Stability is the component of skill that allows for the use of agonist and antagonist muscle groups to maintain balance over the center of gravity. Much of the training for balance is done in positions of "off balance" so that the body can more easily accommodate when challenged from a position of "on" balance. An example of this is the tossing and catching of a weighted ball while standing on a balance board such as a BAPS (biomechanical ankle platform system, CAMP, Jackson, Michigan). One is challenged to maintain upright posture, balance on the BAPS board, while simultaneously attempting to carry out the ball toss.

Force production concepts are familiar to most people. Weight training to improve strength, sprinting to decrease race time, and repetitive jumping to improve vertical leap are examples of force production training techniques. In the gym, this can be accomplished with the bench press. In this exercise, the pectorals are strengthened. Likewise, with the knee extension exercise, quadriceps strength is improved. In both of these, muscle strengthening occurs while muscle fibers are shortening (i.e., undergoing concentric activity).

Force absorption concepts relate to either the action of an antagonistic muscle group to control the activity of its agonist counterpart or the action of the agonist group itself to perform a specific task. In either situation, strengthening occurs while muscle fibers are lengthening (i.e., undergoing eccentric activity). Consider the fact that if it were not for the ability of the shoulder decelerators to slow down a ballplayer's overhand pitch, the upper extremity would propel in a forward direction unchecked except by the anatomic limits of the shoulder's bone, ligament, muscle, and skin—a highly inefficient technique and detrimental to the athlete. There has been a significant deficit in training for force absorption in many rehabilitation protocols, and training programs must increase directives for these techniques.

Stability (balance) and coordination concepts form the foundation for skill training and are the key components for performance success. Integration of neural input from the body's central nervous system into the effector muscle groups allows energy efficient and purposeful motion to occur.

In our discussion we will survey select disabilities of the lower limb and offer guidelines for the management of each. The components of skill will be incorporated into each strategy when appropriate.

FOOT AND ANKLE

Often the foot and ankle complex serves as the first line of contact between the environment and the body, so an athlete's ankle is one of the most frequently injured joints.[23,58] The basic function of the ankle and subtalar joints have been likened to a universal joint.[34] The interaction of these two joints allows for both static and dynamic support of the ankle while each serves to accommodate for a deficiency in the other. A practitioner should evaluate each of them separately when developing a rehabilitation program. Too often an athlete injures an ankle and is told, "ice and rest it and it will be OK." We must not assume that all ankle sprains are minor and will simply "get better": 25% to 40% of ankle sprains have associated chronic disability and instability.[5] This kind of injury is most common in runners.[5,18] It is rare to treat an athlete who has never sustained an ankle sprain at one time or another.

In general, most injuries to the ankle follow acute trauma, but up to 30% of injuries are related to overuse.[18] Overuse injuries often are more difficult to treat because the associated anatomy usually is more negatively affected and the psyche of the athlete does not allow enough down time to recoup. One of the most challenging athletes to treat is a dedicated runner. It is important for the clinician to be inventive and imaginative when choreographing a treatment plan for this group. The so-called "runner's high" is a strong force that resists keeping a runner off his or her feet.

The rehabilitation strategies for treating foot and ankle disabilities largely overlap. In common to most is a period of rest, ice, compression, and elevation (RICE). The specifics of each of these have been described in the chapter on spine rehabilitation. One difference in treating the ankle and foot is the length of time for the period of rest. In treating the foot and ankle complex for a sprain or strain, a protracted period of relative rest may be required before the patient returns to aggressive weight bearing. Because the foot and ankle are under constant stress in the gait cycle, two weeks is probably a conservative guide to restricting "normal" activities and protecting this complex. However, weight bearing, for even the most severe sprains, may be beneficial because it can reduce inflammation and decrease pain. Even the most minor sprains and strains take approximately 6 weeks to heal, and this must be considered when deciding on the appropriate time for relative rest. It is a good idea to keep the foot and ankle protected with a supportive device, at least throughout this early healing phase.

Rehabilitation of the foot and ankle is essentially the same regardless of complaint. The basic problems are strains (Achilles tendon, posterior tibial tendon, extensor hallucis longus tendon), sprains (anterior and posterior talofibular ligament, calcaneofibular ligament, deltoid ligament), hyperpronation syndrome, plantar fasciitis, peroneal tendon dislocation, heel pain (plantar fasciitis, retrocalcaneal bursitis, tendo-Achilles bursitis), seronegative spondyloarthropathies (bone tumor, tarsal tunnel syndrome, calcaneal disorders, sciatica), turf toe, and fractures.

Sprains are classified as grades I through III, as indicated in Tables 44-1 and 44-2[3,5,34] with grade I being the most mild and grade III more severe. Grade I usually signifies a small tear of ligamentous structures with minimal pain and disability. Grade III signifies a relatively unstable structure (for example, greater than 3 mm side-to-side anterior displacement on anterior drawer test, or greater than 10° talar tilt on stress radiography for anterior talofibular ligament sprain) with significant pain and disability. Weight bearing for all three phases is guided by pain and swelling. As soon as the patient is able to bear weight, and when swelling has subsided, progress toward full weight bearing can begin. Use of an ankle support should continue for at least 3 to 4 weeks after the injury to foster ligamentous healing, including collagen proliferation and maturation. To reduce stress on injured ligaments or muscles, a wedge can be added to footwear. For Achilles tendinitis, a heel wedge can be added. It should be of sufficient height to free the Achilles from gait-cycle stresses. A ⅜-inch felt pad could elevate the heel sufficiently to lessen stress on the Achilles tendon.[31] For posterior tibial tendinitis, a medial wedge can be added. For flexor hallucis tendinitis, a rigid plantar splint is beneficial in limiting motion of the great toe. For acute strains these are worn until symptoms subside, and for chronic strains their use may be more protracted.

Hyperpronation syndrome (dynamic pronation, i.e. the foot that "flattens" as one transfers from heel strike to foot flat in the gait cycle) and plantar fasciitis often are present simultaneously, and the former may indeed cause the latter. Hyperpronation syndrome, which is noted by increased medial drift of the ankle complex (forefoot abduction) on weight bearing, is a relatively common

TABLE 44-1 Practical Universal Classification of Sprains/Strains

Grade	Symptoms[a]	Signs	Stability	Anatomy[b]
1	pain—0–2 edema—0–2 tenderness—0–2 swelling—0–2 disability—0–2 function loss—0–2	Stable	≤20% fibers torn; internal micro damage (micromechanical dissociation) with full continuity	
2	pain—3 edema—3 swelling—3 tenderness—3 solid endpoint disability—3 function loss—4 ecchymosis 30%–50%	unstable	20%–70% fibers torn; mechanical dissociation with partial loss of continuity	
3	pain—4 edema—4 swelling—4 tenderness—4 no/mushy endpoint disability—4 function loss—4 ecchymosis 70%–90% palpable mass–strain only palpable gap	unstable	≥70% fibers torn; total rupture	

Note: Pain, tenderness, swelling, edema, and function loss are graded on a 0-to-4 scale: 0, absent; 1, minimal; 2, mild; 3, moderate; 4, severe.
[a]Injuries seen during the golden period have no or minimal pain, swelling, ecchymosis, or tenderness.
[b]Sprain: ligament fibers are torn; strain: muscle–tendon unit is torn.
From Birrer RB: Ankle injuries. In Birrer RB (ed): Sports Medicine for the Primary Care Physician, 2nd ed. Boca Raton, FL, CRC, 1994, p 310.

cause of foot and ankle pain. It is not likened to pes planus, or the fixed flat foot. A person with hyperpronation syndrome maintains a medial longitudinal arch, with the foot not in contact with the floor, but tends to lose or flatten this arch when bearing weight. This repetitive motion tends to stretch the plantar surface and produce pain and disability. Knee pain, particularly of the patellofemoral joint, is sometimes caused by hyperpronation. It is clearly understood that the valgus knee drift that accompanies foot pronation is certainly a factor in patellofemoral syndrome. In addition to stretching the plantar soft tissues, hyperpronation tends to stretch the posterior tibial tendon. The eventual fraying and/or rupture of this tendon can be directly associated with this excess pronation.

The best method for evaluating loss of posterior tibial function is the single heel rise test.[28] For this test the

TABLE 44-2

Classification of Acute Ankle Sprains

Grade	Precipitating Injury	Findings
I	Stepping off curb; stepping on rock; alighting from vehicle; other low-level activity	Little functional deficit; patient can walk without limping and can hop on ankle; swelling minimal and localized; tenderness localized over ATL; may be isolated partial rupture of ATL
II	Misstep while running; inversion sprain while descending stairs; other higher-level activities	Some functional loss; patient may be unable to hop on ankle and walks with a limp; localized lateral swelling; localized tenderness around ATL and possibly calcaneofibular ligament; possible rupture of ATL and tearing of calcaneofibular ligament
III	Vigorous force during footstrike while ankle is plantar-flexed and internally rotated	Patient prefers crutches to weight bearing; diffuse pain and swelling; usually complete rupture of ATL and calcaneofibular ligament; anterior and lateral laxity

ATL, anterior talofibular ligament.
From Baker CL, Todd JL: Intervening in acute ankle sprain and chronic instability. J Musculo Med 54:1995.

patient stands on one leg with the knee extended and rises onto the ball of the foot. A positive test is noted if the patient fails to achieve heel rise or if the heel fails to invert. The failure of heel rise is secondary to the gastrocnemius muscle's inability to flex the foot if the tibialis posterior is malfunctioning and fails to set the heel into a locked, varus position. As will be emphasized later in this chapter, the emphasis in treating plantar fasciitis or plantar surface pain should not be on stretching the plantar soft tissues but rather on strengthening the intrinsic foot muscles. Peroneal tendon subluxation occurs after moderate to severe inversion stress or forceful dorsiflexion tears the peroneal retinaculum. The associated tendons are then free to dislocate from their groove.[2] If this occurs, 5 to 6 weeks of compressive strapping is indicated. After this period, if instability persists, surgical stabilization may be necessary.

Systemic etiologies of heel pain must be considered. An example is Reiter syndrome, for which heel pain can be an arthropathy associated with uveitis and urethritis. Treatments are geared toward the primary diagnosis of Reiter syndrome, and rehabilitation strategies are focused on improvement in overall functional performance.

Neurologic entities such as S1 radiculopathy, tarsal tunnel syndrome (posterior tibial nerve entrapment), deep peroneal nerve entrapment, superficial peroneal nerve entrapment, abductor digiti quinti entrapment, and sural nerve entrapment can all be culprits in heel pain. Eliciting the Tinel sign over various nerves can be helpful if entrapment is suspected. In evaluating heel pain, pay close attention to the distribution of pain and note any associated dermatomal or nerve distribution.

The general algorithm for treating foot and ankle pain is shown in Table 44-3. This model, with minor alterations, is applicable to most rehabilitation programs. The first phase in treating foot and ankle injuries consists of pain reduction and control of swelling. Ice should be used liberally and, in foot and ankle disorders, is helpful beyond the depicted first 24 to 48 hours. In general, after any prolonged activity requiring repeated foot–surface contact, ice should be used liberally to control swelling and decrease pain. Pain and swelling can be further controlled with medications and adjunct modalities. Analgesics and nonsteroidal anti-inflammatory drugs (NSAIDs) are recommended. Analgesics must be used with caution because they may mask potentially detrimental instabilities or injuries. They should be given to take the edge off of high-grade injury pain without masking informational signs or symptoms.

In general, the pain associated with most soft-tissue injuries will begin to abate a few days after the injury. If pain persists or progresses, the insult may be more serious than initially thought. For instance, a presumed

TABLE 44-3

Rehabilitation Sequence

- Diagnosis
- RICE
- Range of Motion
- Stretch/Flexibility
- Proprioception
- Gait
- Strength
- Functional Performance

Adapted from Nicholas JA, Strizak AM, Veras G: A study of thigh muscle weakness in different pathological states of the lower extremity. Am J Sports Med 4(6):241, 1976.

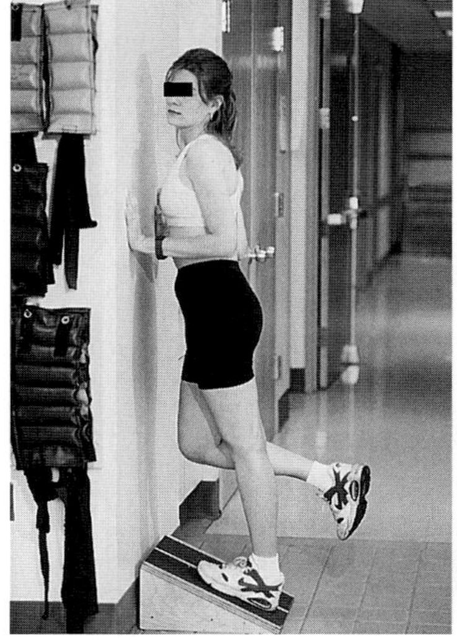

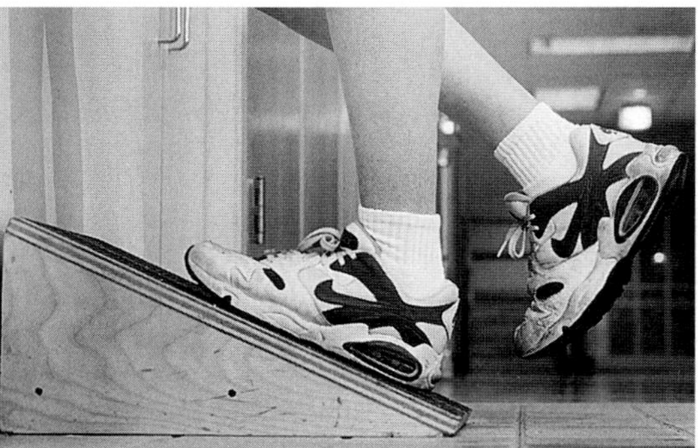

FIGURE 44-1. Standing calf and Achilles stretch. **A** and **B,** Standing on an incline board or on a flat surface, lean forward, keeping the torso and lower extremity straight. The rear leg tries to maintain heel contact with the ground. Hold this stretch for 20 to 30 seconds. Repeat 10 to 15 trials, 3 to 4 times per day.

grade II to III ankle sprain may actually be a subtle fracture. Although x-rays should be routine for many injuries, they are not always taken. A good clinician is aware of subtle changes and lack of progress that alerts him or her to reevaluate an injury.

NSAIDs are useful in reducing edema but must be used with caution. I recommend blood checks (hepatic, renal, and CBC) every 3 months for those taking NSAIDs continuously. I have found approximately 20% of patients, on routine follow-up, with abnormalities on one or more of the above. Modalities such as pulsed ultrasound and electrical stimulation are helpful and should be applied if available. The settings for ultrasound should be 1.5 watts/cm^2 for approximately 7 minutes. This modality can be applied to a submerged limb. In that case the settings are increased to 2.0 watts/cm^2 for 7 minutes. Under water, there is no direct contact of the ultrasound probe with the skin. A distance of approximately one inch should be maintained during its application. Electrical stimulation is useful for edema and pain control. Its intensity is to patient tolerance and it is not used underwater. Positive pole galvanic current is an electrical modality that is very effective for ankle sprains. Contraindications for ultrasound and electrical stimulation are listed in Tables 46-1 and 46-2.

The next phase of rehabilitation emphasizes range of motion. Early ranging is recommended (1 to 2 days after the injury), beginning with active motion. This allows the patient to guide the amount of early motion attempted. If passive motion is emphasized too early, collagen reorganization may be hindered. Once swelling and pain have diminished, more aggressive passive range of motion should commence. Careful measurements should be made of the uninvolved limb to establish range of motion goals for the involved limb. Frequent measurements are made throughout the rehabilitation process to identify ranges that may be lagging. The use of hydrotherapy (cool temperature) allows pain and swelling reduction while increasing range. This can be combined with surgical tubing[52] or muslin. The tubing is placed around the foot and ankle and held with the hands. The patient can then assist in ranging his or her own limb. As pain subsides, the rubber tubing can be used for resistive exercises and in more advanced strengthening techniques. Stretching of the soleus and Achilles tendon is important. These groups are tight in most people and tend to become tighter after injury of the foot and ankle. Figure 44-1 and Figure 44-2 depict a standing calf stretch and Achilles stretch. Each of these stretches is done at least 3 or 4 times per day.

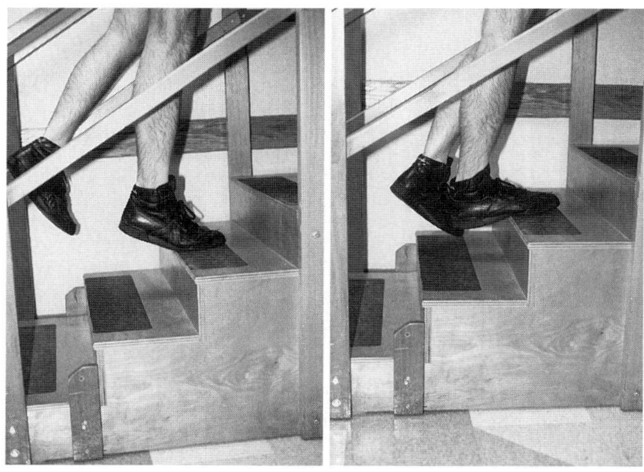

FIGURE 44-2. Standing calf and Achilles stretch. **A** and **B,** With the ball of the foot supported on the edge of a step, slowly lower the heel toward the ground. Hold this for 20 to 30 seconds. Repeat 10 to 15 trials, 3 to 4 times per day.

TABLE 44-4 **Average Proximal Muscle Strength Deficits in Patients with Pathologic Conditions of the Foot and Ankle**

Affected Body Part	Affected vs. Normal Leg Deficit
Hip abductors	31%
Hip adductors	30%
Quadriceps	19%
Hamstrings	26%
Total leg strength	26%

Adapted from Nicholas JA, Strizak AM, Veras G: A study of thigh muscle weakness in different pathological states of the lower extremity. Am J Sports Med 4(6):241, 1976.

During this phase, attention should be paid to the remainder of the musculoskeletal system, particularly the proximal portion of the injured limb. Disabilities of the distal limb often are associated with proximal muscle weakness.[42] The hip abductors have been shown to have a 31% deficit on the involved lower limb side (Table 44-4). This is a significant finding and must be considered in rehabilitation of the limb. This relationship supports the concept that the musculoskeletal system is an interconnected linkage or chain and that when we address any specific region, attention must be placed on the entire system. If we consider all the components of skill training, we can understand why rehabilitation training must involve the entire system.

Proprioception training is important and can be accomplished with the use of a balance board, that is, a BAPS (Fig. 44-3). This type of training reeducates the brain as to where a limb is in space, which capacity is often lost after injury. To maximize proprioception, joint range of motion and local muscle balance must be restored.[19,21] A balance board allows the foot and ankle to range through a full arc of motion in a controlled fashion.

Strengthening the foot and ankle complex is achieved by a variety of exercises. Heel raises can be done on any raised platform while the body is supported on the forefoot. This can be done standing erect (gastroc-soleus group) or with knees bent (isolates the soleus group) (Fig. 44-4). A series of 10 to 20 repetitions repeated three to four times is recommended. As a patient begins to master this exercise, he or she is asked to either wear a weighted vest or hold free weights in the hands (Fig. 44-5).

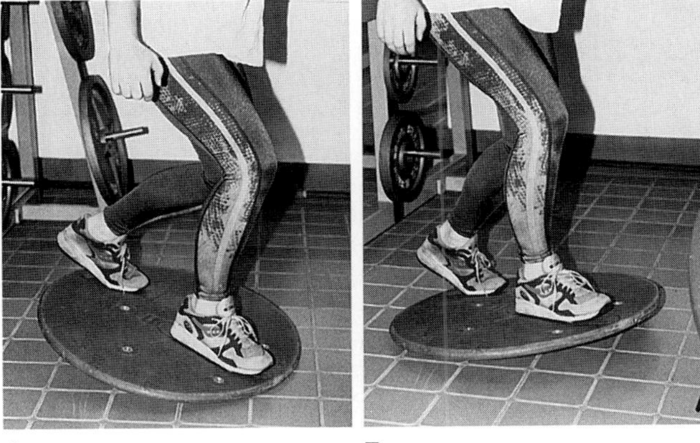

A B

FIGURE 44-3. BAPS for proprioception. **A** and **B,** The involved limb is placed onto the BAPS board and goes through a range of motion in all directions while maintaining contact with the board to increase joint position awareness.

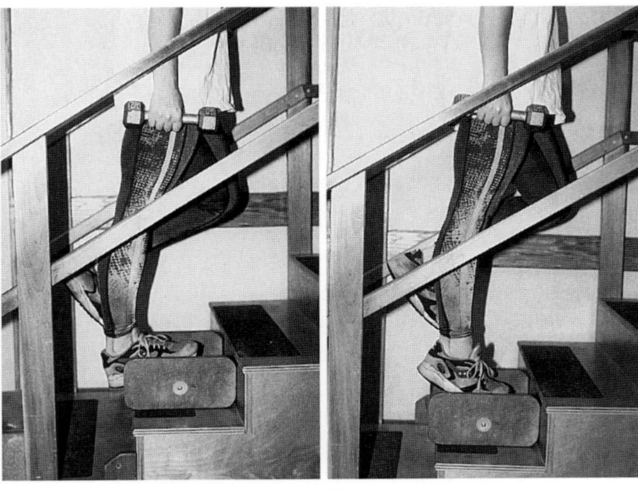

A B

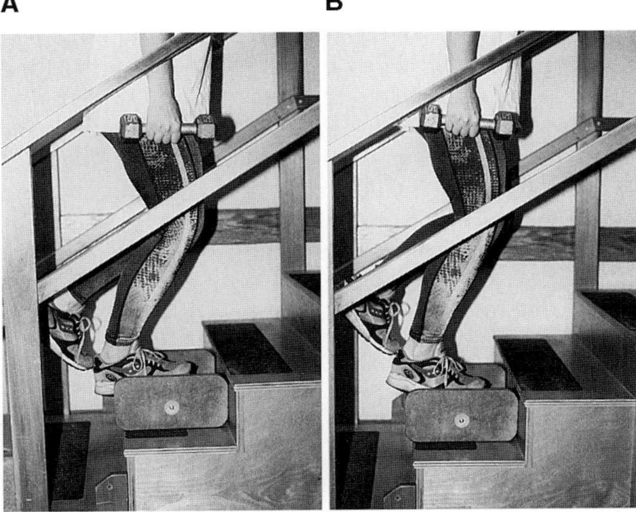

C D

FIGURE 44-4. Standing gastroc-soleus strengthening. **A** and **B,** With the ball of the foot supported on the edge of a step, slowly raise the heel upward. Then slowly lower the heel to neutral. Ten repetitions are done per set. Three or four sets should be done 4 times per day. **C** and **D,** Standing flexed knee soleus strengthening. Same as A and B, but with a flexed knee (approximately 30° to 45°). This technique isolates the soleus muscle, which is important in closed-chain knee extension (posterior pull on tibia relative to femur).

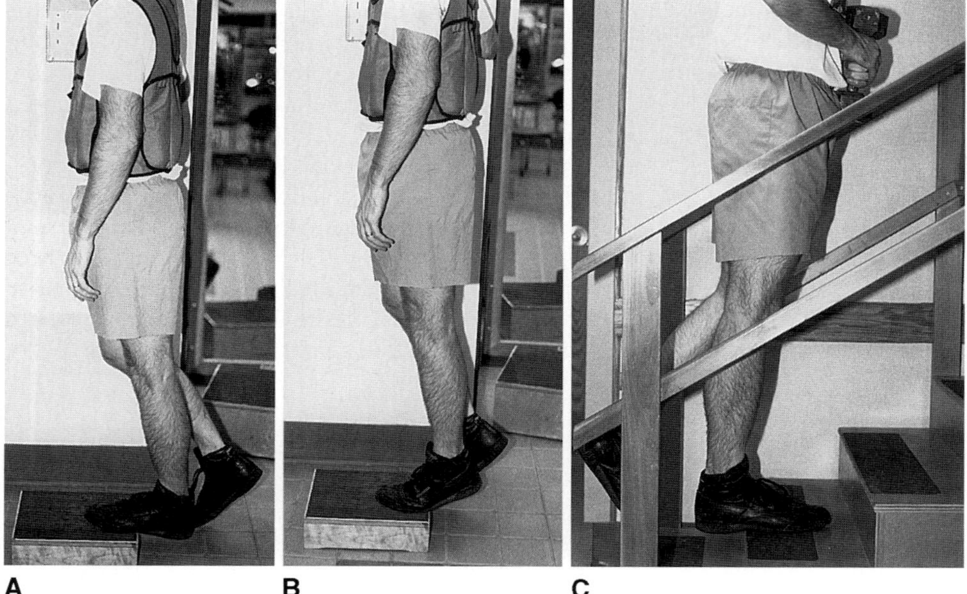

FIGURE 44-5. Gastroc-soleus strengthening with weighted vest. **A** and **B,** Progressively add weight to the vest. The proper amount is enough weight so that you must struggle to complete the tenth repetition of the set. The goal is 10 repetitions per set. Three or four sets should be done 4 times per day. **C,** Gastroc-soleus strengthening holding free weights. Same as A and B but done holding free weights close to the torso.

These weights should be held close to the body to maintain a stable center of gravity.

Writing the letters of the alphabet using the toes as writing instruments is another efficient way of strengthening the foot and ankle complex. To increase the challenge of this exercise, the patient is instructed to wrap rubber tubing such as Thera-Band (The Hygenic Corporation, Akron, Ohio) under the ball of the foot and perform the exercises against the resistance of the rubber (Fig. 44-6). The entire alphabet should be attempted and repeated 2 to 3 times.

The mechanics of forward and backward ambulating place direct stresses on the foot and ankle complex. Forward walking invokes a valgus moment at the knee along with pronation of the foot and ankle complex. Conversely, retro walking causes a varus moment at the knee and supination at the foot–ankle joint. It relates biomechanically to the progression of heel-to-toe mechanics in forward ambulating and toe-to-heel mechanics in retro walking. This exercise is done in an isotonic fashion with resistance offered by the pulling of a weighted sled (Fig. 44-7). Initially start with a load of ½ of the body weight and progress as tolerated. The amount of added weight must not be so much as to alter the mechanics of retro walking. Ask the patient to either strap a belt that is attached to the sled around his or her waist or pull the sled, attached to a cord, with the upper extremities. In both instances, there should be anatomic pelvic tilt and good upper body posture. The weighted sled is pulled a distance of 10 meters (five to ten times) and this sequence is repeated two to three times.

Plantar roll-bar exercises are another method of strengthening the plantar muscle groups. In this exercise, the foot is placed on a roller (roughly 4 inches in diameter) and the patient is asked to grasp the roller with the plantar muscles in a rocking fashion (Fig. 44-8). This is repeated several times and may best be guided by a time frame rather than number of repetitions. For example, the patient should rock over the roller for 5 consecutive minutes.

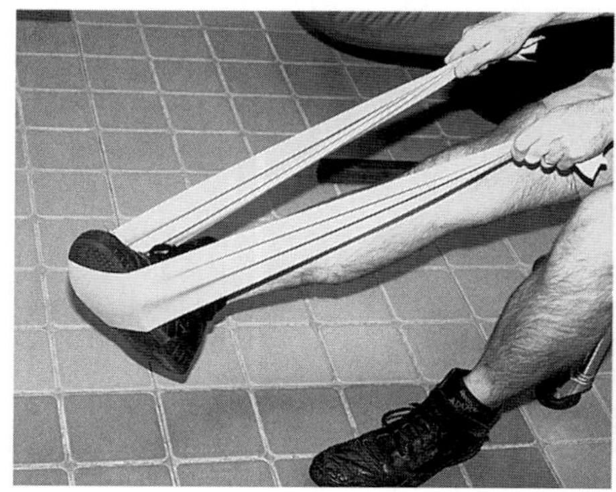

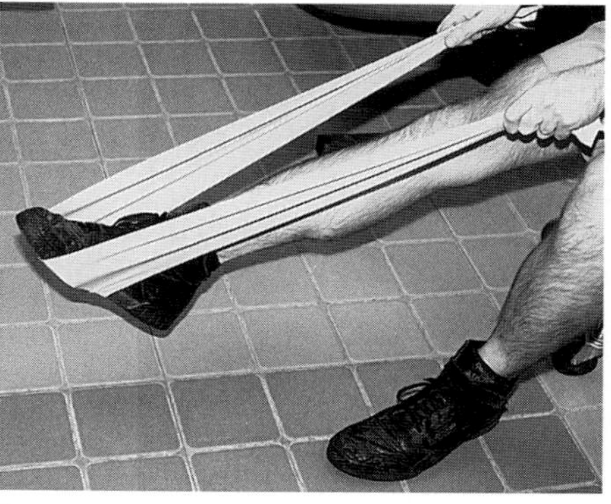

FIGURE 44-6. Thera-Band foot/ankle strengthening. **A** and **B,** Placing a Thera-Band around the ball of the foot, write the letters of the alphabet using the foot as the writing tool. The bands are color-coded to give different resistance when stretched. The exercise is performed by repeating the letters of the alphabet several times or reading printed text and copying the letters with the foot-ankle.

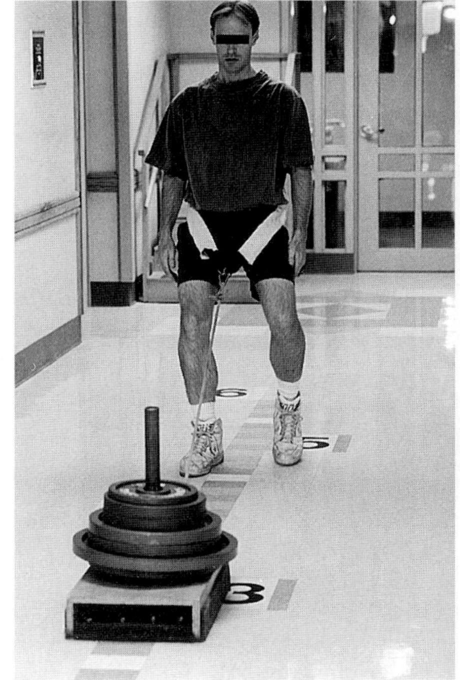

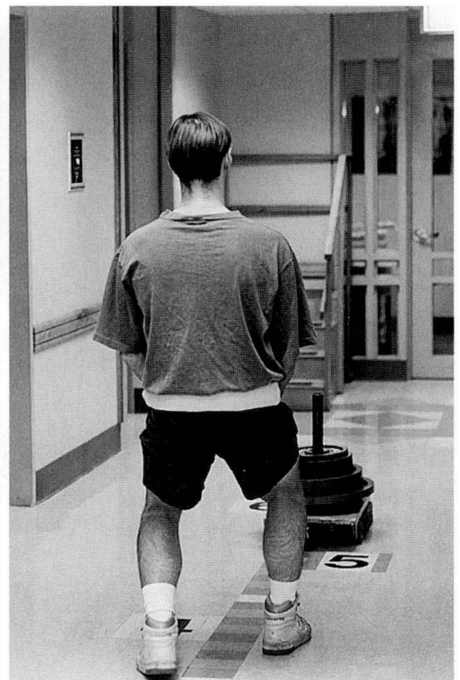

A B

FIGURE 44-7. Retro walking. **A** and **B,** A weighted sled is attached to the body and retro walking is done in a toe-to-heel pattern. Weights are progressively added to the sled. This exercise unloads the patellofemoral joint by increasing the varus movement at the knee.

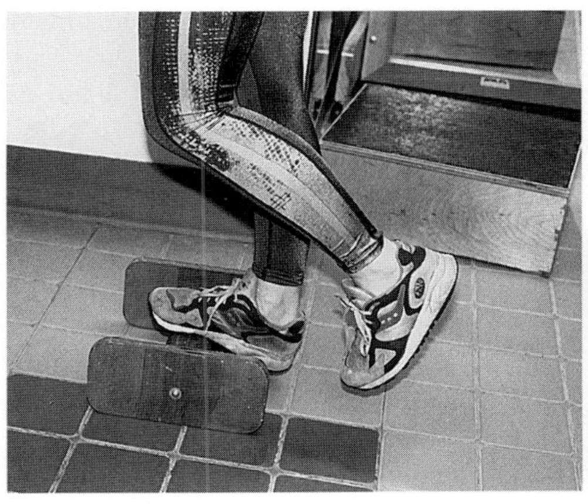

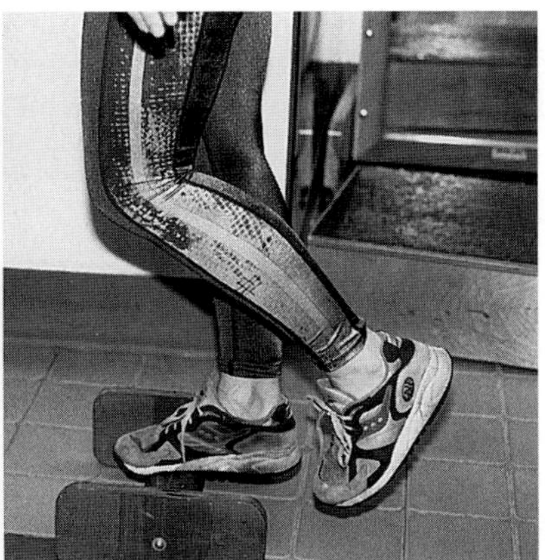

A B

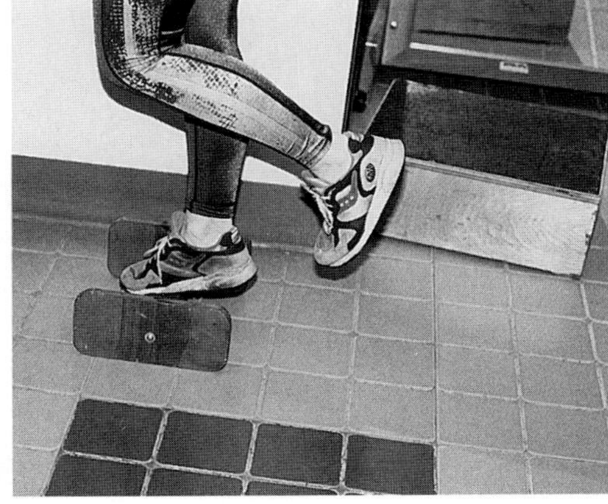

C

FIGURE 44-8. Plantar-roll progressive resistive exercises (PREs). **A, B,** and **C,** While standing, place the foot on a round bar and contract the plantar muscles so as to maintain continuous contact between the foot and the bar. The other leg is flexed and not in contact with the ground. The exercise can be performed by repeating a rocking motion in sets of 30 to 40 repeated 4 to 5 times or, more simply, by repeating the motion for 4 to 5 consecutive minutes. Strengthening of the plantar muscles is important in maintaining upright posture.

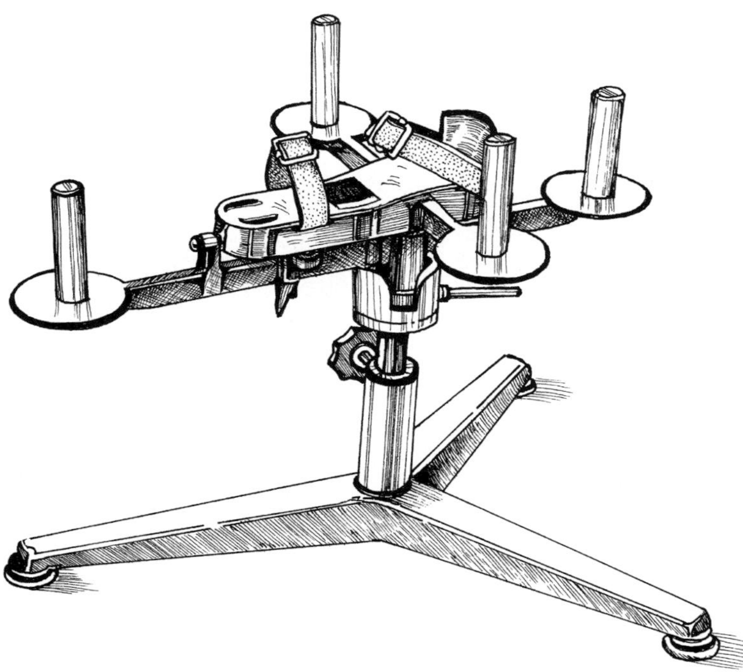

FIGURE 44-9. Elgin ankle exerciser. The patient sits and his ankle is placed in the apparatus. Range-of-motion and strengthening exercises are done.

The Elgin ankle exerciser can be used to increase ankle strength and improve range of motion (Fig. 44-9). The patient places his or her foot and ankle firmly into the device, and weights are added progressively while the patient performs exercise sets. The ankle is ranged to the limits of the motion, that is, the patient achieves maximum dorsiflexion, and then this position is held for 2 seconds before it is returned to neutral. Three sets of 10 to 12 repetitions are done (Fig. 44-10).

More advanced exercises include off-balance weighted ball tossing. This exercise is not used solely to treat the ankle and foot complex but is a key exercise in addressing

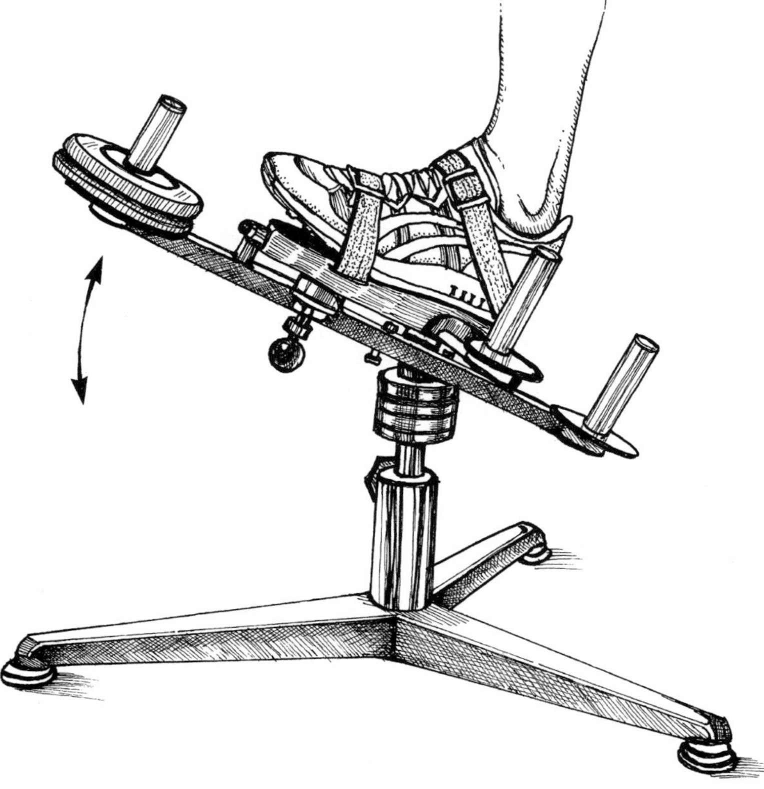

FIGURE 44-10. Elgin ankle exerciser. The patient's foot is placed in the apparatus and, against added weight, moved through a complete range of motion and then held for 2 seconds before returning to neutral. Sets of 10 to 12 repetitions are done 3 or 4 times.

the components of skill. The complex task of maintaining postural control on a rocker board while accomplishing upper extremity acceleration and deceleration training is demonstrated in Figure 44-11. We find this type of multitask challenge very beneficial in our rehabilitation programs. It plays a key role in enhancing proprioception in the ankle and foot complex while challenging the neuromusculoskeletal system.

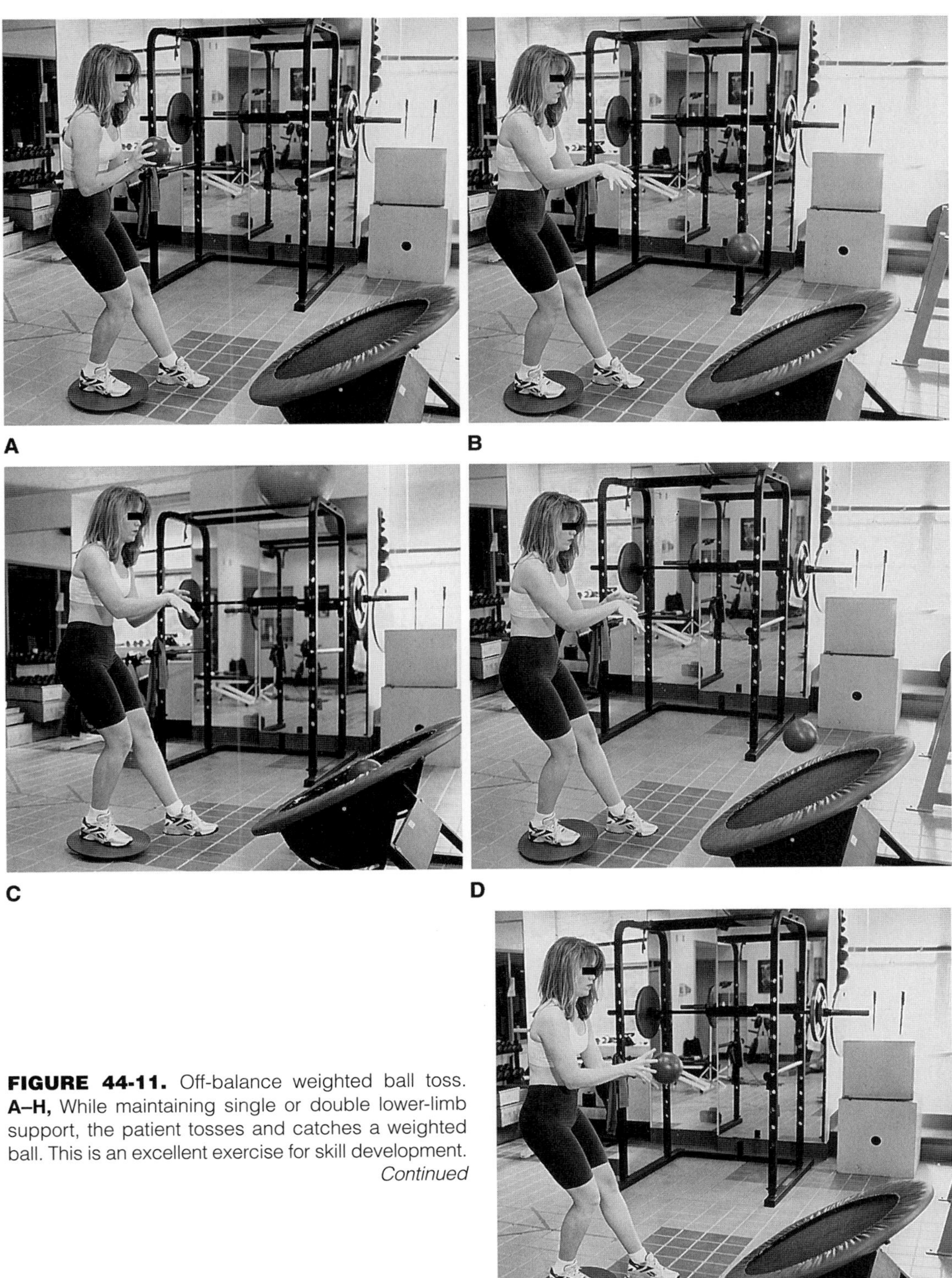

FIGURE 44-11. Off-balance weighted ball toss. **A–H,** While maintaining single or double lower-limb support, the patient tosses and catches a weighted ball. This is an excellent exercise for skill development.
Continued

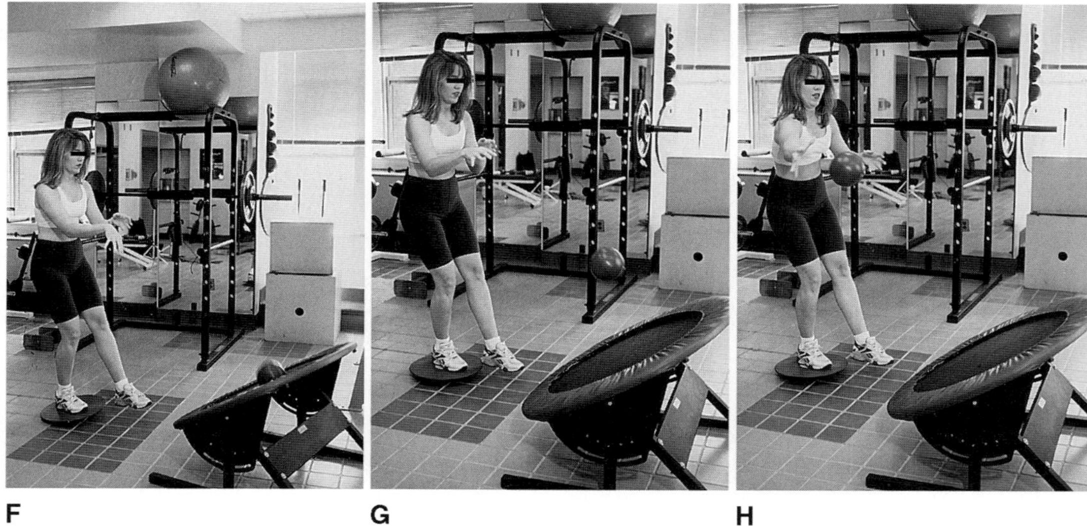

F G H

FIGURE 44-11, cont'd.

The final phase of ankle and foot rehabilitation involves improving agility and speed. To accomplish this, we incorporate forward, lateral, backward, and multidirectional jogs, shuffles, and sprints. Obstacles are strategically placed to challenge the neuromuscular system, which enforces coordination training. Typically, we start with short distances and increase both distance and repetitions. Most gains are achieved by altering the obstacle patterns and timing their completion. We use box patterns and alternate running around and over them (Fig. 44-12). The heights of the boxes are varied to increase the challenge.

The last consideration is footwear. The market is replete with various styles, shapes, contours, heights, and materials of shoe wear. Mann has stated that forces of 2 to 3 times body weight are created at foot-strike during running and jogging.[33] Because it is the first in line to distribute these forces, the ankle and foot complex must be properly protected. The three basic considerations in the construction of athletic footwear are shock absorption qualities, support of the foot, and comfort to the wearer.[38] Each person may express different needs, but all are integral in the management of the ankle and foot.

The shoe is not evaluated as a whole entity but broken down into two basic areas, the rear foot and the forefoot. Each is evaluated separately and has specific characteristics necessary to provide adequate support. The rear foot must have a snug fit and adequate sole surface area to distribute forces, that is, it must possess as large a purchase as possible. A well-fitted heel counter has been shown to decrease resultant forces at heel-strike.[29] In contrast to the primary role of the rear foot (support and shock absorption), the forefoot's main function is support and sole flexibility. The metatarsophalangeal joint undergoes approximately 25° to 30° of dorsiflexion at toe-off, so the sole must be flexible. If not, there is increased incidence of metatarsal stress fracture and gastrocnemius strain.[38]

The use of orthotics to stabilize ankle–foot mechanics, particularly in conditions such as plantar fasciitis and dynamic pronation, has been written about extensively. A range of simple heel cups (to bolster the calcaneal fat pad), to rigid/semirigid full-length inserts, to inverted CAM (controlled ankle motion) boots is used. Controversy often arises as to the proper orthotic, but in our experience there is no clear choice between orthotic inserts and CAM boots. Patient satisfaction with each is about equal. Clearly, a person with recalcitrant signs and symptoms of plantar fasciitis, who has not responded to conservative care with modalities and medications, deserves a trial with an orthotic.

Shockwave therapy is an adjunct for the treatment of plantar fasciitis, but its effectiveness is still debated in the literature.

LEG PAIN

Disorders of the leg are common in sports medicine; their incidence is almost 30%.[11,25,32,46,47] The usual conditions that the clinician should be aware of include strains, shin splints, and stress fractures.

Strains of the leg are fairly common and usually involve the soleus or anterior/posterior tibial tendons. For these isolated instances in the leg, basic conservative treatment is similar to that for any sprain or strain. Ice should be applied liberally, rest prescribed for a short period of time, and NSAIDs and/or analgesics should be given. After pain subsides, a progressive course of stretching and strengthening is indicated. An isolated tear of the proximal portion of the medial gastrocnemius muscle is termed "tennis leg." As originally described

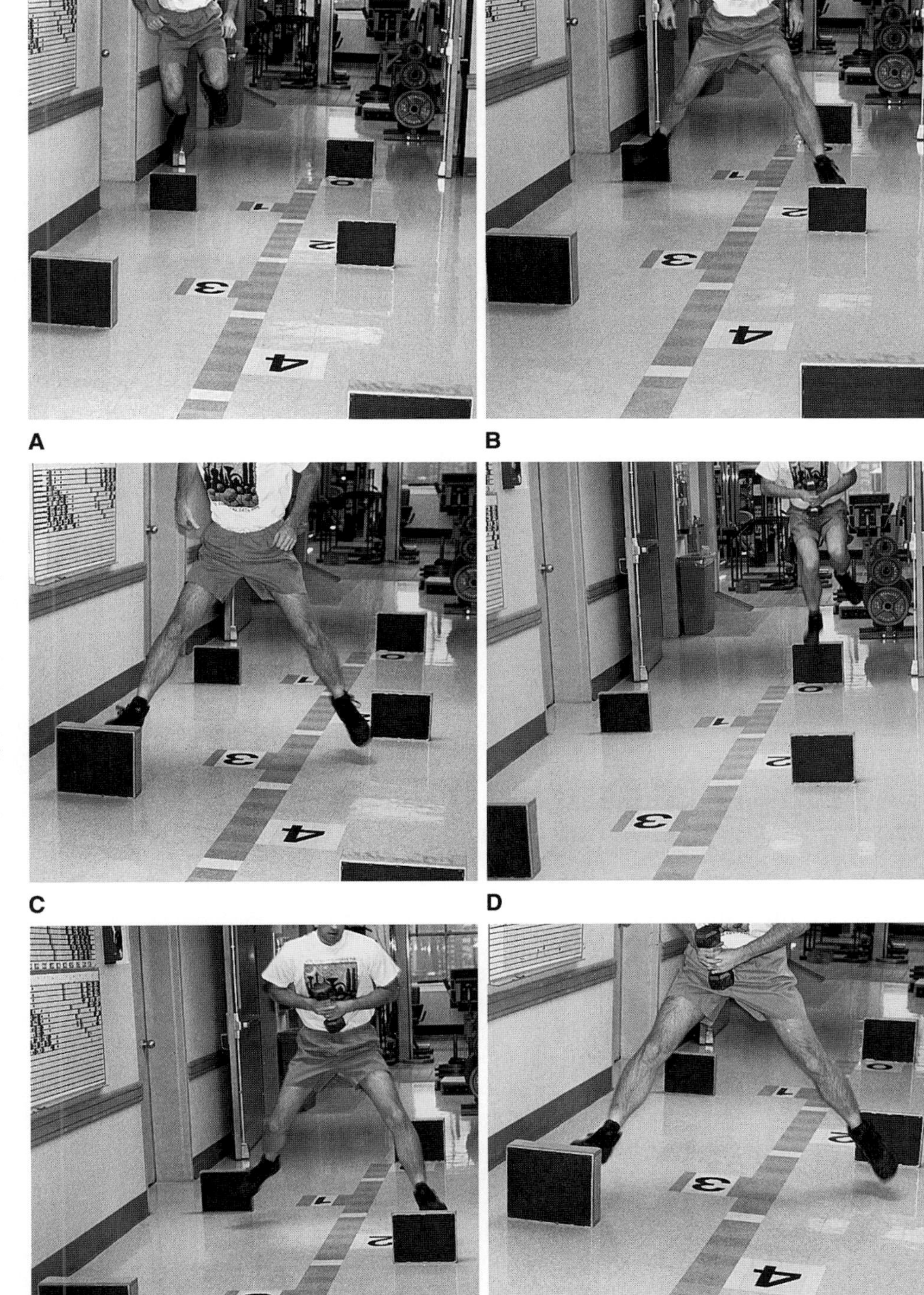

FIGURE 44-12. Agility training. **A–F,** An obstacle course is created that challenges the patient in force acceleration/deceleration, coordination, and balance. As he progresses, timing for completion of the course is monitored. This is an excellent training program for skill development. The pattern of the box layout and the heights of the boxes are alternated on subsequent sessions. **A–C,** without hand weights, **D–F,** with hand weights.

by Powell in 1833, tennis leg was initially thought to be associated with a tear of the plantaris tendon but later was found to be associated with a tear of the medial gastrocnemius.[1,51] Tennis leg typically occurs after a sudden cutting maneuver associated with knee extension and ankle dorsiflexion. Patients feel as though they have received a direct blow to the posterior/proximal part of the leg. On examination, there is often a palpable defect in the region. Treatment includes rest and progressive slow stretching of the leg. Apply a heel lift to unload the gastroc-soleus group during walking. A ⅜- to ½-inch lift is recommended for 2 to 3 weeks.

Shin splints are common and historically are associated with any pain in the lower leg related to overuse.[24] Their location is anterior (lateral tibia) or posterior (medial tibia). When located along the medial tibia the condition is more appropriately termed *medial tibial stress syndrome*.[41,47] Shin splints represent an inflammatory state of the musculotendinous area of the muscles whereas medial tibial stress syndrome represents the same with the addition of periosteal injury. Shin splints are biomechanically correlated to forefoot pronation and the subsequent development of overuse syndromes of the lower extremity.[36] The treatment of shin splints focuses on pain relief, biomechanical correction, and reinjury prevention. Initially, frequent applications of ice (10 to 15 minutes, 3 to 4 times a day), relative rest (no strenuous stretching or contraction of the involved compartment muscles), NSAIDs, analgesics, and taping are used.[5] Orthotics can be considered early if there is evidence of excessive pronation. After the acute phase (2 to 3 days) modalities such as ultrasound can be applied. This will increase local blood flow and expedite tissue healing. A dosage of 1.0 to 1.5 watts/cm^2 is recommended, applied for approximately 5 to 7 minutes.

The next phases of rehabilitation follow the recommendations described for plantar fasciitis. A minor difference would be to more closely focus on eccentric muscle action around the medial ankle joint. The eccentric contraction of the medial soleus is largely responsible for controlling subtalar pronation on heel contact. The patient is advised to refrain from all running for at least 2 or 3 weeks and then gradually begin light jogging over the next 3 or 4 weeks.

Stress fractures are most common in the tibia. Nearly 50% of all stress fractures occur in the tibia.[35] Two differing theories as to the cause of tibial stress fractures somewhat confound the issue of developing rehabilitation strategies, particularly those geared to preventing their occurrence. It is not clear whether muscle weakness or excess contraction causes the fractures. The first theory, proposed by Clement, argues that muscle fatigue reduces the relative shock-absorbing capability of the lower extremities' musculature, predisposing it to fracture.[10] This is noted as an abnormal response to a normal stress. Stanitski and colleagues propose just the opposite.[55] They believe that highly concentrated muscle forces that are repetitively applied to long bones ultimately accumulate to stress fracture. This, in contrast, is noted as a normal response to an abnormal stress.

Once the diagnosis is made, the treatment of stress fractures is essentially rest, reduced weight bearing, and pain management. If the patient has excess pronation, an orthotic should be fabricated. In addition, the clinician must address muscular imbalance and develop training strategies to prevent future insult. In general, focus on stretching the associated inciting musculature, concentrate on cross-friction massage and soft-tissue mobilization. Rest is advised for 4 to 6 weeks and return to competitive sports delayed for about 3 months. Weight bearing is allowed as tolerated throughout the healing phase.

If, however, the fracture occurs on the anterior tibial surface (tension side of the bone), there is potential for delayed or nonunion.[53] This phenomenon has been called the "dreaded black line." An x-ray or fluoroscope will reveal a horizontal fracture line transcending the anterior tibial cortex. If there is evidence of nonunion, weight bearing is limited for at least 4 weeks and surgical drilling may be required.

HIP AND THIGH

Most injuries of the hip and thigh result from overuse or acute trauma. The differential diagnosis of hip pain is rather lengthy and includes disorders such as osteochondritis dissecans, lumbar disk disease, and trochanteric bursitis (see box, Differential Diagnosis of Hip Pain in Athletes).[49] When knee pain is present, the hip should be examined due to the possibility of referred pain from the hip. Often the presenting symptom of a hip disorder is pain in or about the knee. The hip is pivotal in supporting the upper torso above and transmitting the ground reactive forces from below. For this reason it is particularly

CHECKLIST

Differential Diagnosis of Hip Pain in Athletes

Hip dislocation
Hip subluxation with or without acetabulum or labrum injury
Osteochondritis dissecans
Acetabulum or pelvis fracture or stress fracture
Anterior superior iliac spine avulsion
Iliac spine contusion (hip pointer)
Adductor muscle strain
Osteitis pubis
Inguinal hernia
Lateral femoral cutaneous nerve entrapment or injury
Femoral nerve or artery injury
Idiopathic avascular necrosis of the femoral head
Idiopathic chondrolysis
Slipped capital femoral epiphysis
Legg-Calvé-Perthes disease
Metabolic disorders:

- ☐ Sickle cell disease
- ☐ Inflammatory disease
- ☐ Lumbar disk disease
- ☐ Neoplastic abnormalities of the pelvis, acetabulum, or femur
- ☐ Piriformis syndrome
- ☐ Transient synovitis
- ☐ Snapping hip syndrome
- ☐ Trochanteric bursiti

From Pearsall AW: Assessing acute hip injury: Examination, diagnosis, and triage. Am J Sports Med 23(6):40, 1995.

vulnerable to injury. Soft-tissue injuries including sprains/strains, bursitis, and contusions are all treated conservatively. Degenerative changes of the hip are treated with joint stress reduction, corticosteroid injection, or surgery. Neurologic factors must not be forgotten and should be considered in evaluating hip and thigh pathology, especially when there is weakness, atrophy, or progressive radiating pain.

Strains of the hip and thigh usually involve the hip flexors, extensors, adductors, or abductors. The mechanism of injury probably is acute trauma or overuse, and the patient typically has a clear idea of when and how the injury occurred. Injury is often postexertional, and the local region palpates very tender. Hip flexor tendinitis is associated with iliopsoas and rectus femoris dysfunction. A common finding in those, typically females, with unexplained hip pain may be related to anatomic considerations. This may be related to the common finding of synovitis on MRI in those with unexplained hip pain. Possibly the wider pelvic diameter in females predisposes to increased biomechanical stress across the hip, leading to discomfort. Over a period of time, those in this category typically have spontaneous resolution of pain; however, it has a fair chance for recurrence. In those with injury-associated hip pain, isotonic or eccentric overuse is the usual culprit. Rehabilitation strategies are thus geared to restoring flexibility and strength (isotonic and eccentric) to the associated muscle groups. After a brief period of rest, modalities (ultrasound), and, if warranted, NSAIDs (because the pain associated with acute muscle strain is partly caused by an inflammatory response[30]), the patient should begin active exercise focusing on the groin and anterior thigh muscles. Groin stretching is done in various ways; these are depicted in Figure 44-13. The anterior thigh muscles are addressed similarly, as shown in Figure 44-14. Figures 44-15 and 44-16 show hip extensor and abductor stretches.

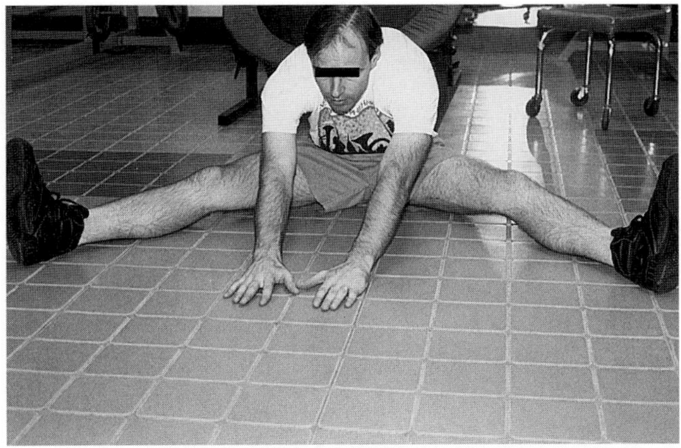

A

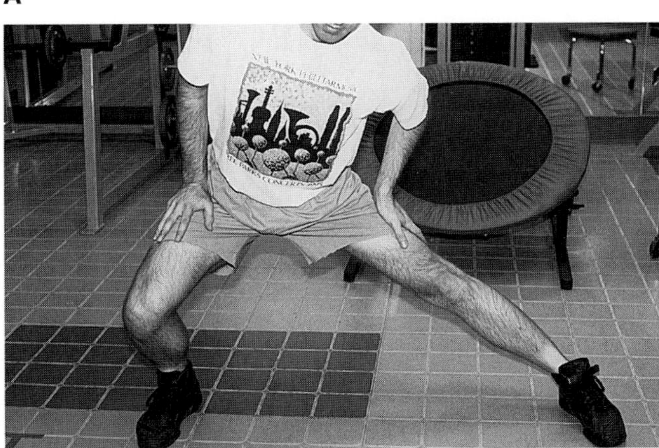

B

FIGURE 44-13. Groin stretch. **A,** Sit with the lower extremities abducted maximally, then lean forward by flexing at the waist. Hold the position for 20 to 30 seconds and repeat several times. **B,** Squat and abduct the lower extremity of the groin to be stretched. Then lean over this limb, place your ipsilateral hand on the waist, and thrust it into adduction. Hold this position for 20 to 44 seconds. It is important not to bounce the area being stretched but to maintain a slow, sustained stretch.

Stretches can be made more efficient if the technique of muscle energy is used. If our goal is to increase stretch of the hamstring muscles, we might ask our patient to place his or her extended lower extremity onto a table as he or she stands alongside (Fig. 44-17). The patient then leans forward over the lower limb and achieves stretch on the hamstrings. The axis of motion for leaning forward should be through the hips, not the lumbar spine. Typically, one will find much greater difficulty leaning forward through the hip axis than when leaning through the lumbar spine axis. Incorporating the concept of muscle energy can improve stretch while increasing flexibility. Stand next to an examining table and ask your patient to lie down on the table and place his or her lower limb on your shoulder (Fig. 44-18). You should then firmly grasp the patient's distal thigh and ask the patient to push downward onto your shoulder. The amount of force exerted by the patient is submaximal and the type of contraction is isometric. (I prefer to allow the patient to slightly overpower me, which may avert any sudden exertional stress, with a potential risk of muscle injury or tearing, that a prolonged isometric contraction may have.) The contraction should be held for a count of 5 to 6 seconds. After completion, the degree of straight leg raise is increased by elevating the patient's limb more cephalad. The entire sequence is then repeated two or three times, each time increasing the degree of hip flexion and hamstring stretch. This technique allows for increased flexibility by "fatigue stretching" the target muscle group. The hamstring group fatigues from repeated contraction, allowing greater excursion with less resistance of the muscles. It would not be surprising to find associated trigger points in the setting of strains, and these must be identified and treated.

Strengthening exercises of the hip region are focused on the same groups we discussed for stretching. The emphasis in strengthening is on resistive training.

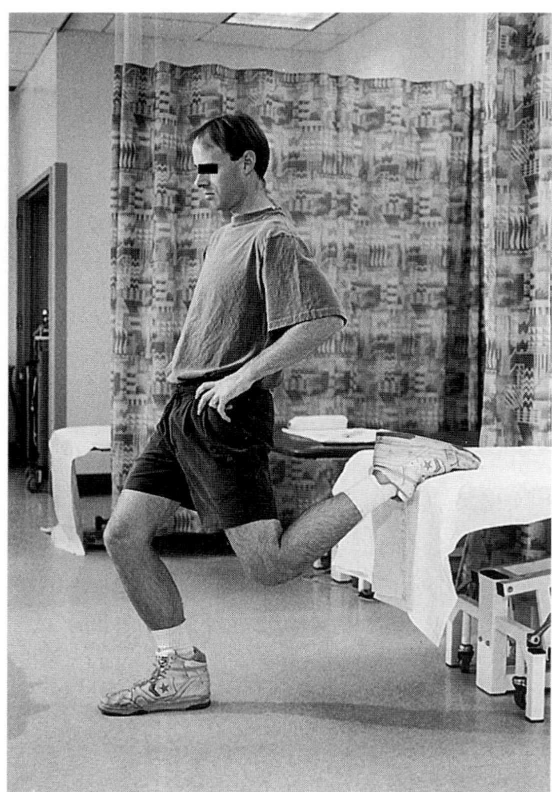

FIGURE 44-14. Quadriceps stretch. Stand and place the back of the foot onto a table behind you. Try not to hyperflex the knee. While maintaining erect posture, perform a posterior pelvic tilt that should, if you are doing the stretch correctly, produce a feeling of stretch on the anterior thigh group. Hold this for 20 to 30 seconds and repeat several times.

Figure 44-19 illustrates several exercises that strengthen the hip region.

Whereas strains are thought to occur at the musculotendinous junction,[43] contusions can be seen anywhere along the musculotendinous unit. Contusions are best treated with ice and compressive dressings. Gradual return to play is allowed, but in the best of all scenarios, healing of a torn muscle (strain) takes a minimum of 6 weeks. The rehabilitation program for subacute and chronic contusions is similar to that for strains.

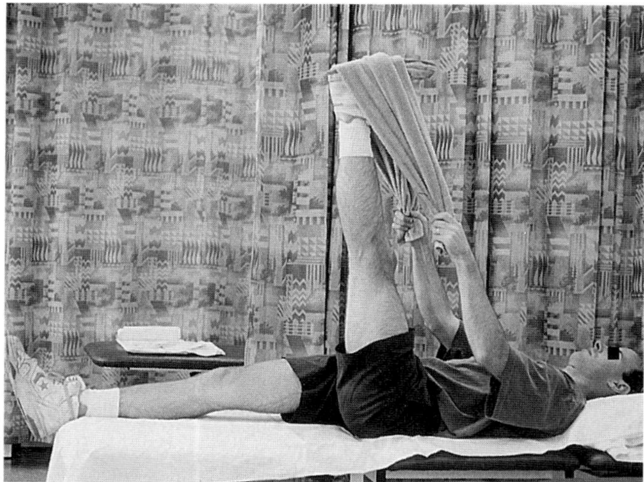

FIGURE 44-15. Assisted hip extensor stretch supine (hamstrings). A towel is used to stretch the hamstring group while the patient is lying down.

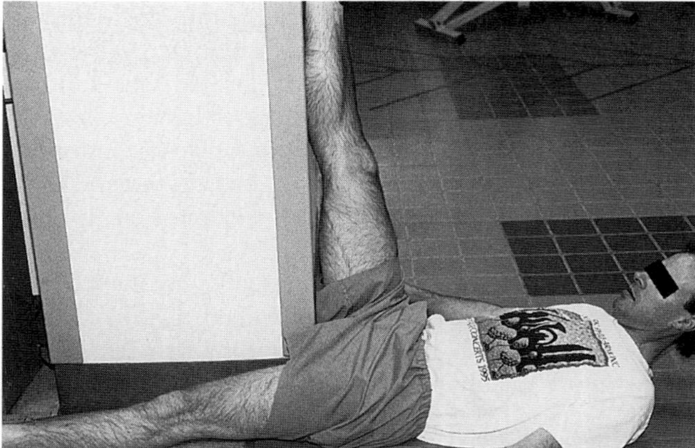

FIGURE 44-16. Wall hamstring stretch. This is best done lying on the floor in a doorway. The leg to be stretched is placed on a wall while the other leg may, if needed, be placed in the doorway. This allows the buttocks to approach the wall and affords the opportunity for the greatest stretch of the hamstrings. As the exercise progresses, the limb is placed, little by little, further up the wall by scooting the buttocks closer to the wall. Hip abductor stretch technique is depicted in Figure 44-36.

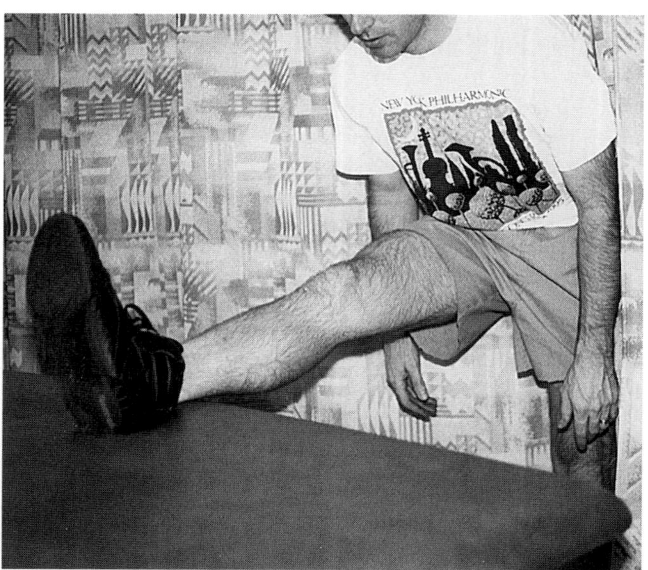

FIGURE 44-17. Standing hamstring stretch. The leg to be stretched is placed onto an adjacent table and the hip is slowly flexed. The cervico-thoracic-lumbar spine remains fairly straight during this maneuver. The stretches in Figures 44-15, 44-16, and 44-17 are held for 20 to 30 seconds and repeated several times. Be careful not to hyperextend the knee when doing these stretches. This could lead to patellofemoral symptoms.

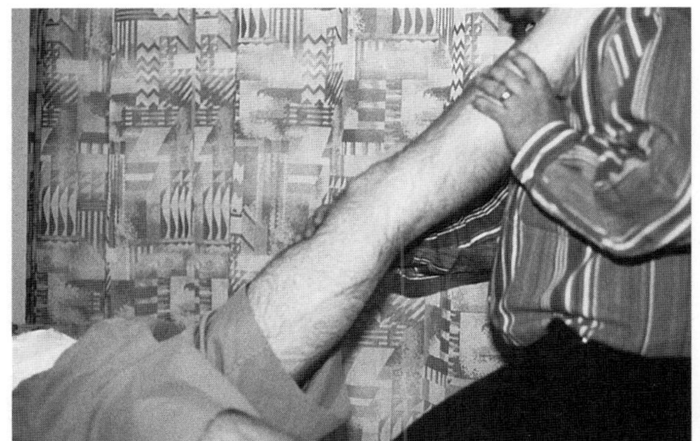

A

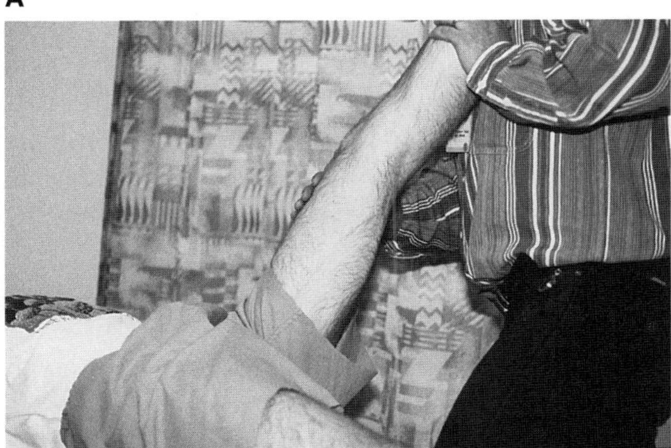

B

FIGURE 44-18. Muscle energy hamstring stretch. **A** and **B,** The patient lies down and places an extended leg on the hands and shoulder of the examiner. He or she attempts to hyperextend the hip against resistance offered by the examiner. The contraction is held for 5 seconds and released. The leg is then flexed further by the examiner and the cycle is repeated.

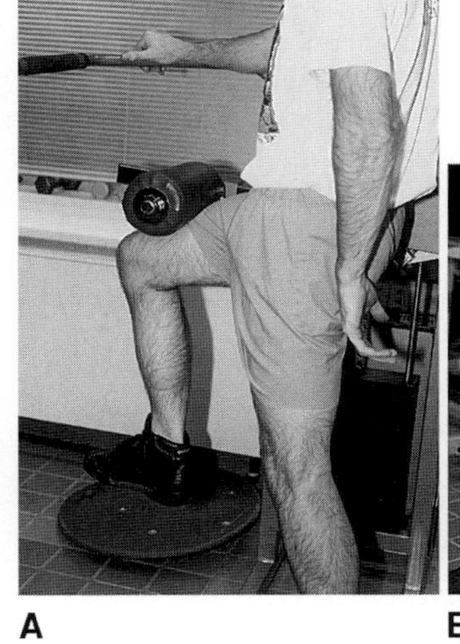

A

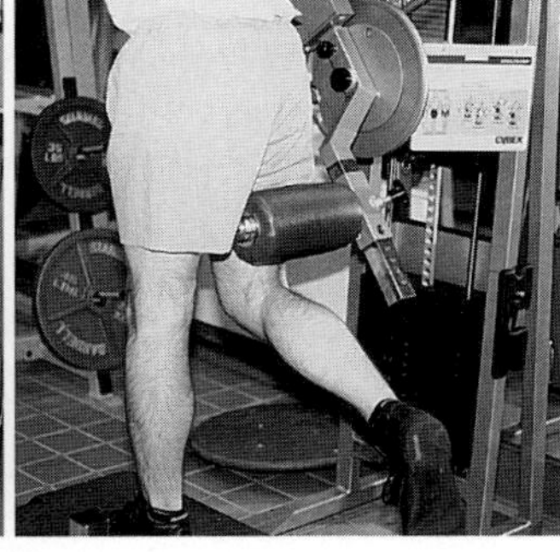

B

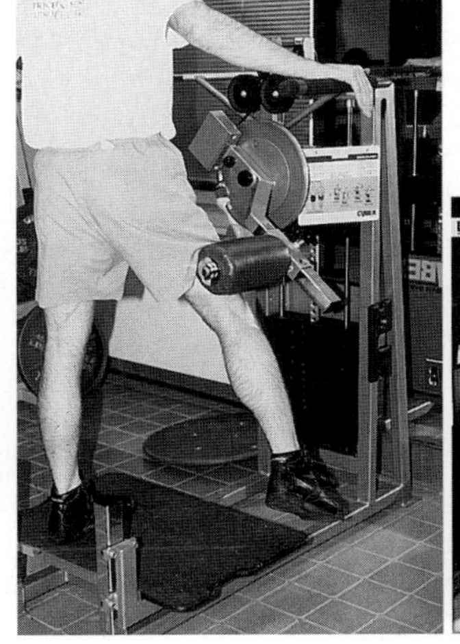

C

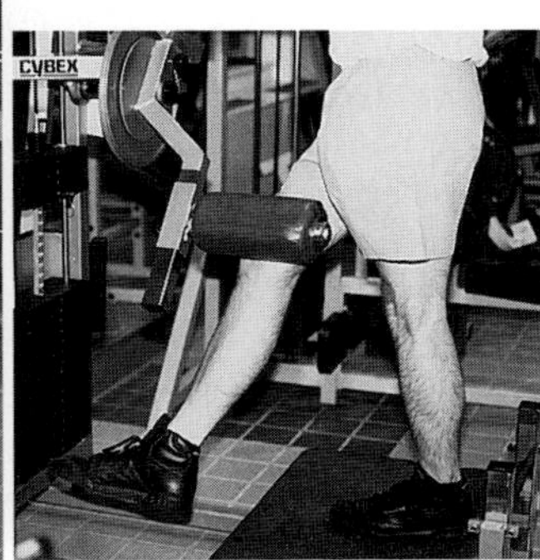

D

FIGURE 44-19. Hip group strengthening. **A–D,** Place the bolster pad above the knee and perform sets of ten repetitions 3 to 4 times. The exercise should be carried through a complete range of motion. To increase stability, the upper limbs can hold onto the support bars. **A,** hip flexors; **B,** hip extensors; **C,** hip abductors; **D,** hip adductors.

Bursitis of the hip, particularly trochanteric bursitis, is fairly common and particularly debilitating. It seems rather easy to diagnose but often can be confused with tendinitis of the external hip rotators. Pain from injury of external hip rotators mimics trochanteric bursitis due to a sharing of common anatomy. The insertion of these muscles onto the greater trochanter makes tendinitis of this group present in a similar manner as trochanteric bursitis. If a course of ice, NSAIDs, and relative rest does not alleviate symptoms, an injection of a steroid and anesthetic into the trochanteric bursa may be helpful (methylprednisolone, 40 mg with 1% lidocaine, 1 to 2 cc).

Degenerative arthritis of the hip is a common, painful disability that progresses, leading to functional loss. Much has been written addressing the affect of joint stresses and the progression or regression of degenerative changes. Joint forces are said to be 2.6 times body weight in single-leg standing and up to five times body weight in running.[39] Rehabilitation strategies in treating an arthritic hip are adapted toward pain relief, joint unloading, and improvement of overall function.

Pain relief is mainly achieved with NSAIDs. Again, be cognizant of the side effects of these medications since patients often take them for a long time. Joint unloading may be the key to offering symptomatic relief of degenerative arthritis. The use of an assistance device such as a cane can help. The literature supports using the cane in the contralateral hand to the most symptomatic hip. Pauwels has stated that the use of a cane in the contralateral hand will greatly reduce force on the ipsilateral femoral head.[48] When the body's center of gravity is in front of the second sacral vertebra directly in the center of the pelvis, weight to the lower extremities is equally distributed to each femoral head. This assumption is made if the distance from the body's center to each hip is equidistant, that is, if the lever arms are equal. If a person leans to either side, the center of gravity also shifts to that side, increasing the relative lever arm to the contralateral side and decreasing the lever arm to the ipsilateral side. On the contralateral side, the hip abductor muscles fire to reposition the body's center of gravity toward midline. This generates significant force across the contralateral hip. If a patient uses a cane on the ipsilateral side, contralateral hip abductor firing is reduced and stress decreased across the contralateral hip. The cane creates a force that acts in the same direction as the contralateral hip abductor muscles.[12]

Another mechanism of hip joint stress reduction is a direct result of the force created by the cane. We have stated that when one leans to the ipsilateral side, the contralateral hip abductors fire and create excessive stress across the contralateral hip. However, the effect on the ipsilateral hip is a reduction in joint stress. This is due to both a shorter lever arm on the ipsilateral side and a mechanical advantage whereby the ipsilateral hip abductor muscles fire less because of the relative hip abduction created by the upper torso's leaning over the lower torso. These concepts explain why we recommend use of a cane in the hand opposite the most involved hip, and why a patient has a propensity to lean over the degenerative hip.

Aqua therapy is beneficial in treating degenerative joints because stress across the joints is relieved by the body's buoyancy in water. Resistive exercises can be done with minimal joint compression when a body is submerged. Exercises range from walking in place (which on land can be extremely painful) to flutter-kicking and aerobic conditioning. A practitioner must be careful when preparing an exercise program for a degenerative joint. There is a misconception that degenerative arthritis and osteoporosis are one and the same. Although the two often coexist, they are separate and distinct entities. Degenerative arthritis is manifest by an overproduction of bone and osteoporosis by the production of weakened bone. As the two entities are different, so too are their rehabilitation and exercise programs. Whereas the patient with degenerative arthritis benefits from the buoyant, stress-reducing effect of water, the osteoporotic patient benefits most from careful loading of the joints, attained by on-land exercises. The deficit in the osteoporotic patient is in the bony matrix, and bone is best strengthened with resistive exercises.

The next consideration in treating the degenerative joint is in ergonomic activity of daily living (ADL) efficiency. Educating patients for proper biomechanical principles often is successful, not so much for pain relief, but for functional improvement. The basic principle is simple. If a patient learns to shorten the effective axial lever arm of each lower extremity, activities of daily living become easier. An example of this is an evaluation of the biomechanics a person uses to arise from a lying-down position. We have viewed and videotaped several patients arising from a prone position. The way a person usually accomplishes this is to thrust the upper torso in front and immediately raise the leg or legs straight. This is followed by a rotational action at the hips and lumbosacral spine, to carry the lower extremities over the bed or exam table. The legs and feet are carried through an arc and are eccentrically controlled by the associated muscles until the feet rest on the floor. The stress across the hips is directly related to the length of the lower extremities and the distance of the distal-most segment from the hip. The accumulated forces across the hip can be significantly reduced when the lower extremities are flexed as a person rises. Also, using the arms and hands to help the upper torso rise increases ergonomic efficiency (Fig. 44-20).

When one notes persistent groin pain that is associated with a twisting injury, a sports hernia may be evident. This entity involves injury to one or more of the following structures: the conjoint tendon, transversalis fascia, or ilioinguinal nerve. Discomfort is noted in the

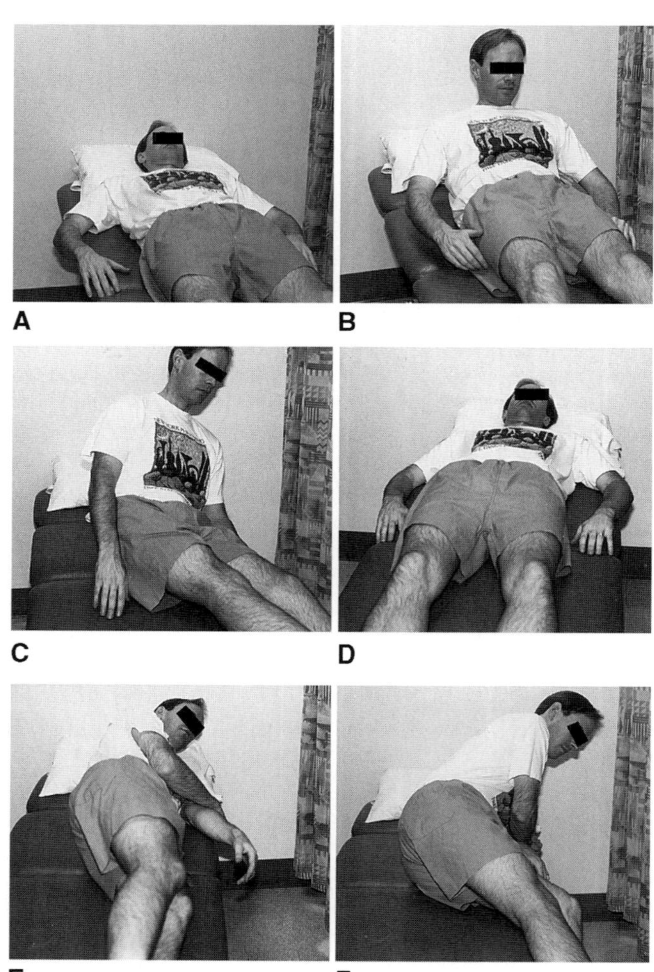

FIGURE 44-20. Ergonomics of getting up. **A–C** demonstrates poor ergonomic efficiency when arising from a supine position, as compared to **D–F,** which illustrates a more efficient method. The stress on the low back is decreased in **D–F**.

inguinal and inner thigh region and is increased with positions of pelvic rotation. Also, when the ilioinguinal nerve is stressed, pain may radiate into the labia or scrotum. It is often a diagnosis of exclusion, but ultrasonography is often a reliable tool when it detects bladder evagination into or through the transversalis fascia. The efficacy of ultrasound is enhanced in that it is a dynamic study and when the patient performs a Valsalva maneuver, the intraabdominal and pelvic pressures highlight the anatomic defect. Symptoms related to the sports hernia may resolve with conservative care including use of analgesic and/or anti-inflammatory preparations; however, the treatment for the sports hernia is usually surgical.

KNEE

The knee is one of the largest joints in the body and accounts for one third of sports injuries clinically evaluated.[5] The most common injury seen is tendinitis. This four-bone, three-joint structure is very mobile and has drawn significantly increased attention in sports-related injuries. From simple strains to total joint arthroplasty, the disabilities affecting the knee present an array of therapeutic options for rehabilitation protocols.

In this section, we will focus specifically on rehabilitation options. Sprains, strains, and tendinitis are common disorders of the knee. The most common injuries affect the anterior/posterior cruciate ligaments, medial/lateral collateral ligaments, capsule, quadriceps, hamstrings, iliotibial band, and patella tendon. The anterior cruciate ligament sprain/tear has become the rehabilitation challenge of the new age. In the not-too-distant past, recovery after ACL surgery was destined to be greater than one year. Although full recovery, physical and psychological, may still take approximately one year, functional success now is seen at a much shorter time. Today, physicians routinely discharge patients within a few months after surgery, giving them the green light for athletic participation. The trend to accelerate rehabilitation protocols began with Shelbourne in the 1980s.[54] In evaluating noncompliant postoperative patients, he found that those who progressed at their own accelerated pace did not as a group suffer adverse effects. Many programs have been developed since with varying rates of progression. Our program has fluctuated between a 4- to 7-month time frame. It is unfortunate, but true, that many patients search for a rehabilitation facility with the promised time frame for completion as a pivotal determining factor. I spend hours counseling patients and trying to redirect their focus. Using our components of skill as the foundation for our training program, patients are encouraged to concentrate on functional outcomes rather than time frames.

Our postoperative training program is addressed by four phases (see box, Post-Op ACL Rehabilitation). Phase I, Early Functional, incorporates weeks 1 and 2. The emphasis is on pain/edema reduction, gaining functional range of motion, achieving normal gait mechanics, balance control, and achieving independent ambulating. We allow full available range of motion within the first few days after surgery. Weight bearing is as tolerated. Retro walking while pulling a nonweighted sled is started in the first phase (Fig. 44-21). This technique is particularly useful for strengthening the

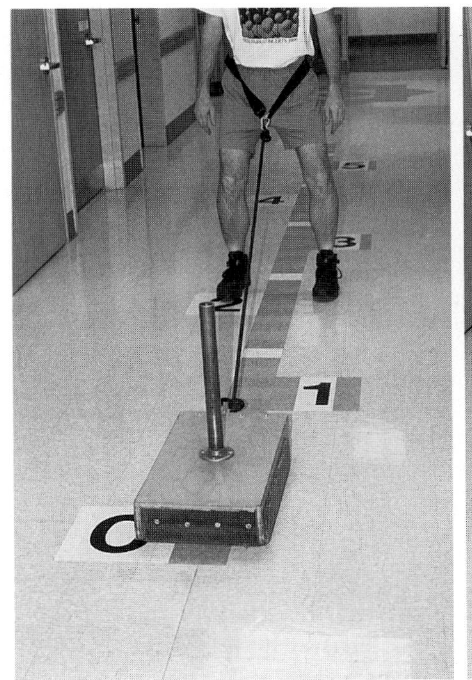

A

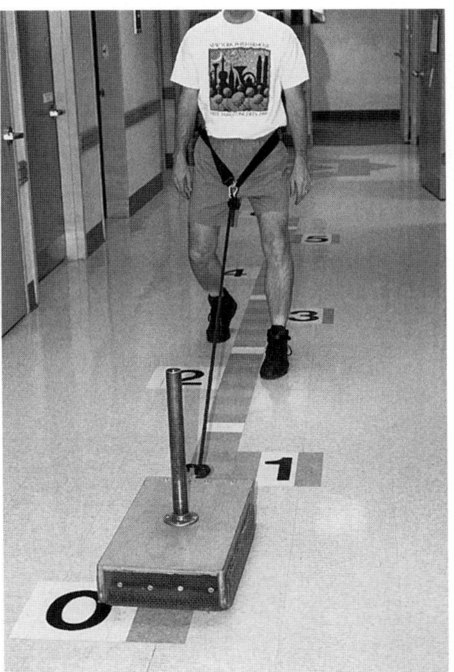

B

FIGURE 44-21. Retro walking pulling a nonweighted sled. **A** and **B,** Retro walking is useful to unload the knee and relieve patellofemoral forces while strengthening the lower extremities.

CHECKLIST

Post-Op ACL Rehabilitation

Phase I—Early Functional (Weeks 1–2)
Goals:

1. Attaining full (involved knee) extension/flexion
2. Pain/edema reduction
3. Ambulation without assistive device
4. Normal gait-cycle mechanics
5. Early balance control
6. Baseline values for uninvolved limb training program, including 10 rep max testing (leg press), and isokinetics

PO Day 1

- ☐ Bledsoe 0°–60° for ambulation, increased excursion as knee ROM increases (sleep with brace locked in full extension until attaining comfortable extension)
- ☐ CPM 0°–60° or as tolerated started in recovery room, twice/day for 2 hours each session. Continued daily CPM until attaining 90° active knee flexion, increased CPM daily, approximately 10 (more if tolerated)
- ☐ Ice for 20 minutes every 1–2 hours
- ☐ Ambulating bearing weight as tolerated with brace on, using axillary crutches
- ☐ Beginning patella mobilization when drain removed
- ☐ Electrical stimulation to decrease pain/effusion, and for quadriceps/hamstrings co-contraction
- ☐ Passive extension 4–5 times/day (passive knee extension with use of bolster or pillow under ankle)
- ☐ Heel slides
- ☐ Supine wall slides with operated limb supported by nonoperated limb
- ☐ Pain medication
- ☐ Standing knee extension (soleus, hamstrings, quadriceps)
- ☐ Gait training

PO Day 2

- ☐ Continuing above as needed
- ☐ Hamstring isometrics 0°–90°
- ☐ Active quadriceps/hamstrings co-contraction (hamstrings by first pushing heel into table followed by pushing knee into table)
- ☐ Ambulating stairs
- ☐ Attempting SLR with brace locked at 0° (all directions, may remove brace if good quad control)
- ☐ Full passive extension
- ☐ Sitting hip flexion

PO Days 3–7

- ☐ Continuing above as needed
- ☐ Retro walking: start with no load, progress to pulling weighted sled, increase load in subsequent weeks
- ☐ Calf raises
- ☐ BAPS sitting, progress to standing
- ☐ Multi-hip–to involved limb
- ☐ Active flexion (full arc), active extension 90°–0° (or as tolerated)
- ☐ Prone hangs
- ☐ Quadriceps isometrics at varied degrees of knee flexion
- ☐ Standing wall slide to 30° knee flexion
- ☐ Stationary bicycle: start with comfortable seat to promote flexion, most force through nonoperated extremity; increases seat height in subsequent sessions
- ☐ Teaching home stretching for quadriceps, hamstrings, gastroc
- ☐ Bilateral standing knee bend 0°–30°
- ☐ Bilateral standing balance exercises, i.e., sidestepping, marching, line walking in parallel bars
- ☐ Forward propulsion of rolling chair using alternating lower extremities

PO Days 8–14

- ☐ Continuing as above
- ☐ Resisted knee flexion prone
- ☐ Full active range of motion
- ☐ Multi-hip bilateral lower limbs (AP/Lat)
- ☐ Step-ups without weights (add weights and height gradually)

Continued

CHECKLIST

Post-Op ACL Rehabilitation—cont'd

- ☐ Unilateral knee bends (0°–30°), be aware of patellofemoral signs and symptoms
- ☐ Unilateral balance standing
- ☐ Resisted SLR (without brace if good quad control) resistance applied proximal to knee
- ☐ Beginning (closed-chain) leg press (begin with short arc) and targeted range of motion to increase proprioception
- ☐ D/C crutches
- ☐ Multi-hip in all directions

Phase II—Progressive Functional (Weeks 3–9)
Goals:

1. D/C post-op brace: begin knee sleeve with patella cut out
2. Achieving symmetric balance proprioception of bilateral lower limbs
3. Maximizing neuromotor development of all muscle groups

Weeks 3–4
- ☐ Continuing as above
- ☐ D/C post-op brace when knee stable (good quad control), switch to sleeve with patella cut out (when sutures removed)
- ☐ Progressing to medicine ball toss on weighted stool
- ☐ Unilateral standing medicine ball toss
- ☐ Pool activities: FAROM, underwater flutter kicking with knees flexed and motion occuring at hips
- ☐ Cable column with locked knee or brace in full extension. Must have good quad control. Begin flexion and extension. Progress to abduction/adduction (be more cautious with those patients who have meniscal and MCL/LCL involvement)
- ☐ Relaxed knee dead lifts
- ☐ Forward and backward fast walking
- ☐ Short step closed-chain step machine (low resistance)

Weeks 5–6
- ☐ Continuing as above
- ☐ Progressing to PREs for knee extension. Begin with cuff weight for involved leg. Perform this exercise with cuff weight until patient can do at least 20 lbs
- ☐ Ball toss on rocker board (double support, single support)
- ☐ Standing cable column (flex, extend, abd, add) with multi-joint motion, BLE (including knee)

Weeks 7–8
- ☐ Continuing as above
- ☐ Begin progression of lateral activities: ski simulator, lateral stepping, lateral shuffles, and slide board
- ☐ Simulated running using cable column
- ☐ Crossover stepping; progress to cariocas as tolerated
- ☐ Modified posterior lunge to 45° flexion, weight on lead leg

Weeks 8–10
- ☐ Continuing as above
- ☐ Standing bicycle with high resistance
- ☐ Initiating plyometrics: mini-jumps on leg press at approximately 30% of body weight
- ☐ Lunges (modified range of motion)

Phase III—Functional (Weeks 10–16)
Goal:

1. Mastering functional tasks of desired physical activity

Weeks 10–15
- ☐ Progressing to mini-jumps in the hallway
- ☐ Initiating depth jumping and hopping as tolerated
- ☐ Beginning sport-specific activity
- ☐ Evaluating light jogging

Week 16
- ☐ Leaping
- ☐ KT 2000, isokinetic evaluation (repeat isokinetics every month until side to side for quads adequate, i.e., 10%. Hams should be symmetric)
- ☐ Video analysis of functional performance, i.e., running, jumping

Continued

CHECKLIST

Post-Op ACL Rehabilitation—cont'd

Phase IV—Return to Sport (4–6 months)
Goals:

1. Isokinetic values to exceed baseline uninvolved limb values
2. Normal performance on functional testing
3. Pain alleviation
4. No effusion with sport-specific exercises
5. KT 2000 4 mm side-to-side
6. Return to sport
7. Adaption to accelerator and decelerator forces and changes of direction
8. Development of power

Functional brace if:
KT 5 mm side-to-side
Pain on sport-specific activity
Patient chooses so

* Throughout program, patients undergo intense, uninvolved lower-extremity and bilateral upper-extremity training program as well:

Onset
Performing Cybex evaluation on sound limb
Performing baseline functional testing and periodic 10 rep max testing
Strength Assessment

The patient's maximal lifting capabilities will be assessed in order to assign the optimal training loads necessary to induce maximal strength gains. The patient will determine the most weight that can be safely lifted ten times in a given exercise. This value will be considered his ten repetition maximum (10 RM)

The 10 RM–value represents 75% of a patient's total lifting capacity and is useful in establishing training workloads for specific exercises. This test is currently administered in the following exercises: knee bends, step-ups, leg extensions, and stiff-leg dead lifts. The 10 RM–test, however, is appropriate for any exercise involving multiple sets with a distinct number of repetitions.

lower extremity while unloading the patellofemoral joint. It causes a supination moment at the subtalar joint while the knee goes into varus.

Phase II, Progressive Functional, includes weeks 3 through 9. During this phase the post-op brace is usually discontinued. Neuromotor developmental training enters full swing to prepare for sport-specific training. Progressive resistive training of the quadriceps begins around postoperative week (POW) 5 or 6. We use various modes of resistive training to maximize efficiency by training the nervous system to solve problems. Knee extensions using ankle weights challenge the system in a different way from performing knee extensions using a cable column (Fig. 44-22). With progressive weight training, our strategy is to impose greater responsibility on the entire body while tasks are attempted. For greater coordination and balance, we ask a patient to stand and balance (single or double support) on a BAPS or rocker board rather than sitting in a chair to perform biceps curls. These techniques, which are the foundation of motor learning, are the forerunners of skill development. Motor learning strategies integrate the afferent, perceptive, and efferent functions of the mind and body that govern posture and movement.[45] Before progressing to Phase III we begin to emphasize force-absorption strategies.

It is well known that we all seem to focus on gaining strength to improve force production—to be able to throw a baseball harder, to kick a football farther, to jump higher, and to sprint faster. But when one looks more closely, a few questions surface. Why are there so many knee injuries in basketball players? Why are there so many rotator cuff ailments in baseball pitchers? Why do golfers strain their quadratus lumborum and rhomboid muscles? The common link among all three is the probable mechanism of injury: poor force absorption or inefficient deceleration of the agonist muscle group. McNair, studying landing characteristics in normal and ACL-deficient knees noted that ACL-deficient knees were not adept at force absorption.[37] Our focus is primarily on accepting forces rather than producing them.

Consider the martial art aikido. It isn't unusual for a 95-pound aikido player to accept the challenge of and dominate a 230-pound attacker. Certainly the attacker is larger and may be more powerful, at least for force production, but the aikido player is functionally stronger.

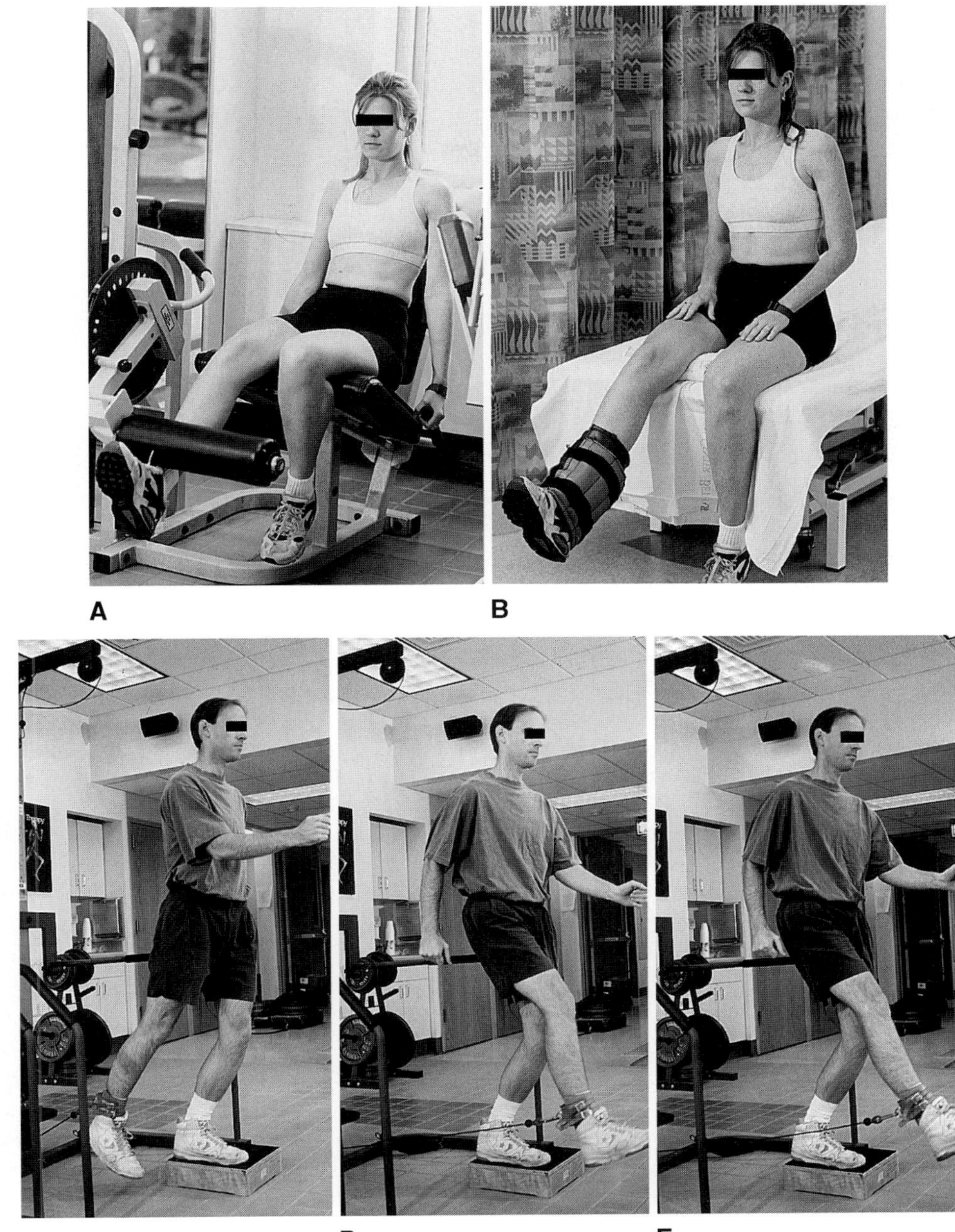

FIGURE 44-22. Quadriceps strengthening. Open-chain strengthening is performed when the distal aspect of the exercising limb is not in direct contact with an external source; and closed-chain strengthening is performed when the distal aspect of the exercising limb is in direct contact with an external source. This, a rather confusing issue, is clarified if one thinks in terms of **perpendicular** and **axial** load when speaking of **open**- and **closed**-chain, respectively. With the quadriceps, a perpendicular load exercise is one in which the majority of forces passes through (anterior-posterior or posterior-anterior) the tibio-femoral joint. An axial load exercise is one in which the majority of forces passes through (cephalad-caudad or caudad-cephalad) the tibio-femoral joint. If you want to spare undue stress across the ligaments of the knee, axial loading is more appropriate, and when trying to spare undue stress on the articular surfaces of the knee, perpendicular loading is more appropriate. **A–E** depict open-chain quadriceps exercises and **F–H** depict closed-chain quadriceps exercises. **A,** Seated supported knee extension. **B,** Seated unsupported knee extension (requires more intrinsic balance and coordination than A). **C–E,** Standing cable column knee extension (requires more balance and coordination than A or B).

Continued

He or she summates forces from within with the absorbed forces from the attacker. The aikido player actually uses the strength of an opponent to overpower the opponent. By skillfully maneuvering the body, the player can internalize extrinsic forces and put them to productive use. In essence, the aikido player is skilled and masters force absorption. In our training sessions, we try to achieve similar skill. For example, we employ box jumping (Fig. 44-23). The focus is not so much on the height of ascent achieved but rather the technique of descent. With video analysis, frame-by-frame sequences can be reviewed to identify weakness in landing. This has been extremely helpful and the combination of off-balance and force-absorption training has made the most significant positive impact on functional testing scores.

The next phase in our rehabilitation program (Phase III) is the Functional (POW 10 to 16) period. Jogging begins and the focus is on sport-specific activities. There is an extension of the activities from Phase II. The last phase (IV) begins with POW 16 and spans approximately 2 months. It involves more advanced techniques of pivoting and leaping. At completion of this phase, the athlete is usually ready to undergo functional testing to evaluate for return to sport. Functional testing is performed at approximately 4 to 6 months postoperative and assesses five parameters before return to sports.

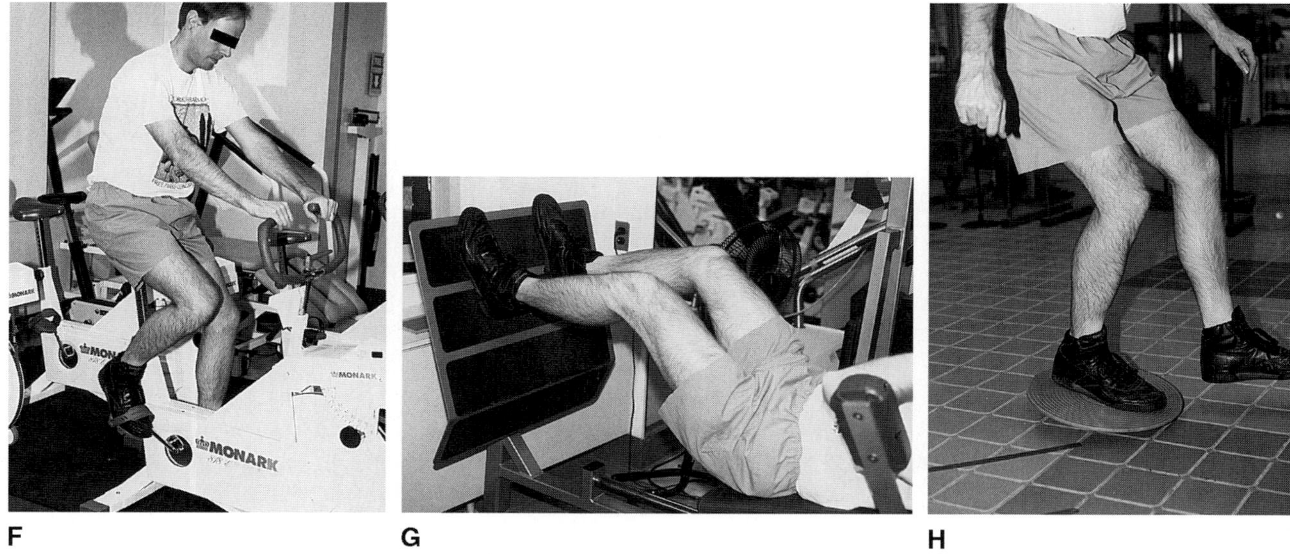

F G H

FIGURE 44-22. cont'd. F, Stationary bicycle. **G,** Leg press (be careful not to hyperflex/extend the knee). **H,** Knee bend. The above should be done in sets of ten repetitions, 4 to 5 times. Be careful not to hyperextend the knee in the above exercises; this could lead to patellofemoral symptoms.

A B C D

E F

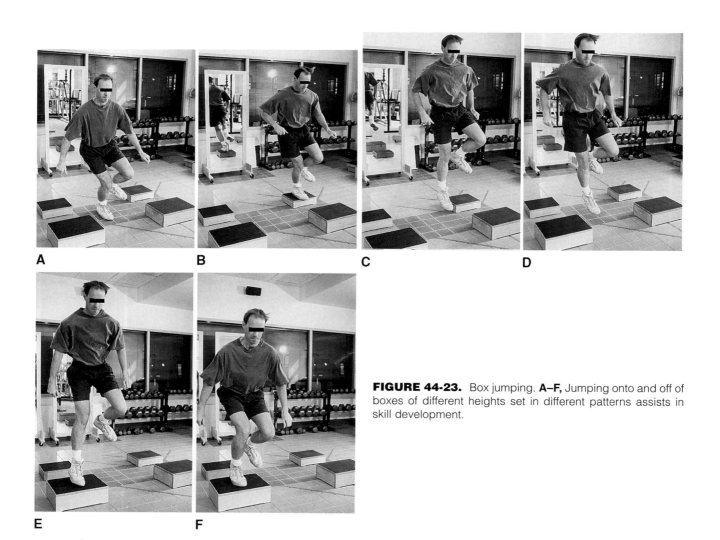

FIGURE 44-23. Box jumping. **A–F,** Jumping onto and off of boxes of different heights set in different patterns assists in skill development.

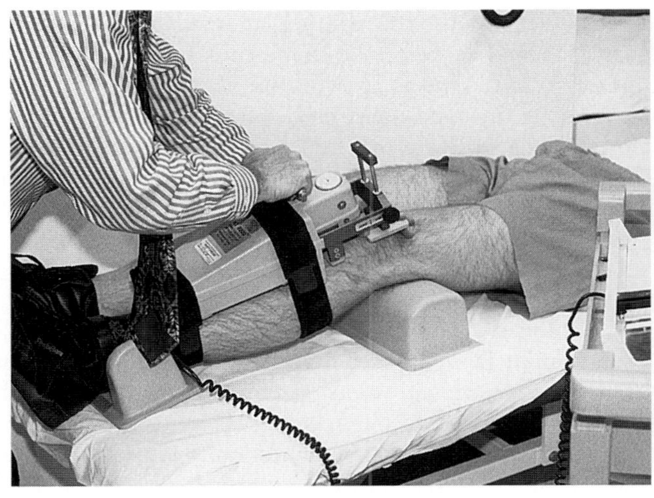

A

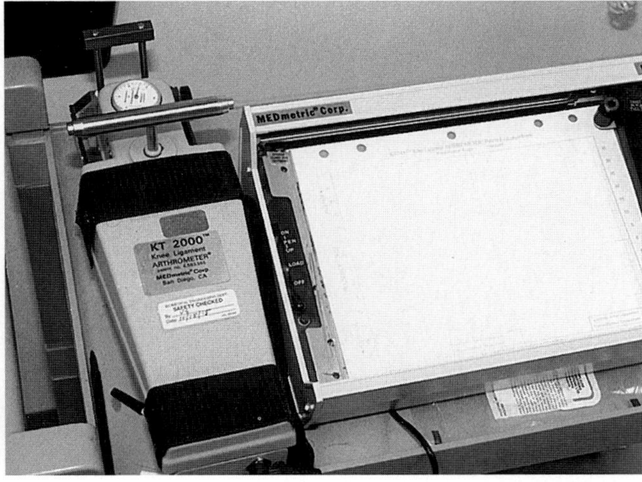

B

FIGURE 44-24. KT 2000 Arthrometer. **A** and **B,** The patient lies down with the distal thigh placed on a bolster. The knee will be flexed approximately 20°. The inferior aspect of the patella should be aligned with the superior aspect of the bolster. The arthrometer is secured to the leg with two Velcro straps. Several trials are then performed measuring anterior and/or posterior excursion of the tibia with reference to the femur. The plotter graph quantifies the excursions that measure millimeters of anterior/posterior movement of the tibia relative to the femur on the x axis and force of anterior/posterior pull or push respectively of the arthrometer on the y axis.

These include KT 2000 arthrometry, isokinetic strength testing, Noyes hop testing, hop-n-stop testing, and a subjective outcome questionnaire. To test static integrity of the ACL graft, we use KT arthrometry (MEDmetric, San Diego, California) (Fig. 44-24). Anterior and posterior excursion of the tibia relative to the femur is measured at 15, 20, or 30 pounds of anterior force at 20 pounds of posterior force. We closely track side-to-side comparisons at 30 pounds of anterior force. We accept differences of less than 4 mm side to side as "normal." Isokinetic testing for peak torque (strength), endurance, and power are evaluated in side-to-side analysis and for comparison of current values to pretraining sound-limb values (patients routinely are tested within the first week of the rehabilitation program for baseline sound-limb values). Speeds of 60° and 180° are employed (Fig. 44-25). The Noyes hop test is performed (Fig. 44-26).[44] This is a series of hops including single hop, triple hop, crossover hop, and 6-m hop for time. Eighty-five percent symmetry is acceptable, meaning that the operated limb must perform at 85% or better of the unoperated, sound limb. Currently the Modified Cincinnati ACL questionnaire is used to correlate subjective perceptions. The final challenge is the hop-n-stop test (Fig. 44-27). This

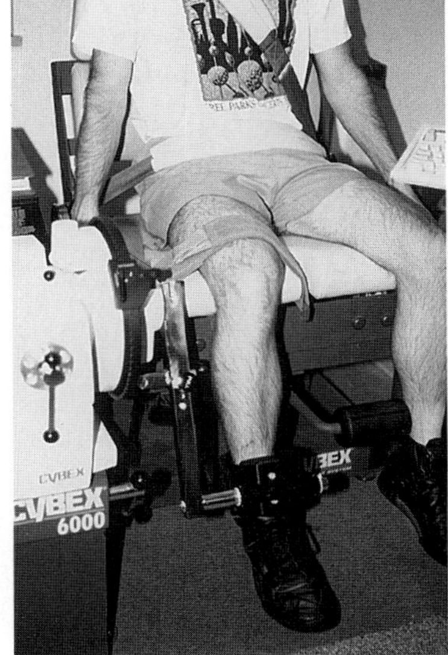

A

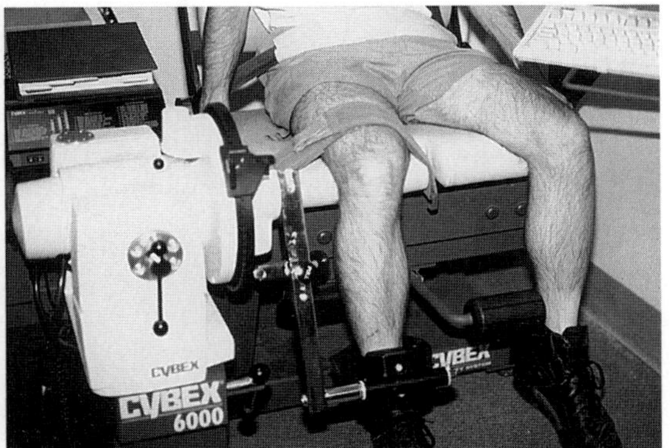

B

FIGURE 44-25. Isokinetic testing. **A** and **B,** Baseline evaluation of sound limb and periodic testing for comparison between limbs serves as a training guide. It is particularly useful for the force-production component of skill training.

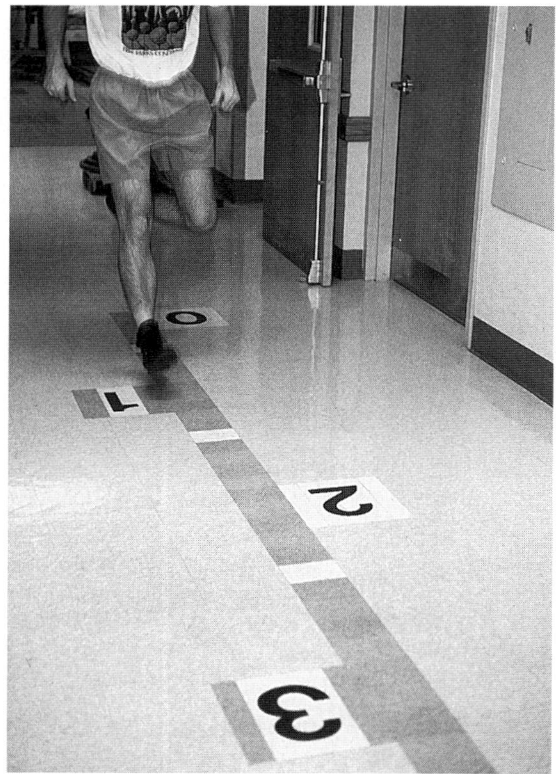

FIGURE 44-26. Noyes hop test.

was developed at our training facility and its full description is in publication. The test evaluates force production and absorption while assessing a patient's ability to perform the pivot-shift maneuver during a functional activity.

There are certain caveats to remember during the ACL training program. There is a direct correlation between anterior knee pain (patello femoral syndrome) and the amount of loaded knee flexion allowed. If one squats with a heavy load, and the knee is flexed beyond 65° to 75°, results reveal a higher incidence of anterior knee pain. The best take-home message for managing anterior knee pain is to avoid its occurrence. If it does appear, it must be identified and treated early. If not, there likely will be protracted pain. In the acutely painful stage, a short course of anti-inflammatory medication and ice massage is helpful. Once pain is identified, patients should be instructed to limit the amount of knee flexion during squatting. A patient can continue to add weight but should not flex the knees beyond 65° to 75°.

Another concern many express is the effect that aggressive training has on the ACL graft. It is commonly thought that excess terminal extension of the involved knee will stretch the graft. Most aggressive rehabilitation programs allow early full active range of motion (FAROM), without specific limitation on terminal extension. Beynnon studied ACL stress by placing a transducer on 12 healthy volunteers' ligaments.[4] He found that certain ranges of motion caused more stress on the ACL than others. Our KT 2000 data, radiographic assessment, and subjective functional scales do not show positive evidence for graft stretching. Data for our current protocol are similar to those when we were limiting terminal extension.

Bracing is an issue that is becoming more controversial. In the recent past a patient with ACL surgery could expect to wear some sort of knee support for most athletic activities. There was a three-phase system: post-op brace, rehabilitation brace, functional brace. (There is a fourth, which is the prophylactic brace, but it is not directly related to the postoperative scheme described here.) More recently, the decision as to whether or not to brace has become less simple. The ultimate usefulness of a knee brace depends on its ability to protect the ligamentous structures.[6] This raises the question of whether a particular knee needs external support enough to safely perform without one. Also, are the limb muscles strong enough to dynamically protect the knee, thereby

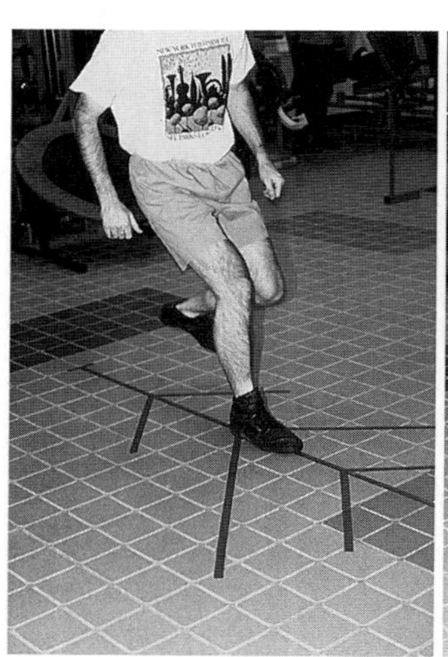

A

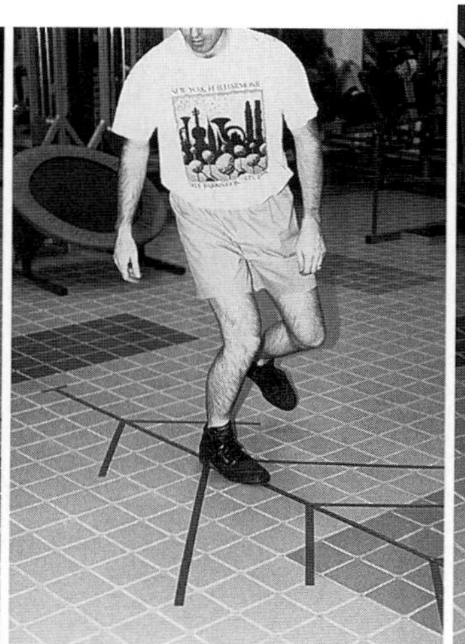

B

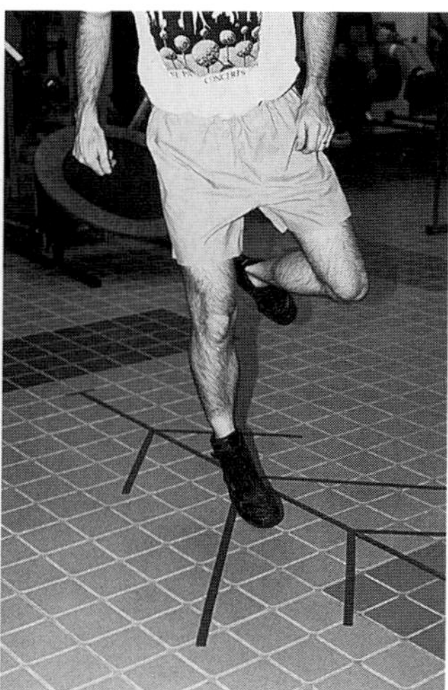

C

FIGURE 44-27. Hop-n-stop test. **A, B,** and **C,** Functional test of force absorption, production, balance, and coordination. It incorporates the pivot-shift phenomenon.

negating the need for a brace? Tibone and others reported prolonged hamstring firing in the postsurgical (weight-bearing) limb of an ACL-deficient patient. This prolonged firing is natural as the hamstrings work synergistically to stabilize an ACL-deficient knee.[56]

The literature is replete with investigative opinions on bracing. Johnston and Paulos investigated prophylactic lateral knee braces, and their conclusion was that no clear scientific or clinical consensus could be reached regarding the efficacy of these braces.[27] Likewise, rehabilitation and functional braces have shown varied results with tibia–femur shear stress. The notion of brace-related proprioceptive feedback has been reviewed. Although I believe that braces add proprioceptive feedback, there are several opposing opinions.[9,57] In one review, bracing did not alter electromyographic activity nor did it change firing patterns, compared to nonbracing. All muscles showed similar changes in activity, suggesting that bracing did not have proprioceptive influence.

At our center, we prescribe a hinge brace, which is worn for the first 2 to 3 weeks after surgery. Except for a knee sleeve, no other bracing is considered for 5 or 6 months, when we test function. Based on the combined results of these tests, we determine the need for bracing. Generally, if KT 2000 scores are less than 4 mm to 5 mm side to side, and quadriceps and hamstring strengths are within 20% and 10% side to side, respectively, no brace is recommended. However, the single most important determinant in applying a brace is patient choice. Even with excellent functional scores, if the patient desires a brace, one should be prescribed. In selecting a brace, a patient may consider some basic points: the brace should be lightweight (14 to 18 ounces), comfortable, nonintrusive on athletic performance, and economically reasonable.

Our conservative (nonsurgical) training program is very similar to the postoperative program. The length of training is shorter (2 to 3 months) because the early phase of the program proceeds more rapidly. Our goals and emphases are essentially the same. One significant difference is in strength training (force production and absorption), in which the hamstrings are a major focus. The dynamic ability of the hamstring group, particularly the lateral, to assist in posterior displacement of the tibia in relation to the femur is emphasized. The posterior cruciate ligament (PCL) rehabilitation program is not as well developed. Many centers have structured protocols, but the relative number of patients with this injury is significantly less than those with anterior cruciate ligament injuries. The training sequence provides slightly more protection against extrinsic forces in the early stages. Post-op bracing persists for 4 to 6 weeks, with initial settings at minimal (on weight bearing) free motion. Hamstring strengthening is avoided (if possible) until about POW 6. The emphasis is on strengthening the quadriceps, with progression to functional training starting at 3 months. The box, Posterior Cruciate Ligament (PCL) Rehabilitation, illustrates the training progression.

Medial and lateral collateral ligament sprains are usually treated conservatively. Medial collateral ligament sprains are graded I to III. The classification is outlined in Table 44-5. Training for low-grade sprains (I) progresses more quickly than training for high-grade sprains (III). Tables 44-6 and 44-7 outline conservative regimens for medial collateral sprains. Lateral collateral ligament sprains are treated much the same way, with care taken not to gap the lateral joint line. For third-degree sprains, surgical intervention is sometimes required, and the

CHECKLIST

Posterior Cruciate Ligament (PCL) Rehabilitation

Postoperative Day 1
- ☐ Brace locked at 0°
- ☐ Continuous passive motion 5:60°
- ☐ Ambulation bearing weight as tolerated with crutches
- ☐ Ice, elevation
- ☐ Quadriceps sitting, straight leg raise, ankle pumps
- ☐ Electrical stimulation prn to quadriceps

Postoperative Days 2–7
- ☐ Brace open for available range of motion
- ☐ Isometric hip abduction/adduction
- ☐ Passive knee flexion
- ☐ Multi-angle quadriceps isometrics
- ☐ Patellar mobilization
- ☐ Toe raises (extended knee)
- ☐ Reverse stool slides

Postoperative Weeks 2–7
- ☐ Stationary bicycle as tolerated
- ☐ Balance training
- ☐ Pool walking
- ☐ Adding weight to previous exercises
- ☐ Mini–knee bends (no more than 50°)
- ☐ Sitting range of motion (POW 3–4)
- ☐ Hamstring curls (POW 7) with light weights
- ☐ Fitter (POW 7)

Postoperative Weeks 8–13
- ☐ Nordic Track
- ☐ Jogging (POW 12–13)
- ☐ Step-ups
- ☐ Step machine—short arc (POW 10–12)

Postoperative Weeks 14–16
- ☐ Sport-specific training
- ☐ Light running
- ☐ Endurance training

Postoperative Week 17 to 6 Months
- ☐ Agility drills
- ☐ Running
- ☐ Plyometrics

TABLE 44-5 Classification of Medial Collateral Ligament Injury at 30° of Flexion

First-degree injury	No laxity, firm endpoint
Second-degree injury	5 mm laxity, firm endpoint
Third-degree injury	5 mm laxity, soft endpoint

From Nicholas JA, Hershman EB (eds): The Lower Extremity and Spine in Sports Medicine, 2nd ed. St. Louis, Mosby–Year Book, 1995, p 832.

length of postoperative immobilization varies. Usually a rigid cast is applied for 2 to 3 weeks for the surgically repaired medial collateral ligament.

The menisci are frequently injured. This is understandable considering their role in joint stabilization, shock absorption, and weight bearing. Forty percent to 60% of the weight transferred across the knee is carried by the menisci. Conservative treatment of diagnosed meniscal tears is somewhat effective. A program design emphasizing open-chain (perpendicular load) and short arc closed-chain (axial load) exercises can dynamically stabilize the knee. Once pain control is achieved and swelling reduced, patients who successfully complete a conservative program are quite satisfied. In addition to closed-chain progressive resistive exercises, functional activities including Nordic Track, slide board, and roller board help to maximize performance (Fig. 44-28).

TABLE 44-6 Treatment of First-Degree Medial Collateral Ligament Injuries

Stage I	Ice Knee immobilizer Full weight bearing with crutches Isometric exercises
Stage II (as pain and swelling subside)	Discontinuing immobilizer Discontinuing crutches Range-of-motion exercises Hip flexor and abductor strengthening Closed-chain exercises Adduction strengthening with resistance proximal to knee
Stage III (as range of motion returns)	Progressive resistance exercises Isokinetic exercise Proprioceptive training Functional rehabilitation

Thoughout the program, aerobic, well-leg, and upper-body conditioning are continued.
From Nicholas JA, Hershman EB (eds): The Lower Extremity and Spine in Sports Medicine, 2nd ed. St. Louis, Mosby–Year Book, 1995, p 832.

TABLE 44-7 Treatment of Second-Degree Medial Collateral Ligament Injuries

Stage I	Ice Compression Knee immobilizer Partial weight bearing with crutches Isometric exercises
Stage II (as acute symptoms resolve)	Gentle range of motion Progression to full weight bearing in brace Quadriceps setting Straight leg raising Closed-chain exercises Hip flexor and adductor strengthening Hip adduction strengthening with resistance proximal to knee
Stage III (when 90° of flexion is present)	Continuation of range-of-motion program Exercise bicycle Isokinetic program (high speed) Beginning proprioceptive training
Stage IV (when full range of motion is present)	Progessive resistance exercises in flexion Isokinetic program (full) Exercise bicycle
Stage V (full painless range of motion)	Running in brace Functional program (progressive)

Thoughout the program, aerobic, well-leg, and upper-body conditioning are continued.
From Nicholas JA, Hershman EB (eds): The Lower Extremity and Spine in Sports Medicine, 2nd ed. St. Louis, Mosby-Year Book, 1995, p 833.

For postoperative meniscal injuries, the number of meniscal tears currently being treated by repair vs. resection is growing. Long-term follow-up data on outcomes of meniscal repair are unavailable, but a decrease in the high incidence of degenerative changes, which are seen in meniscectomy, is anticipated. It is reported that degenerative changes are seen in the joints after meniscectomy as early as 3 months after surgery.[13] If meniscal repair proves a successful salvage procedure, the functional benefits will be very rewarding.

Rehabilitation after meniscal repair historically has been a slower process than after meniscectomy, but more aggressive programs now are being advocated (Table 44-8). After meniscectomy, patients are allowed to bear weight as tolerated. Riding a stationary bicycle is encouraged. The liberal application of ice helps to decrease effusion and pain. It is important to let the

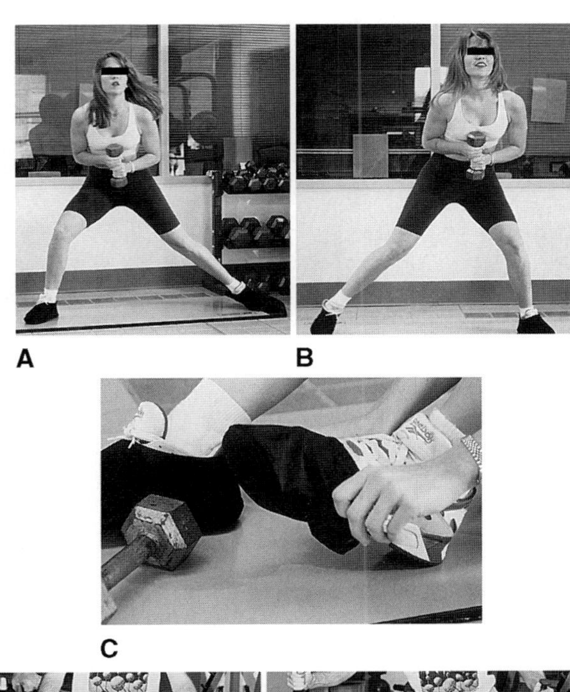

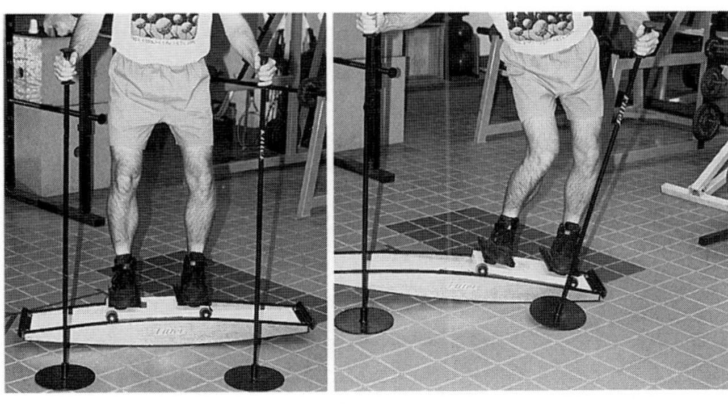

FIGURE 44-28. Slide and roller board. **A** and **B,** The slide board is an effective conditioning device that can be combined with upper-body techniques including hand-held weight or ball toss. The boards have various lengths and are easily stored. **C,** Cloth booties are worn to decrease friction while gliding on the board. Treatment sessions are based upon time on board rather than number of slides. **D** and **E,** The roller board is a good device to begin lateral agility training. It offers proprioceptive feedback and strengthens the lower extremities in general.

TABLE 44-8 Rehabilitation After Meniscectomy/Repair

Postoperative week 1	Ambulation bearing weight as tolerated Ice prn Range of motion as tolerated Bicycle for range of motion (high seat)
Postoperative weeks 2–4	Short arc closed-chain (axial load) exercise 0°–30° Open-chain (perpendicular load) exercises with light weights Bicycle
Postoperative weeks 5–8	Progression to functional exercises and sport-specific exercises

From Nicholas JA, Hershman EB (eds): The Lower Extremity and Spine in Sports Medicine, 2nd ed. St. Louis, Mosby–Year Book, 1995, p 833.

patient know of potential degenerative changes. Avoidance of excessive impact loading onto the knees is important. Modification of activities like running should be discussed. Swimming is encouraged. Exercises to stretch and strengthen the associated muscles are emphasized.

For the patient undergoing meniscal repair, many advocate a more conservative protocol.[16] This would include limited weight bearing for 4 to 6 weeks after surgery (Table 44-9). Range of motion is also limited for the first 6 weeks. Resistive exercises are delayed until the third month after surgery and returning to competitive sports until 4 or 5 months after surgery. The more aggressive rehabilitation program for meniscal repair closely follows the guidelines for meniscectomy. The major difference is the ability of the patient to continue athletic performance, including impact absorption, because of the returned integrity of the meniscus. The details of this program are similar to those of postoperative ACL rehabilitation.

Osteoarthritis (OA) of the knee is one of the most frequently occurring musculoskeletal diseases.[40] After the spine and the hip, the knee is the site most often affected.[8] Approximately 10% of persons older than 65 (a greater number of females than males) have symptomatic OA of the knee.[8] Before embarking on a specific rehabilitation program, careful evaluation of the entire musculoskeletal system should be made. Aberrations elsewhere can predispose or directly influence a person to the development of OA. An example is the person who pronates at the subtalar joint. As previously stated, this causes a valgus stress on the knee and loads the lateral compartment. If the patient has heel spurs or plantar fasciitis, anterior knee pain can occur because of

TABLE 44-9 Meniscal Repair

Postoperative weeks 0–6	Partial weight bearing Range of motion 0°–90°
Postoperative weeks 6–12	Progression to weight bearing as tolerated Progressive weight training Endurance training Progression to full range of motion

increased load onto the quadriceps in avoidance of heel-strike. This predisposes to quadriceps tendinitis and increased anterior joint stress.

A patient's first step in OA treatment is to modify activity and avoid being overweight. Loaded knee flexion extension activities, particularly those with large impact, should be avoided. Occupations that require prolonged squatting are detrimental and are associated with symptomatic OA. Obesity is a precursor to OA of the knee, and weight loss may prevent the development of symptoms.[14] Remember that stress across the joint is a factor of body weight, and forces across the knee range from 1 to 7 times body weight (depending on the activity, e.g., there are higher forces with running).

Pharmacologic management includes acetominophen and NSAIDs. There are many NSAIDs to chose from; they are listed in the discussion on spine rehabilitation. Careful attention must be paid to GI, liver, and kidney function when using NSAIDs. A low dosage of tricyclic antidepressants can be used for the management of OA. Patients with OA who complain of prolonged morning stiffness often do not sleep well. These people may sleep and feel better after taking tricyclics.[15] Commonly used preparations include amitriptyline, starting at 25 mg/day and progressing to 75 mg/day. I ask for baseline electrocardiograms on patients with known cardiac arrhythmia or those with compromised cardiac status. Tricyclics can have untoward effects on the PR interval, and arrhythmia may be induced. The cardiogram is periodically checked throughout the course of administration of the tricyclic. Corticosteroids, taken orally or parenterally, are minimally effective for OA. The route of choice is intraarticular. I use triamcinolone hexacetonide, 20 mg, or methylprednisolone acetate, 40 mg. Care should be taken in administering repeated doses because they may speed the degenerative process.

Exercises to treat OA focus on joint preservation. Initially, isometric exercises are done. These can be supine straight leg raising, or against the fixed resistance of a belt (Fig. 44-29). Isotonic exercises are performed and focused in the pain-free arc. Isokinetic exercises are particularly useful because the speed and direction of motion can be carefully monitored (Fig. 44-30). Exercises must be done regularly; a minimum of three times a week is required. Daily routines should be considered if time allows. To simplify things, each exercise should have a fixed number of repetitions and consist of three sets. Figure 44-31 illustrates exercises for OA.

For more advanced cases of OA, total joint arthroplasty may be recommended. This procedure has been one of the most successful joint replacement procedures in terms of morbidity and patient satisfaction. The rehabilitation program after total knee arthroplasty initially focuses on restoring functional range of motion. This is accomplished with hands-on ranging by a therapist along with a continuous passive motion (CPM) device (Fig. 44-32). Benefits of CPM include improved range of motion[26] and earlier independent mobility. The use of electrical stimulation has been shown to improve motion after total knee arthroplasty, particularly by decreasing extensor lag.[20] Patients are typically hospitalized for 4 to 7 days and continue their exercises at home. A stationary bicycle is very effective for gaining knee motion and obtaining an aerobic workout. Ambulating is done as tolerated, typically with an assistance device (such as a cane) for a few weeks. There is persistent swelling about the knee, which lasts for approximately 6 months. Patients should be alerted to expect this normal finding. Greatly increased swelling may not be normal. It could signify overuse but may be a sign of infection. Patients should

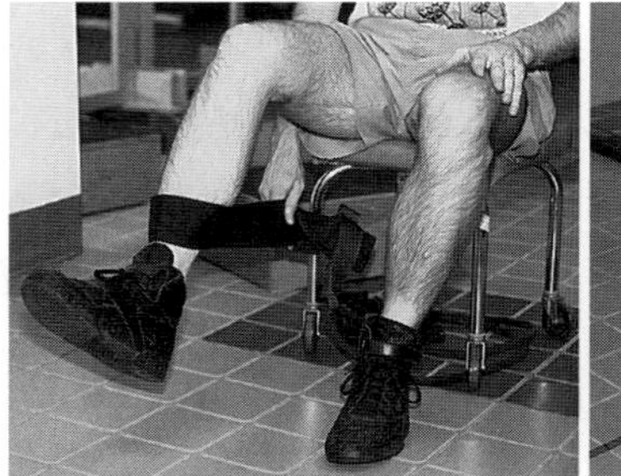
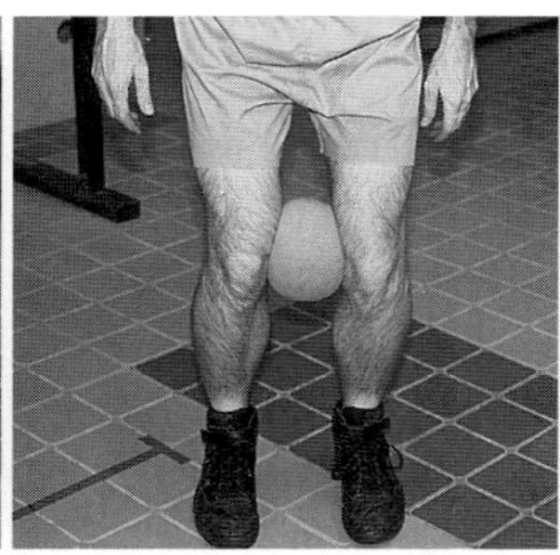

A B

FIGURE 44-29. Isometric knee exercise. **A,** A simple belt can be used to effectively isometrically strengthen the periarticular muscles of the knee. The contractions should be held for 3 to 4 seconds and repeated. Patients should be cautioned not to forcibly exhale with mouth and nostrils closed and to limit this exercise if there is a significant cardiac history. **B,** A ball could be squeezed between the knees to effect an isometric contraction.

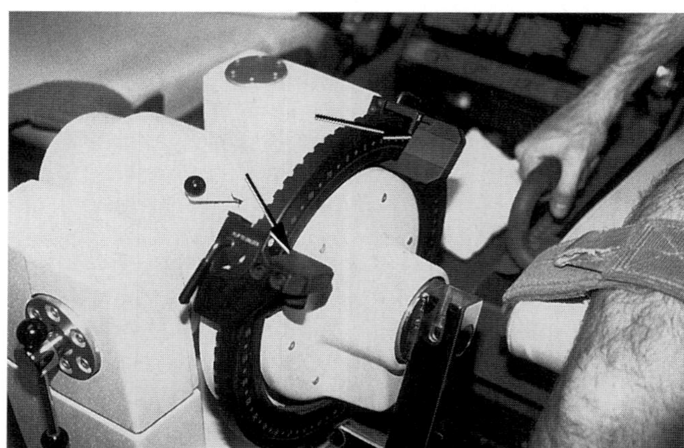

FIGURE 44-30. Isokinetics with limited range of motion. After securing a limb into the device, a limited range of motion can be set by adjusting the mechanical blocks as shown on the dynamometer. Specific joint arcs can be protected with this device. For example, if there is pain on knee flexion beyond 60°, limiting the range to less than 60° can avoid the painful arc.

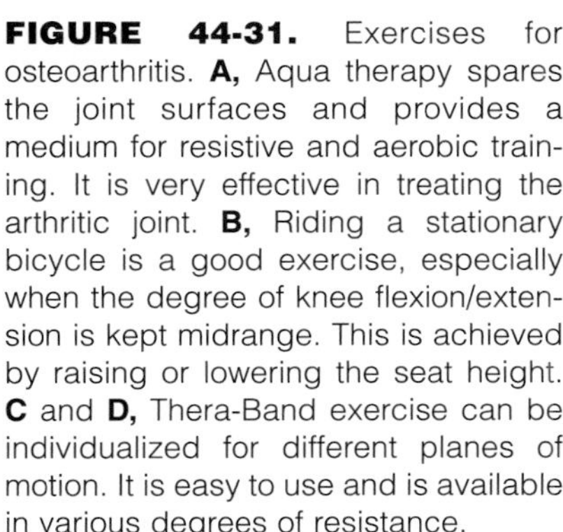

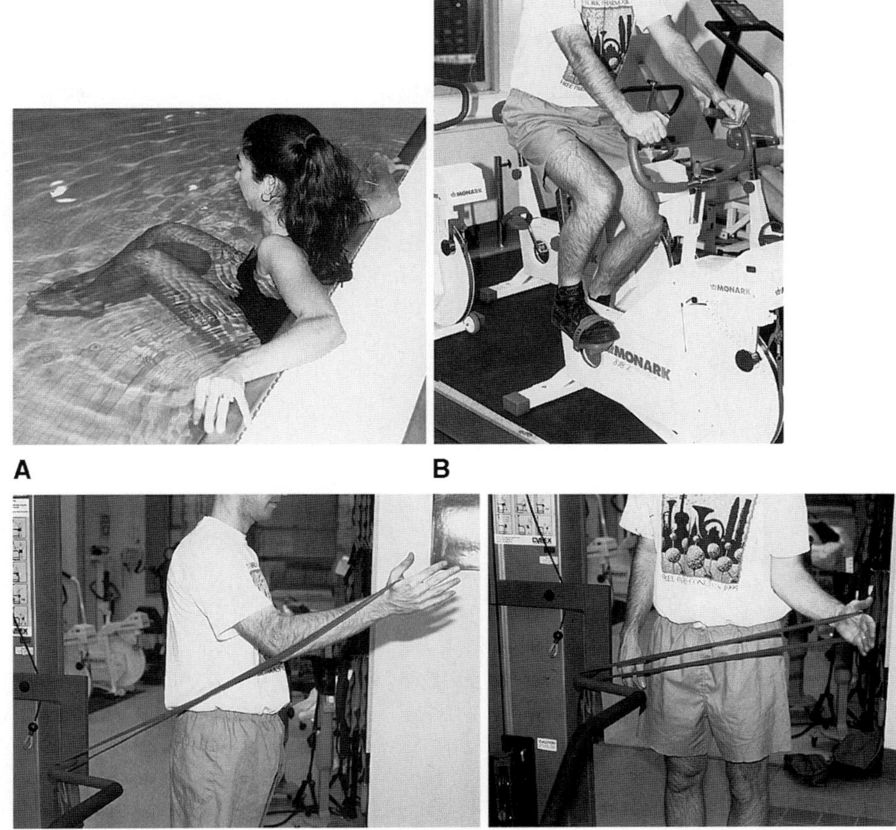

FIGURE 44-31. Exercises for osteoarthritis. **A,** Aqua therapy spares the joint surfaces and provides a medium for resistive and aerobic training. It is very effective in treating the arthritic joint. **B,** Riding a stationary bicycle is a good exercise, especially when the degree of knee flexion/extension is kept midrange. This is achieved by raising or lowering the seat height. **C** and **D,** Thera-Band exercise can be individualized for different planes of motion. It is easy to use and is available in various degrees of resistance.

call their surgeon if any significant change occurs, such as sudden loss of motion, fever, drainage, or erythema.

The associated musculature is strengthened the same way as for OA. Guidelines for activity limitation are unclear at this time. A recent review of younger (younger than 55 years of age) patients after total knee replacement showed their increased ability to tolerate load on the prosthetic knee. We advise patients to limit impact on the postsurgical knee, but we encourage physical activity. Doubles tennis is preferred to singles. Running on solid ground is not recommended. Swimming is encouraged. The patient should expect to feel encouraged sometime between 6 weeks and 6 months after surgery. The activities severely hindered before surgery can then become feasible.

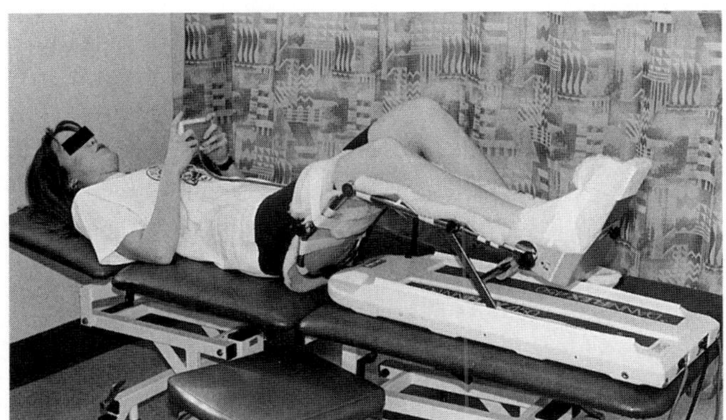

FIGURE 44-32. Continuous passive motion (CPM). The limb is mechanically ranged at predetermined degrees of motion. CPM assists in attaining increased motion in the involved joint.

Tendinitis

Anterior knee pain is one of the most usual musculoskeletal complaints, having a number of possible etiologies. Patella tendinitis and patellofemoral syndrome (PFS) are two common diagnoses. Patella tendinitis, "jumper's knee,"[7] is usually seen in athletic activities requiring forceful eccentric muscle contractions or repeated flexion and extension of the knee.[50] The most common presentation is pain at the inferior pole of the patella. It can also occur at the tibial tubercle and at the superior pole of the patella. Pain is common after physical exercise and when ascending or descending stairs.

The biomechanics of this complex are important to understanding the mechanism of injury and subsequent development of appropriate rehabilitation strategies. The forces on the patella—the quadriceps tendon above and the patella tendon below—are not equally distributed during muscle contraction.[50] During closed-chain activities (landing from a jump), the ratio of quadriceps tendon tension to patella tendon tension increases with increasing knee flexion; but during open-chain activities (seated knee extension), the ratio of quadriceps tendon tension to patella tendon tension increases with knee extension.[17] When the quadriceps undergoes eccentric contraction, significantly increased force is transmitted to the patella tendon. The treatment of patella tendinitis begins with a brief period of rest, use of ice, ultrasound, and NSAIDs.

Before a patient begins rehabilitative exercises, a general warm-up is recommended. Riding a stationary bicycle for 15 to 20 minutes with low resistance and an elevated seat height is a good way to begin. Stretching the quadriceps and hamstrings is next. Strengthening the associated muscles, particularly the eccentric knee extensors, will best prepare the knee to successfully absorb impact. This can be done through progressive step-downs (Fig. 44-33). The patient should progress to short jump-downs from varied heights (Fig. 44-34). In addition, lunges, isokinetic quadriceps eccentrics, and hamstring isotonics should be performed. Starting weights should not be excessive. The patient should be able to complete 10 repetitions with relative ease. As recovery progresses, the workout weight should be such that the patient struggles to lift it 10 times.

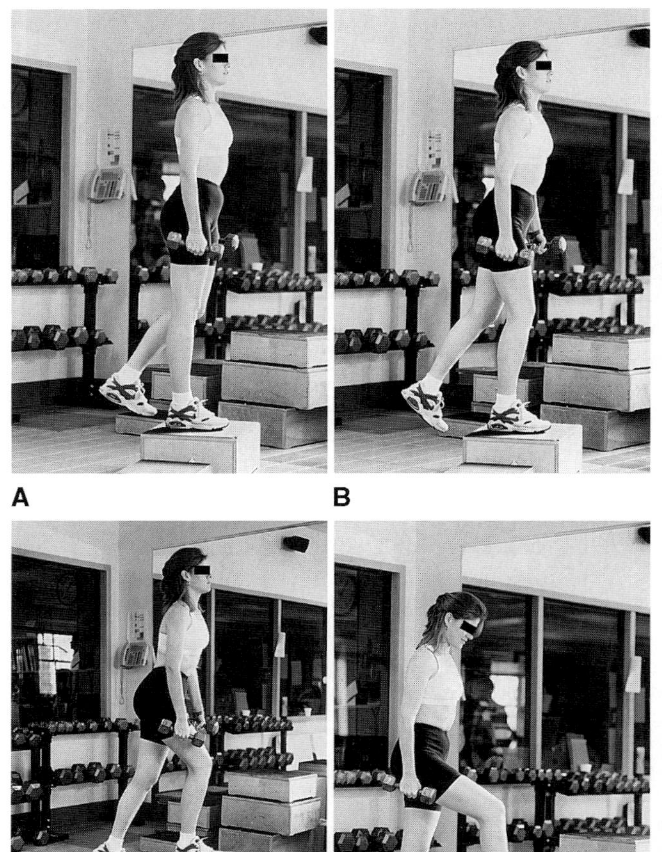

FIGURE 44-33. Step-downs. **A–D,** To effectively train the limb to absorb force, controlled step-downs are done. This is to support the weight of the body while progressively increasing velocity. As the patient begins to master the technique, the force of impact is distributed through the muscles in a very synchronous way. Weight can be added to increase the mass that the limbs must support.

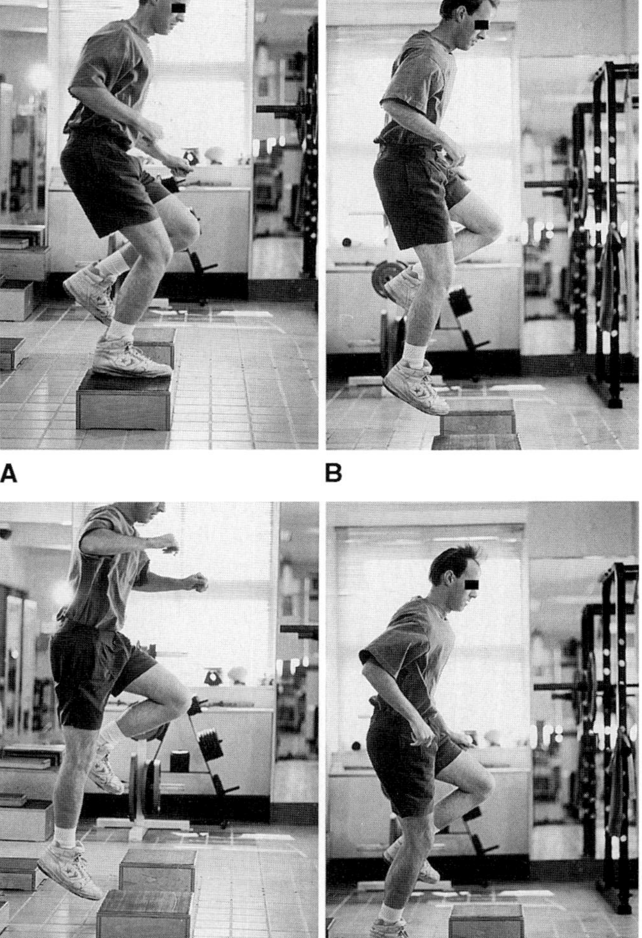

FIGURE 44-34. Jump-downs. **A–D,** The progression from step-downs is to jump-downs. The patient jumps to the floor from varied heights and must control the landing by allowing a springing-type motion at the joints to distribute the forces of impact.

Patellofemoral syndrome is probably the most common presentation of anterior knee pain. Much has been written about this syndrome, both its manifestations and treatment. It often remains a diagnostic and therapeutic dilemma. The biomechanics of the patellofemoral joint are constantly being researched and evaluated. The basic understanding in treating this syndrome is that the patellofemoral relationship is altered; this incongruence sets the stage for the associated signs and symptoms.

The treatment paradigm mimics many of those we have discussed in this chapter. The first step is to remove the inciting event, which is achieved with a brief period of rest. The adjunct treatments of ice, NSAIDs, ultrasound, and electrical stimulation are followed. At our center we approach this disorder as if the patella were an object freely floating in the anterior compartment of the knee, desperately searching for a niche to call home. The knee is a large joint and is acted on by muscles asymmetrically, which lays the foundation for maltracking and malalignment. Rehabilitation entails stretching and strengthening the associated muscles in a way that most closely creates symmetry for force vectors around the patella. At the same time, we try to reduce perpendicular loads across the patellofemoral joint, to salvage the joint surfaces. The training progression is carried out over a 2- to 3-month period.

Figure 44-35 depicts the techniques used to rehabilitate a patient with patellofemoral syndrome. As with patella

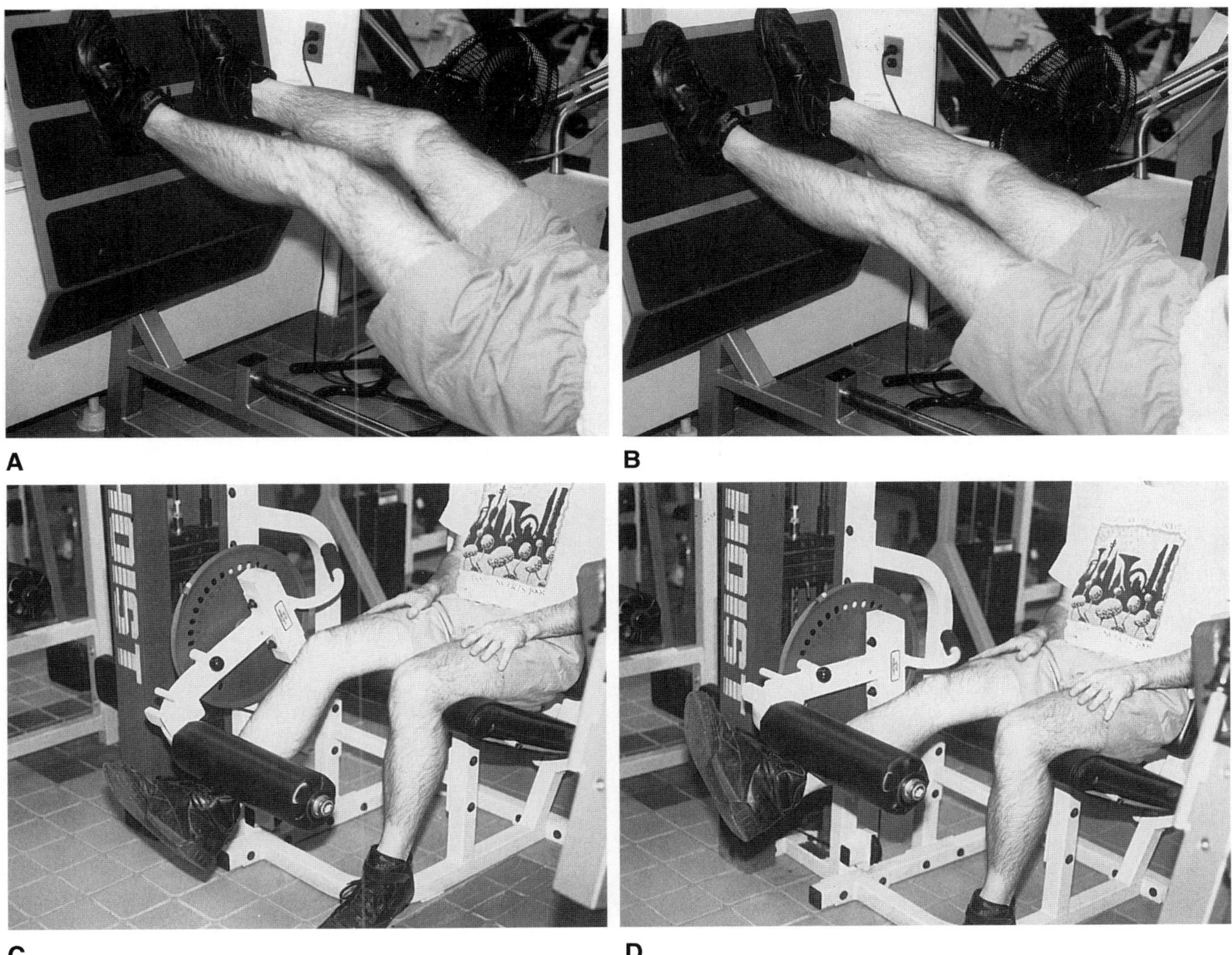

FIGURE 44-35. Patellofemoral exercises. **A–N,** Terminal knee extensions. Starting with closed-chain (axial load, **A, B**) in the range of 30° to 0° and progressing to open-chain (perpendicular load, **C, D**), these exercises are effective in strengthening the quadriceps while sparing undo patellofemoral stresses. **E,** Towel grab—to increase supinator strength and prevent excessive subtalar pronation, this is a very effective exercise. The towel is grabbed with the forefoot and attempts are made to pick it up with the toes. **F,** McConnell taping—a technique to realign a maltracking patellar. Tape is applied to the knee, attempting to place the patella in a more congruent position with respect to the femur. Hopefully, the tape will maintain proper contact to allow the patella to track more anatomically.

Continued

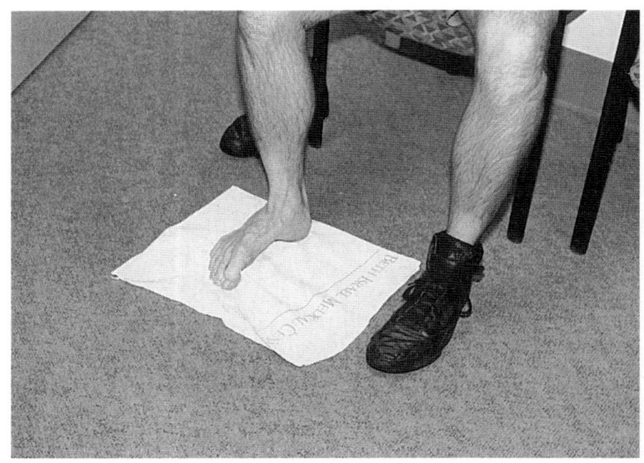

E

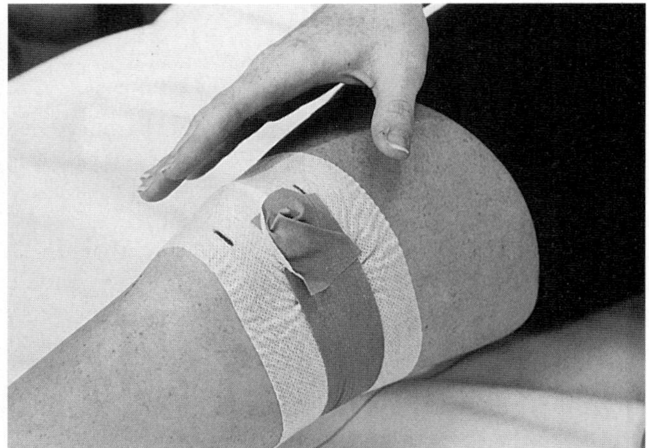

F

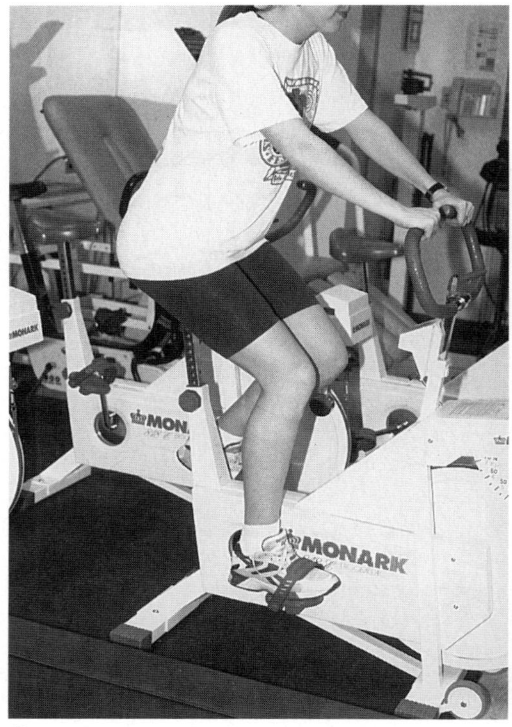

G

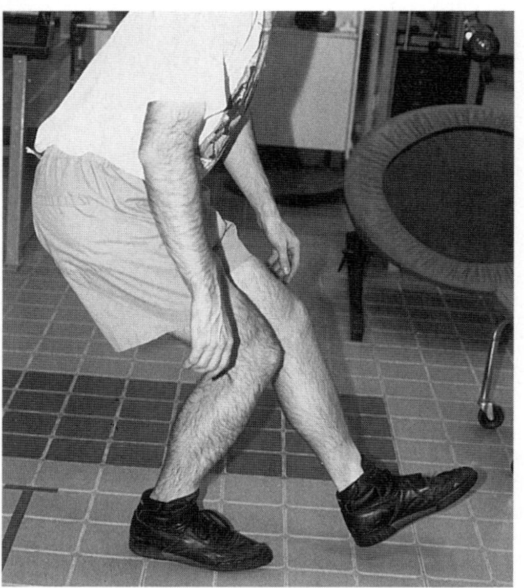

H

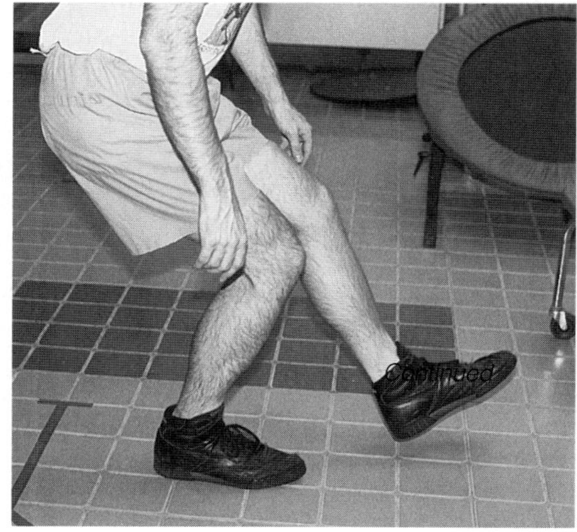

I

FIGURE 44-35, cont'd. **E,** Towel grab—to increase supinator strength and prevent excessive subtalar pronation, this is a very effective exercise. The towel is grabbed with the forefoot and attempts are made to pick it up with the toes. **F,** McConnell taping—a technique to realign a maltracking patellar. Tape is applied to the knee, attempting to place the patella in a more congruent position with respect to the femur. Hopefully, the tape will maintain proper contact to allow the patella to track more anatomically. **G,** High seat bicycle. Set seat height to prevent knee flexion beyond 50° to 55°. Pedal resistance should be low. Time exercise to pedal for 20 to 30 minutes 1 to 2 times/day. **H** and **I,** Short-arc knee bends. Standing firmly on a single leg, flex knee to maximum of 50° to 55°. Upright posture must be maintained. Multiple sets are performed.

Continued

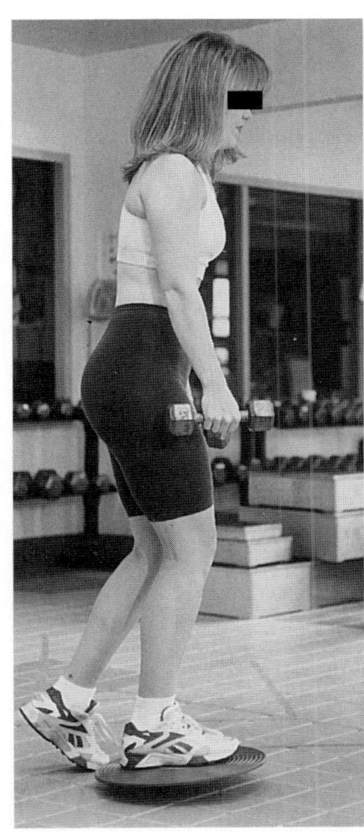

J

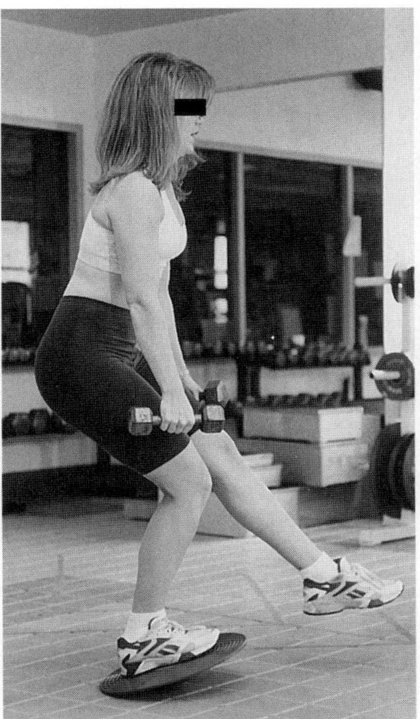

K

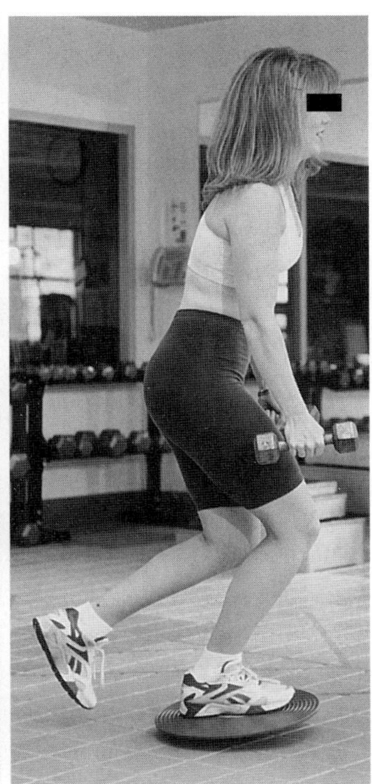

L

M

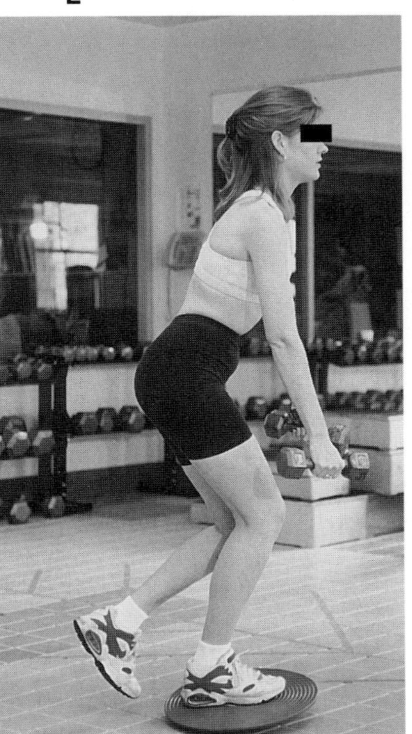

N

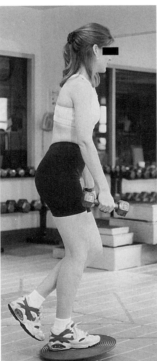

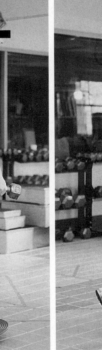

FIGURE 44-35, cont'd. J–N, To further challenge the patient, knee bends can be performed on a balance board.

Continued

tendinitis, patellofemoral syndrome is influenced by the activities occurring at other joints, such as when the subtalar joint pronates and there is an associated valgus moment at the knee. This then increases the Q angle and promotes maltracking. Retro walking in a toe-to-heel gait causes subtalar supination and results in a varus moment at the knee that acts to decrease the Q angle (and unload the patellofemoral joint). If a person pronates excessively, it is important to consider the use of orthotics. Sleeves and braces are advocated for the knee. There are many braces on the market that manufacturers claim are effective in treating PFS. None stands alone as a clear choice, and research continues to evaluate the role of bracing in PFS. In general, most practitioners attempt

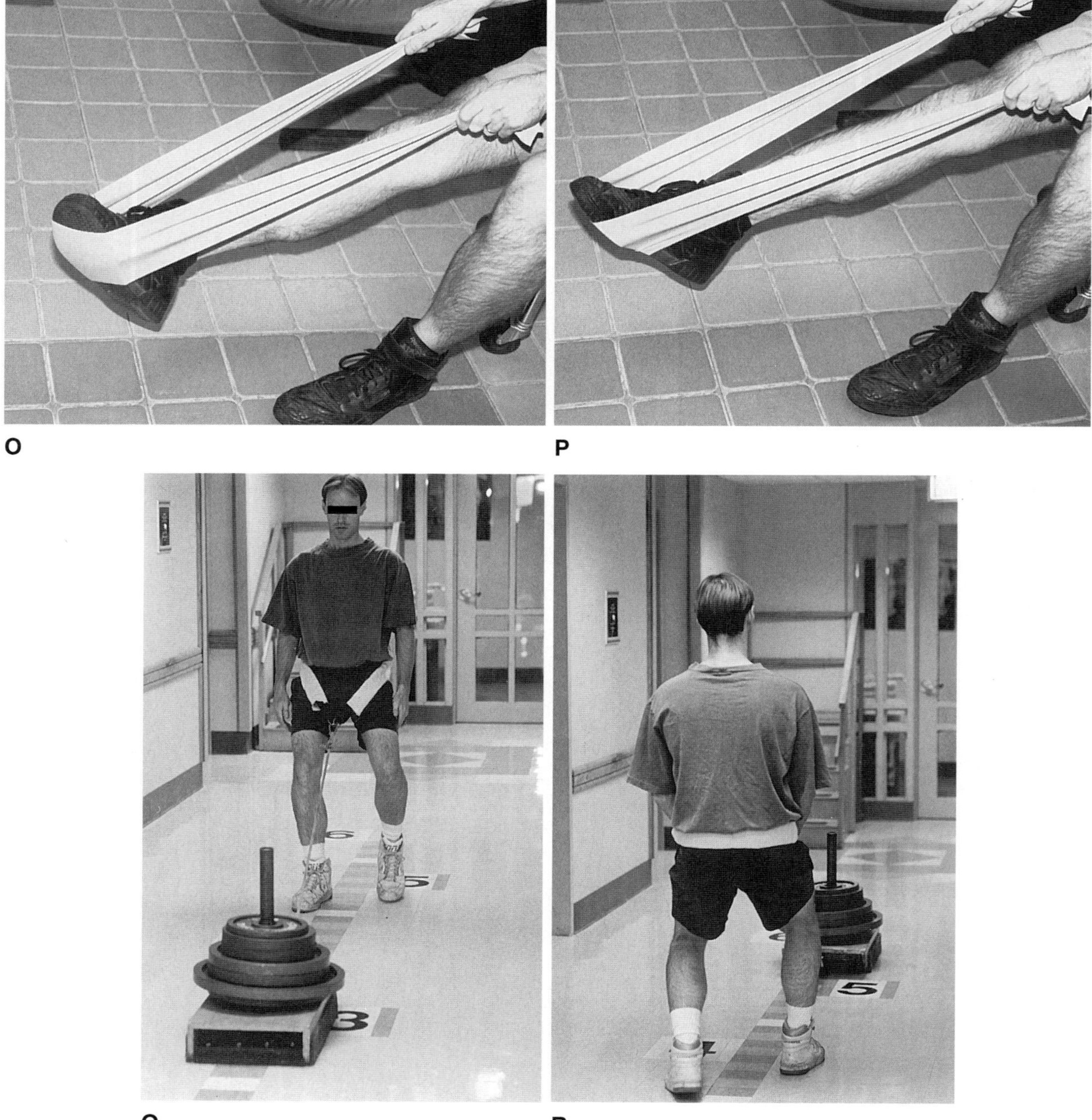

FIGURE 44-35, cont'd. O and **P,** Thera-Band alphabets—see Figure 44-6 for description. **Q** and **R,** Retro walking—see Figure 44-7 for description.

Continued

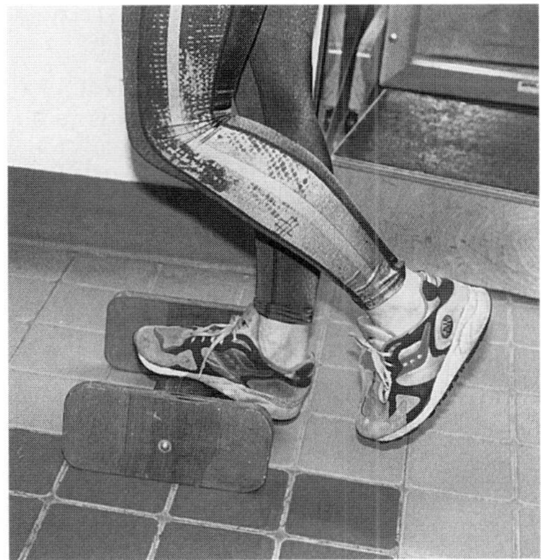

S

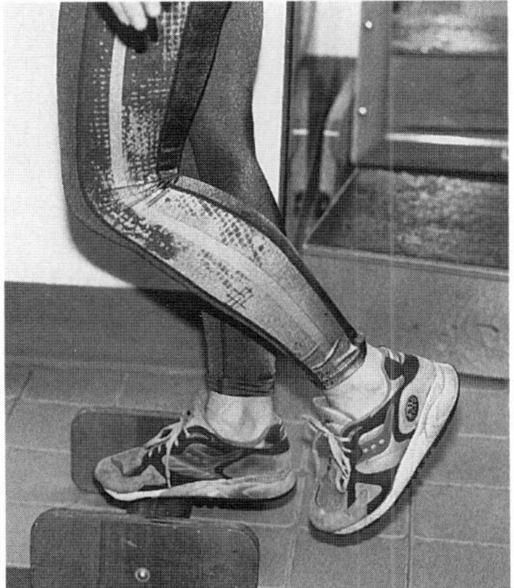

T

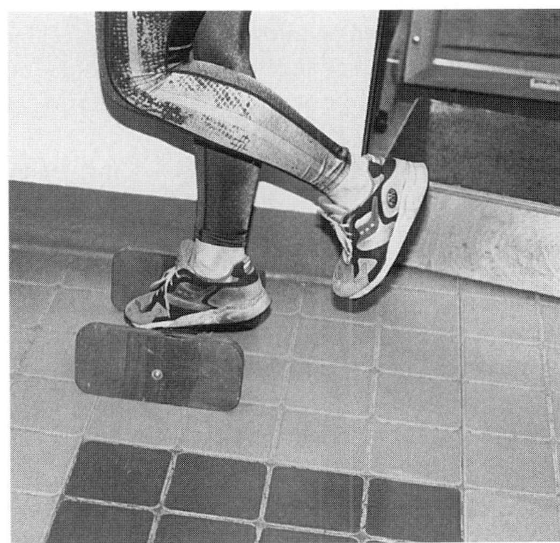

U

FIGURE 44-35, cont'd. **S**, **T**, and **U**, Plantar-roll bar exercises—see Figure 44-8 for description.

to align the patella centrally between the femoral condyles. McConnell taping uses directed taping sequences. These unload the patellofemoral joint during training sessions.

Iliotibial band friction syndrome is a condition that usually manifests itself as pain over the lateral femoral condyle. It is common in runners, especially those who run on uneven terrain. It is thought to occur secondarily to translocation of the iliotibial band (ITB) from anterior to posterior as a runner goes from knee extension to knee flexion. It is proximally related to the tensor fascia lata at the fascia of the gluteus maximus. Treatment of this syndrome includes rest, ice, NSAIDs, ultrasound, stretching of the ITB (Fig. 44-36), and orthotics if there is concomitant foot and ankle pathology. Normal gait causes internal tibial rotation, which is exaggerated if excess ronation occurs. This exaggerated internal tibial rotation will stretch the ITB across the femoral condyle.

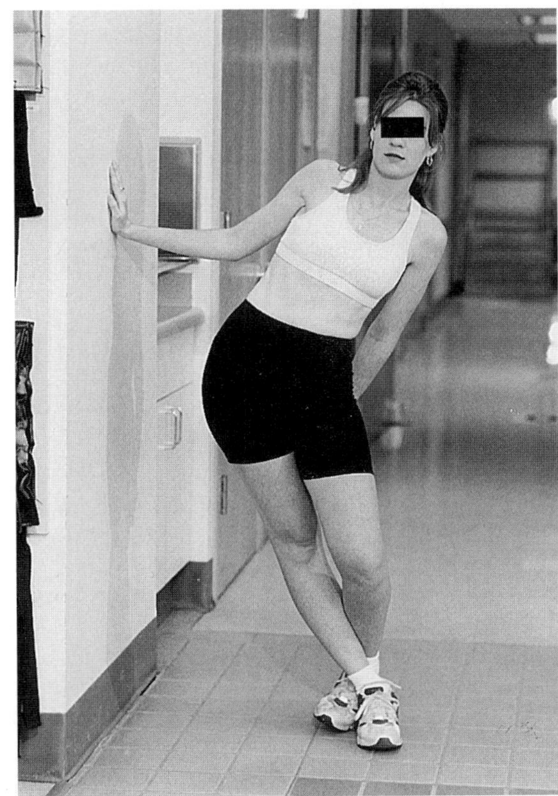

FIGURE 44-36. Iliotibial band stretch. The patient stands, and the limb to be stretched is placed across the body in front of the other limb. The ipsilateral hip is then thrust laterally while the foot maintains contact with the ground. This position is held for 30 seconds.

REFERENCES

1. Arner O, Lindholm A: "What is tennis leg?" Acta Chir Scand 116:73, 1958.
2. Arnheim DD, Prentice WE: The ankle and lower leg. In Smith JM (ed): Principles of Athletic Training, 8th ed. Baltimore, Mosby-Year Book, 1993.
3. Baker CL, Todd JL: Intervening in acute ankle sprain and chronic instability. J Musculoskeletal Med 54, July 1995.
4. Beynnon BD, et al: Anterior cruciate ligament strain behavior during rehabilitation exercises in vivo. Am J Sports Med 23:24–34, 1995.
5. Birrer RB: Ankle injuries. In Birrer RB (ed): Sports Medicine for the Primary Care Physician, 2nd ed. Boca Raton, FL, CRC Press, 1994.
6. Black KP, Raasch WG: Knee braces in sports. In Nicholas JA, Hershman EB (eds): The Lower Extremity and Spine in Sports Medicine, 2nd ed. St. Louis, Mosby-Year Book, 1995.
7. Blazina M, Kerlan R, Jobe F: Jumpers knee. Orthop Clin North Am 4:665–678, 1973.
8. Bradley JD: Nonsurgical option for managing osteoarthritis of the knee. J Musculoskeletal Med 14–26, August 1994.
9. Branch TP, Hunter R, Donath M: Dynamic EMG analysis of the anterior cruciate deficient legs with and without bracing during cutting. Am J Sports Med 17:35, 1989.
10. Clement DB: Tibial stress syndrome in athletes. Am J Sports Med 2:81–85, 1974.
11. Devereaux MD, Lachmann SM: Athletes attending a sports injury clinic—A review. Br J Sports Med 17(4):137–142, 1983.
12. Edwards G: Contralateral and ipsilateral cane usage by patients with total knee or hip replacement. Archives of Phys Med Rehab 67:734, 1986.
13. Fairbank TJ: Knee joint changes after meniscectomy. J Bone Joint Surg 30B:664, 1981.
14. Felson DT, Andrews JJ, Naimark A: Obesity and knee osteoarthritis. The Framingham Study. Ann Intern Med 109:18–24, 1989.
15. Frank RG, Kashani JH, Parker JC, et al: Antidepressant analgesia in rheumatoid arthritis. J Rheumatol 15:1632–1638, 1988.
16. Fu FH, Baratz M: Meniscal injuries. In DeLee JC, Drez D (eds): Orthopaedic Sports Medicine, Principles and Practice, vol. 2. Philadelphia, WB Saunders, 1994.
17. Fulkerson J, Hungerfor D: Disorder of the Patellofemoral Joint, 2nd ed. Baltimore, Williams and Wilkins, 1990.
18. Garrick JG, Requa RK: The epidemiology of foot and ankle injuries in sports. Clin Sports Med 7(1):29–36, 1988.
19. Gary G: Ankle rehabilitation using the ankle disk. Phys Sports Med 6(6):141, 1978.
20. Gotlin RS, et al: Electrical stimulation effect on extensor lag and length of hospital stay after total knee arthroplasty. Arch Phys Med Rehabil 75: 957–959, 1994.
21. Grimes DW, Bennion D, Blusk K: Functional foot reconditioning exercises. Am J Sports Med 6:194, 1978.
22. Higgins JR: Human Movement: An Integrated Approach. St. Louis, Mosby, 1977.
23. Jackson DW, Ashley RL, Powell JW: Ankle sprains in young athletes. Clin Orthop 101:201–215, 1974.
24. Jackson D, Bailey D: Shin splints in the young athlete: A non specific diagnosis. Phys Sports Med 3(3):45, 1975.
25. James SD, Bates BT, Osternig LR: Injuries to runners. Am J Sports Med 6(2):40–50, 1978.
26. Johnson DP, Eastwood DM: Beneficial effects of continuous passive motion after total condylar knee arthroplasty. Ann Royal Col Surg Engl 74:412–416, 1992.
27. Johnston JM, Paulos LE: Prophylactic lateral knee braces. Med Sci Sports Exerc 23(7):783–787, 1991.
28. Johnson KA: Tibialis posterior tendon rupture. Clin Orthop 177:140–147, 1983.
29. Jorgenson U: Body load in heel strike running: The effects of a firm heel counter. Am J Sports Med 18:77, 1990.
30. Kellett J: Acute soft tissue injuries: A review of the literature. Med Sci Sport Exerc 18:489–500, 1986.
31. Leach R, Schepsis A: When hind foot pain slows the athlete. J Musculoskeletal Med 114, April 1992.
32. Lehman WL Jr: Overuse syndromes in runners. Am Fam Physician 29(1):157–161, 1984.
33. Mann, RA: Biomechanics of running. In Mack RP (ed): American Academy of Orthopaedics Surgeons Symposium on the Foot and Leg in Running Sports. St. Louis, Mosby, 1982.
34. Mann RA: Foot and ankle: Biomechanics of the foot and ankle linkage. In DeLee JC, Drez D (eds): Orthopaedic Sports Medicine Principles and Practice. Philadelphia, WB Saunders, 1994.
35. Matheson GO, Clement DB, McKenzie DC, et al: Stress fractures in athletes: A study of 320 cases. Am J Sports Med 15(1):46–58, 1987.
36. McKenzie DC, Clement DB, Taunton JE: Running shoes, orthotics and injuries. Sports Med 2:334–347, 1985.
37. McNair PJ, Marshall RN: Landing characteristics in subjects with normal and anterior cruciate deficient knees. Arch Phys Med Rehab 75:584–589, 1994.
38. Micheli LJ, Vorderer TW, Santopietro F, Sohn R: Athletic footwear and modifications in the lower

extremity and spine. In Nicholas JA, Hershman EB (eds): Sports Medicine, 2nd ed. vol. 1. St. Louis, Mosby-Year Book, 1995.

39. Morris J: Biomechanical aspects of the hip joint. Orthop Clin of North Am 2:33, 1971.
40. Morrey BF: Primary osteoarthritis of the knee: A step wise management plan. J Musculoskeletal Med 79–94, 1992.
41. Mubarak SJ, Gould RN, Lee YF, et al: The medial tibial stress syndrome, a cause of shin splints. Am J Sports Med 10(4):201–205, 1982.
42. Nicholas JA, Strizak AM, Veras G: A study of thigh muscle weakness in different pathological states of the lower extremity. Am J Sports Med 4(6):241, 1976.
43. Nikolao PK, Ribbeck BM, Glisson RR, et al: The effect of muscle architecture on the biomechanical failure properties of skeletal muscle under passive extension. Am J Sports Med 16:7–12, 1988.
44. Noyes FR: The Noyes Knee Rating System. An International Publication of Cincinnati Sports Medicine Research and Education Foundation. Cincinnati, OH, Cincinnati Sports Medicine Center, 1990.
45. Nyland J, Brosky T, Currier D, et al: Review of the afferent neural system of the knee and its contribution to motor learning. JOSPT 19(1):2–8, 1994.
46. Orava S, Jormakka E, Hulkko A: Stress fractures in young athletes. Arch Orthop Trauma Surg 98: 271–274, 1981.
47. Orava S: Stress fractures. Br J Sports Med 14:40–44, 1980.
48. Pauwels F: Der Schenkelhalsbruch ein Mechanisches Problem. Stuttgart, Ferdinand Enke Verlag, 1935.
49. Pearsall AW: Assessing acute hip injury; examination, diagnosis, and triage. Phys Sports Med 23(6): 40, 1995.
50. Pezzullo DJ, Irrgang JJ, Whitney SL: Patellar tendonitis: Jumpers knee. J Sports Rehab 1:56–88, 1992.
51. Powell RW: Lawn tennis leg. Lancet 2:44, 1883.
52. Regan K, Underwood L: Surgical tubing for rehabilitating shoulder and ankle. Phys Sports Med 9:1, 1981.
53. Rogers R, Lipscomb B: Non union stress fractures of the tibia. Am J Sports Med 13:171, 1985.
54. Shelbourne DK: Accelerated rehabilitation after anterior cruciate ligament reconstruction. JOSPT 15(6):256–264, 1992.
55. Stanitski C, McMaster J, Scranton P: On the nature of stress fractures. Am J Sports Med 6(6):391–396, 1978.
56. Tibone JE, et al: Functional analysis of anterior cruciate ligament instability. Am J Sports Med 16:332, 1988.
57. Vailas JC, et al: Dynamic biomechanical effects of functional bracing. Med Sci Sports Exerc (Suppl):582, 1989.
58. Vegso JJ, Harmon LE: Non operative management of athletic ankle injuries. Clin Sports Med 1:85–97, 1982.

45 The Upper Extremity

Nancy Kim, Daniel J. Kane, and Robert S. Gotlin

The lower extremities' predominant role, as they make the motions of running, skating, and jumping, is to maneuver an athlete's body in the environment. The upper extremities, on the other hand, function to actually manipulate the environment. In most sports, athletes use their upper extremities to catch, propel, or guide an object either directly or with an apparatus such as a glove, bat, or racket. In some sports, such as swimming, gymnastics, and pole vaulting, the athletes' upper extremity provides force to move the body. Whereas the lower extremities may put athletes in position to perform a task, the upper extremity often is called on to accomplish the task. The muscles, bones, and joints of the shoulders, elbows, wrists, and hands work as a unit to perform the fine manipulative neuromuscular behavior necessary for the athletes' sport.

The shoulder positions the arm and supplies power intrinsically, using the muscles of the shoulder joint complex, and extrinsically, by harvesting the energy generated by the remainder of the athlete's body. The elbow helps to pre-position the hand and provide force. The wrist and hand are the final common pathway. They not only transmit forces but grip objects and perform fine manipulation.

An athlete's upper extremity can be injured by either macrotrauma or microtrauma. Macrotrauma describes impairment from a single event, such as a blow to the arm during a football tackle. Microtrauma pertains to injuries originating from repetitive movements that result in cumulative pathological conditions. An example of microtrauma is anterior shoulder instability from repeated overhead throwing motions.

The rehabilitation for macrotrauma is relatively straightforward. The clinician should allow sufficient time for healing and then work on regaining lost range of motion, strength, and skill. The rehabilitation of an athlete with an injury from microtrauma is more complex. Essentially, the biomechanics of the athlete must be evaluated to diagnose the disorder. Thus the capable rehabilitative clinician must not only be familiar with the actions of the athlete's muscles, but also the nuances and demands of the athlete's sport. Not until the abnormal flexibility, muscular imbalance, or faulty technique leading to poor biomechanics is addressed and corrected is the task of rehabilitation possible.

This chapter focuses on the rehabilitation of the shoulder, elbow, wrist, and hand. To elaborate on the treatment of each injury of the upper extremity is beyond the scope of this text. Instead, a generalized rehabilitation plan is offered and then applied to each major area of the upper extremity (see box, General Rehab Strategy).

SHOULDER

Joint Mobilization

The focus of an early rehabilitation program for the shoulder emphasizes range of motion rather than strength. Magnusson's conclusions help support the theory that is the basis for this emphasis. He found that professional baseball pitchers actually had weaker arms but greater range of motion than nonpitchers.[37]

There is a time frame for maximal effectiveness in exercises for motion, whereas strengthening exercises are generally effective at most times after an injury. If active exercises begin too soon, muscle soreness can be increased and this pain can limit the recovery of motion. Too much range of motion exercise in one sitting can cause muscle fatigue, soreness, and muscle tightening, so can be counterproductive. Multiple therapies for short durations throughout the day, as opposed to one or two longer therapy sessions, are preferred.

After an injury or surgery, a brief period is allowed for inflammation and swelling to subside. Then passive range of motion exercises are initiated. To restore motion in the shoulder, Codman's pendulum exercises are an excellent early intervention (Fig. 45-1).[13] Before initiating range of motion exercises, warming the area, perhaps with hydrocollator packs, is useful. Heat should be used cautiously within the first five days postsurgery because it may induce hematoma formation.[43]

Continuous passive motion (CPM) may be applied to the joints of the upper extremity, as for the knee, to increase range of motion (Fig. 45-2). Another type of passive range of motion is termed *early passive motion* or EPM (Fig. 45-3).[43] In this technique, the patient completely relaxes the arm that has been operated on, like the arm of a "rag doll." Then an experienced clinician elevates the arm along the scapular plane of motion while supporting its full weight. The clinician also may exert distraction force on the glenohumeral joint. Unlike Neer's description of EPM with the patient standing, we prefer to have the patient lying down. With this modification, once 90° of elevation is obtained, the clinician and

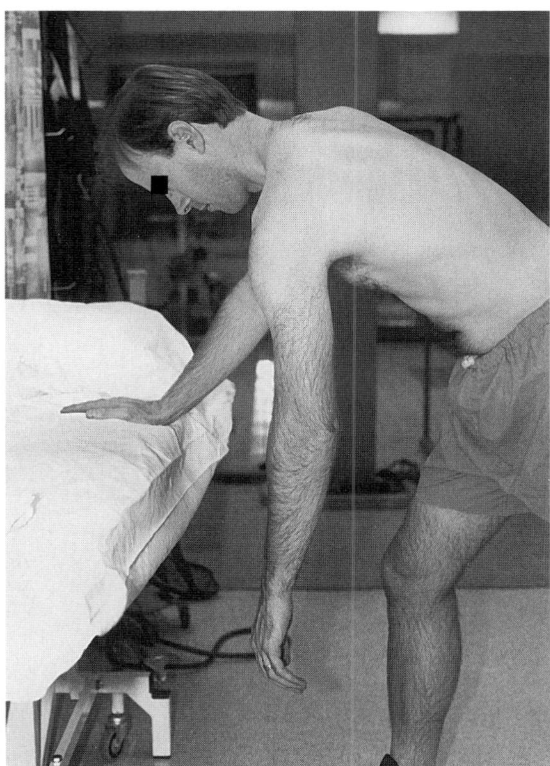

FIGURE 45-1. Passive range of motion exercises. Exercises such as Codman's pendulums are effective in restoring early motion and curtailing the occurrence of adhesions. Gravity will distract the glenohumeral joint and allow free motion. A light weight can be held in the hand to foster this effect.

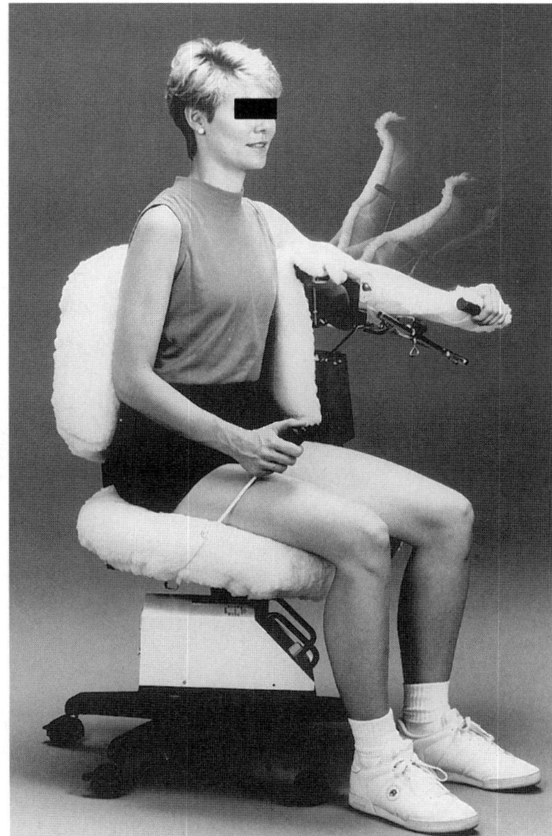

FIGURE 45-2. Continuous passive motion (CPM). Mechanical devices such as CPM are useful in increasing range without the need of an assistant or active participation by the patient. The desired speed and range of motion is set and increased as tolerated. (Smith and Nephew Richards Shoulder CPM pictured. Manufactured by Kinster. Used with permission.)

patient are assisted by gravity in achieving additional range of motion.

The patient ultimately is in charge of his or her own rehabilitation and is taught active assisted range of motion exercises. These can be performed with the uninvolved arm alone, or with a cane, T-bar, pulley, or towel (Fig. 45-4). When muscle soreness has dissipated, active range of motion exercises can begin. These exercises assist the patient in achieving full range of motion (Fig. 45-5).

At our institution, we divide shoulder rehabilitation into phases. In Phase I the patient lies supine and undergoes passive range of motion. Phase II includes active ROM of the shoulder while the patient is supine, and PROM while the patient is sitting or standing. Phase III of the program includes active ROM with the patient in the upright position. This phase progresses toward resistive exercise training.

The scapula also must have full range of motion. Any limitation in scapula range of motion must be addressed. The range of motion can be tested by the lateral scapula slide test or the modified scapular slide test.[15,16,31,34] It can also be measured with a goniometer and testing range of motion with the scapula stabilized and not stabilized using techniques described by Boon.[7] Motion of the glenohumeral joint is accompanied by motion between the scapula and the thoracic vertebrae. Codman defined this as scapulohumeral rhythm.[13] Elevation of the upper extremity requires both glenohumeral and scapulothoracic motions that move synchronously through a 3:2 ratio of glenohumeral motion versus scapular rotation. Poppin investigated the relationship further by studying abduction of the shoulder. On average, it is a 2:1 ratio. However, in the initial phase of abduction, the GH motion predominates and the ratio was found to be 4.4° of GH motion for every degree of ST motion. Then, as the shoulder abducts to greater than 90°, the ratio becomes 1.1° of GH motion for every degree of ST motion.[53] In conclusion, without proper movement of the scapula, glenohumeral motion is limited.

Joint mobilization is effective for lysing adhesions and maintaining or increasing range of motion. Its goal is to restore normal motion to a joint. Early range of motion can prevent the formation of a stiff joint, but restricted movement of the periarticular tissues is common after an

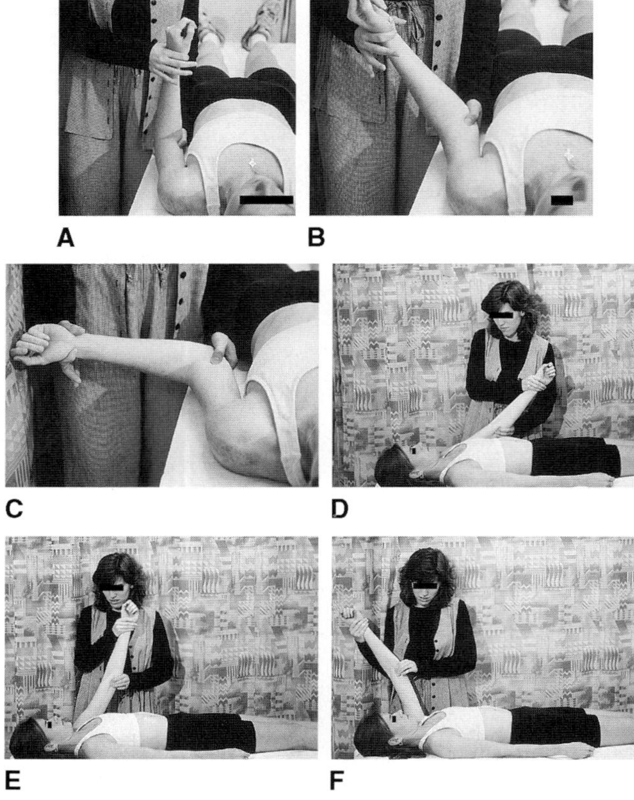

FIGURE 45-3. Early passive motion (EPM). **A–F,** With the patient completely relaxed, the clinician gently distracts the glenohumeral joint and glides it through anatomic range of motion (i.e., flexion in the scapular plane). If the patient is lying down, gravity will assist the motion once 90° forward flexion is achieved.

injury or period of immobilization. Once they become stiff, mild joint adhesions can be lysed with mobilization techniques. These maneuvers consist of a group of skilled passive movements applied to improve soft-tissue and joint mobility. Joint mobilization is based on a sound knowledge of muscle function, arthrokinematics, and osteokinematics (Fig. 45-6).

The effects of passive movements to an injured joint include:

1. Decreases in wound edema and joint effusion[19]
2. Provision of proprioceptive information to the central nervous system, which in turn may interfere with the transmission of pain[19]
3. Stimulation of mechanoreceptors, which may diminish many types of pain[73]
4. Decreases in complications of immobilization
5. Maintenance of tissue homeostasis[19]
6. Reduction in the restrictions of scar tissue[17]
7. Lengthening of an immature scar[1]
8. Proper orientation of collagen fibers[1]
9. Reestablishment of normal active range of motion

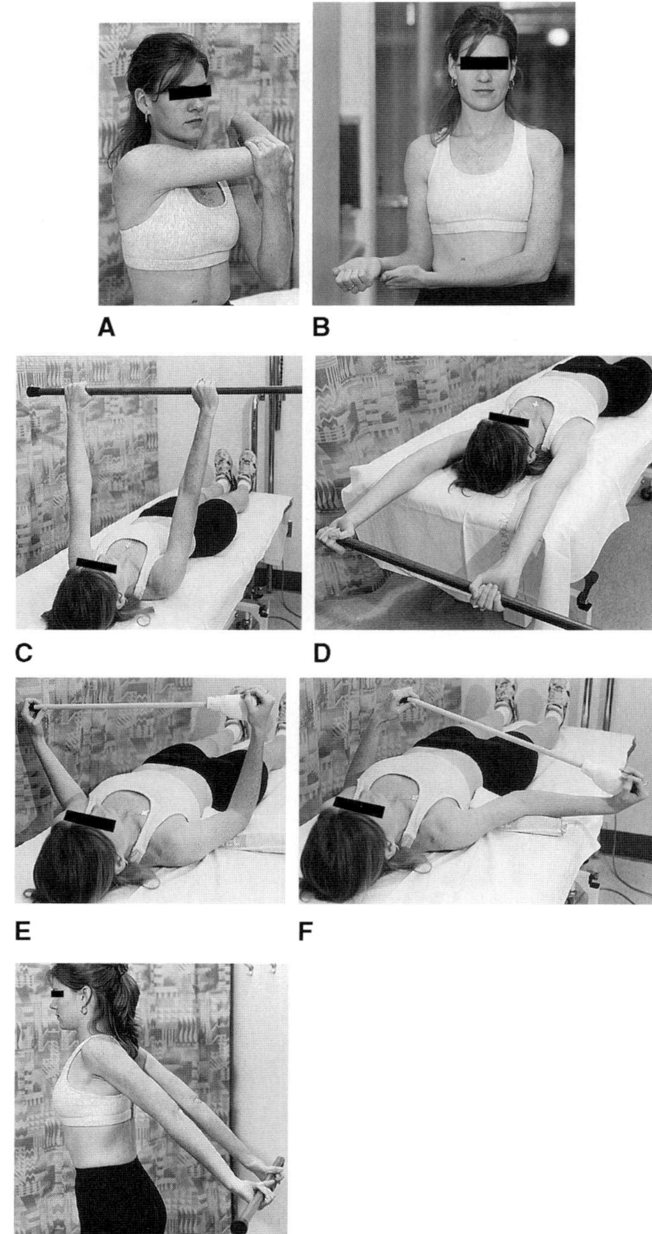

FIGURE 45-4. Active assisted range of motion. **A** and **B,** The involved glenohumeral joint can be ranged with the assistance of the uninvolved limb. **C–G,** A cane or stick is also helpful in increasing forward flexion/extension and internal/external rotation.

10. Breaking of intracapsular adhesions that may have formed during immobilization
11. Enhancement of collagen fiber glide[1]

Mobilization techniques vary.[38] Closely related types of passive movement to a joint include manipulation, articulations, oscillations, distractions, and thrust techniques.[17] Manipulation is described as "the forceful

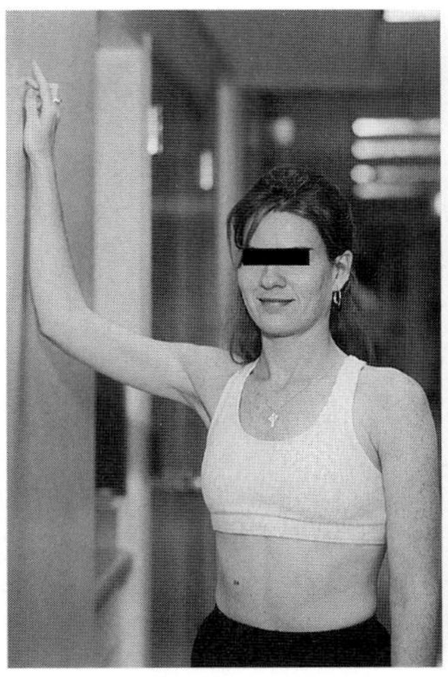
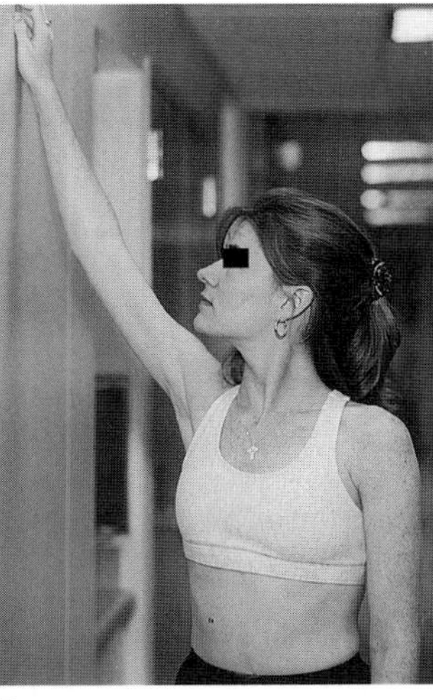

A **B**

FIGURE 45-5. Active range of motion, wall climb. **A** and **B,** On repeated trials, the patient elevates the involved arm by sequentially placing the fingers upward on a wall board, each time trying to raise the arm higher.

passive movement of a joint beyond its active limit of motion." Articulation is passive movement applied in a smooth, rhythmic fashion to stretch contracted muscles, ligaments, and capsules gradually.[65] Oscillatory technique involves passive movements that can be of small or large amplitude and applied anywhere in the range of motion of a joint, whether the joint surfaces are distracted or compressed. Distraction involves stretching a joint capsule by separating the surfaces of the joint. Thrust techniques are of two basic types. You can employ a high velocity, low amplitude or a low velocity, high amplitude technique. The common goal of these is to free restricted joint motion.

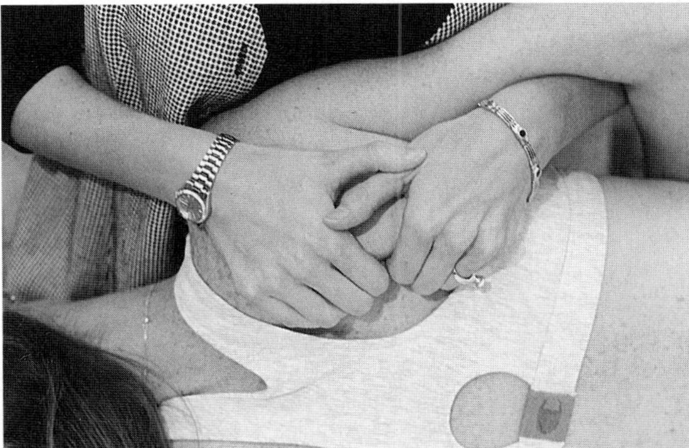

FIGURE 45-6. Joint mobilization. For stiff joints, soft-tissue adhesions can be broken by skilled passive ranging. This technique also establishes normal congruency between the scapula and thoracic cage.

These passive range of motion exercises can be delivered by the clinician to help prevent or treat joint limitations. Sometimes manipulation under anesthesia is indicated to break larger adhesions that may have formed during a period of immobilization. This is a more aggressive technique and can be done under general anesthesia or with a brachial plexus block. Some centers use an interscalene brachial plexus block for the manipulation and leave the catheter in the interscalene space. The patient receives anesthesia via the catheter daily for 2 to 4 days as he or she receives physical therapy, in an effort to retain the motion gained in the operating room.[3]

Closely related to mobilization strategies is the concept of proprioceptive neuromuscular facilitation (PNF) (Fig. 45-7).[36,55] This is a type of neuromuscular mobilization. In this technique, the patient is instructed to contract an antagonist muscle or group of muscles. Immediately following this contraction, the therapist instructs the patient to perform a contraction of the agonist muscle or passively moves the patient's limb in the desired direction, in an effort to increase the range of motion. Theoretically, the preliminary contraction of the range-limiting muscle group (the antagonist) will inhibit its refiring for a short time as it repolarizes. This is called the refractory period. Then the agonist can contract without a co-contraction by the antagonists, via the stretch reflex. Also, while the agonist contracts, the antagonist will be silenced at the spinal level by the principle of reciprocal inhibition. In this way, it is possible to obtain more range of motion in the desired plane. The repeated contractions of the antagonist muscles will fatigue them, reducing their ability to counteract the agonist muscles. This is similar to the theory of muscle energy described in the discussion of spine rehabilitation.

Knott and Voss modified PNF techniques for use around the shoulder.[51] They described four basic diagonal patterns for the shoulder and upper extremity. By facilitating agonist muscles and inhibiting antagonist muscles around the scapula and humerus, dysfunctional movements of the shoulder were eliminated. The result was a more fluent, rhythmic shoulder movement pattern in an effort to obtain full range of motion.

Some patients have difficulty moving their shoulders early in the rehabilitation period. This may be due to pain and anxiety but also could be the result of an inability to contract the muscles around the shoulder effectively. A study by Yishay revealed that pain inhibits shoulder strength.[74] This parallels the findings that neurological inhibition decreases quadriceps function in a painful knee.[18,41,64,72] Therefore, it is important that the patient avoid painful positions during rehabilitation.

Hydrotherapy entails placing a patient in a warm pool of water to neck level. It is felt that the buoyancy effect of the water helps decrease pain around the shoulder joint. Also, the resistance offered by the water translates into sensory and proprioceptive feedback. Typically, PNF

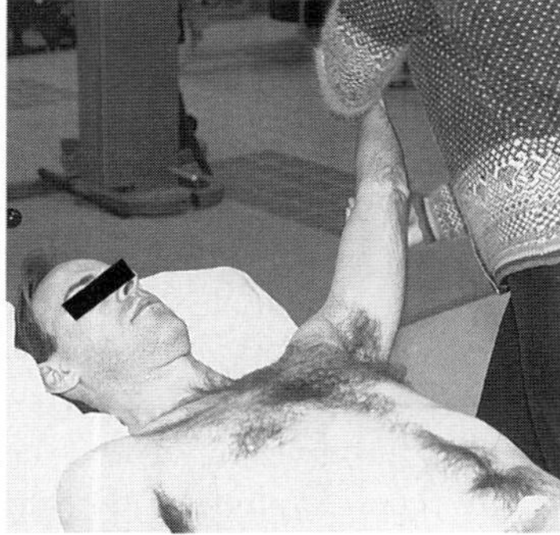

A

B

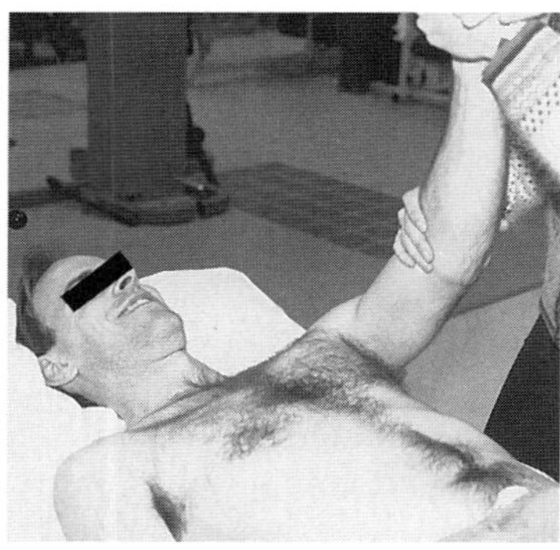

C

FIGURE 45-7. Proprioceptive neuromuscular facilitation. **A, B,** and **C,** In increasing range of motion, the antagonist muscle must not be resistive to the desired movement. Initially, the antagonist muscle is contracted, immediately followed by a contraction of, or passive movement of, the agonist muscle. The antagonist muscle is refractory during the agonist contraction.

shoulder axis patterns are practiced underwater to help achieve greater range of motion and kinetically correct shoulder movements.[63]

Spencer's techniques use gentle, repeated stretching to treat shoulder dysfunction.[51] They are especially useful in adhesive capsulitis and other painful shoulder conditions. Because the patient's scapula is stabilized and not permitted to rotate, the arm should not be ranged past 90° of elevation lest an impingement or rotator cuff disorder be aggravated (Fig. 45-8).

Strengthening

"History does not long entrust the care of freedom to the weak or timid." —D.D. Eisenhower, January 20, 1953 at the Inaugural Address.

Once the patient's range of motion has been sufficiently maximized, rehabilitation focuses on strengthening the shoulder girdle musculature.[11] The shoulder has great freedom of movement, so it is imperative for the muscles around the shoulder to be strong. The muscles of the shoulder girdle have three major functions: stability, force production, and force absorption.

The rotator cuff muscles afford stability of the glenohumeral joint.[68] From a purely structural aspect, the subscapular muscle lies anterior to the glenohumeral joint, thereby helping to prevent subluxation. The same can be said about the teres minor and infraspinatus muscles, posteriorly. The rotator cuff muscles blend with the capsule, and contraction of the muscle produces tension in the capsule and the capsular ligaments. This is referred to as dynamic ligament tension. The biceps brachii also assist with anterior stability, especially in the vulnerable overhead throwing position.[52,54]

The circle concept of stability originally was described for the capsule and ligaments around the glenohumeral joint.[27,57,58,69,71] However, it can be extrapolated to include the muscles of the rotator cuff. The circle concept implies that stability is provided by opposing structures on each side of the joint. For example, the posterior musculature helps prevent anterior subluxation and vice versa. This point is very evident with inferior instability. There are no dynamic inferior stabilizers, therefore we know that the supraspinatus and deltoid muscles are integral in preventing the humeral head from subluxing inferiorly.[8]

Another mechanism by which the rotator cuff muscle affords stability is force coupling. When the rotator cuff muscles contract, they pull the humeral head into the glenoid. This maximizes joint congruity, increases adhesion and cohesion of the joint surfaces, and prevents humeral translation. Any rotator cuff muscle contraction helps center the humeral head within the glenoid, thereby increasing the shoulder's stability. For dynamic stability, it is important that the force couples are properly balanced with synchronized co-contraction to prevent abnormal joint kinematics.

In addition to the rotator cuff, deltoid, and biceps, the scapular stabilizer muscles need to be strengthened.[34,42,49] The glenoid fossa must be positioned correctly to prevent the humeral head from gliding inferiorly. Also, the

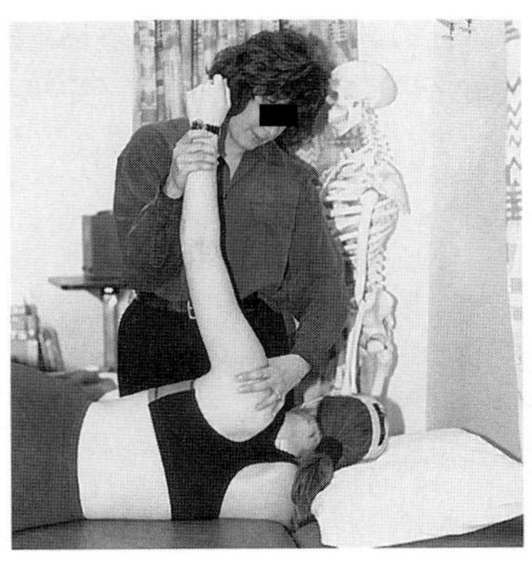
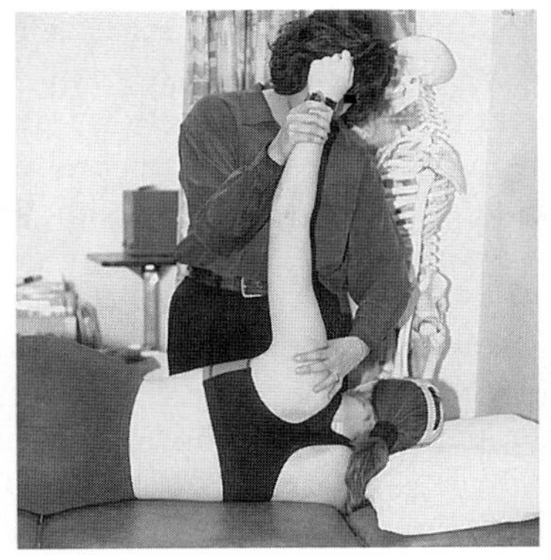
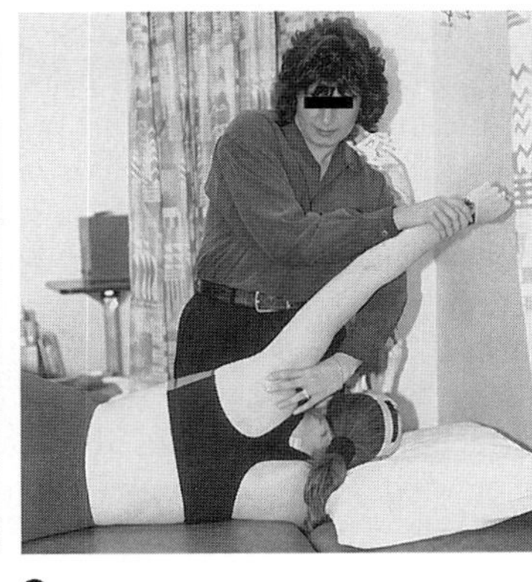

A B C

FIGURE 45-8. Spencer's techniques. **A, B,** and **C,** A series of passive exercises is performed to increase all motions of the glenohumeral joint.

scapulohumeral rhythm allows the rotator cuff muscles to be set properly, which provides the optimum length-tension ratio. If the scapula is unstable, the rotator cuff muscles will not have a strong base of support and will be much less efficient. Therefore it is imperative to strengthen the scapular stabilizers, especially the serratus anterior, trapezius, and the rhomboids (Fig. 45-9).[30] By keeping the glenohumeral joint dynamically stable, we can decrease the likelihood of the development of impingement.

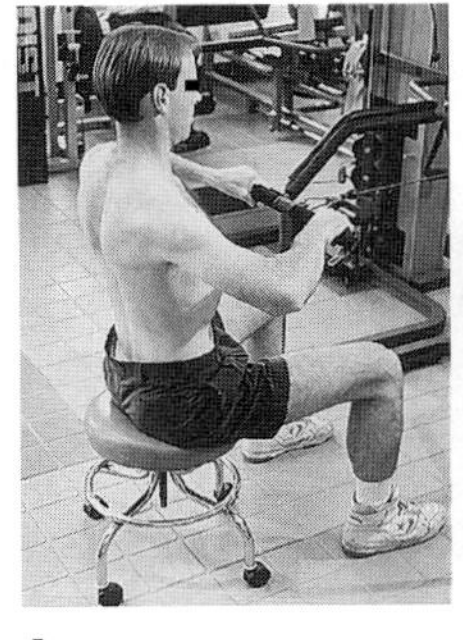
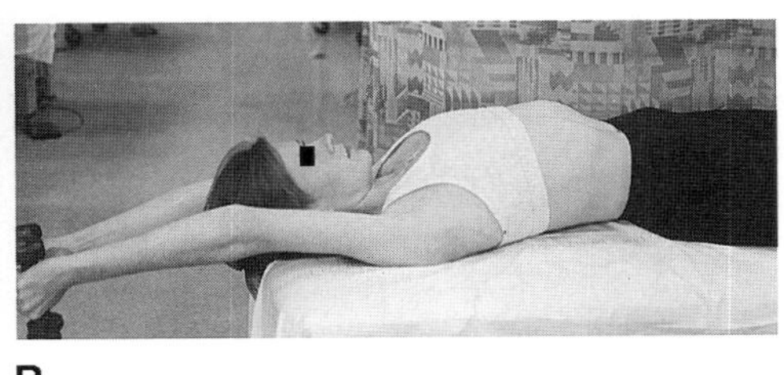

A B

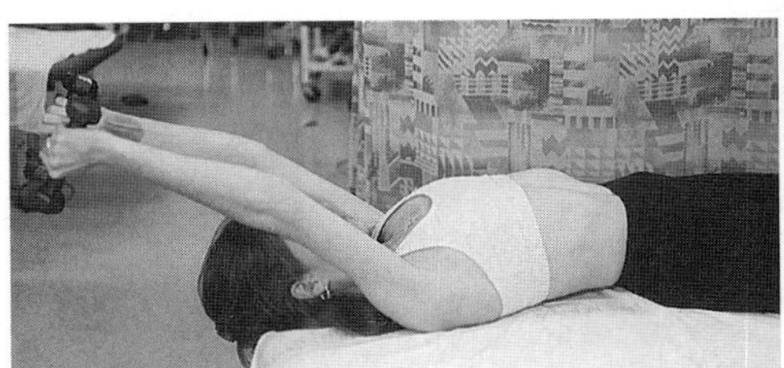
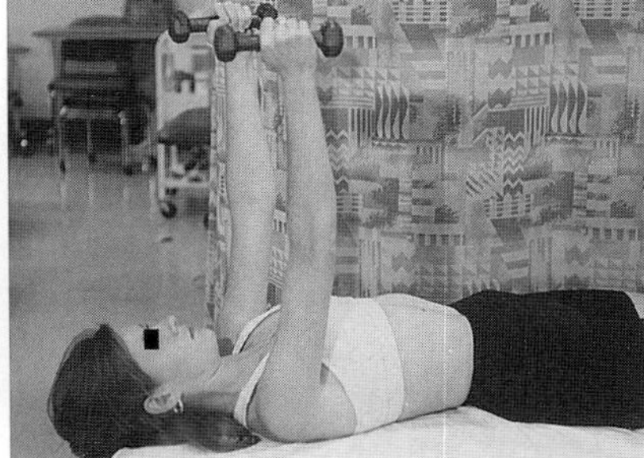

C D

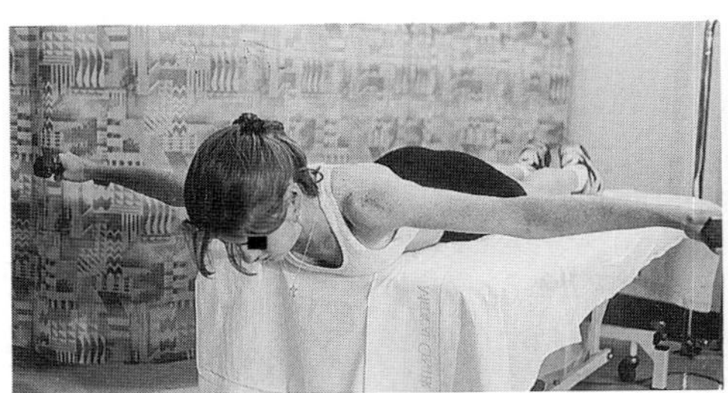
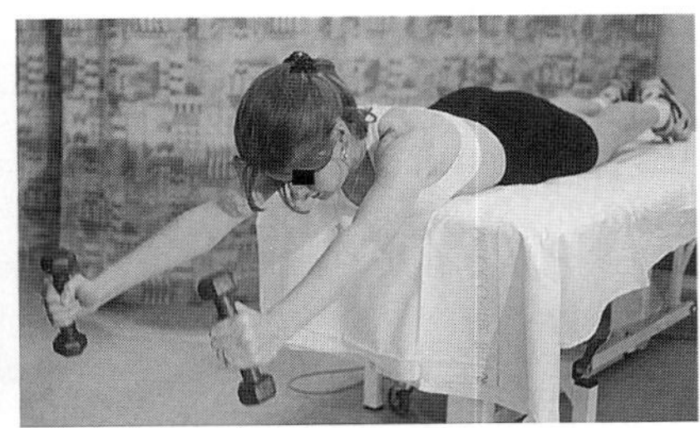

E F

FIGURE 45-9. Scapular stabilizer exercises. **A,** Rhomboid progressive resistive exercise. **B–D,** Serratus anterior progressive resistive exercises. **E** and **F,** Trapezius progressive resistive exercises.

Strong scapular stabilizers, smooth scapulohumeral rhythm, and strong rotator cuff muscles work together in an efficient glenohumeral relationship. When the deltoid contracts, the glenoid fossa acts as a fulcrum and the arm rotates correctly. But when the humeral head depressors are weak, the humeral head does not properly enter the glenoid. Upon contraction of the deltoid, the humeral head migrates superiorly, which narrows the subacromial space and can trigger symptoms of impingement. Smooth scapular motion positions the glenoid properly to maintain an adequate subacromial space. Normal elevation of the acromion is approximately 36° from the neutral position and is achieved in maximum abduction of the arm.[53]

The preceding paragraphs outlined reasons for maximizing the dynamic shoulder stabilizers. This function is essential in providing the foundation for the upper extremities' role in functional performance. Strengthening strategies apply to the use of the arm, forearm, and hand. There are two specific entities: force production and force absorption.

Force production is quite important in sports such as wrestling, weight lifting, and rugby. A larger muscle can produce more tension and therefore produce more force, or torque. However, this does not always translate into better function in other sports. In Wilk's study of professional baseball pitchers, he concluded that there was no significant difference between the dominant and the nondominant throwing arm in internal and external rotator muscle strength.[70] Aldenrink and colleagues reported similar results in their investigation of rotator cuff strength.[2,28,44,59]

Where does the force of the upper extremity originate? We must look at the kinetic chain. For activities like throwing a ball or swinging a golf club, force generation is mainly by ground reaction forces and rotational forces of the trunk and hips. These are guided, increased, and directed by the anterior shoulder muscles' working in concentric fashion. Kibler has compared the shoulder to a funnel.[34] The energy generated by the lower extremities and the trunk is transferred to the upper extremities by the smooth, integrated movement of the stable shoulder. This helps explain why some Little League baseball pitchers can throw a baseball 90 miles per hour and why golfers can drive a golf ball more than 300 yards. Therefore, as part of the rehabilitation program, the hip and trunk activation are also addressed as a part of his therapy guidelines.[35]

The other function of the muscles around the shoulder is force absorption. This can refer to the follow-through of a pitcher's arm when the posterior rotator cuff muscles must contract eccentrically to slow down the upper extremity, or it can refer to an offensive lineman's stopping an oncoming rusher with his arms. Typically, force generation requires a concentric muscular contraction, whereas force absorption requires a strong eccentric effort. We also call these muscle groups accelerators and decelerators, or agonists and antagonists. Typically, an agonist muscle, or group of muscles, will contract to accelerate a body part, and toward the end of the motion the antagonist muscle or muscles will fire eccentrically to decelerate the body part. When both muscle groups are firing simultaneously, it is termed *co-contraction*. If there is a great disparity between the force a body can generate and the force it can absorb, injury may ensue. For example, in the throwing motion, the internal rotators contract to internally rotate the shoulder (along with momentum from the body turn). The external rotators must slow down and control the shoulder's internal rotation to prevent injury.

There are three basic types of muscle-strengthening exercises: (1) isometrics, (2) isotonics, and (3) isokinetics.

Isometric refers to equal length (Fig. 45-10). During this type of contraction, no work is performed. This can be understood when one considers the formula work = force × distance. In an isometric contraction, no net change in muscle length or movement of the body part occurs. Therefore the distance traveled is zero. If work = force × distance, net work must be zero if no distance is traveled. Some clinicians feel that injured joints are inflamed and that undue motion can adversely affect them. Isometrics allow for strengthening muscles around a joint without straining them, so this technique is relatively safe for strengthening muscles around an inflamed joint. Caution must be exercised in performing isometrics when muscles or tendons are injured because high muscle tensions further injure the compromised structures.

Isotonic connotes "equal tension" (Fig. 45-11). In this type of exercise, the load remains constant as the muscle

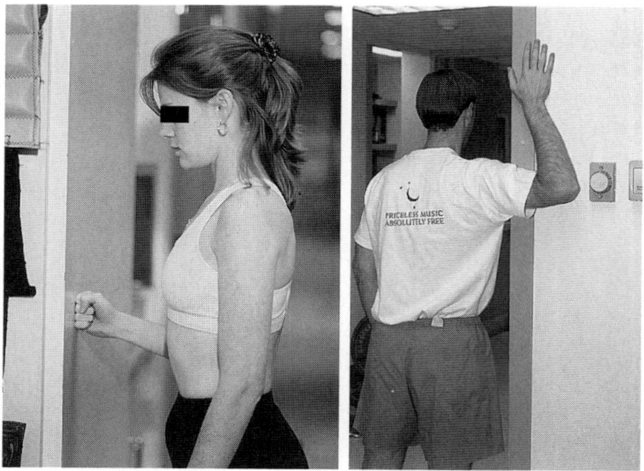

FIGURE 45-10. Isometric exercises. **A** and **B,** This is an excellent exercise when you are trying to strengthen an inflamed joint. A wall acts as a resistive force for isometric training of the shoulder complex. Precaution must be taken with isometric exercises in patients with cardiac compromise.

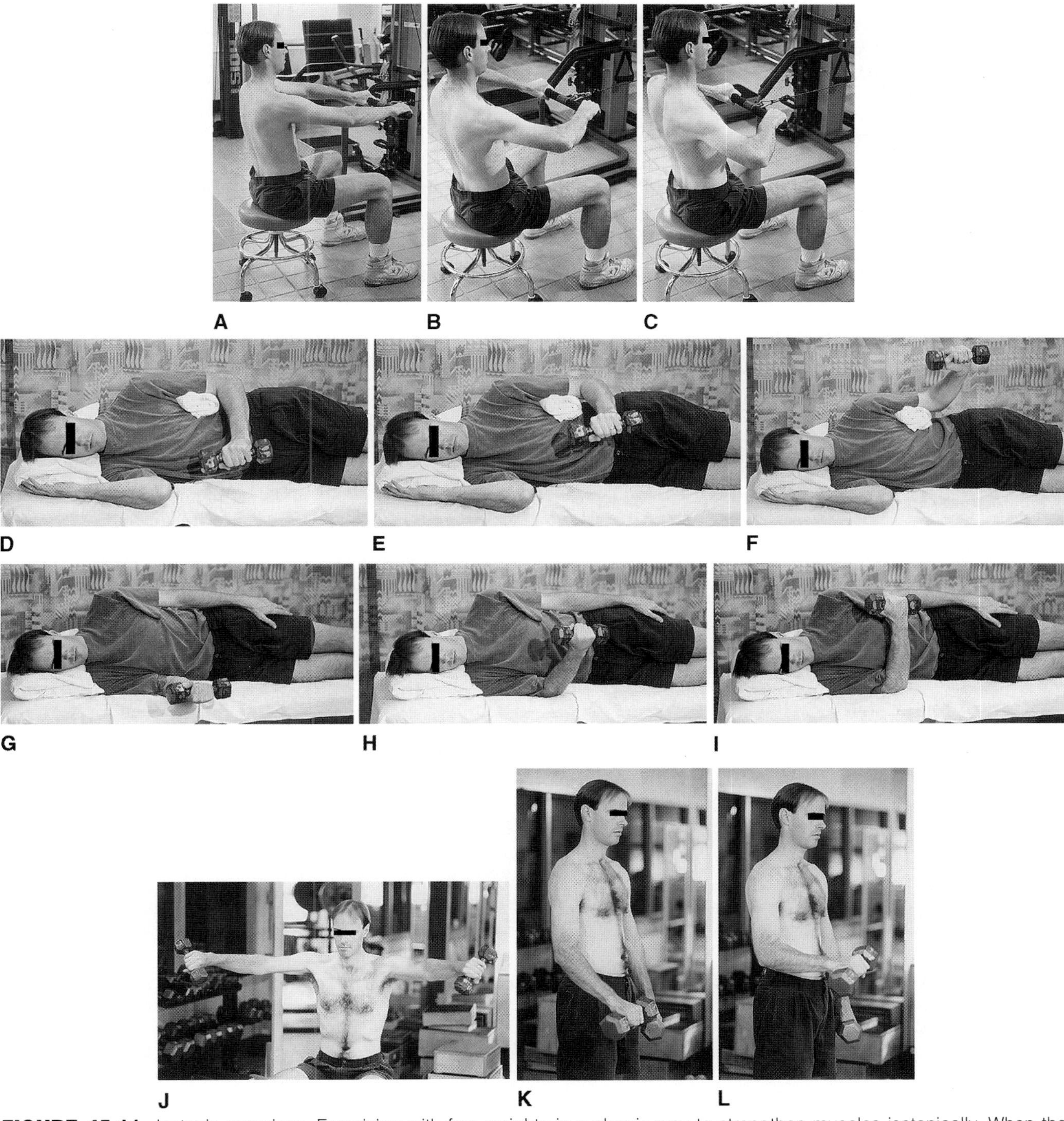

FIGURE 45-11. Isotonic exercises. Exercising with free weights is a classic way to strengthen muscles isotonically. When the muscle lengthens as it contracts, it is termed eccentric and when it shortens as it contracts, it is termed concentric. Progressing from **A–C** depicts concentric contraction of the rhomboids and from **C–A** eccentric contraction. These exercises should be done in sets of 10 repetitions, 3 to 4 times/session. Maximum weight should be that which the patient struggles to lift 10 times. **D–F,** External rotators—lie on uninvolved side and flex involved limb at elbow to 90°. Slowly raise arm into external rotation and lower it. **G–I,** Internal rotators—lie on affected side and flex elbow 90°. Slowly raise arm into internal rotation and lower it. **J,** Supraspinatus—sit on a stool with upper extremities extended. Horizontally rotate the upper extremities approximately 30° anterior in the frontal plane and pronate the forearms. Then lower and raise the upper extremities in the scapular plane, not to rise above eye level. A weight is held in the hands. Starting weight should be that which can be lowered and raised ten times with moderate difficulty. **K** and **L,** Brachioradialis, brachialis—stand with elbows slightly flexed. Forearms are pronated with weights held in each hand. Slowly flex and extend the elbow. *Continued*

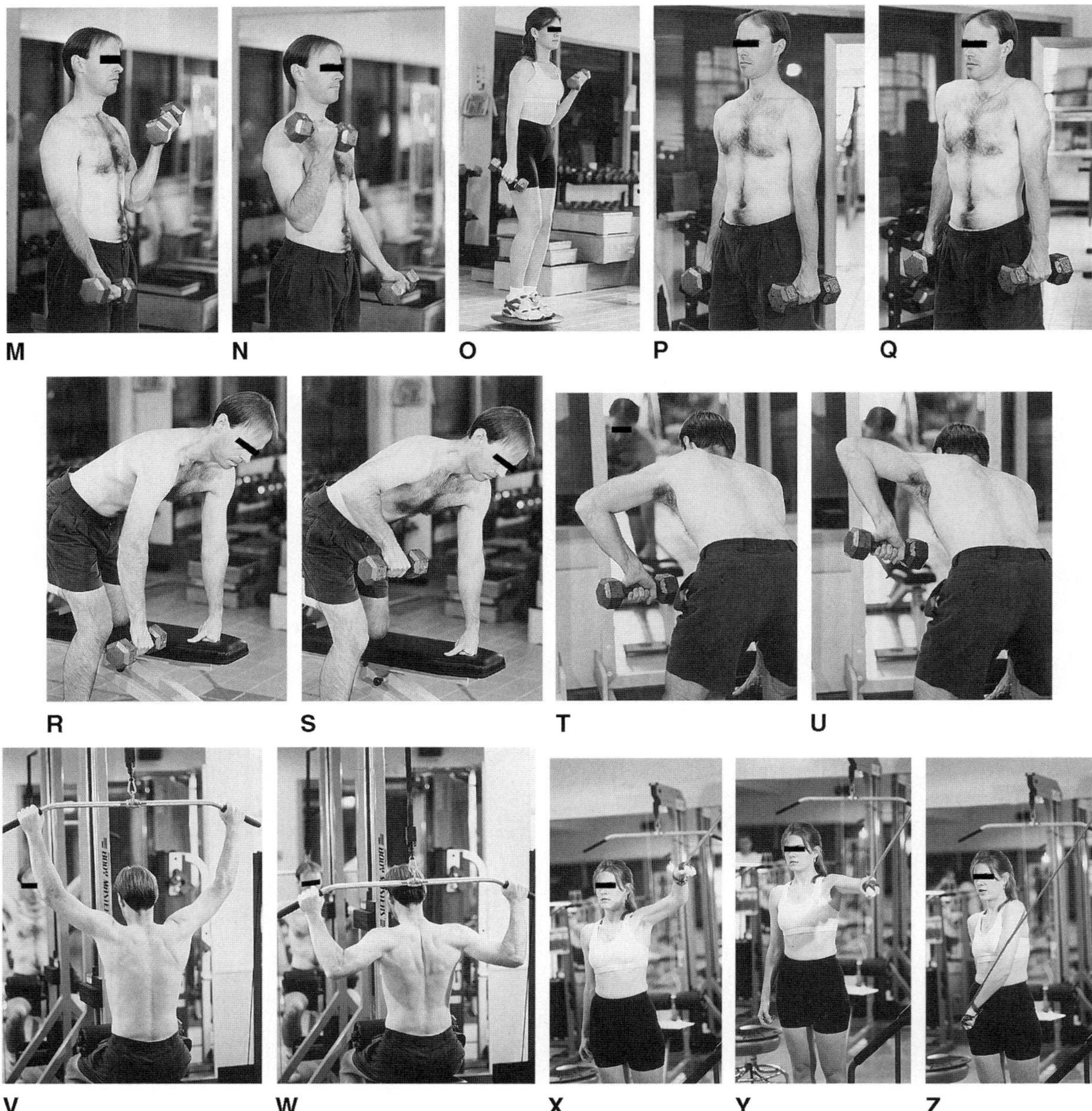

FIGURE 45-11, cont'd. **M** and **N,** Biceps—stand with elbows slightly flexed. Forearms are supinated with weights held in each hand. Slowly flex and extend at the elbow. **O,** Biceps curl on balance board—to add complexity to the biceps strengthening, you can maintain balance on a balance board while performing the exercise. This adds complexity and challenges the nervous system to devise strategies to successfully achieve the task. **P** and **Q,** Shoulder shrug (levator scapulae and trapezius)—stand with upper extremities extended. Shrug shoulder against resistance supplied by hand-held weights. **R–U,** Rows (deltoids, rhomboids, levator scapulae and trapezius)—standing with hips flexed approximately 45°, place unaffected upper extremity on support (table or bench). While holding hand weights, extend the shoulder, maintaining flexion at the elbow. **V** and **W,** Lattisimus dorsi—sitting facing the weight stack, place upper extremities on the weight bar. Slowly lower the bar to the shoulders and then return to starting point. **X–Z,** Shoulder adductors (pectorals)—stand with upper extremity attached to cable column. Slowly pull cable across body maintaining extension at elbow.

Continued

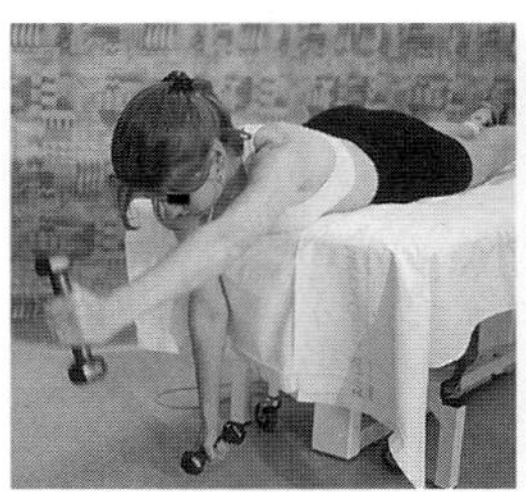
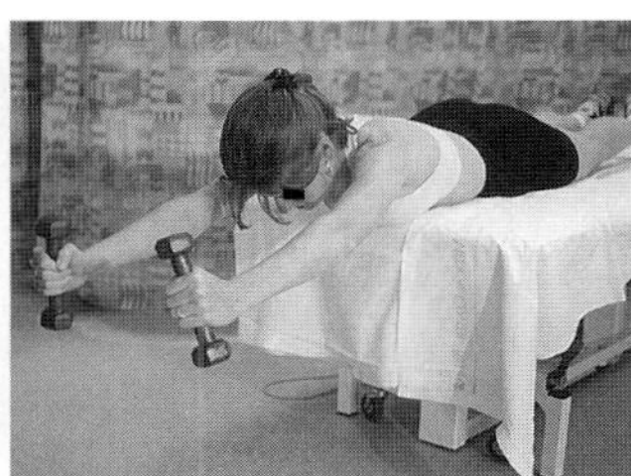
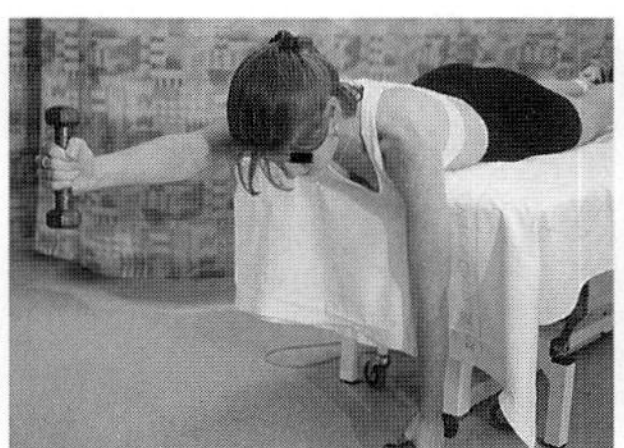
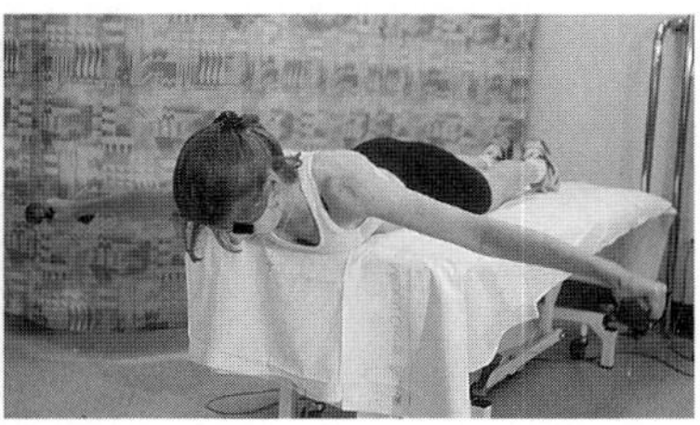

AA BB CC DD

FIGURE 45-11, cont'd. AA–DD, Prone trapezius, deltoids, and levator scapulae—lie prone with head over edge of table. Forward-flex upper extremities while holding hand weights. Alternate raising and lowering each upper extremity. **DD,** Prone deltoids and trapezius—lie prone with head over edge of table. Abduct upper extremities while holding hand weights.

shortens or lengthens. When the muscle shortens, it is termed a *concentric contraction,* and when the muscle lengthens in a controlled fashion, it is termed *eccentric.* Note that equal resistance is not offered throughout the full arc of these exercises. Free weights, weight machines, push-ups, and pull-ups all exercise muscles isotonically in both concentric and eccentric fashions.

Isokinetic connotes "equal velocity or speed" (Fig. 45-12). In this type of exercise the speed of the limb does not change, no matter how much load is applied. Therefore there is maximal resistance throughout the range of the exercise. This is not the case with isotonic exercise. Isokinetic exercise can be performed either concentrically or eccentrically.

Most exercises are beneficial, but each one has its limitations. No one type of exercise has proven to be universally superior. All have a place in the strengthening of an athlete.[40]

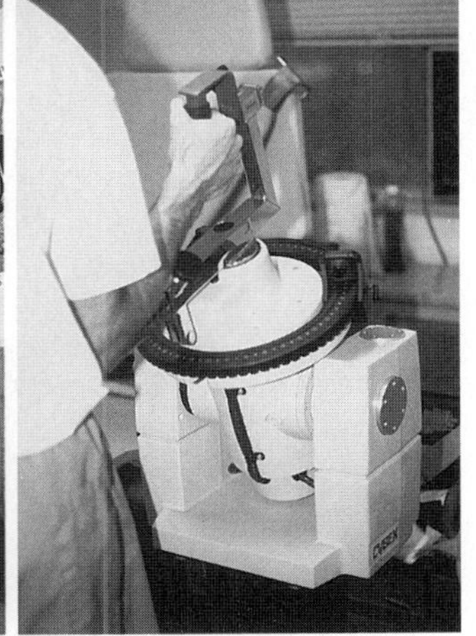

A B

FIGURE 45-12. Isokinetic exercises. **A** and **B,** This form of exercise is speed-dependent and gives maximum resistance throughout the range of motion. The limb is usually secured in the equipment, so this is a very good controlled-motion exercise. The movement of the limb will be guided by the range of the machine; this is thought to be a very safe exercise.

Another way to differentiate strengthening exercises involves open–kinetic chain versus closed–kinetic chain exercise.[71] In closed–kinetic chain or CKC exercise, the distal segment of the limb to be exercised is relatively fixed, whereas in open–kinetic chain exercise the distal segment of the limb to be exercised is free to move. An example of closed–kinetic chain exercise is the push-up, whereas an open–kinetic chain would be the biceps curl. The advantage of closed–kinetic chain exercise is the promotion of muscular co-contraction around the joint, the promotion of a more fluent movement pattern, and increased dynamic joint stability (Fig. 45-13). However, one must not forget that training must include both open and closed kinetic techniques because our daily requirements for motion incorporate both.

We prefer to use the terms *axial* and *perpendicular load* when describing these concepts. Axial load is likened to closed–kinetic chain, and perpendicular load is likened to open–kinetic chain exercises. For descriptive purposes, a closed–kinetic chain exercise (axial load) is one that produces force across a joint line, whereas an open–kinetic chain exercise (perpendicular load) produces force tangent to or along a joint line. For example, if a person does a push-up, an axial load is generated across the elbow joint as she elevates her body from the floor. If someone does a biceps curl, the predominant force is tangent to the elbow joint, and this produces a perpendicular load through the elbow.

There are combined versus isolated movement patterns. Exercises can be performed that concentrate on one individual muscle or on a movement pattern (Fig. 45-14).[67] For instance, the triceps surae muscles can be exercised alone with resisted elbow extension (the scapular stabilizers also are firing to stabilize the origin of the long head of the triceps) or as part of a movement pattern such as the military press. Both types of exercises are beneficial. The weak link in a movement pattern should be strengthened individually so that the stronger muscles in that pattern do not mask the deficit. Gross

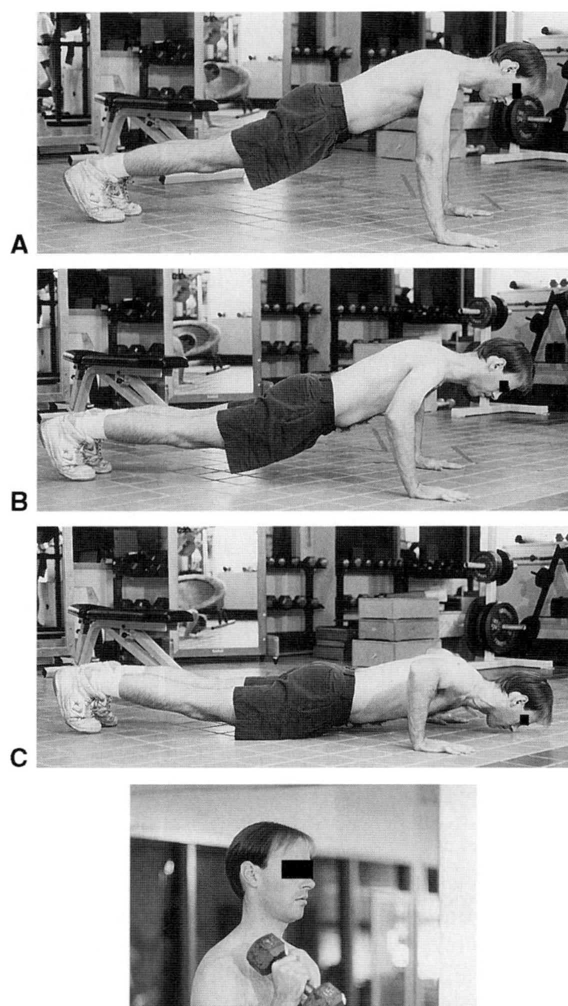

FIGURE 45-13. Closed (axial load)– and open (perpendicular load)–kinetic chain exercises. **A–C,** When forces are primarily generated across a joint, the exercise is predominantly closed (axial load) chain. **D,** If the forces are tangent to the joint, the exercise is open (perpendicular load) chain. The push-up is closed chain and the biceps curl open chain.

movements should be exercised first during a workout. It would be counterproductive to fatigue a muscle that is already the weak link in a movement pattern with a single muscle exercise. When the gross movement is required there would be even greater substitution, and abnormal movement patterns might ensue.

Strength is different from endurance. A muscle can be trained for each. Muscle strength is the maximum force a muscle or group of muscles can exert against resistance.

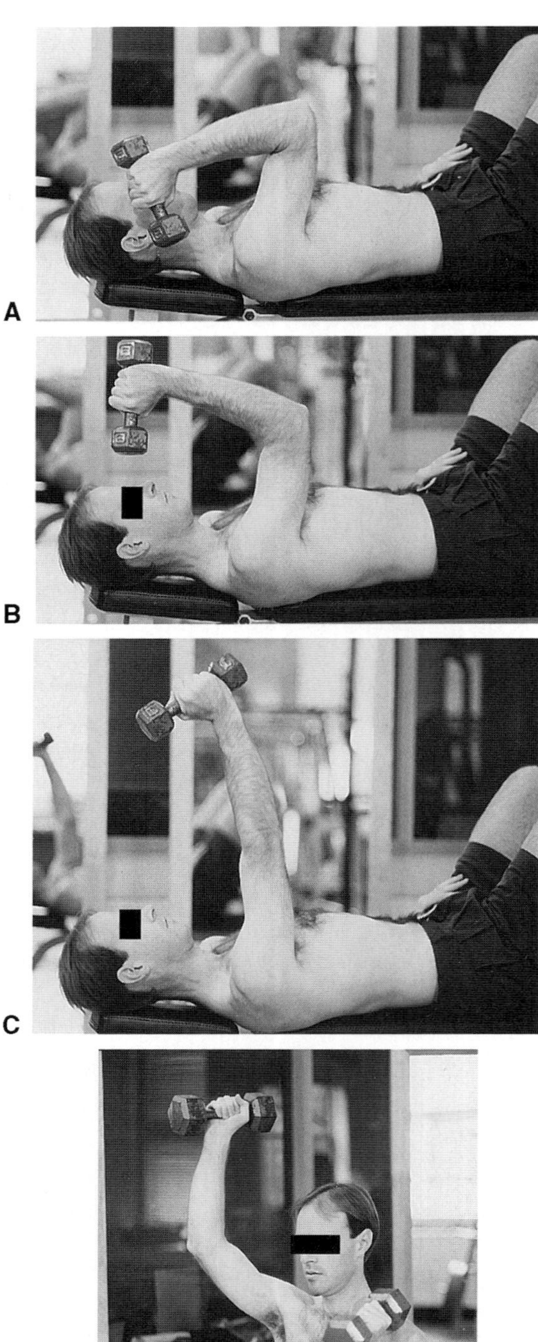

FIGURE 45-14. Combined versus isolated strengthening exercises. A muscle such as the triceps can be strengthened in an isolated fashion as in **A–C.** In **D** the triceps is strengthened in combination with other muscles, such as in the military press. Ten repetitions repeated 3 or 4 times is recommended. The ideal weight is that which the individual must struggle to successfully lift 10 times.

Muscle endurance is the ability to perform repeated contractions of the muscle or muscle groups over an extended period before fatiguing. These elements of physical conditioning are related, so exercises to increase muscle strength may also increase endurance, and vice versa. The principle of overload states that increases in strength occur when muscles are exercised at or near their maximal strength. To increase endurance, exercises at or near maximum repetitions must be done. Classically, to increase strength we use resistance exercises with high loads and low repetitions, and to increase endurance we use low loads at high repetitions. The muscle group will adapt to stresses, so it is imperative that the clinician know the goals of the athlete. To prescribe only endurance-type exercises to a power lifter would be a disservice, as would the prescription of only strengthening exercises to a tennis player who must compete for several hours. A balanced program incorporating strength and endurance training is recommended.

Power

Power = force ÷ time. It denotes a muscle's or a group of muscles' ability to exert a high amount of force in the shortest amount of time. It is sometimes referred to as explosive strength. Plyometric exercise is concerned with developing power (Fig. 45-15). Plyometric exercise involves rapid loading of a muscle followed by a powerful muscle contraction. Plyometrics consist of three phases:

1. Eccentric phase—the muscle is being stretched
2. Amortization phase—the time between eccentric stretch and concentric contraction
3. Concentric phase—the forceful contraction of the agonist

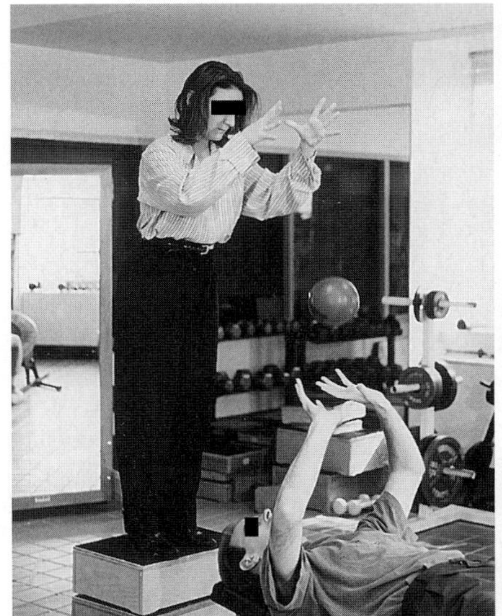
A

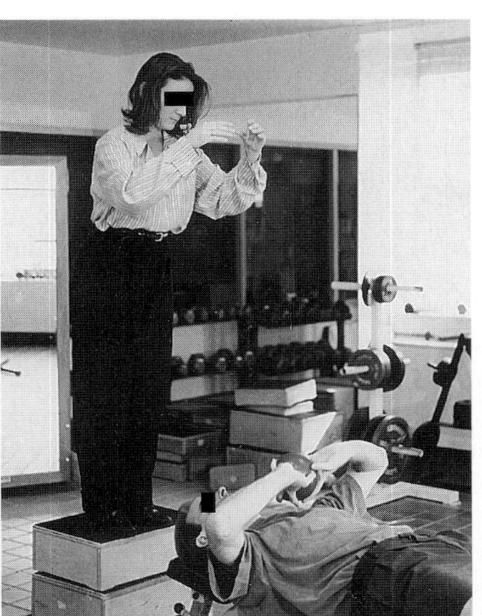
B

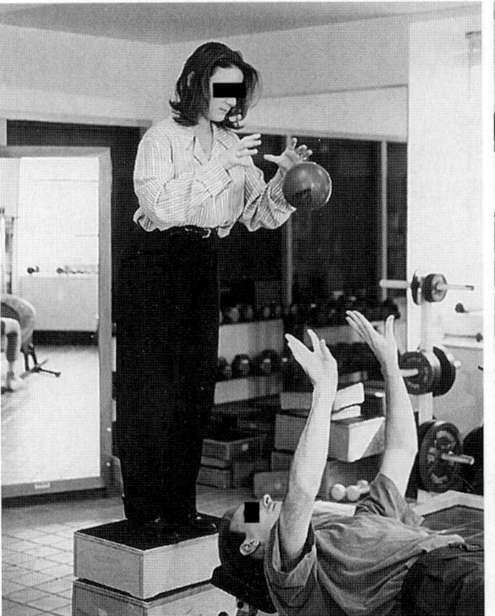
C

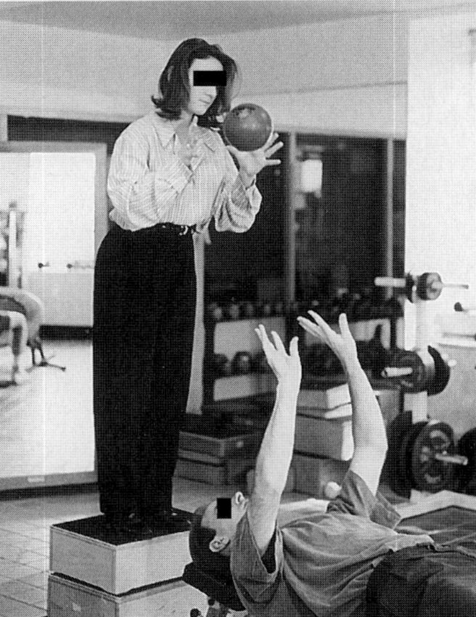
D

FIGURE 45-15. Plyometrics. This sequence demonstrates the initial eccentric preload (**A, B**) followed by the concentric contraction of the agonist group (**C, D**) for the triceps.

This eccentric and concentric coupling is also known as stretch shortening. It makes use of the stretch reflex of the muscle tendon unit. Simply put, the stretch reflex involves the proprioceptors of the body, including the muscle spindle, the Golgi tendon organ, and the joint capsule and ligamentous receptors. When the sensory end-organs are stimulated via a stretch of the muscle, they will activate and transmit an afferent impulse to the spinal cord. This afferent impulse can be either facilitory, from the muscle spindle, or inhibitory, from the Golgi tendon organ. After synapse in the spinal cord, the efferent alphamotor neuron will activate the agonist muscle. The total time of this reflex is 0.3 to 0.5 msec. In addition to the stretch reflex, the recoil action of the soft tissues adds to the power of the agonist contraction. During the eccentric phase, soft tissues are stretched, and at the cessation of the stretch these tissues must return to their original form. Newton's principles state that energy is neither gained nor lost and each action produces an equal and opposite reaction. The energy needed to stretch the soft tissues is stored in those tissues and then transferred and used as elastic dynamic energy to aid the concentric contraction of the agonist.

Force generation of the agonist is highest in plyometrics when the eccentric stretch is rapid and of short range and the period of amortization is minimal. Plyometric exercise attempts to train the neuromuscular system to use the added force supplied by the myotactic reflex and the elastic recoil of the soft tissues. Plyometrics should be employed only after the limb has been strengthened by conventional exercises. Bench jumping is a good example of plyometrics for the lower extremity, whereas traditionally, medicine balls have been used for the upper extremity. As an athlete catches the medicine ball, the momentum of the ball causes an eccentric contraction of the agonist muscles and the athlete quickly tosses the ball away. This can be done with the assistance of a trainer or a trampoline.

Flexibility

Certainly, the shoulder, with its constant mobility, needs to be flexible. In the throwing athlete, flexibility of the internal rotators and external rotators is particularly important. Clinical studies have noted increased risk of shoulder injuries in this population as a result of a decreased internal rotation and increased external rotation.[9,26] Arthrokinematically, tight posterior musculature can cause anterior translation and superior migration of the humerus during the throwing motion. This can lead to anterior instability. Paradoxically, tightness of the anterior shoulder muscles also can create an anterior subluxating force by altering the thrower's proper biomechanics. Therefore stretching the anterior and posterior shoulder musculature is important (Fig. 45-16).[50]

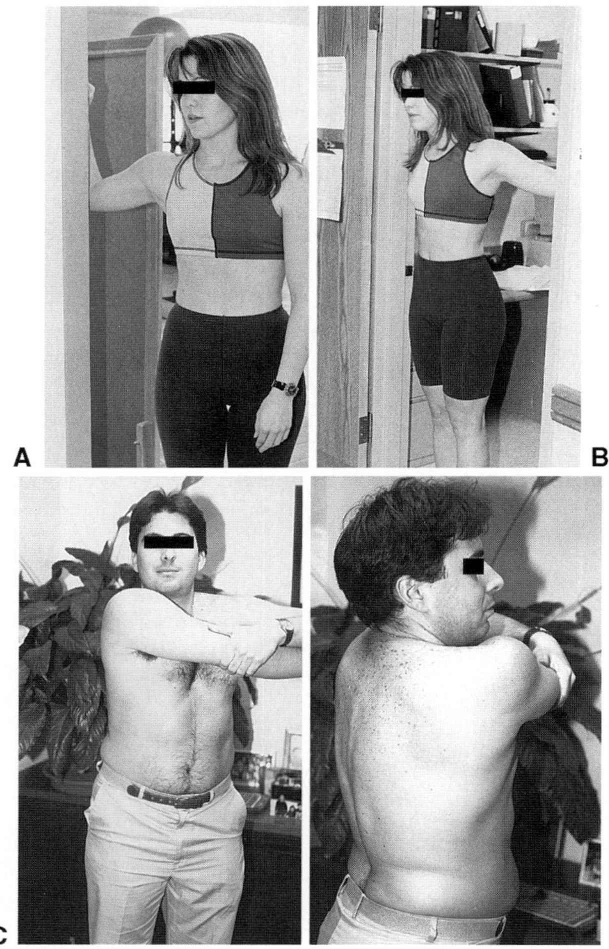

FIGURE 45-16. Stretching of the anterior and posterior shoulder musculature. **A** and **B,** The anterior musculature is stretched to allow increased range of motion and improved flexibility. **C** and **D,** Likewise, the posterior shoulder musculature is stretched. Both of these groups are passively stretched by holding the elongated position for 30 seconds, or we can incorporate muscle-energy techniques, as previously described, to focus particularly on flexibility. If you wish to increase flexibility of the shoulder flexors, the shoulder extensors must be fatigued. This is done with serial 5-second contractions of the shoulder extensors, bringing the shoulder into increased flexion after each one. This promotes improved anterior shoulder flexibility.

Coordination/Neuromotor Control

Once range of motion and strengthening have been addressed, attention can be shifted to coordination and neuromotor control. The movement of an upper limb is not an isolated event. For instance, throwing a baseball involves harvesting energy of the ground reaction and supplementing it via concentric, eccentric, and isometric contractions; of alternating force and duration; of muscles in the feet, leg, pelvis, trunk, shoulder, arm, forearm, and hand. Once the arm is in motion to throw the ball, the body must decelerate and stop, and this requires another pattern of muscular activity. Coordination is the ordered control of the timing, amplitude, and duration of the neuromuscular firing patterns. Coordination requires that the athlete:

1. Know what he or she wants to do
2. Have a neuromotor plan to accomplish his or her goal
3. Be aware of where the body parts are in space (proprioception) and at what speed they are moving (kinesthesia)
4. Know the force, both linear and rotational, his or her muscles can produce and absorb
5. Know the mechanical properties of the object he or she wishes to throw, catch, manipulate, or have manipulated

Proprioneuromuscular facilitation (PNF) exercises assist patients in gaining awareness of their body. Closed–kinetic chain exercises are multijoint activities that assist the athlete in gaining insight into the relationships between different body parts. Sport-specific exercises and practices are a prime way to gain coordination and skill. By performing a task repetitively, the central nervous system may generate patterns or perfect engrams that will enable the athlete to perform a task most efficiently. To increase coordination, we often employ an exercise with multiple tasks. For instance, we will ask an athlete to stand on a BAPS board or slide along a slide board while catching and throwing a medicine ball. As the athlete performs multiple tasks, he or she must develop strategies to coordinate the complex patterns required to achieve a goal. This will assist him or her in achieving maximal skill (Fig. 45-17).

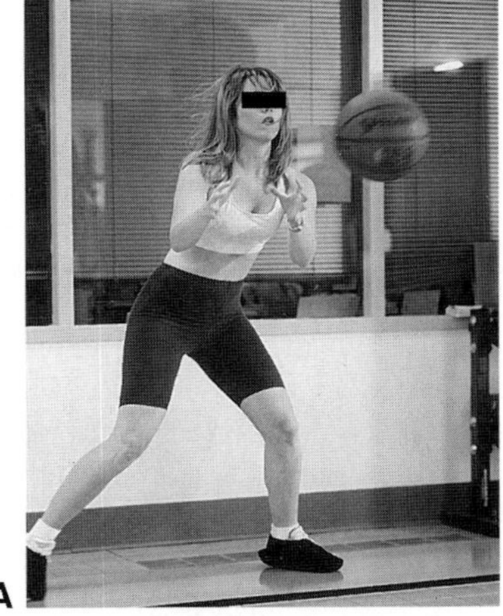
A

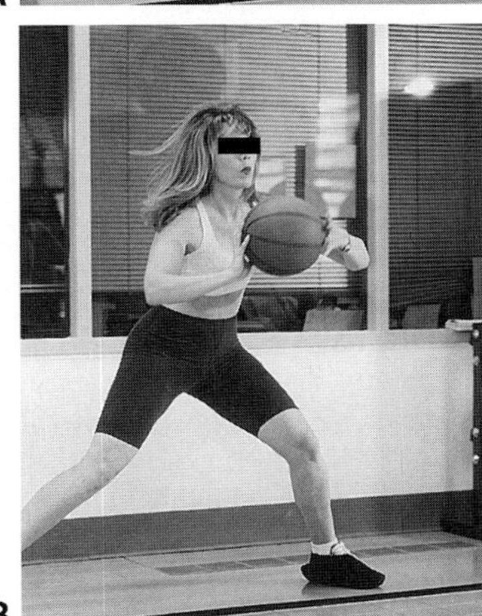
B

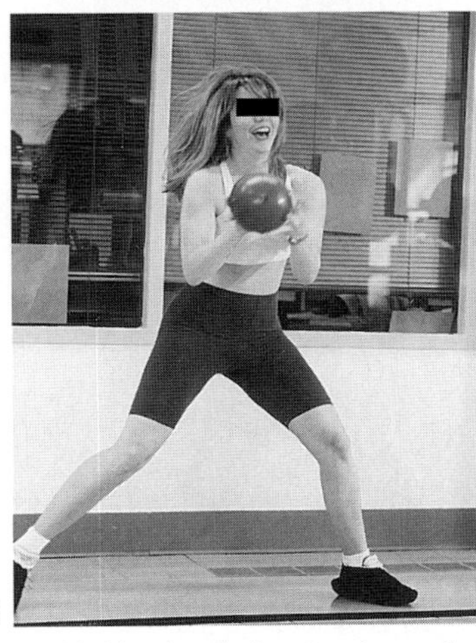
C

FIGURE 45-17. Multitask rehab exercises. **A, B,** and **C,** To focus on coordination and endurance, exercises requiring multiple tasks are beneficial. While gliding laterally on a slide board, toss a medicine ball or weighted ball. During the exercise, the clinician provides feedback to the patient on proper technique. As you begin to master this drill, increase time on the board. Progress is guided by increased time of the exercise (with a consistent or improved pace).

Proprioception

As stated earlier, shoulder stability is provided by static factors, including the bony architecture, the glenoid labrum, low intraarticular pressure, joint surface adhesion, the joint capsule and ligamentous structures, and dynamic structures including the muscles around the glenohumeral joint and the periscapular region.[6,8,12,46-48,62]

Because the peri glenohumeral muscles contract as the humerus nears end-range, the body must have an awareness as to where the humerus is in relation to the glenoid. This is termed *joint position sense*. The knowledge that the limb is moving is termed *kinesthesia*. Proprioception encompasses both joint position sense and kinesthesia.

Sensory feedback from the shoulder to the central nervous system is important for dynamic stability of the shoulder.[4,5,10,20,25,66] The sensory end-organs are found in the muscles and tendons around a joint[60] and in the capsule and ligaments.[60] Afferent impulses will increase when the shoulder nears end-range, then presumably efferent messages are sent to the muscles to reverse the motion of the humerus. This postural change as a response to proprioceptive input is termed *neuromuscular control*.

Research suggests that diminished proprioception is associated with shoulder instability,[60] therefore shoulder rehabilitation must address proprioception. Proprioneuromuscular facilitation exercises, closed–kinetic chain exercises, and plyometric exercises all encourage the patient to appreciate afferent proprioceptive input and develop motor patterns to prevent instability.

Rhythmic stabilization exercises also assist in proprioceptive awareness.[15] In these exercises, the shoulder is placed in a position vulnerable to anterior subluxation, that is, 90° of humeral abduction with 90° of external rotation. A force is applied to the patient's arm to increase the instability, and the patient must counteract that force. With repetition, the patient's proprioception will increase and he or she will better be able to make neuromuscular adjustments (Fig. 45-18).

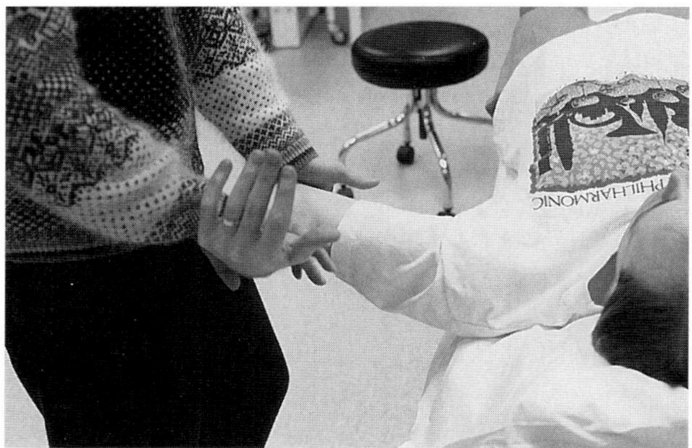

A

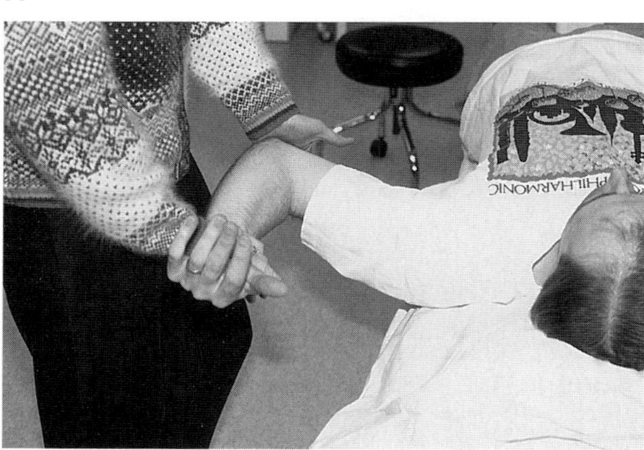

B

FIGURE 45-18. Rhythmic stabilization exercises. **A** and **B**, The patient's shoulder is placed in a vulnerable position (i.e., apprehension), then a gentle destabilizing force is applied by the examiner. The patient must counteract this force to prevent subluxation. The examiner is trying to translocate the humeral head anteriorly while the patient is trying to stabilize it and prevent this action. This exercise assists in developing proprioceptive input to the joint.

The scapulothoracic joint is also involved in movement of the shoulder. An athlete should appreciate the motion of the scapula to perfect smooth glenohumeral movements.

Therapeutic intervention for the most common ailments of the shoulder region (rotator cuff tendinitis, impingement, and instability) includes a short period of rest. A few days usually will suffice. This can be in conjunction with medications such as nonsteroidal anti-inflammatories. People with allergies to these preparations or GI sensitivity are cautioned as to their use. Ice massage or heating modalities are useful, and the choice is largely one of patient preference. The basic guidelines of ice for the first 24 hours followed by intermittent heat can be followed. Range of motion and strengthening exercises are employed.

The initial phase of the rehabilitation emphasizes restoration of maximal range of motion. Care must be taken to remain in the pain-free range of motion and gently progress to overhead exercises as guided by pain. It is most useful to begin these range of motion exercises with the patient supine and progress to sitting and standing. The use of pulleys and sticks can assist in obtaining adequate range of motion (Fig. 45-19). For rotator cuff

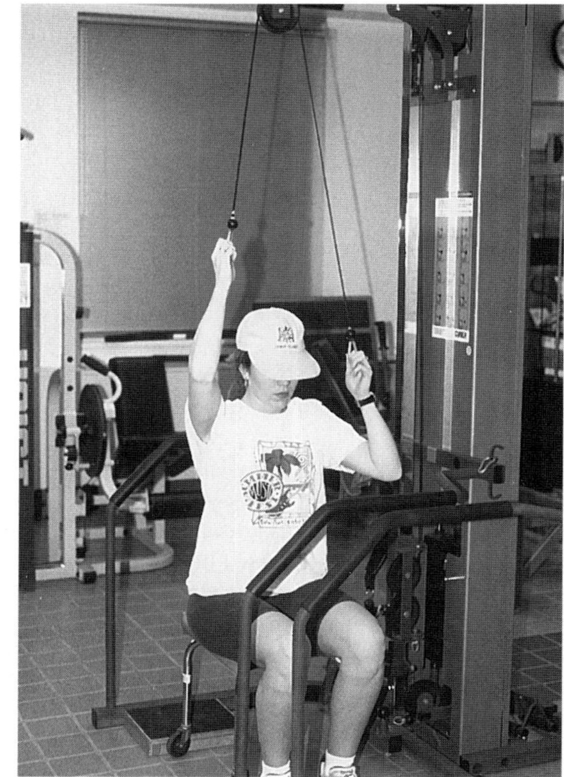

FIGURE 45-19. Overhead pulleys to increase range of motion. Pulleys are useful in increasing range of motion. The uninvolved limb pulls the involved limb through a range of motion. This exercise has been stated to be passive to the injured limb but in reality there is active involvement on the part of the injured limb.

tears and shoulder instabilities that have been corrected surgically, progressive resistive exercises do not begin until about the tenth to twelfth week after surgery.

The use of injection for rotator cuff tendinitis/bursitis is common. After a positive impingement test, a steroid preparation such as methylprednisolone (40 mg) can be injected into the subacromial bursa. If this is successful, it may be repeated in 1 to 2 weeks. The patient should be warned that there may be transient discomfort in the region of the injection and a bit of erythema can be noted on the face. Pain is usually alleviated with one or two doses of a painkiller or anti-inflammatory medicine and the erythema is a "cortisone" effect and abates within 24-48 hours.

CHECKLIST

General Rehab Strategy

1. Rest
   A) Absolute
   B) "Actual" rest
2. Mobility—to decrease effects of immobility
3. Range of motion (ROM)
   A) Passive range of motion (PROM)
   B) Continuous passive range of motion
   C) Active assisted range of motion
   D) Active range of motion
4. Strengthening
   A) For stability
   B) For force production
   C) For force absorption
5. Flexibility
6. Coordination/neuromotor control
7. Proprioception
8. Sport-specific exercise
9. Biomechanics

THE ELBOW

The elbow joint assists in positioning the hand, in production of force, and in force absorption. A common disorder of the elbow is lateral epicondylitis. This is usually an overuse injury that results in microscopic or macroscopic tears in the extensor aponeurosis, most frequently at the origin of the extensor carpi radialis brevis (ECRB) muscle. It is characterized by painful inflammation in the area of the extensor musculature origin. It is aggravated by forceful wrist extension, forearm supination, or passive wrist flexion with forearm pronation. Because the ECRB inserts into the base of the third metacarpal, resisted extension of this digit also may cause elbow discomfort secondary to injury.

By following the hierarchy outlined in the box, General Rehab Strategy, we can properly rehabilitate elbow overuse injury. Initially, rest is indicated, with nonsteroidal anti-inflammatory drugs and proper modalities such as ultrasound with or without cortisone phonophoresis. The liberal use of ice in the acute phase is recommended. For more resistant cases, local steroid injections around the enthesis have been helpful. If these are given, patients must be carefully instructed to rest the arm for approximately one week.

We can use the concept of relative rest by fitting the patient with a lateral forearm counterforce brace.[24,39,61] This brace is worn over the forearm extensor musculature and acts as a fulcrum to prevent excessive strain on the origin of the wrist extensors (Fig. 45-20). The use of the brace allows an athlete to move his or her elbow sooner and therefore decrease the deleterious effects of immobility. We also prescribe a cock-up wrist splint to stabilize the wrist extensors. Flexibility of the wrist and finger extensors plays a role in the development of tennis elbow syndrome. Therefore, a proper stretching program should begin when pain in the area has sufficiently decreased (Fig. 45-21).

A weak muscle is likely to fatigue and be injured. Therefore, strengthening of the wrist and finger extensors, forearm supinators, and, to a lesser extent, all the other muscles of the upper extremities is required. Special attention should be given to the posterior musculature of the shoulder. Injury of these muscles is a good example of the failure of a muscle complex to absorb force. In this case, force is represented by a moving tennis ball's being struck by a moving tennis racket head.

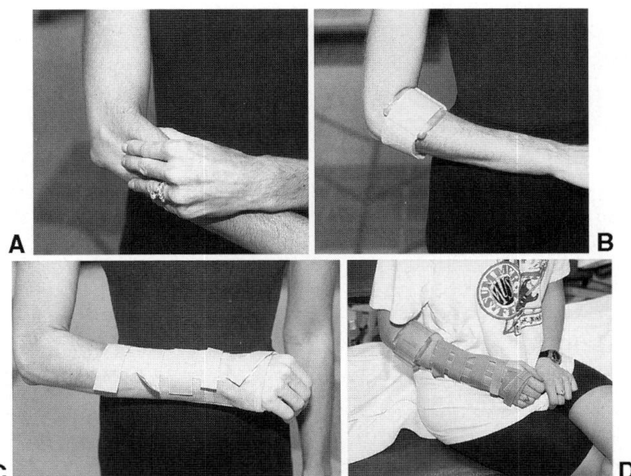

FIGURE 45-20. Lateral forearm counterforce brace (lateral epicondylitis). **A,** To locate the best place to apply the brace, flex the elbow and point the thumb superiorly. Grab the lateral forearm muscles with your thumb and index finger. This area, directly below the elbow, is the site the brace should contact. **B,** The brace, in place, acts to unload the forearm muscles closest to the brace and substitutes a new origin for the muscle (beneath the brace). **C** and **D,** A cock-up splint stabilizes the wrist, which is important because the muscles involved cross this region.

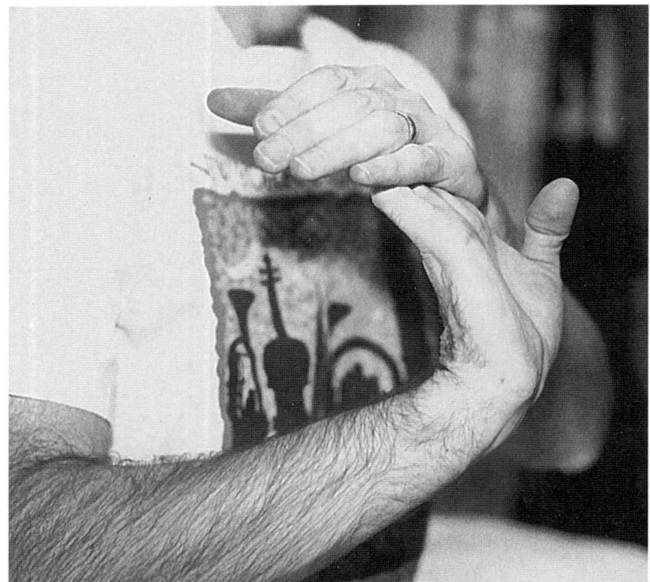

FIGURE 45-21. Stretching the digits and wrist. As the muscles are rested and pain is subsiding, it is important to stretch the associated soft tissues to prevent adhesions and stiff joints.

A strengthening program should include exercises for improving both strength and endurance.

Lateral epicondylitis rehabilitation requires knowledge of the epidemiology of the disease and the proper biomechanics of a tennis swing, specifically the one-handed backhand stroke. It has been shown that improper technique can lead to tennis elbow. Kelley revealed that all of the patients with tennis elbow in their study had at least two of four deviations from proper stroke mechanics.[32] Improper stroke mechanics include: (1) leading elbow with the olecranon pointing toward the net and the shoulder elevated and in internal rotation, (2) wrist flexion in the early phases with an abrupt change to extension, (3) exaggerated wrist pronation, and (4) ball impact on the lower portion of the racket. Schantz and Steiner concluded that a late backhand stroke and off-center contact of a racket are the two basic stresses that lead to tennis elbow.[56]

Studies with electromyography (EMG) and cinematography analysis revealed that injured players had significantly greater activity in the wrist extensors and pronator teres muscles during ball impact and follow-through than did noninjured players.[32] It has been found that decreasing the tension of the racket strings and changing to a larger racket grip helps reduce some of the stresses placed on the extensor origin.[14,21]

The treatment of tennis elbow is incomplete until the clinician treats the presenting condition and advises the patient as to how to avoid the ailment in the future. If the player cannot adjust his or her swing, the player may have to go to a two-handed backhand or slice backhand, both of which require less stress on the wrist extensors. Please note that a proper one-handed backhand places as much stress on the wrist extensors as the two-handed backhand.[22] No differences were found in EMG activity of the wrist extensors between the single-handed and double-handed backhand ground strokes in a study involving elite noninjured tennis players.[22]

Medial epicondylitis, or golfer's elbow, is caused by overload of the wrist flexors and pronators of the arm. The common flexor tendon of the flexor carpi ulnaris, flexor carpi radialis, and palmaris longus becomes inflamed. The overload can be due to either increased duration of muscle activity, increased force, or both. Nirschl postulated that repetitive strains are cumulative and lead to disruption of the muscle-tendon unit.[45] Glazebrook and colleagues, using EMG analysis, found that golfers with medial epicondylitis had a higher mean flexor musculature activity during address and swing phase than did asymptomatic golfers.[23] A player may be trying to exert too much wrist snap to the tennis serve or golf swing.

Often the problem may be an unstable shoulder with inability to transfer energy through the shoulder joint. The player compensates for this lack of force generation in the shoulder by trying to produce force at the elbow and wrist; overloading these muscles causes injury. Treatment is similar to that for lateral epicondylitis but with attention to the wrist flexor musculature. This time a medial forearm counterforce brace is employed. The forearm brace decreases EMG duration and muscle activity in the service and backhand drive of tennis players.[23] Stretching the wrist flexors and pronator teres and strengthening these muscles is paramount. Attention to the shoulder musculature, especially the anterior muscles, is recommended. A wider golf-club grip also may help alleviate symptoms.

WRIST AND HAND

The wrist and hand are the final common pathway for all movements of the upper extremity. Their role may be to provide a powerful grip to an apparatus such as a bat or an oar, or to perform more skillful maneuvers requiring fine manual dexterity, such as pitching a ball. The wrist and hand also may aid in power generation. For this reason, the proper rehabilitation of a wrist or hand injury is essential. Again, use the box on General Rehab Strategy as a guide to rehabilitation.

After an injury, rest is recommended. Fractures, injuries of the ligaments, and tendon tears are immobilized. More rigid casts are preferred to over-the-counter splints. It is prudent to immobilize only the injured wrist and to allow the noninjured hand to carry out its function. This will decrease the deleterious effects of immobility in the intact areas of the hand.

Once movement is allowed, obtaining full range of motion is the primary goal. Active and passive range of motion should be measured separately. Passive range of motion typically is restricted by joint effusions or capsular tightening. Active range of motion, on the other hand, requires excursion of the tendon and may be limited by tendon rupture, inflammation, or constriction of the tendon sheath. A hand goniometer should be used to monitor progress. A large discrepancy between active and passive range of motion may indicate a muscle, tendon, or nerve injury.

Edema in the hand can severely limit range of motion and be quite painful. It can be measured by using volume displacement of water, with a volumetric container. Treatment of edema involves keeping the hand elevated, retrograde massage, and the application of a pressure device (Fig. 45-22). Active range of motion should not be painful. If it is, there may be inflammation. Edema results and ultimately decreases range of motion and prolongs the rehabilitation process. Overzealous rehabilitation sessions may be harmful, so we prefer short but frequent therapy sessions.

After the patient achieves full range of motion, strengthening can begin (Figs. 45-23 and 45-24). This

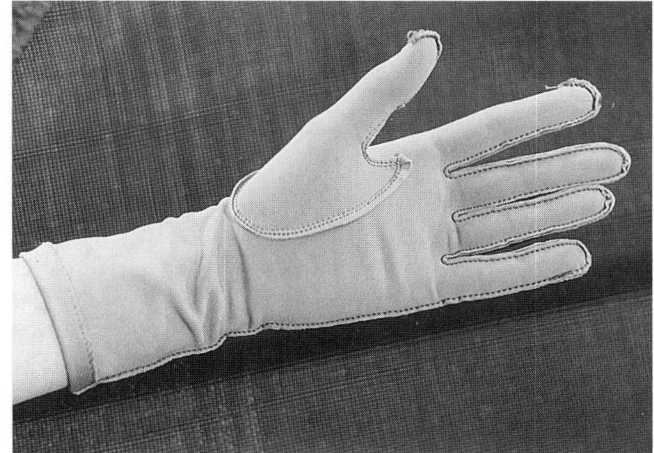

FIGURE 45-22. Compressive garments for edema of the hand/wrist. Application of compressive garment for edema of the hand and wrist. It should have a snug fit and not cause paresthesias in the distal digits. It should be worn as much as possible.

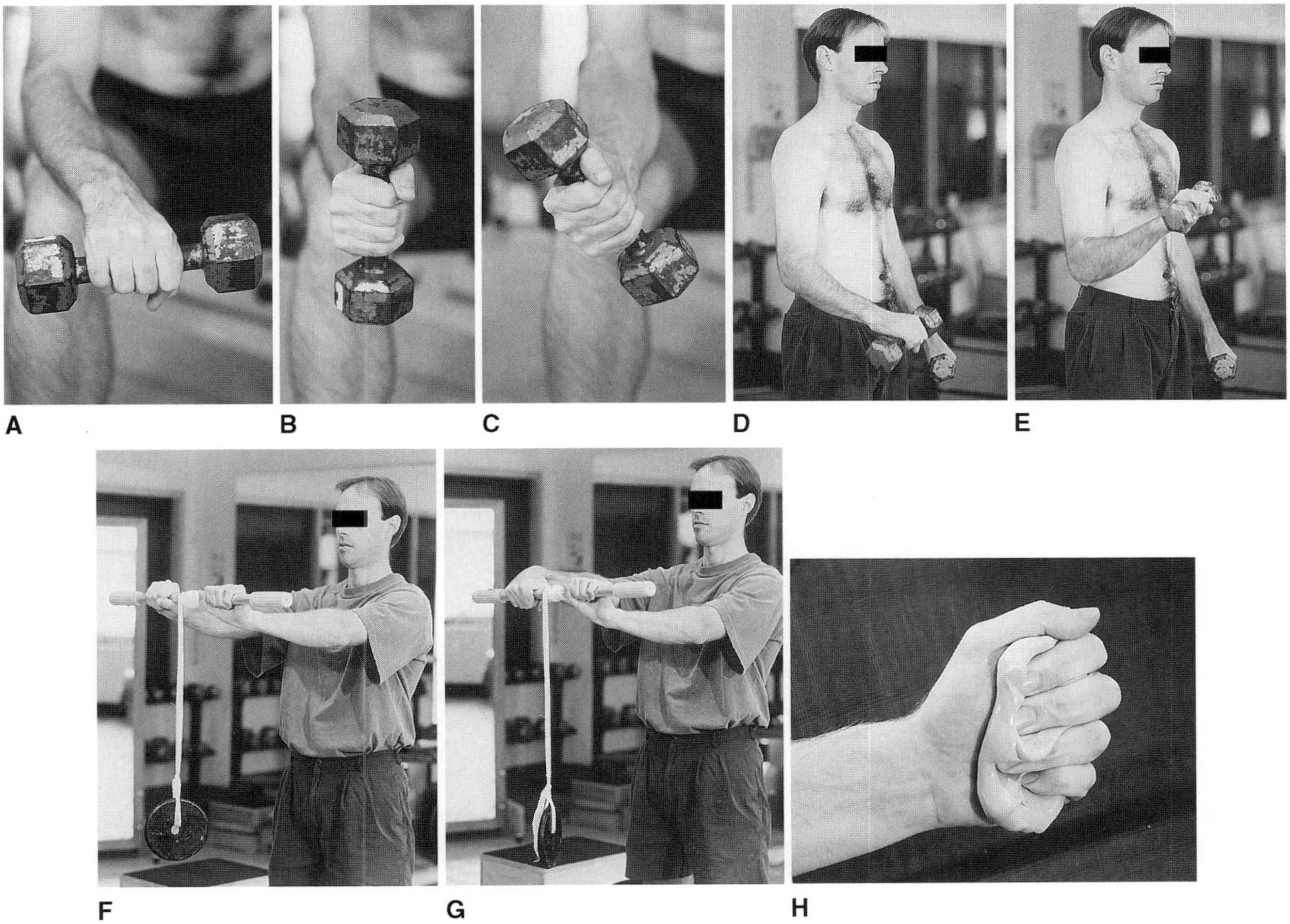

FIGURE 45-23. Strengthening of the wrist/digits. **A–C,** Forearm supinator strengthening, **D** and **E,** wrist extensor strengthening. **F** and **G,** wrist strengthening. The wrist continually flexes and extends to lower and raise the weight attached by cable to the stick. **H,** Theraputty. Continuous gripping and molding of the putty to strengthen the intrinsic hand muscles.

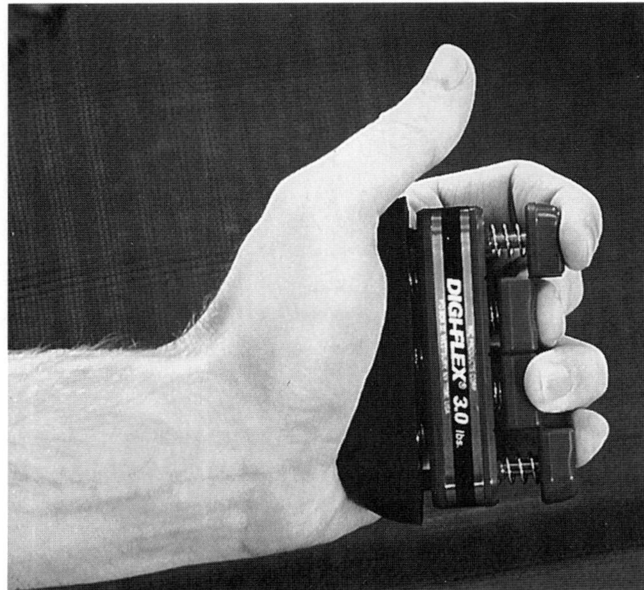

FIGURE 45-24. Dynamometer for grip strength. A device that measures grip strength. The trainee grabs the handle and squeezes it with as much force as possible. The dial on the dynamometer records the strength.

should be of both the fine and gross types. A simple tennis ball or sponge can be used to increase grip strength. Therapeutic putty allows the clinician to titrate the resistance. Some devices can strengthen digits individually. A dynamometer allows the grip strength to be monitored. Keep in mind that the strength generated on the ulnar side of the wrist does indeed represent strength. This is in contrast to the strength that is generated on the radial aspect. That is a precision-type of strength.

Coordination and Neuromotor Control

The long finger flexors are four times as strong as the wrist extensors. When the fingers flex, the wrist will flex unless acted on by the wrist extensors. The co-contraction is necessary for a powerful grip. Therefore, the strengthening of both wrist flexors and wrist extensors should be emphasized. The need for coordination of the hand is evident because the hand carries out fine motor movements. There are numerous dexterity drills to promote coordination of the hand.

Proprioception

Sensory feedback from the fingers is crucial to the athlete in almost all sporting endeavors. Edema in the hand interferes with the sensory end-organs and therefore must be addressed.

Carpal tunnel syndrome is a common ailment affecting the wrist joint, and conservative treatments sometimes prove helpful. One must try to identify the disorder's etiology, if possible, before embarking on a cure. The list of possibilities is lengthy and includes arthritis, pregnancy, diabetes, and hypothyroidism. We try bracing with a neutral alignment cock-up splint, which is worn as much as possible. Also, manual techniques can be tried. The goal of these is to open up the region of the carpal tunnel to decompress it. This can be attempted by opposing the thumb and fifth digit in a repeating series. Vitamin B_6, starting with 50 mg PO every 6 hours and increasing to 100 mg PO every 6 hours is also recommended.[33] Injection with a steroid preparation such as methylprednisone is indicated as a last resort. If symptoms persist, refer the patient for surgical opinion.

REFERENCES

1. Akeson WH, Amiel D, Woo SL-Y: Immobility affects on synovial joints. The pathomechanics of joint contracture. Biorheology 17:95, 1980.
2. Aldenrink G, Kuck D: Isokinetic shoulder strength of high school and college-aged pitchers. JOSPT 7:163–172, 1986.
3. Anthony R, Brown MB: Regional and intermittent anesthesia. Presented at the seminar, Current Concepts in Shoulder Rehabilitation, Columbia-Presbyterian Medical Center, New York, October 29, 1994.
4. Bassett RW, Browne AO, Morrey BS, An KN: Glenohumeral muscle forces and moment mechanics in a position of shoulder instability. J Biomech 23:405–415, 1990.
5. Blasier R, Carpenter J, Huston L: Shoulder proprioception: Effect of joint laxity, joint position and direction of motion. Ortho Review 23(1):45–50, 1994.
6. Blasier RB, Guldberg RE, Rothman EG: Anterior shoulder stability: Contributions of rotator cuff forces and the capsular ligaments in a cadaver model. J Shoulder Elbow Surg 1(3):140–150, 1992.
7. Boon A: Manual scapular stabilization: Its effect on shoulder rotational range of motion. Arch Phys Med Rehabil 81:978–983, 2000.
8. Bowen MK, Warren RF: Ligamentous control of shoulder stability based on selective cutting and static translation experiments. Clin Sports Med 10:757, 1991.
9. Brown L: Upper extremity range of motion and isokinetic strength of the internal and external shoulder rotators in Major League baseball players. Am J Sports Med 16:577–585, 1988.
10. Buchwald JS: Exteroceptive reflexes and movement. Am J Phys Med 46:121, 1967.
11. Burkhead W, Rockwood C: Treatment of instability of the shoulder with an exercise program. JBJS 74A: 890–896, 1992.

12. Cain PR, Mutschler TA, Fu FH, Lee SK: Anterior stability of the glenohumeral joint: A dynamic model. Am J Sports Med 15(2):144–148, 1987.
13. Codman EA: The Shoulder. Boston, Thomas Todd, 1934.
14. Coonrad R, Hooper R: Tennis elbow: Its course, natural history, conservative and surgical management. JBJS 55A:1177–1182, 1973.
15. Davies G, Dickoff-Hoffman D: Neuromuscular testing and rehabilitation of the shoulder complex. JOSPT 18:449–458, 1993.
16. Davies GJ, Heidersceit B, Jones B: Isokinetic testing of scapula-thoracic protraction/retraction and correlation to a modified lateral scapular slide test. Unpublished research, University of Wisconsin-LaCrosse, 1992–1993.
17. Donatelli RA (ed): Mobilization of the shoulder. In Physical Therapy of the Shoulder, 2nd ed. New York, Churchill Livingstone, 1991.
18. Fahrer H, Rentsch HV, Gerber WJ: Effusion and reflex inhibition of the quadriceps. JBJS 70B:635–638, 1988.
19. Frank C, Akeson, WH, Woo S, et al: Physiology and therapeutic value of passive joint motion. Clin Orthop 185:135, 1984.
20. Freeman MAR, Wyke B: The innervation of the knee joint. An anatomical and histological study in the cat. J Anat 101:505, 1967.
21. Gardner R: Tennis elbow: Diagnosis, pathology, and treatment. Clin Orthop 72:248–253, 1970.
22. Giangarra LE, Jobe FW, Perry J: Electromyographic and cinematographic analysis of elbow function in tennis players using single and double handed back hand strokes. Am J Sports Med 21(3):394–399, 1993.
23. Glazebrook MA, et al: Medial epicondylitis. An electromyographic analysis and an investigation of intervention strategies. Am J Sports Med 22(5): 674–679, 1994.
24. Groppel JL, Nirschl RP: A mechanical and electromyographical analysis of the effects of various joint counterforce braces on the tennis player. Am J Sports Med 14:195–200, 1986.
25. Hall LA, McCloskey DI: Detections of movements imposed on finger, elbow and shoulder joint. J Physiol 335:519–533, 1983.
26. Harryman D. Translation of the humeral head on the glenoid with passive glenohumeral motion. J Bone Joint Surg Am 72:1334–1343, 1990.
27. Hawkins RJ: Basic science and clinical application in the athlete's shoulder. Clin Sports Med 10:4, 1991.
28. Ivey FM, et al: Isokinetic testing of shoulder strength: Normal values. Arch Phys Med Rehabil 66:384–386, 1985.
29. Jobe F, Moynes D: Delineation of diagnostic criteria and a rehabilitation program for rotator cuff injuries. AJSM 10:336–339, 1982.
30. Jobe F, Moynes D, Brewster D: Rehabilitation of shoulder joint instabilities. Orthop Clin N Am 18:473–482, 1987.
31. Kamkar A, Irrgang J, Whitney S: Nonoperative management of secondary shoulder impingement syndrome. JOSPT 5:211–224, 1993.
32. Kelley JD, et al: Electromyographic and cinematographic analysis of elbow function in tennis players with lateral epicondylitis. Am J Sports Med 22:359–363, 1994.
33. Keniston RC, Nathan PA, Leklem JE, Lockwood RS: Vitamin B6, vitamin C, and carpal tunnel syndrome: A cross-sectional study of 441 adults. J Occup Environ Med 39(10):949–959, 1997.
34. Kibler WB: Role of the scapula in the overhead throwing motion. Cont Orthop 22:525–532, 1991.
35. Kibler WB, McMullen J, Uhl T: Shoulder rehabilitation strategies, guidelines, and practice. Orthop Clin North Am 32(3):527–538, 2001.
36. Knott M, Voss DE: Proprioceptive Neuromuscular Facilitation. New York, Harper and Row, 1968.
37. Magnusson S, Gleim G, Nicholas J: Shoulder weakness in professional baseball pitchers. Med Sci Sports Exerc 26:5–9, 1994.
38. Maitland GD: Peripheral Manipulation. London, Butterworth, 1970.
39. Meyer NJ, Pennington W, Haines B, Daley R: The effect of the forearm support band on forces at the origin of the extensor carpi radialis brevis: A cadaveric study and review of literature. J Hand Ther 15(2):179–184, 2002.
40. Mont M, Mathur S, et al: Isokinetic concentric versus eccentric training of shoulder rotators with functional evaluation of performance enhancement in elite tennis players. AJSM 22:513–517, 1994.
41. Morrissey MC: Reflex inhibition of the thigh muscles in knee injury: Causes and treatment. Sports Med 7:263–276, 1989.
42. Mosely J, Jobe F, et al: EMG analysis of the scapular muscles during a shoulder rehabilitation program. AJSM 20:128–134, 1992.
43. Neer CS II: Shoulder Reconstruction. Philadelphia, WB Saunders, 1990.
44. Newsham KR, Keith CS, Saunders JE, Goffinett AS: Isokinetic profile of baseball pitchers' internal/external rotation 180, 300, 450 degrees. Med Sci Sports Exerc 30(10):1489-1495, 1998.
45. Nirschl R: Soft tissue injuries about the elbow. Clin Sports Med 5:637–652, 1986.
46. Ovensen J, Nielsen S: Anterior and posterior shoulder instability: A cadaver study. Acta Orthop Scand 57:324–327, 1986.
47. Ovensen J, Nielsen S: Posterior instability of the shoulder: A cadaver study. Acta Orthop Scand 57:436–439, 1986.

48. Ovensen J, Nielsen S: Stability of the shoulder joint. Cadaver study of stabilizing structures. Acta Orthop Scand 56:149–151, 1985.
49. Paine R, Voight M: The role of the scapula. JOSPT 18:386–391, 1993.
50. Pappas A, Zawacki R, McCarthy C: Rehabilitation of the pitching shoulder. AJSM 12:223–235, 1985.
51. Patriqin DA: The evolution of osteopathic manipulative technique: The Spencer technique. J Am Osteopath Assoc 93(4):426, 428, 1993.
52. Pollock RG, Bigliani LU, Flatow EL, et al: The mechanical properties of the inferior glenohumeral ligament. Orthop Trans 14:259, 1990.
53. Poppin NK, Walker PS: Normal and abnormal motion of the shoulder. JBJS 58A:195–201, 1976.
54. Rodosky M, Harner C, Fu F: The role of the long head of the biceps muscle and superior glenoid labrum in anterior stability of the shoulder. Am J Sports Med 22:121–130, 1994.
55. Sady SP, Wortman M, Blanke D: Flexibility training: Ballistic, static or proprioceptive neuromuscular facilitation? Arch Phys Med Rehabil 63(6):261–263, 1982.
56. Schantz P, Steiner C. Tennis elbow: A biomechanical and therapeutic approach. J Am Osteopath Assoc 93(7): 778, 1993.
57. Schwartz RE, O'Brien SJ, Warren RF: Capsular restraints to anterior-posterior motion of the abducted shoulder. A biomechanical study. Orthop Trans 17:727, 1988.
58. Silliman J, Hawkins R: Current concepts and recent advances in the athlete's shoulder. Clin Sports Med 10:693–705, 1991.
59. Sirota SC, Malanga GA, Eischen JJ, Laskowski ER: An eccentric- and concentric-strength profile of shoulder external and internal rotator muscles in professional baseball pitchers. Am J Sports Med 25(1):59–64, 1997.
60. Smith RL, Brunolli J: Shoulder kinesthesia after anterior glenohumeral joint dislocation. Phys Ther 69(2):106–112, 1989.
61. Snyder-Macklin L, Epler M: Effect of standard and aircast tennis elbow bands on integrated electromyography of forearm extensor musculature proximal to the bands. Am J Sports Med 17:278–281, 1989.
62. Soslowsky LJ, Flatow EL, Bigliani LU, et al: Quantitation of in situ contact areas at the glenohumeral joint: A biomechanical study. J Orthop Res 10:524–534, 1992.
63. Speer K, Wickiewicz T, et al: A role for hydrotherapy in shoulder rehabilitation. AJSM 21:850–853, 1991.
64. Spencer JD, Keith CH, Alexander IJ: Knee joint effusion and quadriceps reflex inhibition in man. Arch Phys Med Rehab 65:171–177, 1984.
65. Stoddard A: Manual of Osteopathic Technique. London, Hutchinson Medical Publishers, 1959.
66. Ticker JB, Bigliani LU, Soslowsky LJ, et al: Biomechanical properties of the inferior glenohumeral ligament: A study of fast and slow strain rates. Presented at the Tenth Anniversary Annual Meeting of the American Shoulder and Elbow Surgeons, September 4–7, 1991, Seattle, Washington.
67. Townsend H, Jobe F, Pink M, Perry J: Electromyographic analysis of the glenohumeral muscles during a baseball rehabilitation program. AJSM 19:264–271, 1991.
68. Turkel SJ, Panio MW, Marshall JL, Girgis F: Stabilizing mechanisms preventing anterior dislocation of the glenohumeral joint. JBJS 63A:1208–1217, 1981.
69. Warren RF, Kornblatt IB, Marchand R: Static factors affecting posterior shoulder stability. Orthop Trans 8:89, 1984.
70. Wilk K, Andrews J, et al. The strength characteristics of internal and external rotator muscles in professional baseball pitchers. AJSM 21:61–66, 1993.
71. Wilk K, Arrigo C: Current concepts in the rehabilitation of the athletic shoulder. JOSPT 18:365–378, 1993.
72. Wood L, Ferrell WR, Baxendale RH: Pressures in normal and acutely distended human knee joints and effects on maximal voluntary contractions. Q J Exo Physiol 73:305–314, 1988.
73. Wyke BD: The neurology of joints. Ann R Coll Surg Engl 41:25, 1966.
74. Yishay AB, Zuckerman JD, Gallagher M, Cuomo F: Pain inhibitor of shoulder strength in patients with impingement syndrome. Orthopedics 17:685–688, 1994.

46 The Spine

Robert S. Gotlin, Michael A. Palmer, and Pietro A. Memmo

Low back pain is the most common musculoskeletal disorder of industrialized society, the number one cause of work-related injuries and the most common cause of disability in persons younger than age 45.[1,51] The annual medical costs of treating back pain in the United States are estimated to be $18 billion to $25 billion.[27,66] It is estimated that 90% of adults experience low back pain sometime in their lives, and thus, it is now the second leading cause for visits to primary care physicians, the first being upper respiratory tract infections.[20]

Despite the recent advances in the treatment of spinal disorders, the cause and source of low back pain remain difficult and challenging to diagnose and treat. In fact, 50% of individuals with low back disabilities have no objective findings.[52,76] However, for a practitioner to successfully diagnose and treat spinal disorders, he or she must have an understanding not only of the static anatomy and fundamental physiology of the spine's many interrelated segments, but also a thorough appreciation of functional anatomy, muscle dynamics, principles of force production and absorption, and the chemical environment surrounding the spine.

The field of spine rehabilitation has experienced great strides in therapeutic interventions as technology has advanced. In the past, patients were treated only with passive modalities such as heat and ultrasound. Today patients are exercised back into good health. Rehabilitation strategies are most effective when they are customized to a person's needs. The rehabilitation program should accommodate an individual's lifestyle, needs, training time, and occupation.[71] Although protocol-type treatment algorithms clearly outline progression in a step-by-step structured format, they are inappropriate for many patients. They are useful as generalized therapies and basic guidelines, but practitioners should make every effort to customize and individualize rehabilitation programs.

OVERVIEW

To implement a successful treatment strategy, one must first establish a specific diagnosis of a spinal disorder to uncover the actual pain generator. With this in mind, back pain can be further differentiated into mechanical, facet mediated, discogenic, or neuropathic pain. The most common spinal disorder among athletes, and the cause of over 70% of back problems, is mechanical back pain, which is due to muscle strains, ligament sprains, or microscopic tears. Mechanical back pain is usually localized back pain, affected by axial movements. Facet pain, usually due to degeneration of the facet or zygapophyseal joints, usually presents with a sudden onset, is usually of short duration, is localized in the back (and/or buttock), and is aggravated by extension movements and twisting.[23]

Disk pain has more of a gradual onset, is long lasting, is primarily localized in the back, and is aggravated by flexion or sitting. It is usually caused by degeneration of the intervertebral disk (degenerative disk disease) or from an annular tear.[1]

Nerve root pain is acute or chronic in onset, intermediate in duration, and localizes to an extremity. If the etiology is due to a disk herniation, then symptoms can be aggravated with forward lumbar flexion or sitting, and relieved with lumbar extension or standing. Pain can originate from either mechanical compression of the exiting nerve root into the intervertebral foramen, or from chemical mediators that originate from nuclear disk material itself, which have been found to have inflammogenic properties. Nerve pain can also originate from narrowing of the intervertebral foramen due to spinal stenosis, which in effect strangulates the exiting nerve root upon back extension. Pain is relieved with flexion.

Of course, there are many other pain sources and it is as much a challenge to identify the etiology of dysfunction as it is to develop a treatment paradigm. The reader should keep an open mind when treating spine-related pain since there is often significant overlap in the presentation of pain from different sources.

In this chapter, treatment options for the common afflictions generally seen in the private practitioner's office are discussed.

MUSCLE STRAIN/LIGAMENTOUS SPRAIN

Mechanical back pain, usually due to a muscle strain or ligament sprain, occurs when a person overstretches a muscle or ligament due to undue stress or repetitive injury. It is very common to injure one's spine by performing maneuvers that, on the surface, are rather harmless such as shoveling snow or moving boxes at home. The reason may be lack of the body's accommodation for an action by the driving force of movement, the nervous system. It is the function of muscles to move bones, but it is the nervous system that directs muscle activity. To better understand this, we must understand the concepts defined in "motor learning."[34] This foundation is integral to the thorough knowledge of just how we move. The coordinated motor neurons, firing in frequency, duration, and amplitude, choreograph the movement patterns of our musculoskeletal system. Movements require an adaptation for both force production and force absorption. Otherwise, our motions all would be of the acceleration type without the ability to decelerate. One can clearly appreciate this phenomenon when one considers the act of bending forward at the waist. If it were not for the ability of the thoracolumbar extensor muscles to control this gravity-assisted motion of lumbosacral flexion, as one carried his or her upper torso toward the ground, one would flex in an accelerating manner until the head hit the floor. Obviously, this does not happen, because of the ability of the thoracolumbar extensor muscles to decelerate the flexion motion, preventing the upper torso from thrusting toward the floor. The coordinated effort is under direct control of our central nervous system.

Treatment of the acute strain/sprain is similar to treatment of other body regions, with slight modification. We must remember that most strains/sprains take 4 to 6 weeks to heal and any significant challenge to the area of injury during that time may be detrimental. RICE (rest, ice, compression, and elevation) is often very helpful in the acute stages of healing. Rest should be brief, most often no more than one day. Restoration of mobility is essential and helps to expedite the healing process. Ice can be applied for 10 to 20 minutes (unless the region is excessively erythematous or hypoesthetic) three to four times a day. There is always the question of whether ice or heat is more appropriate.[49] The adage that ice is best for the first 24 to 48 hours and heat for the time after can be followed. Ice and heat, however, seem to offer equal benefit in most spine-related strain/sprain injuries no matter when applied. Either can be applied for 10 to 20 minutes directly over the involved area. Care should be taken, however, not to freeze or burn the area treated.

Compression is typically achieved by bracing, usually using a soft Velcro-type support. It adds stability during the healing phase but should not be a substitute for muscle stabilization. Often compressive wraps become substitutes for training and actually promote future instability. This probably is due to abdominal weakness that results from wearing a support brace for prolonged periods. Although commonly used for extremity strains/sprains, elevation is not typically part of the treatment of strains/sprains in the spine.

Adjunct modalities such as ultrasound and electrical stimulation are useful. Ultrasound can be applied over the paraspinal muscles at 1.5 to 2.0 watts/cm^2 for 7- to 10-minute increments (Fig. 46-1). Two settings may be applied, pulsed or continuous. The pulsed setting acts via mechanical "pumping" and assists in edema reduction by improving drainage from the region. The continuous setting acts as a deep-heating modality and is most focused at the muscle-bone interface. In general, the higher the pulse rate, the more heat production, and the lower the pulse rate, the greater the mechanical pumping effect.

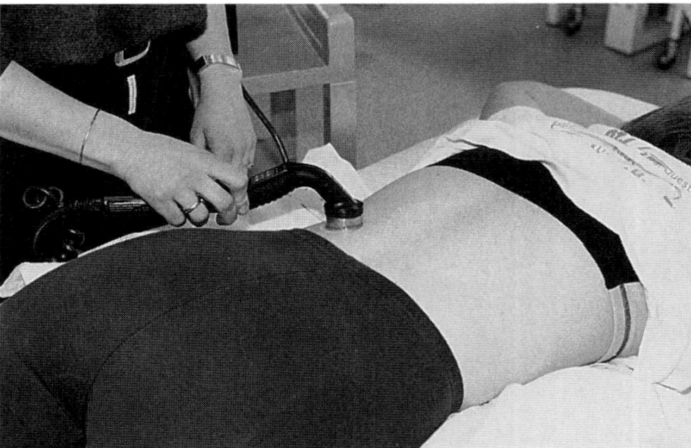

FIGURE 46-1. Ultrasound. A deep-heating modality on continuous setting and a mechanical pumping modality on pulsed setting, this is a very effective adjunct therapy in the treatment of musculoskeletal ailments.

The indications and contraindications for the use of ultrasound are listed in Table 46-1.[40] Electrical current in the form of electrical stimulation can be used to achieve physiologic effects on muscle and body fluid regulation (Fig. 46-2). A common mode of electrical stimulation is galvanic stimulation, which can be of the positive or negative pole. Typically, the positive pole is used in the acute injury phase and the negative pole is used in the chronic injury setting. Positive is helpful in reducing pain and swelling (acute) whereas negative increases blood flow (chronic) and cleanses the region. The indications and contraindications for the use of electrical stimulation are listed in Table 46-2.[40]

TABLE 46-1 Ultrasound

Indications	Muscle spasm Scar tissue Warts
Contraindications	Over: Growing epiphysis, pregnant uterus, bony prominences, ailments of the testes In presence of pacemakers In areas of sensory loss Near metallic implants, orthopedic cement, or healing fractures

From Kahn J: Principles and Practice of Electrotherapy. New York, Churchill Livingstone, 1987.

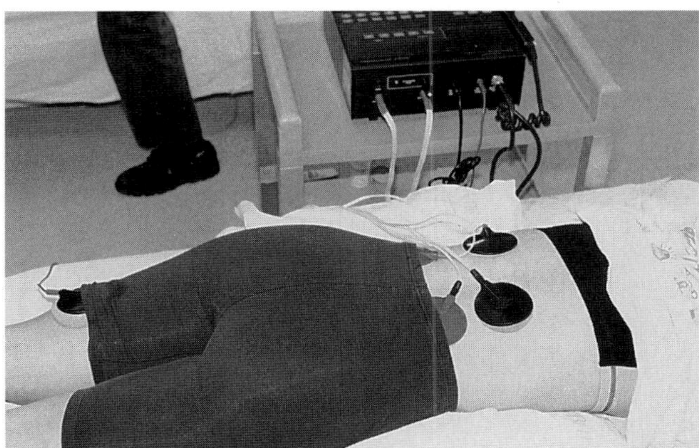

FIGURE 46-2. Electrical stimulation. Electrical current is effective in regulating body-fluid flow and in muscle relaxation and contraction. A dispersive pad is used and placed at a site distant to the active pads or applicator.

In addition to modalities, progressive range of motion and general limbering exercises should be initiated early in the treatment. These could include supine knee-to-chest, standing toe-touching, and side-bending exercises. Nonsteroidal anti-inflammatory or muscle relaxant medications may be beneficial if medically tolerable. Muscle relaxants used for a brief period can assist in increasing mobility once a definitive diagnosis is established, but they should not be overly sedating. Adjunct passive treatments can be used, as with other ailments, to improve motion and decrease pain.

Massage therapy, which has both reflex and mechanical actions, is effective in reducing muscle hypertonicity and increasing venous return. Also, soft-tissue adhesions can be mobilized with strategies such as friction massage. In this technique, the direction of massage is perpendicular or parallel to the muscle fibers, and it helps to increase muscle efficiency.

The next phase in treating strains/sprains includes regaining flexibility or "ease of motion." There are several strategies that are efficacious for improving flexibility. Proprioceptive neuromuscular facilitation (PNF)[73] and muscle energy techniques are both extremely helpful. PNF techniques employ the active contraction of an antagonist muscle, to be immediately followed by a contraction of the related agonist muscle. The active contraction of the agonist muscle is improved secondarily to the antagonist muscle's refractory period, therefore, it is unable to fire and resist the direction of contraction of the agonist. Muscle energy techniques are similar and will be discussed in the following section of the text.

The final stage of healing involves strengthening. This begins once pain is under control, maximum functional range of motion is restored, and flexibility is achieved. It should encompass all associated muscles, particularly those involved in spinal stabilization as described in this chapter under "lumbar stabilization."

TABLE 46-2 Electrical Stimulation

Indications	Muscles that need to be relaxed Muscles that need contracting, simulating active exercise Lack of endorphin production Impaired circulation because of lack of pumping action of muscles Waste products that need clearing away by reticuloendothelial response
Contraindications	Over fresh fractures, to avoid unwanted motion Active hemorrhage Phlebitis Demand-type pacemaker

From Kahn J: Principles and Practice of Electrotherapy. New York, Churchill Livingstone, 1987.

INTERVERTEBRAL DISK DISEASE/MYOFASCIAL PAIN

The intervertebral disk can cause pain either through degeneration (degenerative disk disease) or disk disruption, such as an annular tear, or through a herniation. Clinically, degenerative disk disease can present as localized back and/or myofacial pain. If there is a herniation of the disk, symptoms will further include neuropathic or radicular symptoms, also known as "sciatica," which are classically described as pain radiating into an extremity, with or without associated numbness and tingling. Many authors make a clear distinction between disk disease and myofascial pain, but as it relates to the spine, this distinction is difficult to delineate. In this section, an overview of rehabilitation techniques used to conservatively treat musculoskeletal disorders directly related to the spine is presented, as are recent advances in interventional spine care. As more advances are made in these minimally invasive techniques and more treatment options become available, practitioners will have greater success in restoring a patient's function and reducing pain.[61]

A key element in rehabilitation of the spine is exercise training, which is achieved by gaining adequate control of the dynamic spine forces. Active participation by the patient is essential, and a goal-oriented approach is important. Two factors seem most pressing when a person suffers physical disability: pain control and ability to increase functional performance. Attaining either of these may be enough for some patients, whereas others must attain both. In general, if a patient can be in control of the disability rather than the disability being in control of the patient, the therapeutic intervention undertaken can be considered successful.

As with all rehabilitation programs, goal setting is essential. Spinal disk disease is often painful and physically disabling, and one must clearly establish individualized goals when embarking on the road to optimal health. Pain control is the first concern when treating disk-related disease, and nonsteroidal anti-inflammatory medications are the first line of treatment.[62] Though Saal et al. proposed avoidance of narcotics, muscle relaxants, and sleep hypnotics for the reasons outlined in Table 46-3,[62] muscle relaxants and narcotics have now been shown to be effective when used for acute, well-identified pain flares. All medications carry the risk of harm, particularly when overused or abused. Patients must be educated about the proper indications and usage for medicines. Particular cautions should be taken with muscle relaxants because their mechanism of action is often through the central nervous system. The sedating and mind-altering effects of these can interfere with a patient's mental status. It is therefore recommended that muscle relaxants be used judiciously.

Passive Modalities

In addition to pain medications, passive modalities such as traction, manual techniques, and deep heating modalities can be used. Traction is helpful in both the cervical and lumbar regions. It aids in soft-tissue relaxation and intervertebral disk space widening. There is controversy as to whether, as traditionally applied, traction actually widens the intervertebral disk space, since it is well recognized that the force required for intervertebral distraction is quite large. With this in mind, the following recommendations may be clinically useful. For the cervical spine, try to gradually increase weight up to the target value. Colachis and Strohm have shown that 30 pounds of traction with a slightly flexed cervical spine (24°) can cause vertebral separation.[16] Others have suggested that a minimum of 25 pounds is needed to have vertebral separation.[39]

When receiving cervical spine traction, the patient's head should be slightly flexed and comfortably relaxed. If you are using an automated traction device, be sure your patient has an emergency cutoff switch (one that deactivates the traction toward zero pounds) or access to disengage the device manually. Treatment sessions should last 20 to 30 minutes and can be done two to three times a week. Colachis and Strohm suggest that the optimum time for vertebral separation is 25 minutes.[17]

In the lumbar spine, our target poundage is 60% to 65% of body weight. This type of traction is best done with the patient lying supine and patients should have the same emergency parameters available. The duration of treatment is similar to the cervical spine. Traction can be applied in a continuous manner or intermittently. The decision as to which to use depends largely on patient comfort. Geiringer indicates that both physician and patient preference is most important in deciding between intermittent and continuous traction.[28] When applied intermittently, on/off times can vary. I prefer brief, slow-ramping times, 10 to 15 seconds on and 5 to 7 seconds off. Be aware that the onset of traction may invoke discomfort rather than alleviate it. Individuals with spinal stenosis and disk disease may actually complain of more, rather than less, pain at the onset. The reason for this may be root irritation from column lengthening.

If a patient wishes to use a "home traction device," there are several considerations. First, the most popular of these devices are those that contain water-fillable pouches with an over-the-door suspension apparatus (Fig. 46-3). Second, remember to instruct your patient to face the frame (typically a door) from which the unit is suspended. This traction device too is accompanied by a slight flexion of the cervical spine. Finally, make sure your patient follows all directions carefully. Strict attention must be paid to the amount of water/pounds applied to the spine. Home cervical traction units do not typically allow a patient to apply too much weight because the water (or sometimes sand) container will allow only safe amounts of substance to be added. This is usually 20 to 25 pounds maximum. This, however, may not be enough external weight to achieve sufficient traction. When you consider that part of the applied external weight is negated by the inherent weight of the patient's head (typically 10 to 13 pounds), the resultant net traction force is not enough to promote intervertebral lengthening. For example, if the water bag is filled with 25 pounds of water, and you subtract 10 pounds for the weight of the head, the net traction force is only 15 pounds.

TABLE 46-3 Medication Checklist

Medication	Indications and Use
Nonsteroidal Anti-inflammatory drugs	Useful for anti-inflammatory action and analgesia
Narcotic analgesics	To be avoided because of endorphin blockade and addictive potential
Muscle relaxants	To be avoided because of their central nervous system sedative effects
Sleep hypnotics	To be avoided because of their central nervous system depressive effects
Tricyclic antidepressants	Useful to promote sleep and decrease serotonergic pain stimuli

From Saal J, Dillingham M: Nonoperative treatment and rehabilitation of disk, facet, and soft tissue injuries. In Nicholas J, Hershman E (ed): The Lower Extremity in Spine and Sport Medicine, 2nd ed. St. Louis, Mosby–Year Book, 1995.

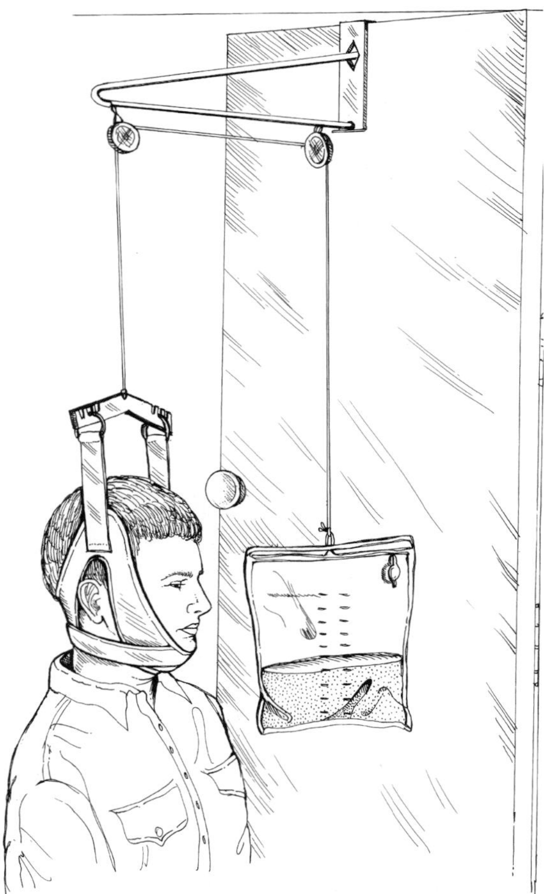

FIGURE 46-3. Cervical spine traction. Home traction devices are somewhat useful in treating cervical spine pathology, but caution must be used when applying the device (see text).

It is important to emphasize to patients that careful application of home cervical traction is paramount. Patients often think, "If some is good then more is better." This certainly is not the case, and patients must be reminded to follow recommended guidelines and not be overzealous. Disregard for this could lead to significant complications. Contraindications and relative contraindications do exist for the use of traction. These are outlined in Table 46-4.[25]

Manual techniques are very helpful in cervical, thoracic, and lumbosacral disk disease. They are particularly useful in treating restrictions of motion, particularly those caused by hypomobility of related joints.

Two other passive modalities utilized to treat spine pain include TENS (transcutaneous electrical nerve stimulation) and deep-heating modalities. TENS is a modality used to reduce pain, especially neuropathic pain.[19] It produces a strong but comfortable current that is thought to provide analgesic effects over the applied areas. The current is delivered from a beeper-like device into small surface pads that are attached to the unit with fine wire (Fig. 46-4).

TABLE 46-4 Traction

Indications	Pain Vertebral separation/disk herniation Muscle hypertonicity Nerve root decompression Disk and facets that need unloading
Contraindications	Malignancy Sepsis Vascular compromise Unstable spine
Precautions	Inflammatory arthropathy Aortic aneurysm Pregnancy Hiatal hernia Vertigo

From Esses, 1995; Greenman PE: Principles of Manual Medicine. Baltimore, Williams and Wilkins, 1989.

Deep-heating modalities are effective for both subjective and physiologic effects. The application of warm packs or ultrasound makes most people subjectively feel better. This may be a placebo effect or related to muscle relaxation. Physiologically, heat increases blood flow, which subsequently increases the body's local metabolic rate. This, in turn, allows a cleansing of metabolic byproducts and accelerates the rate of healing. Heating packs are commercially available and are available in several varieties. Some are operated electrically (dry heat), others have heat-retaining gels (moist heat) (Fig. 46-5). The gel packs are moistened by placing them into hot water, which allows the gel to absorb heat. The pack is then placed over the area to be treated, usually with a towel between the moist pack and the skin's surface. It remains applied for 10 to 20 minutes. The true physiologic effects of this heating modality are often questioned, since heating pads'

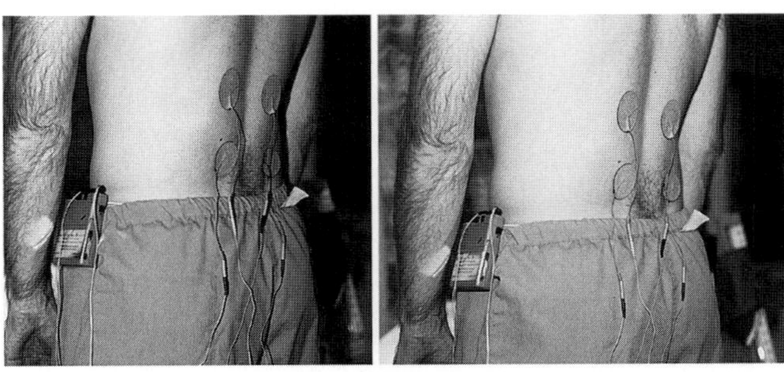

A B

FIGURE 46-4. Transcutaneous electrical nerve stimulation (TENS). **A** and **B,** Electrodes are placed at key sites of pain referral to control transmission of aberrant sensation. The unit is regulated by control dials to increase/decrease intensity and frequency of impulse transmission.

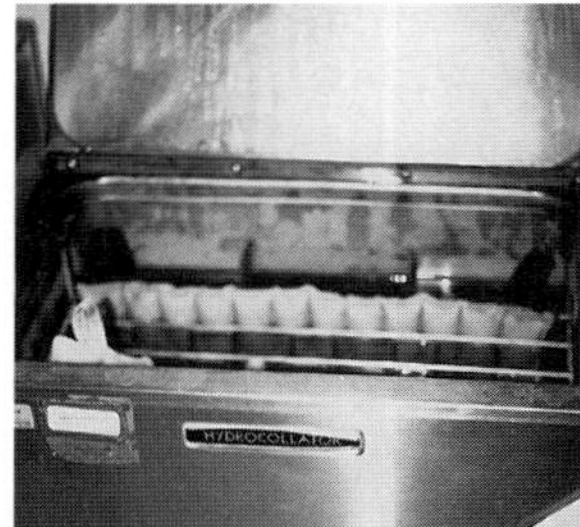

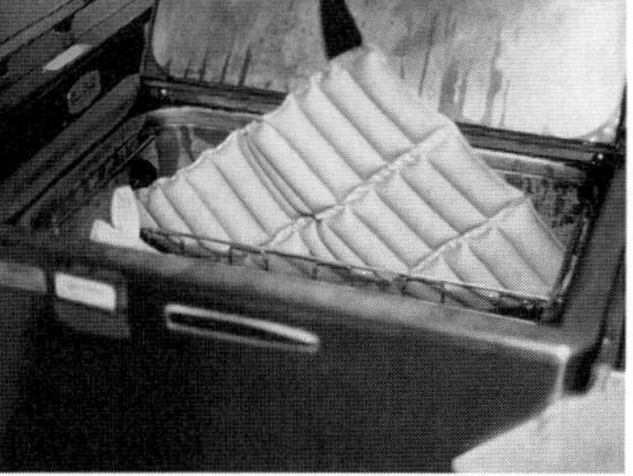

A B

FIGURE 46-5. Heating packs. **A** and **B,** Heating devices are useful to reduce musculoskeletal pain and ease muscle hypertonicity. They are usually applied in the chronic setting of injury but are not restricted to this use only. Application is for 10 to 20 minutes and frequent checks are made to assure comfort (i.e., that the packs are not too hot).

(moist or dry) heat penetrates only into the superficial subcutaneous layers. To achieve deeper heating effects, ultrasound can be used. The indications and contraindications of heat are listed in Table 46-5.[25]

Manual Therapy

Although mentioned here under the category of disk disease, manual therapies are used in treatments of various musculoskeletal disorders.[29] There are several types of manual interventions, ranging from soft-tissue to forceful bony thrusting techniques (Fig. 46-6). An example of soft-tissue intervention is muscle energy (Fig. 46-7). In this strategy the focus is to relax a hypertonic motion-restricting muscle to allow freedom of movement toward the opposite direction of the restrictive muscle's action. As an example, if a patient tries to extend his or her lumbosacral spine but is unable to do so, the reason may be tight abdominal muscles. If the abdominals are not relaxed or do not offer pliability, they will inhibit movement in the opposite direction (extension).

TABLE 46-5 Heat

Indications	Pain and muscle spasm Need for range of motion improvement Pain Lowered metabolic rate
Contraindications	Anesthetic area Obtunded patient Over: gonads, gravid uterus Malignancy Hemorrhagic diathesis Area of poor vascularity

Adapted from Michlovitz SL: Thermal Agents in Rehabilitation. Philadelphia, FA Davis, 1986; Esses SI: Textbook of Spinal Disorders. Philadelphia, Lippincott, 1995.

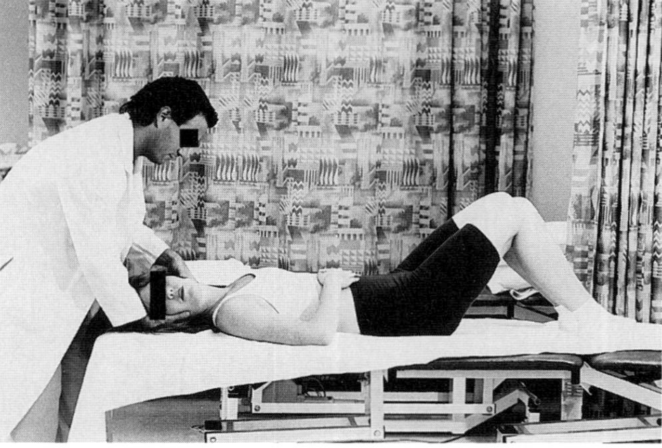

A

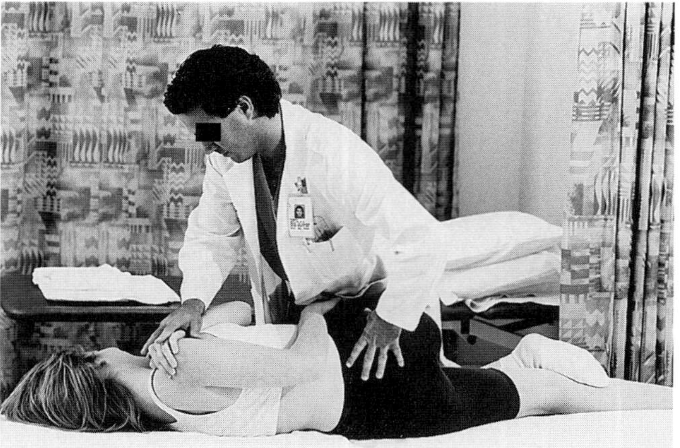

B

FIGURE 46-6. Manipulation-thrusting technique. **A** and **B,** After taking the associated joint to its physiologic limit, a gentle high-velocity, low-amplitude thrust is administered. Before any manipulative procedure, a complete knowledge of contraindications must be familiar (see Table 46-6).

To overcome stiff abdominal muscles, muscle energy techniques can be applied. In this instance, trying to extend the lumbosacral spine will be resisted by the tight abdominals, so stretching the abdominal muscles is impractical. To achieve the desired effect of lumbosacral extension, we attempt to contract the abdominal muscles, usually for a count of 5 to 6 seconds, against resistance (isometric) and then passively extend the lumbosacral spine. The isometric contractions of the abdominals induce muscle fatigue. Then the abdominals no longer resist the lumbar extension movement. The exercise is repeated several times, increasing the amount of lumbosacral extension on each repetition. This is a very effective technique to increase flexibility and relax muscles.

Other manual techniques include craniosacral, counterstrain, and myofascial release. Craniosacral technique was introduced by William G. Sutherland circa 1940. The foundation of his therapy lies in the

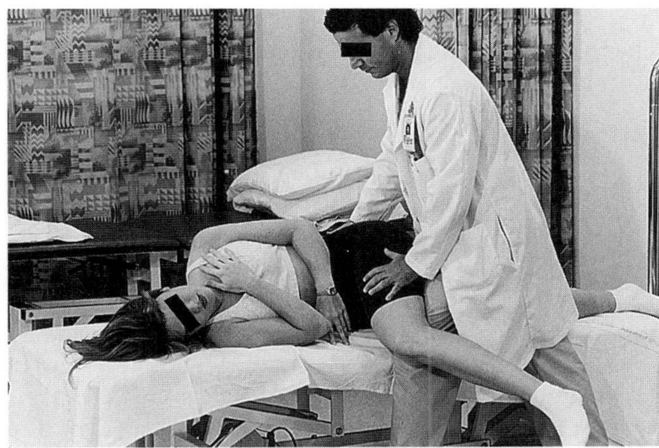

A

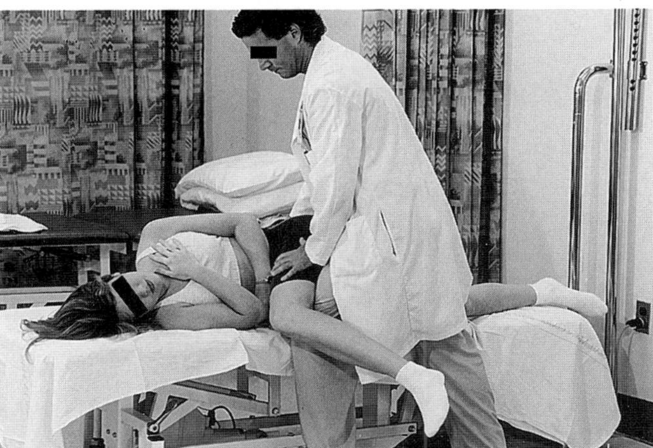

B

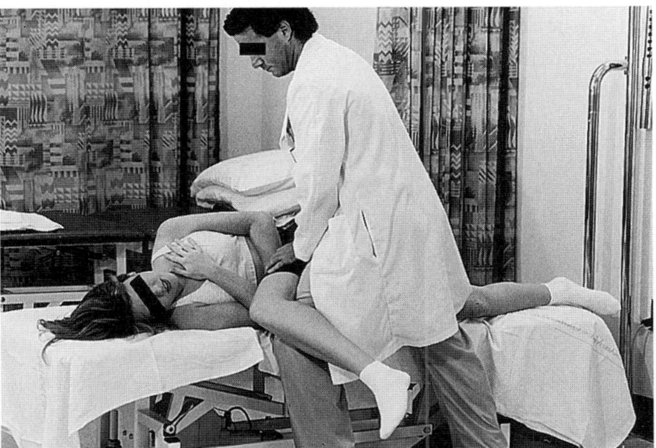

C

FIGURE 46-7. Muscle energy technique. **A, B,** and **C,** Through a series of repetitive contractions of a hypertonic muscle, increased freedom of movement in the opposite direction can be achieved. If the lumbosacral extensors are hypertonic, a series of repeated contractions of these muscles can lead to relaxation and increased freedom of motion in the opposite direction, i.e., lumbosacral flexion.

consistent architecture of the skull's sutures, which maintain mobility during health. When a person is traumatized or ill, this normal mobility is interrupted and restrictions of motion occur. Because the skull is connected to the sacrum by the meninges, restrictions of motion in one will directly influence the other. Hence the name *craniosacral.* Craniosacral technique involves manual pressure exerted onto various key bony regions to free restricted motion. There are a growing number of clinicians who deliver craniosacral therapy. Its indications in musculoskeletal treatments are rather broad and range from simple joint stiffness to complex soft-tissue restrictions.

Counterstrain technique was formally introduced by Lawrence H. Jones in his text entitled *Strain and Counterstrain.*[38] It is believed that spinal pathology has a consistent coinciding muscular reference area that is tender to palpation.[31] These so-called tender spots, when localized, are the monitoring areas for the success of this technique. When a clinician confidently palpates such a tender spot, he or she positions the patient's body in such a way that the tender region under the palpating finger no longer produces discomfort. This position is held for about 90 seconds and the body part is then slowly returned to the pretreatment habitus. Often the pain and discomfort the patient was experiencing in this tender spot no longer exists (Fig. 46-8).

Myofascial release involves massage-like stretching of soft-tissue structures. Its goal is to elongate restricted muscles and soft tissue. Although similar, it is not massage therapy. If muscles are restricting motion and muscle energy technique is being used, myofascial release technique is an excellent adjunct. Bony techniques fall under several names. These include adjustment, manipulation, mobilization, and "cracking." Historically, the chiropractic (DC) profession uses the term "adjustment," osteopathic (DO) physicians "manipulate" the bony segments, and physical therapists (PT) "mobilize" the joints. In recent years allopathic (MD) physicians are more frequently making use of this alternative approach when treating musculoskeletal disorders.

Spray and stretch is a useful technique when treating myofascial pain. In this technique, ethyl chloride or fluori-methane spray is applied to the area being treated to assist in obtaining muscle flexibility. This spray is rather cold when applied to the skin and assists in briefly desensitizing the region sprayed. This allows slow, sustained stretch to be applied to the muscles below the sprayed sites. The spray is aimed at the area of the body where muscles are irritated; while the practitioner sprays in the same direction as the muscle fibers, the patient stretches the muscles.

Another muscle commonly implicated in, but rarely identified when discussing, myofascial pain is the quadratus lumborum. It is a well-recognized source of low back and buttock pain, but only when the examiner knows to

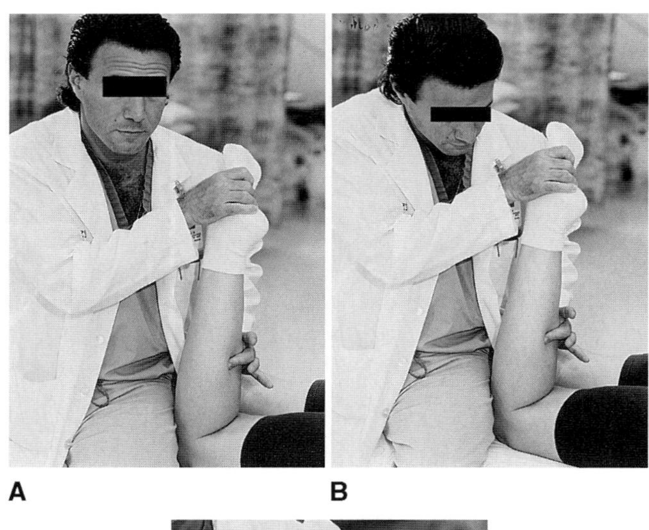

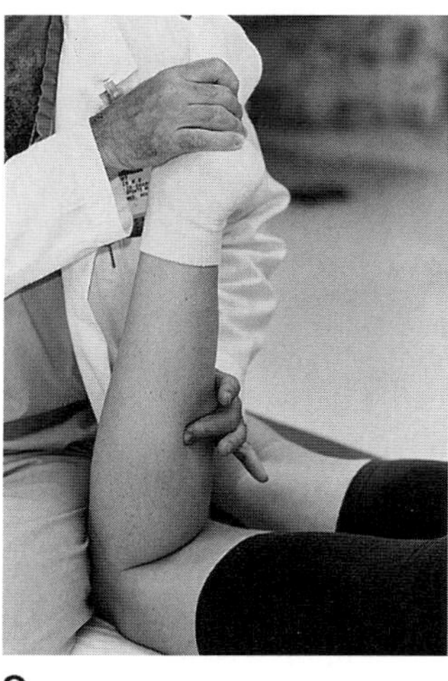

FIGURE 46-8. Counterstrain technique. **A, B,** and **C,** By placing the body in a position that allows relaxation of associated muscles so that an area of palpable tenderness no longer exists, the palpating digit no longer produces tenderness. The position that no longer produces tenderness is held for about 90 seconds. A gastrocnemius point is being treated here.

look for it. This quadrangular-shaped muscle lies beneath the erector spinae muscle group and functions as a lateral flexor–extensor of the lumbar spine, elevator of the pelvis, and depressor of the twelfth rib.[81] One must specifically palpate this muscle when examining a patient. To best identify its painful trigger point areas, the practitioner should place the patient lying with his or her knees flexed in the fetal position. The neck should be comfortably tucked onto the chest, and the patient should take slow, deep breaths. The examiner then gently palpates, with pads of several digits, the region between the erector spinae and the ribs on the raised side of the patient's torso. Palpating with several digits increases the purchase of skin contact so as not to tense the muscles of the patient's back by examining in a probing fashion (Fig. 46-9). If trigger points are present in this muscle, they will be palpated easily with this technique. Muscle energy techniques should be directed at relieving painful areas and should prove very effective.

A particularly useful manual technique is performed with the patient sitting comfortably in a chair with his or her feet firmly placed on the ground. The patient then places his or her arms across the chest and the examiner, standing behind the patient, leans his or her chest onto the patient's upper back (Fig. 46-10). The patient will tilt further toward one side little by little, each time going through a series of isometric contractions back toward midline, against resistance from the examiner. This is repeated several times before performing the same exercise on the opposite side. It can be repeated two or three times on each side. Flexibility/stretching exercise is also useful and includes lateral trunk-bending and toe-touching. Injections are warranted in conjunction with or after failed conservative approaches. These would be administered as described for myofascial pain.

The iliopsoas muscle is said to be a treatable cause of "failed" low back syndrome.[35] This ventral spinal muscle functions as a hip flexor and is thought to be tightened in certain pathologic conditions of the low back. Ingber proposes a "dry" needling technique whereby a 30-gauge, 2.5-inch needle is slowly inserted into the iliopsoas muscle in an attempt to relax the tightened fibers.[35] In this technique, no solution is injected into the trigger point. After the injection, the patient performs a series of lumbosacral extension exercises to stretch the previously tight region.

Aside from myofascial release, more advanced methods of manual medicine should be considered. It is no longer uncommon for physicians to refer patients to practitioners with expertise in manual medicine.[29] Manipulation aims at correcting functional impairment rather than treating pathology. It attempts to restore natural play between body parts so that they can resume normal functioning.[14] Techniques vary from very gentle stretching maneuvers to high-velocity thrusting techniques. There are two commonly accepted thrusting techniques. The first is known as high velocity, low amplitude. This is performed by applying a quick thrust to a bony structure to overcome a restrictive soft-tissue barrier. The second is low-velocity, high-amplitude technique, which implies a slow movement but with force carried over a greater distance.

Several studies have investigated the efficacy of spinal manual medicine. Chiropractic treatment has been shown to provide worthwhile, long-lasting benefits compared to hospital outpatient management.[46] When comparing spinal mobilization (nonrotational) to spinal manipulation/adjustment, Hadler and others found significant improvement in the manipulation/adjustment group.[30] On December 4, 1994, the U.S. Agency for Health Care Policy and Research proposed federal guidelines for the treatment of low back pain. In its

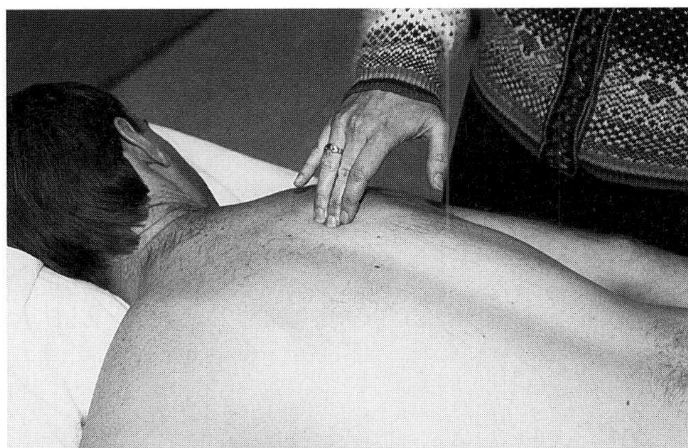

A

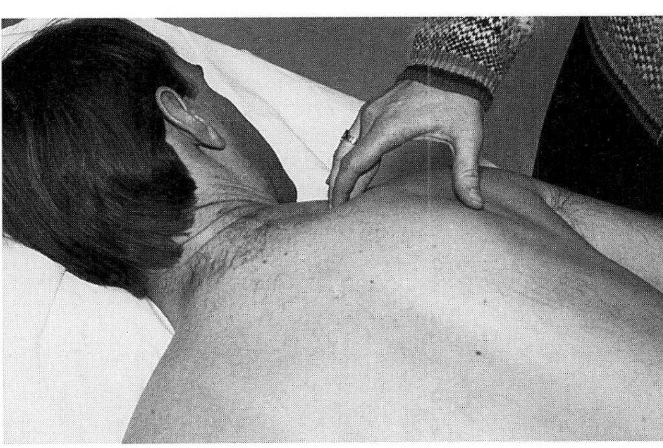

B

FIGURE 46-9. Palpatory technique for trigger points. **A** and **B,** With the pads of 1–2 digits, deep palpation in the direction of muscle fibers reveals "taut" bands. When isolating such, there is a sensation of discomfort.

report, manipulation/adjustments were endorsed and encouraged as a treatment of choice. It should be noted that this recommendation was not inclusive for those with radiculopathy.[1] Also, after one month of unsuccessful manipulation, further diagnostic work-up is indicated. Before performing spinal manipulation/adjustment, one should offer a series of muscle energy therapies to ease the application of thrusting techniques. In this manner, the muscles in the region to be manipulated are made more flexible. Contraindications to manipulation/adjustments do exist and are noted in Table 46-6.[30,37]

Lumbar Stabilization, McKenzie Exercises, and Aquatic Therapy

Two other approaches in the treatment of intervertebral disk disease include lumbar stabilization and McKenzie extension exercises. Lumbar stabilization, as proposed by Saal and others, has gained considerable popularity in the management of disk disease.[61] It is postulated that a

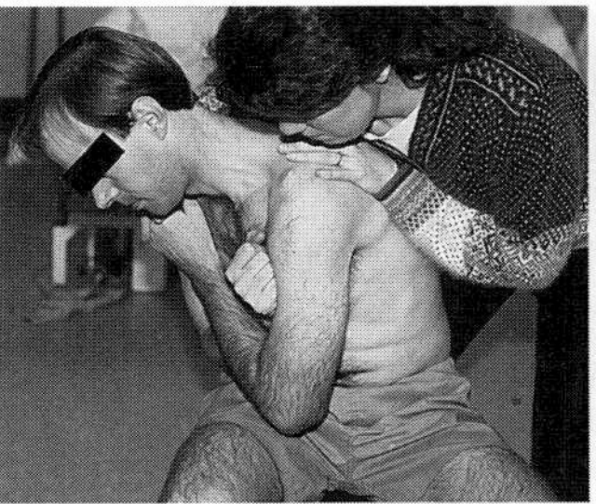

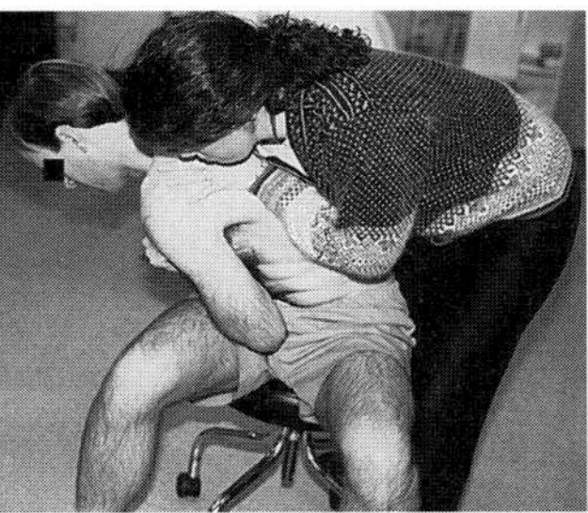

A B

FIGURE 46-10. Muscle energy techniques for quadratus lumborum strain. **A** and **B,** With the patient sitting comfortably and both feet firmly on the ground, the examiner leans over the patient's thoracic spine and passively sidebends/rotates the torso in the direction of the strain. The patient is then instructed to upright the torso to neutral against resistance applied by the examiner's chest. This isometric contraction technique is held for approximately 5 seconds. The resistance is then released and the patient is laterally flexed passively and rotated further to the involved side. The entire process is then repeated. A series of 4 to 5 contraction sets are done. Typically, the same series is done to the opposite side.

well-thought-out and scientifically based program could result in successful conservative treatment for herniated disks. The basic premise of stabilization theory requires a thorough understanding of spinal/vertebral forces and their relationship to biomechanical motion. Attainment of what is described as a "neutral" spine helps to minimize extraneous forces on the spine and associated soft tissues. Neutral spine is that anterior–posterior, medial–lateral, superior–inferior alignment whereby the net forces transmitted through the spine are balanced by increasing the purchase of the vertebral segments.

TABLE 46-6 Manipulation

Indications	Joint restrictions
	Joint immobility
	Nerve root compression
	Psychological stress
Contraindications	Unstable spine
	Cauda equina syndrome
	Systemic anticoagulation
	Rheumatoid arthritis
	Vertebral insufficiency
	Vertebral malignancy
	Myelopathy
	Advanced spondylosis
	Spondyloarthropathies
	Osteoporosis
	Osteomalacia

From Janse J: History of the development of chiropractic concepts: Chiropractic terminology. In Goldstein M (ed): The Research Status of Spinal Manipulation, NINCDC Monograph No. 5, DHEW Pub. No. (NIH) 76-998, 1975.

The increased surface area allows for more evenly distributed forces. When the overall contact areas are increased, the force per unit-area is decreased. This can be accomplished, for example, by pelvic tilts.

One can appreciate this maneuver if attempting the following. While standing, try to thrust the superior border of your iliac crests posteriorly, then tighten your abdominal muscles and squeeze your buttocks together. This maneuver will relax the lumbosacral paraspinal region, and there is usually a feeling of lower back pressure relief if the technique is done correctly. Once a patient can attain and maintain this posture, a fully structured and monitored exercise program can be developed. The exercises are performed with the pelvis in "neutral spine," which assists in maximizing ergonomic efficiency and acts to protect the spinal structures (Fig. 46-11).

In the cervical spine, the natural lordotic curve does not promote optimal bony contact. To begin training, we must establish the position of optimal function (POF). This can take place with slight occipito-atlanto flexion. It is only when the patient feels comfortable with postural adaptations that the appropriate exercise program can begin.

For the lumbar spine, the goal is to train the abdominal, lumbosacral extensor, and buttock muscles while maintaining neutral spine. For the cervical spine, we focus on the posterior cervical paraspinal muscles and the scapula stabilizers (particularly the serratus anterior and rhomboids) to help stabilize the spine. The program has several phases, each with a further progression of exercises. The ultimate goal is relative freedom from pain with increased mobility.[63]

Akin to the stabilization techniques described in the preceding paragraphs, the McKenzie technique of postural control and vertebral stabilization has gained much popularity as well.[45] As proposed by Robin McKenzie, a physiotherapist from New Zealand, this

CHECKLIST

Treatment Phases

Pain Control
- ☐ Back first aid
- ☐ Trial of extension exercises
- ☐ Trial of traction
- ☐ Basic stabilization exercise training
- ☐ NSAIDs
- ☐ Nonnarcotic analgesics
- ☐ Corticosteroids
- ☐ Oral
- ☐ Epidural injection
- ☐ Selective nerve root injection
- ☐ Facet injection

Exercise training
- ☐ Soft tissue flexibility
- ☐ Hamstring musculotendinous unit
- ☐ Quadriceps musculotendinous unit
- ☐ Iliopsoas musculotendinous unit
- ☐ Gastroc-soleus musculotendinous unit
- ☐ External and internal hip rotators

Joint mobility
- ☐ Lumbar spine segmental mobility
- ☐ Hip range of motion
- ☐ Thoracic segmental mobility

Stabilization program
- ☐ Finding neutral position
- ☐ Sitting stabilization
- ☐ Prone gluteal squeezes
- ☐ Supine pelvic bracing
- ☐ Bridging progression
- ☐ Basic position
- ☐ One leg raised
- ☐ Stepping
- ☐ Balance on gym ball

Quadriped
- ☐ With alternating arm and leg movement

Kneeling stabilization
- ☐ Double knee
- ☐ Single knee
- ☐ Lunges
- ☐ Wall slide quadriceps strengthening
- ☐ Position transition with postural control

Abdominal program
- ☐ Curl-ups
- ☐ Dead bugs
- ☐ Diagonal curl-ups
- ☐ Diagonal curl-ups on incline board
- ☐ Straight leg lowering

Gym program
- ☐ Latissimus pull-downs
- ☐ Angled leg press
- ☐ Lunges
- ☐ Hyperextension bench
- ☐ General upper body strengthening exercises
- ☐ Pulley exercises to stress postural control

Aerobic program
- ☐ Progressive walking
- ☐ Swimming
- ☐ Stationary bicycling
- ☐ Cross-country ski machine
- ☐ Running
- ☐ Initially supervised on a treadmill

From Saal JA, Saal JS: Nonoperative treatment of herniated lumbar intervertebral disk with radiculopathy: An outcome study. Spine 14(4):435, 1989.

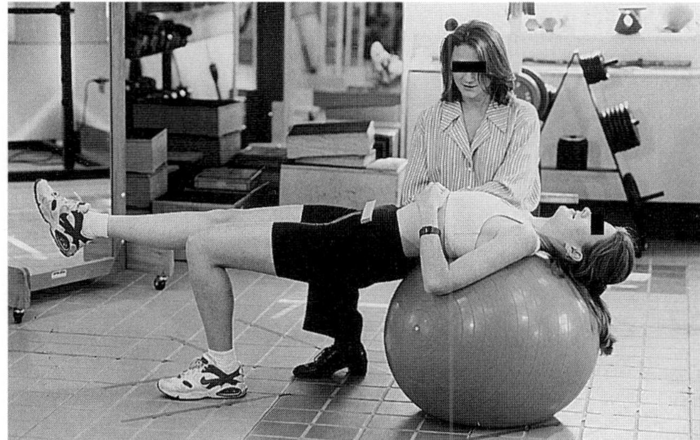

A

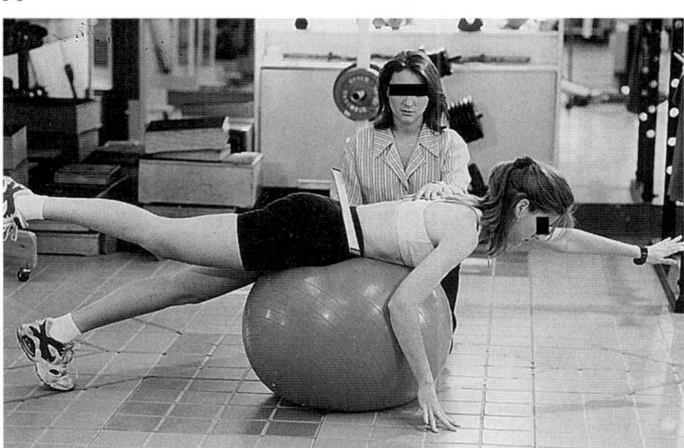

B

FIGURE 46-11. Stabilization in neutral spine. **A, B,** While maintaining neutral spine, a series of exercises are performed. The maintenance of neutral spine is essential during these exercises. A stick or pole can be placed across the lumbar spine to monitor stable pelvic tilt during these exercises.

technique emphasizes extension-type movements to counteract a slumped, biomechanically inefficient posture. Its exercise sequence focuses on restricted versus pathologic movement. An example is noted in the patient who has difficulty extending his or her lumbosacral spine while in a sitting posture. Is this due to tight abdominal muscles or posterior spinal pathology that inhibits the extension movement?

Aquatic therapy is an excellent means for exercises with significant joint load reduction. For the arthritic patient, whose range of motion exercises are more difficult to perform on dry land, aqua therapy becomes an option and preferred choice. From an aerobic perspective, an excellent workout, that spares the joints at the same time, is feasible with water resistance. A detailed regimen of aqua therapy as proposed by Cirullo, who describes a complete stabilization program that unloads the spine and minimizes postexercise edema.[15] Patient compliance often is better than with conventional land exercises. The indications for aqua therapy are varied but can be individualized to treat many musculoskeletal diagnoses.

Minimally Invasive Injection Techniques

Once noninvasive techniques have been tried, interventional techniques may be attempted when treating spine-related pain. In the treatment of myofascial pain, the writings of Travell and Simons clearly define a disease of hyperirritable soft-tissue foci located within the skeletal muscle or its associated fascia.[74] These foci are called "trigger points" and are soft-tissue regions that are very tender to palpation. Inherent to these is a distinct pain-referral pattern when they are stimulated (Fig. 46-12); when palpating a specific trigger point, pain will radiate from the trigger point along a specific path. The muscle that harbors a trigger point contains taut bands which are palpable and often cause a twitch when palpated. These bands tend to tighten and shorten the muscle.[74] The taut band refers pain when tension is placed on it. The treatment for trigger points usually consists of injection with a solution of anesthetic, commonly 1% lidocaine (without epinephrine), in a volume of 5 to 10 cc. When a trigger point is injected, the typical response is a "jump sign." The area will twitch upon needle insertion, which is a good indication that the needle is in the correct location. Once the needle is positioned, it is gently moved in a short range back and forth several times to assist in breaking up the trigger foci. Response to this technique is very positive when you precisely localize a specific trigger point to be injected. The injections can be repeated several times over a few weeks. Skin preparation before injection should follow basic aseptic technique guidelines. It is not uncommon to feel transient soreness several hours after the injections, and patients should be made aware of this. A steroid solution can be added to the injection solution. If this is done, you should limit the frequency of injections (with steroid) to not more than three in 4 to 6 months.

Acupuncture is an alternative injection technique that is rapidly gaining a strong following in the Western world. This ancient Chinese therapy has been practiced for more than 2500 years. It is indicated for pain relief and disease cure. Its followers believe its results occur by restoring the balance between yin (blood) and yang (spirit). These energies flow within the body along fourteen channels or meridians.[47] There are 361 sites (acupuncture points), which, when stimulated by pressure or needle insertion, stimulate innate processes within the body. Researchers argue that acupuncture is a form of neuromodulation. Two theories are proposed. The needles used in acupuncture may stimulate large sensory afferent fibers and suppress pain perception. Or the needle insertion can act as a noxious stimulus and induce intrinsic production of opiate-like substances to control pain.[81]

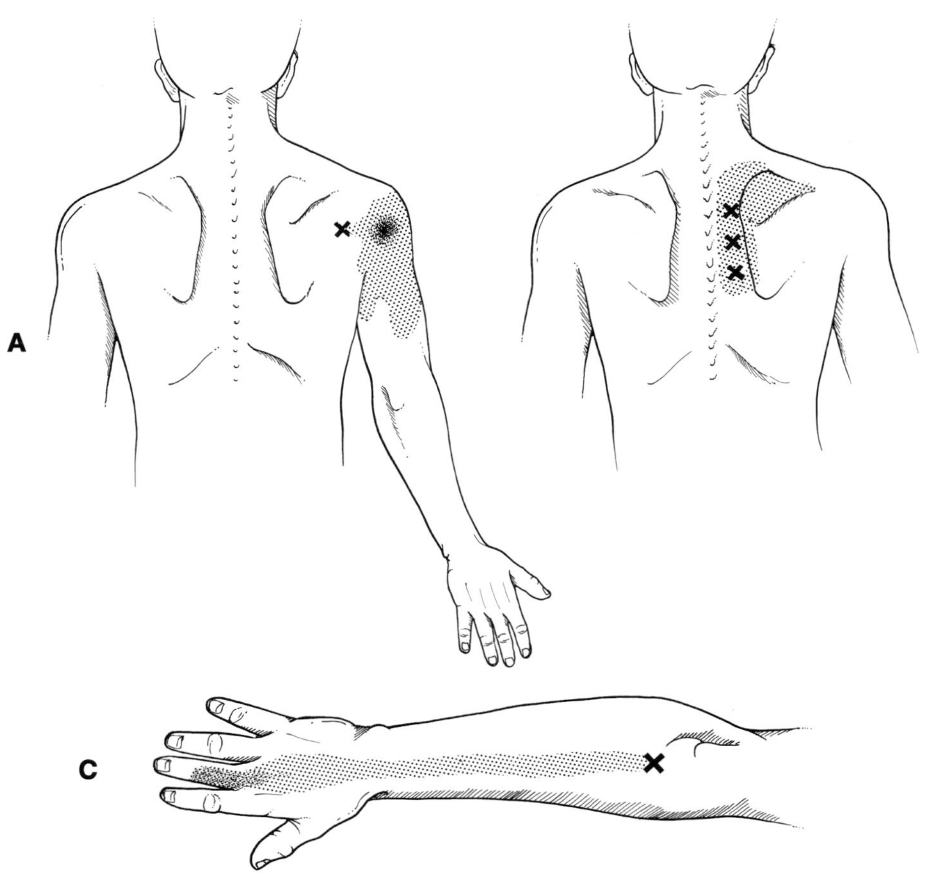

FIGURE 46-12. Trigger points/myofascial pain. Map of trigger points and associated pain referral zones. **A,** Teses minor; **B,** Rhomboid; **C,** Digit extensors. Trigger points are noted by the *X* and pain referral zone by the shaded area.

It has been shown that a significant similarity exists between myofascial trigger points and acupuncture sites.[48] The sensation generated by the use of an acupuncture needle resembles the dull ache often reported by a patient after a trigger point has been injected. Acupuncture can aid in reducing muscle hypertonicity and trigger point sensitivity. Also, it is useful in controlling radicular pain by increasing endorphin levels within the central nervous system.[62] It seems that regardless of the substance injected, the result is likely to be pain relief. The trigger points of myofascial injection may indeed be the same as areas of needle insertion associated with acupuncture.[77] Trigger point therapy is very effective in the management of myofascial pain, and clinicians should be familiar with its application.

More advanced interventional spine procedures have become available in the arsenal to treat back pain. These interventional injection techniques offer a variety of alternatives for the treatment of spine-related back pain. Inclusive are paravertebral nerve blocks, epidural injections, facet joint injections, and sacroiliac injections.[3,5,8,12,24,26,43,58] Such injections should be considered only after a trial of active, hands-on rehabilitation has failed. This is so since more than 80% of spine-related back pain responds favorably to conventional noninvasive treatment. The more advanced injection techniques provide both diagnostic and therapeutic benefits, with short- and long-term efficacy more apparent when patients are properly selected.[3,4,5,8,12,22,24,26,42,68,69] Lutz et al. in 1998 observed that 75% of the 69 patients who received corticosteorid epidural injections reported greater than 50% reduction in pain scores.[44] In another study, Riew et al. prospectively randomized 55 patients scheduled to undergo spine surgery for spinal nerve compression into two groups. Half underwent epidural injections with corticosteroids and lidocaine, the other half with lidocaine alone. Twenty-nine of these 55 patients who had initially requested surgery decided to forego the surgery, due to improved symptoms. Twenty of these 29 patients had received corticosteroids in their injectate.[57] More recently, Vad et al. found that epidural injections offered relief in 84% of the patients studied, who reported greater than 50% improvement even after one year post-injection.[75] Thus, once a decision is made to proceed with these interventions, the delivery of the injectate, usually lidocaine and a corticosteroid, can be achieved with significant precision and low risk through the use of fluorscopic guidance of the needle, along with epidural and joint visualization with contrast medium. Before proceeding to epidural steroid injection, one should consider administration of paravertebral nerve blocks. With this technique, a mixture of anesthetic such as lidocaine is combined with a corticosteroid solution and injected intramuscular approximately 1.5 inches lateral to the spinal column. The injection is given into the region of the deep paraspinal muscles and offers great relief for paraspinal pain. This author has found almost comparable symptom relief with paravertebral nerve block as with epidural steroid injection. In fact, I often reserve the use of epidural injections for those who fail paravertebral nerve block.

The use of steroids in the treatment of either degenerative disk disease or disk herniation is based on the theory that the sensory nerve irritation is due to direct toxic injury, from chemical and inflammatory reactions. It has been postulated that the various pain modulators responsible for localized back pain and/or radicular pain include any one of the following mediators: phospholipase A2, nitric oxide, prostaglandins, leukotrienes, thromboxanes, immunoglobulins such as IgG, IgM, and even tumor necrosis factor alpha.[2,32,51,53,59,60,61] In all, the mainstay of treatment continues to be injections of corticosteroids, which provide a "shotgun" treatment to neutralize these mediators. Corticosteroids inhibit the synthesis and release of pro-inflammatory chemicals, the release of cytokines by immune cells, and neural peptide synthesis. In addition, corticosteroids cause membrane stabilization of the nerve root by suppressing ectopic discharges, partially block immune complexes traversing the basement membrane, and suppress superoxide radicals.[2,10,11,14,22,33,41,70,72,79]

Contraindications do exist, and minor and transient complications can occur with the use of epidural steroids, and the clinician must be aware of these.[9,36] They are outlined in Table 46-7. The most common side effects of the corticosteroids include insomnia, headache, and facial flushing. Though rare, there have been case reports of paralysis due to radicular or vertebal artery infarction from particulate matter found in the corticosteroid itself. Though the use of fluoroscopy does minimize this risk, it can occur and patients should be advised of this rare complication. The above disorders are conservatively managed with manual techniques and injection therapies. Table 46-8 reviews various injection techniques used for advanced pain control.[62]

More invasive techniques such as nucleoplasty may prove effective in treating disk-related spine pain but are much more invasive. In this technique, a probe is inserted intradiscal and the disk contents are reduced, thus reducing the pain associated with disk disease.

SPONDYLOLISTHESIS

The classification of spondylolisthesis as described by Witse, Newman, and McNab, includes six categories:[80]

Type I. Congenital/Dysplastic
Type II. Isthmic
Type III. Degenerative
Type IV. Traumatic
Type V. Pathologic
Type VI. Postsurgical

The most common levels of occurrence are L5–S1 (congenital and isthmic) and L4–L5 (degenerative). The grading of spondylolisthesis is from low grade I through high grade V. These grades are determined by the degree of anterior (anterolisthesis) or posterior (posterolisthesis) movement of the superior vertebrae in reference to the inferior vertebrae. A slip of up to 25% of the width of the inferior endplate by the superior vertebrae is grade I; 25% to 50% slippage is grade II; 50% to 75%, grade III; 75% to 100%, grade IV; and when the superior vertebrae slip entirely off of the inferior vertebrae (spondyloptosis),

TABLE 46-7 Epidural Injections

Indications	Pain Inflammation
Contraindications	In area of congenital anomaly or previous surgery If steriods may unmask an infection Hemorrhagic diathesis Local infection Medicine allergy (to solution being injected)

From Bogduk N, Aprill C, Derby R: Epidural steroid injections. In White AH, Schofferman JA, Goldstein M (eds): Spine Care Diagnosis and Conservative Treatment, vol 1. St. Louis, Mosby–Year Book, 1995.

TABLE 46-8 Advanced Pain Control Methods

Clinical Presentation	Treatment Techniques
Persistent radicular pain	Selective epidural cortisone injection Epidural cortisone injection Acupuncture
Facet joint synovitis and capsular pain	Facet joint cortisone injection
Muscle hypertonicity and trigger point sensitivity	Trigger point injection with local anesthetic Acupuncture
Cervicogenic headaches	Acupuncture Facet joint injection to symptomatic and relevant joints

From Saal J, Dillingham M: Nonoperative treatment and rehabilitation of disk, facet, and soft tissue injuries. In Nicholas J, Hershman E (eds): The Lower Extremity in Spine and Sport Medicine, 2nd ed. St. Louis, Mosby–Year Book, 1995.

grade V. Conservative treatment of this disorder is useful in low-grade slips (grades I and II). This includes lumbosacral flexion exercises, lumbar stabilization, and bracing. I have found that flexion exercises are not as successful in patients with spondylolisthesis who have increased slippage as seen by flexion views radiographically. This subtle sign of instability may exaggerate pain even though the lumbosacral flexion moment tends to unload the painful articular facets. Young people with grade I spondylolisthesis have a 78% success rate in terms of symptom resolution when treated conservatively. For advanced grades, treatment should include the use of a modified Boston brace (worn full-time for 6 months and then weaned over the subsequent 6 months).[56]

Often adult patients fair well when wearing lumbosacral corsets, with or without stays. Stabilization exercises with a flexion bias should be emphasized, because they have been shown to achieve better results in patients with spondylolisthesis.[62] Bracing is most successful when it promotes lumbar flexion and decreases the inherent lordosis. The braces that accomplish this are usually bulky, and many patients reject them. Also, the time commitment for wearing the brace is lengthy and involves most hours of the day. Low-profile designs are preferable but may not be successful in symptomatic relief.

To evaluate the efficacy of exercise protocols addressing the symptoms of spondylolisthesis, one study evaluated 48 patients with grade I slippage.[67] A comparison of lumbar flexion versus extension exercises was done. Flexion exercises consisted of abdominal strengthening, pelvic tilting, and chest-to-thigh positioning. Extension exercises consisted of prone lumbar and hip extension. At a three-year follow-up, 19% of the flexion group had moderate or severe pain as compared with 67% in the extension group. Also, 24% of the flexion group were unable to return to work compared to 61% in the extension group. In our experience, flexion exercises that include pelvic tilting in conjunction with lumbar flexion seem to give symptomatic pain relief. This may be due to unloading of the pars region, which may be the prime pain generator. There have been less successful results with lumbar extension exercises.

Muscle energy technique is also beneficial in this setting when the lumbosacral paraspinal muscles are treated. Through serial contractions, fatigue of the lumbar extensors can assist in unloading the posterior elements. Williams' flexion exercises help to unload the lumbar paraspinal region and strengthen the abdominal muscles. This series of exercises includes single and double knee-to-chest, straight leg raises, and sit-ups. It is recommended that any exercise program be performed at least three times a week and about 30 minutes per session be set aside to complete that day's exercises.

STENOSIS/SPONDYLOSIS

Stenosis and spondylosis (degenerative arthritis) are afflictions everyone fears, especially with advancing age. It must be stated clearly, however, that developing arthritis is not an automatic component of aging. Many elderly people are amazingly free of arthritis and, on the contrary, many younger people are very arthritic. The key to treating arthritis is to clearly diagnose and understand the ongoing pathophysiology. Simply stated, if we are discussing a purely degenerative process, the location of the changes can guide our therapy efforts. If there is a predominance of anterior degenerative changes, our goals are to unload this area by promoting extension exercises. Alternatively, if there is a predominance of posterior changes, our goals are to unload this area and promote flexion exercises. The addition of modalities such as warm packs, ultrasound, and electrical stimulation (applications discussed in a previous section) along with techniques such as muscle energy and soft tissue massage offer symptomatic relief.

Narcotics and nonsteroidal medications are used also (Table 46-9).[64] Recently, we began using individualized videotaping in treating arthritis. This allows us to generate feedback of a patient's biomechanical efficiency, which greatly assists in establishing specific training programs. A patient is initially videotaped performing activities of daily living. There is no coaching or prompting during this session. A standard video camera is sufficient to capture the maneuvers patients frequently perform, and analysis may be done on any standard tape-playing machine (Fig. 46-13). The purpose of the video is to capture the efficiencies and inefficiencies of the biomechanical actions associated with selected tasks. When they review the videotape, the patients usually are amazed. They don't believe they do it "that way." The ergonomic flaws of motion are easily seen.

The most consistent inefficient pattern occurs when a person tries to rise from a lying-down position. Most people "lurch" forward and thrust their bodies to achieve a sitting posture. This, as seen by videotape, is an ergonomically inefficient maneuver. Our goal is to make patients aware of this and, through exercise sessions, correct the inefficiencies. To accomplish this, we re-videotape the same tasks with guidance and prompting. The clinician and patient review both the "before" and the "after" actions and try to reinforce proper biomechanics. A series of exercises is then customized to specifically address the needs of the patient in improving ergonomic efficiency. This process is repeated on several follow-up visits to remind the patient of proper techniques. The results of this intervention have been rewarding. Although we are not addressing any specific pain generator or symptom focus, the overall ability of the patient to do more and walk further is viewed by many as successful treatment.

TABLE 46-9 Nonsteroidal Anti-Inflammatory Drugs: Dosing Suggestion

Generic Name	Brand Name	Starting Dose	Maximum Dose
Short half-life			
Aspirin	650 mg q6h	4000–6000 mg	
Flurbiprofen	Ansaid	50 mg q6h	3000 mg
Ibuprofen	Motrin	400 mg q6h	4200 mg
Ketoprofen	Orudis	50 mg q6–8h	300 mg
Intermediate half-life			
Choline salicylate	Trilisate	1500 mg once, then 1000 mg bid	4000 mg
Diflunisal	Dolobid	1000 mg once, then 500 mg bid	1500 mg
Diclofenac	Voltaren	50 mg q6–8h	225 mg
Etodolac	Lodine	400 mg once, then 200 mg q8h to 300 mg q12h	1200 mg
Nabumetone	Relafen	500 to 750 mg bid	2000 mg
Naproxen	Naprosyn	375 mg q8–12h	1250 mg
Sulindac	Clinoril	100 mg q12h	400 mg
Long half-life			
Piroxicam	Feldene	20 mg q24h	40 mg

From Schofferman JA: Use of medication for pain of spinal origin. In White AH, Schofferman JA, Goldstein M (eds): Spinal Care Diagnosis and Conservative Treatment, vol 1. St. Louis, Mosby–Year Book, 1995.

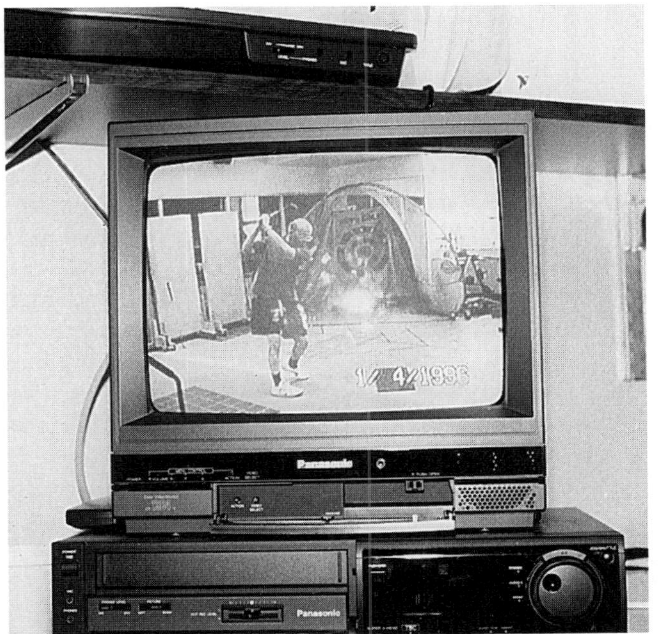

FIGURE 46-13. Video analysis. Ergonomic efficiency is evaluated by videotape to isolate particular deficiencies. These deficiencies are reviewed with the patient and serve as an excellent mechanism of biofeedback. Adjustments for deficiencies are easily accomplished when patients are directly involved in viewing the inefficiencies.

SACROILIAC DYSFUNCTION

A common cause of pain, often described as low back pain, actually arises from dysfunction of the sacroiliac joint. This often-forgotten joint probably plays a significant role in the low back pain scenario. Sacroiliac pathology has been underestimated as a cause of back or sciatic-type pain.[6,18,21,54,65] Very often patients complaining of low back pain point to the posterior superior iliac spine. Sacroiliac pain has been shown to occur in the groin as well as the buttock and posterior proximal thigh.[25,26]

There has been debate for several years as to the role of the sacroiliac joint as a pain generator.[50] The increased interest in sacroiliac pain may be due to advances in spinal imaging techniques, which assist physicians in eliminating pathologic conditions of the disks or canals.[56] Also, evidence does support motion in this unique synovial joint.[78] Treatments for dysfunction of this joint include manual techniques, injection, stabilization, prolotherapy, and muscle energy. Manual medicine has been used by a variety of practitioners offering a myriad of techniques. All have the common goal of restoring normal mechanics to the region. Cassidy and associates reported 90% success in the manipulation of the sacroiliac region.[13]

When provocative injections (usually fluoroscopically guided) reproduce similar pain, infusion of the joint with a combination of water-soluble steroid and anesthetic agent may be effective.[6] In one series, 72 patients underwent sacroiliac (SI) joint injection and achieved 81% successful pain relief at 9 months.[7] Stabilization of the sacroiliac joint is also somewhat successful. Use of one of a variety of sacroiliac belts that are commercially available is recommended. Another technique for treating sacroiliac dysfunction aims to stabilize the joint. By injecting a proliferant solution (one that is said to proliferate collagen-like tissue), unstable joints can be stabilized. Prolotherapy is a technique whereby a hypertonic solution is injected into an area of ligament or tendon insertion onto a bony structure. This agent is said to promote proliferation of collagen-like tissue that acts to stabilize a hypermobile joint. There are two commonly used proliferants. The first consists of 4 ml D50, 2 ml 2% lidocaine, and 6 ml of bacteriostatic water. The second consists of 2.5% phenol, 25% glucose, 25% glycerin, and pyrogen-free water. This solution is then diluted 50% with 0.5% lidocaine. A 0.5 to 0.75 ml solution is injected at each site.[55]

The clinician should be very familiar with the technique of prolotherapy before attempting it, and readings beyond the scope of this text are recommended. Proponents claim very successful results for this technique with spine-related disorders. Muscle energy techniques are useful in treating sacroiliac dysfunction. They act to relax the lumbosacral extensor muscles and to promote symmetric sacroiliac motion. When the physical examination of the sacroiliac joint suggests decreased motion on forward-bending tests, muscle energy techniques are geared toward freeing the restricted joint. To assess sacroiliac motion, the patient stands with his or her feet comfortably separated. The examiner's thumbs are then placed under the posterior and superior iliac spines while the other digits circle the respective iliac crests. The patient is then instructed to bend forward at the waist while the clinician monitors the posterior superior iliac spines for motion. The side that tends to rise superiorly on the forward-bend is thought to be the side of pathology. This is a general guide to establishing the side of sacroiliac dysfunction. It is only a screen, and a complete sacroiliac examination should be done before initiating specific therapies.

SCOLIOSIS

The conservative treatment of scoliosis stresses postural corrections of deformities to limit visceral compromise. There are many schools of thought as to the most appropriate timing for and application of conservative versus surgical intervention in scoliosis. A general guideline is to attempt conservative exercises for curves less than 20°, bracing for curves between 20° and 40°, and surgical intervention for curves greater than 40°. Exercises should be of the lateral-bending rotational type. The direction of strengthening should promote reduction of the scoliotic curve. If bracing is warranted, body jacket–type orthoses are required, and these must be worn for 23 hours a day. An example of such is the Milwaukee brace.

CONCLUSION

Diagnosing and treating spine-related disorders remains a challenge, even for the most experienced clinician. However, if a step-wise approach is used to properly diagnose a spinal condition, a wide array of treatment options are available to conservatively manage these patients.

REFERENCES

1. US Department of Health and Human Services: Acute Low Back Problems in Adults, Clinical Practice Guidelines. Washington, DC, Agency for Health Care Policy and Research (AHCPR), 1994.
2. Andersen KH, Mosdal C: Epidural application of cortico-steroids in low back pain and sciatica. Acta Neurochir 87:52, 1987.
3. April C, Dwyer A, Bogduk N: Cervical zygapophyseal joint pain patterns. A clinical evaluation. Spine 15(6):458, 1990.
4. Benzon HT: Epidural steroid injection for low back pain and lumbosacral radiculopathy. Pain 24: 277–295, 1986.
5. Berman AT, Garbarinbo JL, Fisher SM, Bosacco SJ: The effects of epidural injection of local anesthetics and cortico-steroids on patients with lumbosacral pain. Clin Orthop 188:144, 1984.
6. Bernard TN Jr, Kirkaldy-Willis WH: Recognizing specific characteristics of nonspecific low back pain. Clin Orthop Rel Res 217:266–280, 1987.
7. Bernard TN, Cassidy JD: The sacroiliac joint syndrome. Pathophysiology, diagnosis, and management. In Frymoyer JW (ed): The Adult Spine: Principles and Practice. New York, Raven Press, 1991.
8. Biewen PC: Injection therapy for treatment of low back pain. J Back Musculoskeletal Rehab 1(3): 17–28, 1991.
9. Bogduk N, April C, Derby R: Epidural steroid injections. In White AH, Schofferman JA, Goldstein M (eds): Spine Care Diagnosis and Conservative Treatment. St. Louis, Mosby-Year Book, 1995, pp 327–328.
10. Bullard JR, Houghton FM: Epidural treatment of acute herniated nucleus pulposis. Anesth Analge Curr Res 56:862, 1977.
11. Burn JMB, Langdon L: Lumbar epidural injection for the treatment of chronic sciatica. Rheum Phys Med 10:368, 1970.

12. Bush K, Hillier SA: Controlled study of caudal epidural injections of triamcinolone plus procaine for the management of intractable sciatica. Spine 16:572, 1991.
13. Cassidy JD, Kirkaldy-Willis WH, MacGregor M: Spinal manipulation for the treatment of chronic low back and leg pain. An observational study. In Burger AA, Greenman PE (eds): Empirical Approaches to the Validation of Spinal Manipulation. Springfield, IL, Charles C. Thomas.
14. Chila AG, Jeffries RR, Levin SM: Is manipulation for your practice? Patient Care 77–92, May 1990.
15. Cirullo JA: Orthopaedic Physical Therapy Clinics of North America. Philadelphia, WB Saunders.
16. Colachis SC, Strohm BR: Cervical traction: Relationship of traction time to a varied tractive force with constant angle of pull. Arch Phys Med Rehab 46:815–819, 1965.
17. Colachis SC, Strohm BR: Effect of duration on intermittent cervical traction on vertebral separation. Arch Phys Med Rehab 47:353–359, 1966.
18. Dawn WJ: The sacroiliac joint: An underappreciated pain generator. Am J Orthop 24(6):475, 1995.
19. Deyo RA, Walsh NE, Martin DC, et al: A controlled trial of transcutaneous electrical nerve stimulation (TENS) and exercises for chronic low back pain. N Eng J Med 322(23):1627–1637, 1990.
20. Deyo, RA, Loeser JD, Bigos SJ. Herniated lumbar intervertebral disk. Ann Intern Med 112:598–603, 1990.
21. Don Tigny RL: Function and pathomechanics of the sacroiliac joint. A review. Phys Ther 65(1):35–44, 1985.
22. Dworken GE: Advanced concepts in interventional spine care. J Am Osteopath Assoc 102(9 Suppl 3): S8–S11, 2002.
23. Esses SI: Textbook of Spinal Disorders. Philadelphia, JB Lippincott, 1995.
24. Evans W: Intrasacral epidural injection in the treatment of sciatica. Lancet 2:1225–1227, 1930.
25. Fortin JD, Dwyer AP, West S: Sacroiliac joint: Pain referral maps in proceedings of the North American Spine Society, Boston paper No. 78 Boston, 1992.
26. Freiberg AH, Vinckle TH: Sciatica and the sacroiliac joint. J Bone Joint Surg 16:126–136, 1934.
27. Frymoyer JW, Cats Baril WL: An overview of the incidence and costs of low back pain. Orthop Clin N Am 22:263, 1991.
28. Geiringer SR, Kincaid BK, Rechtien JS: Traction, manipulation, and massage. In DeLisa JA (ed): Rehabilitation Medicine Principles and Practice. Philadelphia, JB Lippincott, 1988.
29. Greenman PE: Principles of Manual Medicine. Baltimore, Williams and Wilkins, 1989.
30. Hadler NM, Curtis P, Gillings DB: A benefit of spinal manipulation as adjunctive therapy for low back pain: A stratified controlled study. Spine 12(7): 703–706, 1987.
31. Hall H: Examination of the patient with low back pain. Bull Rheum Diseases 33(4), 1983.
32. Habtermariam A, Gronblad M, Virri J, et al: Immunocytochemical localization of immunoglobulins in disc herniations. Spine 21(16):1864–1869, 1996.
33. Hickey RF: Outpatient epidural steroid injections for low back pain and lumbosacral radiculopathy. NZ Med J 100:594, 1987.
34. Higgins JR: Human Movement: An Integrated Approach. St. Louis, Mosby-Year Book, 1977.
35. Ingber RS: Iliopsoas myofascial dysfunction: A treatable cause of "failed" low back syndrome. Arch Phys Med Rehab 70:382–384, 1989.
36. Jacobs S, Pullan PT, Potter JM, Shenfield GM: Adrenal suppression following extradural steroids. Anesthesia 38:953, 1983.
37. Janse J: History of the development of chiropractic concepts: Chiropractic terminology. In Goldstein M (ed): The Research Status of Spinal Manipulation. NINCDC Monograph No. 5 DHEW Publication No. (NIH) 76–998, 1975.
38. Jones LH: Strain and Counterstrain. Colorado Springs, CO, American Academy of Osteopathy, 1981.
39. Judovich BD: Herniated cervical disk: A new form of traction therapy. Am J Surg 84:646–656, 1952.
40. Kahn J: Principles and Practice of Electrotherapy. New York, Churchill Livingstone, 1987.
41. KiKuchi S, Have M, Nishqyama K, Ito T: Anatomic and clinical studies of radicular symptoms. Spine 9:23–30, 1984.
42. Kwan O, Fiel J: Critical appraisal of facet joint injections for chronic whiplash. Med Sci Monit 8(8):191–195, 2002.
43. Lewinnek GE, Warfield LA: Facet degeneration as a cause of low back pain. Clin Orthop 213: 216–222, 1986.
44. Lutz GE, Vad VB, Wisneski RJ: Fluoroscopic transforaminal lumbar epidural steroids: An outcome study. Arch Phys Med Rehab 79:1362–1369, 1998.
45. McKenzie R: Treat Your Own Neck. Spinal Publication, Waikanae, New Zealand, 1983.
46. Meade TW, Dyers S, Browne W, et al: Low back pain of mechanical origin: Randomized comparison of chiropractic and hospital outpatient treatment. Brit Med J 300(6737):1431–1436, 1990.
47. Melzak R: Acupuncture and related forms of folk medicine. In Wall PD, Melzak R (eds): Textbook of Pain. New York, Churchill Livingston, 1984.
48. Melzak R, Stillwell DM, Fox ET: Trigger points and acupuncture points for pain: Correlation and implications. Pain 3:3–23, 1977.
49. Michlovitz SL: Thermal Agents in Rehabilitation. Philadelphia, FA Davis, 1986.

50. Mooney V: Understanding, examining for, and treating sacroiliac pain. J Musculoskeletal Med 37–49, July 1993.
51. Mooney V, Saal JA, Saal JS: Evaluation and treatment of low back pain. Clinical Symposium 48(4): 1–32, 1990.
52. Nachemson A: Work for all. Clin Orth Rel Res 179:77–82, 1983.
53. Nygaard OP, Mellgren SI, Osterud B: The inflammatory properties of contained and non-contained lumbar disc herniation. Spine 22:2484–2488, 1997.
54. Pace JB, Nagle D: Piriformis syndrome. West J Med 124:435–439, 1976.
55. Reeves KD: Technique of prolotherapy. In Lennard TA (ed): Physiatric Procedures in Clinical Practice. St. Louis, Mosby-Year Book, 1995.
56. Reynolds JB, Slosar PJ: Spondylolisthesis: Isthmic, congenital, traumatic, and post surgical. In White AH, Schofferman JA (eds): Spine Care Diagnosis and Conservative Treatment. St. Louis, Mosby-Year Book, 1995, p 1285.
57. Riew KD, YinY, Gilula L, et al: Can nerve root injections obviate the need for operative treatment of lumbar radicular pain? A prospective, randomized, controlled, double-blinded study. NASS Proceedings; Annual Meeting, 1999, pp 94–95.
58. Rosen CD, Kahanovitz N, Bernstein R, Viola K: A retrospective analysis of the efficacy of epidural steroid injections. Clin Orthop 228:270–272, 1988.
59. Saal JS: The role of inflammation in the lumbar spine. In Physical Medicine and Rehabilitation: State of the Art Reviews. Neck and Back Pain, vol 4. Philadelphia, Hanley & Belfus, 1990.
60. Saal JS: High levels of inflammatory phospholipase activity in lumbar disc herniations. Spine 15(7): 674, 1990.
61. Saal JS: Human disc PLA2 induces neural injury: A histomorphic study. Poster presentation at the Annual Meeting of Orthopaedic Research Society, 1993, San Francisco, CA.
62. Saal J, Dillingham M: Nonoperative treatment and rehabilitation of disk, facet, and soft tissue injuries. In Nicholas J, Hershman E (eds): The Lower Extremity in Spine and Sport Medicine, 2nd ed. St. Louis, Mosby-Year Book, 1995.
63. Saal JA, Saal JS: Nonoperative treatment of herniated lumbar intervertebral disc with radiculopathy: An outcome study. Spine 14(4):435, 1989.
64. Schofferman JA: Use of medication for pain of spinal origin. In White AH, Schofferman JA (eds): Spinal Care Diagnosis and Conservative Treatment. St. Louis, Mosby-Year Book, 1995, p 519.
65. Schuchmann JA, Cannon CL: Sacroiliac strain syndrome: Diagnosis and treatment. Texas Med 82: 33–36, 1986.
66. Shekelle P, et al: Comparing the costs between provider types of episodes of back pain care. Spine 20:221–227, 1995.
67. Sinaki M, Lutness MP, Ilstrup DM, Chu CP, Gramse RR: Lumbar spondylolisthesis: A retrospective comparison and three year follow-up of two conservative treatment programs. Arch Phys Med Rehab 70:594–598, 1989.
68. Slipman CW, Chow DW: Therapeutic spinal corticosteroid injections for the management of radiculopathies. Phys Med Rehab Clin N Amer 13(3):697–711, 2002.
69. Slipman, CW, et al: Fluoroscopically guided therapeutic sacroiliac joint injections for sacroiliac joint syndrome. Am J Phys Med Rehab 80(6): 425–432, 2001.
70. Snoek W, Weber H, Jorgensen B: Double blind evaluation of extradural methylprednisone for herniated discs. Acta Orthop Scand 48:635–637, 1977.
71. Sweeny T, et al: Cervicothoracic muscular stabilization techniques. In Physical Medicine and Rehabilitation: State of the Art Reviews 4(2):335. Philadelphia, Hanley & Belfus, 1990.
72. Takeshi T, Kouzaburou F, Kuramachi E: Selective lumbosacral radiculopathy and block. Spine 5: 68–77, 1980.
73. Tanigawa MC: Comparison of the hold relax procedure in passive mobilization on increasing muscle length. Phys Ther 32:725–735, 1972.
74. Travell J, Simons D: Low back pain. Post Grad Med 73:2, 1983.
75. Vad VB, Bhat AL, Lutz GE, Cammisa F, Transforaminal epidural steroid injections in lumbosacral radiculopathy: A prospective, randomized study. Spine 27(1):11–16, 2002.
76. Vallfors B: Acute, sub-acute, and chronic low back pain: Clinical symptoms, absenteeism, and working environment. Scand J Rehab Med 11:1–98, 1985.
77. Walsh, et al: Treatment of the patient with chronic pain. In DeLisa J (ed): Rehabilitation Medicine: Principles and Practice. Philadelphia, JB Lippincott, 1993.
78. Weisl H: The movements of the sacroiliac joints, Acta Anatomica 23:80–91, 1955.
79. White AM: Injection techniques for the diagnosis and treatment of low back pain. Orthop Clin N Am 14:553–567, 1983.
80. Witse LL, Newman PH, McNab I: Classification of spondylolysis and spondylolisthesis. Clin Orthop 117:23, 1976.
81. Zohn DA: The quadratus lumborum: An unrecognized source of back pain, clinical and thermographic aspects. Orthop Rev 14(3):163, 1985.

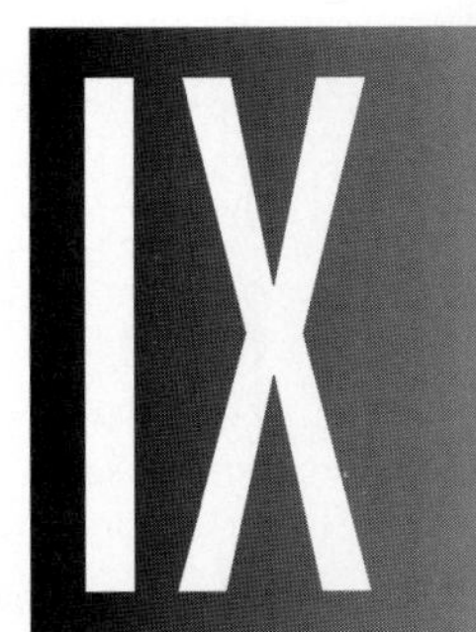

General Information

47 Nutrition

Jacqueline R. Berning

Athletes who eagerly accept high-technology workouts and equipment also need to recognize the importance of diet in enhancing performance quickly, easily, and dramatically. Indeed, no amount of motivation, training, or natural ability will ensure success without proper fuel for the engine. Yet despite the wealth of knowledge regarding nutrition and the specific metabolic needs of the human body in training, not all athletes, coaches, or even dietitians and physicians have bridged the gap between laboratory and clinical research and the practical application of these findings. In today's athletic world of digitizing and rapid rehabilitation, the concern is not only on improving performance but also on using diet and nutrition to maintain an athlete's long-term health for the prevention of injury and illness.

DIETARY HABITS OF ATHLETES

To understand the food consumption habits of athletes, we need to look at the general population. Athletes may be winning gold medals and breaking world records, but many have the same dietary habits as their sedentary counterparts. In general, many eat too much fat and protein at the expense of carbohydrates and fiber. Numerous surveys have shown that the food consumption practices of both male and female athletes are proportionally very similar to the national averages, except for total kilocalorie intake. Recent surveys[3,43] of elite adolescent swimmers revealed that, like other typical Americans, they consumed more fat than carbohydrates in their diets. Furthermore, when they were given a nutrition knowledge test, they did very well on basic nutrition knowledge (of the four food groups) but poorly when it came to choosing foods that were high in a specific nutrient. For example, when swimmers were asked to name a nutritious carbohydrate, in a multiple-choice format, 62% chose an apple, but 38% chose french fries. When asked which food is a good source of protein, 63% chose the correct answer of chicken, but 37% chose oatmeal.

In another survey,[9] of competitive swimmers ages 13 to 20, several misconceptions were reported. For example, over half of them believed that everyone should take supplements, that vitamin E improves performance, B complex vitamins provide energy, and milk consumed the day of competition impairs performance. In a study[36] of male track, baseball, and football teams, only 28% could define *glycogen loading*, 69% did not know which foods were good sources of carbohydrates, and 54% did not know the major functions of vitamins. A nutrition knowledge questionnaire completed by adolescent gymnasts showed that over 50% of the girls could not define the term *complex carbohydrate* and did not know that carbohydrates were an important source of energy for exercise.[30] Instead, 75% of the girls erroneously believed that protein was the best source of energy.

Volleyball players had difficulty with questions on food sources of quality protein and vitamin C, and good sources of energy, carbohydrate loading, and caloric requirements for training.[33] However, they were knowledgeable about the importance of eating a wide variety of foods, vitamin supplements, and the differences between plant oils and animal fats. These findings suggest that most athletes are unable to select the proper balance of foods necessary for the energy demands of their sports. If athletes cannot make informed food choices, they cannot be expected to select a proper diet that is required for peak performance.

DIETARY RECOMMENDATIONS FOR ATHLETES

An athlete's energy and nutrient requirements vary with weight, height, age, sex, and metabolic rate, and with the type, intensity, frequency, and duration of training. The emotional and physical stress of training and competition, combined with hectic travel schedules, also affects intake. As a result, adequate calories and essential nutrients must be planned carefully to meet nutritional requirements for training and health. Depending on the training regimen, athletes need to consume at least 50%, but ideally 60% to 70% of their total calories from carbohydrate. The remaining calories should be obtained from protein (10% to 15%) and fat (20% to 30%). Calories and nutrients should come from a wide variety of foods on a daily basis. The food guide pyramid is an excellent nutrition education tool to teach athletes how to make wise food choices. The food guide pyramid, along with the number of recommended daily servings, is presented in Figure 47-1.

CARBOHYDRATES: FUEL FOR EXERCISE

Carbohydrates provide fuel for the exercising muscles and for the central nervous system. The use of carbohydrates by the skeletal muscles of the body depends on the

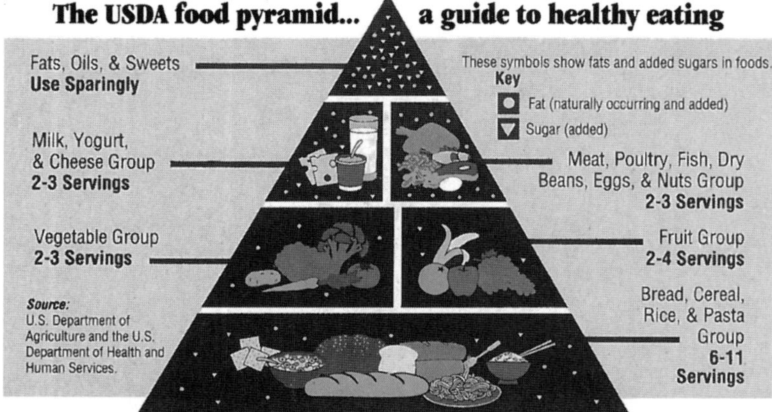

FIGURE 47-1. Food guide pyramid.

TRAINING DIET BASED OFF THE FOOD GUIDE PYRAMID

	2800 CALORIES	3300 CALORIES
MILK	4 OR MORE	4 OR MORE
MEAT	3 OR MORE	3 OR MORE
VEGE	6 OR MORE	8 OR MORE
FRUIT	4 OR MORE	6 OR MORE
GRAIN	16 OR MORE	18 OR MORE

availability of endogenous energy sources and on the intensity and duration of exercise.

Carbohydrate Oxidation

Intensity and duration of exercise have opposite effects on carbohydrate utilization. The portion of energy coming from carbohydrate oxidation increases with the intensity of exercise, whereas it progressively decreases when exercise is prolonged (Fig. 47-2). Training status also can influence the composition of the fuel being oxidized. Indeed, the proportion of carbohydrate being burned is lower in exercise-trained than in untrained individuals at rest.[42] Endurance training increases the capacity of the aerobic pathway in the mitochondria to break down fat for energy. When more fat is burned, less muscle glycogen is used. This glycogen-sparing effect of fat utilization is advantageous during prolonged exercise because muscle glycogen depletion limits performance. Endurance training also increases the capacity of the muscles to store glycogen. Thus endurance training confers a dual performance advantage: the muscle glycogen stores are higher at the onset of exercise, and the athlete depletes them at a slower rate.

Diet composition also can significantly affect the mixture of fuel being oxidized during exercise. If the diet is high in carbohydrate, the athlete will use more glycogen as fuel. Although the goal is to increase the availability of fat as fuel through endurance training, this does not mean that athletes should eat a high-fat diet. Even the leanest athletes store more fat than they will ever need during exercise.

A high-fat diet compromises carbohydrate intake, which lowers muscle glycogen stores and reduces the ability of an athlete to sustain high-intensity exercise.[37] Low muscle glycogen stores also can limit endurance. Thus the ideal diet to ensure optimal muscle glycogen stores supplies less than 30% of total calories as fat and 60% to 70% as carbohydrates.

CARBOHYDRATES AND TRAINING

During endurance exercise that exceeds 90 minutes, such as marathon running, muscle glycogen stores become progressively lower. When they drop to critically low levels, high-intensity exercise cannot be maintained. In practical terms, the athlete is exhausted and must either stop exercising or drastically reduce the pace of exercise. Glycogen depletion may be a gradual process, occurring over repeated days of heavy training, in which muscle glycogen breakdown exceeds its replacement. This also can happen during high-intensity exercise that is repeated several times during competition or training. For example, a distance runner who averages 10 miles a day but doesn't take the time to consume enough carbohydrates in his diet, or the swimmer who completes

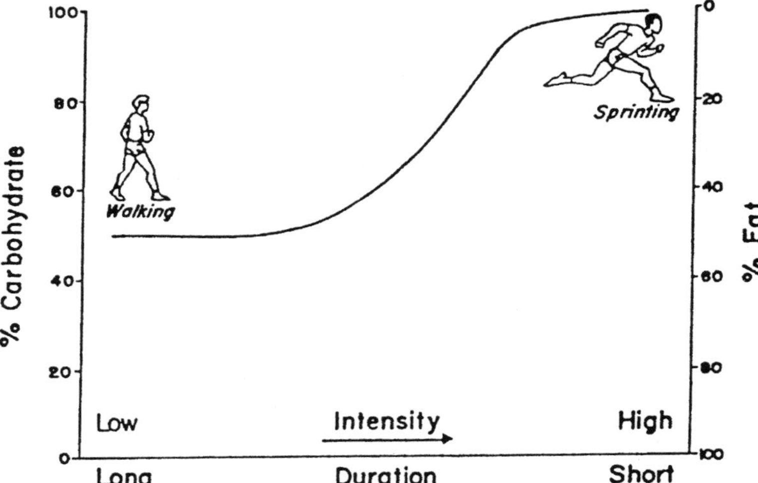

FIGURE 47-2. As exercise intensity increases and duration decreases, the prominent food fuel shifts toward carbohydrates. (From Matthew and Fox: Sports Physiology. Philadelphia, WB Saunders, 1979.)

several interval sets at above her maximal oxygen consumption can both deplete glycogen stores rapidly.

Training Glycogen Depletion

Costill[11] compared glycogen synthesis on a 40% carbohydrate diet to that on a 70% carbohydrate diet during repeated days of 2-hour workouts. On the low-carbohydrate diet, the muscle glycogen stores dropped lower with each successive day of training. After several days of the diet and exercise regimen, the athletes had low muscle glycogen stores and could not exercise at even a moderate intensity. The high-carbohydrate diet provided nearly maximal repletion of the muscle glycogen stores after the strenuous training. The high-carbohydrate diet provided the athletes with muscle glycogen values that remained above 100 mmol/kg, and they were able to continue the heavy training (Fig. 47-3). This study suggests that athletes who fail to consume enough carbohydrates on a daily basis while training will possibly decrease endurance as well as exercise performance. It is suggested that athletes in heavy training should consume a carbohydrate intake of 7 to 10 grams per kilogram of body weight per day to help prevent daily carbohydrate depletion.

Types of Carbohydrate

The type of carbohydrate is another nutritional factor that has been considered to potentially affect carbohydrate metabolism. Unfortunately, research has not provided clear guidance on the issue. One study by Costill et al.[13] compared the effects of simple- and complex-carbohydrate consumption during a 48-hour period after a glycogen-depleting exercise. During the first 24 hours, no differences were found in muscle glycogen synthesis between the two types of carbohydrates; however, at

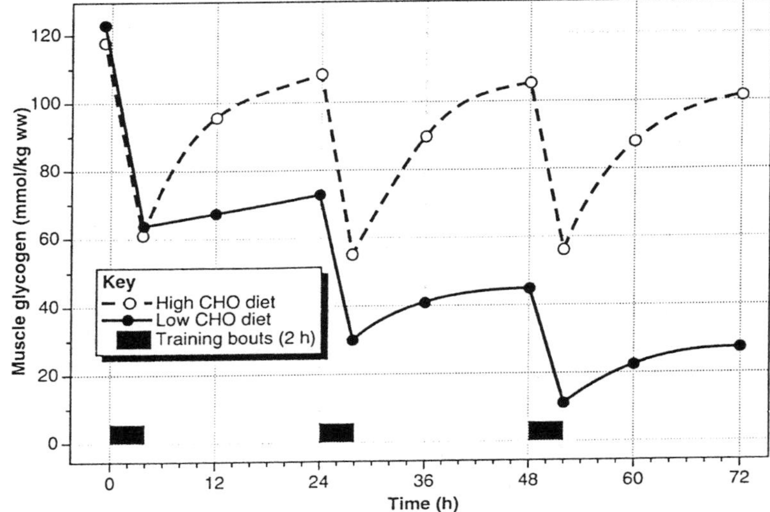

FIGURE 47-3. Muscle glycogen gradually declines when daily running is undertaken while consuming a low-carbohydrate diet. A high-carbohydrate diet allows for daily recovery of muscle glycogen.

48 hours the complex carbohydrates resulted in significantly greater muscle glycogen synthesis than the simple carbohydrates. Recently, Kiens et al.[27] reported that increases in muscle glycogen content were significantly greater during the first six hours after exercise following the intake of simple rather than complex carbohydrates, and that plasma insulin levels were greater following the intake of simple carbohydrates.

Glycemic Index

Coyle[14] and Hargreaves[21] have suggested that part of this conflict over which type of carbohydrate is better may be cleared up if the carbohydrate is considered to be based on its physiologic reaction in the body rather than its structure. They have suggested that carbohydrate foods should be classified according to glycemic index. The glycemic index represents the ratio of the area under the blood glucose curve resulting from the ingestion of a given quantity of carbohydrate food and the area under the glucose curve resulting from the ingestion of the same quantity of white bread.[26] Coyle and Hargreaves recommend that carbohydrates with a moderate to high glycemic index should be consumed after exercise. Indeed, preliminary work by Burke et al.[5] has demonstrated that a diet based on high glycemic index carbohydrate foods promoted greater glycogen storage in 24 hours of recovery after strenuous exercise than an equal amount of carbohydrate eaten in the form of low glycemic index foods. The box Glycemic Index of Various Foods lists foods that are carbohydrate-rich and their respective glycemic indexes.

CHECKLIST

Glycemic Index of Various Foods

High glycemic foods (above 85)
- ☐ Honey, corn syrup
- ☐ Bagels, white bread
- ☐ Cornflakes
- ☐ Raisins
- ☐ Potato (baked, boiled, or mashed)
- ☐ Sweet corn

Moderate glycemic foods (60 to 85)
- ☐ Spaghetti, macaroni
- ☐ Oatmeal
- ☐ Bananas, grapes, oranges
- ☐ Rice
- ☐ Yams
- ☐ Baked beans

Low glycemic foods (less than 60)
- ☐ Apples, applesauce
- ☐ Cherries, dates, figs, peaches, pears, plums
- ☐ Kidney beans, chickpeas, green peas, navy beans, red lentils
- ☐ Whole milk, skim milk, plain yogurt

CARBOHYDRATE INTAKE BEFORE, DURING, AND AFTER EXERCISE

Preexercise Meal

The preevent or pretraining meal serves two purposes. These include keeping the athlete from feeling hungry before and during the exercise bout, and maintaining optimal levels of blood glucose for the exercising muscles during training and competition.

Athletes often train early in the morning without eating. This overnight fast lowers liver glycogen stores and can impair performance, particularly if the exercise regimen involves endurance training.

Carbohydrate feedings before exercise can help restore suboptimal liver glycogen stores, which may be called on during prolonged training and competition. While allowing for personal preferences and psychological factors, the preevent meal should be high in carbohydrates, nongreasy, and readily digested. High-fat, high-protein foods such as steaks, hamburgers, eggs, and hot dogs should be avoided or limited in the preevent meal because fat slows gastric emptying time. Exercising with a full stomach also may cause indigestion, nausea, and possibly vomiting.

How much carbohydrate should the athlete consume in the precompetition meal? Current research suggests that 1 to 4 grams of carbohydrate per kilogram of body weight should be consumed 1 to 4 hours before exercise.[35] To avoid gastrointestinal distress, the carbohydrate content of the meal should be reduced according to how long before exercise it is consumed. For example, it is suggested that 4 hours before the event the athlete consume 4 grams of carbohydrates per kilogram of body weight, whereas 1 hour before the competition the athlete would consume 1 gram of carbohydrate per kilogram of body weight. Table 47-1 lists food examples for preevent meals.

Consuming Sugar before Exercise

Fifteen years ago, Costill et al.[12] suggested that preexercise glucose intake could be associated with hypoglycemia and increased muscle glycogen utilization during exercise. A recent study[22] contradicts this earlier finding. Cyclists consumed 75 grams of glucose or water 45 minutes before cycling to exhaustion. Although the sugar feedings caused high blood insulin and low blood glucose levels, there were no differences in the exercise time to exhaustion between the two trials. Does this mean that endurance athletes should load up on soft drinks and candy before their events? Comparison of the results of the old and new studies suggest that individuals differ in susceptibility to a lowering of blood glucose during exercise. The physiologic and biochemical basis for this difference has not been determined. At this time, therefore, athletes should be advised that consuming

TABLE 47-1

Examples of Preevent Meals and Recommended Carbohydrate Intake Based on Body Weight and Length of Time Before Competition

Body Weight	Carbohydrate Intake Recommendation	Foods to Meet
120 lbs (54.5 kg)	54 grams (1 hour before the event)	2 slices of toast, 1tbsp jam, 8 oz skim milk
	163 grams (3 hours before the event)	2 slices of toast, 2tbsp jam, 8 oz nonfat yogurt, 1/4 cup Grapenuts, 8 oz orange juice
190 lbs (86.4 kg)	86 grams (1 hour before the event)	2 slices of toast, 1 tbsp jam, 8 oz skim milk, 8 oz orange juice
	259 grams (3 hours before the event)	2 English muffins, 3 tbsp jam, 2 c oatmeal, 1 tbsp honey, 1 banana, 8 oz skim milk, 8 oz orange juice

Fatty foods such as potato chips, doughnuts, french fries, and pastries take longer to digest and provide little energy during exercise. Protein foods that are likely to contain high amounts of fat (peanut butter, cheese, and high-fat meats like bacon and ribs) are also more slowly digested. Eating foods high in fat and protein and low in carbohydrate can actually diminish athletic performance. For this reason, it is recommended that athletes eat high-carbohydrate foods like pasta, cereals, bagels, whole grains, fruits, and vegetables.

sugar 30 to 45 minutes before exercise could harm their performance if they are sensitive to a lowering of their blood glucose levels.

Carbohydrate Intake during Exercise

Carbohydrate feedings during endurance exercise lasting longer that 60 minutes may enhance endurance by providing glucose for the muscles to use when their glycogen stores have dropped to low levels.

The liver generally supplies glucose to maintain blood sugar levels for proper functioning of the central nervous system. As the muscles run out of glycogen, they will begin to take up some of the blood glucose, placing a drain on the liver glycogen stores. The longer the exercise session, the greater the utilization of blood glucose by the muscles for energy (Fig. 47-4). Although supplies of blood glucose can be drawn from liver glycogen, muscle glycogen stays in the muscle and cannot provide glucose for the blood. When the liver glycogen is depleted, blood glucose drops. A few athletes will experience central nervous symptoms typical of hypoglycemia (dizziness, nausea, confusion, and partial blackout), but most will note local muscular fatigue and will have to reduce their exercise intensity.

The improved performance associated with carbohydrate feedings probably results from the maintenance of blood glucose levels. The dietary carbohydrate supplies glucose for the muscles at a time when their glycogen stores are diminished. Thus, carbohydrate utilization (and therefore ATP production) can continue at a high rate, and endurance is enhanced.

Fatigue is not prevented by carbohydrate feeding; it is simply delayed. During the final portions of exercise, when muscle glycogen is low and athletes rely on blood glucose for energy, their muscles feel heavy and they must concentrate to maintain exercise at intensities that are ordinarily not stressful when muscle glycogen stores are filled.

How much carbohydrate should an athlete consume during exercise to improve endurance? The available

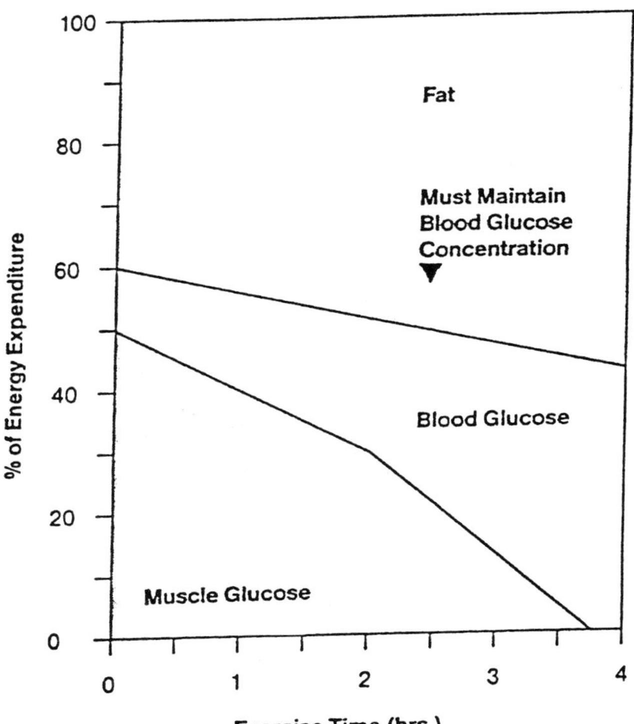

FIGURE 47-4. Sources of energy during prolonged cycling at 70% of maximal oxygen uptake. It is important to maintain blood glucose for prolonged exercise because it becomes the primary source of carbohydrate around the 2- to 2½-hour mark. (From Coyle EF: Carbohydrates and athletic performance. Gatorade sports science exchange 1(7), Oct. 1988.)

evidence suggests that athletes should take in 25 to 30 grams of carbohydrate every 30 minutes.[16,15] This amount can be obtained through either carbohydrate-rich foods or fluids. Drinking 8 ounces of a sports drink containing 6% to 7% carbohydrate every 15 minutes provides this amount of carbohydrate and also aids in hydration.

Carbohydrates after Exercise

On an average, only 5% of the muscle glycogen used during exercise is resynthesized each hour following exercise. Accordingly, at least 20 hours are required for complete restoration after exhaustive exercise, provided approximately 600 grams of carbohydrate are consumed. Ivy et al.[25] studied glycogen repletion following exercise. When 2 grams of carbohydrate per kilogram was consumed immediately after exercise, muscle glycogen synthesis was 15 mmol/kg. When the carbohydrate feeding was delayed for 2 hours after exercise, muscle glycogen synthesis was cut by 66% to 5 mmol/kg. By 4 hours after exercise, total muscle glycogen synthesis for the delayed feeding was still 45% slower than for the feeding given immediately after exercise.

This means that delaying carbohydrate intake for too long after exercise will reduce muscle glycogen and that glycogen resynthesis can be elevated when carbohydrates are consumed immediately after exercise. The current recommendations are to consume around 100 grams of carbohydrate within a 30-minute window postexercise to maximize muscle glycogen synthesis. Many athletes find it difficult to consume food immediately after exercise. Usually when body or core temperature is elevated, appetite is depressed and it becomes difficult to consume carbohydrate-rich foods. Many athletes find it easier and simpler to drink their carbohydrates than to eat them. A sports drink rich in carbohydrates after a hard practice will not only provide the necessary carbohydrates for glycogen synthesis but also help with hydration.

Zawadski and colleagues[45] followed up on the Ivy study and found that not only does consuming carbohydrates immediately after exercise help restore muscle glycogen stores faster, but adding protein with the 100 grams of carbohydrate will increase the glycogen resynthesis rate. It appears that this amount of protein with the 100 grams of carbohydrate elicits a greater insulin response and therefore activates glycogen synthase, the enzyme responsible for glycogen storage. The box Foods That Contain 100 Grams of Carbohydrate and Protein lists some examples of foods that contain about 100 grams of carbohydrate and protein that could be used immediately after exercise.

CHECKLIST

Foods That Contain 100 Grams of Carbohydrate and Protein

Consumption of the following foods increases muscle glycogen synthesis:

- ☐ One bagel with peanut butter and ⅔ cup raisins
- ☐ One cup of low-fat yogurt, one banana, and a cup of orange juice
- ☐ One turkey sandwich on whole-wheat bread with a cup of applesauce
- ☐ Spaghetti with meat sauce and garlic bread
- ☐ Eight ounces of skim milk, one apple, one orange, two slices of bread, and three pancakes
- ☐ Twelve ounces of a carbohydrate-loading drink and a bagel

PROTEIN

Proteins are a group of structural and regulatory molecules, each made up of a specific combination of 20 different amino acids. Eight of these amino acids cannot be synthesized in the body and therefore must be supplied by the diet if body proteins are to be synthesized. Generally, dietary intake of most athletes exceeds even the highest recommendation.

Because protein, especially the branched-chain amino acid leucine, is used as a metabolic fuel during exercise, much controversy surrounds the need for protein in exercising individuals.[6,29] There are now sufficient data to suggest that protein requirements do vary with the type and intensity of exercise performed and the total energy consumed.

Protein Needs for Endurance Athletes

Early work by Yoshimura[44] and Gontzea[20] illustrated a fall in nitrogen balance in response to beginning a moderate endurance exercise program, suggesting an increased need for protein under these conditions. However, this decline corrected itself within two weeks of the start of exercise without dietary intervention. Butterfield and Calloway[8] confirmed the transient nature of the decline in nitrogen balance with initiation of an exercise program like those proposed in programs to improve health and fitness. They found that nitrogen balance was more positive after the adaptation than before, suggesting that the protein intake requirement for nitrogen equilibrium in individuals performing moderate endurance exercise may actually be lower than that of the sedentary population, provided energy intake is adequate.

More recent work suggests that individuals who exercise at a higher intensity have protein needs that might be greater.[41,31] Meredith et al.[31] conducted a classic nitrogen balance regression assessment of trained male runners exercising daily at 75% of their $\dot{V}O_2max$ and have estimated protein requirements of 0.94 g/kg/bw/day.

Protein need in exercise is dependent on energy intake. Butterfield[7] demonstrated that feeding as much as 2 grams of protein/kg/bw/day to men running 5 or 10 miles a day at 65% to 75% of their $\dot{V}O_2max$ is insufficient to maintain nitrogen balance when energy intake is inadequate by as little as 100 kcal/day. This points out the important role that calories play in sparing protein. Protein will be used as an energy source if calories are insufficient.

Protein Needs for Resistance Exercise

For bodybuilders or individuals who are interested in increasing body mass, the mythology of increased protein needs is rampant. Weight lifters consume anywhere from 1.2 to 3.4 grams of protein/kg/bw/day. Most of this protein is in the form of supplements. The basis for this practice is word of mouth and traditions that have not been substantiated by scientific studies. The traditional thinking among bodybuilders and weight lifters is that the more protein consumed, the bigger the muscles.

Since 1991 sufficient data have accumulated to allow division of the study of protein needs with resistance exercise into two areas: the need for maintenance (minimum protein required to accomplish nitrogen equilibrium) and the need for increasing lean tissue (positive nitrogen balance). Tarnopolsky et al.[40] showed that experienced bodybuilders could maintain nitrogen equilibrium on intakes similar to those required by sedentary controls. However, the high protein intakes used to generate their regression lines may have resulted in overestimation of protein requirements.

Requirements for maintenance of nitrogen balance under circumstances of beginning a resistance exercise program may depend on the intensity of the exercise performed. Tarnopolsky et al.[41] have estimated protein requirements in young novice male bodybuilders exercising 6 days a week for 1.5 hours a day to be 1.5 grams/kg/bw/day. Energy intake is not reported in Tarnopolsky's paper. Hickson[24] found no change in nitrogen excretion with the initiation of a program of 30 minutes of lifting 3 times a week at an intensity of about 50% of maximum capacity when subjects were consuming 0.8 grams of protein/kg/bw/day, the RDA for protein for adults.

Recently, Butterfield and colleagues have attempted to establish the relevance of added protein in the accretion of lean tissue in recreational weight lifters.[6] They found that when energy intake exceeded need by 400 kcal, increasing nitrogen intake from requirement (mean = 10 g N/day) to 1.5 times requirement (mean = 15 g N/day) had no significant effect on nitrogen retention. Any improvement in nitrogen balance seen with increased energy and protein intake was explained by the energy contribution of the protein.

Nutritional Implications

If protein need for exercising people is slightly more than that for sedentary individuals, the usual protein intake of the population will more than meet these needs. Reports of food intake in athletes and nonathletes consistently indicate that protein represents from 12% to 20% of total energy intake, or 1.2 to 2 g protein/gk/bw/day. The exception to the rule is small, active women who consume a low-energy intake in conjunction with an exercise or training program. These women may consume close to the RDA for protein, but if the data of Butterfield are correct, this value in conjunction with the restricted energy intake may be inadequate to maintain lean mass.

Consuming more protein than the body can use should be avoided. When athletes consume diets that are high in protein, they compromise their carbohydrate status and therefore may affect their ability to train and compete at peak performance. The National Research Council also points out that protein foods often are also high in fat; consumption of excess protein creates difficulty in maintaining a low-fat diet. In addition, the hypercalciuric effect of high-protein diets is still considered by some a significant factor in calcium balance, and until the controversy is settled a conservative approach is advised.

Amino Acid Supplementation

Protein or amino acid supplementation in the form of powders or pills is not necessary and should be discouraged. Taking large amounts of protein or amino acid supplements can lead to dehydration, loss of urinary calcium, weight gain, and stress on the kidney and liver.[38] Taking amino acids singly or in combination, such as arginine and lysine, may interfere with the absorption of certain essential amino acids.[38] An additional concern is that substituting amino acid supplements for food may cause deficiencies of other nutrients found in protein-rich foods, such as iron, niacin, and thiamine. Athletes and coaches need to realize that amino acid supplements taken in large doses have not been tested in human subjects and no margin of safety is available. It is important for the health professional to develop a strategy to effectively approach and discuss supplement use with both athletes and coaches.[2]

FAT

Even though maximal performance is impossible without muscle glycogen, fat also provides energy for exercise. Fat is the most concentrated source of food energy and supplies more than twice as many calories (9 kcal/gm) by weight as protein (4 kcal/g) or carbohydrate (4 kcal/g). Fat provides essential fatty acids, which are necessary for cell membranes, skin, hormones, and transporting fat-soluble vitamins. The body has total glycogen stores (both muscle and liver) that equal about 2500 calories, whereas each pound of body fat supplies 3500 calories. This means that an athlete weighing 74 kg (163 pounds) with 10% body fat has 16.3 pounds of fat, which equals 57,000 calories.

Fat is the major, if not most important, fuel for light to moderate intensity exercise. Although fat is a valuable metabolic fuel for muscle activity during longer-term aerobic exercise, and performs many important functions in the body, no attempt should be made to consume more fat. In addition, athletes who consume a high-fat diet typically consume fewer calories from carbohydrates. Simonsen and his colleagues[37] had elite rowers consume either 40% of their calories from fat or 20% of their calories from fat and then compared the two diets on power output and speed. Afterward, they performed muscle biopsies and found that the rowers who consumed the low-fat, high-carbohydrate diet had more muscle glycogen. Rowers on the high-fat, low-carbohydrate diet had moderate levels of muscle glycogen and actually were able to complete the workout sets. However, when it came to power output and faster speeds, the athletes who consumed the lower-fat, higher-carbohydrate diets had significantly more power and speed. This has important implications for athletes in muscular endurance sports that require a burst of power, such as rowing, swimming, gymnastics, figure skating, judo, boxing, or any sport in which some energy will need to be generated by the anaerobic pathway. Following a low-fat, high-carbohydrate diet is also important for health reasons, because a high-fat diet has been associated with cardiovascular disease, obesity, diabetes, and some kinds of cancer.[28]

Types of Fat

Fats are categorized as either saturated or unsaturated (including monounsaturated and polyunsaturated) because they have differing chemical structures and, as a result, different effects on bodily function and health. Saturated fats are solid at room temperature, are derived mainly from animal sources, and tend to raise blood levels of cholesterol. Unsaturated fats are liquid at room temperature, found mainly in plant sources, and tend to decrease blood cholesterol. Palm and coconut oil are exceptions. They are unsaturated fats and are liquid at room temperature; however, they tend to raise blood levels of cholesterol.

Athletes need to recognize the many sources of hidden fat in foods. Fat is present, but not separately visible, in dairy products such as cheese, ice cream, and whole milk, and in bakery items, granola bars, french fries, avocados, chips, nuts, and many highly processed foods. The other dietary sources are more clearly visible, such as margarine, butter, mayonnaise, salad dressing, oil, and meats with high marbling of fat.

It is recommended that athletes should consume 20% to 30% of their calories from fat. Aside from decreasing overall calories, limiting consumption of dietary fat is the first step toward losing excess body fat. Doing so eliminates excess calories but not nutrients. Suggestions for reducing fat intake are listed in Table 47-2.

VITAMINS AND MINERALS

Vitamins and minerals are food components that serve as coenzymes in the metabolic reactions that release energy, transport and consume oxygen, and maintain cell integrity. Because of these important functions, their use as ergogenic aids has been highly touted, although there is little scientific evidence to document their effect. The need for these food components in exercise has been reviewed recently by Haymes[23] and Clarkson,[10] with the

TABLE 47-2 Fat Substitutions

Instead of:	Try:
Whole milk	Skim milk
Cheddar, Jack, or Swiss cheese	Part-skim mozzarella, string, low-fat cottage cheese, or other cheese that contains less than 5 grams of fat per ounce
Ice cream	Ice milk or low-fat/nonfat frozen yogurt
Butter or margarine	Jam, yogurt, ricotta cheese, light or nonfat cream cheese
Sour cream	Low-fat yogurt, light sour cream, blender-whipped cottage cheese
Bacon	Canadian bacon or bacon bits
Ground beef	Extra lean ground beef or ground turkey
Fried chicken	Baked chicken without the skin
Doughnuts and pastries	Bagels, whole-grain homemade breads, muffins, and quick breads
Apple pie	Baked or raw apples
Chocolate candy or bars	Jelly beans, hard candy, licorice
Cookies, cakes, brownies	Vanilla wafers, ginger snaps, graham crackers, fig bars

consensus that unless an individual is deficient in a given nutrient, supplementation with that nutrient does not have a major effect on performance.

Nutrients at Risk

Nutrients at risk in the athletic population are similar to those of concern for the general population. In other words, just because you are an athlete does not mean that you need special amounts of any vitamin or mineral. The nutrients that are of concern for the general population and athletes include folate, vitamin B^6, calcium, and zinc. Because many women athletes are also vegetarians, iron and, perhaps, vitamin B^{12} may be of specific concern to them. Components that protect against free radical attack will be discussed.

Free Radicals and Exercise

Exercise is thought to increase the production of superoxide radicals consequent to the increased rate of oxygen utilization in the mitochondria.[17] The nutrients involved in these complex reactions include vitamins C, E, and A as beta-carotene (which acts as an antioxidant), and zinc, copper, manganese (which occur as various forms of superoxide dismutase), iron as a catalase, and selenium as glutathione peroxidase.[1]

Although the research data for exercising humans remain controversial, several investigators conclude that the increased superoxide radical production that accompanies repeated bouts of exercise is adequately buffered by shifts in the existing systems and results in no deleterious permanent changes.

Vitamin Supplementation

Because athletes often are looking for an edge, something that will give them an advantage, many turn to supplements in the form of pills, powders, and magical elixirs in an effort to make the body perform at its best. Unfortunately, many self-proclaimed experts are eager to convince athletes that their products will improve athletic performance by improving muscle contractions, preventing weight gain, enhancing strength, or supplying energy—just to name a few. These "experts" may insist that athletes' fatigue and muscle soreness are due to a vitamin or mineral deficiency. In fact, when there is a nutritional reason for fatigue, it is usually a lack of calories and/or carbohydrates.

Vitamins can be divided into two groups—water soluble and fat soluble. Vitamins A, D, E, and K are soluble in fat, whereas vitamin C and the B complex vitamins are soluble in water. Table 47-3 lists all of the vitamins, their physiologic functions, and major food sources.

Fat-soluble vitamins are stored in body fat, principally in the liver. Excess accumulation of fat-soluble vitamins, particularly vitamins A and D, can produce serious toxic effects. Although excess of most water-soluble vitamins is typically excreted, some may pose toxicity problems, particularly if they are taken at a pharmacologic level. Large amounts of niacin, for example, can cause burning or tingling, a skin rash, nausea, and diarrhea.[38] High doses of niacin also interfere with fat mobilization and increase glycogen depletion.[38] Vitamin B^6 can cause nervous system damage when taken at high doses. In 1983, seven women consumed more than 2000 mg of B^6 in supplement form for 2 months because they had been told that this amount would help them cure the edema associated with premenstrual syndrome (PMS). The women developed numbness in their feet, then lost sensation in their hands, then became unable to work. They may have suffered irreversible nerve damage. At last report, although the symptoms had been clearing up after withdrawal from the supplements, they had not completely disappeared.

Athletes need to understand that more is not always better. The National Academy of Sciences has established recommended dietary allowances (RDAs) for vitamins and minerals as a guide for determining nutritional needs.[32] The RDA is the daily amount of a nutrient recommended for practically all healthy individuals, in promoting optimal health. It is not a minimal amount needed to prevent disease symptoms—a large margin of safety is added in. Even though it has been shown that a severely inadequate intake of certain vitamins can impair performance, it is unusual for an athlete to have such deficiencies. Even marginal deficiencies do not appear to markedly affect the ability to exercise efficiently.

Minerals

Minerals perform a variety of functions in the body. Whereas some are used to build tissue, such as calcium and phosphorus for bones and teeth, others are important components of hormones, such as iodine in thyroxine. Iron is critical for the formation of hemoglobin, which carries oxygen within the red blood cells. Minerals also are important for regulation of muscle contractions and body fluids, conduction of nerve impulses, and regulation of normal heart rhythm.

Minerals are divided into two groups. The first is referred to as macrominerals, and they are needed in amounts of from 100 mg to 1 g. These include calcium, phosphorus, magnesium, sodium, potassium, chloride, and sulfur. The others fall under the category of trace minerals: copper, iodine, zinc, cobalt, fluoride, and selenium. Food sources and the physiologic functions for each mineral are listed in Table 47-4.

Vitamins

TABLE 47-3

Vitamin	Main Function	Good Sources
A	Maintenance of skin, bone growth, vision, teeth	Eggs, cheese, margarine, milk, carrots, broccoli, squash, spinach
D	Bone growth and maintenance of bones	Milk, egg yolk, tuna, salmon
E	Prevents oxidation of polyunsaturated fats	Vegetable oils, whole-grain cereal, bread, dried beans, green leafy vegetables
K	Blood clotting	Cabbage, green leafy vegetables, milk
Thiamine B^1	Energy-releasing reactions	Pork, ham, oysters, breads, cereals, pasta, green peas
Riboflavin B^2	Energy-releasing reactions	Milk, meat, cereals, pasta, mushrooms, dark green vegetables
Niacin	Energy-releasing reactions	Poultry, meat, tuna, cereal, pasta, bread, nuts, legumes
Pyridoxine B^6	Metabolism of fats, proteins, formation of red blood cells	Cereals, bread, spinach, avocados, green beans, bananas
Cobalamin B^{12}	Formation of red blood cells, functioning of nervous system	Meat, fish, eggs, milk
Folacin	Assists in forming proteins, formation of red blood cells	Dark green leafy vegetables, wheat germ
Pantothenic acid	Metabolism of proteins, carbohydrates, fats, formation of hormones	Bread, cereals, nuts, eggs, dark green vegetables
Biotin	Formation of fatty acids, energy-releasing reactions	Egg yolk, leafy green vegetables
C	Maintenance of bones, teeth, blood vessels, collagen	Citrus fruits, tomato, strawberries, melon, green pepper, potato

Iron

The iron status of athletes, particularly female athletes, is of concern because occurrence of low serum iron (ferritin, iron, and hematocrit) has been observed.[39] Reasons for these low levels may be due to inadequate dietary intake, low bioavailability of iron, or high rates of iron loss.[39] Females are at an increased risk for iron deficiency not only because of increased physiologic need, but because of sometimes lower caloric intakes. In addition, many athletes, particularly females, are vegetarians. In one report, 43% of the female distance runners studied were modified vegetarians and consumed less than 200 grams of meat per week.[4]

Although dietary intake of iron is tied to caloric intake, iron absorption depends on the bioavailability of the iron. Meats contain heme-iron, which is highly bioavailable and, therefore, a more absorbable source of iron. Heme-iron also enhances the absorption of the non–heme-iron found in plant foods such as leafy greens, legumes, cereals, whole grains, and enriched breads. Combining these foods with a source of vitamin C can significantly enhance the absorption of iron—for example, orange juice with an iron-enriched cereal, or pasta in combination with broccoli, tomatoes, and green peppers.

Regular monitoring of iron levels in athletes, including biochemical evaluations and dietary assessments, is recommended to ensure optimal performance.

Calcium

Osteoporosis is a major health concern, especially for women. Although the disease has been regarded as an elderly women's problem, young females, especially those who have had interrupted menstrual function, may be at risk for decreased bone mass. Although there is still much to be discovered about the cause of osteoporosis, three major risk factors have been identified: hormonal status, particularly estrogen deficiency; calcium consumption; and physical activity.

Bone mass is attained until the age of 35 to 40 years; however, peak bone mass is obtained between the ages of 14 and 24. The amount of bone mass a woman has by age 35 strongly influences her susceptibility to fractures in later years. Therefore it is important that young women consume calcium throughout the peak bone-mass years and through early adulthood.

Minerals

TABLE 47-4

Vitamin	Main Function	Good Sources
Calcium	Formation of bones, teeth, nerve impulses, blood clotting	Cheese, sardines, dark green vegetables, clams, milk
Phosphorus	Formation of bones, teeth, acid-base balance	Milk, cheese, meat, fish, poultry, nuts, grains
Magnesium	Activation of enzymes, protein synthesis	Nuts, meats, milk, whole-grain cereal, green leafy vegetables
Sodium	Acid-base balance, body water balance, nerve function	Most foods except fruit
Potassium	Acid-base balance reactions, body water balance, nerve function	Meat, milk, many fruits, cereals, vegetables, legumes
Chloride	Gastric juice formation, acid-base balance	Table salt, seafood, milk, meat, eggs
Sulfur	Component of tissue, cartilage	Protein foods
Iron	Component of hemoglobin and enzymes	Meats, legumes, eggs, grains, dark green vegetables
Zinc	Component of enzymes, digestion	Milk, shellfish, wheat bran
Iodine	Component of thyroid hormone	Fish, dairy products, vegetables, iodized salt
Copper	Component of enzymes, digestion	Shellfish, grains, cherries, legumes, poultry, oysters, nuts
Manganese	Component of enzymes, fat synthesis	Greens, blueberries, grains, legumes, fruit
Fluoride	Maintenance of bone, teeth	Water, seafood, rice, soybeans, spinach, onions, lettuce
Chromium	Glucose and energy metabolism	Fats, meats, clams, cereals
Selenium	Functions with vitamin E	Fish, poultry, meats, grains, milk, vegetables

The National Institutes of Health (NIH) recommends that premenopausal adult women consume 1000 mg of calcium per day. Postmenopausal women who are not on estrogen should consume 1500 mg of calcium per day. Although calcium levels have been recommended for women, the Health and Nutrition Examination Survey (HANES) found that 50% of all females age 15 and over consume less than 75% of the RDA of 1200 mg, and that three quarters of women over 35 consume less than the RDA of 800 mg.

Athletic Amenorrhea. Some women who exercise strenuously stop menstruating, a condition known as athletic amenorrhea. It is associated with many factors, such as nutritional inadequacy, physical stress, energy drain, and acute and chronic hormonal alterations.[34]

Although the specific cause of athletic amenorrhea is unknown and may vary among women, it appears to coincide with decreased estrogen production. Because estrogen deficiency is an important risk factor for the development of osteoporosis, amenorrhea may predispose female athletes to early-onset osteoporosis and fractures. Spinal bone mass has been found to be lower in amenorrheic women runners than in eumenorrheic women runners.[18] Especially disturbing is the fact that further follow-up of these women indicated that bone mineral density remained well below the average for their age group four years after the resumption of normal menses.[19]

Women with athletic amenorrhea should consult a physician to rule out any serious medical problems, and all amenorrheic women should be consuming 1500 mg of calcium per day.

After consultation with a physician, several strategies may be recommended to promote the resumption of menses. These include estrogen replacement therapy, weight gain, diet modification, and reduced training.

Regardless of menstrual history, most female athletes need to increase their calcium intake to meet the RDA for calcium. Low-fat and nonfat dairy products, such as nonfat and low-fat milk, yogurt, cottage cheese, and other low-fat cheeses, are excellent sources of dietary calcium.

CONCLUSION

Nutrition plays a critical role in athletic performance, and sponsors of organized sport programs need to realize that if they educate their athletes to make wise food choices, the chances of optimal athletic performance increase. Athletes, parents, coaches, and sports medicine professionals should not fall prey to nutrition misinformation and fads just because they have had no formal training in nutrition. Using a qualified sports nutritionist as part of a sports medicine program will help athletes compete at their best.

REFERENCES

1. Benedich A: Exercise and free radicals effect of antioxidant vitamins. Med Sport Sci 32:59–78, 1991.
2. Berning JR: The facts and fallacies of sports nutrition: How athletes can evaluate nutrition claims. In Berning JR, Steen SN (eds): Sports Nutrition for the Nineties: The Health Professional's Handbook. Gaithersberg, MD, Aspen Publishers, 1991.
3. Berning JR, Troup JP, VanHandel PJ, et al: The nutritional habits of young adolescent swimmers. Int J Sport Nutr 1:3, 240–248, 1991.
4. Brooks SM, Sanborn CF, Albrecht BH, Wagner WW: Diet in athletic amenorrhea. Lancet 1:559, 1984.
5. Burke LM, Collier GR, Hargreaves M: Muscle glycogen storage following prolonged exercise: Effect of glycemic index of carbohydrate feeding. J Appl Physiol 75:1019–1023, 1993.
6. Butterfield GE: Amino acids and high protein diets. In Lamb DR, Williams MH (eds): Perspectives in Exercise Science and Sports Medicine, vol 4, Ergogenic Enhancement of Performance in Exercise and Sport. Ann Arbor, MI, Brown and Benchmark, 1991.
7. Butterfield GE: Whole body protein utilization in humans. Med Sci Sports Exerc 19:S157–S165, 1987.
8. Butterfield GE, Calloway DH: Physical activity improves protein utilization in young men. Brit J Nutr 51:171–184, 1984.
9. Campbell ML, McFadyen KL: Nutritional knowledge, beliefs and dietary practices of competitive swimmers. Can Home Econom J 34:47, 1984.
10. Clarkson PM: Vitamins and trace minerals. In Lamb DR, Williams MH (eds): Perspectives in Exercise Science and Sports Medicine, vol 4, Ergogenic Enhancement of Performance in Exercise and Sport. Ann Arbor, MI, Brown and Benchmark, 1991.
11. Costill DL, Bowers K, Branam G, Sparks K: Muscle glycogen utilization during prolonged exercise on successive days. J Appl Physiol 31:834–838, 1977.
12. Costill DL, Coyle EF, Dalsky G, et al: Effects of elevated plasma FFA and insulin on muscle glycogen usage during exercise. J Appl Physiol 43:695–699, 1977.
13. Costill DL, Sherman WM, Fink WJ, et al: The role of dietary carbohydrate in muscle glycogen resynthesis after strenuous running. Am J Clin Nutr 34: 1831–1836, 1981.
14. Coyle EF: Timing and method of increased carbohydrate intake to cope with heavy training, competition, and recovery. J Sport Sci 9:29–52, 1991.
15. Coyle EF, Coggan AR, Hemmert MK, Ivy JL: Muscle glycogen utilization during prolonged strenuous exercise when fed carbohydrate. J Appl Physiol 61:165–172, 1986.
16. Coyle EF, Hagberg JM, Hurley BF, et al: Carbohydrate feeding during prolonged strenuous exercise can delay fatigue. J Appl Physiol 55: 230–235, 1983.
17. Davies KJA, Quinantilla AT, Brooks GA, Packer L: Free radical and tissue damage produced by exercise. Biochem Biophys Res Comm 107:1198–1205, 1982.
18. Drinkwater BL, Nilson K, Chestnut CH: Bone mineral content of amenorrheic and eumenorrheic athletes. N Eng J Med 311:277–281, 1984.
19. Drinkwater BL, Nilson K, Ott S, Chestnut CH: Bone mineral density after resumption of menses in amenorrheic athletes. JAMA 256:380–382, 1986.
20. Gontzea I, Sutzesco P, Dumtrache S: The influence of muscular activity on nitrogen balance and on the need of man for protein. Nutr Reports Int 10:35–43, 1974.
21. Hargreaves M: Carbohydrate and exercise. J Sport Sci 9:17–28, 1991.
22. Hargreaves M, Costill DL, Fink WJ, et al: Effect of pre-exercise carbohydrate feedings on endurance cycling performance. Med Sci Sports Exerc 19: 33–36, 1987.
23. Haymes EM: Vitamin and mineral supplementation to athletes. Int J Sport Med 1:146–169, 1991.
24. Hickson JF, Wolinsky I, Divarnik JM: Repeated days of body building exercise do not enhance urinary excretions from untrained young adult males. Nutr Res 10:723–730, 1990.
25. Ivy JL, Datz AL, Cutler CL, et al: Muscle glycogen synthesis after exercise effect of time of carbohydrate ingestion. J Appl Physiol 64:1480–1485, 1988.
26. Jenkins DJA, Woolever JMS, Thorne MJ, et al: The relationship between glycemic response, digestibility and factors influencing the dietary habits of diabetics. Am J Clin Nutr 40:1175–1192, 1989.
27. Kiens B, Raben AB, Valeur AK, Richter EA: Benefit of dietary simple carbohydrates on the early post exercise muscle glycogen repletion in athletes. Med Sci Sports Exerc 22(S4):88, 1990.
28. Krause ME, Mahan CK: Food Nutrition and Diet Therapy, 7th ed. Philadelphia, WB Saunders, 1984.
29. Lemon PWR: Protein and amino acid needs of the strength athlete. Int J Sport Nutr 1:127–145, 1991.
30. Loosli AR, Benson J, Gillien DM, Bourdet K: Nutrition habits and knowledge in competitive adolescent female gymnasts. Phys and Sports Med 14: 118, 1986.
31. Meredith CN, Zachin MJ, Fontera WR, Evan WJ: Dietary protein requirements and body protein metabolism in endurance trained men. J Appl Physiol 66:2850–2856, 1981.

32. National Research Council: Recommended Dietary Allowances, 10th ed. Washington, DC, National Academy Press, 1990.
33. Perron M, Endres J: Knowledge, attitudes and dietary practices of female athletes. J Am Diet Assoc 85:573, 1985.
34. Sanborn CF, Albrech BH, Wagner WW: Athletic amenorrhea, lack of association with body fat. Med Sci Sports Exerc 19:207–212, 1987.
35. Sherman WM, Brodowicz G, Wright DA, et al: Effects of 4-hour pre-exercise carbohydrate feedings on cycling performance. Med Sci Sports Exerc 12:598–604, 1989.
36. Shoaf LR, McClellan PD, Birskovich KA: Nutrition knowledge, interests and information sources of male athletes. J Nutr Education 18:243, 1986.
37. Simonsen JC, Sherman WM, Lamb DL, Dernbach AR, et al: Dietary carbohydrate, muscle glycogen, and power output during rowing training. J Appl Physiol 70(4):1500–1505, 1991.
38. Slavin J: Protein needs for athletes. In JR Berning, Steen SN (eds): Sports Nutrition for the Nineties: The Health Professional's Handbook. Gaithersberg, MD, Aspen Publisher, 1991.
39. Synder AC, Dvorak LL, Roepke JB: Influence of dietary iron on measures of iron status among female runners. Med Sci Sports Exerc 21:7–10, 1989.
40. Tarnopolsky MA, Lemon PWR, Macdougall JD, Atkinson SA: Effect of body building exercise on protein requirements. Can J Sports Sci 15:225, 1991.
41. Tarnopolsky MA, MacDougall JD, Atkinson SA: Influence of protein intake and training status on nitrogen balance and lean body mass. J Appl Physiol 64:187–193, 1988.
42. Tremblay A, Fontaine E, Nadeau A: Contribution of post-exercise increment in glucose storage to variations in glucose-induced thermogenesis in endurance athletes. Can J Physiol Pharmacol 63: 1165–1169, 1985.
43. Van Handel PJ, Cells KA, Bradley PW, Troup JP: Nutritional status of elite swimmers. J Swim Res 1:27–31, 1984.
44. Yoshimura H: Adult protein requirements. Fed Proc 20:103–110, 1961.
45. Zawadski KM, Yaspelkis BB, Ivy JL: Carbohydrate-protein complex increases the rate of muscle glycogen storage after exercise. J Appl Physiol 72(5):1854–1859, 1992.

48 Fluid Balance

Gilbert B. Cushner and Fred D. Cushner

In 490 BC, the Greeks were victorious at the Battle of Marathon. To deliver the historic news, a soldier in full armor ran 22 miles to Sparta, only to collapse and die after delivering his important message.[70] Fortunately, the role of the messenger has been replaced by more modern methods of communication, and a new emphasis on fluid balance and hydration has developed in this era of triathlons and "iron man" competitions.

The need for fluid replacement in competitive athletes, to help maximize performance and reduce the incidence of heat-associated disorders, has been emphasized only in the last 25 years. Even in the early 1950s, it was common dogma that "to run a complete marathon without any fluid replacement was regarded as the ultimate aim of most runners."[71] A 1969 paper by Wyndham and Strydom[99] stimulated modern interest in fluid replacement during exercise. The writers found correlation between the degree of dehydration and rectal temperature and deduced that avoidance of dehydration might prevent heat injury during exercise. This interest, in turn, has produced an enormous commercial outpouring of sports drinks promoted as being superior to water replacement alone.

In this chapter, the pathophysiology of temperature regulation and dehydration is reviewed and exercise-associated medical disorders are discussed. At the end of this chapter, specific recommendations for fluid, electrolyte, and carbohydrate replacement before, during, and after exercise are given.

THERMOREGULATION

Approximately 70% to 80% of energy generated by the working muscle is released as heat.[65,89] As oxygen consumption increases, heat generation also increases, and thermal regulation is needed to control the increased heat production. Unlike lizards and other creatures that rely on the sun's heat to raise their body temperatures to a level that allows for physical activity, humans are warm-blooded animals (homeotherms) and require a relatively constant internal body temperature that is usually in excess of the ambient temperature.[65] As reviewed by Sawka,[83] core temperatures may become elevated from 0.1° to 0.4° for each percent decrease in body weight under a variety of conditions. Without the body's intact heat loss mechanism, a 1% centigrade increase in body temperature could take place every 5 minutes, with death occurring within 20 minutes.[13] With mild to moderate ambient temperatures, conduction, convection, and radiation may be sufficient; but when the environmental temperature is higher than the skin temperature, or in the competing athlete, the most critical thermoregulatory mechanism remains the evaporation of sweat.

Thermoregulation is monitored by thermoreceptors in the skin and body core and then regulated by the hypothalamus. This is a fragile regulatory center, one in which even minor dehydration adversely affects the hypothalamus function. Cohen et al.[17] concluded that even a deficiency as low as 1.2% could lead to thermoregulatory dysfunction. Man's thermoregulatory function can best be studied by example. Let us examine the "Gatorade Iron Man World Championship Triathlon," an event that includes a 2.4-mile swim, followed by a 112-mile bicycle ride, and ending in a full marathon run of 26.2 miles. According to Santi and Gonzales,[86]

> A triathlon typically starts with a morning swim. In cold water, heat loss is rapid, but the response is partially offset by the intense muscular activity. The participants emerge from the water and begin the bicycle stage, perhaps along a winding coastal highway, alternating exposure to sun and shade, wind and calm, as well as the air flow created by the speed of their own motion. As the morning progresses, the sun rises higher in the sky, increasing both air temperature and solar radiation. As the ground heats, wind movement, directed as up-and-down slow breezes, and more gentle winds change in strength and direction. Along the coast, the air tends to be humid, limiting the cooling value of body sweat. At the end of the cycle ride, the participants begin a marathon, generally running on more level terrain under the afternoon sun as air temperatures reach their daily maximum. In the warmer air, away from the ocean's moisture, sweat evaporates more readily, allowing more heat to be lost. For the slower participants, the sunlight wanes at sunset and they will continue their run into the night, either benefiting from the absence of direct sunlight and cooler air temperatures, or becoming chilled due to the combination of colder air and radiant heat loss.

This passage summarizes the four mechanisms of heat transfer that are produced during athletic activity. These include conduction, such as the conduction of heat to the surrounding cooler water, and convective cooling, which occurs during the bicycle portion of the event. Solar radiation takes place during the entire event, and the most critical thermoregulatory mechanism remains the evaporation of sweat.

SWEATING AND DEHYDRATION

As monitored by the anterior hypothalamus, increases in core temperature that exceed the set point result in stimulation of sympathetic cholinergic nerves that stimulate the 2 to 4 million sweat glands in the human skin to produce sweat.[85] Also, skin blood flow accelerates because of raised skin temperature and as a result of central sympathetic control. This helps increase heat loss through sweat evaporation.

Human sweat is a hypotonic solution with an osmolality of between 80 and 185 mOsm/L. For comparison, normal plasma osmolality is 302 mOsm/L. During heavy sweating, observed water loss is greater than electrolyte loss. Therefore the greatest need is to replace the body's water loss rather than to replace the electrolytes.[20]

The sweat rate is proportional to not only the rate of energy expanded but also the rate of work performed. White et al.[97] evaluated the effect of competition on body fluid losses. With 2½ hours of activity in relatively mild conditions, the average body weight loss was found to be 3.25%. Sweat rate during exercise is influenced by multiple factors (see box, Factors Affecting the Sweat Rate in Athletes) including acclimation, hydration, aerobic fitness, and clothing of the athlete. External factors include temperature, humidity, and air velocity. The sweating athlete can produce up to 1.8 liters of sweat and can dissipate all the exercise-generated heat. The sweat rate, however, on occasion can rise as high as 2 to 3 L/hr.[7,21] The highest sweating rate reported in the literature was 2.7 L/hr, measured for Alberto Salazar during the 1984 Olympic marathon.[7]

As dehydration occurs, the sweat rate decreases or stays the same.[71] A rise in serum osmolality and serum sodium correlates with the rise in esophageal temperature[64] and may be the stimulation for any reduction in sweating that occurs at high levels of dehydration.[55] The highest sweat rate takes place during prolonged, high-intensity exercise in the heat. Therefore sweating is a vital thermoregulatory response that occurs at the expense of both intra- and extracellular compartments. If intake cannot keep pace with losses, dehydration will occur. Dehydration will definitely limit the capacity for work and the health of athletes. A practical example would be the finish of a 1984 women's marathon, when Gabrielle Anderson-Scheris staggered her way around the final lap showing signs of hyperthermia and dehydration.[65] Dehydration has been shown to result in decreases in anaerobic capacity, muscle endurance, maximal aerobic power, and physical work capacity.[84] The effects are not limited to physical measurements—the ability to do mental tasks is also impaired.[37]

CHECKLIST

Factors Affecting the Sweat Rate in Athletes

Aerobic fitness
Hydration status
Environmental temperature and humidity
Air velocity
Radiant heat load
Type of clothing
Intensity of exercise

PHYSIOLOGIC RESPONSE TO DEHYDRATION

The body responds to dehydration in a variety of ways, some of which are positive and protect the physiologic homeostasis, others of which have a deleterious effect on the organism. Primary changes include gastrointestinal, cardiovascular, and hormonal adaptation (see box, Gastrointestinal, Cardiovascular, and Hormonal Responses to Dehydration).

Gastrointestinal Changes

Dehydration decreases gastric emptying,[68] impeding the rate of rehydration. In contrast, intestinal resorption probably increases with a declining blood volume.[88]

CHECKLIST

Gastrointestinal, Cardiovascular, and Hormonal Responses to Dehydration

Gastrointestinal Changes

1. Decreased gastric emptying
2. Increased intestinal absorption

Cardiovascular Changes

1. Restoration of plasma volume by fluid movement
2. Decreased stroke volume
3. Increased heart rate
4. Decreased central blood volume
5. Decreased central venous pressure
6. Decreased cardiac filling pressure
7. Decreased cardiac output
8. Decreased splanchnic & renal blood flow

Hormonal Changes

1. Increased vasopressin
2. Increased renin, angiotensin II, and aldosterone activity

Symptoms related to diminished gastric emptying include nausea, bloatedness, and a general gastrointestinal distress.[79]

Cardiovascular Changes

The plasma volume falls when exercise is initiated, influenced by the type, the intensity, and the posture adopted.[26] With a fall in plasma volume, plasma osmolality increases[32] as well as plasma viscosity.[94] This is aggravated by fluid loss until fluid movement from the intracellular space and glycogen breakdown[84] tends to restore it. As is to be expected with a fall in plasma volume, there is a decreased central blood volume,[84] decreased central venous pressure,[52] and decreased cardiac output. Blood flow is redistributed from inactive tissues (e.g., digestive organs, liver, and kidney) into the central blood volume.[82] In spite of the decreased renal blood flow, no change in renal function is observed with dehydration of less than 4% of body weight.[46,47] Heart rate also increases with dehydration,[4,14,39,62,90] and stroke volume is reduced. However, if fluid intake prevents dehydration, cardiac output and stroke volume do not fall,[40] and heart rate remains elevated. This suggests that dehydration is not the only cause of exercise-induced tachycardia.

Hormonal Changes

During prolonged exercise, plasma concentrations of the fluid- and electrolyte-regulating hormones increase, specifically, vasopressin, renin, and aldosterone.[5,11,33,95] Vasopressin secretion from the posterior pituitary gland can be influenced by plasma osmolality, blood volume, and various chemical mediators, all of which operate in the dehydrated state. A plasma osmolality of 280 mmol/kg is considered to be the threshold level at which osmoreceptors trigger vasopressin release.[81] Even in the presence of decreased plasma osmolality, a decrease in effective circulating blood volume will cause vasopressin release. Baroreceptors are located in many areas of the circulatory system, but the left atrial receptor seems to be the most important, responding to smaller changes in volume as its arterial counterpart.[91] The renin–angiotensin system described previously also participates in vasopressin release with angiotensin II having a stimulatory role.[93] Vasopressin increases the water permeability of collecting ducts, resulting in water absorption and producing a maximally concentrated urine.

Renin is a proteolytic enzyme stored and synthesized in the juxtaglomerular apparatus in the wall of afferent glomerular renal arteriolae. Renin is secreted in response to decreased renal perfusion, increased plasma osmolality, and hypovolemic stimulation of beta-adrenergic neurons.[31] The enzyme cleaves to angiotensinogen (renin substrate), an α_2-globulin synthesized in the liver to produce the decapeptide angiotensin I. Angiotensin I is rapidly split by the angiotensin enzyme in the lungs and other tissues to form the octapeptide angiotensin II. As already described, angiotensin II stimulates vasopressin release and causes an increase in aldosterone secretion. Potassium release by the active muscle fibers also stimulates release of this mineralocorticoid hormone. Aldosterone promotes active sodium absorption and excretion of potassium in its major target organs (kidney, colon, and salivary glands). Although these changes begin early in exercise by the movement of up to 13% of fluid into muscle, they continue to operate as sweat-induced fluid loss persists, conserving water and sodium.

RISK FACTORS FOR HEAT-INDUCED ILLNESSES

Although dehydration secondary to sweating is the most important factor in heat-induced illness, there are other conditions that may play a significant role. These include obesity, age, previous heat injury, hypertension, and a variety of drugs (Table 48-1). Deserving special mention are diuretics. Diuretic use, although discouraged, is currently practiced by athletes, not only to weigh in at an appropriate level for sports such as wrestling and boxing, but also in attempts to conceal illegal drug or substance use during urine testing. Diuretics are currently banned by the National Collegiate Athletic Association (NCAA) and the International Olympic Committee Medical Commission. Diuretic use is dangerous not only because of dehydration effect, but also because of secondary electrolyte imbalances such as hypokalemia and hypomagnesemia. Not only can the fluid loss from diuretics cause a larger loss of plasma volume than that caused by voluntary exercise, but it is also usually accompanied by potassium and magnesium losses of a far greater magnitude than we observe with exercise. In conjunction

TABLE 48-1 The Mechanism of Action of Various Drugs on the Thermoregulatory System

Drug	Mechanism
Thyroid hormone (excess)	Excessive heat production
Amphetamines	Excessive heat production
Haloperidol	Decreased thirst
Antihistamines	Decreased sweating
Phenothiazines	Decreased sweating
Diuretics	Sodium and fluid loss
Beta-blockers	Decreased sweating
Benztropine mesylate	Decreased sweating

with self-induced vomiting or laxative abuse, the potential for an electrolyte imbalance is accentuated.

For many reasons, obesity can be a significant risk factor. Much of this increased risk is secondary to the obese athlete's inability to tolerate heat as well as thinner athletes. The specific heat of adipose tissue, compared to lean body mass, leads to an increased heat production. Thermoregulation in the obese patient is also decreased secondarily to altered sweating and decreased sweat gland production.[89] Other risk factors include age. Children appear to be at increased risk because of a less effective thermoregulatory system.[89] Prior heat stroke also can be a risk factor for heat-induced illness.

ENVIRONMENTAL RISK FACTORS FOR HEAT-INDUCED ILLNESSES

Not only is an athlete's thermoregulation mechanism important, but environmental factors also play a role in the development of heat-induced injuries. Ambient temperature, humidity, air velocity, and radiating heat sources are important in determining conditions that may prove harmful to the athlete. Although these factors may be announced by the local weather services, they may be different at the actual athletic site. Therefore, measurements should be made before the start of the event to accurately predict the risk of heat-induced illnesses.

To evaluate temperature, humidity, air movement, and radiating heat, the wet-bulb globe temperature (WBGT) is calculated as follows:

$$\begin{aligned} \text{WBGT} = {} & (0.1 \times \text{ambient dry-bulb temperature}) \\ & + (0.2 \times \text{black-globe temperature}) \\ & + (0.7 \times \text{wet-bulb temperature}) \end{aligned}$$

The black globe (a black toilet-tank float with a thermometer inside) measures the radiant heat and the wet bulb, minus the dry bulb, measures relative humidity when both bulbs are exposed to similar air movement. As can be seen from the preceding formula, 70% of the WBGT comes from the humidity level. A relative humidity of 60% or greater indicates that sweat evaporation will occur only if significant air movement is present. If a wet-bulb temperature is greater than 75° F (24° C), rest periods every 30 minutes are advised; and at wet-bulb temperatures over 76° F (24.4° C), only light exercise should be performed.[89]

A WBGT below 65° F (18° C) indicates a low risk, and temperatures of 74° F to 82° F (23° C to 28° C) constitute a high risk.[89] No activities should be performed with a WBGT value greater than 90. By monitoring the relative humidity as well as the WBGT, modifications in sporting events can be made to decrease the relative risk to participating athletes.

EXERCISE-ASSOCIATED ILLNESSES

The incidence of heat-related illnesses is unknown. Many of the incidents occur and are treated with simple hydration, whereas the more catastrophic illnesses make local newspaper headlines. In this section we will discuss both heat- and dehydration-induced illnesses (muscle cramps, exertional heat injury, heat exhaustion, and heat stroke) and those associated illnesses in which dehydration probably does not play a role (exercise-associated collapse and hyponatremia).

Muscle Cramps

Muscle cramps, although often painful, are the most benign of the injuries described as heat-induced injuries. These cramps occur in the large muscle groups such as the hamstrings or gastrocnemius muscles.[1] This cramping is thought to be secondary to an impaired circulation in the exercising muscle. Because only a few muscle bundles are involved at a time, the pain is noted to "wander" as different muscle bundles are affected. This circulation defect is thought to be secondary to dehydration. A decrease in serum sodium and chloride also may be associated with the development of muscle cramps.

Treatment of muscle cramps begins with prevention. Attention to hydration before, during, and after an athletic event decreases the incidence of muscle cramps. Proper conditioning and heat acclimatization also serve to prevent the onset of muscle cramps. If these muscle cramps develop, the exercise should be stopped and oral hydration initiated. The athlete should be placed in a supine position to increase blood flow to the muscles involved. Massage of the affected muscle groups also may help to relieve symptoms, and improved conditioning may serve to decrease the occurrence of a repeat episode of cramping.

Exertional Heat Injury and Heat Exhaustion

Exertional heat injury is really heat exhaustion in the setting of athletic competition. These conditions are a continuing spectrum culminating in the severe, and often fatal, heat stroke. Heat exhaustion can occur in any athlete who participates in activities that lead to profuse sweat loss. This sweat loss can occur during the activity itself or during time spent exposed to sunlight; an example is the shot-putter on a track-and-field team who has only short periods of sustained athletic activity but is exposed to the elements during the day's events. Heat exhaustion is the most common form of heat intolerance noted.

Symptoms of heat exhaustion include nausea, headache, ataxia, dizziness, and muscle weakness.[24] Rectal temperature may rise as the body's thermoregulatory system fails to compensate for the increased heat production. Cutaneous flushing with profuse sweating may be noted. An elevated temperature as high as 104° F may be present.

The focus of treatment for heat exhaustion is rehydration and reduction of the body's temperature. The athlete first should be moved away from direct sunlight into a shady area. This will help to reduce the body temperature. Placing ice bags in the area of the great vessels also serves to decrease the body's temperature. Toweling dry and fanning the athlete may be helpful. Rectal temperature should be monitored for a rapidly rising core temperature—an early indication of heat stroke. Treatment of heat exhaustion includes hydration of the athlete. This should be performed as early as possible. Fluids can be given via the oral route, with a goal of 1 to 2 L over a 2- to 4-hour period.[89] Intravenous fluids should be initiated if the patient is unconscious or otherwise unable to tolerate oral hydration. Hydration should continue until preathletic body weight is obtained and polyuria is present. Once heat exhaustion occurs, a high recurrence rate can be noted. Senay[87] studied military reservists and noted an 8.5% hospital readmission rate 2 to 3 days after the initial heat illness event.

Water is the first fluid choice provided to the athlete with heat exhaustion. Controversy does exist as to the benefit of adding glucose to the rehydration fluid.[59,77] Glucose may be of value if glycogen storage in the muscles and liver is felt to be depleted.

Heat Stroke

Heat stroke is the second-most common cause of death in the athlete. Although many animals will decrease their running and activity levels as body temperatures increase, humans in a quest for victory will often ignore these natural protective mechanisms. As the body temperature rises above 106° F, heat stroke is said to occur. The presenting symptom of heat stroke is hypovolemic shock in the setting of a markedly elevated core temperature. Profuse sweating may be present,[41] and neurologic symptoms such as irritability, aggression, and delirium may occur. Heat stroke is a medical emergency with a mortality rate estimated to be 50% to 70%.[6] It is not the degree of hyperthermia but rather the duration of sustained hyperpyrexia and unconsciousness that is the most important prognostic factor for heat stroke. Because a shortened length of hyperpyrexia is critical, an early diagnosis and treatment are urgent. Misdiagnosis may be made, including that for encephalitis, meningitis, dysentery, hepatitis, malaria, epilepsy, and conversion reaction,[10,49] leading to a delay in treatment. Therefore, a high index of suspicion must be maintained for any athlete who collapses during physical activity. Measurement of rectal temperature may aid in the early diagnosis of this condition.

Treatment of heat stroke begins with the cooling of the patient. As for the patient with heat exhaustion, the athlete is moved to a shaded area, and ice bags are placed near the great vessels. Fanning and massage are initiated to aid in the lowering of the core temperature.[6] Although immersion in ice water may induce a sudden drop in the body's core temperature,[16] it also causes vasoconstriction. Vasoconstriction and shivering have a negative effect on subsequent heat loss. Hubbard and others[45] have used niacin to help counteract vasoconstriction that occurs with ice immersion, but the use of niacin remains experimental at this time.

Rehydration and cardiac support should be provided early. Blood pressure should be monitored, as should urine output, and a catheter should be placed as needed. Beta-adrenergic drugs may be needed to increase cardiac output, but alpha-adrenergic drugs should not be used because they may hamper skin perfusion and, therefore, hamper heat transfer. Hospital monitoring for 24 to 36 hours is recommended, to observe for complications associated with heat stroke. Individual system, as well as multisystem, involvement may occur as a result of heat stroke. In 10% to 35% of patients, acute renal tubular necrosis may develop.[50] Liver involvement such as lobular necrosis and marked cholestasis[51] also can occur. In a study by Senay,[87] 40 out of 42 patients readmitted for heat exhaustion had an increased SGOT level. This may be a marker for the severity of heat injury, but further experimentation needs to be done. A malabsorption syndrome may develop if the gastrointestinal tract has an ischemic event at the time of the heat stroke.

EXERCISE-ASSOCIATED DISEASES WITHOUT DEHYDRATION

Exercise-Associated Collapse

For a long time, runners who were thought to have suffered from dehydration were treated with IV fluids.[2,29,42–44,56,58,75,98] Recent studies have shown that collapsing runners are not more likely to be hyperthermic or dehydrated than their noncollapsing peers.[72,73,80] In fact, IV fluids seem to retard recovery.[30] Noakes[71] has proposed a postural hypotension caused by fluid displacement to the muscles of the lower extremities as a most likely cause. Rational therapy, therefore, would include elevation of the pelvis and legs, and this has been proven to be effective.[38]

Hyponatremia

With the exception of one case reported in a marathon runner,[67] all reports of symptomatic hyponatremia have occurred in endurance athletes participating in triathlon or ultramarathon events.[34,35,44,74] A variety of neurologic symptoms has been reported, including convulsions and coma. Serum sodium is less than 125 mEq/L, and normal to increased blood volumes are compatible with the observation that these athletes have had excessive fluid intake, rather than increased sodium losses.

Noakes[71] has postulated three possible etiologies that operate in combination to cause hyponatremia. The syndrome of inappropriate antidiuretic hormone (SIADH) may be present, with expanded blood volume failing to shut off ADH secretion but appropriately shutting off aldosterone. The latter is associated with increased urinary sodium loss, contributing to the hyponatremia state.

A second possible cause is a disturbed regulation of the extracellular volume, so that the normal relationship between the volume and its sodium chloride content is lost; and, possibly, a third space phenomenon of sodium moving into the unabsorbed fluid in the large bowel may contribute. Since most athletes are "reluctant" drinkers and more prone to develop voluntary dehydration, the "avid" drinkers are a small subset who may develop hyponatremia if associated with over 6 hours of fluid replacement exceeding 1.3 L/hr.[71]

PREVENTION OF HEAT ILLNESSES

As for any disease process, the best form of treatment for heat illness is prevention. Because of increased awareness of exertion-induced injuries, as well as more formal sports medicine education, the importance of proper hydration in the athlete is being stressed. It is now common knowledge that water breaks are not to be considered "a sign of weakness" for the training athlete.[53]

Hydration is the first line of prevention against heat-induced injuries. Proper hydration begins before the start of a sports event. The athlete should be well hydrated at the beginning of the competition. During the event, hydration should be stressed despite the absence of thirst. A subjective feeling of thirst occurs only after 2% to 3% of body weight is lost. At this point athletic performance is already impaired.[89] Because athletes will not voluntarily replace all fluids lost,[10] the guidelines of 12 oz of fluid for every 20 minutes of exercise should be followed. The sweat rate is proportional to body mass.[17] Fluid requirements for a middle linebacker will be much different from those of a female gymnast. Because some sports (soccer, rugby) have only one break, at halftime, the intermission is not long enough for adequate replenishment of fluids. Coaches should agree before the start of the game to divide the game into quarters, thereby providing proper rehydration time during extreme weather conditions.

As a guide to fluid replacement after exercise, athletes can provide a rough estimate by weighing themselves nude before the event and then following the event. One pound of weight loss equals approximately one pint of fluid that needs to be replenished after exercise.[89]

Proper clothing is essential for the prevention of heat-induced illnesses. In heat and humidity, uniforms should be lightweight, with as much skin exposure as possible, to facilitate perspiration. Sports such as soccer and rugby, which are played in both the cool and warmer months, should have heavier- and lighter-weight uniforms to accommodate the extremes of temperatures present at game time during both seasons. Football players should remove their helmets when on the sidelines to facilitate heat dissipation. Of course, running in sauna suits or multiple sweatshirts to "make weight" is a dangerous practice that should be discouraged.

Proper conditioning and acclimatization to local weather conditions are other factors that can reduce the incidence of heat-associated illnesses. It is well known that both training and acclimatization will confer some protection against heat illness. Although adaptation is most marked when conditioning is carried out in the heat, some benefit will also be achieved at moderate temperatures. Training expands the blood volume, contributing to better cardiac output. Physiologic changes with acclimatization include increased skin blood flow at a given core temperature, increased sweat protection, decreased rate of glycogen utilization, and more dilute sweat production.[89] In the adult, maximal sweat acclimatization can be achieved in 8 to 12 days with as little as 30 minutes of intense exercise daily. Despite optimal heat acclimatization, no athlete can develop complete immunity to heat illness.[89] Adequate hydration is still essential to minimize the risk of exercise-associated dehydration illnesses.

SPECIFIC RECOMMENDATIONS FOR FLUID, CARBOHYDRATE, AND ELECTROLYTE REPLACEMENT

Sports drinks have become big business in the world of athletics today. Millions of dollars are spent in advertising each year on such products. Corporate institutions such as Pepsi (All Sport) and Coca Cola (Powerade) have introduced their versions of sports drinks to compete with the long-standing Gatorade Corporation. The question remains: Do these products offer an advantage over just plain cold water? We will evaluate this question in the following section, and guidelines to fluid replacement for specific athletic events will also be detailed.

All sports drinks are not created equal. Table 48-2 shows the contents of several popular sports drinks as provided by their nutritional labels. Formulation is different not only in their sodium content but also in their carbohydrate content. Therefore, caloric amounts also may be varied for these drinks. Johnson et al.[48] evaluated several sports drinks and found no difference between the various formulations and their abilities to prevent dehydration or electrolyte imbalance. There was no difference noted in sweating or athletic performance. Johnson[48] and other authors[97] concluded that the sports products may be beneficial according to their palatability, thereby encouraging a more or less voluntary oral hydration.

TABLE 48-2

Composition of Various Sports Drinks

Beverage (8 oz)	CHO (g)	Na (mg)	K (mg)
Gatorade	14	110	30
Powerade	19	55	30
All Sport	22	55	55
Coca Cola	13	16.3	0
Water	0	trace	trace

As suggested by Gisolfi and Duchman,[36] choice of replacement fluids depends on the intensity and the length of the event. We have divided our discussion into short events (less than 1 hour), intermediate events (1 to 3 hours), and prolonged events (in excess of 3 hours). In Table 48-3, the choice of fluid replacement and the need for carbohydrate/electrolyte replacement are summarized for all three types of events.

Short Events (Less Than 1 Hour)

Short events include team sports such as cycling and essentially all track events. Sports in these categories have an intensity level between 75% and 100% VO_2max. Preexercise hydration for this sports category depends on the intensity of the exercise expected and the state of hydration of the athlete. Either no fluids are necessary or the use of 300 to 500 cc of a 6% to 10% carbohydrate solution is deemed appropriate. The latter is required so as to avoid glycogen depletion in a highly intense athletic event. Otherwise, water only would be appropriate to ensure that the patient enters the event hydrated.

During events there is a rationale for replacing all fluids to attenuate any rise in core temperature. In contrast to other species, only humans develop voluntary dehydration when given free access to fluid during exercise.[3,9,15,28,92] A significant dehydration (2% of body fluid loss) occurs before thirst is perceived, resulting in voluntary dehydration with exercise. A water deficiency of 3% reduces maximum aerobic power in a temperate climate.

TABLE 48-3

Guidelines for Fluid Hydration for Mild, Moderate, and Severe Activity Levels

	Duration of Exercise		
	1 hour	**1–3 hours**	**Over 3 hours**
Exercise Intensity	75%–100% VO_2 maximum	60%–90% VO_2 maximum	30%–70% VO_2 maximum
Events	Teamsports, some cycling events	Soccer, marathon	Ultramarathon, triathlon, most track events
Formula			
Preevent	30–50 g CHO or H_2O	H_2O	H_2O
Fluid Volume			
Preevent	300–500 cc	300–500 cc	300–500 cc
During exercise	500–1000 cc	500–1000 cc/hr will meet CHO need 800–1600 cc/hr will meet fluid need	500–1000 cc/hr will meet CHO fluid requirements of most
Rationale			
Preevent	CHO—only for events that produce glycogen depletion in less than 1 hour	H_2O—to encourage fat metabolism (see text) and combat dehydration	H_2O—to encourage fat metabolism (see text) and combat dehydration
During exercise	H_2O—to prevent rise in core temperature	CHO—to replete glycogen stores Fluid—to prevent rise in core temperature Na^+, Cl^- will promote CHO and fluid absorption and enhance palatability	CHO—to replete glycogen stores Fluid—to prevent rise in core temperature Na^+, Cl^- will promote CHO and fluid absorption, enhance palatability, and prevent hyponatremia

In hotter environments, a 2% deficiency will show some reduction. We suggest that, for fluid replacement, approximately half of the sweat rate, which is 500 to 1000 cc in most athletes, should be replaced. Gastric volume does play a role in gastric emptying. The larger the volume, the greater the gastric emptying rate, up to 600 cc.[23]

Cool liquids were preferred at one time because of enhanced gastric emptying, but more recent studies have cast doubt on the importance of liquid temperature.[63] In a similar vein, there is probably no effect from carbonation, although earlier studies suggested that increased emptying[63] was present with carbonated fluids.

Is there any need to add carbohydrate or salt to sports drinks during exercise lasting less than one hour? Sweat is hypotonic, and using a 3 L/hr sweat rate, no more than 120 mg of sodium loss will occur within 1 hour. As calculated by Gisolfi and Duchman,[36] a serum sodium would exceed 136 mEq/L after 1 hour of exercise. Therefore, no use of sodium is necessary in short events except to increase the palatability of the beverage and perhaps facilitate fluid absorption,[36] although the latter is not substantiated.[66,96]

The evidence for glucose replacement is unclear. There is documentation by earlier authors of the possibility of delayed gastric emptying related to carbohydrate concentration, but this has not been substantiated in more recent studies.[27] No carbohydrate should be added in short exercise. Heat[76] and high-intensity exercises[23] also delay emptying. Glucose polymers have been studied to see if, in theory, the decreased osmolality for the same carbohydrate content causes increased fluid and substrate to reach the small intestine. The results have been variable,[63] but polymer has been found to empty more slowly. Fructose should be avoided because of increased GI problems.[61]

In summary, the use of electrolyte and carbohydrate solutions offers no improvement in plasma volume or electrolyte concentrations for short-event competition. The question of whether they might perhaps improve performance is equivocal.

Intermediate Events of 1 to 3 Hours' Duration

Intermediate-length events (soccer games, rugby games, and marathons) take place for the majority of well-trained athletes. An exercise intensity of 65 to 90 VO_2max is achieved in this sports category.

Preevent hydration for this class of athletic events would include 300 to 500 cc of water to ensure adequate hydration at the start of competition. Early in the event, fat metabolism should be promoted, and the inclusion of carbohydrated drinks might cause increased carbohydrate metabolism and glycogen deposition, leading to premature fatigue.[36] In contrast to the short events, longer events can result in hypoglycemia, hypovolemia, hyperthermia, dehydration, and glycogen depletion.[25,38,78] There is no question that adequate fluid replacement is necessary in events that last for 1 to 3 hours. Between 800 and 1600 cc of fluid, including carbohydrate, can definitely enhance performances, since glycogen stores are reduced.[57,60] Is sodium necessary in these events? The answer is probably "No." The sodium level would probably rise to 130 mEq/L, or even a little higher, since some fluid enters the cells.

Potassium Replacement

Potassium ranges from 1 to 15 mEq/L in sweat and does not increase with the sweat rate.[19] Some data suggest that there are significant losses,[8,54] but this is not supported.[18] On the other hand, potassium facilitates rehydration of the intracellular fluid (ICF) compartment,[12,69] and glucose causes secretion of potassium in the liver. Therefore, to prevent any potential losses, 3 to 5 mEq/L of potassium should be included in a sports drink for an extended event.

Magnesium Replacement

The likelihood of hypomagnesemia secondary to magnesium losses in sweat is an unlikely phenomenon.[89] Maximum losses based on a concentration of 0.02 to 0.05 mmol/L will result in only a 1% decrease in total body content.[22] Magnesium should be replaced for the average daily intake of 10 to 15 mmol/L/day. As emphasized before, magnesium and potassium losses are more accentuated when athletes have used diuretics.

Fluid Replacement During Recovery

The goals of fluid replacement during recovery should be storage of glycogen and restoration of fluid and sodium balance. Appropriate solutions should contain 40 mEq/L of sodium, with the fluid rate adjusted to replace losses and supply 25 to 50 g of carbohydrates every 2 hours.

SUMMARY

The body has adapted to a variety of conditions to avoid elevations in temperature during exercise, particularly in hot environments. However, elevations in core temperatures can have severe consequences, and failed defense mechanisms can result in deadly dehydration if appropriate fluid and electrolyte needs are not addressed during competition. The need for fluid replacement and, on occasion, carbohydrate and electrolyte replacement has been summarized in this chapter. It varies, of course, with the intensity and the duration of the exercise plan. A number of exercise-induced illnesses can be prevented, or at least appropriately treated, if the sports physician is aware of the consequences and the possibilities.

The need for a comprehensive approach to fluid and electrolyte balance in competitive athletes has been emphasized only in the last 25 years and the approach probably will become better developed over the next decade.

REFERENCES

1. Adams WC, Fox RH, Fry AJ, McDonald IC: Thermoregulation during marathon running in cool, moderate, and hot environments. J Appl Physiol 38: 1030–1037, 1975.
2. Adner MM, Scarlet JJ, Casey J, et al: The Boston Marathon medical care team: Ten years of experience. Phys Sports Med 16:99–106, 1988.
3. Adolph EF: Measurement of water drinking in dogs. Am J Physiol 125:75–86, 1939.
4. Adolph EF: Physiology of Man in the Desert. New York, Interscience Publishers, 1947.
5. Altenkirch HU, Gerzer R, Kirsch KA, et al: Effect of prolonged physical exercise on fluid regulating hormones. Eur J Appl Physiol 61:209–213, 1990.
6. Appenzeller O, Atkinson R: Sports Medicine: Fitness, Training, Injuries. Baltimore, Urban and Schwarzenberg, 1981.
7. Armstrong LE, Hubbard RW, Jones BH, Daniels JT: Preparing Alberto Salazar for the heat of the 1984 Olympic Marathon. Phys Sports Med 3:73–81, 1986.
8. Armstrong LE, Hubbard RW, Szlyk PC, et al: Voluntary dehydration and electrolyte losses during prolonged exercise in the heat. Aviat Space Environ Med 56:765, 1985.
9. Arnauld E, duPont J: Vasopressin release and firing of supraoptic neurosecreting neurones during drinking in the dehydrated monkey. Pflugers Arch 394:195–201, 1982.
10. Bar-Or O, Dotan R, Inbar O, et al: Voluntary hypohydration in 10–12 year old boys. J Appl Physiol; Respir Environ Exerc Physiol 48:104–108, 1980.
11. Brandenberger G, Condas V, Follenius M, Kahn KM: The influence of the initial state of hydration on endocrine response to exercise in the heat. Eur J Appl Physiol 58:674–679, 1989.
12. Brigs AP, Koechig I: Some changes in the composition of blood due to the injection of insulin. J Biol Chem 58: 721–730, 1923.
13. Brotherhood JR: The nutritional stresses consequent to thermoregulation in athletes. Proc Nutrition Soc Australia 6:123–125, 1981.
14. Candas V, Libert JP, Brandenberger G: Thermal and circulatory responses during prolonged exercise at different levels of hydration. J Physiol (Paris) 83: 11–18, 1988.
15. Choshniak I, Wittenberg C, Saham D: Rehydrating Bedouin goats with saline: Rumen and kidney function. Physiol Zool 60:373–378, 1987.
16. Clowes GHA Jr, O'Donnell TF Jr: Heat stroke. N Engl J Med 291:564, 1974.
17. Cohen I, Mitchell D, Seider R, et al: The effect of water deficit on body temperature during rugby. S Afr Med J 60:11–14, 1981.
18. Costill DL: Muscle metabolism and electrolyte balance during heat acclimation. Acta Physiol Scand 128:111, 1986.
19. Costill DL: Sweating: Its composition and effects on body fluids. In Milvey P (ed): The Marathon Physiologic, Medical, Epidemiological, and Psychological Studies. New York, NY Academy of Science, 1977.
20. Costill DL: Water and electrolyte requirements during exercise. Clin Sports Med 3(3):639–648, 1984.
21. Costill DL, Cote E, Fink W: Muscle water and electrolytes following varied levels of dehydration in man. J Appl Physiol 40:6–11, 1976.
22. Costill DL, Miller JM: Nutrition for endurance sport: Carbohydrate and fluid balance. Int J Sports Med 1:2–14, 1980.
23. Costill DL, Saltin B: Factors limiting gastric emptying during rest and exercise. J Appl Physiol 37:679–683, 1974.
24. Costrini AM, Pitt HA, Gustafson AB, et al: Cardiovascular and metabolic manifestations of heat stroke and severe heat exhaustion. Am J Med 66:296–302, 1979.
25. Coyle EF, Coggan AR, Hemmert MK, Ivy SL: Muscle glycogen utilization during prolonged strenuous exercise when fed carbohydrates. J Appl Physiol 61:165–172, 1986.
26. Coyle EF, Hamilton M: Fluid replacement during exercise: Effects on physiologic homeostasis and performance. In Gisolfi CV, Lamb DR (eds): Perspectives in Exercise Science and Sports Medicine, vol 3, Fluid Homeostasis During Exercise. Indianapolis, IN, Benchmark Press, 1990.
27. Davis JM, Lamb DR, Burgess WA, et al: Accumulation of deuterium oxide in body fluids after ingestion of D_2O labelled beverages. J Appl Physiol 63:2060–2066, 1987.
28. Dill DB: Physiologic Effects of hot Climates and Great Heights: Life, Heat and Altitude. Cambridge, MA, Harvard University Press, 1938.
29. Eichner ER: Sacred cows and straw men. Phys Sports Med 19:24, 1991.
30. Ellis D, Verdile V, Heller M, et al: The effectiveness of the addition of intravenous hydration of oral hydration in post-marathon patients. Med Sci Sports Exerc 22(Suppl): S101, 1990.
31. Fitzsimons JT: The Physiology of Thirst and Sodium Appetite. New York, Cambridge University Press, 1979.

32. Fortney SM, Wenger CB, Bove JR, Nadel ER: Effect of hyperosmolality on control of blood flow and sweating. J Appl Physiol 57:1688–1695, 1984.
33. Freund BJ, Claybaugh JR, Hashiro GM, et al: Exaggerated ANF responses to exercise in middle-aged vs. young runners. J Appl Physiol 71:2518–2527, 1991.
34. Frizzell RT, Lang GH, Lowance DC, Latham SR: Hyponatremia and ultra marathon running. JAMA 255:772, 1986.
35. Gisolfi CV, Copping JR: Thermal effects of prolonged treadmill exercise in the heat. Med Sci Sports 6:108–113, 1974.
36. Gisolfi CV, Duchman, SM: Guidelines for optimal replacement beverages for different athletic events. Med Sci Sports Exerc 24(6):679–687, 1992.
37. Gopinathan PM, Pichan G, Sharma VM: Role of dehydration in heat-stress induced variation in mental performance. Arch Environ Health 43: 15–17, 1988.
38. Gough KJ: Why marathon runners collapse (letter). S Afr Med J 30:461, 1991.
39. Greenleaf JE, Castle BL: Exercise temperature regulation in man during hypohydration and hyperhydration. J Appl Physiol 30:847–853, 1971.
40. Hamilton MC, Gonzalez-Alonso J, Montain S, Coyle EF: Fluid replacement and glucose infusion during exercise cardiovascular drift. J Appl Physiol 71:871–877, 1991.
41. Hart LE, Egier BP, Shimizv AG: Exertional heat stroke: The runner's nemesis. Can Med Assoc J 122:1144–1150, 1980.
42. Hiller WDB: Current and Future Research: Report on the Ross Symposium on Medical Coverage of Endurance Athletic Events. Columbus, OH, Ross Laboratories, 1987.
43. Hiller WDB, O'Toole ML, Laird RH: Hyponatremia and ultra marathons (letter). JAMA 256:213, 1986.
44. Hiller WDB, O'Toole ML, Fortess EE, et al: Medical and physiologic considerations in triathalons. Am J Sports Med 15:164–167, 1987.
45. Hubbard RW, Armstrong LE, Young AJ: Rapid hypothermia subsequent to oral nicotinic acid ingestion and immersion in warm (30 degrees C) water (letter). Am J Emerg Med 6:316–317, 1988.
46. Irving RA, Noakes TD, Burger SC, et al: Plasma volume and renal function during and after ultramarathon running. Med Sci Sports Exerc 22:581–587, 1990.
47. Irving RA, Noakes TD, Raine RI, Van Zyl-Smit R: Transient oliguria with renal tubular dysfunction after a 90 km running race. Med Sci Sports Exerc 22:756–761, 1990.
48. Johnson HL, Nelson RA, Consolazio CF: Effects of electrolyte and nutrient solutions on performance and metabolic balance. Med Sci Sports Exerc 20(1):26–33, 1988.
49. Keren G, Shonfeld Y, Sohar E: Prevention of damage by sport activity in hot climates. J Sports Med 20:452–459, 1980.
50. Kew MC, Abrahams C, Seftel HC: Chronic interstitial nephritis as a consequence of heat stroke. Q J Med 39:189, 1970.
51. Kew MC, Berson I, et al: Liver damage in heat stroke. Am J Med 49:192, 1970.
52. Kirsch KA, Von Amelin AH, Wicke HJ: Fluid control mechanisms after exercise dehydration. Eur J Appl Physiol 47:191–196, 1981.
53. Knochel JP: Dog days and siriasis: How to kill a football player. JAMA 233(6):513–515, 1975.
54. Knochel JP, Dotin LN, Hamburger RJ: Pathophysiology of intense physical conditioning in a hot climate. J Clin Invest 51:242–255, 1972.
55. Ladell WSS: The effects of water and salt intake upon the performance of men working in hot and humid environments. J Physiol 127:11–46, 1955.
56. Laird RH: Medical complications during the ironman triathlon world championship 1981–1984. Ann Sports Med 3:113–116, 1987.
57. Lamb DR, Brodowicz GR: Optimal use of fluids of varying formulations to minimize exercise induced disturbances in homeostasis. Sports Med 3:247–274, 1986.
58. Lind RH: The Western States 100 Mile Run, Report on the Ross Symposium on Medical Coverage of Endurance Athletic Events. Columbus, OH, Ross Laboratories, 1987.
59. Mallard D, Owen KC, Kregel P, et al: Exercise physiology and medicine: Effects in ingesting carbohydrate beverages during exercise in heat. Med Sci Sports Exerc 18:568–575, 1986.
60. Maughan R: Carbohydrate-electrolyte solutions during prolonged exercise. In Lamb DR, Williams MH (eds): Perspectives in Exercise Science and Sports Medicine, Ergogenics: Enhancement of Performance in Exercise and Sport. Indianapolis, IN, Benchmark Press, 1991, pp 35–85.
61. Maughan RJ, et al: Fluid replacement in sport and exercise—a consensus statement. Br J Sports Med 27:34–35, 1993.
62. Maughan RJ, Fenn CE, Gleeson M, Leiper JB: Metabolic and circulatory responses to the ingestion of glucose polymer and glucose/electrolyte solutions during exercise in man. Eur J Appl Physiol 56: 356–362, 1987.
63. Maughan RJ, Noakes TD: Fluid replacement and exercise stress: A brief review of studies on fluid replacement and some guidelines for the athlete. Sports Med 12:16–31, 1991.
64. Montain SJ, Coyle EF: The influence of graded dehydration on hyperthermia and cardiovascular

drift during exercise. J Appl Physiol 73:1340–1350, 1992.

65. Murray R: Nutrition for the marathon and other endurance sports: Environmental stress and dehydration. Med Sci Sports Exerc 24(9 Suppl): 319–323, 1992.
66. Murray R: The effects of consuming carbohydrate-electrolyte beverages on gastric emptying and fluid absorption during and following exercise. Sports Med 4:322–351, 1987.
67. Nelson PB, Robinson AG, Kapoor W, Rinaldo J: Hyponatremia in a marathon runner. Phys Sports Med 16(10):78, 1988.
68. Neufer PD, Young AJ, Sawka MN: Gastric emptying during exercise: effects of heat stress and hypodehydration. Eur J Appl Physiol 58:433–439, 1989.
69. Nielsen B, Sjogaard G, Ugelvig J, et al: Fluid balance in exercise dehydration and rehydration with different glucose-electrolyte drinks. Eur J Appl Physiol 55:318–325, 1986.
70. Noakes TD: Exercise-induced heat injury in South Africa. S Afr Med J 47:1968–1972, 1973.
71. Noakes TD: Fluid replacement during exercise. Exerc Sport Sci Rev 21:297–330, 1993.
72. Noakes TD: Sacred cows revisited. Phys Sports Med 19:49, 1991.
73. Noakes TD, Berlinski N, Solomon E, Weight LM: Collapsed runners: Blood biochemical change after IV fluid therapy. Phys Sports Med 19:70–81, 1991.
74. Noakes TD, Goodwin W, Rayner BL, et al: Water intoxication: A possible complication during endurance exercise. Med Sci Sports Exerc 17:370, 1985.
75. Novak D: Ironman Canada Triathlon Championship: Medical Coverage of an Ultra Distance Event, Report on the Ross Symposium on Medical Coverage of Endurance Athletic Events. Columbus, OH, Ross Laboratories, 1987.
76. Owen MD, Kregel KC, Wall PT, Gisolfi CV: Effects of ingesting carbohydrate beverages during exercise in the heat. Med Sci Sports Exerc 18:568–575, 1986.
77. Pinorka RW, Robinson S, Gay UL, Manalis RS: Preacclimatization of men to heat by training. J Appl Physiol 20: 379–389, 1965.
78. Pugh LG, Corbett JL, Johnson RH: Rectal temperatures, weight losses and sweat rates in marathon running. J Appl Physiol 23:347–352, 1967.
79. Rehrer NJ, Beckers EF, Brouns F, et al: Effects of dehydration on gastric emptying and gastrointestinal distress while running. Med Sci Sports Exerc 22:790–795, 1990.
80. Roberts WO: Exercise-associated collapse in endurance events: A classification system. Phys Sports Med 117:49–59, 1989.
81. Robertson GL, Berl T: Water metabolism. In Bremer BM, Rector FC Jr (eds): The Kidney, 3rd ed. Philadelphia, WB Saunders, 1986.
82. Rowell LB: Human cardiovascular adjustments to exercise and thermal stress. Physiol Rev 54:75–159, 1974.
83. Sawka MN: Physiologic consequences of hypohydration: Exercise performance and thermoregulation. Med Sci Sports Exerc 24:657–670, 1992.
84. Sawka MN, Pandolf KB: Effects of body water loss on physiologic function and exercise performance. In Gisolfi CV, Lamb DR (eds): Perspectives in Exercise Science and Sports Medicine, vol 3, Fluid Homeostasis During Exercise. Indianapolis, IN, Benchmark Press, 1990.
85. Sawka MN, Wenger CB: Physiologic responses to acute exercise-heat stress. In Pandolf KB, Sawka MN, Gonzolez RR (eds): Human Performance Physiology and Environmental Medicine at Terrestrial Extremes. Indianapolis, IN, Benchmark Press, 1988.
86. Schultz SG, Curran PF: Coupled transport of sodium and organic solutes. Physiol Rev 50:637–718, 1970.
87. Senay LC: Effects of exercise in the heat on body fluid distribution. Med Sci Sports Exerc 11:42–48, 1979.
88. Sjovall H, Abrahamsson H, Westlander G, et al: Intestinal fluid and electrolyte transport in man during reduced circulating blood volume. Gut 27:913–918, 1986.
89. Squire DL: Heat illness–fluid and electrolyte issues for pediatric and adolescent athletes. Ped Clin N Am 37:1085–1109, 1990.
90. Strydom NB, Benade AJS, Van Rensburg AJ: The state of hydration and the physiologic responses of men during work in the heat. Aust J Sports Med 7:28–33, 1975.
91. Sved AF: Central neural pathways in baroceptor control of vasopressin secretion. In Schrier, RW (ed): Vasopressin. New York, Raven, 1985.
92. Thrasher TN, Nistal-Herrera JF, Keil LC, Ramsay DJ: Satiety and inhibition of vasopressin secretion and drinking in dehydrated dogs. Am J Physiol 240:E394–E401, 1981.
93. Usberti M, Federico S, Cianciaruso B and others: Effects of angiotensin II on plasma ADH, PGE^2 synthesis and water excretion in normal man. Am J Physiol 248:F254–F259, 1985.
94. Vanderwalle H, Lacombe C, Lelievre JC Poirot C: Blood viscosity after a 1-h submaximal exercise with and without drinking. Int J Sports Med 9:104–107, 1988.
95. Wade CE, Freund BJ: Hormonal control of blood volumes during and following exercise. In Gisolfi CV, Lamb DR (eds): Perspectives in Exercise

Science and Sports Medicine, vol 3, Fluid Homeostatis During Exercise. Indianapolis, IN, Benchmark Press, 1990.
96. Wheller KB, Banwell JG: Intestinal water and electrolyte flux of glucose-polymer electrolyte solutions. Med Sci Sports Exerc 18:436–439, 1986.
97. White J, Ford MA: The hydration and electrolyte maintenance properties of an experimental sports drink. Br J Sports Med 17(1):51–58, 1983.
98. Winslow EBJ: The Chicago Marathon, Report on the Ross Symposium on Medical Coverage of Endurance Athletic Events. Columbus, OH, Ross Laboratories, 1987.
99. Wyndham CH, Strydom NB: The danger of an inadequate water intake during marathon running. S Afr Med J 43:893–896, 1969.

49 Substance Abuse

Dennis J. Gleason

Substance abuse among athletes is a major concern for medical personnel. To review the major aspects of this issue, this chapter is divided into four sections: attitudes and influences resulting in substance abuse among athletes; "roid rage"; symptoms of substance abuse in athletes; and substance abuse prevention.

ATTITUDES AND INFLUENCES

There is tremendous interest in athletics in the United States today, and, some may argue, an overemphasis on "winning at all costs," not only in collegiate and professional sports but also at the high school and grade school levels. Pressures exist among athletes to do whatever it takes to win. Consequently, there is interest among some athletes in investigating drugs that may enhance performance. Recent reports of Olympic athletes banned from international competition as a result of failing routine drug tests confirm the fact that there are strong influences on athletes to find ways to use drugs to enhance performance. Many athletes believe the reports that certain drugs may increase athletic performance by as much as 15% and consider their use in spite of known long-term health hazards.[4]

Weight loss drugs frequently taken by athletes as a stopgap measure to lose weight quickly to make a particular weight classification or to fool the coach into believing that they are in good shape have proven to be deadly. Too often the athlete will be looking for the quick fix. Currently the biggest culprit being used to lose weight fast is the drug ephedra. This drug, which is banned by the International Olympic Committee, the National Football League, the National Basketball Association, and the National Hockey League, but not by Major League Baseball, is unfortunately available and easy to buy in over-the-counter diet pills. The one being the most used by athletes now is a product called Xenadrine RFA-1, and it is currently being investigated in the untimely deaths of a Major League Baseball player, a National Football League player, and a major college football player. This weight loss syndrome is adding to the pressure young athletes already are experiencing. In summary, both cultural and competitive pressures can influence athletes and contribute to the problem of substance abuse in sports medicine.

"ROID RAGE"

One of the most common substances being abused by athletes is anabolic steroids. These chemical derivatives of testosterone are used medically in the treatment of some blood disorders, cancers, and other illnesses.[1] Anabolic steroids also contribute to the increase of muscle mass, which improves strength and power.[2] For this reason, there is considerable interest in them as performance-enhancing drugs.

The long-term side effects of anabolic steroids include liver cancer, prostate cancer, and abnormal sperm production.[2] These long-term side effects are frequently overlooked by the athlete whose primary goal is short-term increase in muscle mass. Other side effects of anabolic steroids include severe acne, hair loss, atrophy of the testicles, and increased moodiness.[4] One of the most serious side effects of the steroids, especially in younger athletes, is sudden outbursts of aggressive and violent behavior, frequently referred to as "roid rage." The real problem with the use of steroids is that they do "work." Anabolic steroids do increase muscle mass relatively quickly but, at higher doses, certainly contribute to the development of psychological changes.[2,4] Aggressive behavior may manifest itself in the classroom as discipline problems since the young athlete is unable to control these outbursts on or off the playing field. Such behavior is a warning sign of substance abuse and will be addressed in the next section of this chapter. A videotape entitled *The Downfall of Sports and Drugs*, produced by the National Parents Resource Institute for Drug Education, offers a dramatic example of the signs and symptoms of roid rage.[3]

SYMPTOMS AND WHEN TO MAKE A REFERRAL

The symptoms of substance abuse in the athlete often are subtle, therefore it is sometimes difficult to establish the diagnosis. It is important for medical personnel, athletic coaches, and trainers to be familiar with subtle signs of substance abuse because often younger athletes will be more inclined to discuss problems with these professionals than with their parents.

One major sign of substance abuse is wide mood swings, including both elation and depression. These are illustrated graphically in Figure 49-1. The straight line represents the stresses of normal daily living, including the pressures placed on athletes by their peers,

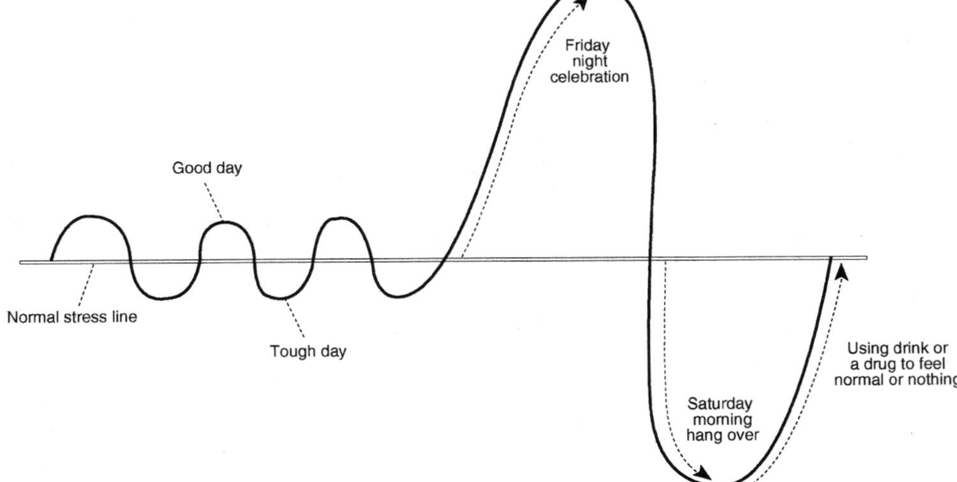

FIGURE 49-1. The normal mood swings of everyday activities and the excessive mood swings that may be indicative of substance abuse.

schoolwork, teachers, and parents. The higher and lower curves represent larger stresses and unusual occurrences in the athlete's life. Wide variations in mood may be an indication of substance abuse. Poor performance in academic work and inability to maintain commitments in school or part-time employment are early warning signs of possible substance abuse. In addition to missing classes or practices and a drop in the student's grades, other signs of substance abuse may include changes in groups of friends, withdrawal and secretiveness, unfinished schoolwork, and excessive lateness for school or sporting events. These signs may be more readily recognized by an athlete's parents. As soon as they recognize these signs and symptoms, the school, parents, and/or medical personnel should consider referral of the athlete to an appropriate mental health expert.

Once the suspicion of substance abuse is raised, appropriate referral for treatment is mandatory. In a school or university setting, there often are programs established by the administration that may include a guidance counselor to offer the first step of an appropriate referral for substance abuse. If the suspicion is raised by a trainer or team physician, this avenue of referral would be the first logical step. Many educational facilities have policies and procedures in place that review in student handbooks the appropriate mechanism for making such a referral. Outside the academic realm, sources of referral include the local chapters of Alcoholics Anonymous or the National Substance Abuse Council. These agencies have a wide variety of services available to both adults and students and provide counseling and intervention programs. The essential step for the primary care medical provider is to recognize the possibility of substance abuse and make an appropriate referral to a medical professional who is capable of treating the problem.

PREVENTION

Perhaps the most important step in the prevention of substance abuse among athletes is to recognize that it does exist. Hence, the most important strategy is education. Administration, coaches, and parents should address the possibilities of substance abuse in both preseason gatherings and team meetings for school-age athletes. Specifically, parents need to be educated and involved in the process. Among athletes at the collegiate and professional levels, addressing the issues of substance abuse must be done in open team-level forums. Zero tolerance must be the policy for all athletes under the age of 21.

Team sports should have specific team policies regarding substance abuse among team members. Again, the most important aspect is an open discussion of the possibilities of substance abuse. One strategy for decreasing the opportunity for substance abuse can be for parent or booster club groups to provide postgame parties for athletes and their families in a safe, controlled environment, so that they can celebrate without excesses of drugs or alcohol.

Probably the most effective program for the prevention of substance abuse is a clear statement, reemphasized periodically, of team policies regarding substance abuse. These policies are to be adhered to not only by the team members but by the coaching staff as well, since coaches and trainers often are positive role models for student athletes.

CONCLUSION

The best program for prevention of substance abuse among athletes is an open and direct discussion of the problems and tendencies that lead to drug abuse, a consistent review of policies and procedures, and an understanding by the team members that drug and alcohol abuse simply will not be tolerated. For athletes in whom substance abuse is suspected, early referral to an appropriate medical professional is essential for successful treatment.

REFERENCES

1. Dolan EF Jr: Drugs in Sports. New York, Franklin Watts, 1986.
2. Lukas SE: Steroids. Springfield, NJ, Enslow Publishers, 1994.
3. National Parents Resource Institute for Drug Education: The downfall of sports and drugs. Capitol Heights, MO, National Audiovisual Center (videotape), 1988.
4. Yesalis CE: Anabolic Steroids in Sports and Exercise. Champaign, IL, Human Kinetics, 1993.

50 Infectious Diseases

David C. Helfgott

Exercise has an integral role in the maintenance of our society's health and well-being. Mainly because of the salutary effects of exercise on the cardiovascular system, and its role in weight reduction and enhancing muscle strength and tone, athletes are considered healthier than the population who do not exercise. Also, participation in athletics requires a degree of strength and endurance that persons with acute and chronic diseases do not typically possess. However, acute infections are common in everyday life in both the healthy and the sick. Therefore, issues such as susceptibility to infection during exercise training and the effects of acute infection on training and physical performance are of special concern to the athlete. Athletes also are exposed to certain contagious diseases simply by their close proximity to each other. Infections may be transmitted via skin contact, respiratory secretions, and other body fluids. The fear of contracting contagious diseases and minimizing the risk of doing so also are important issues to athletes.

EFFECTS OF EXERCISE ON IMMUNE CELLS AND MEDIATORS

Several studies examining the effects of exercise and athletic training on the body's natural defenses against infection have been performed. These investigations mostly focus on changes in the number and function of the cells and mediators of the immune system. In assessing the conclusions from these studies, it is important to note that the subjects are mostly males and that their level of fitness within and across studies varies greatly. In addition, the intensity and duration of the exercises employed vary significantly across studies.

Polymorphonuclear leukocyte concentration rises immediately after exercise.[1,17,21,22,34,52,56,59,65] This increase is short-lived, and granulocyte numbers return to baseline values within 45 minutes.[17,52] Foster et al. demonstrated that the less fit the participant and the more intense the exercise, the higher the degree of granulocyte increase.[22] Two to four hours after intense exercise, there is a second rise in the concentration of polymorphonuclear leukocytes.[31,52] The increase in granulocyte concentration has been attributed to several factors, including hemoconcentration, catecholamine release resulting in demargination of leukocytes, and cortisol release resulting in demargination and subsequent delayed remargination of white blood cells.[58] However, a few studies refute the premise that granulocyte concentrations increase after exercise. Hanson and Flaherty[32] reported no change in granulocytes in athletes after a 13 km run, and Gray et al. noted no change in this leukocyte subset after anaerobic exercise.[27]

In addition to granulocyte number, granulocyte function after exercise has been studied. Schaefer et al. demonstrated that elastase, a product of polymorphonuclear leukocyte degranulation, increased 16% in male subjects after a 2000 m jog and increased almost four-fold after a 10,000 m jog.[56] Lewicki et al. found that neutrophil adherence and bactericidal activity decreased in well-trained cyclists but not in untrained males after maximal exercise.[43] In addition, resting measurements of neutrophil adherence were lower in trained than in untrained subjects, and the phagocytic activity of neutrophils increased after exercise in untrained males but did not change after exercise in the well-trained cyclists.[43]

Many studies demonstrate that total lymphocytes increase immediately after exercise,[1,5,17,18,27,34,52,59,67] but other studies report absolute numbers of lymphocytes unchanged[20,33,65] or decreased[16,31] when measured after exercise. Analysis of lymphocyte subpopulations reveals similar discrepancies among published reports. Most demonstrate numbers of B lymphocytes increasing after exercise,[5,27,34,40,62,67] though others refute this.[17,33] Similarly, numbers of T lymphocytes appear to mostly increase,[5,17,27,32,34,40,52,67] however, as a percentage of total lymphocytes, they appear to decrease.[17,27,40,67] Natural killer (NK) cells, another lymphocyte subset, seem to play an important role in recognizing malignant cells, as well as in antiviral immunity,[51] and there are conflicting data regarding changes in their number after exercise. Deuster et al. described an increase in NK cell number, and as a percentage of total lymphocytes, after maximal treadmill exercise;[17] Hoffman-Goetz demonstrated that after significant exercise the number of NK cells rises, then falls to below baseline within 2 hours and returns to baseline within 24 hours.[37] However, Haq et al. measured a decrease in the concentration of NK cells, and as a percentage of total lymphocytes, in subjects after a 42 km marathon.[33]

Studies of lymphocyte function are equally inconclusive. Lymphocyte transformation in response to antigenic stimulation in vitro has been shown to decrease[21,34] and increase[56,59] after exercise. Cytokines, the mediators released from mononuclear leukocytes that affect a myriad of metabolic and immune functions, have been measured after exercise. Serum "endogenous pyrogen" (interleukin-1 plus other inflammatory cytokines) activity increased immediately after moderate bicycle exercise,[10] and interleukin-1 activity after antigenic stimulation of peripheral blood mononuclear cells in vitro increased in marathon runners after a race.[65] The effect of exercise on other cytokines also has been studied.[30] NK cell activity was found to decrease after maximal exercise and remain depressed compared to baseline for almost one day.[7]

Serum immunoglobulins appear to change little after exercise;[19] however, several groups have noted changes in secretory IgA concentrations in saliva with training and after exercise. Tomasi et al. found that salivary IgA levels in United States National cross-country skiers were lower than in controls and that marathon skiing lowered their salivary IgA levels even more.[63] In well-trained cyclists, there was no difference in salivary IgA levels compared to controls; however, these levels significantly fell after two hours of cycling.[44]

EFFECTS OF EXERCISE ON SUSCEPTIBILITY TO INFECTION

Despite well-documented, albeit sometimes contradictory, alterations in immune mechanisms with exercise and training, the correlation between these changes and susceptibility to infection is unclear. The transient perturbations in immune cell number and function that occur immediately after exercise and return to baseline within hours are unlikely to have long-term clinical consequences. However, whether or not one's "resistance" to infection can be affected for a short time by exercise, and whether or not conditioning results in more chronic changes in resting state immunity, remain open to investigation.

In a study of the incidence of upper respiratory tract infections in marathoners, one third of the runners reported such symptoms within two weeks after a race, compared with 15% of age-matched controls.[49] The symptoms lasted more than three days in 80% of the marathoners, but these symptoms were self-reported and were not documented by medical personnel. Nieman[47] studied marathoners during training for the Los Angeles marathon and found that those who ran at least 60 miles weekly reported twice as many upper respiratory tract infections as those who ran less than 20 miles a week. Compared to the runners who did not run in the marathon but were similarly trained, those who completed the marathon reported six times as many upper respiratory tract infections. On the other hand, Nieman[48] had previously reported a trend toward fewer infectious episodes in runners training for a half-marathon compared to runners training for shorter 5 km or 10 km races. The stress of training and competition may contribute to susceptibility to infection; persons with greater psychologic stress have been shown to be more likely to develop upper respiratory tract infections when challenged with intranasal aerosolized virus.[14]

There are other data to suggest that athletes may have increased susceptibility to infection and that exercise may worsen active viral infection. In several college outbreaks of viral meningitis (which occurs most frequently in autumn), the attack rate for the college football team was much higher than the general student attack rate.[45] In two of these outbreaks, although several athletes required hospitalization, there were no hospitalizations in the infected nonathletes. In one outbreak, the longer the athletes continued heavy exercise, the longer they remained symptomatic. In a poliomyelitis outbreak at a boarding school in 1973, all of the infected students were athletes.[66]

Ongoing physical activity despite acute illness also has been reported to exacerbate the course of poliomyelitis in several studies,[38,54,55] and monkeys exercised during incubation for poliomyelitis developed worse paralysis than did nonexercised animals.[42] Similarly, murine studies demonstrated that coxsackievirus myocarditis was more severe and was associated with increased mortality in exercised versus nonexercised mice.[25,39,50,62] With regard to bacterial infections studied, Cannon and Kluger showed that exercise training improved the survival rate in rats subsequently infected with *Salmonella typhimurium*,[11] but Friman and colleagues demonstrated that rats with tularemia fared worse if they were subsequently exercised.[24]

EFFECTS OF INFECTION ON ATHLETIC PERFORMANCE

Several studies demonstrate that infection decreases athletic performance capacity. Subjects experimentally infected with plasma from a patient harboring the virus that causes sandfly fever had diminished muscle strength and exercise endurance during fever.[15] Similar observations have been made during pyrogen-induced fever[28] and malaria in humans.[36] Friman's group[23] tested muscle strength in patients with viral diseases just after illness and in healthy controls who were put to bed rest for one week and then similarly tested. Muscle strength was significantly decreased after illness compared to strength 4 months later in the subjects, whereas no change was seen in the control group between initial and subsequent testing. Bengtsson[2] also demonstrated that exercise capacity was diminished during convalescence from acute infection.

INFECTIONS COMMON IN ATHLETES

Transmission of contagious diseases is facilitated in athletes by their contact with each other and the environment (dirt, locker room floors, swimming pools) in the course of training and competition, as well as by teammates sharing beverages and towels. Most of the infections that are more common to athletes than the nonathletic population are therefore dermatologic;

however, isolated outbreaks of systemic illnesses among teammates have been reported.

There have been several outbreaks of viral meningitis on college campuses, between August and October, which have involved a disproportionate number of football players.[45] Sharing water from common cups or a water bucket was documented as a cause of increased transmission among football players at two of the campuses and, presumably, similar factors and close contact among teammates facilitated viral transmission in the other teams. At the College of the Holy Cross, 93% of the football team became infected with viral hepatitis in 1969.[46] This outbreak, which involved only football players, was linked to an infected water supply used to irrigate the practice field and provide drinking water at the field.

Swimmer's Ear (Otitis Externa)

Otitis externa is a common infection involving the external auditory canal, which results from exposure to fresh water or swimming pools. Repeated exposure may result in desquamation of the epithelium of the external ear canal, with subsequent infection of this abnormal skin. Symptoms and signs include itching in the ear, pain in the ear exacerbated by pulling on the pinna, and redness and swelling, sometimes with purulence, involving the external canal. The most common organism that causes this infection is *Pseudomonas aeruginosa*, although other bacteria may be etiologic. Treatment should be with topical antibiotic drops, which include neomycin and polymyxin B; systemic antibiotics usually are unnecessary.

Impetigo

Impetigo is a bacterial infection of the epidermis caused by *Streptococcus pyogenes* and much less commonly by *Staphylococcus aureus*, which presents itself as vesiculopustular lesions that rupture and form thick, yellow crusts.[61] This infection is easily communicable and is transmitted in swimming pools, by direct contact, and by sharing towels and athletic equipment. Swimmers and wrestlers are therefore especially susceptible.[3] Diagnosis is made by gram stain and/or culture of the vesicle fluid or base of a crusted lesion. Treatment should be with an antistreptococcal systemic antibiotic such as penicillin, clindamycin, or erythromycin, which is superior to topical treatment for this infection. In rare cases, acute glomerulonephritis may occur secondary to impetigo. Athletes should not participate in sports activities until the lesions have completely healed.

Folliculitis

Folliculitis is characterized by small, erythematous papulopustular lesions originating within hair follicles. *Staphylococcus aureus* is usually the etiologic organism; however, folliculitis from swimming pools, whirlpools, and hot tubs is caused by *Pseudomonas aeruginosa*. Outbreaks from these exposures occur when pH and chlorine levels are inadequate. Swimming pools should be maintained at a pH of 7.2 to 8.2 with chlorine levels at 0.4 to 1.0 mg/L, and hot tubs should have chlorine levels of 2.0 to 5.0 mg/L to prevent outbreaks of pseudomonas folliculitis.[41] Antibiotics are usually unnecessary because the folliculitis is typically self-limited.

Furunculosis

Furuncles are abscesses caused by *Staphylococcus aureus* that arise at the site of hair follicles, usually preceded by folliculitis. A furuncle begins as a tender, erythematous nodule that becomes fluctuant and usually spontaneously drains purulent material.[61] Sometimes clinical drainage is necessary, but usually the application of warm soaks results in spontaneous drainage. If a surrounding cellulitis is present, systemic antibiotic therapy with an antistaphylococcal penicillin, clindamycin, or erythromycin should be used. Some individuals develop recurrent furunculosis for unknown reasons; attempts at control and prevention with multiple systemic and topical antibiotics and meticulous skin and clothing care have had limited success. An outbreak of furunculosis occurred among basketball and football players at a Kentucky high school in 1986–1987; the risk of infection was higher in players who had a skin injury and in players who had skin exposure to other players with furuncles.[60]

Herpes Gladiatorum (Herpes Simplex)

Herpes simplex is a viral infection transmitted by direct contact with infected skin lesions, which occur as vesicles on an erythematous base. Herpes simplex typically appears on the face and genitalia, but lesions can occur anywhere that affected skin is contacted. Several days after vesicle formation the lesions break and become crusted before disappearing in about a week. Herpes gladiatorum describes this infection in wrestlers: they are the athletes most commonly affected by herpes simplex virus because of the constant skin contact between competitors. The initial infection may be associated with fever, malaise, and headache. Recurrences can be triggered by physical or emotional stress. Diagnosis is made by recognizing the clusters of typical lesions and by the revealing of multinucleated giant cells by Tzanck preparation of the base of a lesion. Although the lesions are self-limited, treatment with acyclovir can shorten the time of viral shedding and of visible lesions by a day or two. For individuals with frequent recurrences, prophylaxis with acyclovir (400 mg twice daily) has been demonstrated to significantly decrease their number of outbreaks.[53] Athletes with herpes simplex infection should not participate in contact sports while lesions are present.

Molluscum Contagiosum

Molluscum contagiosum is a viral infection transmitted by skin-to-skin or fomite-to-skin contact.[3] The characteristic lesions are multiple flesh-colored umbilicated papules that are most commonly found on the trunk, thigh, or groin areas. Characteristic appearance or skin biopsy is required for diagnosis; the lesions will resolve spontaneously, but treatment is accomplished by curettage or destruction of the skin lesions. Athletes with these lesions should not participate in contact sports.

Cutaneous Warts

Warts are hyperkeratotic papules of the epithelium caused by papillomaviruses. Athletes are more susceptible to warts because these viruses are more likely to invade at sites of calluses.[57] Plantar warts occur on the plantar aspect of the feet, and pressure causes the lesions to be flatter than common warts. Common warts are exophytic and occur mostly on the hands and fingers.[6] The virus is inoculated via direct skin contact or via fomites such as floors and equipment. The incubation period from exposure to development of a cutaneous wart is about 6 months.[57] Although spontaneous resolution of warts typically occurs, they can be present for years.

Superficial Fungal Infections

Superficial fungal infections of the skin are usually caused by the dermatophytes *Trichophyton rubrum* and *Trichophyton mentagrophytes*. These organisms are the etiologic agents in athlete's foot (tinea pedis) and jock itch (tinea cruris), which are the most common dermatophytoses of athletes. Infection is facilitated by increased moisture from sweat in these areas and is acquired on locker room floors and from towels and clothing harboring the fungus. Infection can spread from foot to groin as a person towels off or dresses. Tinea pedis has pruritic and sometimes painful scaling or blisters, usually in the webs of the toes, and can lead to onychomycosis (nail tinea). Tinea cruris occurs in the groin and on the upper thighs and produces pruritic, erythematous, scaling patches. Treatment is with topical antifungal agents; terbinafine twice daily for one week is probably the most efficacious.[4] Prevention is most effective and consists of using only clean, dry towels and clothing, protective footwear in the locker room, and putting on socks before underclothing and trousers. Onychomycosis is extremely difficult to treat, requiring a prolonged course of systemic antifungal therapy. The imidazoles, fluconazole and itraconazole, recently have been proven to be relatively safe and effective in treating onychomycosis, but hepatic toxicity may limit their use in some patients.

Other fungi also may cause dermatophytoses in athletes. Ringworm, or tinea corporis, is characterized by annular erythematous lesions mostly on the back, shoulders, and neck,[57] and is caused by *T. rubrum*, *T. mentagrophytes*, or *T. tonsurans*. Tinea corporis gladiatorum refers to this infection in wrestlers, in whom several outbreaks have been documented.[13] Tinea versicolor occurs typically on the torso and arms of swimmers and is caused by *Malassezia furfur*. The lesions are lightly colored scaling patches that are generally nonpruritic and are treated with 2% selenium sulfide.[3]

THE SPECIAL CASE OF HUMAN IMMUNODEFICIENCY VIRUS

Recent disclosures by several professional athletes who tested positive for human immunodeficiency virus (HIV) have attracted significant attention to issues surrounding the HIV-positive athlete. Athletes have repeated physical contact with teammates and opponents and may sustain a bleeding laceration in the course of competition. Fear of HIV infection has fueled an ongoing debate as to the usefulness and ethical propriety of mandatory HIV testing of athletes.[9]

HIV is transmitted via infected blood and blood products, by sexual exposure, and by perinatal transmission. There has been no documentation that the virus is transmitted by sweat or saliva. In evaluating the risk of HIV transmission for health care workers after occupational exposure, studies support a transmission rate of 0.2% to 0.5% after percutaneous injuries with contaminated devices.[26] For any individual worker, the risk of acquiring HIV after such an injury appears to be related to the volume of blood exposure and the depth of the injury.[12] The risk of transmission to health care workers with mucocutaneous exposure to HIV may be half that of percutaneous injuries, and there have been no reported HIV conversions in health care workers with only intact skin exposure.[35] The likelihood of hepatitis B or C transmission after percutaneous injury is 10 to 100 times as likely as is HIV transmission.[26] Extrapolating these data to possible exposure of an athlete to the blood from an HIV-infected athlete, the likelihood of HIV transmission would seem to be anywhere between 0 and 0.25%. The prevalence of HIV infection in the population depends on the population studied, but the prevalence rate in applicants to the U.S. military between 1985 and 1989 was 0.13%.[8]

Athletes would seem to have a much greater risk of acquiring HIV off the playing venue than on it. Despite this, a report of HIV transmission presumed to be the result of a sports injury has been reported.[64] In this particular case there was bloody wound contact between an HIV-positive and an HIV-negative (one year previously) athlete in a soccer match, and no other explanation could be found to account for the HIV-negative athlete's seroconversion. Prudence dictates that any athlete who suffers a bleeding injury should be removed from competition until the bleeding stops and the wound is appropriately covered.

PREVENTION OF INFECTION IN ATHLETES

Some simple guidelines can minimize the risk of infection in athletes in the course of training and strenuous exercise. Because it is unclear how exercise-caused alterations in immune mechanisms affect the risk of clinical infection, the usual recommendations such as good nutrition, adequate sleep, and efforts to minimize stress may help to reduce the risk of infection. It is clear that acute infection compromises athletic performance and that certain infections may be exacerbated by strenuous exercise; therefore, it is wise to avoid such exercise and athletic competition during an acute infection.

Athletes can acquire communicable diseases from each other and the environment. Avoidance of sharing beverages, athletic equipment, and towels; attention to good foot care; and enforcement of nonparticipation in contact sports by athletes with communicable skin diseases can minimize transmission of these infections.

Immunizations are important in preventing communicable diseases. After the initial childhood diphtheria-pertussis-tetanus series, diphtheria-tetanus boosters should be administered routinely every ten years, but if a person suffers a wound involving potentially contaminated soil or debris, a tetanus toxoid booster should be given if it has not been administered within five years.[29] Two measles-mumps-rubella vaccinations are required because about 5% of recipients will not respond to the first measles vaccination.[29] The second vaccine is not always given at the recommended 4 to 6 years of age, so athletes should have proof of two vaccinations or evidence of measles immunity. Because they are in such close contact with one another, and because influenza would severely hamper their athletic performance, athletes who participate in winter sports may choose to receive annual influenza vaccinations.

REFERENCES

1. Ahlborg B, Ahlborg G: Exercise leukocytosis with and without beta-adrenergic blockade. Acta Med Scand 187:241–246, 1970.
2. Bengtsson E: Working capacity and exercise electrocardiogram in convalescents after acute infectious diseases without cardiac complications. Acta Med Scand 154:359–373, 1956.
3. Bergfeld WF: Dermatologic problems in athletes. Primary Care 11:151–160, 1984.
4. Bergstresser PR, Elewski B, Hanifin J, et al: Topical terbinafine and clotrimazole in interdigital tinea pedis: A multicenter comparison of cure and relapse rates with 1- and 4-week treatment regimens. J Am Acad Dermatol 28:648–651, 1993.
5. Bieger WP, Weiss M, Michel G, Weicker H: Exercise-induced monocytosis and modulation of monocyte function. Int J Sports Med 1:30–36, 1980.
6. Bonnez W, Reichman RC: Papillomaviruses. In Mandell GL, Bennett JE, Dolin R (eds): Principles and Practice of Infectious Diseases, 4th ed. New York, Churchill Livingstone, 1995.
7. Brahmi Z, Thomas JE, Park M, et al: The effect of acute exercise on natural killer-cell activity of trained and sedentary human subjects. J Clin Immunol 5:321–328, 1985.
8. Brundage JF, Burke DS, Gardner LI, et al: Tracking the spread of the HIV infection epidemic among young adults in the United States: Results of the first four years of screening among civilian applicants for U.S. military service. J Acquir Immune Defic Syndr 3:1168–1180, 1990.
9. Calabrese LH, Haupt HA, Hartman L: HIV and sports: What is the risk? Phys Sports Med 21: 173–180, 1993.
10. Cannon JG, Kluger MJ: Endogenous pyrogen activity in human plasma after exercise. Science 220:617–619, 1983.
11. Cannon JG, Kluger MJ: Exercise enhances survival rate in mice infected with *Salmonella typhimurium.* Proc Soc Exp Biol Med 175:518–521, 1984.
12. Case-control study of HIV seroconversion in health-care workers after percutaneous exposure to HIV-infected blood: France, United Kingdom, and United States, January 1988-August 1994. MMWR 44:929–933, 1995.
13. Cohen BA, Schmidt C: Tineal gladiatorum. N Engl J Med 327:820, 1992.
14. Cohen S., Tyrrell DAJ, Smith AP: Psychological stress and susceptibility to the common cold. N Engl J Med 325:606–612, 1991.
15. Daniels WL, Sharp DS, Wright JE, et al: Effects of virus infection on physical performance in man. Military Med 150:8–14, 1985.
16. Davidson RJL, Robertson JD, Maughan RJ: Haematological changes due to triathalon competition. Br J Sports Med 12:159–161, 1986.
17. Deuster PA, Curiale AM, Cowan ML, Finkelman FD: Exercise-induced changes in populations of peripheral blood mononuclear cells. Med Sci Sports Exerc 20:276–280, 1988.
18. Edwards AJ, Bacon TH, Elms CA, et al: Changes in the populations of lymphoid cells in human peripheral blood following physical exercise. Clin Exp Immunol 58:420–427, 1984.
19. Eichner ER: Infection, immunity, and exercise: What to tell patients? Phys Sports Med 21:125–135, 1993.
20. Eskola J, Ruuskanen E, Soppi E, et al: Effect of sports stress on lymphocyte transformation and antibody formation. Clin Exp Immunol 32:339–345, 1978.
21. Eskola J, Soppi E, Viljanen K, et al: Effect of sport stress on lymphocyte transformation and antibody formation. Clin Exp Immunol 32:339–345, 1978.

22. Foster NK, Martyn JB, Rangno RE, et al: Leukocytosis of exercise: Role of cardiac output and catecholamines. J Appl Physiol 61:2218–2223, 1986.
23. Friman G: Effect of acute infectious disease on isometric muscle strength. Scand J Clin Lab Invest 37:303–308, 1977.
24. Friman G, Ilback N-G, Beisel WR, Crawford DJ: Effects of strenuous exercise on *Francisella tularensis* in rats. J Infec Dis 5:706–714, 1982.
25. Gatmaitan BG, Chason JL, Lerner AM: Augmentation of the virulence of murine coxsackievirus B-3 myocardiopathy by exercise. J Exp Med 131: 1121–1136, 1970.
26. Gerberding JL: Management of occupational exposures to blood-borne viruses. N Engl J Med 332:444–451, 1995.
27. Gray AB, Smart YC, Telford RD, et al: Anaerobic exercise causes transient changes in leukocyte subsets and IL-2R expression. Med Sci Sports Exerc 24: 1332–1338, 1992.
28. Grimby G: Exercise in man during pyrogen-induced fever. Scand J Clin Lab Invest (Suppl 67) 14:1–112, 1962.
29. Guide for Adult Immunization, 3rd ed. Philadelphia, American College of Physicians, 1994.
30. Haahr PM, Pedersen BK, Fomsgaard A, et al: Effect of physical exercise on in vitro production of interleukin-1, interleukin-6, tumor necrosis factor-alpha, interleukin-2, and interferon gamma. Int J Sports Med 12:223–227, 1991.
31. Hansen JB, Wilsgard L, Osterud B: Biphasic changes in leukocytes induced by strenuous exercise. Eur J Appl Physiol 62:157–161, 1991.
32. Hanson PG, Flaherty DK: Immunological responses to training in conditioned runners. Clin Sci 60: 225–228, 1981.
33. Haq A, Al-Hussein K, Lee J, Al-Seidairy S: Changes in peripheral blood lymphocyte subsets associated with marathon running. Med Sci Sports Exerc 25: 186–190, 1993.
34. Hedfors E, Holm G, Ohnell B: Variations of blood lymphocytes during work studied by cell surface markers, DNA synthesis and cytotoxicity. Clin Exp Immunol 24:328–335, 1976.
35. Henderson DK, Fahey BJ, Willy M, et al: Risk for occupational transmission of human immunodeficiency virus type 1 (HIV-1) associated with clinical exposures: A prospective evaluation. Ann Intern Med 113:740–746, 1990.
36. Henschel A, Taylor HL, Keys A: Experimental malaria in man. I. Physical deterioration and recovery. J Clin Invest 29:52–59, 1950.
37. Hoffman-Goetz L, Simpson JR, Cipp N, et al: Lymphocyte subset responses to repeated submaximal exercise in men. J Appl Physiol 68:1069–1074, 1990.
38. Horstmann DM: Acute poliomyelitis: Relation of physical activity at the time of onset to the course of the disease. J Am Med Assoc 142:236–241, 1950.
39. Ilback N-G, Fohlman J, Friman G: Exercise in Coxsackie B3 myocarditis: Effects on heart lymphocyte subpopulations and the inflammatory reaction. Am Heart J 117:1298–1302, 1989.
40. Keast D, Cameron K, Morton AR: Exercise and the immune response. Sports Med 5:248–267, 1988.
41. Kramer MH, Herwaldt BL, Craun GF, et al: Surveillance for waterborne-disease outbreaks: United States, 1993–1994. MMWR 45(SS-1):1–30, 1996.
42. Levinson SO, Milzer A, Lewin P: Am J Hygiene 42:204–213, 1945.
43. Lewicki R, Tchorzewski H, Denys A, et al: Effect of physical exercise on some parameters of immunity in conditioned sportsmen. Int J Sports Med 8:309–314, 1987.
44. Mackinnon LT, Chick TW, Van As A, et al: Decreased secretory immunoglobulins following intense endurance exercise. Sports Training Med Rehab 1:209–218, 1989.
45. Moore M, Baron RC, Filstein MR, et al: Aseptic meningitis and high school football players: 1978 and 1980. J Am Med Assoc 249:2039–2042, 1983.
46. Morse LJ, Bryan JA, Hurley JP, et al: The Holy Cross college football team hepatitis outbreak. J Am Med Assoc 219:706–708, 1972.
47. Nieman DC, Johanssen LM, Lee JW, et al: Infectious episodes in runners before and after the Los Angeles Marathon. J Sports Med Phys Fitness 30:316–328, 1990.
48. Nieman DC, Johanssen LM, Lee JW: Infectious episodes in runners before and after a roadrace. J Sports Med Phys Fitness 29:289–296, 1989.
49. Peters EM, Bateman ED: Ultramarathon running and upper respiratory tract infections: An epidemiological survey. S Afr Med J 64:582–584, 1983.
50. Reyes MP, Lerner AM: Interferon and neutralizing antibody in sera of exercised mice with coxsackie B-3 myocarditis. Proc Soc Exp Biol Med 151: 333–338, 1976.
51. Ritz J: The role of natural killer cells in immune surveillance. N Engl J Med 320:1748–1749, 1989.
52. Robertson AJ, Ramesar CRB, Potts RC, et al: The effect of strenuous physical exercise on circulating blood lymphocytes and serum cortisol levels. J Clin Lab Immunol 5:53–57, 1981.
53. Rooney JF, Straus SE, Mannix ML, et al: Oral acyclovir to suppress frequently recurrent herpes labialis: A double blind, placebo-controlled trial. Ann Intern Med 118: 268–272, 1993.
54. Russell WR: Paralytic poliomyelitis: The early symptoms and the effect of physical activity on the course of the disease. Br Med J 1:465–471, 1949.

55. Russell WR: The pre-paralytic stage and the effect of physical activity on the severity of paralysis. Br Med J 2:1023–1029, 1947.
56. Schaefer RM, Kokot K, Heidland A, Plass R: Jogger's leukocytes (letter). New Engl J Med 316: 223–224, 1987.
57. Sevier TL: Infectious disease in athletes. Med Clin N Am 78:389–412, 1994.
58. Simon HB: The immunology of exercise: A brief review. J Am Med Assoc 252:2735–2738, 1984.
59. Soppi E, Varjo P, Eskola J, et al: Effect of strenuous physical stress on circulating lymphocyte number and function before and after training. J Clin Lab Immunol 8:43–46, 1982.
60. Sosin DM, Gunn RA, Ford WL, et al: An outbreak of furunculosis among high school athletes. Am J Sports Med 17:828–832, 1989.
61. Swartz MN: Cellulitis and subcutaneous tissue infections. In Mandell GL, Bennett JE, Dolin R (eds): Principles and Practice of Infectious Diseases, 4th ed. New York, Churchill Livingstone, 1995.
62. Tilles JG, Elson SH, Shaka JA, et al: Effects of exercise on coxsackie A-9 myocarditis in adult mice. Proc Soc Exp Biol Med 117:777–778, 1964.
63. Tomasi TB, Trudeau FB, Czerwinski D, et al: Immune parameters in athletes before and after strenuous exercise. J Clin Immunol 2:173–178, 1982.
64. Torre D, Sampietro C, Ferraro G, et al: Transmission of HIV-1 infection during sports injury (letter). Lancet 335:1105, 1990.
65. Weight LM, Alexander D, Jacobs P: Strenuous exercise: Analagous to the acute phase response? Clin Sci 81:677–683, 1991.
66. Weinstein L: Poliomyelitis—a persistent problem. N Engl J Med 288:370–372, 1973.
67. Yu DTY, Clements J, Pearson CM: Effect of corticosteroids on exercise-induced lymphocytosis. Clin Exp Immunol 28:326–331, 1977.

51 Sports Psychology

Ulla Kristiina Laakso

RECOGNITION OF THE PROBLEM

Comprehensive medical care for athletic patients today must incorporate the psychological as well as the physical aspects of management. Approaching the patient and athlete as a whole has given rise to an entirely new field called sports psychology. Although the field has experienced tremendous growth in the past 25 years, it is still afforded little attention in the standard psychiatry and psychology textbooks and even in sports medicine texts. The fact that people are concerned about their psychological as well as their physical well-being is reflected in the veritable explosion of self-help, fitness, and self-improvement books and manuals, along with the appearance of workshops, seminars, and various support organizations. In fact, the need to "keep fit" has spawned an entirely new kind of social interaction. Social lives often revolve around various sports, recreational, and fitness activities. The rapidly growing phenomenon of health and fitness clubs, running clubs, biking and skiing clubs, and other sports-related social groups has, in turn, had a ripple effect in the economy in terms of fitness gear, clothing, and other related paraphernalia. Sports-related injuries that cause absence from work also have an effect on the economic environment.

Coaches, trainers, and teachers all have become increasingly familiar with the importance of psychological training of athletes to enhance their performance and maximize their achievements. Virtually all professional teams, and many college teams, routinely employ the services of a sports psychologist for consultation on a regular basis. Sexual harassment and abuse of female athletes has been acknowledged. The relationship between coach and athlete is vulnerable to the abuse of trust, and professional policies are addressing this issue. The International Society of Sports Psychology (ISSP) has recommended measures to be taken to address aggression and violence in sports. These include education of young athletes in the ethics of fair play.

Most players have some familiarity with specific psychological techniques and strategies to enhance their performance. These are various forms of "psyching up" for a particular event. They range from forms of ritualistic behavior such as wearing the same "lucky" pair of socks to a more logical type of behavior such as eating a specific kind of meal before performing. Beneath the surface of these benign mannerisms and activities, one finds that these actions are well rooted in the field of sports psychology.

Coaches have been using psychological motivation for decades, for example, in the use of "pep talks." This type of psychological motivation is used to enable athletes to increase their concentration, enhance their reflexes, and focus their attention. It also helps to alleviate and displace anxiety and nervousness before the sporting event. It helps to put the athlete in the proper mood for participation and optimizes his or her performance. The coaching staff and players use psychological techniques such as self-talk, imagery, and cognitive restructuring. The same motivators that enhance athletic performance can be adapted and applied to the rehabilitation process following an injury.

It may be conceded that most athletes who are injured, including recreational players and elite professionals, may recover without any need for formal psychological intervention. However, as the stakes for achievement in sports grow higher and higher in terms of social implication and commercial worth, every avenue must be pursued to ensure a rapid and satisfactory recovery.

THE SPORTS, HEALTH, AND FITNESS EXPLOSION

Decades of epidemiologic research on how lifestyle factors affect the morbidity of chronic illnesses paved the way to the current exercise and fitness boom. Work began in the 1950s by fitness pioneers such as Ernst Wynder at the American Health Foundation, Nathan Pritikin at the Pritikin Longevity Institute, and Dean Ornish. Once it was shown that heart disease could be reversed by comprehensive lifestyle changes, it led to more public awareness of the benefits of physical fitness. These researchers showed the benefits of regular exercise on cardiovascular disease, weight reduction, cancer, and even in lowering cholesterol. Exercise became an important adjunct to smoking cessation and therefore has had a role in the prevention of smoking-related cancers. Exercise also has had a beneficial effect on diabetic patients and those with arthritis and other diseases.

The benefits of exercise affect not only our physical being but also our mental and emotional state. Today every kind of stress reduction program invariably includes some form of exercise. These range from vigorous running to simple meditation, yoga, and breathing exercises. Because there are more people exercising, there has been an increase in sports-related injuries. This has caused an acute awareness of how to prevent these injuries, in the form of adequate warm-up and significant physical, mental, and academic preparation for a sport.

Exercise stimulates secretion of naturally produced hormones called endorphins that have a euphoric effect at moderate levels. Over-secretion has been implicated in so-called exercise addiction, in which the act of exercise itself becomes the dominant part of a person's life. In the same way that the primary care physician has always been the traditional person to whom the family could go for advice, the practitioner has once again become the storehouse for information on fitness, a very important part of patients' lives. This physician often is called on to give recommendations for exercise planning, injury prevention, weight reduction, and for an overall program of physical fitness, including the physiologic and psychological aspects. To this end, the practitioner must be prepared to intervene psychologically on the patients' behalf. The injured recreational athlete, like the professional one, may require a flexible, safe, and alternative exercise plan during recovery, to boost morale and provide continuity in the exercise regime. This is often referred to as "something for the head." Although the physician's main attention may be on treating the injury, the discontinuation of exercise routines can have a significant negative consequence for the patient's emotional and psychological condition.

The field of sports psychology has become a subdiscipline of the broader field of psychology and also has evolved into an academic discipline. Through the ever-growing body of publications and conferences, information reaches a wide and varied audience. There has been a rapid proliferation of books dealing with the subject of sports psychology. "Performance enhancement" as it applies to different sports is the main focus of these books. Sports psychologists have correlated certain personality traits with varying degrees of athletic success and motivation. In addition, certain character features have been shown to be not compatible with sustained satisfactory athletic performance. There are personality traits that are likely to cause an undesirable amount of anxiety and even lead to depression. This, of course, has a negative effect on athletic performance. Psychology reveals a direct relationship between mental health and sports performance. We now know that a number of mental skills and cognitive functions can be trained, as can motor skills. Programs in this specific area are already in place at all levels of competitive sports, including professional teams, college and high school teams, and in Olympic and international competition.

The core area of performance enhancement is anxiety management using cognitive skills. A variety of mental phenomena influence athletic performances. These include arousal, attention, concentration, imagery, and altered states of consciousness. Cognitive skill training uses techniques such as self-talk, thought stopping, mental rehearsal, and imagery. There is also emphasis on a holistic approach to this subject, an example of which is the program developed by the Performance Enhancement Center at the Military Academy at West Point. Various psychological instruments have been used to measure emotional states and their relationship to athletic performance. Tests such as the Sports Competitive Anxiety Test (SCAT) have found wide acceptance among sports psychology researchers.[27] Anxiety and stress management techniques have employed performance curves related to confidence, stress, and even arousal. In these "inverted U" theories, optimal performance is found at moderate levels of confidence, stress, and arousal. On the other hand, performance is relatively impaired by either too little or too much of these emotions. A variety of techniques stem from this concept, including progressive muscle relaxation, biofeedback, and autogenic training.

THE ROLE OF THE PRIMARY CARE PHYSICIAN

The Good Listener

The benefits of having a "good listener" to hear our troubles and difficulties at times are well known. Primary care physicians should try to develop an empathetic style of listening and communicating with athletes, especially at the time of an injury. The physician needs to carefully screen every statement made by the athlete who is describing an ailment or injuries, paying attention to the specific language the patient is using. A determination must be made as to whether the patient is exaggerating or perhaps even minimizing the symptoms. It is not uncommon for the high-performance athlete to want to trivialize his or her injury "for the good of the team." On the other hand, some athletes might exaggerate the injury for secondary gain, reflecting perhaps a fear of performance or some other psychological entity. The physician must determine whether or not the patient's description and language are appropriate and whether the emotions associated with the injury are in the expected range.

Interviewing Techniques

Evaluating the athlete's psychological profile requires some specific skills and techniques. Not only must the physician be an empathetic listener, but also the physician's body language and eye contact must convey the message that the practitioner is interested in whatever the athlete is going to share with him or her. It is strongly recommended that this encounter be conducted with the physician sitting down, a comfortable distance away from the patient. It has been clearly shown that the patient perceives the interview as lasting longer and being more thorough if the physician is sitting down rather than standing up. It also is important to have as much privacy as possible. Exploration of psychological issues is a delicate and private matter. It should not be conducted in a public environment.

The physician needs to convey to the patient that he or she can be trusted with sensitive psychological material and that it will not be shared unless the patient consents. Appropriate body language helps facilitate the conveyance of this message. Even a simple nodding of the head or a neutral comment such as "I understand," or "that is normal," can ingratiate the physician to the patient and facilitate communication. This will further enhance the likelihood of the patient's opening up with his or her true feelings. If the patient perceives the feedback or body language as even mildly critical or judgmental, it is likely to cause the patient to feel disappointment and thereby shut down the communication between them. It is recommended that the physician ask open-ended questions that cannot be answered merely with a "yes" or a "no." This allows the athlete to reveal more, and it fosters a rapport between the patient and the physician. Using the patient's own words to reframe responses, comments, and questions has proven to be a valuable technique. It reassures the patient that he or she has indeed been heard.

It must be remembered that many athletes are perfectionists and therefore they may regard their health situations very negatively and pessimistically. When explaining the nature of an injury to a patient, the physician certainly must be honest with the patient but also should be careful not to take away the hope of recovery when at all possible. To this end, it is helpful to emphasize and reemphasize the treatment possibilities and the progress that the patient has made so far. The injured athlete is likely to welcome the physician's knowledge about some of the psychological techniques available. The athlete may be hesitant to ask about relaxation training, biofeedback, or meditation if he or she perceives the physician as being closed-minded. Often the injured athlete welcomes an adjunct therapy from outside the traditional medical venue. Such techniques, when used individually or in combinations, enhance athletic performance and improve the rehabilitation process.

INJURY: PSYCHOLOGICAL IMPLICATIONS AND ATHLETES' PERCEPTIONS

Following a serious injury, athletes will typically experience three phases of reaction. During the initial phase, the athlete is likely to express denial and disbelief. Denial may be so strong that the athlete is ready to continue to play despite warnings that the injury may worsen. Disbelief may cause the injured patient to seek several professional opinions.

During the second phase, the patient exhibits a variety of negative emotions. Those likely to surface include anger, anxiety, frustration, depressed mood, insomnia, poor concentration, and disruption of usual activities. These psychological reactions slow treatment and rehabilitation. The athlete's anxiety and frustration often are more difficult to deal with than the actual injury. During this phase, the physician needs a great deal of patience. The athlete's frustration may impair his or her ability to listen to professional advice.

The third phase includes acceptance and adaptation. During this phase, the injured athlete comes to terms with the injury and its consequences. The physician can help the patient to adjust to the new medical information and find reasons for hope and optimism. Helping the athlete to reach this phase is important in reducing the length of the rehabilitation and recuperation process. Some of the patient's previous activities may be resumed and some goals may be revised. Some of the goals may have to be given up. The physician should demonstrate compassion, support, and helpfulness. Cognitive behavioral stress management has been shown to help prevent injuries and shorten recovery time.[30]

THE ATHLETE'S PERCEPTION OF INJURY

The primary care physician working with injured athletes will witness a variety of reactions to injuries. Sometimes an athlete may exhibit lack of concern, indifference, or even detachment over an injury. Further exploration of these observations may show that the athlete is actually relieved at being excused from competitive activities because the athlete fears that his or her poor performance or loss in competition might result in embarrassment. The athlete also may welcome having the "safe" excuse for further sub-optimal performances.

Another athlete may totally catastrophize an injury. This athlete may feel that all is lost and may hold rigidly to a single explanation for the injury. There may be paranoid thoughts expressed toward training practices, coaches, team leadership, or even another player. The primary care physician needs to be aware of this kind of maladaptive reaction and poor insight to the injury at hand. If the athlete is unable to view the injury from a more flexible perspective, the athlete's psychological state will be a roadblock to recovery and rehabilitation. The athlete may decide that his or her recovery will be "exactly the same" as that of a fellow athlete whose recovery has been sub-optimal.

The primary care physician needs to remember that a host of other factors influence the rehabilitation process, including whether or not the doctor is perceived as open and helpful. The patient may mask pain and physical symptoms. Marital problems and other social problems, low expectation of support from others, and lack of religious faith appear to influence the rehabilitation process. Patients with a history of psychological problems and a high anxiety level are more likely to have impaired recovery.[25,26] Low ego strengths lead to poor coping skills at the time of injury. These coping skills are put under considerable demands. Patients with a history of substance and alcohol abuse predictably have problems in recovery. The athlete with more concerns of all kinds is vulnerable to slow rehabilitation. Athletes may perceive injury as a punishment or they may read special meaning into the injury. Parental views of health, injury, and overall coping in life can influence, on an unconscious level, the athlete's coping mechanisms.[10]

There is a wide range of ways in which athletes can cope with illness and injury. To cope effectively with stress, one must make a conscious effort to do so and seek and obtain help from others. Important parts of the coping mechanism are the ego's unconscious adaptive mechanisms. These include altruism, humor, suppression, anticipation, and sublimation. They are called mature defenses. A less mature defense, such as denial, is also common in severe circumstances.

WARNING SIGNS OF PSYCHOLOGICAL IMPAIRMENT

As in the general population, the athlete's signs of psychological impairment and disturbance can be quite subtle. Often the athlete and his or her family, coach, and training staff may have little suspicion that anything is amiss. The skilled observer, however, can sort out some of the cardinal warning signs of psychological illness, which can respond to intervention. Common types of psychological disturbances include depression, anxiety, bipolar disorder (manic–depressive illness), panic disorder, and obsessive–compulsive disorder. It is not uncommon for patients and athletes so affected to question whether these symptoms represent "weakness" in their will and character. The physician can help to reassure the patient that these conditions are not rare.

Depression

The physician can assure the athlete that depression can affect anyone at any time, including children and adolescents. Depression can have multiple causes, including genetic patterns. The tendency to have mood disorders does run in families. Illnesses, infections, some medications, and substance abuse also can cause depression.[10] The social and work settings, with interpersonal conflicts, can prompt depressive symptoms. Certainly, personality traits may increase the likelihood of depression. These include being highly self-critical and seeing things as "black or white" or "either–or". In addition, individuals who tend to be dependent or passive seem to be more prone to depression.[10]

The physician may observe a wide range of symptoms, including physical complaints for which no physical cause is found. The athlete may complain of sleep disturbances including insomnia, hypersomnia, or early morning awakening with inability to fall back to sleep. There may be complaints of chronic fatigue and lack of usual energy. The athlete may tell about unexplained backaches, headaches, or similar pains. There may be reports of digestive upsets including nausea, indigestion, stomach pain, constipation, or diarrhea. Other symptoms of depression include changes in attitude and behavior. The athlete, coaching staff, or the physician may observe slowed-down behavior, poor grooming and dress, neglected responsibilities, missed practices and matches, and irritability. The athlete may report loss of appetite or the opposite, an increased appetite with significant weight gain. He or she may not be able to concentrate. The athlete may report different emotions and changed perceptions, including feelings of emptiness, emotional flatness, or feeling "blue" or "down in the dumps." The patient is likely to report inability to find pleasure in his or her usual activities. He or she may experience complete loss of, or a diminished, sexual desire, as well as feelings of hopelessness and helplessness. Feelings of guilt, exaggerated self-blame, and sad ruminations with loss of self-esteem are further symptoms of depression. Preoccupation with death, suicidal thoughts, and suicidal gestures or threats are clear signals of depression.

There are three main types of depression, which sometimes occur in combination. Dysthymia is a milder form of depression. It may last for years, so that a person may have forgotten any different mood state. This person may describe the "introverted" mood even as a part of his or her personality. This type of chronic mild depression will prevent the person's achieving his or her full potential. Sometimes a more severe form of depression can be superimposed on dysthymia, and then it is called double depression. The third type, major depression, commonly starts rather suddenly, precipitated by a crisis, a change, or a loss. Symptoms usually are severe enough to interfere with work or social functioning. This type of depression may last for a few months or become chronic, lasting even years. A person may have repeated episodes of major depression during his or her lifetime. The phenomenon of repeated episodes is actually more common than is a single episode.

Treatment of Depression. For depression, as for most illnesses, early intervention works best. Combinations of different methods may be the approach of choice. Psychotherapy, the traditional talking therapy, still remains an important part of the treatment, but may not be adequate alone, and is often supplemented with drug therapy. The goal of psychotherapy is to understand underlying causes and to map out depressive patterns of thinking. The cognitive-behavioral theorists led by Aaron Beck[19] explain that the depressed person has cognitive dysfunctions regarding himself, others, and the future. For example, depressed people are likely to view themselves as worthless, inadequate, and undesirable. Others, as well as the world in general, are seen as negative, demanding, and defeating. Consequently, the depressed person expects failure and, therefore, punishment. The future is viewed as a continuation of deprivation, suffering, and inevitable failure. Psychotherapy addresses these cognitive-depressive errors and goes further in providing support and help in finding solutions.

Pharmacological agents most commonly used today in the treatment of depression include fluoxetine (Prozac), sertraline (Zoloft), paroxetine (Paxil), Citalopram (Celexa), escitalopram (Lexapro), bupropion (Wellbutrin), venlafaxine (Effexor), and mirtazepam (Remeron). The older antidepressant classes, which include tricyclic and heterocyclic antidepressants and MAO inhibitors, are less often used by primary care physicians because of their various and complex side effects.

Anxiety Disorders

Although anxiety may be used as a term in the general sense, it actually includes many specific disorders, including generalized anxiety disorder, anxiety disorders caused by general medical conditions, acute stress disorder, panic disorder (with or without agoraphobia), specific phobia, social phobia, obsessive–compulsive disorder, post-traumatic stress disorder, and substance-induced anxiety disorder.

The patient reports anxiety and worry, which he or she may have difficulty in controlling. The patient is likely to complain of restlessness, feeling "on edge," being easily fatigued, feeling irritable, and difficulty in concentrating. He or she may report muscle tension and sleep disturbances. In acute stress disorder, a person has been exposed to a traumatic event in which he or she may have experienced or witnessed an episode that involved a serious injury, or the patient may have been threatened by death or serious injury. The person's response involves intense fear, helplessness, and horror. This is followed by a subjective sense of numbness—detachment or absence of emotional responsiveness. There may be feelings of "being in a daze," feelings of derealization and depersonalization, and inability to recall important aspects of the trauma. The traumatic event is re-experienced in recurrent images, thoughts, dreams, illusions, flashbacks, and a sense of reliving the experience when reminded of it. There is an avoidance of stimuli that remind the patient of the trauma. Anxiety symptoms, hypervigilance, and exaggerated startle response are part of the clinical picture. When the symptoms last longer than four weeks, the disorder is called post-traumatic stress disorder.

Treatment of Anxiety Disorders. Before making a diagnosis of generalized anxiety disorder, a physician needs to rule out medical diagnoses and evaluate the patient for other possible psychiatric conditions. One must of course exclude the normal anxiety state so common before engaging in athletic competition or artistic performance. Antianxiety medications including benzodiazepines can be prescribed on an as-needed basis. They also can be given as a standing dose for a period of time while other psychotherapeutic approaches are implemented. However, physicians need to keep in mind that benzodiazepines may impair alertness and thus negatively affect athletic performance. Commonly used for treatment is a class of antidepressants called selective serotonin reuptake inhibitors (SSRIs), such as sertraline (Zoloft), paroxetine (Paxil), citalopram (Celexa), escitalopram (Lexapro), and the noradrenergic serotonergic dual uptake inhibitor venlafaxine (Effexor). Buspirone (Buspar) is a nonbenzodiazepine antianxiety drug with a delayed onset of action. It may be a better choice for athletes because it does not share the problems of the benzodiazepines, including drowsiness and the possible development of physical dependency during longer periods of use. Beta-adrenergic blocking agents such as propranolol (Inderal) have been used successfully to treat peripheral symptoms of anxiety, including rapid heartbeat and tremor. These have been especially effective for performing artists experiencing "stage fright."

Acute stress disorder and post-traumatic stress disorder usually are treated with antidepressant medications. These include serotonin uptake inhibitors such as fluoxetine (Prozac) and sertraline (Zoloft), as well as paroxetine (Paxil), bupropion (Wellbutrin), venlafaxine (Effexor), and citalopram (Celexa), escitalopram (Lexapro), and mirtazepam (Remeron). Sometimes antipsychotic medications like risperidone (Risperdal) or olanzapine (Zyprexa), quetiapine (Seroquil), and ziprazidone (Geodon) are required for effective treatment. Other effective medications, including the tricyclics imipramine (Tofranil) and amitriptyline (Elavil), and the monoamine oxidase inhibitor phenelzine (Nardil), are rarely used today. These drugs should be given only by an experienced psychopharmacologist who supervises the patient closely. Drug interactions and serious, even fatal, side effects have been reported and observed with MAO inhibitors.

Within the broad category of anxiety disorders lies the phobic conditions, including social phobias and specific-object phobias. The treatment of phobias can be behavioral as well as pharmacological. In the behavioral technique called systematic desensitization, the patient is exposed to the anxiety-provoking stimuli, starting from the least frightening and proceeding to the most frightening. Furthermore, a relaxation technique is taught, to be practiced when the patient confronts anxiety-causing stimuli. In another technique called flooding, the patient is exposed to the phobic stimulus either in actuality or through imagination for as long as the patient can tolerate the fear or as long as it takes not to feel the fear any longer. SSRIs such as paroxetine (Paxil), sertraline (Zoloft), fluoxetine (Prozac), escitalopram (Lexapro), and the dual uptake inhibitor venlafaxine (Effexor) are used to treat social anxiety.

Bipolar Spectrum Disorders

This broad category includes various types of mood fluctuations. Bipolar I disorder is characterized by prominent mood swings, mania, and depression, interspersed with normal moods. Symptoms of the "highs" include feelings of exaggerated competence, very much increased energy, and hyperactivity. The patient may report no need for sleep and reduced appetite. There are likely to be racing thoughts, rapid speech, irritability, grandiose feelings, and lack of good judgment, often leading to recklessness in different areas of behavior. The length of these different phases can be variable. Obviously, this disorder must be differentiated from the normal elation of victory and the normal sadness and frustration of athletic defeat. Manic–depressive illness may occur in more subtle forms. Once diagnosed, it is best treated by a mental health specialist familiar with the range of mood stabilizers and antidepressant medications.

Bipolar I disorder is likely to run in families, and it appears to be equally common in men and women.[10] The first episode appearing in men is usually a manic episode, whereas in women the first episode is more likely to be a major depressive episode. This disorder is a recurrent disorder and more than 90% who experience a manic episode will have more episodes in the future. In addition, the intervals between episodes tend to become shorter with time.

Another form of cyclical mood disorders is Bipolar II disorder, which is characterized by recurrent major depressive episodes with milder hypomanic episodes. It also has been shown to have a clear familial pattern of inheritance. Cyclothymic disorder is a chronic cyclical mood disturbance that includes episodes of hypomania and mild depression. People with these cyclical mood disorders feel as if they are on an emotional roller coaster. At one moment, they feel on top of the world, with overconfidence and multiple plans, yet during the depressive periods they feel worthless and hopeless, with little interest in the future.

Treatment of Bipolar Spectrum Disorders. Lithium remains the prototypical drug for bipolar disorder. However, other mood stabilizers are available, including valproate (Depakote), lamotrigine (Lamictal), olanzapine (Zyprexa), and carbamazepine (Tegretol). Successful treatment of cyclical mood disorders requires the detailed exploration of the patient's psychiatric history, proper medical work-up, good knowledge of psychopharmacology, and ongoing monitoring for potential side effects. Certain mood stabilizers, such as lithium, require ongoing blood level monitoring on a routine basis. Overall, the treatment of bipolar disorders is more complicated than that of depression. Often physicians need to combine several psychotropic drugs to obtain a satisfactory result. Other biologic treatments include vagal nerve stimulation and transcranial magnetic stimulation.

Panic Disorder

In panic disorder, the essential features are unexpected panic attacks followed by persistent worries of having another attack. The patient reports palpitations, pounding heart, sweating, trembling, or shaking. There may be a sensation of shortness of breath or a feeling of smothering or choking, accompanied by chest pain or discomfort, nausea, abdominal distress, dizziness, unsteadiness, and lightheadedness. There may be feelings of unreality or feelings of being detached from oneself. Fear of losing control or "going crazy" or fear of dying are the symptoms that are likely to bring the patient to an emergency room or to seek immediate medical attention. Panic disorders may be accompanied by agoraphobia, in which the patient avoids being in places or situations from which egress or escape may be difficult or embarrassing, or in which help may not be available. These locations and situations typically include being outside the home alone, being in a crowd, on a bridge, or traveling in a bus, train, or car. This disorder commonly leads the patient to seek multiple medical consultations, including visits to the emergency room, cardiologists, pulmonary specialists, and gastroenterologists. Despite repeated assurance and many medical tests, the patient is likely to remain uncertain and frightened. Panic disorder may occur infrequently or up to several times a day. It may occur as either a full-blown panic attack or as a "limited-symptom" attack.

Panic disorder has been known to evolve into a major depressive episode and even to suicide ideation.[7] Athletes commonly experience "panic" before an upcoming sporting event, but these episodes are usually short-lived and disappear once the competition has begun.

Treatment of Panic Disorder. The principal treatment approach to panic disorder is pharmacological. Serotonin uptake inhibitors such as fluoxetine (Prozac), starting in small doses, have become a common treatment. Tricyclic antidepressants (TCAs) and monoamine oxidase inhibitors (MAOIs) have also been shown to be effective. The benzodiazepine alprazolam (Xanax) in sufficient and multiple daily doses is effective treatment. Most psychopharmacologists prefer using benzodiazepines only in the initial phase of treatment until the antidepressant medications take effect. It must be stressed that because of the variable reactions of patients to the initial drug dosage and because of serious drug interactions and side effects, the primary care physician might consider referral to a specialist once the diagnosis of panic disorder is made.

Obsessive–Compulsive Disorder (OCD)

Obsessive–compulsive disorder was previously thought to be rather rare. However, recent community studies have estimated a lifetime prevalence of approximately 2.5%.[10]

This is a disorder that is likely to cause embarrassment and shame. The patient usually tries to hide or camouflage the unwanted and senseless behaviors involved. The essential features of obsessive–compulsive disorder are recurrent obsessions or compulsions that cause marked distress and significant impairment. Obsessions are recurrent and persistent thoughts, impulses, or images that are experienced at some time during the disturbance. They are intrusive and inappropriate and cause anxiety and distress. These are not simply excessive worries about real-life problems. The patient attempts to ignore or neutralize the impulses with some other thoughts or actions. The patient recognizes that the obsessional thoughts, impulses, or images are a product of his or her own mind. Compulsions are repetitive behaviors (for example, hand washing, tapping, ritualistic touching) or mental acts (for example, praying, counting, repeating words silently) that the person feels driven to perform in response to an obsession or according to a rule that must be applied rigidly. These behaviors or mental acts are aimed at preventing or reducing distress or preventing some dreaded event or situation. This type of behavior can be seen in a mild form with various types of ritualistic behavior in sports, for example, wearing the same pair of socks during a successful period of competition, or the ritualistic movements before batting the ball in baseball or shooting a free throw in basketball. In this context, the behaviors should not be considered senseless, but rather a means of increasing concentration on the athletic task. These behaviors, of course, require no treatment.

Obsessive–compulsive patients may demonstrate biologic abnormalities in an electroencephalogram (EEG), sleep EEG, computed tomography (CT scan) of the brain, and neuroendocrine studies.[22] These abnormalities may be found in the left hemisphere. Some of the neurological abnormalities are similar to those found in depression.

Treatment of Obsessive–Compulsive Disorder. The most common treatment approach today to obsessive–compulsive disorder is the combination of behavioral therapy with effective psychopharmacologic agents. The drug clomipramine (Anafranil) was the first truly effective agent in the treatment of OCD. Newer agents include serotonin uptake inhibitors such as fluoxetine (Prozac) and fluvoxamine (Luvox). The serotonin uptake inhibitors have surpassed clomipramine in popularity because of their more favorable side-effect profile. Behavioral techniques can be effective, but they require a high degree of motivation and are time consuming.

SPECIAL CIRCUMSTANCES

The Child Athlete

The injured child athlete requires special attention. Serious competitive child athletes often miss many conventional childhood activities. Emotional and physical challenges of the relentless training routine are likely to take their toll. Peer relationships are particularly important during childhood in the development of healthy self-esteem, and the child athlete commonly feels isolated and lonely. Rebellion against strict athletic discipline surfaces from time to time. The child athlete may be reminded of significant family sacrifices and of the big changes in family life caused by his or her rigorous training routines and travel requirements. A child's athletic career may require temporary parental separation and consequently cause feelings of guilt. The child athlete is constantly aware of the high stakes, including potential future financial rewards. Child athletes also may be reminded of the financial sacrifices and investment by their parents in their present and future athletic careers.

When dealing with the injured child athlete, the physician often is called on to treat the emotional consequences to the entire family. At times, parents may disagree with each other about the treatment recommendations and proposed rehabilitation plan, leading to a true family crisis. In these instances, the rehabilitation process can be enhanced by consultation with an experienced child therapist or family therapy counselor. Rehabilitation of the child athlete requires perseverance and always some form of family counseling. Overanxious and overinvolved parents may, at times, impair the rehabilitation process and confuse decision making. A child whose parents are living only for their child's achievements and victories is bound to feel anger and resentment. These emotions can lead to feelings of guilt if the athlete thinks he or she is not living up to parental expectations. The harsh training schedule may be experienced as physical punishment and as a demand to please others. There is always a danger of ambitious parents projecting their own values onto the athletic youngster. Parents may need to be reminded that their child's chronological age may not reflect his or her psychological readiness to take on adult pressures.

The Female Athlete

The successful female athlete by necessity must have characteristics that traditionally have been considered masculine. These include intense determination to win, aggressiveness, and competitiveness that often encompass the "killer instinct." The male athlete's masculinity is fortified by winning, whereas the female athlete is likely to feel torn between athletic achievement and societal expectations of femininity. Frequently, the female athlete experiences depression while struggling with these conflicting issues. Some gender traits such as emotionality may be cultural, but others such as aggression may have a biological basis. Some studies have looked into the relationship between the female athlete and the onset of menstrual function.[8,28] Menarche in the United States occurs at 12.6 years of age. Studies of elite competitive athletes and dancers have shown a clear delay in menarche of up to two or more years.[22] The cause of this is multifactoral. The onset of menarche is dependent upon the maturation of the hypothalamus-pituitary-ovarian axis. Furthermore, a minimum requirement of body fat is needed for the onset of menarche. It appears that 17% body fat is a minimum prerequisite. If a rigorous training regimen decreases the percentage of body fat to below a critical level, menarche may be delayed. Another important factor in delaying menarche seems to be the impaired nutritional state prompted by repeated dieting and starvation efforts starting at an early age. It is obvious that rigorous athletic training may have a profound effect on body systems.

Eating Disorders

Although eating disorders are generally associated with females, more recent knowledge also shows a significant involvement of males. Given the rigors of training and the need to be at "optimal" body weight for strength and endurance, the athlete, male or female, is at high risk for these disorders. The intense preoccupation with weight in our culture affects as many as 10% of adolescent girls and young women.[21] These figures are far higher in sports that emphasize the importance of thinness.[4]

For many young people, dieting and excessive exercising becomes a way of coping with life and a distraction from the stress with which they cannot cope. Our Western culture emphasizes thinness as a virtue. This is reflected in our fashions and in our advertising. Many women, and increasing numbers of men, consequently feel that thinness is the outward manifestation of overall success in life. The need for thinness among athletes, especially figure skaters, gymnasts, and ballet dancers, increases their risk for eating disorders.

Anorexia Nervosa (Anorexia). Biological factors have been implicated in the syndrome of anorexia.[14] Researchers believe that severe dieting leads to emotional stress and to various hormonal imbalances present in anorexia. It is felt, however, that these may be the result of anorexia rather than the cause of it. A number of psychological factors have been associated with anorexia. Fear of growing up and fear of adult responsibilities often are seen as the root of the problem. The goal of being "the best" is shared by many people with eating disorders as well as by athletes. It is agreed that food is not the central issue; however, anorectics feel that control over food intake represents control over various aspects of their lives. Eating disorders become a way to express control over life, which may seem to be out of control.

Often this disorder is seen as rebellion against parental standards that may be too high. Typically, anorexic patients have not had major problems before adolescence. The patient is often described as a model child with good behavior at home and at school. Usually dieting begins with a change such as puberty or leaving home for school or college. Dieting makes the patient feel good about herself or himself, and it creates a feeling of control in a changing environment. Little by little, food and fat phobia becomes the most important thing in life.

Often, exhausting exercise is added. There may be rigid rules regarding exercise schedule and intensity. Food intake may be contingent upon having completed a self-imposed daily exercise regimen.

Bulimia Nervosa (Bulimia). Bulimia nervosa is characterized by binge eating and purging. During a binge, a person may consume large quantities of food in a short period of time. The purging part of bulimia is getting rid of the food consumed during a binge. This includes self-induced vomiting, periods of starvation, severe diets, and the use of laxatives, diuretics, and vigorous exercise. Typically, people with bulimia are young women for whom weight, dieting, and food in general are extremely important. They are usually of normal weight but harbor a distorted image of their bodies. They are likely to be perfectionists like anorectics and they are usually also high achievers.[13,16,32] Bulimic women are overly concerned about their looks and body weight and about being accepted by their peers. They feel out of control with eating and emotionally insecure and lonely. They usually lack confidence and have low self-esteem. Commonly, they feel inadequate in their relationships. A person with bulimia uses food to cope with conflicting emotions. Often the binge–purge cycle starts with diet as a means to improve self-esteem. Dieting, however, is likely to lead to craving for rich, highly caloric foods. This is likely to cause overeating as a response to attempts to starve. Overeating also is used to alleviate anxiety, anger, frustrations, loneliness, and a variety of complicating emotions. Guilt and fear following binges and purging are discovered as an ideal solution against gaining weight. Soon a person is feeling out of control and locked in a vicious binge–purge cycle. Often substance abuse and depression accompany bulimia nervosa.[23]

Increasing numbers of bulimics fall into a category of exercise bulimics. In this group, rigorous and rigid exercise has replaced purging. There is a preoccupation with maintenance of frequently exaggerated exercise routines. Social pursuits and relationships become secondary to exercise. Often exercise bulimics describe a feeling that they are "addicted" to exercise and that they feel out of control if they are prevented from exercising or have to cut short a planned exercise routine. This represents a pathological entity that, on the surface, is difficult to distinguish from the dedicated exercise enthusiast. A red flag should rise when the patient displays inordinate resistance to discontinuing an exercise regimen while an injury heals. If the patient appears highly agitated, anxious, and irrational when given medical advice to suspend exercise even after repeated explanations, the diagnosis of exercise bulimia should be considered.

People with eating disorders suffer several hormonal consequences. Anorectics can suffer from impaired or even complete lack of menstruation (amenorrhea). This has serious consequences in the patient's hormonal status, thereby leading to osteoporosis, abnormally low body temperature, anemia, and even cardiac arrhythmias.[20,31] Repeated binging and purging can cause erosion of dental enamel, esophagitis, and even gastric rupture. Depression is a very common consequence of eating disorders. The feeling of poor control over weight and the sensation of hunger often lead to feelings of hopelessness, helplessness, and despair. The treating physician must be vigilant for these depressive symptoms. Suicidal ideation is an issue among the eating-disorder population.

To say that the treatment of eating disorders is difficult would be an understatement. Because eating disorders are often chronic serious illnesses, it is advisable to seek help or second opinions from mental health professionals specializing in the treatment of eating disorders. Hospitalization of a patient is usually reserved for immediately life-threatening consequences of anorexia or bulimia or active suicidal preoccupations. The younger the patient, the more important is the need for family therapy to bring about a successful outcome. The mortality rate of eating disorders may exceed 10% because of medical complications and suicides.[10] Suicidal ideation always warrants psychiatric referral. Complex psychological factors have been found to contribute to the development of eating disorders, including family enmeshment, rigidity, overprotectiveness, inability to express emotions, and overemphasis on achievements in life. Although advances in psychopharmacology have added to the drug armamentarium for treating depression and urges to binge and purge, individual psychotherapy combined with family therapy remains the cornerstone of the treatment of eating disorders. Early intervention with a specialist is recommended to improve clinical outcomes. Sadly, many adolescents with eating disorders have harbored symptoms for several years before coming for treatment, and denial of the problem is quite common in families of such a patient. Problems centering around food and eating can appear from generation to generation in families.[15]

DRUGS, SUBSTANCE ABUSE, AND THE ATHLETE

The athlete, like any other member of society, is subject to the temptations and weaknesses that we all face every day. The athlete may feel especially pressured because his or her performance is constantly being judged and evaluated. In addition to being subject to the influence of alcohol and "recreational" drugs, the athlete may become interested in drugs that can enhance athletic performance, such as anabolic steroids and stimulants. Drug use and substance abuse by athletes, in its worst form, has led to fatalities caused by either the ordinary type of "overdose" or unique medical conditions such as coronary artery spasm, ventricular arrhythmia, myocardial infarctions, and sudden death syndrome. Certain drugs also can precipitate seizures and cerebrovascular accidents. The widespread use of performance-enhancing drugs has led to random and routine checking during athletic sporting events.

Cocaine

The initial effect of cocaine is usually pleasurable. It produces a feeling of well-being and increased self-confidence. There is also a sense of being more energetic and more alert. The psychological effects of cocaine include euphoria, increased libido, enhanced vigor, feelings of grandiosity, aggression, and manic excitement. These qualities have led athletes to use it in the competitive setting for performance enhancement. It has been reported that up to 18% of high school athletes have used cocaine at least once.[6] The use of this drug among elite female athletes is reported at up to 3%,[12] and it has been implicated as one of the most popularly used illegal drugs in the National Football League.

Cocaine use and abuse has become an increasingly common and serious problem in the United States. The alkaloid drug found in the leaves of the coca plant is readily available and can be purchased in an inexpensive form called "crack" cocaine. This highly concentrated chemically reconstituted cocaine is extremely addictive. It is commonly smoked and its effects are felt in less than 10 seconds. Cocaine stimulates the central nervous system. It dilates the pupils and elevates the heart rate, blood pressure, respiratory rate, and body temperature. Cocaine abuse can lead to several organic syndromes, including intoxication, withdrawal, delirium, and delusional disorders. Inhalation of cocaine on a chronic basis can cause serious ulceration of the mucous membranes of the nasal passages. Cocaine intoxication is likely to result in paranoid ideations, increased libido, ringing in the ears, and bizarre syndromes of behavior such as organizing common objects into pairs.[10] Disorientation and violent behavior are seen in states of delirium. Another unusual phenomenon, called formication, can occur, leading a person to believe that insects or animals are crawling under his skin. Cocaine is appealing for athletes because of its initial pleasurable effect and the production of a feeling of well-being and increased self-confidence with a sense of being more alert and energetic.

Alcohol

Athletes are no more immune to the appeal of alcohol than is the general population of the United States. Approximately three quarters of adult Americans consume some form of alcohol on a regular basis.[5] It remains the main substance abused by teenagers. It is not surprising that alcohol use has been reported by up to 88% of the athletic population.[1] The physician must maintain a high index of suspicion for alcohol abuse. It is extremely difficult to detect, especially when an athlete's performance is not impaired. It should be remembered that alcohol experimentation begins at an early age. The use of alcohol is attractive to adolescents and teenagers because it creates feelings of independence and rebellion, causing excitement for them and helping in their quest to overcome nervousness.

Alcohol abuse can lead to various chemical presentations, including intoxication, idiosyncratic intoxication, uncomplicated alcohol withdrawal, withdrawal delirium, hallucinations, amnestic disorder, and even dementia. These syndromes present unique characteristic symptoms and diagnostic criteria.

In alcohol intoxication, we may see familiar adaptational behavioral changes, including disinhibition, aggression, labile moods, poor judgment, and impairments in occupational or social functioning. All of these characteristics may be accompanied by slurred speech, lack of coordination, unsteady gait, nystagmus, and flushed facies. In uncomplicated alcohol withdrawal, there is a coarse tremor of the hands, tongue, or eyelids. This follows cessation or reduction of heavy and prolonged consumption. Further signs include nausea or vomiting, weakness and malaise, tachycardia, sweating, and increased blood pressure. There is anxiety, irritability, and perhaps transient hallucinations or illusions, insomnia, and headaches. The more serious clinical picture is alcohol withdrawal delirium, more commonly known as delirium tremens (DTs). The syndrome includes delirium, autonomic hyperactivity, visual or tactile hallucinations, sensory disturbances, lethargy, and hyperexcitability.[10] It usually follows within 7 days after a person stops or reduces the alcohol intake. This serious condition requires symptomatic treatment, hydration, bedrest, and benzodiazepines such as chlordiazepoxide (Librium). In alcohol hallucinosis, the patient develops auditory or visual hallucinations, usually within 48 hours after cessation or reduction of heavy drinking. These persistent and vivid hallucinations occur in a clear sensorium. This disorder can occur in any age group in people who are dependent on alcohol. Naltrexone (Revia), an opioid antagonist, is helpful in reducing and sometimes preventing drinking. This agent may be preferable to the older drug disulfram (Antabuse). The latter will cause unpleasant physical symptoms if any amount of alcohol is consumed while the person is taking the drug.

Marijuana

Marijuana is one of the oldest drugs, used throughout centuries as an intoxicant and as a medical adjunct. This drug is called by its various slang names including pot, grass, smoke, reefer, weed, tea, and Mary Jane. The drug itself comes from the hemp plant *Cannabis sativa*, containing over 400 chemical substances. The cannabis is primarily responsible for the mind-altering properties of marijuana. Its major psychoactive component is tetrahydrocannabinol, known as THC. Cannabis can be smoked in a pipe, rolled into a cigarette as a tobacco-like mixture, or even eaten, as in a baked cookie. Marijuana affects the cardiovascular system and the central nervous system. In low doses, it can temporarily relieve tension, boredom, or depression and produce a feeling of relaxation and well-being as well as sleepiness. In higher doses, it leads to impairment of short-term memory, altered sense of time, and distortions in sensorium. There also may be loss of balance and difficulties in following a logical thought process. When marijuana is used in high doses, it can lead to unpleasant feelings of anxiety, loss of insight, panic reactions, and paranoia. Psychotic symptoms with hallucinations and delusions may occur. When habitual users stop using the drug, they are likely to experience anxiety and depression as withdrawal phenomena.

Marijuana poses a particular hazard to the young athlete because it interferes with normal maturation and the process of growing up. Youngsters involved with marijuana are likely to have a limited range of interests and show apathy and indifference in their pursuit of athletic goals. An athlete who is at one time enthusiastic about a sport but then rapidly becomes apathetic should be evaluated for the possibility of marijuana use. Although marijuana is frequently considered rather innocuous, it has been implicated as possibly leading to exposure to a variety of drugs, each stronger and "better." Research has shown that marijuana smoke contains large amounts of carcinogens.[19] Reportedly, 36% of athletes have experimented with this drug and an estimated 3% use it on a regular basis.

Anabolic Steroids

These drugs, developed in the 1930s, are compounds related to the male sex hormone testosterone. The enticement of taking steroids for an athlete is that they induce a rapid increase in muscle mass, bulk, and strength. Androgenic steroids are widely used by athletes, bodybuilders, and power lifters. However, the current understanding of the effects of anabolic steroids on athletic performance remains limited. Testosterone does not improve endurance athletic performance. It may, however, improve performance in power lifting.[3] Power lifters are at higher risk of premature death from causes such as myocardial infarction, neoplasms, and suicide than is a control population.[29] Prevention of substance abuse including anabolic agents must start early, be sex-specific, and be team-centered, involving peer educators, coaches, and strength trainers.[18] The perils of steroid use in sports are now well publicized and should be quite familiar to players, trainers, coaches, and administrators. The psychological effects for both sexes include aggressive behavior, personality changes, combativeness, mood swings, depression, and even psychoses. The use of anabolic steroids has been universally banned and prohibited in competitive sports except for the treatment of specific diseases. Detoxification or withdrawal after long-term steroid use may be quite difficult medically and psychologically.

If substance abuse in any form is suspected or confirmed, a thorough psychiatric evaluation is indicated. Many psychiatric conditions predispose the patient to substance abuse because unpleasant mood states are easily medicated with alcohol or drugs. Early intervention is crucial, before the athlete and his or her performance suffer or the athlete has acquired well-entrenched drug habits.

Growth Hormones

Various studies have shown no evidence that human growth hormone increases muscle strength in athletes.[9] With present testing methods, growth hormone doping is undetectable.[33]

Doping of Athletes

The traditional doping agents, stimulants and anabolic steroids, are detectable in urine. However, athletes are turning now to other doping agents, which are not easily detected in urine samples. These include blood transfusion, endogenous stimulation of red blood cell production altitude, or using hypoxic rooms, erythropoetin (EPO), EPO gene therapy or EPO mimitics, allosteric effectors of hemoglobin, and blood substitutes, such as modified hemoglobin solutions and perfluorochemicals.[17] In 1999, the World Anti-Doping Agency (WADA) was formed, prompted by international concern about the banned performance-enhancing drugs (PEDs) used by athletes. Its main function is to control the use of PEDs, testing and developing new tests to detect doping.[11]

Over-the-Counter Drugs and Supplements

Over-the-counter sports supplements include creatinine, androstenedione, dehydroepiandrosterone (the popular precursors of testosterone), and chromium. Though all these supplements are popular, data do not support manufacturers' claims.[24]

Another concern is the abuse of pain-reducing drugs. The use of nonsteroidal anti-inflammatories among high school football players is common. Recent studies show that one of seven players uses NSAIDs daily.[34] Ephedra, a naturally occurring herbal substance, is considered by the FDA as a dietary supplement and is often marketed for weight loss and performance enhancement. The alkaloids of ephedra stimulate dopamine and norepinephrine release. Minor side effects include tachycardia, nausea, heartburn, trauma, sweating, and insomnia. Serious side effects include hypertension, hemorrhagic strokes, seizures, and death. Psychiatric side effects of ephedra include euphoria, agitation, depression, and psychosis.

REFERRAL TO A MENTAL HEALTH SPECIALIST: ABSOLUTE INDICATIONS

The athlete's career can be severely curtailed or impaired by untreated emotional problems. The pressure of vigorous training, demanding competition, and constant judging and evaluating can push any preexisting emotional problem to the surface. Significant emotional problems may warrant referral immediately to a mental health professional or at least a consultation or second opinion.

Severe depression or a depression that has not adequately responded to the prescribed antidepressant treatment regimen requires psychiatric referral. The same applies to panic disorder and obsessive–compulsive disorder. The latter two disorders usually respond very well to medications; however, the patient needs a practitioner with firm expertise and familiarity with these conditions and the drugs that are used to treat them. Untreated cases will lead to loss of athletic careers and may even cause suicidal preoccupation.

Suicidal ideations always warrant psychiatric referral. Most suicide victims suffer from mental illness, mood disorders, alcoholism, or drug abuse. Suicide is more common among males than females. Risk factors for suicide include depression and bipolar disorders, as well as schizophrenia, anxiety disorders, alcoholism, drug abuse, personality disorders, and serious physical illnesses. Suicide is much more common in patients who have previously attempted it.[2]

Psychosis is another absolute indication for referral. In the psychotic state, patients commonly express paranoid ideation and delusions, and many have hallucinatory experiences. This state can be dangerous and may eventually lead to violent behavior, homicide, or suicide. This requires immediate specialized professional treatment. Substance abuse is also an absolute indication for referral to a specialist in that field or a mental health specialist.

Patients must be referred to a mental health specialist if the initial treatment plan proposed and implemented by the primary care physician has not successfully treated the problem. Lack of response to a medication regimen is also an indication for referral. When in doubt, a second opinion to determine whether a mental disorder is present is always warranted. Needless to say, if a patient or a family member requests a mental health evaluation, it should be considered quite seriously.

Another situation in which referral to a mental health specialist is essential is when a devastating, potentially career-ending injury occurs to an elite athlete. In these situations, early intervention will help the athlete put the injury in perspective and prepare for the future.

It should also be remembered that in today's health care society, especially within the guidelines of managed care, the "mental health specialist" can be a physician, psychologist, psychiatric nurse, or social worker.

SUPPORT GROUPS

Patients with psychiatric diagnoses such as substance abuse, anorexia, bulimia, depression, obsessive–compulsive disorder, and others can benefit from interaction with peers who share the same diagnosis. Once the diagnosis is established, in addition to the routine psychological care given to a patient, referral to an appropriate support group should be made. To obtain the most up-to-date pertinent information on these support groups, inquiries should be made to the local branch of the American Psychiatric Association or the American Psychological Association.

SUMMARY

The primary care physician treating athletes and sports injuries should remember three important steps in maintaining proper mental health: (1) preventive vigilance, (2) early diagnosis, and (3) early intervention. Implementing these recommendations will enhance successful outcomes.

REFERENCES

1. Anderson WA, McKeag DB: The Substance Use and Abuse Habits of College Student Athletes. Mission, Kan, NCAA, 1995.
2. Beck H, Resnick LP, Letieri DJ (eds): The Prediction of Suicide. Bowie, Md, Charles Press, 1974.
3. Bhasin S, Woodhouse L, Stower TW: Proof of the effect of testosterone on skeletal muscle. J Endocrinol 170:27–38, 2001.
4. Byrne S, McLean N: Elite athletes: Effects of the pressure to be thin. J Sci Med Sport Jun 5(2):80–94, 2002.
5. Calahan D, Cisin IH, Crossley HM: American Drinking Practices: A National Survey of Behavior and Attitudes, Monograph No. 6. New Brunswick, NJ, Rutgers University Center of Alcohol Studies, 1969.
6. Clement DB: Drug use survey: Results and conclusions. Phys Sports Med 11(9):64–67, 1983.
7. Conyell W, Noyes R Jr, Howe JD: Mortality among out-patients with anxiety disorders. Am J Psychiatry 143:508–510, 1983.
8. Dale E, Gerlach D, Willhote A: Menstrual dysfunction in distance runners. Obstet and Gynecol 54:47, 1979.
9. Dean H: Does exogenous growth hormone improve athletic performance? Clin J Sport Med 12(4): 250–253, 2002.
10. Diagnostic and Statistical Manual of Mental Disorders, 4th ed (DSM-IV). Washington, DC, American Psychiatric Association, 1994.
11. Donovan RJ, Egger G, Kapernick V, Mendoza J: A conceptual framework for achieving performance enhancing drug compliance in sport. Sports Med 32(4):269–284, 2002.
12. Duda M: Female athletes: Targets for drug abuse. Phys Sports Med 14:142–146, 1986.
13. Fairborn CG: A cognitive behavioral approach to the treatment of bulimia. Psychological Med 11:707–711, 1988.
14. Fava M, Copeland PM, Schweigher V, Herzog DB: Neurochemical abnormalities of anorexia nervosa and bulimia nervosa. Am J Psychiatry 146(9): 963–971, 1989.
15. Garshon ES, et al: Anorexia nervosa and major affective disorders associated in families (preliminary report). In Guze SR, Earls FJ, Barnett JE (eds): Childhood Psychopathology and Development. New York, Raven Press, 1983.
16. Garver DM, Garfinkel PE, Schwartz D, Thompson M: Cultural expectation of thinness in women. Psychol Rep 47:483–491, 1980.
17. Gaudard A, Varlet-Marie E, Bressolle F, Audran M: Drugs for increasing oxygen and their potential use in doping: A review. Sports Med 33(3): 187–212, 2003.
18. Goldberg L, MacKinnon DP, Elliot DL, et al: Adolescent training and learning to avoid steroids program preventing drug use and promoting health behaviors. Arch Pediatric Adolsc Med 154(4): 332–338, 2000.
19. Grinspon L: Marijuana. Harvard Medical School Mental Health Letter 4(5), 1987.
20. Halmi KA, Falk JR: Common psychological changes in anorexia nervosa. Intl J of Eating Dis 1:16–27, 1981.
21. Brownell KD, Foreyt JP: Handbook of eating disorders. New York, Basic Books, 1986.
22. Jennke MA: Obsessive compulsive disorder. Comp Psych 24:99, 1983.
23. Johnson C, Larson R: Bulimia: An analysis of moods and behavior. Psychosomatic Med 44:341–351, 1982.
24. Kaplan HI, Sadock BJ: Comprehensive Textbook of Psychiatry, 5th ed, vol 1. Baltimore, Williams and Wilkins, 1989.
25. Kenkare ZN, Federman DG: Over the counter sports supplements: What clinicians need to know. Comp Ther 28(2):148–154, 2002.
26. Kerr G, Cairns L: The relationship of selected psychosocial factors to athletic injury occurrence. J Sport Ex Phys 10(2):167–173, 1988.

27. Kerr G, Fowley B: The relationship between psychological factors and sports injuries. Sports Med 6:1988.
28. Martens R: Sport Competition Anxiety Test. Champaign, IL, Human Kinetics, 1977.
29. Menstrual changes in athletes: A round table. Phys Sports Med 9(11):99–112, 1981.
30. Parssinen M, Kusala U, Vartianen, et al: Increased premature mortality of competitive power lifters suspected to have used anabolic agents. Int J Sports Med 22(3):225–227, 2000.
31. Perna FM, Antoni MH, Baum A, et al: Cognitive behavioral stress management effects on injury and illness among competitive athletes: A randomized clinical trial. Ann Behav Med 25(1):66–72, 2003.
32. Silverman JA: Anorexia nervosa: Clinical and metabolic observations. Intl J Eating Disorders 2:159–166, 1983.
33. Vigersy RA: Anorexia Nervosa. New York, Raven Press, 1977.
34. Wallace JD, Cuneo RC, Baxter R, et al: Responses of the growth hormone (GH) and insulin-like growth factor axis to exercise, GH administration, and GH withdrawal in trained adult males: A potential test for GH abuse in sport. J Clin Endocrinol Metab 84(10):3591–3601, 199.
35. Warner DC, Schnepf G, Barrett MS, et al: Prevalence, attitudes and behaviors related to the use of nonsteroidal anti-inflammatory drugs (NSAIDS) in student athletes. J Adolesc Health 30(3):150–153, 2002.

BIBLIOGRAPHY

Anderson WA, Albrect RR, McKeag DB, et al: A national survey of alcohol and drug use by college athletes. Phys Sports Med 19(2):91–104, 1991.

Anthony J: Psychological aspects of exercise. Clin Sports Medicine 10:171–180, 1991.

Ashe AR: A Hard Road to Glory. New York, Warner Books, 1988.

Athletic Training and Sports Medicine, 2nd ed. Rosemont, Ill, American Academy of Orthopaedic Surgeons, 1991.

Birrer R (ed): Sports Medicine for the Primary Care Physician, 2nd ed. Boca Raton, Fla, CBC Press, 1994.

Borgen JS, Corbin CB: Eating disorders among female athletes. Phys Sports Med 15(2):19, 1987.

Clark K, Parr R (eds): Evaluation and Management of Eating Disorders: Anorexia, Bulimia and Obesity. Champaign, Ill, Life Enhancement Publications, 1988.

Diagnostic and Statistical manual of Mental Disorders, 4th ed (DSM-IV). Washington, DC, American Psychiatric Association, 1994.

Dick RW: Eating disorders in NCAA athletes. Athletic Training 26:136, 1991.

Haupt HA: Drugs in athletes. Clin Sports Med 8(3):561–582, 1989.

Jonas AP, Sickles PT, Lombardo JA: Substance abuse, Clinic Sports Med 1992.

Kaplan HI, Sodock BJ, eds: Comprehensive Handbook of Psychiatry, 5th ed. Baltimore, MD, Williams and Wilkins, 1989.

Kuipers H, Kazer H: Overtraining in elite athletes. Sports Med 6:79–92, 1988.

Loucks AB, Vartukaitis J, Cameran JL, et al: The reproductive system and exercise in women. Med Sci Sports Exerc 24(65):5288–5293, 1992.

Lynch GA: Athletic injuries and the practicing sports psychologist: Practical guidelines for assisting athletes. Sports Psychologist 2:161–1678, 1988.

Marks IM: Fears, Phobias and Rituals. Oxford, Oxford University Press, 1987.

Mellion MB: Sports Medicine Secrets. Philadelphia, Hanley and Belfus, 1994.

Micheli LJ: Sports wise: An Essential Guide for Young Athletes, Parents and Coaches. Boston, Houghton Mifflin, 1990.

Olgilvie BC: The child athlete: Psychological implications of participation in sport. Am Acad Polit Soc Sci 445:47–58, 1979.

Paglin JS: Anxiety and sports performance. Exerc Sports Sci Rev 20:243–274, 1992.

Raglin JS: Exercise and mental health: Beneficial and detrimental effects. Sports Med 9(6):323–329, 1990.

Shanegold MM, Mirkin G, eds: Women and Exercise: Physiology and Sports Medicine. Philadelphia, FA Davis, 1988.

Silva JM, Weinberg RS: Psychological Foundation of Sports. Champaign, Ill, Human Kinetics, 1984.

Sinoll FL, Smith RE: Psychology of the young athlete—stress related maladies and remedial approaches. Ped Clinics North Am 37:1021–1046, 1990.

Smith AM, Scotts G, Wiese DM: The psychological effects of sports injuries. Sports Med 9(6):352–369.

Tutko T, Tosi U: Sports Psychiatry. New York, Tacher/Pedigree Books, 1976.

Weinberg RS: The Mental Advantage. Champaign, Ill, Leisure Press, 1988.

Wells C: Women, Sports and Performance. Champaign, Ill, Human Kinetics, 1991.

Wichmann S, Markin DR: Exercise excess: Treating patients addicted to fitness. Phys Sports Med 20:193–200, 1992.

Wiese DM, Weiss MR: Psychological rehabilitation and physical injury: Implications for the sports medicine team. Sports Psychol 1:318–330, 1987.

Williams JM: Applied Sports Psychology—Personal Growth to Peak Performance, 2nd ed. Mayfield, 1993.

Walker SH: Winning: The Psychology of Competition. New York, WW Norton, 1986.

52 Sport for the Athlete with a Physical Disability

Kenneth J. Richter, Michael S. Ferrara, and Susan M. Kaschalk

Sport opportunities for athletes with disabilities have been increasing every year. The nature and type of injuries that occur to these athletes are not as widely known as are those for athletes without disabilities. The purpose of this chapter is to inform the reader of sporting opportunities available, specific medical concerns, and typical injury patterns among athletes with physical and sensory disabilities.

Sport is of immense therapeutic value; its object is to optimize physical and psychologic equilibrium for the enjoyment of daily life.[30] An estimated 2 to 3 million athletes with physical and mental disabilities are involved annually in athletic competition within the United States.[4,16] A large number of people with disabilities also are involved in recreational and leisure sports. The range of activities for athletes with disabilities includes a variety of recreational and competitive activities. Sporting opportunities are available even for those with the most involved disabilities.

BENEFITS OF SPORT

Knowledgeable physicians realize the need for physical activity for disabled people.[12] They recognize that persons with disabilities can successfully participate and compete in a wide range of recreational and competitive pursuits, from boccie to swimming to marathons. Sometimes athletes with a disability can participate with their able-bodied peers in interscholastic and intercollegiate activities. Depending on the activity, slight modification may be needed in equipment for the person to participate. On the other hand, unique sporting events such as goal ball for the blind have been established and are increasingly available (Fig. 52-1).

A special thanks to Marie Laidler for her dedication and assistance.

Active participation in sports is generally associated with positive outcomes for people with disabilities.[67,68] It has been reported that involvement in competitive sports has a beneficial affect on disabled athletes' social interactions at home, helps them make friends, and improves their physical coordination, strength, endurance, and self-confidence.[38]

SCOPE OF SPORTS FOR THE DISABLED

The sports movement for athletes with disabilities started with military programs after World War II. The large number of injured veterans used sport and related activities for rehabilitation. By the 1970s, involvement in sports grew to the extent that exercise and fitness programs were available to most people with disabilities. The Amateur Sports Act of 1978 detailed the rights for United States amateur athletes, including athletes with disabilities. This law was a major step forward in legitimizing sports for the disabled.

In 1979 the United States Olympic Committee (USOC) formed a category (Group E) under its authority for athletes with disabilities. The category now comprises Wheelchair Sports, USA (WSUSA); USA Deaf Sports Federation (USADSF); the National Disability Sports Alliance (NDSA); the Special Olympics International (SOI); Disabled Sports USA (DSUSA); the Dwarf Athletic Association of America (DAAA); and the United States Association for Blind Athletes (USABA). There also are two organizations that serve a large number of athletes but are not members of the USOC. They are the National Wheelchair Basketball Association (NWBA) and the United States Les Autres Sports Association (USLASA). The box Sport Organizations for Athletes with Disabilities lists the addresses for each organization.

The USOC Group E category has been renamed the Disabled in Sports Organizations (DSO). The Committee on Sports for the Disabled (COSD) was developed by the USOC for all DSOs. The membership of the committee includes two individuals from each organization and one of each must be disabled. At least 20% of the COSD membership must comprise active athletes. The USADSF, WSUSA, DSUSA, USABA, National Disability Sport Alliance (NDSA—formerly the USCPAA), DAAA, and SOI are current members of the COSD.

The international sports movement for the disabled moved toward cross-disability, or integrated, competition in 1992 with the formation of the International Paralympic Committee (IPC). The current philosophy of the IPC is cross-disability, or sport-specific, competition, although there are concerns with this approach.[64] It would allow athletes with all types of disabilities to compete against each other in major competitions, that is, World Championships and Paralympics. The 2000 Paralympics in Sydney, Australia, was the largest sports

CHECKLIST

Sport Organizations for Athletes with Disabilities

USA Deaf Sports Federation (USADSF)
3607 Washington Blvd., Ste. 4
Odgen, UT 84403

Disabled Sports USA (DSUSA)
451 Hungerfored Dr., Ste. 100
Rockville, MD 20850

Dwarf Athletic Association of America (DAAA)
418 Willow Way
Lewisville, TX 75067

National Disability Sports Alliance (NDSA)
(Formerly USCPAA)
25 W. Independence Way
Kingston, RI 02881

National Wheelchair Basketball Association
(NWBA)
1710 Queensbury Loop
Winter Garden, FL 34787

Special Olympics International (SOI)
1325 G Street NW, Ste. 500
Washington, DC 20005

United States Association for Blind Athletes
(USABA)
33 N. Institute Street
Brown Hall, Suite 015
Colorado Springs, CO 80903

United States Les Autres Sports Association
(USLASA)
9207 Baber Dr.
Houston, TX 77095

Wheelchair Sports, U.S.A. (WSUSA)
3595 E. Fountain Boulevard, Suite L-1
Colorado Springs, CO 80910

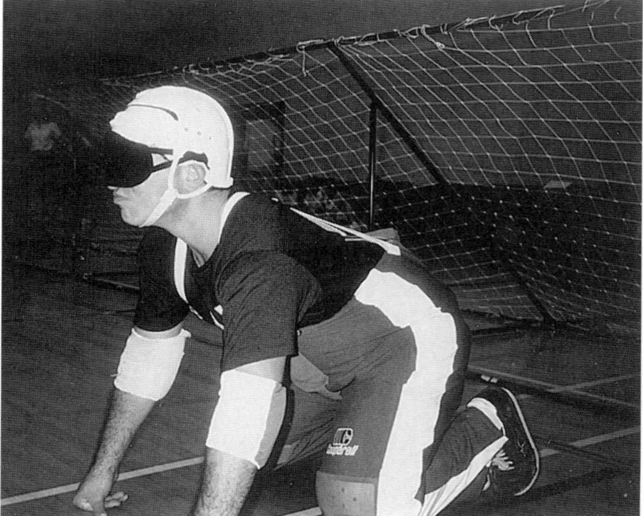

FIGURE 52-1. Athlete with a visual impairment playing goal ball.

event for athletes with disabilities, with almost 4000 competitors and 1.16 million paid spectators and 300 million television viewers.[72] The Paralympics, which has become the second largest multisport event in the world (second only to the summer Olympics), were held in Sydney, Australia, in 2000, shortly after the conclusion of the Olympic Games (Fig. 52-2). Although this is positive, the elite competition of the Paralympics has also brought problems. Ten athletes were disqualified from power sports in Sydney for testing positive for anabolic steroids.

PHYSICIAN CONCERNS

Physicians sometimes fail to promote sport as a life option for people with disabilities because they lack awareness of sport opportunities available. There is a broad spectrum of sport options, ranging from casual recreational events to elite sports such as the Paralympics. Having a disability, even a severe disability, does not prevent a person from being an athlete even on the world-class, elite level.

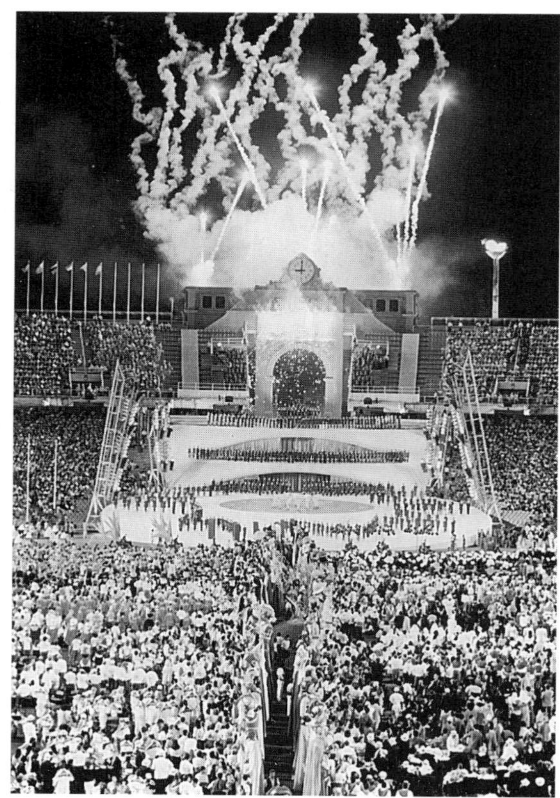

FIGURE 52-2. Opening ceremonies, Paralympics, Barcelona, 1992.

Opportunities for competition are available through various classification schemes.[66] Classification has long been an acceptable practice in the sports world for the able-bodied, with systems of gender, weight, age, and performance. Classification in sport is even more essential for the disabled.[66] Although there are some controversies regarding classification,[43,44,64] it should provide athletes with disabilities an equitable starting point for athletic competition.[73] It should not be assumed that an individual with an above-the-knee amputation cannot be a world-class high jumper, or a person with spastic athetoid quadriplegia caused by cerebral palsy cannot be a world-class swimmer.

Frequently, we have observed problems with precompetition evaluation. Physicians may make one of two mistakes. They may assume that sport for athletes with a disability cannot be very rigorous or risky, therefore anyone can compete. The other error is assuming that athletes with a disability are so fragile that any competition should be prohibited. Sports physicians must evaluate potential athletes objectively and fairly to accurately apprise them of any potential risks yet not needlessly prevent them from participating. To do this effectively requires knowledge both of sports medicine and of the specific disability that an individual may have.

PHARMACOLOGIC CONCERNS

It is not unusual for athletes with disabilities to use prescribed medications such as muscle relaxants or medications for asthma, seizures, hyperactivity, and other conditions. Physicians and involved allied medical personnel should be aware of the indications, contraindications, side effects, and synergistic effects of using multiple medications.

Some athletes may be using antiseizure medicines that are known to have significant cognitive effects and to decrease the attention span of the athlete.[61] There are three drugs commonly used to control seizures. They can be placed on a continuum based on the severity of their side effects, which range from mild to potentially severe.[61] The usual medications for seizures include phenobarbital, phenytoin, and carbamazepine; to a lesser extent, valproic acid also is being used. Carbamazepine may be the preferred medication for disabled athletes,[61] because it may have the fewest side effects and should not adversely affect athletes' performance. New medications with fewer side effects such as Gabapentin are being used more frequently now for some seizures and other neurological conditions.[7]

It is very important to stress compliance with a medication's prescribed dosage. Athletes, particularly those involved in national or international travel, may have their usual schedules disrupted and therefore forget to take a medication. An athlete needs to keep a proper blood level of any prescribed drug to maintain desired effects. The athlete should keep the medicine always available, for example, by carrying it on his or her person while traveling, so that a dose is not missed. Do not adjust or change medications before major competitions or events. This may upset the equilibrium that the athlete has obtained with a particular medication. If a drug must be changed, monitor blood levels and look for physical changes or side effects, such as nystagmus and ataxia with the antiseizure drugs, that may occur from the new medicine. Most important is to remember that the goal is the clinical response, not the serum drug level. If the athlete is seizure free, even with subtherapeutic levels, increasing the dose will more likely just increase side effects, not lessen the rise of future seizures.[36,77] Refractory epilepsy requires the expertise of an experienced epileptologist.[69]

Physicians need to be aware of an important principle when treating athletes with seizures. In aerobic athletic activities the incidence of seizures usually decreases.[61] As a person exercises aerobically, he or she tends to develop a metabolic acidosis, which is compensated for by hyperventilation. This results in a lower hydrogen ion concentration (pH), which tends to stabilize neuromembranes (Fig. 52-3). There are few cases in which an athlete experiences seizure activity during sporting events. If there is a question about seizures occurring during exercise, do a stress test with EEG to see if there is any seizure activity.[53]

A physician evaluating an athlete with seizures for competition may need to be made aware of the effect seizures could have, not only on the athlete but also on fellow competitors. For example, if a cyclist has a seizure while riding in the peloton in a mountain road race, it

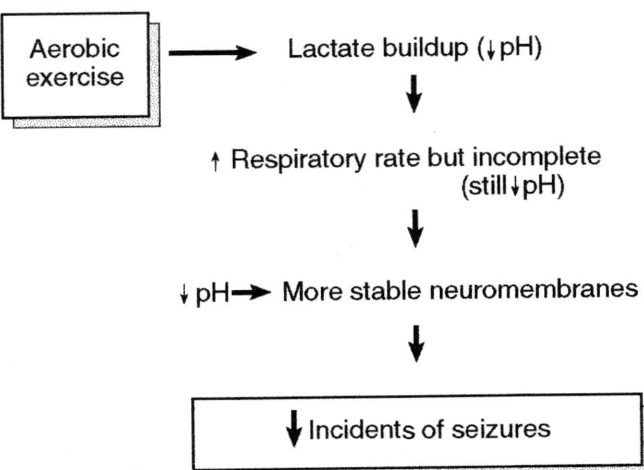

FIGURE 52-3. Algorithm of relationship between exercise and incidence of seizure.

could cause serious injuries to nearby riders. However, if the athlete is in good seizure control, there is not a high risk. Keep in perspective that physicians are always making this kind of judgment as to whether or not people with seizures can drive a car, which with good control is legally permitted in every state.

With most antiseizure medications there is some cognitive dysfunction. Therefore, athletes on these medications often will need to have more time to focus their attention before an athletic competition. The athlete and coach need to be advised of this so that they can incorporate appropriate mental preparation strategies. Remember proper first aid for a generalized tonic-clone seizure. During the seizure, keep the person prone and safe, remove eyeglasses, loosen any clothing around the neck, do not restrain the person, and never place anything in the person's mouth. After the seizure, turn the person to the side to prevent aspiration and monitor until completely awake.[77]

TEMPERATURE REGULATION

Exposure to heat and cold may provide unique challenges for athletes with disabilities.[3,6,42,45,59] Some athletes may not be able to tolerate normal environmental conditions as well as can athletes without disabilities. This intolerance is due to decrease in sensory awareness, sympathetic nervous system dysfunction, and a deficient body mechanism for warming and cooling.[1] The problem typically affects the athlete with spinal cord injury, but it also may be prevalent in athletes with disabilities such as cerebral palsy, obesity, and Down syndrome.[56]

Heat Intolerance

Athletes with spinal cord injuries tend to be more susceptible to heat injuries. Quadriplegics and those with a spinal cord lesion above the eighth thoracic level are particularly vulnerable to heat stress.[13,19,70] These athletes do not sweat or have effective vasodilation below the level of the spinal cord injury, thus there is no effective mechanism for body cooling. Specific drugs (tranquilizers, diuretics, alcohol, sympathomimetics, anticholinergics, and thyroid replacement drugs) may predispose the athlete to problems with heat.[21] Further, athletes with high blood pressure, diabetes, and sweat gland dysfunction may have an increased incidence of heat illness.[56]

Prevention. Given the probability of heat illness for athletes with disabilities, prevention is a major issue. Limit practice and competitive sessions when the temperature is greater than 85° F and the humidity is higher than 70%. High temperature and humidity will not allow efficient cooling of the body through heat dissipation and normal sweating.[3]

All athletes should be encouraged to drink plenty of fluids. The disabled athlete should hydrate the body as much as possible before any event and should consume 1 to 2 cups of water every 10 to 15 minutes during competition or training.[19] Athletes who use a wheelchair should be encouraged to attach a water bottle to the wheelchair while training.

Pay particular attention to athletes with a swallowing disorder. This is sometimes manifested by drooling in an upper motor neuron–type of condition such as cerebral palsy. These athletes may not only have a difficult time taking in fluid, but may also have a significant fluid loss from the saliva. They need to be counseled to drink frequently before they sense any problem, use swallowing strategies, and to monitor the volume and color of their urine output.

The use of shade, light clothing, and hats is recommended. Sunscreens should be applied whenever the athlete will be exposed to the sun for prolonged periods. The athlete with a spinal cord injury may be at an increased risk for sunburn because of decreased sensory awareness.[65] Special attention should be paid to athletes who will be required to remain in the sun for a long time. They should be encouraged to move to a shaded and cooler area before and after competition. Meet organizers should provide tents and other shade to which the athletes can escape from the sun.

HYPOTHERMIA

An athlete's ability to tolerate the cold is based on several factors: level of fitness, percent of body fat, and environmental conditions such as the wind chill factor and wetness. Normal mechanisms for heat production by the body, such as shivering, goose-bump production, and circulatory shunting, may not take place in athletes with a spinal injury. Air temperature around 50° F may produce problems for athletes with quadriplegia.[19,20] However, in water, which has a much higher specific heat, a temperature much below 90° F may be problematic to a quadriplegic. Athletes having prolonged exposure require careful monitoring.[47]

Prevention

Physicians and other allied medical personnel should investigate the athlete's medical history before he or she participates in winter sports. Prior episodes of hypothermia may predispose the athlete to further problems in a cold environment. Also, certain medications or medical conditions may predispose the athlete to temperature regulation problems in the cold.[47]

Athletes should be encouraged to wear appropriate clothing in cold weather. Cotton and other fabrics that absorb moisture are advised for the inner layers of clothing. Additional layers should be added or deleted to maintain proper body heat. Hats should be worn because a large amount of heat is lost through the head.

All wet clothing should be removed immediately after the exercise session. This will eliminate postexercise chilling. Careful attention should be given to those athletes with communicative or cognitive disorders who may not be able to relate symptoms of hypothermia. Special awareness of environmental conditions also should be considered.

AUTONOMIC DYSREFLEXIA

Autonomic dysreflexia (AD) is a condition seen in athletes with a spinal injury at the T6 level or higher, which causes involvement of the splanchnic nerves.[22] The splanchnic nerves control peripheral vascular resistance, which is the primary determinant of blood pressure. AD is a massive sympathetic discharge of the splanchnic nerves with resultant hypertension. There may be a corresponding bradycardia as the baroreceptors cause an increase in vagal output, which can affect the heart rate but is not effective in lowering the blood pressure.[22] The usual cause of AD in over 90% of cases is a distended bladder; in approximately 9% the cause is a distended bowel, and other causes can be anything from ingrown toenails to appendicitis, or anything that particularly causes a sacral input.[62]

It appears that AD may be a performance-enhancing technique called *boosting*. Athletes with high-level spinal injuries deliberately induce autonomic dysreflexia, which has been shown in the laboratory to improve performance.[8] Athletes need to be cautioned about the dangers,[71] which include death. This technique is banned by the IPC.

Prevention

The chief prevention strategy for autonomic dysreflexia is to make sure that the athlete's bladder and rectum are emptied before he or she begins physical activity.

Recognition

The symptoms of AD may include sudden hypertension, bradycardia, increased sweating, severe headache, and goose flesh. However, athletes with quadriplegia may not demonstrate bradycardia because of their injured sympathetic nervous system.[22]

Treatment

When autonomic dysreflexia occurs, the athlete should be placed in an upright position to take advantage of orthostatic changes, then the bladder should be drained and, if necessary, the bowel emptied carefully, using lidocaine gel as a lubricant. Approximately 99% of cases are relieved with this treatment. Caution must be used when interpreting the blood pressure because it normally will be low in quadriplegics, with systolic blood pressure less than 100 mm/Hg. The use of drug therapy is rarely indicated. When it is needed, acute antihypertensive agents can be administered; however, one must be careful of rebound hypotension.

INJURY PATTERNS AMONG ATHLETES WITH DISABILITIES

Several authors[5,42,48] characterized the common injuries suffered by athletes with disabilities. They listed abrasions, contusions, strains, and carpal tunnel syndrome, and described methods for the prevention and care of these injuries.

Health care providers should realize that injuries are to be expected in sports and should be addressed promptly and appropriately. Practitioners should evaluate, treat, and rehabilitate disabled athletes as they would any well-conditioned athlete. An injury may mean a decrease in training and conditioning level, thus a reduction in motivation. The goal of the physician should be to restore strength and function as quickly and safely as possible so that the athlete can resume activity.

GENERAL INJURY INVESTIGATIONS

Sports for the disabled have been considered to place the athlete with a disability at an increased risk of injury.[33] However, researchers have provided documentation for the theory that the percentage of injuries is no higher than for athletes without disabilities.[4,25,46,63] This theory is further substantiated by the Athletes with Disabilities Injury Registry (ADIR), an epidemiologic investigation that determined an injury rate of 7.23 injuries per 1000 athlete exposures for 12 months.[26] This injury rate is within the normative values reported in literature for athletes without disabilities.

Typically, medical professionals treat problems such as minor illnesses, dehydration, and sprains and strains at major competitions for disabled athletes. Richter[62] found that the majority of injuries to athletes with cerebral palsy at the 1988 Paralympics were minor and acute in nature. The shoulder, low back, and knee were the most common injury locations. At the 1990 World Championships and Games for the Disabled held in Assen, Holland, illnesses were the most common injury reported to the U.S. medical staff. Illnesses are not unexpected because of the drastic environmental, diet, stress, and sleep pattern changes that occur from international travel and competition.

In 1989, a cross-disability retrospective injury survey was administered to athletes from the WSUSA, USABA, and USCPAA. For the WSUSA athletes, the highest percentage of injuries were in the upper extremity, with the

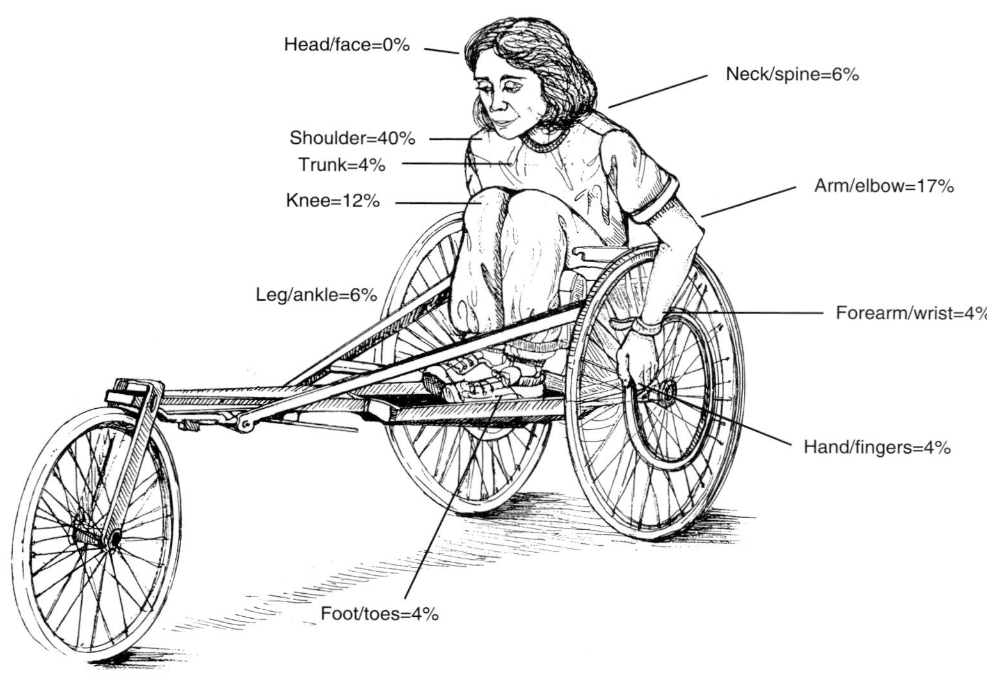

FIGURE 52-4. Injury incidence in athlete with spinal cord injury/wheelchair user.

shoulder accounting for 40% of the total injuries, as seen in Figure 52-4. The USABA athletes had a high percentage of injuries in the shoulder and leg/ankle complex, as presented in Figure 52-5. The shoulder, hand/finger, knee, and leg/ankle were the most frequently involved body locations for the USCPAA athlete, as shown in Figure 52-6. Each disability manifests itself with different effects and demands on the body. Accordingly, a specific injury prevention program, as opposed to a general program, needs to be designed for each organization.

In the following sections, common injuries that are specific to each type of disability are described. Prevention strategies and common methods for the treatment of these injuries will be presented.

WHEELCHAIR ATHLETES

Athletes with disabilities experience injuries that are specific to the demands and risks of their sports. Track, road racing, and basketball have the potential for the

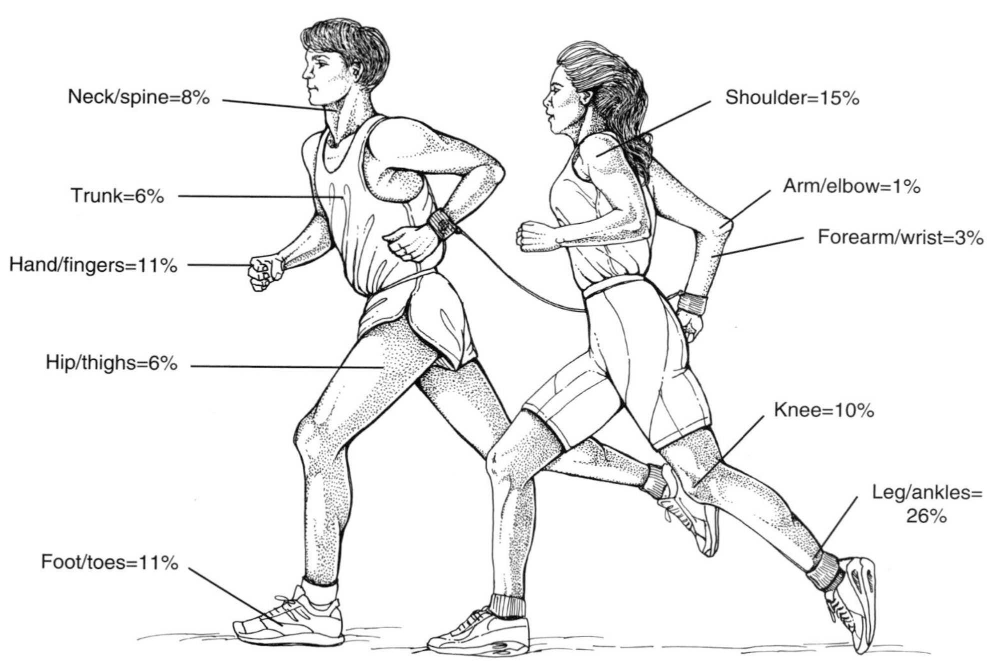
Neck/spine=8%
Shoulder=15%
Trunk=6%
Arm/elbow=1%
Forearm/wrist=3%
Hand/fingers=11%
Hip/thighs=6%
Knee=10%
Leg/ankles=
26%
Foot/toes=11%

FIGURE 52-5. Injury incidence in athlete with a visual impairment.

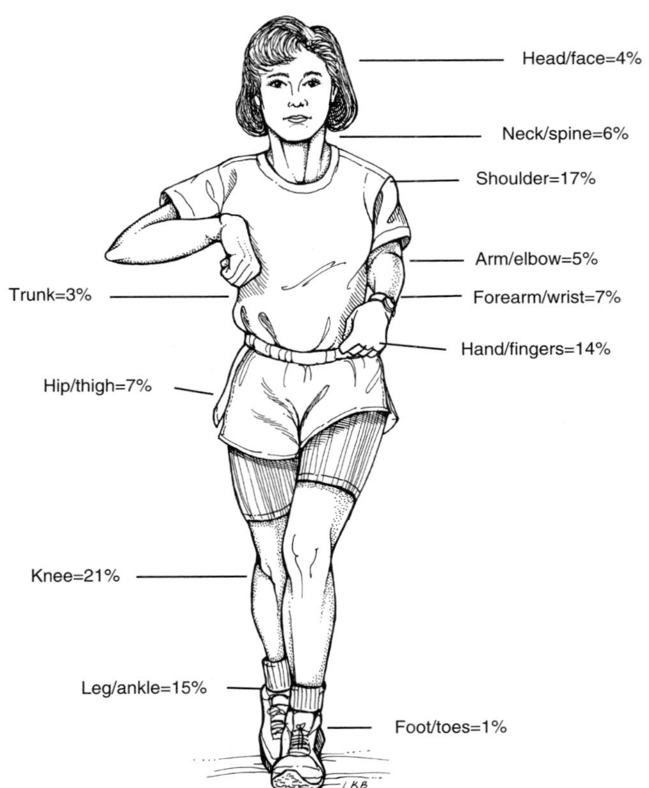

FIGURE 52-6. Injury incidence in athlete with cerebral palsy (ambulatory).

highest incidence of injuries. Curtis and Dillon[16] found a relationship between injuries and the number of hours trained per week and age of wheelchair athletes. The participants in the 21- to 30-year-old age group suffered the highest number of injuries of any age group. Ferrara and Davis[25] found that 50% of the injuries in an athletic wheelchair population were strains and muscular injuries of the upper extremity.

Hand and Finger Injuries

Hand and finger injuries are not uncommon in wheelchair athletes. Because the hands are used continuously for propulsion, blisters of the fingers and thumbs may develop. Thick calluses may form over the first and second digits and the palm of the hand from the repetitive contact with the hand rim. However, the elbow and upper arm also are frequent places where blisters occur.

A wheelchair design change of a drop in the seat height to allow for a lower center of gravity may contribute to more injuries. This decreased seat height places the elbow and upper arm in contact with the wheel, where a friction burn may occur. Blisters of the fingers and hand are a potential problem for infection and painful fissures. Further, fractures of the metacarpal bones and phalanges are possible from falls and collisions with other wheelchairs. Thumb fractures may occur if the digit slips off of the hand rim and gets caught in the spokes of the wheel. Basketball and other such contact activities place the athlete at risk of fracture.

Prevention. Prevention of blisters is a matter of protective devices and proper use of the wheelchair. Many wheelchair athletes use specially designed gloves with protective taping in the region of high friction at the point of contact with the hand rim (Fig. 52-7). They also may place protective pads (knee pads, socks, etc.) in the elbow and upper arm region to reduce the potential of injury from the wheel.

The hands and other high-friction areas should be cleaned frequently and calluses filed to reduce skin layers. For any athlete who has numbness and tingling in the hand and fingers, carpal tunnel syndrome should be considered. This can be diagnosed by electromyography (EMG) and mild cases treated with neutral position wrist splints.

Shoulder Injuries

Wheelchair propulsion requires forceful and repetitive motion applied to the hand rim. Researchers have estimated that for some athletes, the hand is in contact with the hand rim for 270°.[28] This repeated stress is on the athlete's anterior chest and shoulder muscles. The use of the arm to propel the wheelchair requires repetitive motion by the shoulder, elbow, and wrists. The rotator cuff may develop overuse injuries such as impingement and painful arch syndrome, and bicipital tendinitis.

Prevention. Many shoulder injuries could be prevented through the use of strength and flexibility exercises and a carefully monitored training program. The posterior musculature, especially the external rotators and scapular adductors, needs to be strengthened. This will help to achieve a balance with the often-overdeveloped anterior

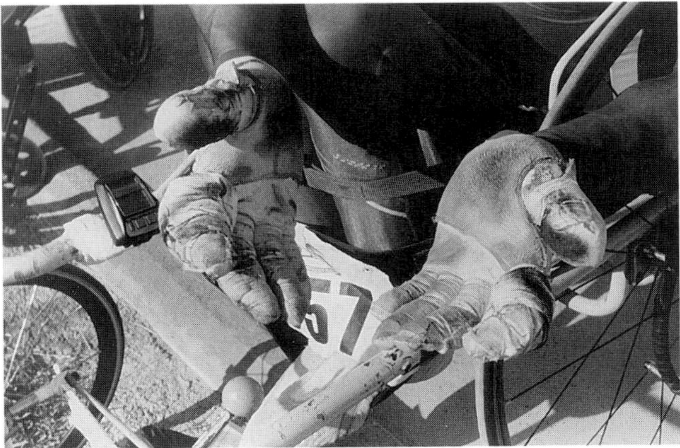

FIGURE 52-7. An example of the wear and tear on hands and gloves of a wheelchair athlete.

shoulder musculature.[8,9] A static flexibility program for all ranges of motion of the shoulder should be instituted, particularly for the anterior muscles and the rotator cuff. Careful monitoring of the training program and alteration of activity could reduce the number and incidence of chronic shoulder injuries.

Management. Treatment of chronic and acute shoulder injuries should follow conventional treatment patterns. Ice, rest, and nonsteroidal anti-inflammatory medications are particularly effective. To maintain cardiovascular fitness of the athlete, alternative exercise should be prescribed.

AMPUTEE ATHLETES

Stump Problems

The athlete who has an amputation is subject to the same injuries and stress as the athlete without a disability. Additionally, the amputee may be subject to irritations and stress at the junction with the prosthetic device. This problem particularly occurs with lower-limb prostheses. It is characterized by redness and irritation at the prosthesis–skin interface.

Prevention. The athlete normally knows when a skin irritation or breakdown from the stump is beginning. These problems can be prevented by a proper fit and maintenance of the prosthetic device. Protective padding at the end of the prosthesis or friction-eliminating material such as NuSkin over irritated areas may aid in the healing process. An excessively loose or tight fit will increase the stress at the junction.

Various materials have been used between the skin and the socket to reduce the stress from vigorous athletic activity. The materials have included gels, soft fabrics, and foam padding. Advances in prosthetic design, development, and fit have reduced the number of prosthesis-related problems. The new knee prosthetic device allows for a truer knee range of motion and less rotational stress, plus the added feature of a plantar flexion to absorb the forces transmitted from the ground during heel strike.

Management. Protective padding of the end of the prosthesis and cleansing at the irritated area aids the healing process for a stump injury. In advanced cases, the athlete may have to temporarily discontinue use of the prosthesis and reduce athletic participation.

INJURIES TO ATHLETES WITH CEREBRAL PALSY

Muscle Strains and Miscellaneous Conditions

There are varying degrees of cerebral palsy that range from severe to barely perceptible spasticity. Muscular problems can be caused by the influence of spasticity on the muscle. Many individuals with cerebral palsy have had Achilles tendon surgery and hamstring surgery to allow for a greater degree of range of motion. This surgical intervention may cause a decrease in the active muscle units for a muscular contraction, hence an imbalance between the agonist and antagonist muscles may exist.

Seizures are an infrequent problem during sports for individuals with cerebral palsy. Richter[61] stated that 1 out of 87 athletes with cerebral palsy had a minor seizure incident at the 1988 Paralympic Games. Fifteen percent of the athletes with cerebral palsy had a history of seizures.

Prevention. Prevention of muscular injuries is facilitated by flexibility and strength-training programs. It is important that the physician who is treating the athlete with cerebral palsy work with the available range of motion to maintain and restore motion that may be lost because of contractures and spasticity. Proprioceptive neuromuscular facilitation (PNF) stretching appears to be particularly effective when used in conjunction with static stretching programs. Strength training of sport-specific muscles to achieve a muscular balance and improve performance also is indicated (Fig. 52-8).[18,50]

Management. The management of a muscle strain should follow the typical treatment pattern. Ice is particularly helpful, not only because of its anti-inflammatory properties, but also because prolonged use may decrease

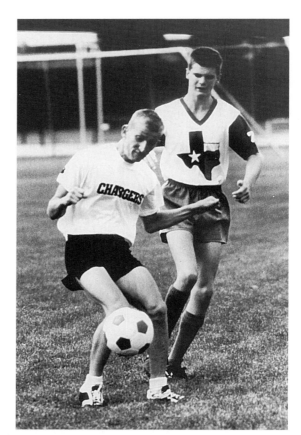

FIGURE 52-8. Athletes with cerebral palsy playing soccer.

spastic tone.[15] Stretching must be slow and steady because quick movements will trigger the muscle spindles, causing a reflex shortening. The stretch must be comfortable enough to be held for at least thirty seconds, but preferably for over two minutes.[76] Key areas of spastic tightness include the shoulder internal rotators, hip flexors, and ankle plantar flexors. If anti-inflammatory medication is prescribed, the physician should be aware of possible drug interactions with antiseizure drugs or other medicine that the athlete may be taking.

Falls

Falls usually are seen in the USCPAA Class V (diplegic) and Class VI (athetoid) competitions. Although not a common problem leading to injury, falls from a loss of balance and coordination may occur. However, most athletes are able to catch and brace themselves for a fall, thus reducing the severity of the injury.

INJURIES TO ATHLETES WHO ARE VISUALLY IMPAIRED

Barrier Problems

The athlete with a visual impairment may not have visual cues in relation to road surface and condition and various barriers such as walls, curbs, and other competing athletes. Many events, such as track and tandem cycling, employ a guide runner to assist the athletes who are visually impaired.

Lower Extremity Injuries

The athlete with a visual impairment tends to have a higher proportion of lower extremity injuries. Ferrara[24] found that 26% of the injuries were to the leg/ankle, 11% to the foot/toes, and 10% to the knee. This could be due to improper training techniques and overuse mechanisms.

There also are biomechanical considerations that can contribute to the increased percentage of lower extremity injuries. Changes in stepping frequency, stride length, prolonged stance time, and excessive braking and acceleration forces have been documented.[24] The athlete with a visual impairment may expend more energy when performing the same tasks as the athlete without a visual impairment; therefore, the athlete is more likely to fatigue quickly. A higher incidence of overuse of the lower extremity may result.

Prevention. Monitoring the training program to eliminate overuse is extremely important. Other considerations for prevention involve the selection of a matched (physiologically and biomechanically) guide runner to maintain an even pace and stride length. The inappropriate selection of the guide runner could hinder the training of an athlete with a visual impairment. Training periodization should be instituted to allow for recovery time and decrease the potential for injury.

SPECIAL OLYMPIANS

Special Olympics International provides athletic competition for athletes with mental impairment and offers a number of sporting opportunities including track, field, ice skating, gymnastics, floor hockey, and skiing. There is a heightened awareness of athletes with Down syndrome, the most recognizable form of mental retardation because of the physical appearance of people with this disability. However, orthopedic problems that particularly afflict athletes with Down syndrome may not be familiar to medical personnel. The typical medical problems include pes planus, patellar instability, and atlantoaxial instability.[34]

Cervical Spine Instability

In 1983, Special Olympics International issued a directive to all medical personnel, coaches, parents, and athletes restricting participation of athletes with Down syndrome until they had received medical examinations for atlantoaxial instability. The sudden concern was due to a finding of collagen and ligamentous laxity in a number of athletes. Researchers have estimated a prevalence of 10% to 20%[14,17,32,52] for cervical spine instability. The ligament laxity and bony abnormality can be completely asymptomatic, or it can result in a variety of symptoms, including weakness of the extremity, neck pain, and deterioration of ambulatory skills.

Prevention. The Special Olympics general rules now restrict participation by these athletes in activities that could produce “hyperextension, hyperflexion, or direct pressure on the upper spine.”[52] Radiographic evidence demonstrating normal atlantoaxial stability and no bony abnormalities must be presented for the athlete to be allowed to participate without any sport restrictions. Permanent sport restrictions are placed on athletes who demonstrate positive radiographic evidence.

Diagnosis. Atlantoaxial instability is detected by radiographic findings in conjunction with a physical examination. Radiographic examination should include the anterior–posterior, lateral, flexion–extension, and odontoid views of the spine. Longitudinal radiographic examinations should be performed to detect any changes in spinal stability.

Management. There are several treatment options available to those with spinal instability. Obviously, the restriction of activities that would increase the risk of spinal injury is indicated. Those activities that result in axial loading, hyperflexion, or hyperextension mechanisms are contraindicated. Spinal fusions may be performed to stabilize the joint in persons with symptomatic dislocations.

MULTIPLE SCLEROSIS

Multiple sclerosis is an upper motor neuron lesion of fluctuating clinical presentation. It has an often-unpredictable clinical course. It is important for athletes with multiple sclerosis to not become overfatigued and particularly to not increase core body temperature, both of which may lead to an exacerbation of the condition.[54] Swimming is a good sport for people with MS because the relatively cool water temperature with its high specific heat (skin temperature is usually 91° F) tends to cool the athlete and prevent a rise in body core temperature. In particular, these athletes need to be counseled to not participate in sports during hot weather, which could be very detrimental to them.

ASTHMA

Asthma is a common disorder; over 15% of the U.S. Olympic Team in Los Angeles has asthma or exercise-induced asthma (EIA).[58,75] Athletes can deal with asthma by avoiding times of high pollution, such as during the heat of the day when the ozone level is up and traffic pollution may be higher. They should warm up slowly for long periods of time, such as 15 minutes, gradually increasing the workload. This permits bronchial dilation to occur. It helps to exercise in humid air. Dry, cold air tends to increase the likelihood of bronchial spasm. Swimming is often an excellent exercise for asthmatics.

The inhalation of long-acting bronchodilators such as salbutamol is very effective in preventing an acute bronchial spasm. For chronic asthma, the use of anti-inflammatories, inhaled steroids such as nedocromil sodium, and leukotriene-receptor antagonists such as montelukast are often effective.[74] Elite athletes using prescribed inhaled steroids need to notify the USOC.

DIABETES

Physicians have been aware for years of the positive benefits of exercise for diabetics. Exercise has been a key component in proper management of diabetic care, along with proper diet and regularly scheduled medication.[31] Exercise can increase insulin sensitivity and decrease adipose tissue, which leads to better control of the known diabetic patient and may help prevent the onset of type II diabetes.[27,35,57] Physicians should be aware of complications and risks that can occur when diabetics exercise. One of the frequent complications for insulin-dependent diabetic athletes is hypoglycemia.[60]

A hypoglycemia attack may occur because too much insulin is present or not enough calories have been taken in. Most frequently, hypoglycemia is the result of escalated absorption of insulin that has been injected into an active muscle. This is especially true when short-acting insulin is being used. The best injection sites are the buttocks and abdomen.[31] Insulin requirements can change. Insulin may need to be decreased one to two units and/or carbohydrate intake may need to be increased by 10 to 15 grams for every half-hour of exercise.[51] For prolonged activity, 5 to 20 grams of carbohydrates should be consumed for every 20 minutes of activity. The diabetic should be encouraged to eat approximately 30 to 60 minutes before beginning an exercise program. Blood sugar should be monitored before and after the completion of an exercise bout because exercise can lower blood sugar levels for 24 to 48 hours following an exercise session.[27]

If hypoglycemia occurs during exercise, the athlete should ingest a high-glucose drink or food and perhaps discontinue the activity.[31] The athlete should be encouraged always to carry glucose and proper identification during exercise and, if blood sugars are unstable, not to exercise alone.

Diabetic patients should be encouraged to wear proper footwear and practice good foot hygiene. Often it is helpful to alternate footwear, that is, have several pairs of good shoes, to redistribute pressure points. Injuries to the foot, such as blisters or infection, should be treated immediately.

Though diabetic complications and exercise have not been fully researched, it is suggested that excessive activity may worsen nephropathy and retinopathy.[11,35,57] If retinopathy is present, the diabetic athlete should avoid prolonged isometrics or heavy resistance training.[31]

Some authors suggest that autonomic neuropathy may predispose individuals to arrhythmias and that extreme activity may precipitate a cardiac event in those with cardiac disease.[11] Individuals with diabetes who are interested in participating in sport should have a complete physical exam including a cardiac evaluation.[11,57] Also, note must be made that the diabetic athlete taking a beta-blocker may not be able to adequately experience the symptoms of hypoglycemia and/or angina, and that exercise in excess heat may lead to problems from dehydration, which must be rigorously prevented.[51]

OBESITY

Obesity, which is described as a body mass index (BMI) equal to or greater than 30,[29,49] is prevalent in American society. The goal of exercise for the obese individual is to increase caloric expenditure to decrease health problems such as cardiovascular disease, diabetes, and joint problems.[14,23,37,41,49] Even if there is no change in an individual's weight, exercise may be helpful in such things as normalizing hypertension induced by obesity.[10] A high level of success is noted for obese individuals who follow an exercise regimen that increases caloric expenditure when joined with a diet program that decreases caloric intake.[2,40] Appropriate types of exercise for the obese include walking, recumbent cycling, using a stair-climber or rowing machine, and water exercise. Exercise at a low intensity may be an effective technique in decreasing fat stores. At lower intensity levels, the lipid mobilizing system provides energy, but the carbohydrate system functions during intense exercise. After intense exercise there is a lipid to carbohydrate shift, but the obese athlete may have difficulty performing at an intense level. The more conditioned the athlete, the more the athlete can mobilize the fat stores. Exercise in water is often a good choice for conditioning because of the buoyancy of the water and absence of elevated body temperature, but not for weight loss, when compared to land exercises.[55]

Excess weight puts additional strain on the joints in the spine and lower extremity. It is suggested that obesity contributes to the development of osteoarthritis in the hips.[37,41,49] Each step taken by an individual puts three times the body weight through the joints of the lower extremity. Just a 10-pound weight loss decreases joint stress by 30 pounds. An individual with an elevated BMI has a twofold to fivefold increase in risk of needing a total hip arthroplasty due to osteoarthritis.[10] Although more intense exercise may have more health benefits,[39] physicians should encourage sedentary individuals that the greatest health benefit may actually be for people who go from no exercise to any form of exercise.

REFERENCES

1. American Academy of Orthopedic Surgeons: Athletic Training and Sports Medicine. Parkridge IL, The Academy, 1991.
2. Bennett WI: Beyond overeating. N Engl J Med 332:673–674, 1995.
3. Benzinger TH: Heat regulation: Homeostasis of central temperature in man. Physiol Rev 671–759, 1969.
4. Birrer RB: The Special Olympics: An injury overview. Phys Sports Med 12:95–97, 1985.
5. Bloomquist LE: Injuries to athletes with physical disabilities: Prevention implications. Phys Sports Med 14:97, 1986.
6. Bouchchama A, Knochel JP: Medical progress: Heat stroke. N Engl J Med 346:1978–1988, 2002.
7. Brodie MJ, Dickter MA: Drug therapy: Antiepileptic drugs. N Engl J Med 334:168–175, 1966.
8. Burnham R, Wheeler G, Bhambhani Y, et al: Intentional induction of autonomic dysreflexia among quadriplegic athletes for performance enhancement: Efficacy, safety, and mechanism of action. Clin J Sport Med 4:1–10, 1994.
9. Burnham RS, May L, Nelson E, et al: Shoulder pain in wheelchair athletes: The role of muscle imbalance. Am J Sport Med 21:238–242, 1993.
10. Carroll JF, Kyer CK: Exercise training in obesity lowers blood pressure independent of weight change. Med Sci Sports Exerc 34(4):596–601, 2002.
11. Chipkin SR, Klugh SA, Chasan-Taber L: Exercise and diabetes. Cardiology Clin 19(3):489–505, 2001.
12. Clark MW: Competitive sports for the disabled. Am J Sports Med 8:366–369, 1980.
13. Colachis SC III, Otis SM: Thermal regulation and fever in SCI. Am J PM&R 74(2):114–119, 1995.
14. Committee on Sports Medicine: Atlanto-axial instability in Downs Syndrome. Orthop Clin North Am 74:152–154, 1984.
15. Corcos DM, Gottlieb GL, Penn RD, et al: Movement deficits caused by hyperexcitable stretch reflexes in spastic humans. Brain 109:1043–1058, 1986.
16. Curtis KA, Dillon DA: Survey of wheelchair athletic injuries: Common patterns and prevention. Paraplegia 23:170–175, 1985.
17. Diamond LS, Lynne KD, Sigman B: Orthopedic disorders in patients with Down's syndrome. Orthop Clin North Am 12:57–71, 1981.
18. Dodd KJ, Taylor NF, Damiano DL: A systematic review of the effectiveness of strength-training programs for people with cerebral palsy. Arch Phys Med Rehabil 72:1157–1164, 2002.
19. Downey JA, Chiodi HP, Darling RC: Central temperature regulation in the spinal man. J Appl Physiol 22:91–94, 1967.
20. Downey JA, Miller JM, Darling RC: Thermoregulatory responses to deep and superficial cooling in spinal man. J Appl Physiol 27:209–212, 1969.
21. Downey RJ, Downey JA, Newhouse E, et al: Hyperthermia in a quadriplegic: Evidence for a peripheral action of haloperidol in malignant neuroleptic syndrome. Chest 101:1728–1730, 1992.
22. Erickson RP: Autonomic hyperreflexia: Pathophysiology and medical management. Arch Phys Med Rehabil 61:431–440, 1980.
23. Fenster CP, et al: Obesity, aerobic exercise and vascular disease: The role of oxidant stress. Obes Res 10(9):964–968, 2002.
24. Ferrara MS, et al: The injury experience of the competitive athlete with a disability: prevention implications. Med Sci Sports Exerc 24(2):184–188, 1992.
25. Ferrara MS, Davis R: Injuries to elite wheelchair athletes. Paraplegia 28:335–341, 1990.
26. Ferrara MS, Buckley WE: Athletes with disabilities injury registry. APAQ 13:50–60, 1996.
27. Flood L, Constance A: Diabetes and exercise safety. Am J Nursing 102(6):47–55, 2002.
28. Gehlsen GM, Davis RW, Bahmonde R: Intermittent velocity and wheelchair performance characteristics. APAQ 7:219–230, 1990.

29. Gilmore J. Body mass index and health. Health Rep 11(1):31–43, 1999.
30. Guttmann L: The importance of sport and recreation for the physically handicapped. In Leon AS, Amundson G (eds): Proceedings of the First International Conference on Lifestyle and Health, Minneapolis, 1979.
31. Horton ES: Role and management of exercise in diabetes mellitus. Diabetes Care 11(2):201–211, 1988.
32. Hreidarsson S, Magram G, Singer H: Symptomatic atlantoaxial dislocation in Down Syndrome. Pediatrics 69:568–571, 1982.
33. Huberman G: Organized sports activities with cerebral palsy. Adoles Rehabil Lit 37:103–106, 1976.
34. Hudson PB: Preparticipation screening of Special Olympics Athletes. Phys Sports Med 16:97–104, 1988.
35. Kahn, BB: Lilly lecture 1995. Glucose transport; Pivotal step in insulin action. Diabetes 45(11): 1644–1654, 1996.
36. Kammerman S, Waserman L: Seizure disorders: Part 2 treatment. West J Med 175:184–188, 2001.
37. Karlson EW, et al: Total hip arthroplasty due to osteoarthritis: The importance of age, obesity and other modifiable risk factors. Am J Med 114(2): 158–159, 2003.
38. Kleiber DA, et al: Involvement with special recreation associations: Perceived impacts in early adulthood. Ther Rec J 24:32–44, 1990.
39. Lee I, Hsieh C, Paffenbarger RS Jr: Exercise intensity and longevity in men. JAMA 273:1179–1184, 1995.
40. Leibel RL, Rosenbaum M, Hirsch J: Changes in energy expenditure resulting from altered body weight. NEJM 332: 621–628, 1995.
41. Lievense AP, et al: Influence of obesity on the development of osteoarthritis of the hip; A systemic review. Rheumatology (Oxford) 41(10):1155–1162, 2002.
42. Magnus BC: Sports injuries, the disabled athlete, and the athletic trainer. Ath Train 22:305–310, 1987.
43. McCann BC: Medical classification: Art, science, or instinct? Sport'n Spokes 5:12–14, 1980.
44. McCann BC: The medical disability specific classification system in sports. In Steadward RD, Nelson ER, Wheeler GD (eds): Vista '93 — The Outlook. Edmonton, Canada, Rick Hansen Centre, 1994, pp 224–229.
45. McCann BC: Thermoregulation in spinal cord injury: The challenge of the Atlanta Paralympics. Spinal Cord 34(7):433–436, 1996.
46. McCormick DP: Injuries in handicapped alpine ski racers. Phys Sports Med 13:93–97, 1985.
47. Menard MR, Hahn G: Acute and chronic hypothermia in a man with spinal cord injury: Environmental and pharmacologic causes. Arch Phys Med Rehabil 72:421–424, 1991.
48. Modorski JB, Curtis KA: Wheelchair sports medicine. Am J Sports Med 12:128–132, 1984.
49. Mokdad AH, et al: Prevalence of obesity, diabetes and obesity related health risk factors 2001. JAMA 289(1):76–79, 2003.
50. Mushett CA, Wyeth DO, Richter, KJ: Cerebral palsy, traumatic brain injury, and stroke. In Goldberg B (ed): Sports and exercise for children with chronic health conditions. Champaign IL, Human Kinetics, 1995.
51. Nathan DM, Madnek SF, Delahanty L: Programming pre-exercise snacks to prevent post-exercise hypoglycemia in intensively treated insulin-dependent diabetics. Ann Intern Med 102(4):483–486, 1985.
52. Official Special Olympics Summer Sports Rules, No 6: Participation by individuals with Downs Syndrome who suffer from the atlantoaxial dislocation condition. Washington D.C., 1992, revised 1995.
53. Ogunytmi A, et al: Seizures induced by exercise. Neurology 38:633–634, 1988.
54. Olgiati R, Jacquet J, di Prampero PE: Energy cost of walking and exertional dyspnea in multiple sclerosis. Am Rev Respir Dis 134:1005–1010, 1986.
55. Pate RR, et al: Guidelines for Exercise Testing and Prescription: ACSM, 4th ed. Philadelphia, Lea & Febiger, 1991.
56. Pickering GW: The vasomotor regulation of heat loss from the human skin in relation to external temperature. Heart 115–135, 1932.
57. Pierce NS: Diabetes and exercise. Br J Sports Med 33(3):161–172, 1999.
58. Pierson WE, Voy RO: Exercise-induced bronchospasm in the XXIII Summer Olympic games. NE & Reg Allergy Pro 9(3):209–213, 1988.
59. Randall WC, et al: Central peripheral factors in dynamic thermoregulation. J Appl Physiol 18:61–64, 1963.
60. Richter EA, Ruderman NB, Schneider SH: Diabetes and exercise. Am J Med 70:201, 1981.
61. Richter KJ: Seizures in athletes. J Osteo Sports Med 3:19–23, 1989.
62. Richter KJ: Hypertensive crisis—autonomic hyperreflexia (Letter). NEJM 324(14):994, 1991.
63. Richter KJ, et al: Injuries in world class cerebral palsy athletes of the 1988 Seoul, Korea Paralympics. J Osteo Sports Med 7:15–18, 1991.
64. Richter KJ, et al: Integrated swimming classification: A faulted system. APAQ 9:5–13, 1992.
65. Secondorf R, Randall WC: Thermal reflex sweating in normal and paraplegic man. J Appl Physiol 16:796–800, 1961.
66. Sherrill C, Adams-Mushett C, Jones JA: Classification and other issues in sports for the blind, cerebral palsied, les autres, and amputee athlete. In Sherrill C (ed): Sports and Disabled Athletes. Champaign IL, Human Kinetics, 1986.

67. Sherrill C, Hinson M, Gench B, et al: Self-concepts of disabled youth athletes. Perceptual Motor Skills 70:1093–1098, 1990.
68. Sherrill C, Rainbolt W: Self actualization profiles of male able-bodied and cerebral palsied athletes. APAQ 5(2):108–119, 1988.
69. Siddiqui A, Keab R, Weale ME, et al: Association of multidrug resistance in epilepsy with a polymorphism in the drug-transporter gene ABCBI. N Eng J Med 348(15):1442–1448, 2003.
70. Simon E: Temperature regulation: The spinal cord as a site of extra hypothalamic thermoregulatory functions. Rev Physiol Biochem Pharmacol 71:1–76, 1974.
71. Steadward, et al: Vista '93. Edmonton, Canada, Rick Hansen Centre, 1993, pp 242–247.
72. Sydney 2000 Paralympic Games Post Games Report – IPC.
73. Tweedy SM. Biomechanical consequences of impairment; A taxonomically valid basis for classification – United Disability Athletics System. Res Quarterly Exer and Sport March 2003.
74. Udem BJ, Lichtenstein LM: Drugs used in the treatment of asthmas. In Hardman JG, Limibiria LE (eds): Goodman and Gilman's The Pharmacological Basis of Therapeutics, 10th ed. New York, McGraw-Hill, 2001.
75. Voy RO: US Olympic committee experience with exercise-induced bronchospasm, 1984. Med Sci Sport Exerc 18(3):328–330, June 1986.
76. Wolf SE: Morphological and functional considerations for therapeutic exercises. In Basmajian JV (ed): Therapeutic Exercise, 4th ed. Baltimore, Williams & Wilkins, 1984.
77. Woo E, Chan YM, Yu YL, et al: If a well-stabilized patient has a sub-therapeutic antiepileptic drug level, should the dose be increased? A randomized prospective study. Epilepsia 29:129–139, 1988.

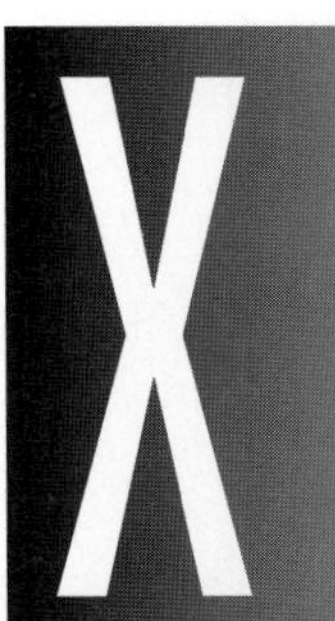

The Team Physician

53 Credentials and Responsibilities for Team Physicians

Edward C. Brown III, W. Norman Scott, and Giles R. Scuderi

Many medical professionals across the spectrum of medical care share a common interest in sports medicine and the medical care of athletes. The medical team assembled to provide care for athletic teams reflects this broad interest and may include medical physicians, orthopedic surgeons, athletic trainers, physical therapists, nutritionists, and other allied health personnel. Sports medicine is not the domain of any one specialty and the care of athletes is only enhanced when it includes the contribution of all medical professionals.

Although the role of the team physician may vary depending on the type of team, the location, team management, and other factors, the team physician's first responsibility is the safety and well-being of each athlete. Until recently, an agreed upon framework of qualifications and responsibilities for team physicians had not been established. In an effort to address the lack of clearly defined qualifications and duties for team physicians, representatives from six major professional medical organizations concerned about clinical sports medicine published the Team Physician Consensus Statement in 1999.[15] These organizations were the American Academy of Family Physicians (AAFP), the American Academy of Orthopaedic Surgeons (AAOS), the American College of Sports Medicine (ACSM), the American Medical Society for Sports Medicine (AMSSM), the American Orthopaedic Society for Sports Medicine (AOSSM),[5] and the American Osteopathic Academy of Sports Medicine (AOASM).

The objective of the Team Physician Consensus Statement is to provide physicians, school administrators, team owners, the general public, and individuals who are responsible for decision making regarding the medical care of athletes and teams with guidelines for choosing a qualified team physician and an outline of the duties expected of a team physician. Ultimately, by educating decision makers about the need for a qualified team physician, the goal is to ensure that athletes and teams are provided the very best medical care. One survey of high school football teams in southern California found that only 71% of responding high schools had a designated team physician.[16]

The Team Physician Consensus Statement establishes the definition of the team physician and outlines a team physician's qualifications, duties, and responsibilities. It also contains strategies for the continuing education of team physicians.

TEAM PHYSICIAN DEFINITION

The team physician must have an unrestricted medical license and be an M.D. or D.O. who is responsible for treating and coordinating the medical care of athletic team members.[15] The principal responsibility of the team physician is to provide for the well-being of individual athletes, enabling each to realize his or her full potential. The team physician should possess special proficiency in the care of musculoskeletal injuries and medical conditions encountered in sports. The team physician also must actively integrate medical expertise with other health care providers, including medical specialists, athletic trainers, and allied health professionals. The team physician must ultimately assume responsibility within the team structure for making medical decisions that affect the athlete's safe participation.

CREDENTIALS

The American Board of Family Practice has offered credentialing to nonsurgical physicians, primarily family practitioners, in sports medicine since 1993 with the Certificate of Added Qualification (CAQ). The eligibility criteria include primary certification in the fields of family practice, internal medicine, emergency medicine, or pediatrics, and the completion of a one-year ACGME-approved (Accreditation Council for Graduate Medical Education) fellowship in sports medicine. These nonsurgical fellowships are sponsored by various training programs in family practice, internal medicine, emergency medicine, and pediatrics and there are currently approximately 74 ACGME-accredited[1] and 20 nonaccredited[11] available fellowships. Since 1993, 1190 diplomates have received the Certificate of Added Qualification and 54 diplomates passed the most recent examination in April 2003.[4]

One of the major landmarks regarding credentialing within the realm of sports medicine is the recent approval on March 20, 2003, by the American Board of Medical Specialties of the subspecialty of orthopedic sports medicine, which can be viewed as the operative counterpart to the nonsurgical physicians' credential. The application for subspecialty certification was brought by the

American Board of Orthopaedic Surgery on behalf of the American Orthopaedic Society of Sports Medicine.

The lasting impact of this decision is unknown at this time but it has clearly placed the American Academy of Orthopaedic Surgeons at odds with the American Orthopaedic Society of Sports Medicine, the American Board of Orthopaedic Surgery, and the American Board of Medical Specialties.[3] Since 1989, the American Academy of Orthopaedic Surgery has stated an explicit position opposing Certificates of Added Qualification (CAQs) or subspecialty certification in orthopaedic surgery. The Academy Fellowship reaffirmed this position in 1990, 1994, 1996, and 2000, and the AAOS Board of Directors sent of strong letter of opposition in May 2001 upon recommendation of the Board of Councilors.[3]

Currently, any ACGME residency-trained orthopaedist can practice orthopedic sports medicine. According to the latest AAOS census data, 44% of all practicing orthopedic surgeons claim a special interest in orthopedic sports medicine.[2] Depending on their training, education, and experience, orthopedists will have different levels of proficiency and comfort in caring for each of the areas that encompass sports medicine.

Today there approximately 95 fellowship programs that offer specialized training in orthopedic sports medicine to approximately 200 individuals annually, which represents roughly one third of the number of orthopedic residents that graduate each year. Of these fellowships, more than half (55) are ACGME accredited.[3] These programs offer additional knowledge and skill to the fellow, but a common high standard of education among the fellowships has not been established. A higher and formal standard of certification in orthopedic sports medicine is unlikely to encourage more institutions to establish a program and may even result in some programs closing if they cannot or do not want to fulfill the requirements.

Subspecialty certification is meant to establish educational standards, not standards in the practice of orthopedic sports medicine. Certification in orthopedic sports medicine means that an orthopedist has achieved a level of proficiency in each of the areas comprising orthopedic sports medicine as prescribed by the American Board of Orthopaedic Surgery. Certification does not reflect an exclusive knowledge or skill pertaining to an anatomic region or given procedure within orthopedics. In a statement by the AOSSM in 2000, it was declared that the AOSSM strongly supports the right and ability of all orthopedists, regardless of postgraduate training and education, to provide sports medicine services in the team, clinical, and surgical settings. Additionally, certification cannot be used as a criterion for AOSSM membership or full participation in the society.[3]

The credentialing process for subspecialty certification in orthopedic sports medicine is to be administered by the American Board of Orthopaedic Surgery. Requirements for certification in orthopedic sports medicine have been established by the American Board of Orthopaedic Surgeons.[2] These requirements include:

1. Must be a diplomate of the American Board of Orthopaedic Surgery and have been actively practicing orthopedic sports medicine for at least two years in the same location, following completion of any formal education.
2. Must have a current, full and unrestricted license to practice medicine in the United States, a United States jurisdiction, or a Canadian province, or be engaged in full-time practice in the United States Federal Government, for which licensure is not required.
3. Must have an ethical standing in the profession and a moral and professional status in the community that is acceptable to the Board.
4. Must be actively involved in the practice of medicine, as indicated by holding full operating privileges in a hospital or surgery center approved by the Joint Commission on Accreditation of Health Care Organizations or the Canadian equivalent.
5. Applicants must submit a list of cases of sports medicine surgeries managed during a consecutive 12-month period, within the two years preceding the application. Sports medicine surgery includes procedures associated with injuries or conditions that are related to or interfere with exercise, sports participation, or a physical lifestyle. The case list must include at least 125 sports medicine cases, 75 of which must be arthroscopic cases. A maximum of 6 nonoperative cases may be submitted. Nonoperative cases are those that require significant evaluation such as pain problems or those that require extensive rehabilitation. Nonoperative cases must be documented with consultation reports.
6. In addition, 50 of the cases must be in the following categories:

    I. Knee
        A. Tibiofemoral
            1. Ligament (reconstructioin, repair, realignment)
            2. Tendon (repair, reconstruction, debridement)
            3. Meniscus (repair, replacement)
            4. Articular cartilage (repair, replacement)
            5. Bone (osteotomies, fractures about the knee)
        B. Patellofemoral
            1. Ligament (realignment, repair, reconstruction)
            2. Tendon (repair, debridement, reconstruction)
            3. Cartilage (chondral or osteochondral repair)
            4. Bone (fractures)
    II. Shoulder
        A. Glenohumeral
            1. Ligament (open or arthroscopic stabilization)
            2. Tendon (tendon ruptures or tears, tendonopathy)

3. Cartilage (debridement, repair: excludes arthroplasty)
4. Bone (fractures, dislocations)

B. Acromioclavicular
1. Ligament (repair, reconstruction, realignment)
2. Cartilage (debridement, resection)
3. Bone (fractures: intraarticular, extraarticular)

III. Elbow
A. Ligament (reconstruction, repair, realignment)
B. Tendon (repair, reconstruction, debridement)
C. Cartilage (repair, replacement, debridement)
D. Bone (fractures: intraarticular and extraarticular)

IV. Foot and Ankle
A. Ligament (realignment, repair, reconstruction)
B. Tendon (repair, reconstruction, realignment)
C. Cartilage (repair, replacement, debridement)
D. Bone (fractures and dislocations)

7. Must submit the prescribed application form and all the specified supporting documents pertaining thereto and pay the established fees.
8. Must pass any and all examinations prescribed by the American Board of Orthopaedic Surgery.

Candidates who do not fulfill the practice requirements in requirement 6 may petition the Credentials Committee of the Board for individual consideration. This consideration will take into account contributions and dedication to the discipline of orthopedic sports medicine such as teaching, publication, administration, and research.

The certification process in orthopedic sports medicine will likely begin in 2005 or 2006. Certification will be achieved through a one-day written examination offered by the ABOS. For an initial 5-year period, any individual who meets the criteria may sit for the examination. After 5 years, all applicants must have completed one year of training in an ACGME-accredited orthopedic sports medicine program or Canadian equivalent.

The qualifications of a team physician proposed from the Team Physician Consensus Statement predated the American Board of Medical Specialties recognition of the subspecialty of orthopedic sports medicine. Once certification becomes available within this new specialty, it is possible to envision a future effect on the qualifications for team physicians and orthopaedic surgeons.

QUALIFICATIONS

The Team Physician Consensus Statement outlined a specific set of necessary qualifications and an additional set of desirable skills or experience for team physicians. The primary concern of team physicians continues to be to provide the best medical care for athletes at all levels of participation. To this end, the Consensus Statement delineates the following qualifications necessary for all team physicians:

1. Have an M.D. or D.O. in good standing, with an unrestricted license to practice medicine.
2. Possess a fundamental knowledge of emergency medicine regarding sporting events.
3. Be trained in cardiopulmonary resuscitation (CPR).
4. Have a working knowledge of trauma, musculoskeletal injuries, and medical conditions affecting the athlete.

In addition, it is desirable for team physicians to have clinical training and experience and administrative skills in some or all of the following:

1. Specialty board certification.
2. Continuing medical education in sports medicine.
3. Formal training in sports medicine (fellowship training, board recognized subspecialty in sports medicine [formerly known as a certificate of added qualification in sports medicine]).
4. Additional training in sports medicine.
5. Fifty percent or more of practice involving sports medicine.
6. Membership and participation in a sports medical society.
7. Involvement in teaching, research, and publications in sports medicine.
8. Training in advanced cardiac life support.
9. Knowledge of medical/legal, disability, and worker's compensation issues.
10. Media skills training.

RESPONSIBILITIES

The world of the team physician at the highest levels of competitive amateur and professional athletics has changed significantly over the past decade. Legal, financial, and insurance issues and the resultant ethical issues dominate much of the commentary in the recent literature.[6,7,9,10,13] Some team physicians have discontinued their relationships with athletic teams due to inability to obtain or afford malpractice insurance or to afford expensive contracts with professional teams in exchange for rights to medical care and marketing.[7,9] However, even in the high-pressure world of high-performance athletics, team physicians must act professionally and maintain ethical principles.

The origins of a code of medical ethics and concerns for a patient's welfare and the appropriate behavior of the physician date back to the ancient Code of Hammurabi circa 1750 BC and the Hippocratic Oath of the fourth century BC and are a grand part of the heritage of medicine.[8]

The American Medical Association (AMA) first issued a specific statement regarding professional responsibility of the physician in sports medicine, Code E-3.06, as part of its *Current Opinion of the Council on Ethical and Judicial*

Affairs of the AMA in June 1983, which was updated in June 1994.[12] It states:

> Physicians should assist athletes to make informed decisions about their participation in amateur and professional contact sports which entail risks of bodily injury.
>
> The professional responsibility of the physician who serves in a medical capacity at an athletic contest or sporting event is to protect the health and safety of the contestants. The desire of spectators, promoters of the event, or even the injured athlete that he or she not be removed from the contest should not be controlling. The physician's judgment should be governed only by medical considerations.

The American Academy of Orthopaedic Surgeons developed guidelines for ethical behavior to address the demands of contemporary orthopedic practice. In part derived from the *Current Opinion of the Council on Ethical and Judicial Affairs of the American Medical Association*, the AAOS developed the *Principles of Medical Ethics and Professionalism in Orthopaedic Surgery* and the *Code of Medical Ethics and Professionalism for Orthopaedic Surgeons*, which were initially adopted in 1988 and were directed to the concerns of specific interest to orthopedic surgeons.[8] The *Code of Medical Ethics and Professionalism for Orthopaedic Surgeons* includes articles regarding the physician–patient relationship, personnel conduct, conflicts of interest, maintenance of competence, relationships with orthopedic surgeons, nurses, and allied health personnel, relationships with the public, general principles of care, research and academic responsibilities, and community responsibility.[8]

Although this document provides ethical practice guidelines for orthopedic surgeons, the Team Physician Consensus Statement directly addresses and specifically outlines the duties of a team physician.

Duties of a Team Physician

The team physician must be willing to commit the necessary time and effort to provide care for the team and athlete.[15] In addition, the team physician must develop and maintain a current, appropriate knowledge base of the sports(s) for which he or she is accepting responsibility. The duties for which the team physician has ultimate responsibility include the following:

1. Medical management of the athlete
   a. Coordinate pre-participation screening, examination, and evaluation
   b. Manage injuries on the field
   c. Provide for medical management of injury and illness
   d. Coordinate rehabilitation and return to participation
   e. Provide for proper preparation for safe return to participation after an illness or injury
   f. Integrate medical expertise with other health care providers, including medical specialists, athletic trainers, and allied health professionals
   g. Provide appropriate education and counseling regarding:
      i. Nutrition
      ii. Strength and conditioning
      iii. Ergogenic aids
      iv. Substance abuse
      v. Other medical problems that could affect the athlete
   h. Provide for proper documentation and medical record keeping
2. Administrative and logistical duties
   a. Establish and define the relationships of all involved parties
   b. Educate athletes, parents, administrators, coaches, and other necessary parties of concerns regarding the athletes
   c. Develop a chain of command
   d. Plan and train for emergencies during competition and practice
   e. Address equipment and supply issues
   f. Provide for proper event coverage
   g. Assess environmental concerns and playing conditions

The multi-disciplinary sports medicine committee also created additional consensus statements to provide guidance for team physicians regarding important specific issues faced in the medical management of athletes. These included The Team Physician and Return-to-Play Issues Consensus Statement, The Team Physician and Conditioning of Athletes for Sports Consensus Statement, and Sideline Preparedness for the Team Physician Consensus Statement.[14]

CONCLUSION

The Team Physician Consensus Statement provides language defining the qualifications of a team physician and outlines the duties and responsibilities inherent in the position. The successful team physician at any level of athletic competition can utilize these guidelines. The safety and well-being of athletes remains the first responsibility of the team physician. In addition to the medical management of the athlete, the team physician also has administrative and logistical duties that require excellent communication and organizational skills.

One of the major developments within sports medicine is the recently approved subspecialty of orthopedic sports medicine in March 2003. The anticipated time frame for offering of this Certificate of Added Qualification to qualifying orthopedic surgeons is in 2005 or 2006. The future impact of this subspecialty qualification within the realm of sports medicine is not known at this time.

REFERENCES

1. The Accreditation Council for Graduate Medical Education, Chicago, IL. Sports Medicine Fellowship Listings for 2003, www.acgme.org.
2. The American Academy of Orthopaedic Surgeons, Rosemont, IL. 2002 Census Data, www.aaos.org.
3. American Academy of Orthopaedic Surgery Bulletin Magazine 51(3):13–14, 2003.
4. The American Board of Family Practice, Lexington, KY. Personnel Communication, Statistics for 2003.
5. The American Orthopaedic Society of Sports Medicine, Rosemont, IL, www.aossm.org.
6. Apple D: Team physician: Bad ethics, bad business, or both? Orthopedics 25(1):25–26, 2002.
7. Capozzi JD, Rhodes R: Ethics in practice: Advertising and marketing. JBJS-A 82(11):1668–1669, 2000.
8. Code of Medical Ethics and Professionalism for Orthopaedic Surgeons. Rosemount, IL, American Academy of Orthopaedic Surgeons, 1988.
9. Dodd M: Malpractice crisis hits sports. USA Today March 10, 2003:C1–2.
10. Matheson GO: Can team physicians buy credibility? Physician Sportsmed 29(12):1–2, 2001.
11. The Physician and Sports Medicine, Minneapolis, MN. Sports Medicine Fellowship Listings for 2003, www.physsportsmed.com/fellows.
12. Recent opinions of the Judicial Council of the American Medical Association. JAMA 251(16): 2078–2079, 1984.
13. Rubin A: Team physician or athlete's doctor? Physician Sportsmed 26(7):1–2, 1998.
14. Sideline preparedness for the team physician: Consensus statement. Med Sci Sports Exerc 33(5):846–849, 2001.
15. Team Physician Consensus Statement. Med Sci Sports Exerc 32(4):877–878, 2000. Copyright © 1999 American Academy of Family Physicians, American Academy of Orthopaedic Surgeons, American College of Sports Medicine, American Medical Society for Sports Medicine, American Orthopaedic Society of Sports Medicine, and American Osteopathic Academy of Sports Medicine.
16. Vangsness CT, Hunt T, Uram M, Kerlan RK: Survey of health care coverage of high school football in southern California. Am J Sports Med 22(5): 719–722, 1994.

54 Medicolegal Issues

Andrew H. Patterson

Liability issues have been a constant concern to all health care professionals since the late 1960s, when there was a steady and dramatic increase in the frequency of liability claims and in the severity of their results. This increase in legal action affected not only physicians and others providing health care but also manufacturers of sports equipment. Indeed, some companies chose to close their doors rather than try to continue to function in a climate in which liability costs had risen so precipitously.

The issues of professional liability and the obvious inequities of our current system have been well covered in other forums. The extensive statistics compiled by the Physician Insurers Association of America (PIAA) and the Medical Liability Mutual Insurance Company (MLMIC), a physician-owned New York company, do not present a clear picture of the sources of professional liability in sports medicine. However, there do seem to be common elements in liability suits that occur with regularity. The health care professional's awareness of these factors will help avoid litigation, the ideal goal, or at least help make lawsuits easier to defend.

PATIENT ANGER

A serious, unexpected injury that, in the best of hands, may lead to a poor result can generate considerable anger on the part of a patient or the patient's family. There have been a number of cases in which a physician was sued only after litigation against the person responsible for the injury failed or yielded limited results.

Anger over an injury sustained in a sports event may be directed toward the opposing players, coaches, or even the officials. The organization sponsoring the event or the facility in which it took place can also become the object of hostility. Physicians and trainers should be careful not to say anything that might inflame a potentially volatile situation. One ill-advised comment about an individual or organization can come back to haunt the person who made it. The physician's responsibility is to render the best possible medical care; under no circumstances should the physician make a comment that can reinforce or fuel anger. The result of a careless statement may well have the unanticipated effect of turning the patient's anger against the physician.

Furthermore, the physician should never be tempted to give legal advice. If asked for advice regarding a prospective lawsuit, he should respond that he is not qualified to give such advice and will not do so.

COMMUNICATION AND FOLLOW-UP

Because of the nature of sports medicine and marked variations in the quality of care immediately available at an athletic event, communication is extremely important. Typically, a patient injured on the athletic field receives emergency care at the site, further care in an emergency room setting, and definitive care from a private physician in the appropriate specialty.

A lack of communication among the caregivers may lead to a preventable disaster. Better communication might well have saved the leg of one 13-year-old boy injured on the playing field. The boy underwent "a reduction of a dislocated knee" on the field. The real injury, a completely displaced fracture of the distal proximal tibial epiphysis, was not diagnosed until it was too late. First a splint and later a full cast masked the fracture, which was perfectly reduced. A laceration of the popliteal artery was diagnosed too late to salvage a viable extremity. Even though either diagnosis should have raised real concern regarding an arterial injury, it is clear from a review of this case that more direct communication would have been extremely valuable.

Individuals involved in primary care of athletes should try to arrange to have their findings transmitted to at least the next-level caregiver. This is especially important when the injury is serious. Obviously, this sharing of information is relatively simple in small towns but more difficult in large cities. One suggested solution is to require that the sponsoring entity of the sporting event obtain a legible and reasonably complete record of any initial findings and tentative diagnoses. This record could then be supplied to the physician rendering subsequent care.

DEALING WITH COACHES, FAMILIES, AND ATHLETES

In an ideal world a physician would be responsible only to individual patients. In the real world, however, coaches, trainers, parents, or other family members may well become involved. Furthermore, the amount of potential outside interference can vary greatly with the level of competition. The overwhelming majority of coaches would rather rest a player than risk further injury, but a small number will insist that an athlete "play hurt." This attitude of stoicism is unfortunately reinforced when the news media praise professional athletes who play despite significant injuries. Although such an attitude may be appropriate at the professional level, it should never be allowed when youngsters at or below high school level are involved.

The desire to win can be carried much too far. One of my patients was a 12-year-old pitcher who could not extend his arm beyond 40°. When I suggested that he stop pitching, his parents stormed out of the office, pulling their son along. A physician has no control over this kind of behavior. It is important, however, to remember that the physician's first duty is to the patient, and that caution is frequently the best approach to treatment. Trainers and coaches can help reinforce treatment plans, especially since they often know the young athlete better than the physician does. However, they should not be permitted to override the physician's judgment if the risk of a more serious injury exists. The physician who allows emotional appeals and demands from others to overrule a carefully thought-out treatment decision may very well end up as defendant in a lawsuit.

EMERGENCY CARE AND EQUIPMENT

Financial considerations always limit the availability of both emergency equipment and transportation, especially at lower levels of competition. Even though serious injuries occur rarely, it is important for physicians who provide primary care at sports events to insist on a reasonable plan to secure care for a seriously injured athlete. At a high school football game I attended, a player with a devastating knee injury (that required extensive surgery) lay on the sidelines through halftime and the entire second half. Although he had an excellent recovery, the initial management of this injury was far from ideal. The covering physician must also keep in mind the fact that adequate primary care and prompt, safe transportation can be life saving in a few cases. A balance between providing maximum care for a seriously injured athlete and the practical considerations of having sophisticated equipment on hand at all times will probably never be found. Despite this, it is the responsibility of the covering physician (who is, after all, the ultimate patient advocate) to insist on the best compromise possible. Certainly, everything that can be provided at a reasonable cost should be available. If an injury is aggravated by inadequate primary care, the physician will probably be caught in the crossfire of a future lawsuit.

EVALUATION OF THE SPORTS FACILITY

It is highly unlikely that any physician can ever influence the design or choice of the facility provided for an athletic event. The physician can, however, identify conditions within the facility that increase the risk of serious injury by simply conducting a brief tour during the warm-up period before the event. The physician should consider the placement of sideline benches, which can usually be changed easily. Control of players on the sidelines not only will reduce the possibility of injury, but may very well reduce the incidence of fights and personal fouls. Immovable barriers and other obstructions near or adjacent to a playing field or indoor court should be carefully marked and well padded. Although physicians should not be sued because of inadequate physical facilities, a primary physician should make every effort to identify potential problem areas and to suggest reasonable corrections that will prevent injuries. The investment of a few minutes of time in reviewing safety conditions can pay great dividends.

55 Legal Issues in Sports Medicine

David L. Herbert

A variety of major legal concerns face those who provide primary medical care services for athletes. The legal system is frequently called on to resolve a variety of sports medicine issues related to preparticipation examinations of athletes; clearance or return-to-play decisions; training and conditioning of athletes; mismatching of athletes; examination, diagnosis, treatment, and rehabilitation of athletes; drug testing; compliance with the bloodborne pathogen rule; emergency response considerations; and many other issues. These issues are frequently examined and analyzed in publications that report on relevant practice developments and in actual case filings and decisions.[18] Although one chapter cannot provide a thorough discussion of all of these practice concerns,[7] a close examination of one selected sports medicine issue should be of benefit to those in primary care.

During the last 10 to 15 years, the practice of medicine has been inundated by the development and publication of practice guidelines for medical care providers. These guidelines, often referred to as standards, consensus statements, or parameters of practice, have been developed by a number of professional associations, various governmental agencies, and many respected authorities. At last count, there were more than 20,000 of these statements.[5]

Despite the proliferation of such statements, many medical care practitioners have resisted this movement. A number of providers have even criticized the trend as mandating that physicians provide medical care according to a "cookbook-type recipe" that allows little room for implementing the "art" of medicine.[8] Notwithstanding criticism of the trend, efforts to standardize medical care have increased exponentially because of efforts to standardize care, reduce the likelihood of untoward events, minimize claims and suits, lower costs, limit defensive medical care practices, and provide clear benchmarks for expected care, standardization will continue.

Even if this approach to medical care practice is a form of cookbook-type medicine, providers should remember, as others have stated, that every great chef (and every competent physician) starts with some recipe that is enhanced by personalized attention and the blending of various spices that add to the final product.[15] Although enhancements in medicine may be based on "intelligent reasoning and clinical intuition"[15] rather than spices, there must be some basic protocol available to caregivers. Otherwise, there will be nothing to enhance through individualized care.

In this regard, sports medicine is not different from other branches of medicine. As of the end of 2002, over 100 sports medicine standards or guidelines statements have been developed and published by a number of respected professional associations.[9] These include standards dealing with preparticipation examinations,[16] the management of sports-related concussions,[3] and the treatment of HIV-infected athletes through compliance with the bloodborne pathogen standard.[1]

New heat-safety guidelines for football players have recently been published[13] along with an important standards statement by the National Strength and Conditioning Association (NSCA) that addresses a whole host of sports medicine issues.[14]

Like other health care practitioners, sports medicine physicians must be aware of relevant standards statements and use them to enhance their care of athlete-patients. However, it may be that many practitioners in sports medicine, like their counterparts in other medical care areas, do not know or fully appreciate the benefits of guidelines in their own practices. Based on recent research findings as well as actual litigations, providers may run certain medicolegal risks in addition to creating unnecessary risks for their patients if such practitioners do not heed these standards statements. Despite the foregoing, some providers are even moving beyond standards statements and are providing care on an optimum basis. For example, some providers are now conducting preparticipation screenings of entire athletic teams with echocardiograms to provide care beyond that specified by standards.[2] Sometimes these efforts arise out of responses to intramural events which some believe could be avoided by more intense or higher medical practices.[17]

In the litigation following the 1990 death of Loyola Marymount University star basketball player Hank Gathers, certain of his heirs cited the 16th Bethesda Conference guidelines[12] in challenging the courtside care that was provided to Gathers following his collapse during a nationally televised basketball game.[6] The plaintiffs contended in their detailed, 52-page complaint against, among others, Gathers' sports medicine physicians, that Gathers, who was suffering from hypertrophic cardiomyopathy, was not properly treated and that he died as a consequence of negligent care. The lawsuit, which sought $32.5 million in damages, was settled for a substantial amount.[4] The suit did, however, represent one of the first times that practice guidelines were actually cited in court filings to allege negligence in the care of a patient. More recently, the 26th Bethesda Conference guidelines[19] were cited by Northwestern University, in litigation related to the exclusion of an athlete from participation,[11] to support rather than to challenge a sports medicine care decision.

It is clear from these two high-profile cases that standards statements can have an impact in the medical–legal arena even at the onset of litigation and long before experts are deposed. Standards statements may be used either as a sword, to attack sports medicine care, or as a shield, to protect against an attack. The application of standards as a weapon (an inculpatory device) or as a shield (an exculpatory device) may not, however, be available to practitioners who do not know or understand the standards and the potential use of those standards.

In an effort to determine if and how practice parameters are used in the medicolegal setting, researchers from three respected institutions recently surveyed almost 1000 attorneys who pursue medical malpractice claims on behalf of patients. They also reviewed over 250 malpractice claim files from two medical malpractice insurance carriers.[10] Their summary and analysis of this information sought to determine how practice guidelines are used in claims and litigation, for what purposes, and with what results. Interestingly, the researchers determined that, although attorneys and malpractice insurers currently make only moderate use of standards statements, it appears, at least to the plaintiffs' bar, that the use of statements is increasing. The researchers also determined that statements are used more often to challenge the care rendered to patients than to defend care. The researchers noted, however, that when a provider followed and cited a practice guideline to support specific care, plaintiffs' attorneys were less likely to pursue malpractice claims or lawsuits on behalf of their clients.

As a corollary to the foregoing findings, there is both an upside and a downside to the development, publication, and dissemination of practice guidelines. If physicians use standards statements in their care of athlete-patients and support the care provided with standards statements, they may insulate themselves from litigation, and even claims that allege substandard care. If, however, sports medicine caregivers ignore standards or do not use them to improve patient care, harm will result to patients and physicians alike. The sword will harm both patient and physician, to the detriment of sports medicine and the medical profession as a whole. Sports medicine practitioners should concentrate on using standards statements as a shield to protect against their use as a sword.

REFERENCES

1. American Academy of Pediatrics: Policy statement: Human immunodeficiency virus [acquired immunodeficiency syndrome (AIDS) virus] in the athletic setting. AAP News 6:18, 1991.
2. An exercise in prevention: Echos for all. AMA News 24, November 27, 2000.
3. Colorado Medical Society: Guidelines for the Management of Concussion in Sports, Colorado Medical Society, Sports Medicine Committee, 1991.
4. Gathers case resolved. Sports Medicine Standards and Malpractice Reporter 4(2):27, 1992.
5. Healthcare Standards Directory. Plymouth Meeting, PA, ECRI, 2002.
6. Herbert: The death of Hank Gathers: An examination of the legal issues. Sports Medicine Standards and Malpractice Reporter 2(3):45, 46–47, 1990.
7. Herbert DL: Legal Aspects of Sports Medicine, 2nd ed. Canton, OH, PRC Publishing, 1995.
8. Herbert D: Practice guidelines take center court: How to limit liability. Physician and Sports Medicine 24(3):81–83, 1996.
9. Herbert D: The Sports Medicine Standards Book. Canton, OH, Professional Reports, 1992, suppl 1993.
10. Hyams AL, Brandenburg, Lipsitz, et al: Practice guidelines and malpractice litigation: A two way street. Ann Intern Med 122(6):450–455, 1995.
11. Knapp v. Northwestern University, et al, Case No. 95–C–6454 (N.D. Ill., E.D., filed 1995). The defendants' answer to the plaintiff's complaint.
12. Mitchell JH, Maron BJ, Epstein SE: 16th Bethesda Conference: Cardiovascular abnormalities in the athlete; recommendations regarding eligibility for competition. J Am Coll Cardiol 6(6):1186–1232, 1986.
13. New Heat Safety Guidelines for Football. Sports Medicine Standards and Malpractice Reporter 16(5):69, 2002.
14. NSCA Standards and Guidelines at http://nsca://nsca.lift.org/publications/standards.htm, analyzed in Herbert DL: New Standards and Guidelines from the National Strength and Conditioning Association (NSCA). The Exercise Standards and Malpractice Reporter 15(5):75, 2001.
15. Roberts: Practice guidelines, a positive perspective. Physician and Sports Medicine 24(3):86, 1996.
16. Smith, Kovan, Rich, et al: Preparticipation Physical Evaluation, 2nd ed. Minneapolis, MN, American Academy of Family Physicians, American Academy of Pediatrics, American Medical Society for Sports Medicine, American Orthopaedic Society for

Sports Medicine, American Osteopathic Academy of Sports Medicine, 1997.

17. Some young athletes to undergo more intense preparticipation screening. The Sports Medicine Standards and Malpractice Reporter 13(3):47, 2001.
18. See The Sports Medicine Standards and Malpractice Reporter, a quarterly newsletter examining legal, professional, and standards issues related to sports medicine care published by PRC Publishing, of Canton, Ohio.
19. The 26th Bethesda Conference: Recommendations for determining eligibility for competition in athletes with cardiovascular abnormalities. Med Sci Sports Exerc S227–S283, 1994.

Index

Note: Page numbers followed by f refer to figures; page numbers followed by t refer to tables.

D

H

J

K